Medical Microbiology

SIXTH EDITION

Medical Microbiology

Patrick R. Murray, PhD
Chief, Microbiology Service
Department of Laboratory Medicine
National Institutes of Health Clinical Center
Bethesda, Maryland

Ken S. Rosenthal, PhD
Professor
Department of Integrative Medical Sciences
Northeastern Ohio Universities Colleges of Medicine and Pharmacy
Rootstown, Ohio

Michael A. Pfaller, MD
Emeritus Professor
Pathology and Epidemiology
University of Iowa College of Medicine and College of Public Health
Iowa City, Iowa

MOSBY

ELSEVIER

1600 John F. Kennedy Blvd.
Ste 1800
Philadelphia, PA 19103-2899

Medical Microbiology, 6th Edition   ISBN: 978-0-323-05470-6

Notice

Knowledge and best practice in this field are constantly changing. As new research and experience broaden our knowledge, changes in practice, treatment and drug therapy may become necessary or appropriate. Readers are advised to check the most current information provided (i) on procedures featured or (ii) by the manufacturer of each product to be administered, to verify the recommended dose or formula, the method and duration of administration, and contraindications. It is the responsibility of the practitioner, relying on their own experience and knowledge of the patient, to make diagnoses, to determine dosages and the best treatment for each individual patient, and to take all appropriate safety precautions. To the fullest extent of the law, neither the Publisher nor the Authors assume any liability for any injury and/or damage to persons or property arising out of or related to any use of the material contained in this book.

The Publisher

Patrick R. Murray's role as author of this book was carried out in his private capacity, and his contribution does not reflect official support or endorsement by the National Institute of Health or the Department of Health and Human Services.

Library of Congress Cataloging-in-Publication Data
Murray, Patrick R.
  Medical microbiology / Patrick R. Murray, Ken S. Rosenthal, Michael A. Pfaller. – 6th ed.
    p. ; cm.
  Includes bibliographical references and index.
  ISBN 978-0-323-05470-6
  1. Medical microbiology. I. Rosenthal, Ken S. II. Pfaller, Michael A. III. Title.
  [DNLM: 1. Microbiology. 2. Microbiological Techniques. 3. Parasitology. QW 4 M983m 2009]
  QR46.M4683 2009
  616.9′041–dc22   2008020047

Publishing Director: Linda Belfus
Acquisitions Editor: William Schmitt
Developmental Editor: Katie DeFrancesco
Publishing Services Manager: Linda Van Pelt
Project Manager: Priscilla Crater
Designer: Karen O'Keefe Owens

Printed in Canada
Last digit is the print number: 9 8 7 6 5 4 3 2 1

To all who use this textbook, that they may benefit from its use as much as we did in its preparation.

Preface

Medical microbiology can be a bewildering field to the novice. We are faced with many questions when learning microbiology. How do I learn all the names? Which infectious agents cause which diseases? Why? When? Who is at risk? Is there a treatment? However, all these concerns can be reduced to one essential question: What information do I need to know that will help me understand how to diagnose and treat an infected patient?

Certainly, there are a number of theories about what a student needs to know and how to teach it, which supposedly validates the plethora of microbiology textbooks that have flooded the bookstores in recent years. Although we do not claim to have the one right approach to teaching medical microbiology (there is truly no one perfect approach to medical education), we have founded the revisions of this textbook on our experience gained through years of teaching medical students, residents, and infectious disease fellows as well as on the work devoted to the five previous editions. We have tried to present the basic concepts of medical microbiology clearly and succinctly in a manner that addresses different types of learners. The text is written in a straightforward manner with, it is hoped, uncomplicated explanations of difficult concepts. **Details** are summarized in tabular format rather than in lengthy text, and there are colorful illustrations for the visual learner. **Clinical Cases** provide the relevance that puts reality into the basic science. **Important points** are emphasized in **boxes** to aid the student, especially in their review; and the **study questions,** including **Clinical Cases,** address relevant aspects of each chapter.

Our understanding of microbiology and immunology is rapidly expanding with new and exciting discoveries in all areas. Expansion of knowledge could also lead to expansion of the book. We used our experience as authors and teachers to choose the most important information and explanations for inclusion in this textbook. Each chapter has been carefully updated and expanded to include new, medically relevant discoveries. In each of these chapters, we have attempted to present the material that we feel will help the student gain a clear understanding of the significance of the individual microbes and their diseases.

With each edition of *Medical Microbiology* we refine and update our presentation. The obvious changes with this sixth edition include the addition or reorganization of many new summary boxes, tables, clinical photographs, and original clinical cases. The inclusion of **Clinical Cases** is a new feature in the edition that we believe the students will find particularly interesting and instructive. We feel these are useful teaching aids for the students and the most efficient way to present this complex subject. We have reorganized the basic microbiology section. The expanded mycology section reflects the increased role of fungi in infectious diseases, particularly in the immunocompromised host. The student will also find discussions of important new pathogens (e.g., avian influenza virus) and old pathogens associated with new diseases (e.g., *Staphylococcus aureus* responsible for community-acquired skin and soft tissue infections). Finally, the student is provided with access to the Student Consult website, which provides links to additional reference materials and clinical photographs. A new feature on the website is the addition of more than 200 **practice exam questions** that will help the student assess their mastery of the subject matter and prepare for their Board exams.

To Our Future Colleagues: The Students

How can the student digest what appear to be innumerable facts? On first impression, success in medical microbiology would seem to depend on memorization. Although memorization is an important part of any medical discipline, understanding the basic principles and developing a system for storing this information will help and can be applied to the future of newly discovered diseases and microbes. We suggest that the student concentrate on learning what is important by **thinking like a physician and treating each microbe and its diseases as if it were a patient**. Continue to ask seven basic questions as you approach this material: Who? Where? When? Why? Which? What? and How? For example: Who is at risk for disease? Where does this organism cause infections (both body site and geographic area)? When is isolation of this organism important? Why is this organism able to cause disease? Which species and genera are medically important? What diagnostic tests should be performed? How is this infection managed? Each organism that is encountered can be systematically examined. Know the specifics about how the organism grows, the virulence properties of the organism, and the diseases it causes; understand the epidemiology of infections; know what specimens should be collected and the basic identification tests that should be performed; and be familiar with preventive and therapeutic strategies. Learn three to five words or phrases that are associated with the microbe— words that will stimulate your memory (**trigger words**) and organize the diverse facts into a logical picture. Develop **alternative associations**. For example, this textbook presents organisms in the systematic taxonomic structure (frequently called a "bug parade," but which the authors think is the easiest way to introduce the organisms). Take a given virulence property (e.g., toxin production) or type of disease (e.g., meningitis) and list the organisms that share this property. Pretend that an imaginary patient is infected with a specific agent and create the case history. Explain the diagnosis to the imaginary patient and also to your future professional colleagues. In other words, do not simply attempt to memorize page after page of facts; rather, use techniques that stimulate your mind and challenge your understanding of the facts presented throughout the text.

No textbook of this magnitude would be successful without the contributions of numerous individuals. We are grateful for the valuable professional help and support provided by the staff at Elsevier, particularly William Schmitt, Katie DeFrancesco, and Priscilla Crater. We also want to thank the many students and professional colleagues who have offered their advice and constructive criticism throughout the development of this sixth edition of *Medical Microbiology*.

Patrick R. Murray, PhD
Ken S. Rosenthal, PhD
Michael A. Pfaller, MD

Contents

Introduction

Introduction to Medical Microbiology

Imagine the excitement felt by the Dutch biologist Anton van Leeuwenhoek in 1674 as he peered through his carefully ground microscopic lenses at a drop of water and discovered a world of millions of tiny "animalcules." Almost 100 years later, the Danish biologist Otto Müller extended van Leeuwenhoek's studies and organized bacteria into genera and species according to the classification methods of Carolus Linnaeus. This was the beginning of the taxonomic classification of microbes. In 1840 the German pathologist Friedrich Henle proposed criteria for proving that microorganisms were responsible for causing human disease (the "germ theory" of disease). Robert Koch and Louis Pasteur confirmed this theory in the 1870s and 1880s with a series of elegant experiments proving that microorganisms were responsible for causing anthrax, rabies, plague, cholera, and tuberculosis. Other brilliant scientists went on to prove that a diverse collection of microbes was responsible for causing human disease. The era of chemotherapy began in 1910, when the German chemist Paul Ehrlich discovered the first antibacterial agent, a compound effective against the spirochete that causes syphilis. This was followed by Alexander Fleming's discovery of penicillin in 1928, Gerhard Domagk's discovery of sulfanilamide in 1935, and Selman Waksman's discovery of streptomycin in 1943. In 1946, the American microbiologist John Enders was the first to cultivate viruses in cell cultures, leading the way to the large-scale production of virus cultures for vaccine development. Thousands of scientists have followed these pioneers, each building on the foundation established by his or her predecessors, and each adding an observation that expanded our understanding of microbes and their role in disease.

The world that van Leeuwenhoek discovered was complex, consisting of protozoa and bacteria of all shapes and sizes. However, the complexity of medical microbiology we know today rivals the limits of the imagination. We now know that there are thousands of different types of microbes that live in, on, and around us—and hundreds that cause serious human diseases. To understand this information and organize it in a useful manner, it is important to understand some of the basic aspects of medical microbiology. To start, the microbes can be subdivided into the following four general groups: viruses, bacteria, fungi, and parasites, each having its own level of complexity.

Viruses

Viruses are the smallest infectious particles, ranging in diameter from 18 to 600 nanometers (most viruses are less than 200 nm and cannot be seen with a light microscope). Viruses typically contain either deoxyribonucleic acid (DNA) or ribonucleic acid (RNA) but not both; however, some viral-like particles do not contain any detectable nucleic acids (e.g., prions; see Chapter 66), while the recently discovered Mimivirus contains both RNA and DNA. The viral nucleic acids and proteins required for replication and pathogenesis are enclosed in a protein coat with or without a lipid membrane coat. Viruses are true parasites, requiring host cells for replication. The cells they infect and the host response to the infection dictate the nature of the clinical manifestation. More than 2000 species of viruses have been described, with approximately 650 infecting humans and animals. Infection can lead either to rapid replication and destruction of the cell or to a long-term chronic relationship with possible integration of the viral genetic information into the host genome. The factors that determine which of these takes place are only partially understood. For example, infection with the human immunodeficiency virus, the etiologic agent of the acquired immunodeficiency syndrome (AIDS), can result in the latent infection of CD4 lymphocytes or the active replication and destruction of these immunologically important cells. Likewise, infection can spread to other susceptible cells, such as the microglial cells of the brain, resulting in the neurologic manifestations of AIDS. Thus the diseases caused by viruses can range from the common cold to gastroenteritis to fatal catastrophes such as rabies, Ebola, smallpox, or AIDS.

response is often too late or too slow. To improve the human body's ability to prevent infection, the immune system can be augmented either through the passive transfer of antibodies present in immune globulin preparations or through active immunization with components of the microbes (antigens). Infections can also be controlled with a variety of chemotherapeutic agents. Unfortunately, many microbes can alter their antigenic complexion (**antigenic variation**) or develop resistance to even the most potent antibiotics. Thus the battle for control between microbe and host continues, with neither side yet able to claim victory (although the microbes have demonstrated remarkable ingenuity). There clearly is no "magic bullet" that has eradicated infectious diseases.

Diagnostic Microbiology

The clinical microbiology laboratory plays an important role in the diagnosis and control of infectious diseases. However, the ability of the laboratory to perform these functions is limited by the quality of the specimen collected from the patient, the means by which it is transported from the patient to the laboratory, and the techniques used to demonstrate the microbe in the sample. Because most diagnostic tests are based on the ability of the organism to grow, transport conditions must ensure the viability of the pathogen. In addition, the most sophisticated testing protocols are of little value if the collected specimen is not representative of the site of infection. This seems obvious, but many specimens sent to laboratories for analysis are contaminated during collection with the organisms that colonize the mucosal surfaces. It is virtually impossible to interpret the testing results with contaminated specimens, because most infections are caused by endogenous organisms.

The laboratory is also able to determine the antimicrobial activity of selected chemotherapeutic agents, although the value of these tests is limited. The laboratory must test only organisms capable of producing disease and only medically relevant antimicrobials. To test all isolated organisms or an indiscriminate selection of drugs can yield misleading results with potentially dangerous consequences. Not only can a patient be treated inappropriately with unnecessary antibiotics, but also the true pathogenic organism may not be recognized among the plethora of organisms isolated and tested. Finally, the in vitro determination of an organism's susceptibility to a variety of antibiotics is only one aspect of a complex picture. The virulence of the organism, site of infection, and patient's ability to respond to the infection influence the host-parasite interaction and must also be considered when planning treatment.

Summary

It is important to realize that our knowledge of the microbial world is evolving continually. Just as the early microbiologists built their discoveries on the foundations established by their predecessors, we and future generations will continue to discover new microbes, new diseases, and new therapies. The following chapters are intended as a foundation of knowledge that can be used to build your understanding of microbes and their diseases.

Basic Principles of Medical Microbiology

Bacterial Classification, Structure, and Replication

Bacteria, the smallest cells, are visible only with the aid of a microscope. The smallest bacteria (*Chlamydia* and *Rickettsia*) are just 0.1 to 0.2 μm in diameter, whereas larger bacteria may be many microns in length. A newly described species is hundreds of times larger than the average bacterial cell and is visible to the naked eye. Most species, however, are approximately 1 μm in diameter and are therefore visible with the use of the light microscope, which has a resolution of 0.2 μm. In comparison, animal and plant cells are much larger, ranging from 7 μm (the diameter of a red blood cell) to several feet (the length of certain nerve cells).

Differences between Eukaryotes and Prokaryotes

Cells from animals, plants, and fungi are **eukaryotes** (Greek for "true nucleus"), whereas bacteria and blue-green algae belong to the **prokaryotes** (Greek for "primitive nucleus"). In addition to lacking a nucleus and other organelles, the bacterial chromosome differs from the human chromosome in several ways. The chromosome of a typical bacterium such as *Escherichia coli* is a single, double-stranded, circular molecule of deoxyribonucleic acid (DNA) containing approximately 5 million base pairs (or 5000 kilobase [kb] pairs), an approximate length of 1.3 mm (i.e., nearly 1000 times the diameter of the cell). The smallest bacterial chromosomes (from mycoplasmas) are approximately a fourth of this size. In comparison, humans have two copies of 23 chromosomes, which represent 2.9×10^9 base pairs 990 mm in length. Bacteria use a smaller ribosome, the 70S ribosome, and in most bacteria a meshlike peptidoglycan cell wall surrounds the membranes to protect them against the environment. Bacteria can survive and in some cases grow in hostile environments in which the osmotic pressure outside the cell is so low that most eukaryotic cells would lyse, at temperature extremes (both hot and cold), with dryness, and with very dilute and diverse energy sources. Bacteria have evolved their structures and functions to adapt to these conditions. These and other distinguishing features are depicted in Figure 2-1 and outlined in Table 2-1. Several of these distinctions provide the basis for antimicrobial action.

Bacterial Classification

Bacteria can be classified by their macroscopic and microscopic appearance, by characteristic growth and metabolic properties, by their antigenicity, and finally by their genotype.

Macroscopic and Microscopic Distinction

The initial distinction between bacteria can be made by growth characteristics on different nutrient and selective media. The bacteria grow in colonies, each colony like a city of as many as a million or more organisms. The sum of their characteristics provide the colony with distinguishing characteristics such as color, size, shape, and smell. The ability to resist certain antibiotics, ferment specific sugars (e.g., lactose, to distinguish *E. coli* from *Salmonella*), to lyse erythrocytes (hemolytic properties), or to hydrolyze lipids (e.g., clostridia lipase) can also be determined using the appropriate growth media.

The microscopic appearance, including the size, shape and configuration of the organisms (cocci, rods, curved, or spiral) and their ability to retain the Gram stain (gram-positive or gram-negative) are the primary means for distinguishing the bacteria. A spherical bacterium, such as *Staphylococcus*, is a coccus; a rod-shaped bacterium, such as *Escherichia coli*, is a bacillus; and the snakelike treponeme is a spirillum. In addition, *Nocardia* and *Actinomyces* species have branched filamentous appearances similar to those of fungi. Some bacteria

Prokaryote

Eukaryote

Figure 2–1. Major features of prokaryotes and eukaryotes.

form aggregates, such as the grapelike clusters of *Staphylo-coccus aureus* or the diplococcus (two cells together) observed in *Streptococcus* or *Neisseria* species.

Gram stain is a rapid, powerful, easy test that allows clin-icians to distinguish between the two major classes of bacteria, develop an initial diagnosis, and initiate therapy based on inherent differences in the bacteria (Figure 2-2). Bacteria are heat fixed or otherwise dried onto a slide, stained with **crystal violet** (Figure 2-3), a stain that is precipitated with **iodine**, and then the unbound and excess stain is removed by washing with the acetone-based **decolorizer** and water. A red counter-stain, **safranin**, is added to stain any decolorized cells. This process takes less than 10 minutes.

For **gram-positive bacteria**, which turn **purple**, the stain gets trapped in a thick, cross-linked, meshlike struc-ture, the peptidoglycan layer, which surrounds the cell. **Gram-negative bacteria** have a thin peptidoglycan layer that does not retain the crystal violet stain, so the cells must be counterstained with safranin and turned red (Figure 2-4). A mnemonic device that may help is "P-PURPLE-POSITIVE."

Due to degradation of the peptidoglycan, Gram stain is not a dependable test for bacteria that are starved (e.g., old or stationary phase cultures) or treated with antibiotics.

Bacteria that cannot be classified by Gram stain include mycobacteria, which have a waxy outer shell and are distinguished with the acid-fast stain, and mycoplasmas, which have no peptidoglycan.

Metabolic, Antigenic, and Genetic Distinction

The next level of classification is based on the metabolic signature of the bacteria, including requirement for anaero-bic or aerobic environments, requirement for specific nutri-ents (e.g., ability to ferment specific carbohydrates or use different compounds as a source of carbon for growth), and production of characteristic metabolic products (acid, alcohols) and specific enzymes (e.g., staphylococcal catalase). Automated procedures for distinguishing enteric and other bacteria have been developed; they analyze the growth in different media and their microbial products and provide a numerical biotype for each of the bacteria.

A particular strain of bacteria can be distinguished using antibodies to detect characteristic antigens on the bacteria (**serotyping**). These serologic tests can also be used to identify organisms that are difficult (*Treponema pallidum*, the organism responsible for syphilis) or too dangerous (e.g., *Francisella*, the organism that causes tularemia) to grow in the lab, are associated with specific disease syn-dromes (e.g., *Escherichia coli* serotype O157, responsible for hemorrhagic colitis), or need to be identified rapidly (e.g., *S. pyogenes*, responsible for streptococcal pharyngitis). Serotyping is also used to subdivide bacteria below the species level for epidemiologic purposes.

The most precise method for classifying bacteria is by analysis of their genetic material. New methods distinguish bacteria by detection of specific characteristic DNA sequences. These techniques include **DNA hybridization, polymerase chain reaction (PCR) amplification**, and related techniques described in Chapter 16. These genetic techniques do not require living or growing bacteria and can be used for rapid detection and identification of slow-growing organisms, such as mycobacteria and fungi, or analysis of pathology samples of even very virulent bacteria. The technology is now available for rapid analysis of the nucleic acid sequence of specific segments or the entire bacterial chromosome. The most common application of this technique is analysis of sequences of ribosomal DNA to detect the highly conserved sequences that identify a family or genus and the highly variable sequences that distinguish a species or subspecies. It has also been used to define the evolutionary relationship among organisms and to identify organisms that are difficult or impossible to grow. Various other methods that have been used, primarily to classify organisms at the subspecies level for epidemiologic inves-tigations, include: **plasmid analysis, ribotyping**, and **anal-ysis of chromosomal DNA fragments**. In recent years the technical aspects of these methods have been simplified to the point that most clinical laboratories use variations of these methods in their day-to-day practice.

Table 2–1. Major Characteristics of Eukaryotes and Prokaryotes

Characteristic	Eukaryote	Prokaryote
Major groups	Algae, fungi, protozoa, plants, animals	Bacteria
Size (approximate)	>5 μm	0.5-3.0 μm
Nuclear Structures		
Nucleus	Classic membrane	No nuclear membrane
Chromosomes	Strands of DNA diploid genome	Single, circular DNA haploid genome
Cytoplasmic Structures		
Mitochondria	Present	Absent
Golgi bodies	Present	Absent
Endoplasmic reticulum	Present	Absent
Ribosomes (sedimentation coefficient)	80S (60S + 40S)	70S (50S + 30S)
Cytoplasmic membrane	Contains sterols	Does not contain sterols
Cell wall	Present for fungi; otherwise absent	Is a complex structure containing protein, lipids, and peptidoglycans
Reproduction	Sexual and asexual	Asexual (binary fission)
Movement	Complex flagellum, if present	Simple flagellum, if present
Respiration	Via mitochondria	Via cytoplasmic membrane

Modified from Holt S: In Slots J, Taubman M (eds): Contemporary Oral Microbiology and Immunology. St Louis, Mosby, 1992.

Bacterial Structure

Cytoplasmic Structures

The cytoplasm of the bacterial cell contains the DNA chromosome, mRNA, ribosomes, proteins, and metabolites (see Figure 2-4). Unlike eukaryotes, the **bacterial chromosome** is a single, double-stranded circle that is contained not in a nucleus, but in a discrete area known as the **nucleoid**. Histones are not present to maintain the conformation of the DNA, and the DNA does not form nucleosomes. **Plasmids**, which are smaller, circular, extrachromosomal DNAs, may also be present. Plasmids are most commonly found in gram-negative bacteria, and although not usually essential for cellular survival, they often provide a selective advantage: many confer resistance to one or more antibiotics.

The lack of a nuclear membrane simplifies the requirements and control mechanisms for the synthesis of proteins. Without a nuclear membrane, transcription and translation are coupled; in other words, ribosomes can bind to the mRNA, and protein can be made as the mRNA is being synthesized and still attached to the DNA.

The **bacterial ribosome** consists of 30S + 50S subunits, forming a 70S ribosome. This is unlike the eukaryotic 80S (40S + 60S) ribosome. The proteins and RNA of the bacterial ribosome are significantly different from those of eukaryotic ribosomes and are major targets for antibacterial drugs.

The **cytoplasmic membrane** has a lipid bilayer structure similar to the structure of the eukaryotic membranes, but it contains no steroids (e.g., cholesterol); mycoplasmas are the exception to this rule. The cytoplasmic membrane is responsible for many of the functions attributable to organelles in eukaryotes. These tasks include electron transport and energy production, which are normally achieved in the mitochondria. In addition, the membrane contains transport proteins that allow the uptake of metabolites and the release of other substances, ion pumps to maintain a membrane potential, and enzymes. The inside of the membrane is lined with actin-like protein filaments, which help determine the shape of the bacteria and the site of septum formation for cell division. These filaments determine the spiral shape of the treponemes.

Cell Wall

The structure (Table 2-2), components, and functions (Table 2-3) of the cell wall distinguish gram-positive from gram-negative bacteria. Cell wall components are also unique to bacteria, and their repetitive structures elicit innate protective immune responses in humans.

A

Peptidoglycan

Teichoic acid

Lipoteichoic acid

Cell wall

Cytoplasmic membrane

Structural and enzymatic proteins

B

Lipopolysaccharide

Pore (porin proteins)

Outer membrane

Periplasmic space

Cytoplasmic membrane

Nutrient-binding protein

Carrier protein

Peptidoglycan

Lipoprotein

Figure 2—2. Comparison of the gram-positive and gram-negative bacterial cell walls. **A,** A gram-positive bacterium has a thick peptidoglycan layer that contains teichoic and lipoteichoic acids. **B,** A gram-negative bacterium has a thin peptidoglycan layer and an outer membrane that contains lipopolysaccharide, phospholipids, and proteins. The periplasmic space between the cytoplasmic and outer membranes contains transport, degradative, and cell wall synthetic proteins. The outer membrane is joined to the cytoplasmic membrane at adhesion points and is attached to the peptidoglycan by lipoprotein links.

The important differences in membrane characteristics are outlined in Table 2-4. Rigid **peptidoglycan (murein)** layers surround the cytoplasmic membranes of most prokaryotes. The exceptions are *Archaeobacteria* organisms (which contain pseudoglycans or pseudomureins related to peptidoglycan) and mycoplasmas (which have no cell walls). Because the peptidoglycan provides rigidity, it also helps to determine the shape of the particular bacterial cell. Gram-negative bacteria are also surrounded by outer membranes.

Gram-Positive Bacteria

A gram-positive bacterium has a *thick, multilayered cell wall consisting mainly of peptidoglycan* (150 to 500 Å) surrounding the cytoplasmic membrane (Figure 2-5). The peptidoglycan is a meshlike exoskeleton similar in function to the exoskeleton of an insect. Unlike the exoskeleton of the insect, however, the peptidoglycan of the cell is sufficiently porous to allow diffusion of metabolites to the plasma membrane. A new model for peptidoglycan suggests that the glycan extends out from the plasma membrane like bristles which are cross-linked with short peptide chains. The **peptidoglycan is essential** for the structure, for

replication, and for survival in the normally hostile conditions in which bacteria grow.

The peptidoglycan can be degraded by treatment with **lysozyme**. Lysozyme is an enzyme in human tears and mucus, but is also produced by bacteria and other organisms. Lysozyme degrades the glycan backbone of the peptidoglycan. Without the peptidoglycan, the bacteria succumb to the large osmotic pressure differences across the cytoplasmic membrane and lyse. Removal of the cell wall produces a **protoplast** that lyses unless it is osmotically stabilized.

The gram-positive cell wall may also include other components such as teichoic and lipoteichoic acids and complex polysaccharides (usually called **C polysaccharides**). The M protein of streptococci and R protein of staphylococci also associate with the peptidoglycan. **Teichoic acids** are water-soluble, anionic polymers of polyol phosphates, which are covalently linked to the peptidoglycan and essential to cell viability. **Lipoteichoic acids** have a fatty acid and are anchored in the cytoplasmic membrane. These molecules are common surface antigens that distinguish bacterial serotypes and promote attachment to other bacteria and to specific receptors on mammalian cell surfaces (adherence). Teichoic acids are important factors in virulence.

Figure 2—3. Gram-stain morphology of bacteria. **A,** The crystal violet of Gram stain is precipitated by Gram iodine and is trapped in the thick peptidoglycan layer in gram-positive bacteria. The decolorizer disperses the gram-negative outer membrane and washes the crystal violet from the thin layer of peptidoglycan. Gram-negative bacteria are visualized by the red counterstain. **B,** Bacterial morphologies.

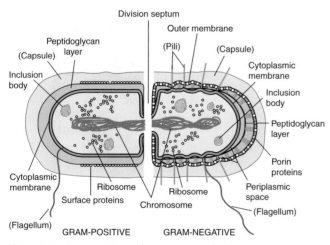

Figure 2—4. Gram-positive and gram-negative bacteria. A gram-positive bacterium has a thick layer of peptidoglycan (filling the purple space) (*left*). A gram-negative bacterium has a thin peptidoglycan layer (single black line) and an outer membrane (*right*). Structures in parentheses are not found in all bacteria. Upon cell division the membrane and peptidoglycan grow toward each other to form a division septum to separate the daughter cells.

Table 2—2. Bacterial Membrane Structures

Structure	Chemical Constituents
Plasma membrane	Phospholipids, proteins, and enzymes involved in generation of energy, membrane potential, and transport
Cell Wall	
Gram-positive bacteria	
Peptidoglycan	Glycan chains of GlcNAc and MurNAc cross-linked by peptide bridge
Teichoic acid	Polyribitol phosphate or glycerol phosphate cross-linked to peptidoglycan
Lipoteichoic acid	Lipid-linked teichoic acid
Gram-negative bacteria	
Peptidoglycan	Thinner version of that found in gram-positive bacteria
Periplasmic space	Enzymes involved in transport, degradation, and synthesis
Outer membrane	Phospholipids with saturated fatty acids
Proteins	Porins, lipoprotein, transport proteins
LPS	Lipid A, core polysaccharide, O antigen
Other structures	
Capsule	Polysaccharides (disaccharides and trisaccharides) and polypeptides
Pili	Pilin, adhesins
Flagellum	Motor proteins, flagellin
Proteins	M protein of streptococci (as an example)

GlcNAc, N-Acetylglucosamine; LPS, lipopolysaccharide; MurNAc, N-acetylmuramic acid.

Lipoteichoic acids are shed into the media and the host and although weaker, they can initiate innate protective responses similar to endotoxin.

Gram-Negative Bacteria

Gram-negative cell walls are more complex than gram-positive cell walls, both structurally and chemically (see Figure 2-2). Structurally, a gram-negative cell wall contains two layers external to the cytoplasmic membrane. Immediately external to the cytoplasmic membrane is a *thin peptidoglycan layer*, which accounts for only 5% to 10% of the gram-negative cell wall by weight. There are *no teichoic or lipoteichoic acids* in the gram-negative cell wall. External to the peptidoglycan layer is the **outer membrane**, which is unique to gram-negative bacteria. The area between

Table 2–3. Functions of the Bacterial Envelope

Function	Component
Structure	
Rigidity	All
Packaging of internal contents	All
Bacterial Functions	
Permeability barrier	Outer membrane or plasma membrane
Metabolic uptake	Membranes and periplasmic transport proteins, porins, permeases
Energy production	Plasma membrane
Motility	Flagella
Mating	Pili
Host Interaction	
Adhesion to host cells	Pili, proteins, teichoic acid
Immune recognition by host	All outer structures
Escape from host immune recognition	Capsule, M protein
Medical Relevance	
Antibiotic sensitivity	Peptidoglycan synthetic enzymes
Antibiotic resistance	Outer membrane

Table 2–4. Membrane Characteristics of Gram-Positive and Gram-Negative Bacteria

Characteristic	Gram-Positive	Gram-Negative
Outer membrane	—	+
Cell wall	Thicker	Thinner
LPS	—	+
Endotoxin	—	+
Teichoic acid	Often present	—
Sporulation	Some strains	—
Capsule	Sometimes present	Sometimes present
Lysozyme	Sensitive	Resistant
Antibacterial activity of penicillin	More susceptible	More resistant
Exotoxin production	Some strains	Some strains

LPS, Lipopolysaccharide.

the external surface of the cytoplasmic membrane and the internal surface of the outer membrane is referred to as the **periplasmic space**. This space is actually a compartment containing components of transport systems for iron, proteins, sugars and other metabolites, and a variety of hydrolytic enzymes that are important to the cell for the breakdown of large macromolecules for metabolism. These enzymes typically include proteases, phosphatases, lipases, nucleases, and carbohydrate-degrading enzymes. In the case of pathogenic gram-negative species, many of the lytic virulence factors, such as collagenases, hyaluronidases, proteases, and β-lactamase, are in the periplasmic space.

The gram-negative cell wall is also traversed by different transport systems, including the Type I, II, III, IV, and V secretion devices. Transport systems provide mechanisms

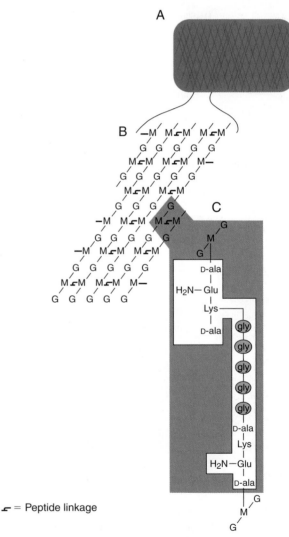

= Peptide linkage

Figure 2–5. General structure of the peptidoglycan component of the cell wall. **A,** The peptidoglycan forms a meshlike layer around the cell. **B,** The peptidoglycan mesh consists of a polysaccharide polymer that is cross-linked by peptide bonds. **C,** Peptides are cross-linked through a peptide bond between the terminal D-alanine (D-ala) from one chain and a lysine (Lys) (or another diamino amino acid) from the other chain. A pentaglycine bridge (gly5) expands the cross-link in *Staphylococcus aureus* (as shown).

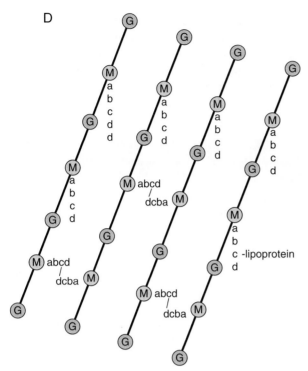

Figure 2–5. cont'd D, Representation of the *Escherichia coli* peptidoglycan structure. Diaminopimelic acid, the diamino amino acid in the third position of the peptide, is *directly linked* to the terminal alanine of another chain to cross-link the peptidoglycan. Lipoprotein anchors the outer membrane to the peptidoglycan. G, *N*-acetylglucosamine; Glu, D-glutamic acid; gly, glycine; M, lyglysine; *N*-acetylmuramic acid. (**A-C** redrawn from Talaro K, Talaro A: Foundations in Microbiology, 2nd ed. Dubuque, Iowa, Wm C Brown, 1996; **D** redrawn from Joklik KJ, et al: Zinsser Microbiology. Norwalk, Conn, Appleton & Lange, 1988.)

for the uptake and release of different metabolites and other compounds. The Type III secretion device is a major virulence factor for some bacteria, with a complex structure that traverses both the inner and outer membranes and can act as a syringe to inject proteins into other cells.

As mentioned previously, outer membranes (see Figure 2-2) are unique to gram-negative bacteria. The outer membrane is like a stiff canvas sack around the bacteria. *The outer membrane maintains the bacterial structure and is a permeability barrier to large molecules* (e.g., proteins such as lysozyme) *and hydrophobic molecules* (e.g., some antimicrobials). It also provides protection from adverse environmental conditions such as the digestive system of the host (important for *Enterobacteriaceae* organisms). The outer membrane has an asymmetric bilayer structure that differs from any other biologic membrane in the structure of the outer leaflet of the membrane. The inner leaflet contains phospholipids normally found in bacterial membranes. However, the outer leaflet is composed primarily of **lipopolysaccharide (LPS)**. Except for those LPS molecules in the process of synthesis, the outer leaflet of the outer membrane is the only location where LPS molecules are found.

LPS is also called **endotoxin**, a powerful stimulator of innate and immune responses. LPS is shed from the

bacteria into the media and host. LPS activates B cells and induces macrophage, dendritic, and other cells to release interleukin-1, interleukin-6, tumor necrosis factor, and other factors. LPS induces fever and can cause shock. The **Shwartzman reaction** (disseminated intravascular coagulation) follows the release of large amounts of endotoxin into the bloodstream. *Neisseria* bacteria shed large amounts of a related compound, lipooligosaccharide (**LOS**), resulting in fever and severe symptoms.

The variety of proteins found in gram-negative outer membranes is limited, but several of the proteins are present in high concentration, resulting in a total protein content that is higher than that of the cytoplasmic membrane. Many of the proteins traverse the entire lipid bilayer and are thus transmembrane proteins. A group of these proteins is known as **porins** because they form pores **that allow the diffusion of hydrophilic molecules less than 700 Da in mass through the membrane.** *The porin channel allows passage of metabolites and small hydrophilic antibiotics.* The outer membrane also contains structural proteins, receptor molecules for bacteriophages, and other ligands and components of transport and secretory systems.

The outer membrane is connected to the cytoplasmic membrane at **adhesion sites** and is tied to the peptidoglycan by **lipoprotein**. The lipoprotein is covalently attached to the peptidoglycan and is anchored in the outer membrane. The adhesion sites provide a membranous route for the delivery of newly synthesized outer membrane components to the outer membrane.

The outer membrane is held together by divalent cation (Mg^{+2} and Ca^{+2}) linkages between phosphates on LPS molecules and hydrophobic interactions between the LPS and proteins. These interactions produce a stiff, strong membrane that can be disrupted by antibiotics (e.g., polymyxin) or by the removal of Mg and Ca ions (chelation with ethylenediaminetetraacetic acid [EDTA] or tetracycline). Disruption of the outer membrane weakens the bacteria and allows the permeability of large, hydrophobic molecules. The addition of lysozyme to cells with a disrupted outer membrane produces **spheroplasts**, which like protoplasts are osmotically sensitive.

External Structures

Some bacteria (gram-positive or gram-negative) are closely surrounded by loose polysaccharide or protein layers called **capsules**. In cases in which it is loosely adherent and nonuniform in density or thickness, the material is referred to as a **slime layer**. The capsules and slime layers are also called the **glycocalyx**. *Bacillus anthracis*, the exception to this rule, produces a polypeptide capsule. The capsule is hard to see in a microscope, but its space can be visualized by the exclusion of India ink particles.

Capsules and slimes are unnecessary for the growth of bacteria, but are very important for survival in the host. *The capsule is poorly antigenic and antiphagocytic and is a major* virulence factor (e.g., *Streptococcus pneumoniae*). The capsule can also act as a barrier to toxic hydrophobic molecules, such as detergents, and can promote **adherence** to other bacteria or to host tissue surfaces. For *Streptococcus mutans*, the dextran and levan capsules are the means by which the bacteria attach and stick to the tooth enamel. Bacterial strains lacking a capsule may arise during growth under laboratory conditions, away from the selective pressures of the host, and are therefore less virulent. Some bacteria (e.g., *Pseudomonas aeruginosa*) will produce a polysaccharide **biofilm** under certain conditions, which establishes a bacterial community and protects them from antibiotics and host defenses. Another example of a biofilm is tooth plaque produced by *Streptococcus mutans*.

Flagella are ropelike propellers composed of helically coiled protein subunits (**flagellin**) that are anchored in the bacterial membranes through hook and basal body structures and are driven by membrane potential. Bacterial species may have one or several flagella on their surfaces, and they may be anchored at different parts of the cell. Flagella provide motility for bacteria, allowing the cell to swim (**chemotaxis**) toward food and away from poisons. Bacteria approach food by swimming straight and then tumbling in a new direction. The swimming period becomes longer as the concentration of chemoattractant increases. The direction of flagellar spinning determines whether the bacteria swim or tumble. Flagella also express antigenic and strain determinants.

Fimbriae (pili) (Latin for "fringe") are hairlike structures on the outside of bacteria; they are composed of protein subunits (**pilin**). Fimbriae can be morphologically distinguished from flagella, because they are smaller in diameter (3 to 8 nm versus 15 to 20 nm) and usually are not coiled in structure. Generally, several hundred fimbriae are arranged peritrichously (uniformly) over the entire surface of the bacterial cell. They may be as long as 15 to 20 μm, or many times the length of the cell.

Fimbriae promote adherence to other bacteria or to the host (alternative names are *adhesins*, *lectins*, *evasins*, and *aggressins*). As an adherence factor (**adhesin**), fimbriae are an important virulence factor for colonization and infection of the urinary tract by *E. coli*, *Neisseria gonorrhoeae*, and other bacteria. The tips of the fimbriae may contain proteins (lectins) that bind to specific sugars (e.g., mannose). **F pili (sex pili)** bind to other bacteria and are a tube for transfer of large segments of bacterial chromosomes between bacteria. These pili are encoded by a plasmid (F).

Bacterial Exceptions

Mycobacteria have a peptidoglycan layer (slightly different structure), which is intertwined with and covalently attached to an arabinogalactan polymer and surrounded by a waxlike lipid coat of mycolic acid (large α-branched β-hydroxy fatty acids), cord factor (glycolipid of trehalose and two mycolic acids), wax D (glycolipid of 15 to 20 mycolic acids and sugar), and sulfolipids. These bacteria are described as **acid-fast staining**. The coat is responsible for virulence and is antiphagocytic. *Corynebacterium* and *Nocardia* organisms also produce mycolic acid lipids. The **mycoplasmas** are also exceptions, in that they have no peptidoglycan cell wall and incorporate steroids from the host into their membranes.

Structure and Biosynthesis of the Major Components of the Bacterial Cell Wall

The cell wall components are large structures made up of polymers of subunits. This type of structure facilitates their synthesis. Like astronauts building a space station, bacteria face problems assembling their cell walls. Synthesis of the peptidoglycan, LPS, teichoic acid, and capsule occurs on the outside of the bacteria, away from the synthetic machinery and energy sources of the cytoplasm and in an inhospitable environment. For both the space station and the bacteria, prefabricated precursors and subunits of the final structure are assembled in a factory-like setting on the inside, attached to a structure similar to a conveyor belt, brought to the surface, and then attached to the preexisting structure. For bacteria, the molecular conveyor belt–like structure is a large hydrophobic phospholipid called **bactoprenol (undecaprenol, [C_{55} isoprenoid])**. The prefabricated precursors must also be activated with high-energy bonds (e.g., phosphates) or other means to power the attachment reactions occurring outside the cell. For gram-negative bacteria, the outer membrane components are delivered through adhesion sites.

Peptidoglycan (Mucopeptide, Murein)

The peptidoglycan is a rigid mesh made up of ropelike linear polysaccharide chains cross-linked by peptides. The polysaccharide is made up of repeating disaccharides of **N-acetylglucosamine (GlcNAc, NAG, G)** and **N-acetylmuramic acid (MurNAc, NAM, M)** (Figure 2-6; see Figure 2-5).

A tetrapeptide is attached to the MurNAc. The peptide is unusual, because it contains both D and L amino acids (D amino acids are not normally used in nature), and the peptide is produced enzymatically rather than by a ribosome. The first two amino acids attached to the MurNAc may vary for different organisms.

The diamino amino acids in the third position are essential for the cross-linking of the peptidoglycan chain. Examples of diamino amino acids include lysine and diaminopimelic and diaminobutyric acids. The peptide cross-link is formed between the free amine of the diamino amino acid and the D-alanine in the fourth position of another chain. *S. aureus* and other gram-positive bacteria use an amino acid bridge (e.g., a glycine$_5$ peptide) between these amino acids to lengthen the cross-link. The precursor form of the peptide has an extra D-alanine, which is released during the cross-linking step.

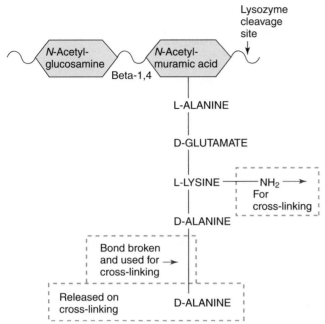

Figure 2–6. Precursor of peptidoglycan. The peptidoglycan is built from prefabricated units that contain a pentapeptide attached to the MurNAc. The pentapeptide contains a terminal D-alanine-D-alanine unit. This dipeptide is required for cross-linking the peptidoglycan and is the basis for the action of β-lactam and vancomycin antibiotics.

The peptidoglycan in gram-positive bacteria forms multiple layers and is often cross-linked in three dimensions, providing a very strong, rigid cell wall. In contrast, the peptidoglycan in gram-negative cell walls is usually only one molecule (layer) thick. The number of cross-links and the length of the cross-link determine the rigidity of the peptidoglycan mesh. The site where **lysozyme** cleaves the glycan of the peptidoglycan is shown in Figure 2-6.

Peptidoglycan Synthesis

Peptidoglycan synthesis occurs in five steps (Figure 2-7). First, inside the cell glucosamine is enzymatically converted into MurNAc and then energetically activated by a reaction with uridine triphosphate (UTP) to produce uridine diphosphate-*N*-acetylmuramic acid (UDP-MurNAc). Second, the UDP-MurNAc-pentapeptide precursor is assembled in a series of enzymatic steps.

Third, the UDP-MurNAc pentapeptide is attached to the **bactoprenol** "conveyor belt" in the cytoplasmic membrane through a pyrophosphate link, with the release of uridine monophosphate (UMP). GlcNAc is added to make the disaccharide building block of the peptidoglycan. Some bacteria (e.g., *S. aureus*) add a pentaglycine or another chain to the diamino amino acid at the third position of the peptide chain to lengthen the cross-link. Fourth, the bactoprenol molecule translocates the disaccharide:peptide precursor to the outside of the cell. The GlcNAc-MurNAc disaccharide

is then attached to a peptidoglycan chain, using the pyrophosphate link between itself and the bactoprenol as energy to drive the reaction by enzymes called **transglycosylases**. The pyrophosphobactoprenol is converted back to a phosphobactoprenol and recycled. **Bacitracin** blocks the recycling. Fifth, outside the cell but near the membrane surface, peptide chains from adjacent glycan chains are cross-linked to each other by a peptide bond exchange (**transpeptidation**) between the free amine of the amino acid in the third position of the pentapeptide (e.g., lysine), or the *N*-terminus of the attached pentaglycine chain, and the D-alanine at the fourth position of the other peptide chain, releasing the terminal D-alanine of the precursor. This step requires no additional energy, because peptide bonds are "traded."

The cross-linking reaction is catalyzed by membrane-bound **transpeptidases**. Related enzymes, DD-**carboxypeptidases**, remove unreacted terminal D-alanines to limit the extent of cross-linking. The transpeptidases and carboxypeptidases are called **penicillin-binding proteins (PBPs)**, because they are targets for penicillin and other β-lactam antibiotics. *Penicillin* and related **β-lactam antibiotics** resemble the "transition state" conformation of the D-ALA-D-ALA substrate when bound to these enzymes. **Vancomycin** binds to the D-ALA-D-ALA structure to block these reactions. Different PBPs are used for extending the peptidoglycan, creating a septum for cell division and curving the peptidoglycan mesh (cell shape). Peptidoglycan extension and crosslinking is necessary for cell growth and division.

The peptidoglycan is constantly being synthesized and degraded. **Autolysins** such as lysozyme are important for determining bacterial shape. Inhibition of synthesis or the cross-linking of the peptidoglycan does not stop the autolysins, and their action weakens the mesh and leads to cell lysis and death. New peptidoglycan synthesis does not occur during starvation, which leads to a weakening of the peptidoglycan and a loss in the dependability of the Gram stain.

An understanding of the biosynthesis of peptidoglycan is essential in medicine, because these reactions are unique to bacterial cells and hence can be inhibited with little or no adverse effect on host (human) cells. As indicated above, a number of antibacterials target one or more steps in this pathway (see Chapter 20).

Teichoic Acid

Teichoic and **lipoteichoic acid** are polymers of chemically modified ribose or glycerol connected by phosphates (Figure 2-8). Sugars, choline, or D-alanine may be attached to the hydroxyls of the ribose or glycerol, providing antigenic determinants. These can be distinguished by antibodies and may determine the bacterial serotype. Lipoteichoic acid has a fatty acid and is anchored in the membrane. Teichoic acid is synthesized from building blocks using the

Figure 2–7. Peptidoglycan synthesis. **A,** Peptidoglycan synthesis occurs in the following three phases: (1) Peptidoglycan is synthesized from prefabricated units constructed and activated for assembly and transport inside the cell. (2) At the membrane the units are assembled onto the undecaprenol phosphate conveyor belt, and fabrication is completed. (3) The unit is translocated to the outside of the cell, where it is attached to the polysaccharide chain, and the peptide is cross-linked to finish the construction. *S. aureus* utilizes a pentaglycine bridge in the cross-link. Such a construction can be compared with the assembly of a space station. **B,** The cross-linking reaction is a transpeptidation. *E. coli* uses a direct cross-link between D-alanine and lysine. One peptide bond (produced inside the cell) is traded for another (outside the cell) with the release of D-alanine. The enzymes that catalyze the reaction are called D-*alanine, D-alanine transpeptidase-carboxypeptidases*. These enzymes are the targets of β-lactam antibiotics and are called penicillin-binding proteins. (© *American Society of Clinical Pathologists. Reprinted with permission.*)

bactoprenol in a manner similar to that of peptidoglycan. Teichoic acid and some **surface proteins** (e.g., Protein A from *S. aureus*) are secreted from the cells and are enzymatically attached to the *N*-terminus of the peptide of peptidoglycan.

Lipopolysaccharide

LPS (endotoxin) *consists of three structural sections: Lipid A, core polysaccharide (rough core), and O antigen* (Figure 2-9). Lipid A is a basic component of LPS and is essential for bacterial viability. *Lipid A is responsible for the endotoxin activity*

Ribitol-Teichoic Acid
(*Staphylococcus*)

A

Glycerol Teichoic Acid
(*Lactobacillus*)

B

Figure 2–8. Teichoic acid. Teichoic acid is a polymer of chemically modified ribitol (**A**) or glycerol phosphate (**B**). The nature of the modification (e.g., sugars, amino acids) can define the serotype of the bacteria. Teichoic acid may be covalently attached to the peptidoglycan. Lipoteichoic acid is anchored in the cytoplasmic membrane by a covalently attached fatty acid.

Figure 2–9. The lipopolysaccharide of the gram-negative cell envelope. **A,** Segment of the polymer showing the arrangements of the major constituents. Each LPS molecule has one Lipid A and one polysaccharide core unit but many repeats of O antigen. **B,** Structure of Lipid A of *Salmonella typhimurium*. **C,** Polysaccharide core. **D,** Typical O-antigen repeat unit *(S. typhimurium)*. *(Redrawn from Brooks GF, Butel JS, Ornston LN: Jawetz, Melnick and Aldenberg's Medical Microbiology, 19th ed. Norwalk, Conn, Appleton & Lange, 1991.)*

of LPS. It has a phosphorylated glucosamine disaccharide backbone with fatty acids attached to anchor the structure in each outer membrane. The phosphates connect LPS units into aggregates. One carbohydrate chain is attached to each disaccharide backbone and extends away from the bacteria. The core polysaccharide is a branched polysaccharide of 9 to 12 sugars. Most of the core region is also essential for LPS structure and bacterial viability. The core region contains an unusual sugar, 2-keto-3-deoxy-octanoate (KDO), and is phosphorylated. Divalent cations link the phosphates of the LPS and core to strengthen the outer membrane. The O antigen is attached to the core and extends away from the bacteria. It is a long, linear polysaccharide consisting of 50 to 100 repeating saccharide units of 4 to 7 sugars per unit. Lipooligosaccharide, which is present in *Neisseria* species, lacks the O-antigen portion of LPS and is readily shed from the bacteria. The shorter O antigen makes *Neisseria* more susceptible to host mediated complement control.

LPS structure is used to classify bacteria. The basic structure of lipid A is identical for related bacteria and is similar for all gram-negative **Enterobacteriaceae.** The core region is the same for a species of bacteria. The O antigen distinguishes serotypes (strains) of a bacterial species. For example, the O157:H7 serotype identifies the *E. coli* agent of hemolytic-uremic syndrome.

The lipid A and core portions are enzymatically synthesized in a sequential manner on the inside surface of the cytoplasmic membrane. The repeat units of the O antigen are assembled on a bactoprenol molecule and then transferred to a growing O-antigen chain. The finished O-antigen chain is transferred to the core lipid A structure. The LPS molecule is translocated through adhesion sites to the outer surface of the outer membrane.

Cell Division

The replication of the bacterial chromosome also triggers the initiation of cell division (Figure 2-10). The production of two daughter bacteria requires the growth and extension of the cell wall components, followed by the production of a septum (cross wall) to divide the daughter bacteria into two cells. The septum consists of two membranes separated by two layers of peptidoglycan. Septum formation is initiated at midcell, at a site defined by protein complexes affixed to a protein filament ring that lines the inside of the cytoplasmic membrane. The septum grows from opposite sides toward the center of the cell, causing cleavage of the daughter cells. This process requires special transpeptidases (PBPs) and

Figure 2—10. Electron photomicrographs of gram-positive cell division (*Bacillus subtilis*) (*left*) and gram-negative cell division (*Escherichia coli*) (*right*). Progression in cell division from top to bottom. CM, cytoplasmic membrane; CW, cell wall; N, nucleoid; OM, outer membrane; S, septum. Bar = 0.2 µm. (*From Slots J, Taubman MA: Contemporary Oral Biology and Immunology. St Louis, Mosby, 1992.*)

other enzymes. For streptococci, the growth zone is located at 180 degrees from each other, producing linear chains of bacteria. In contrast, the growth zone of staphylococci is at 90 degrees. Incomplete cleavage of the septum can cause the bacteria to remain linked, forming chains (e.g., streptococci) or clusters (e.g., staphylococci).

Spores

Some gram-positive, but never gram-negative, bacteria, such as members of the genera *Bacillus* (e.g., *Bacillus anthracis*) and *Clostridium* (e.g., *Clostridium tetani* or *botulinum*) (soil bacteria), are spore formers. Under harsh environmental conditions, such as the loss of a nutritional requirement, these bacteria can convert from a **vegetative state** to a **dormant state**, or **spore**. The location of the spore within a cell is a characteristic of the bacteria and can assist in identification of the bacterium.

The spore is a dehydrated, multishelled structure that protects and allows the bacteria to exist in "suspended animation" (Figure 2-11). It contains a complete copy of the chromosome, the bare minimum concentrations of essential proteins and ribosomes, and a high concentration of **calcium bound to dipicolinic acid**. The spore has an inner membrane, two peptidoglycan layers, and an outer keratin-like protein coat. The spore looks refractile (bright) in the microscope. The structure of the spore protects the genomic DNA from intense heat, radiation, and attack by most enzymes and chemical agents. In fact, bacterial spores are so resistant to environmental factors that they can exist for centuries as viable spores. Spores are also difficult to decontaminate with standard disinfectants.

Depletion of specific nutrients (e.g., alanine) from the growth medium triggers a cascade of genetic events (comparable to differentiation) leading to the production of a spore. Spore mRNA are transcribed, and other mRNA are turned off. Dipicolinic acid is produced, and antibiotics and toxins are often excreted. After duplication of the chromosome, one copy of the DNA and cytoplasmic contents (**core**) are surrounded by the cytoplasmic membrane, the peptidoglycan, and the membrane of the septum. This wraps the DNA in the two layers of membrane and peptidoglycan that would normally divide the cell. These two layers are surrounded by the **cortex**, which is made up of a thin inner layer of tightly cross-linked peptidoglycan surrounding a membrane (which used to be the cytoplasmic membrane) and a loose outer peptidoglycan layer. The cortex is surrounded by the tough, **keratin-like protein coat**, which protects the spore. The process requires 6 to 8 hours for completion.

The germination of spores into the vegetative state is stimulated by disruption of the outer coat by mechanical stress, pH, heat, or another stressor and requires water and a triggering nutrient (e.g., alanine). The process takes approximately 90 minutes. After the germination process begins, the spore will take up water, swell, shed its coats, and produce one new

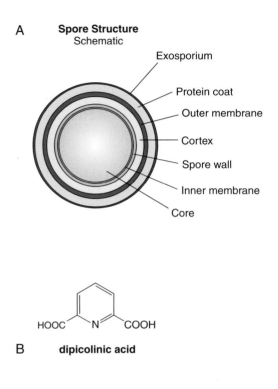

A **Spore Structure**
Schematic

- Exosporium
- Protein coat
- Outer membrane
- Cortex
- Spore wall
- Inner membrane
- Core

B **dipicolinic acid**

HOOC — N — COOH

C Free endospore

Figure 2–11. A, Structure of a spore. **B,** High concentrations of dipicolinic acid in the spore bind calcium and stabilize the contents. **C,** Sporogenesis, the process of endospore formation.

vegetative cell identical to the original vegetative cell, thus completing the entire cycle. Once germination has begun and the spore coat has been compromised, the spore is weakened, vulnerable, and can be inactivated like other bacteria.

Questions

1. How does each of the differences between prokaryotes and eukaryotes influence bacterial infection and treatment (see Table 2-1)?

2. How do the differences between gram-positive and gram-negative cell walls influence the cells' clinical behavior, detection, and treatment?

3. List the cell wall components that contribute to virulence by protecting the bacteria from immune responses. List those that contribute to virulence by eliciting toxic responses in the human host.

4. When peptidoglycan synthesis is inhibited, what processes kill the bacteria? List the precursors that would build up within the bacteria if recycling of bactoprenol were inhibited by penicillin, vancomycin, or bacitracin.

5. Why are spores more resistant to environmental stresses?

6. The laboratory would like to selectively eliminate gram-positive bacteria from a mixture of gram-positive and gram-negative bacteria. Which of the following procedures would be more appropriate and why or why not?
   a. Treatment with ethylenediaminetetraacetic acid (a divalent cation chelator)
   b. Treatment with mild detergent
   c. Treatment with lysozyme
   d. Treatment with transpeptidase
   e. Treatment with ampicillin (a hydrophilic β-lactam antibiotic)

Bibliography

Bower S, Rosenthal KS: Bacterial cell walls: The armor, artillery and Achilles heel. Infect Dis Clin Practice 14:309-317, 2006.

Daniel RA, Errington J: Control of cell morphogenesis in bacteria: Two distinct ways to make a rod-shaped cell. Cell 113:767-776, 2003.

Lutkenhaus J: The regulation of bacterial cell division: A time and place for it. Curr Opin Microbiol 1:210-215, 1998.

Meroueh SO, et al: Three-dimensional structure of the bacterial cell wall peptidoglycan. Proc Natl Acad Sci USA 103(12):4404-4409, 2006.

Nanninga N: Morphogenesis of *Escherichia coli*. Microbiol Mol Biol Rev 62:110-129, 1998.

Talaro K: Foundations in Microbiology, 6th ed. New York, McGraw-Hill, 2008.

Willey J, Sherwood L, Woolverton C: Prescott/Harley/Klein's Microbiology, 7th ed. New York, McGraw-Hill, 2007.

Bacterial Metabolism and Genetics

Bacterial Metabolism

Metabolic Requirements

Bacterial growth requires a source of energy and the raw materials to build the proteins, structures, and membranes that make up and power the cell. Bacteria must obtain or synthesize the amino acids, carbohydrates, and lipids used as building blocks of the cell.

The minimum requirement for growth is a source of carbon and nitrogen, an energy source, water, and various ions. The essential elements include the components of proteins, lipids and nucleic acids (C, O, H, N, S, P), important ions (K, Na, Mg, Ca, Cl) and components of enzymes (Fe, Zn, Mn, Mo, Se, Co, Cu, Ni). **Iron** is so important that many bacteria secrete special proteins (siderophores) to concentrate iron from dilute solutions, and our bodies will sequester iron to reduce its availability as a means of protection.

Oxygen (O_2 gas), although essential for the human host, is actually a poison for many bacteria. Some organisms, such as *Clostridium perfringens*, which causes gas gangrene, cannot grow in the presence of oxygen. Such bacteria are referred to as **obligate anaerobes**. Other organisms, such as *Mycobacterium tuberculosis*, which causes tuberculosis, require the presence of molecular oxygen for metabolism and growth and are therefore referred to as **obligate aerobes**. Most bacteria, however, grow in either the presence or the absence of oxygen. These bacteria are referred to as **facultative anaerobes**. Aerobic bacteria produce superoxide dismutase and catalase enzymes which can detoxify hydrogen peroxide and superoxide radicals that are the toxic byproducts of aerobic metabolism.

Growth requirements and metabolic byproducts may be used as a convenient means of classifying different bacteria. Some bacteria, such as certain strains of *Escherichia coli* (a member of the intestinal flora), can synthesize all the amino acids, nucleotides, lipids, and carbohydrates necessary for growth and division, whereas the growth requirements of the causative agent of syphilis, *Treponema pallidum*, are so complex that a defined laboratory medium capable of supporting its growth has yet to be developed. Bacteria that can rely entirely on inorganic chemicals for their energy and source of carbon (CO_2) are referred to as autotrophs (lithotrophs), whereas many bacteria and animal cells that require organic carbon sources are known as heterotrophs (organotrophs). Clinical microbiology laboratories distinguish bacteria by their ability to grow on specific carbon sources (e.g., lactose) and the end products of metabolism (e.g., ethanol, lactic acid, succinic acid).

Metabolism, Energy, and Biosynthesis

All cells require a constant supply of energy to survive. This energy, typically in the form of adenosine triphosphate (ATP), is derived from the controlled breakdown of various organic substrates (carbohydrates, lipids, and proteins). This process of substrate breakdown and conversion into usable energy is known as **catabolism**. The energy produced may then be used in the synthesis of cellular constituents (cell walls, proteins, fatty acids, and nucleic acids), a process known as **anabolism**. Together these two processes, which are interrelated and tightly integrated, are referred to as **intermediary metabolism**.

The metabolic process generally begins with hydrolysis of large macromolecules in the external cellular environment by specific enzymes (Figure 3-1). The smaller molecules that are produced (e.g., monosaccharides, short peptides, and fatty acids) are transported across the cell membranes into the cytoplasm by active or passive transport mechanisms specific for the metabolite. These mechanisms may use specific carrier or membrane transport proteins to help concentrate metabolites from the medium. The metabolites are converted via one or more pathways to one common, universal intermediate, **pyruvic acid**. From pyruvic acid the carbons may be channeled toward energy production or the synthesis of new carbohydrates, amino acids, lipids, and nucleic acids.

CATABOLISM

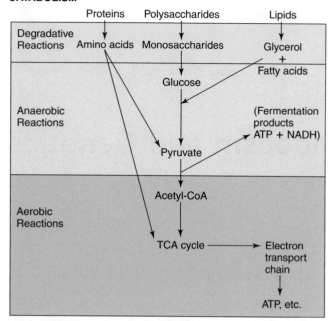

Figure 3–1. Catabolism of proteins, polysaccharides, and lipids produces glucose, pyruvate, or intermediates of the tricarboxylic acid (TCA) cycle and, ultimately, energy in the form of adenosine triphosphate (ATP) or the reduced form of nicotinamide-adenine dinucleotide (NADH).

Metabolism of Glucose

For the sake of simplicity, this section presents an overview of the pathways by which glucose is metabolized to produce energy or other usable substrates. Instead of releasing all the molecule's energy as heat (as for burning), the bacteria break down the glucose in discrete steps to allow the energy to be captured in usable forms. *Bacteria can produce energy from* glucose by—in order of increasing efficiency—fermentation, anaerobic respiration (both of which occur in the absence of oxygen), or aerobic respiration. Aerobic respiration can completely convert the six carbons of glucose to CO_2 and H_2O plus energy, whereas two- and three-carbon compounds are the end products of fermentation. For a more complete discussion of metabolism, please refer to a textbook on biochemistry.

Embden-Meyerhof-Parnas Pathway

Bacteria use three major metabolic pathways in the catabolism of glucose. Most common among these is the **glycolytic**, or Embden-Meyerhof-Parnas (EMP), pathway (Figure 3-2) for the conversion of glucose to pyruvate. These reactions, which occur under both **aerobic** and **anaerobic** conditions, begin with activation of glucose to form glucose-6-phosphate. This reaction, as well as the third reaction in the series, in which fructose-6-phosphate is converted to fructose-1,6-diphosphate, requires 1 mole of ATP per mole of glucose and represents an initial investment of cellular energy stores.

Energy is produced during glycolysis in two different forms, chemical and electrochemical. In the first, the high-energy phosphate group of one of the intermediates

Figure 3–2. Embden-Meyerhof-Parnas (EMP) glycolytic pathway results in conversion of glucose to pyruvate. ADP, adenosine diphosphate; ATP, adenosine triphosphate; iPO4, inorganic phosphate; NAD, nicotinamide adenine dinucleotide; NADH, reduced form of NAD.

in the pathway is used under the direction of the appropriate enzyme (a **kinase**) to generate **ATP** from adenosine diphosphate (ADP). This type of reaction, termed **substrate-level phosphorylation**, occurs at two different points in the glycolytic pathway (i.e., conversion of 3-phosphoglycerol phosphate to 3-phosphoglycerate and 2-phosphoenolpyruvic acid to pyruvate). Four ATP molecules per molecule of glucose are produced in this manner, but two ATP molecules were used in the initial glycolytic conversion of glucose to two molecules of pyruvic acid, resulting in a net production of two molecules of ATP.

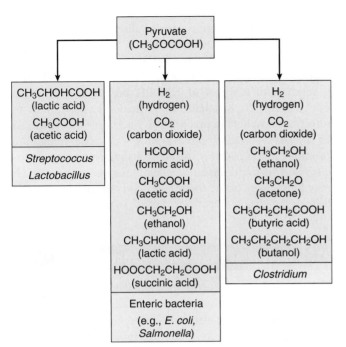

Figure 3—3. Fermentation of pyruvate by different microorganisms results in different end products. The clinical laboratory uses these pathways and end products as a means of distinguishing different bacteria.

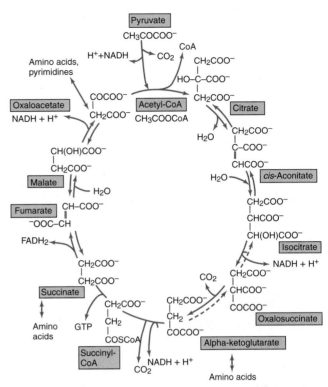

Figure 3—4. Tricarboxylic acid cycle occurs in aerobic conditions and is an amphibolic cycle. Precursors for the synthesis of amino acids and nucleotides are also shown. CoA, coenzyme A; $FADH_2$, flavin adenine dinucleotide; GTP, guanosine triphosphate.

The reduced form of **nicotinamide-adenine dinucleotide (NADH)** that is produced represents the second form of energy, which may then be converted to ATP by a series of oxidation reactions.

In the absence of oxygen, substrate-level phosphorylation represents the primary means of energy production. The pyruvic acid produced from glycolysis is then converted to various end products, depending on the bacterial species, in a process known as **fermentation**. Many bacteria are identified on the basis of their fermentative end products (Figure 3-3). These organic molecules, rather than oxygen, are used as electron acceptors to recycle the NADH, which was produced during glycolysis, to NAD. In yeast, fermentative metabolism results in the conversion of pyruvate to ethanol plus carbon dioxide. Alcoholic fermentation is uncommon in bacteria, which most commonly use the one-step conversion of pyruvic acid to lactic acid. This process is responsible for making milk into yogurt and cabbage into sauerkraut. Other bacteria use more complex fermentative pathways, producing various acids, alcohols, and often gases (many of which have vile odors). These products lend flavors to various cheeses and wines and odors to wound and other infections.

Tricarboxylic Acid Cycle

In the presence of oxygen, the pyruvic acid produced from glycolysis and from the metabolism of other substrates may be completely oxidized (controlled burning) to water and CO_2 using the tricarboxylic acid (TCA) cycle (Figure 3-4), which results in production of additional energy.

The process begins with the oxidative decarboxylation (release of CO_2) of pyruvate to the high-energy intermediate, acetyl coenzyme A (acetyl CoA); this reaction also produces two NADH molecules. The two remaining carbons derived from pyruvate then enter the TCA cycle in the form of acetyl CoA by condensation with oxaloacetate, with the formation of the six-carbon citrate molecule. In a stepwise series of oxidative reactions the citrate is converted back to oxaloacetate. The theoretical yield from each pyruvate is 2 moles of CO_2, 3 moles of NADH, 1 mole of flavin adenine dinucleotide ($FADH_2$), and 1 mole of guanosine triphosphate (GTP).

The TCA cycle allows the organism to generate substantially more energy per mole of glucose than is possible from glycolysis alone. In addition to the GTP (an ATP equivalent) produced by substrate-level phosphorylation, the NADH and $FADH_2$ yield ATP from the electron transport chain. In this chain the electrons carried by NADH (or $FADH_2$) are passed in a stepwise fashion through a series of donor-acceptor pairs and ultimately to oxygen (**aerobic respiration**) or other terminal electron acceptor (nitrate, sulfate, carbon dioxide, ferric iron) (**anaerobic respiration**).

Anaerobic organisms are less efficient at energy production than aerobic organisms. Fermentation produces only 2 ATP molecules per glucose, whereas aerobic metabolism with electron transport and a complete TCA cycle can generate as much as 19 times more energy (38 ATP molecules) from the same starting material (and it is much less

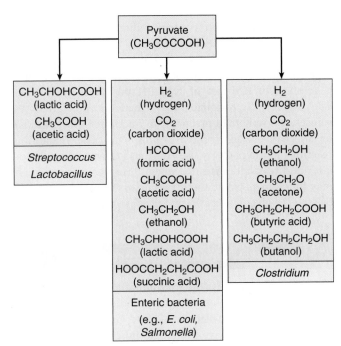

Figure 3—3. Fermentation of pyruvate by different microorganisms results in different end products. The clinical laboratory uses these pathways and end products as a means of distinguishing different bacteria.

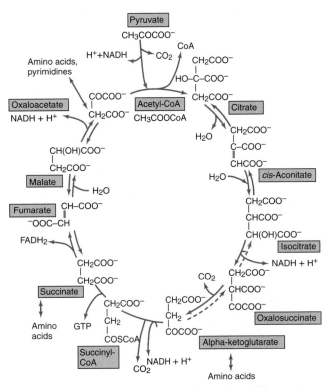

Figure 3—4. Tricarboxylic acid cycle occurs in aerobic conditions and is an amphibolic cycle. Precursors for the synthesis of amino acids and nucleotides are also shown. CoA, coenzyme A; FADH$_2$, flavin adenine dinucleotide; GTP, guanosine triphosphate.

The reduced form of **nicotinamide-adenine dinucleotide (NADH)** that is produced represents the second form of energy, which may then be converted to ATP by a series of oxidation reactions.

In the absence of oxygen, substrate-level phosphorylation represents the primary means of energy production. The pyruvic acid produced from glycolysis is then converted to various end products, depending on the bacterial species, in a process known as **fermentation**. Many bacteria are identified on the basis of their fermentative end products (Figure 3-3). These organic molecules, rather than oxygen, are used as electron acceptors to recycle the NADH, which was produced during glycolysis, to NAD. In yeast, fermentative metabolism results in the conversion of pyruvate to ethanol plus carbon dioxide. Alcoholic fermentation is uncommon in bacteria, which most commonly use the one-step conversion of pyruvic acid to lactic acid. This process is responsible for making milk into yogurt and cabbage into sauerkraut. Other bacteria use more complex fermentative pathways, producing various acids, alcohols, and often gases (many of which have vile odors). These products lend flavors to various cheeses and wines and odors to wound and other infections.

Tricarboxylic Acid Cycle

In the presence of oxygen, the pyruvic acid produced from glycolysis and from the metabolism of other substrates may be completely oxidized (controlled burning) to water and CO$_2$ using the tricarboxylic acid (TCA) cycle (Figure 3-4), which results in production of additional energy.

The process begins with the oxidative decarboxylation (release of CO$_2$) of pyruvate to the high-energy intermediate, acetyl coenzyme A (acetyl CoA); this reaction also produces two NADH molecules. The two remaining carbons derived from pyruvate then enter the TCA cycle in the form of acetyl CoA by condensation with oxaloacetate, with the formation of the six-carbon citrate molecule. In a stepwise series of oxidative reactions the citrate is converted back to oxaloacetate. The theoretical yield from each pyruvate is 2 moles of CO$_2$, 3 moles of NADH, 1 mole of flavin adenine dinucleotide (FADH$_2$), and 1 mole of guanosine triphosphate (GTP).

The TCA cycle allows the organism to generate substantially more energy per mole of glucose than is possible from glycolysis alone. In addition to the GTP (an ATP equivalent) produced by substrate-level phosphorylation, the NADH and FADH$_2$ yield ATP from the electron transport chain. In this chain the electrons carried by NADH (or FADH$_2$) are passed in a stepwise fashion through a series of donor-acceptor pairs and ultimately to oxygen (**aerobic respiration**) or other terminal electron acceptor (nitrate, sulfate, carbon dioxide, ferric iron) (**anaerobic respiration**).

Anaerobic organisms are less efficient at energy production than aerobic organisms. Fermentation produces only 2 ATP molecules per glucose, whereas aerobic metabolism with electron transport and a complete TCA cycle can generate as much as 19 times more energy (38 ATP molecules) from the same starting material (and it is much less

GLYCOLYSIS

Figure 3—5. Aerobic glucose metabolism. The theoretical maximum amount of ATP obtained from one glucose molecule is 38, but the actual yield depends on the organism and other conditions.

smelly) (Figure 3-5). Anaerobic respiration uses organic molecules as electron acceptors, which produces less ATP for each NADH.

In addition to the efficient generation of ATP from glucose (and other carbohydrates), the TCA cycle provides a means by which carbons derived from **lipids** (in the form of acetyl CoA) may be shunted toward either energy production or the generation of biosynthetic precursors. Similarly, the cycle includes several points at which **deaminated amino acids** may enter (see Figure 3-4). For example, deamination of glutamic acid yields α-ketoglutarate, whereas deamination of aspartic acid yields oxaloacetate, both of which are TCA cycle intermediates. The TCA cycle therefore serves the following functions:

1. It is the most efficient mechanism for the generation of ATP.
2. It serves as the final common pathway for the complete oxidation of amino acids, fatty acids, and carbohydrates.
3. It supplies key intermediates (i.e., α-ketoglutarate, pyruvate, oxaloacetate) for the ultimate synthesis of amino acids, lipids, purines, and pyrimidines.

The last two functions make the TCA cycle a so-called **amphibolic cycle** (i.e., it may function in the anabolic and the catabolic functions of the cell).

Pentose Phosphate Pathway

The final pathway of glucose metabolism considered here is known as the **pentose phosphate pathway**, or the **hexose monophosphate shunt**. The function of this pathway is to provide nucleic acid precursors and reducing power in

the form of nicotinamide-adenine dinucleotide phosphate (reduced form) (**NADPH**) for use in biosynthesis. In the first half of the pathway, glucose is converted to ribulose-5-phosphate, with consumption of 1 mole of ATP and generation of 2 moles of NADPH per mole of glucose. The ribulose-5-phosphate may then be converted to ribose-5-phosphate (a precursor in nucleotide biosynthesis) or alternatively to xylulose-5-phosphate. The remaining reactions in the pathway use enzymes known as **transketolases** and **transaldolases** to generate various sugars, which may function as biosynthetic precursors or may be shunted back to the glycolytic pathway for use in energy generation.

The Bacterial Genes and Expression

The bacterial genome is the total collection of genes carried by a bacterium, both on its chromosome and on its extra-chromosomal genetic elements, if any. Genes are sequences of nucleotides that have a biologic function; examples are protein-structural genes (**cistrons**, which are coding genes), ribosomal ribonucleic acid (RNA) genes, and recognition and binding sites for other molecules (promoters and operators). Each genome contains many **operons**, which are made up of **genes**. Eukaryotes usually have two distinct copies of each chromosome (they are therefore diploid). Bacteria usually have only one copy of their chromosomes (they are therefore **haploid**). Because bacteria have only one chromosome, alteration of a gene (mutation) will have a more obvious effect on the cell. In addition, the structure of the bacterial chromosome is maintained by polyamines, such as spermine and spermidine, rather than by histones.

Bacteria may also contain **extrachromosomal genetic elements** such as **plasmids** or **bacteriophages** (bacterial viruses). These elements are independent of the bacterial chromosome and in most cases can be transmitted from one cell to another.

Transcription

The information carried in the genetic memory of the DNA is transcribed into a useful **messenger RNA (mRNA)** for subsequent translation into protein. RNA synthesis is performed by a **DNA-dependent RNA polymerase**.

The process begins when **sigma factor** recognizes a particular sequence of nucleotides in the DNA (the **promoter**) and binds tightly to this site. Promoter sequences occur just before the start of the DNA that actually encodes a protein. Sigma factors bind to these promoters to provide a docking site for the **RNA polymerase**. Some bacteria encode several sigma factors to allow transcription of a group of genes under special conditions, such as heat shock, starvation, special nitrogen metabolism, or sporulation. Once the polymerase has bound to the appropriate site on the DNA, RNA synthesis proceeds with the sequential addition of ribonucleotides complementary to the sequence in the DNA. Once an entire gene or group of genes (**operon**) has been transcribed, the RNA polymerase dissociates from the DNA, a process mediated by signals within the DNA. The bacterial, DNA-dependent RNA polymerase is inhibited by rifampin, an antibiotic often used in the treatment of tuberculosis. The **transfer RNA (tRNA),** which is used in protein synthesis, and **ribosomal RNA (rRNA),** a component of the ribosomes, are also transcribed from the DNA.

Promoters and operators control the expression of a gene by influencing which sequences will be transcribed into messenger RNA (mRNA). **Operons** are groups of one or more structural genes expressed from a particular promoter and ending at a transcriptional terminator. Thus all the genes coding for the enzymes of a particular pathway can be coordinately regulated. Operons with many structural genes are **polycistronic.** The *E. coli lac* operon includes all the genes necessary for lactose metabolism, as well as the control mechanisms for turning off (in the presence of glucose) or turning on (in the presence of galactose or an inducer) these genes only when they are needed. The *lac* operon includes a repressor sequence, a promoter sequence, and structural genes for the β-galactosidase enzyme, a permease, and an acetylase (Figure 3-6). The *lac* operon is discussed later in this chapter.

Translation

Translation is the process by which the language of the **genetic code**, in the form of mRNA, is converted (translated) into a sequence of amino acids, the protein product. Each amino acid word and the punctuation of the genetic code is written in a set of three nucleotides, known as a **codon**. There are 64 different codon combinations encoding the 20 amino acids, the 20 amino acids plus start and termination codons. Some of the amino acids are encoded by more than one triplet codon. This feature is known as the *degeneracy of the genetic code* and may function in protecting the cell from the effects of minor mutations in the DNA or mRNA. Each tRNA molecule contains a three-nucleotide sequence complementary to one of the codon sequences. This tRNA sequence is known as the **anticodon**; it allows base pairing and binds to the codon sequence on the mRNA. Attached to the opposite end of the tRNA is the amino acid that corresponds to the particular codon—anticodon pair.

The process of protein synthesis (Figure 3-7) begins with the binding of the 30S ribosomal subunit and a special initiator tRNA for formyl methionine (fmet) at the methionine codon (AUG) start codon to form the **initiation complex**. The 50S ribosomal subunit binds to the complex to initiate mRNA synthesis. The ribosome contains two tRNA binding sites, the **A (aminoacyl) site** and the **P (peptidyl) site**, each of which allows base pairing between the bound tRNA and the codon sequence in the mRNA. The tRNA corresponding to the second codon occupies the A site. The amino group of the amino acid attached to the A site forms a peptide bond with the carboxyl group of the amino acid in the P site in a reaction known as **transpeptidation**, and the empty tRNA in the P site (uncharged tRNA) is released from the ribosome. The ribosome then moves down the mRNA exactly three nucleotides, thereby transferring the tRNA with attached nascent peptide to the P site and bringing the next codon into the A site. The appropriate charged tRNA is brought into the A site, and the process is then repeated. Translation continues until the new codon in the A site is one of the three termination codons, for which there is no corresponding tRNA. At that point the new protein is released to the cytoplasm and the translation complex may be disassembled, or the ribosome shuffles to the next start codon and initiates a new protein. The ability to shuffle along the mRNA to start a new protein is a characteristic of the 70S bacterial but not of the 80S eukaryotic ribosome. This has implications for the synthesis of proteins for some viruses.

The process of protein synthesis by the 70S ribosome represents an important target of antimicrobial action. The aminoglycosides (e.g., streptomycin and gentamicin) and the tetracyclines act by binding to the small ribosomal subunit and inhibiting normal ribosomal function. Similarly the macrolide (e.g., erythromycin) and lincosamide (e.g., clindamycin) groups of antibiotics act by binding to the large ribosomal subunit.

Control of Gene Expression

Bacteria have developed mechanisms to adapt quickly and efficiently to changes and triggers from the environment. This allows them to coordinate and regulate the expression of genes for multicomponent structures or the enzymes of one or more metabolic pathways. For example, temperature change could signify entry into the human host and indicate the need for a global change in metabolism and up-regulation of genes important for parasitism or virulence. Many bacterial genes are controlled at multiple levels and by multiple methods.

A coordinated change in the expression of many genes, as would be required for sporulation, occurs through use of a different **sigma factor** for the RNA polymerase. This would change the specificity of the RNA polymerase and allow mRNA synthesis for the necessary genes while ignoring unnecessary genes. Bacteria might produce more than six different sigma factors to provide global regulation in response to stress, shock, starvation, or to coordinate production of complicated structures such as flagella.

Coordination of a large number of processes on a global level can also be mediated by small molecular activators, such as cyclic adenosine monophosphate (cAMP). Increased cAMP levels indicate low glucose levels and the need to utilize alternative metabolic pathways. Similarly, the increased concentration of specific small molecules produced by individual bacteria is used to turn on virulence genes when a sufficient number of bacteria are present. This process is called **quorum sensing**. The trigger for biofilm production by *Pseudomonas* spp. is triggered by a critical concentration of *N*-acyl homoserine lactone (AHL)

Figure 3–6. A, The lactose operon is transcribed as a polycistronic messenger RNA (mRNA) from the promoter (P) and translated into three proteins: β-galactosidase (Z), permease (Y), and acetylase (A). The *lac* I gene encodes the repressor protein. **B,** The lactose operon is not transcribed in the absence of an allolactose inducer, because the repressor competes with the RNA polymerase at the operator site (O). **C,** The repressor, complexed with the inducer, does not recognize the operator because of a conformation change in the repressor. The lac operon is thus transcribed at a low level. **D,** *Escherichia coli* is grown in a poor medium in the presence of lactose as the carbon source. Both the inducer and the CAP-cAMP complex are bound to the promoter, which is fully "turned on," and a high level of *lac* mRNA is transcribed and translated. **E,** Growth of *E. coli* in a poor medium without lactose results in the binding of the CAP-cAMP complex to the promoter region and binding of the active repressor to the operator sequence, because no inducer is available. The result will be that the *lac* operon will not be transcribed. ATP, adenosine triphosphate; CAP, catabolite gene-activator protein; cAMP, cyclic adenosine monophosphate.

produced when sufficient numbers of bacteria (a quorum) are present. Activation of toxin production and more virulent behavior by *S. aureus* accompanies the increase in concentration of a cyclic peptide.

To coordinate the expression of a more limited group of genes, such as for a specific metabolic process, the genes for the necessary enzymes would be organized into an **operon**. The operon would be under the control of a promoter or repressor DNA sequence that can activate or turn off the expression of a gene or a group of genes to coordinate

production of the necessary enzymes and allow the bacteria to react to changes in concentrations of nutrients. The genes for some virulence mechanisms are organized into a **pathogenicity island** under the control of a single promoter to allow their expression under appropriate (to the bacteria) conditions. The many components of the Type III secretion devices of *E. coli*, *Salmonella*, or *Yersinia* are grouped together within a pathogenicity island.

Transcription can also be regulated by the translation process. Unlike eukaryotes, the absence of a nuclear membrane in prokaryotes allows the ribosome to bind to the mRNA as it is being transcribed from the DNA. The position and speed of ribosomal movement along the mRNA can affect the presence of loops in the mRNA and the ability of the polymerase to transcribe new mRNA. This allows control of gene expression at both the transcriptional and translational levels.

Initiation of transcription may be under positive or negative control. Genes under **negative control** are expressed unless they are switched off by a **repressor protein**. This repressor protein prevents gene expression by binding to a specific DNA sequence called the **operator**, blocking the RNA polymerase from initiating transcription at the promoter sequence. Inversely, genes whose expression is under **positive control** are not transcribed unless an active regulator protein, called an **apoinducer**, is present. The apoinducer binds to a specific DNA sequence and assists the RNA polymerase in the initiation steps by an unknown mechanism.

Operons can be **inducible or repressible**. Introduction of a substrate (**inducer**) into the growth medium may induce an operon to increase the expression of the enzymes necessary for its metabolism. An abundance of the end products (**co-repressors**) of a pathway may signal that a pathway should be shut down or repressed by reducing the synthesis of its enzymes.

The lactose (*lac*) operon responsible for the degradation of the sugar lactose is an inducible operon under positive and negative regulation (see Figure 3-6). Normally the bacteria use glucose and not lactose. In the absence of lactose

the operon is repressed by the binding of the repressor protein to the operator sequence, thus impeding the RNA polymerase function. In the absence of glucose, however, the addition of lactose reverses this repression. Full expression of the *lac* operon also requires a protein-mediated, positive-control mechanism. In *E. coli* a protein called the **catabolite gene-activator protein** (CAP) forms a complex with cyclic adenosine monophosphate (cAMP), acquiring the ability to bind to a specific DNA sequence present in the promoter. When glucose decreases in the cell, cAMP increases to promote usage of other sugars for metabolism. The CAP-cAMP complex enhances binding of the RNA polymerase to the promoter, thus allowing an increase in the frequency of transcription initiation.

The tryptophan operon (**trp operon**) contains the structural genes necessary for tryptophan biosynthesis and is under dual transcriptional control mechanisms (Figure 3-8). Although tryptophan is essential for protein synthesis, too much tryptophan in the cell can be toxic; therefore its synthesis must be regulated. At the DNA level the repressor protein is activated by an increased intracellular concentration of tryptophan to prevent transcription. At the protein synthesis level, rapid translation of a "test peptide" at the beginning of the mRNA in the presence of tryptophan promotes the formation of a double-stranded loop in the RNA, which terminates transcription. The same loop is formed if no protein synthesis is occurring, a situation in which tryptophan synthesis would similarly not be required. This regulates tryptophan synthesis at the mRNA level in a process termed **attenuation**, in which mRNA synthesis is prematurely terminated.

The expression of the components of virulence mechanisms are also coordinately regulated from an operon. Simple triggers, such as temperature, osmolarity, pH, nutrient availability, or the concentration of specific small molecules, such as oxygen or iron, can turn on or turn off the transcription of a single gene or a group of genes. *Salmonella* invasion genes within a pathogenicity island are turned on by high osmolarity and low oxygen, conditions present in the gastrointestinal tract. *E. coli* senses its exit from the gut of a host by a drop in temperature and inactivates its adherence genes. Low iron levels can activate expression of hemolysin in *E. coli* or diphtheria toxin from *Corynebacterium diphtheriae*, potentially to kill cells and provide iron. Quorum sensing for virulence factors of *S. aureus* and biofilm production by *Pseudomonas* spp. were discussed above.

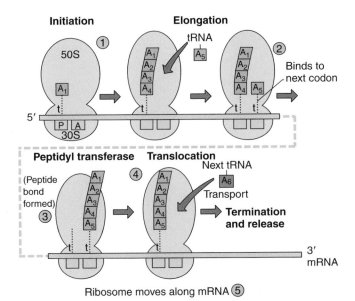

Figure 3—7. Bacterial protein synthesis. *1*, Binding of the 30S subunit to the messenger RNA (mRNA) with the formylmethionine transfer RNA (fmet-tRNA) at the AUG start codon allows assembly of the 70S ribosome. The fmet-tRNA binds to the peptidyl site (P). *2*, The next tRNA binds to its codon at the A site and "accepts" the growing peptide chain. *3*, *4*, Before translocation to the peptidyl site. *5*, The process is repeated until a stop codon and the protein are released.

Replication of DNA

The bacterial chromosome is a storehouse of information by which the characteristics of the cell are defined and all cellular processes are carried out. It is therefore essential that this molecule be duplicated without errors. Replication of the bacterial genome is triggered by a cascade of events linked to the growth rate of the cell. Replication of

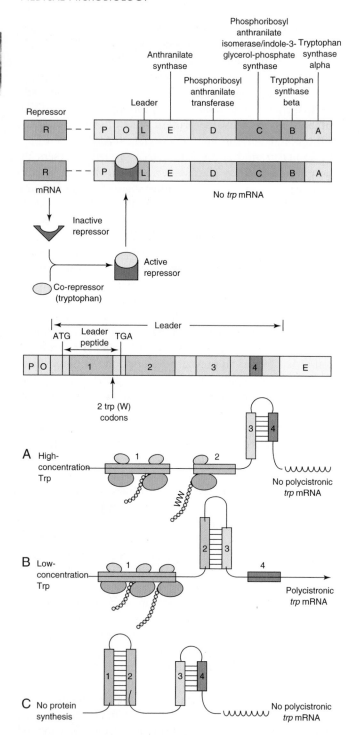

Figure 3—8. Regulation of the tryptophan (*trp*) operon. **A,** The *trp* operon encodes the five enzymes necessary for tryptophan biosynthesis. This *trp* operon is under dual control. **B,** The conformation of the inactive repressor protein is changed after its binding by the co-repressor tryptophan. The resulting active repressor (R) binds to the operator (O), blocking any transcription of the *trp* mRNA by the RNA polymerase. **C,** The *trp* operon is also under the control of an attenuation-antitermination mechanism. Upstream of the structural genes are the promoter (P), the operator, and a leader (L), which can be transcribed into a short peptide containing two tryptophans (W), near its distal end. The leader mRNA possesses four repeats (1, 2, 3, and 4), which can pair differently according to the tryptophan availability, leading to an early termination of transcription of the *trp* operon or its full transcription. In the presence of a high concentration of tryptophan, regions 3 and 4 of the leader mRNA can pair, forming a terminator hairpin, and no transcription of the *trp* operon occurs. However, in the presence of little or no tryptophan the ribosomes stall in region 1 when translating the leader peptide because of the tandem of tryptophan codons. Then regions 2 and 3 can pair, forming the antiterminator hairpin and leading to transcription of the *trp* genes. Finally, the regions 1:2 and 3:4 of the free leader mRNA can pair, also leading to cessation of transcription before the first structural gene *trp*E. A, adenine; G, guanine; T, thymidine.

bacterial DNA is initiated at a specific sequence in the chromosome called *OriC*. The replication process requires many enzymes, including an enzyme (**helicase**) to unwind the DNA at the origin to expose the DNA, an enzyme (**primase**) to synthesize primers to start the process, and the enzyme or enzymes (**DNA-dependent DNA polymerases**) that synthesize a copy of the DNA, but only if there is a primer sequence to add to and only in the 5′ to 3′ direction.

New DNA is synthesized **semiconservatively**, using both strands of the parental DNA as templates. New DNA synthesis occurs at **growing forks** and proceeds **bidirectionally**. One strand (the leading strand) is copied continuously in the 5′ to 3′ direction, whereas the other strand (the lagging strand) must be synthesized as many pieces of DNA using RNA primers (Okazaki fragments). The lagging-strand DNA must be extended in the 5′ to 3′ direction as its template becomes available. Then the pieces are ligated together by the enzyme DNA ligase (Figure 3-9). To maintain the high degree of accuracy required for replication, the DNA polymerases possess "proofreading" functions, which allow the enzyme to confirm that the appropriate nucleotide was inserted and to correct any errors that were made. During log-phase growth in rich medium, many initiations of chromosomal replication may occur before cell division. This process produces a series of nested bubbles of new daughter chromosomes, each with its pair of growth forks of new DNA synthesis. The polymerase moves down the DNA strand, incorporating the appropriate (complementary) nucleotide at each position. Replication is complete when the two replication forks meet 180 degrees from the origin. The process of DNA replication puts great torsional strain on the chromosomal circle of DNA; this strain is relieved by **topoisomerases** (e.g., gyrase), which supercoil the DNA. Topoisomerases are essential to the bacteria and are targets for the quinolone antibiotics.

Bacterial Growth

Bacterial replication is a coordinated process in which two equivalent daughter cells are produced. For growth to occur, there must be sufficient metabolites to support the synthesis of the bacterial components and especially the nucleotides for DNA synthesis. A cascade of regulatory events (synthesis of key proteins and RNA), much like a countdown at the Kennedy Space Center, must occur on schedule to initiate a replication cycle. *However, once it is initiated, DNA synthesis must run to completion, even if all nutrients have been removed from the medium.*

Chromosome replication is initiated at the membrane, and each daughter chromosome is anchored to a different portion of membrane. Bacterial membrane, peptidoglycan synthesis, and cell division are linked together such that inhibition of peptidoglycan synthesis will also inhibit cell division. As the bacterial membrane grows, the daughter chromosomes are pulled apart. Commencement of chromosome replication also initiates the process of cell division, which can be visualized by the start of septum formation between the two daughter cells (Figure 3-10; see also Chapter 2). New initiation events may occur even before completion of chromosome replication and cell division.

Depletion of metabolites (starvation) or a buildup of toxic byproducts (e.g., ethanol) triggers the production of chemical **alarmones**, which causes synthesis to stop, but degradative processes continue. DNA synthesis continues until all initiated chromosomes are completed, despite the detrimental effect on the cell. Ribosomes are cannibalized for deoxyribonucleotide precursors, peptidoglycan and proteins are degraded for metabolites, and the cell shrinks. Septum formation may be initiated, but cell division may not occur. Many cells die. Similar signals may initiate **sporulation** in species capable of this process (see Chapter 2).

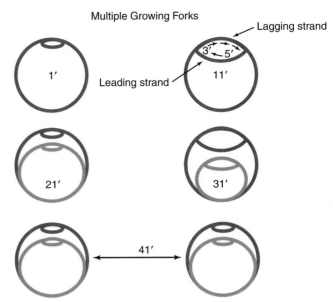

Figure 3—9. Bacterial DNA replication. New DNA synthesis occurs at growing forks and proceeds bidirectionally. DNA synthesis progresses in the 5' to 3' direction continuously (leading strand) or in pieces (lagging strand). Assuming it takes 40 minutes to complete one round of replication, and assuming new initiation every 20 minutes, initiation of DNA synthesis precedes cell division. Multiple growing forks may be initiated in a cell before complete septum formation and cell division. The daughter cells are "born pregnant."

Figure 3—10. Bacterial cell division. Replication requires extension of the cell wall and replication of the chromosome and septum formation. Membrane attachment of the DNA pulls each daughter strand into a new cell.

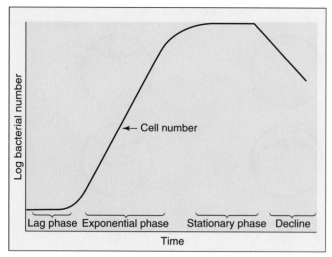

Figure 3–11. Phases of bacterial growth, starting with an inoculum of stationary-phase cells.

Population Dynamics

When bacteria are added to a medium, they require time to adapt to the new environment before they begin dividing (Figure 3-11). This hiatus is known as the **lag phase** of growth. During the **log or exponential phase**, the bacteria will grow and divide with a **doubling time** characteristic of the strain and determined by the conditions. The number of bacteria will increase to 2^n, in which n is the number of generations (doublings). The culture eventually runs out of metabolites, or a toxic substance builds up in the medium; the bacteria then stop growing and enter the **stationary phase**.

Bacterial Genetics

Mutation, Repair, and Recombination

Accurate replication of DNA is important to the survival of the bacteria, but mistakes and accidental damage to the DNA occurs. Despite efficient DNA repair systems, mutations and alterations to the DNA do occur. Most of these mutations have little effect on the bacteria or are detrimental, but some mutations may improve the chances of survival of the bacteria when challenged by the environment, the host, or therapy.

Mutations and Their Consequences

A mutation is any change in the base sequence of the DNA. A single base change can result in a **transition** in which one purine is replaced by another purine, or in which a pyrimidine is replaced by another pyrimidine. A **transversion**, in which, for example, a purine is replaced by a pyrimidine and vice versa, may also result. A **silent mutation** is a change at the DNA level that does not result in any change of amino acid in the encoded protein. This type of mutation occurs because more than one codon may encode an amino acid. A **missense mutation** results in a different amino acid being inserted in the protein, but this may be a **conservative mutation** if the new amino acid has similar properties (e.g., valine replacing alanine). A **nonsense mutation** changes a codon encoding an amino acid to a stop codon (e.g., TAG [thymidine-adenine-guanine]), which will cause the ribosome to fall off the mRNA and end the protein prematurely. **Conditional mutations**, such as **temperature-sensitive mutations**, may result from a conservative mutation which changes the structure or function of an important protein at elevated temperatures.

More drastic changes can occur when numerous bases are involved. A small deletion or insertion that *is not in multiples of three* produces a **frameshift mutation**. This results in a change in the reading frame, usually leading to a useless peptide and premature truncation of the protein. **Null mutations**, which completely destroy gene function, arise when there is an extensive insertion, deletion, or gross rearrangement of the chromosome structure. Insertion of long sequences of DNA (many thousands of base pairs) by recombination, by transposition, or during genetic engineering can produce null mutations by separating the parts of a gene and inactivating the gene.

Many mutations occur spontaneously in nature (e.g., by polymerase mistakes); however, physical or chemical agents can also induce mutations. Among the physical agents used to induce mutations in bacteria are heat, which results in deamination of nucleotides; ultraviolet light, which causes pyrimidine dimer formation; and ionizing radiation, such as x-rays, which produce very reactive hydroxyl radicals that may be responsible for opening a ring of a base or causing single- or double-stranded breaks in the DNA. Chemical mutagens can be grouped into three classes. **Nucleotide-base analogues** lead to mispairing and frequent DNA replication mistakes. For example, incorporation of 5-bromouracil into DNA instead of thymidine allows base pairing with guanine instead of adenine, changing a T-A base pair to a G-C base pair. **Frameshift mutagens**, such as polycyclic flat molecules like ethidium bromide or acridine derivatives, insert (or intercalate) between the bases as they stack with each other in the double helix. These intercalating agents increase the spacing of successive base pairs, destroying the regular sugar-phosphate backbone and decreasing the pitch of the helix. These changes cause the addition or deletion of a single base and lead to frequent mistakes during DNA replication. **DNA-reactive chemicals** act directly on the DNA to change the chemical structure of the base. These include nitrous acid (HNO_2) and alkylating agents, including nitrosoguanidine and ethyl methane sulfonate, which are known to add methyl or ethyl groups to the rings of the DNA bases. The modified bases may pair abnormally or not at all. The damage may also cause the removal of the base from the DNA backbone.

Repair Mechanisms of DNA

A number of repair mechanisms have evolved in bacterial cells to minimize damage to DNA. These repair mechanisms can be divided into the following five groups:

1. **Direct DNA repair** is the enzymatic removal of damage, such as pyrimidine dimers and alkylated bases.

2. **Excision repair** is the excision of a DNA segment containing the damage, followed by synthesis of a new DNA strand. Two types of excision-repair mechanisms, generalized and specialized, exist.
3. **Recombinational** or **postreplication repair** is the retrieval of missing information by genetic recombination when both DNA strands are damaged.
4. The **SOS response** is the induction of many genes (approximately 15) after DNA damage or interruption of DNA replication.
5. **Error-prone repair** is the last resort of a bacterial cell before it dies. It is used to fill in gaps with a random sequence when a DNA template is not available for directing an accurate repair.

Gene Exchange in Prokaryotic Cells

Many bacteria, especially many pathogenic bacterial species, are promiscuous with their DNA. The exchange of DNA between cells allows the exchange of genes and characteristics between cells, thus producing new strains of bacteria. This exchange may be advantageous for the recipient, especially if the exchanged DNA encodes antibiotic resistance. The transferred DNA can be integrated into the recipient chromosome or stably maintained as an extrachromosomal element (**plasmid**) or a bacterial virus (**bacteriophage**) and passed on to daughter bacteria as an autonomously replicating unit.

Plasmids are small genetic elements that replicate independently of the bacterial chromosome. Most plasmids are circular, double-stranded DNA molecules varying from 1500 to 400,000 base pairs. However, *Borrelia burgdorferi*, the causative agent of Lyme disease, and the related *Borrelia hermsii* are unique among all eubacteria because they possess linear plasmids. Like the bacterial chromosomal DNA, plasmids can autonomously replicate and as such are referred to as **replicons**. Some plasmids, such as the *E. coli* F plasmid, are **episomes**, which means that they can integrate into the host chromosome.

Plasmids carry genetic information, which may not be essential but can provide a selective advantage to the bacteria. For example, plasmids may encode the production of antibiotic resistance mechanisms, bacteriocins, toxins, virulence determinants, and other genes that may provide the bacteria with a unique growth advantage over other microbes or within the host (Figure 3-12). The number of copies of plasmid produced by a cell is determined by the particular plasmid. The copy number is the ratio of copies of the plasmid to the number of copies of the chromosome. This may be as few as one in the case of large plasmids or as many as 50 in smaller plasmids.

Large plasmids (20 to 120 kb), such as the **fertility factor F** found in *E. coli* or the resistance transfer factor (80 kb), can often mediate their own transfer from one cell to another by a process called **conjugation** (see the section

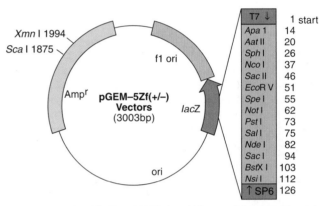

Figure 3–12. Plasmids. The pBR322 plasmid is one of the plasmids used for cloning DNA. This plasmid encodes resistance to ampicillin (Amp) and tetracycline (Tet) and an origin of replication (ori). The multiple cloning site in the pGEM plasmid provides different restriction enzyme cleavage sites for insertion of DNA within the β-galactosidase gene (*lacZ*). The insert is flanked by bacteriophage promoters to allow directional messenger RNA expression of the cloned sequence.

on conjugation later in this chapter). These conjugative plasmids encode all the necessary factors for their transfer. Other plasmids can be transferred into a bacterial cell by means other than conjugation, such as transformation or transduction. These terms are discussed later in the chapter.

Bacteriophages are bacterial viruses. These extrachromosomal genetic elements can survive outside of a host cell, because a protein coat protects the nucleic acid genome (which may be DNA or RNA). Bacteriophages infect bacterial cells and either replicate to large numbers and cause the cell to lyse (**lytic infection**) or in some cases **integrate** into the host genome without killing the host (the **lysogenic state**), such as the *E. coli* bacteriophage lambda. Some lysogenic bacteriophages carry toxin genes (e.g., corynephage beta carries the gene for the diphtheria toxin). Bacteriophage lambda remains lysogenic as long as a repressor protein is synthesized and prevents the phage

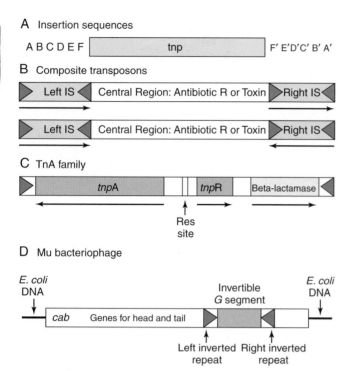

A Insertion sequences

A B C D E F | tnp | F' E' D' C' B' A'

B Composite transposons

Left IS | Central Region: Antibiotic R or Toxin | Right IS

Left IS | Central Region: Antibiotic R or Toxin | Right IS

C TnA family

| tnpA | | tnpR | Beta-lactamase |

Res
site

D Mu bacteriophage

E. coli
DNA

Invertible
G segment

E. coli
DNA

cab | Genes for head and tail

Left inverted
repeat

Right inverted
repeat

Figure 3–13. Transposons. **A,** The insertion sequences code only for a transposase (*tnp*) and possess inverted repeats (15 to 40 base pairs) at each end. **B,** The composite transposons contain a central region coding for antibiotic resistances or toxins flanked by two insertion sequences (IS), which can be either directly repeated or reversed. **C,** Tn3, a member of the TnA transposon family. The central region encodes three genes—a transposase (tnpA), a resolvase (tnpR), and a β-lactamase—conferring resistance to ampicillin. A resolution site (Res site) is used during the replicative transposition process. This central region is flanked on both ends by direct repeats of 38 base pairs. **D,** Phage-associated transposon is exemplified by the bacteriophage mu.

from becoming unintegrated in order to replicate and exit the cell. This reaction can be triggered if the host cell DNA is damaged by radiation or by another means or if the cell can no longer make the repressor protein, a signal that the host cell is unhealthy and is no longer a good place for "freeloading."

Transposons (jumping genes) are mobile genetic elements (Figure 3-13) that can transfer DNA within a cell, from one position to another in the genome, or between different molecules of DNA (e.g., plasmid to plasmid or plasmid to chromosome). Transposons are present in prokaryotes and eukaryotes. The simplest transposons are called *insertion sequences* and range in length from 150 to 1500 base pairs, with inverted repeats of 15 to 40 base pairs at their ends and the minimal genetic information necessary for their own transfer (i.e., the gene coding for the transposase). Complex transposons carry other genes, such as genes that provide resistance against antibiotics. Transposons sometimes insert into genes and inactivate those genes. If insertion and inactivation occur in a gene that encodes an essential protein, the cell dies.

Some pathogenic bacteria use a transposon-like mechanism to coordinate the expression of a system of virulence factors. The genes for the activity may be grouped together in a **pathogenicity or virulence island**, which is surrounded by transposon-like mobile elements, allowing them to move within the chromosome and to other bacteria. The entire genetic unit can be triggered by an environmental stimulus (e.g., pH, heat, contact with the host cell surface) as a way to coordinate the expression of a complex process. For example, the SPI-1 island of *Salmonella* encodes 25 genes that allow the bacteria to enter nonphagocytic cells.

Mechanisms of Genetic Transfer between Cells

The exchange of genetic material between bacterial cells may occur by one of three mechanisms (Figure 3-14): (1) **conjugation**, which is the mating or quasisexual exchange of genetic information from one bacterium (the donor) to another bacterium (the recipient); (2) **transformation**, which results in acquisition of new genetic markers by the incorporation of exogenous or foreign DNA; or (3) **transduction**, which is the transfer of genetic information from one bacterium to another by a bacteriophage. Once inside a cell, a **transposon** can jump between different DNA molecules (e.g., plasmid to plasmid or plasmid to chromosome).

Transformation

Transformation is the process by which bacteria take up fragments of naked DNA and incorporate them into their genomes. Transformation was the first mechanism of genetic transfer to be discovered in bacteria. In 1928, Griffith observed that pneumococcus virulence was related to the presence of a surrounding polysaccharide capsule and that extracts of encapsulated bacteria producing smooth colonies could transmit this trait to nonencapsulated bacteria, normally appearing with rough edges. Griffith's studies led to Avery, MacLeod, and McCarty's identification of DNA as the transforming principle some 15 years later.

Gram-positive and gram-negative bacteria can take up and stably maintain exogenous DNA. Certain species are naturally capable of taking up exogenous DNA (such species are then said to be competent), including *Haemophilus influenzae, Streptococcus pneumoniae, Bacillus* species, and *Neisseria* species. Competence develops toward the end of logarithmic growth, some time before a population enters the stationary phase. Most bacteria do not exhibit a natural ability for DNA uptake. Chemical methods or electroporation (the use of high-voltage pulses) can be used to introduce plasmid and other DNA into *E. coli* and other bacteria.

Conjugation

Conjugation occurs with most, if not all, eubacteria. Conjugation usually occurs between members of the same or related species, but has also been demonstrated to occur between prokaryotes and cells from plants, animals, and fungi. Conjugation occurs for *E. coli*, bacteroides,

TRANSFORMATION

Donor cell | Cell lysis; release of DNA fragments | DNA enters recipient cell and integrates into DNA

TRANSDUCTION

Transducing phage containing donor genomic DNA | Cell lysis; release of phages | Phage infects recipient cell; donor DNA integrates into recipient DNA

CONJUGATION

Genomic DNA | Genomic DNA

Plasmid DNA

Free plasmid moves from donor to recipient cell via sex (F) pilus

Sex pilus

Integrated plasmid (episome) promotes transfer of genomic DNA, which integrates into recipient DNA

TRANSPOSITION

Transposon with inverted repeats

Donor site

gene A gene B′   gene B′ gene C

Recipient site

Figure 3—14. Mechanisms of bacterial gene transfer. *(From Rosenthal KS, Tan J: Rapid Reviews Microbiology and Immunology. St. Louis, Mosby, 2002.)*

enterococci, streptococci, streptomycetes, and clostridia. Many of the large conjugative plasmids specify colicins or antibiotic resistance.

Genetic transfer in *E. coli* was first reported by Lederberg and Tatum in 1946, when they observed sexlike exchange between two mutant strains of *E. coli* K12. Conjugation results in one-way transfer of DNA from a donor (or male) cell to a recipient (or female) cell through the **sex pilus**. Conjugative R (antibiotic resistance) for gram-positive bacteria, such as streptococci, streptomycetes, and clostridia, are brought together by the presence of an adhesin molecule on the surface of the donor cell instead of pili.

The mating type (sex) of the cell depends on the presence (male) or absence (female) of a conjugative plasmid, such as the **F plasmid** of *E. coli*. The F plasmid is defined as conjugative because it carries all the genes necessary for its own transfer, including the ability to make sex pili and to initiate DNA synthesis at the transfer origin (OriT) of the plasmid. The F plasmid transfers itself, converting recipients into F+ male cells. If a fragment of chromosomal DNA has been incorporated into the plasmid, it is designated an F prime (F′) plasmid. When it transfers into the recipient cell, it carries that

fragment with it and converts it into an F′ male. If the F plasmid sequence is integrated into the bacterial chromosome, the cell is designated an Hfr (high frequency recombination) cell.

The DNA that is transferred by conjugation is not a double helix but a single-stranded molecule. Mobilization begins when a plasmid-encoded protein makes a single-stranded, site-specific cleavage at the OriT. The nick initiates rolling circle replication, and the displaced linear strand is directed to the recipient cell. The transferred single-stranded DNA is recircularized and its complementary strand synthesized. Integration of an F plasmid into the bacterial chromosome generates an Hfr cell. Conjugation results in transfer of a part of the plasmid sequence and some portion of the bacterial chromosomal DNA. Because of the fragile connection between the mating pairs, the transfer is usually aborted before being completed such that only the chromosomal sequences adjacent to the integrated F are transferred. Artificial interruption of a mating between an Hfr and an F⁻ pair has been helpful in constructing a consistent map of the *E. coli* chromosomal DNA. In such maps the position of each gene is given in minutes (based on 100 minutes for complete transfer at 37° C), according to its time of entry into a recipient cell in relation to a fixed origin.

Transduction

Genetic transfer by transduction is mediated by bacterial viruses (bacteriophages), which pick up fragments of DNA and package them into bacteriophage particles. The DNA is delivered to infected cells and becomes incorporated into the bacterial genomes. Transduction can be classified as **specialized** if the phages in question transfer particular genes (usually those adjacent to their integration sites in the genome) or **generalized** if the selection of the sequences is random because of accidental packaging of host DNA into the phage capsid.

Generalized transducing particles should contain primarily bacterial DNA and little or no phage DNA. For example, the P1 phage of *E. coli* encodes a nuclease that degrades the host *E. coli* chromosomal DNA. A small percentage of the resultant phage particles package the DNA fragments into their capsids. The encapsulated DNA, instead of phage DNA, is injected into a new host cell, where it can recombine with the homologous host DNA. Generalized transducing particles are valuable in the **genetic mapping** of bacterial chromosomes. The closer two genes are within the bacterial chromosome, the more likely it is that they will be co-transduced in the same fragment of DNA.

Recombination

Incorporation of extrachromosomal (foreign) DNA into the chromosome occurs by recombination. There are two types of recombination: homologous and nonhomologous. **Homologous (legitimate) recombination** occurs between closely related DNA sequences and generally substitutes one sequence for another. The process requires a set of enzymes produced (in *E. coli*) by the *rec* genes. **Nonhomologous (illegitimate) recombination** occurs between dissimilar DNA sequences and generally produces insertions or deletions or both. This process usually requires specialized (sometimes site-specific) recombination enzymes, such as those produced by many transposons and lysogenic bacteriophages.

Generation of Vancomycin-Resistant *Staphylococcus aureus* by Multiple Genetic Manipulations

Until recently, vancomycin was the last-resort drug for *S. aureus* strains resistant to beta lactam (penicillin-related) antibiotics (e.g., methicillin resistant *S. aureus* [MRSA]). *S. aureus* acquired the vancomycin resistance gene during a mixed infection with *Enterococcus faecalis* (Figure 3-15). The gene for the vancomycin resistance gene was contained within a **transposon** (TN1546) on a multiresistance conjugative plasmid. The plasmid was probably transferred by **conjugation** between *E. faecalis* and *S. aureus*. Alternatively, after lysis of the *E. faecalis*, *S. aureus* acquired the DNA by **transduction** and became **transformed** by the

new DNA. The transposon then jumped from the *E. faecalis* plasmid, **recombined**, and **integrated** into the *S. aureus* multiresistance plasmid, and the *E. faecalis* DNA was degraded. The resulting *S. aureus* plasmid encodes resistance to beta lactams, vancomycin, trimethoprim, and gentamycin/kanamycin/tobramycin antibiotics and to quaternary ammonium disinfectants and can transfer to other *S. aureus* strains by **conjugation**. (For more information, refer to Weigel in the bibliography at the end of the chapter.)

Genetic Engineering

Genetic engineering, also known as recombinant DNA technology, uses the techniques and tools developed by the bacterial geneticists to purify, amplify, modify, and express specific gene sequences. The use of genetic engineering and "cloning" has revolutionized biology and medicine. The basic components of genetic engineering are: (1) **cloning and expression vectors**, which can be used to deliver the DNA sequences into receptive bacteria and amplify the desired sequence; (2) the **DNA sequence** to be amplified and expressed; (3) **enzymes**, such as **restriction enzymes**, which are used to cleave DNA reproducibly at defined sequences (Table 3-1) and **DNA ligase**, the enzyme that links the fragment to the cloning vector.

Cloning and expression vectors must allow foreign DNA to be inserted into them, but still must be able to replicate normally in a bacterial or eukaryotic host. Many types of vectors are currently used. Plasmid vectors, such as pUC, pBR322, and pGEM (Figure 3-16), are used for DNA fragments up to 20 kb. Bacteriophages, such as lambda, are used for larger fragments up to 25 kb. More recently, **cosmid** vectors have combined some of the advantages of plasmids and phages for fragments up to 45 kb.

Most **cloning vectors** have been "engineered" to have a site for insertion of foreign DNA; a means of selection of the bacteria that have incorporated any plasmid (e.g., antibiotic resistance); and a means of distinguishing the bacteria that have incorporated those plasmids which contain inserted DNA. **Expression vectors** have DNA sequences to facilitate their replication in bacteria and eukaryotic cells and also the transcription of the gene into mRNA.

The DNA to be cloned can be obtained by purification of chromosomal DNA from cells, viruses, or other plasmids or by selective amplification of DNA sequences by a technique known as *polymerase chain reaction* (PCR). (PCR is explained further in Chapter 16.) Both the vector and the foreign DNA are cleaved with restriction enzymes (see Figure 3-16). Restriction enzymes recognize a specific palindromic sequence and make a staggered cut, which generates sticky ends, or a blunt cut, which generates blunt ends (see Table 3-1). Most cloning vectors have a sequence called the **multiple cloning site** that can be cleaved by many restriction enzymes. Ligation of the vector with the DNA fragments generates a molecule called **recombinant DNA** that is capable of replicating the inserted sequence.

Figure 3—15. Genetic mechanisms of evolution of methicillin and vancomycin resistant *Staphylococcus aureus*. Vancomycin resistant enterococcus (VRE) (*in red*) contains plasmids with multiple antibiotic resistance and virulence factors. During coinfection a methicillin resistant *Staphylococcus aureus* (MRSA) may have acquired the enterococcal resistance plasmid (e-plasmid) by transformation (after lysis of the enterococcal cell and release of its DNA) or more likely, by conjugation. A transposon in the e-plasmid containing the vancomycin resistance gene jumped out and inserted into the multiple antibiotic resistance plasmid of the MRSA. The new plasmid is readily spread to other *S. aureus* bacteria by conjugation.

The total number of recombinant vectors obtained when cloning all the fragments that result from cleavage of chromosomal DNA is known as a **genomic library**, because there should be at least one representative of each gene in the library. An alternative approach to cloning the gene for a protein is to convert the mRNA for the protein into DNA using a retrovirus enzyme called *reverse transcriptase* (RNA-dependent DNA polymerase) to produce a complementary DNA (cDNA). A **cDNA library** represents the genes that are expressed as mRNA in a particular cell.

Table 3—1. Common Restriction Enzymes Used in Molecular Biology

Microorganism	Enzyme	Recognition Site
Acinetobacter calcoaceticus	AccI	5′ G T|(A/C) (C/T)|A C C A (T/G) (G/A)|T G
Bacillus amyloliquefaciens H	BamHI	5′ G|G A T C C C C T A G|G
Escherichia coli RY13	EcoRI	5′ G|A A T T C C T T A A|G
Haemophilus influenzae Rd	HindIII	5′ A|A G C T T T T C G A|A
H. influenzae serotype c, 1160	HincII	5′ G T (C/T)|(C/A) A C C A (G/A)|(G/T) T G
Providencia stuartii 164	PstI	5′ C T G C A|G G|A C G T C
Serratia marcescens	SmaI	5′ C C C|G G G G G G|C C C
Staphylococcus aureus 3A	Sau3AI	5′|G A T C C T A G|
Xanthomonas malvacearum	XmaI	5′ C|C C G G G G G G C C|C

Figure 3—16. Cloning of foreign DNA in vectors. The vector and the foreign DNA are first digested by a restriction enzyme. Insertion of foreign DNA into the *lacZ* gene inactivates the β-galactosidase gene, allowing subsequent selection. The vector is then ligated to the foreign DNA, using bacteriophage T4 DNA ligase. The recombinant vectors are transformed into competent *Escherichia coli* cells. The recombinant *E. coli* cells are plated onto agar containing antibiotic, an inducer of the *lac* operon, and a chromophoric substrate that turns blue in cells having plasmid but not insert; those cells with plasmid containing the insert remain white.

The recombinant DNA is then transformed into a bacterial host, usually *E. coli*, and the plasmid-containing bacteria are selected for antibiotic resistance (e.g., ampicillin resistance). The library can then be screened to find an *E. coli* clone possessing the desired DNA fragment. Various screening techniques can be used to identify the bacteria containing the appropriate recombinant DNA. The multiple cloning site used for inserting the foreign DNA is often part of the *lacZ* gene of the *lac* operon. Insertion of the foreign DNA into the *lacZ* gene inactivates the gene (acting almost like a transposon) and prevents the plasmid-directed synthesis of β-galactosidase in the recipient cell, which results in white bacterial colonies instead of blue colonies if β-galactosidase were able to cleave an appropriate chromophore.

Genetic engineering has been used to isolate and express the genes for useful proteins such as insulin, interferon, growth hormones, and interleukin in bacteria, yeast, or even insect cells. Large amounts of pure immunogen for a vaccine can be prepared without the need to work with the intact disease organisms.

The development of a vaccine against hepatitis B virus represents the first success of recombinant DNA vaccines approved for human use by the U.S. Food and Drug Administration. The hepatitis B surface antigen is produced by the yeast *Saccharomyces cerevisiae*. In the future it may be sufficient to inject plasmid DNA capable of expressing the desired immunogen (DNA vaccine) into an individual to let the host cells express the immunogen and generate the immune response. Recombinant DNA technology has also become essential to laboratory diagnosis, forensic science, agriculture, and many other disciplines.

Questions

1. How many moles of ATP are generated per mole of glucose in glycolysis, the TCA cycle, and electron transport? Which of these occur in anaerobic conditions and in aerobic conditions? Which is most efficient?

2. What products of anaerobic fermentation would be detrimental to host (human) tissue (e.g., *C. perfringens*)?

3. If the number of bacteria during log phase growth can be calculated by the following equation:

$$N_t = N_0 \infty 2^{t/d}$$

in which N_t is the number of bacteria after time (t), t/d is the amount of time divided by the doubling time, and N_0 is the initial number of bacteria, how many bacteria will be in the culture after 4 hours if the doubling time is 20 minutes and the initial bacterial inoculum contained 1000 bacteria?

4. What are the principal properties of a plasmid?

5. Give two mechanisms of regulation of bacterial gene expression. Use specific examples.

6. What types of mutations affect DNA, and what agents are responsible for such mutations?

7. Which mechanisms may be used by a bacterial cell for the exchange of genetic material? Briefly explain each mechanism.

8. Discuss the applications of molecular biotechnology to medicine, including contributions and uses in diagnoses.

Bibliography

Alberts B: Molecular Biology of the Cell, 4th ed. New York, Garland, 2002.

Berg JM, Tymoczko JL, Stryer L: Biochemistry, 6th ed, New York, WH Freeman, 2006.

Lewin B: Genes IX. Sudbury, Mass, Jones and Bartlett, 2007.

Lodish H, et al: Molecular Cell Biology, 6th ed. New York, WH Freeman, 2007.

Nelson DL, Cox M: Lehninger Principles of Biochemistry, 4th ed. New York, Worth, 2004.

Patel SS, Rosenthal KS: Microbial adaptation: Putting the best team on the field. Infect Dis Clin Pract 15:330-334, 2007.

Watson JD, et al: Molecular Biology of the Gene, 4th ed. Menlo Park, Calif, Benjamin-Cummings, 1987.

Weigel LM, et al: Genetic analysis of a high-level vancomycin-resistant isolate of *Staphylococcus aureus*. Science 302:1569-1571, 2003.

Viral Classification, Structure, and Replication

Viruses were first described as "filterable agents." Their small size allows them to pass through filters designed to retain bacteria. Unlike most bacteria, fungi, and parasites, **viruses are obligate intracellular parasites** that depend on the biochemical machinery of the host cell for replication. In addition, *reproduction of viruses occurs by assembly of the individual components rather than by binary fission* (Boxes 4-1 and 4-2).

The simplest viruses consist of a genome of deoxyribonucleic acid (DNA) or ribonucleic acid (RNA) packaged in a protective shell of protein and for some viruses a membrane (Figure 4-1). Viruses lack the capacity to make energy or substrates, cannot make their own proteins, and cannot replicate their genome independently of the host cell. To use the cell's biosynthetic machinery, the virus must be adapted to the biochemical rules of the cell.

The physical structure and genetics of viruses have been optimized by mutation and selection to infect humans and other hosts. To do this, the virus must be capable of transmission through potentially harsh environmental conditions, must traverse the skin or other protective barriers of the host, must be adapted to the biochemical machinery of the host cell for replication, and must escape elimination by the host immune response.

Knowledge of the structural (size and morphology) and genetic (type and structure of nucleic acid) features of a virus provides insight into how the virus replicates, spreads, and causes disease. The concepts presented in this chapter are repeated in greater detail in the discussions of specific viruses in later chapters.

Classification

Viruses range from the structurally simple and small parvoviruses and picornaviruses to the large and complex poxviruses and herpesviruses. Their names may describe viral characteristics, the diseases they are associated with, or even the tissue or geographic locale where they were first identified. Names such as **picornavirus** (*pico*, "small"; *rna*, "ribonucleic acid") or **togavirus** (*toga*, Greek for "mantle," referring to a membrane envelope surrounding the virus) describe the structure of the virus. The name **retrovirus** (*retro*, "reverse") refers to the virus-directed synthesis of DNA from an RNA template, whereas the *poxviruses* are named for the disease smallpox, caused by one of its members. The **adenoviruses** (*adeno*ids) and the **reoviruses** (*r*espiratory, *e*nteric, *o*rphan) are named for the body site from which they were first isolated. Reovirus was discovered before it was associated with a specific disease, and thus it was designated an "orphan" virus. Norwalk virus is named for Norwalk, Ohio; coxsackievirus is named for Coxsackie, New York; and many of the togaviruses, arenaviruses, and bunyaviruses are named after African places where they were first isolated.

Viruses can be grouped by characteristics such as disease (e.g., hepatitis), target tissue, means of transmission (e.g., enteric, respiratory), or vector (e.g., arboviruses; arthropod-borne virus) (Box 4-3). *The most consistent and current means of classification is by physical and biochemical characteristics, such as size, morphology (e.g., presence or absence of a membrane envelope), type of genome, and means of replication* (Figures 4-2 and 4-3). DNA viruses associated with human disease are divided into seven families (Tables 4-1 and 4-2). The RNA viruses may be divided into at least 13 families (Tables 4-3 and 4-4).

Virion Structure

The units for measurement of virion size are nanometers (nm). The clinically important viruses range from 18 nm (parvoviruses) to 300 nm (poxviruses) (Figure 4-4). The latter are almost visible with a light microscope and

Box 4—1. Definition and Properties of a Virus

Viruses are filterable agents.
Viruses are obligate intracellular parasites.
Viruses cannot make energy or proteins independently of a host cell.
Viral genomes may be RNA or DNA but not both.
Viruses have a naked capsid or an envelope morphology.
Viral components are assembled and do not replicate by "division."

Box 4—2. Consequences of Viral Properties

Viruses are not living.
Viruses must be infectious to endure in nature.
Viruses must be able to use host cell processes to produce their components (viral messenger RNA, protein, and identical copies of the genome).
Viruses must encode any required processes not provided by the cell.
Viral components must self-assemble.

Figure 4—1. Components of the basic virion.

Box 4—3. Means of Classification and Naming of Viruses

Structure: size, morphology, and nucleic acid (e.g., picornavirus [small RNA], togavirus)
Biochemical characteristics: structure and mode of replication*
Disease: encephalitis and hepatitis viruses, for example
Means of transmission: arbovirus spread by insects, for example
Host cell (host range): animal (human, mouse, bird), plant, bacteria
Tissue or organ (tropism): adenovirus and enterovirus, for example

*This is the current means of taxonomic classification of viruses.

Figure 4—2. The DNA viruses and their morphology. The viral families are determined by the structure of the genome and the morphology of the virion.

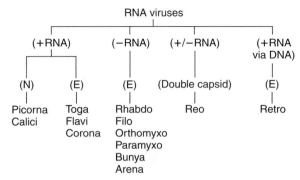

Figure 4—3. The RNA viruses, their genome structure, and their morphology. The viral families are determined by the structure of the genome and the morphology of the virion. E, enveloped; N, naked capsid.

are approximately one fourth the size of *Staphylococcus* bacteria. *Larger virions can hold a larger genome that can encode more proteins, and they are generally more complex.*

The **virion** (the virus particle) consists of a nucleic acid **genome** packaged into a protein coat (**capsid**) or a membrane (**envelope**) (Figure 4-5). The virion may also contain certain essential or accessory enzymes or other proteins to facilitate initial replication in the cell. Capsid or nucleic acid–binding proteins may associate with the genome to form a **nucleocapsid**, which may be the same as the virion or surrounded by an envelope.

The genome of the virus consists either of DNA or RNA. The DNA can be single or double stranded, linear or circular. The RNA can be either positive sense (+) (like messenger RNA [mRNA]) or negative sense (−) (analogous to a photographic negative), double stranded (+/−) or ambisense (containing + and − regions of RNA attached end to end). The RNA genome may also be segmented into pieces, with each piece encoding one or more

Table 4—1. Families of DNA Viruses and Some Important Members

Family	Members*
POXVIRIDAE†	*Smallpox virus*, vaccinia virus, monkeypox, molluscum contagiosum
Herpesviridae	*Herpes simplex virus* types 1 and 2, varicella-zoster virus, Epstein-Barr virus, cytomegalovirus, human herpesviruses 6, 7, and 8
Adenoviridae	*Adenovirus*
Papilloma viridae	*Papilloma virus*
Polyoma viridae	*JC virus*, BK virus, SV40
Hepadnaviridae	*Hepatitis B virus*
Parvoviridae	*Parvovirus B19*, adeno-associated virus

*The italicized virus is the important, or prototype, virus for the family.
†The size of type is indicative of the relative size of the virus.

Table 4-2. Properties of Virions of Human DNA Viruses

Family	Genome*			Viron	
	Molecular Mass × 10^6 Daltons	Nature	Shape	Size (nm)	DNA Polymerase[†]
Poxviridae	85-140	ds, linear	Brick-shaped, enveloped	300 × 240 × 100	+[‡]
Herpesviridae	100-150	ds, linear	Icosahedral, enveloped	Capsid, 100-110 Envelope, 120-200	+
Adenoviridae	20-25	ds, linear	Icosahedral	70-90	+
Hepadnaviridae	1.8	ds, circular[§]	Spherical, enveloped	42	+[‡‖]
Polyoma and papilloma viridae	3-5	ds, circular	Icosahedral	45-55	—
Parvoviridae	1.5-2.0	ss, linear	Icosahedral	18-26	—

ds, Double-stranded; ss, single-stranded.
*Genome invariably a single molecule.
[†]Polymerase encoded by virus.
[‡]Polymerase carried in the virion.
[§]Circular molecule is double-stranded for most of its length but contains a single-stranded region.
[‖]Reverse transcriptase.

Table 4-3. Families of RNA Viruses and Some Important Members

Family[†]	Members*
PARAMYXOVIRIDAE	Parainfluenza virus, Sendai virus, *measles virus*, mumps virus, respiratory syncytial virus, metapneumovirus
ORTHOMYXOVIRIDAE	*Influenza virus* types A, B, and C
CORONAVIRIDAE	*Coronavirus*, SARS (severe acute respiratory syndrome)
Arenaviridae	*Lassa fever virus*, Tacaribe virus complex (Junin and Machupo viruses), lymphocytic choriomeningitis virus
Rhabdoviridae	*Rabies virus*, vesicular stomatitis virus
Filoviridae	*Ebola virus*, Marburg virus
Bunyaviridae	*California encephalitis virus*, LaCrosse virus, sandfly fever virus, hemorrhagic fever virus, Hanta virus
Retroviridae	Human T-cell leukemia virus types I and II, *human immunodeficiency virus*, animal oncoviruses
Reoviridae	*Rotavirus*, Colorado tick fever virus
Picornaviridae	Rhinoviruses, *poliovirus*, echoviruses, coxsackievirus, hepatitis A virus
Togaviridae	*Rubella virus*; western, eastern, and Venezuelan equine encephalitis virus; Ross River virus; Sindbis virus; Semliki Forest virus
Flaviviridae	*Yellow fever virus*, dengue virus, St. Louis encephalitis virus, West Nile virus, hepatitis C virus
Caliciviridae	*Norwalk virus*, calicivirus
Delta	Delta agent

*The italicized virus is the important or prototype virus for the family.
[†]The size of the type is indicative of the relative size of the virus.

Table 4—4. Properties of Virions of Human RNA Viruses

Family	Genome* Molecular Mass × 10⁶ Daltons	Nature	Shape*	Virion Size (nm)	Polymerase in Virion	Envelope
Paramyxoviridae	5-7	ss, −	Spherical	150-300	+	+
Orthomyxoviridae	5-7	ss, −, seg	Spherical	80-120	+	+
Coronaviridae	6-7	ss, +	Spherical	80-130	−	+†
Arenaviridae	3-5	ss, −, seg	Spherical	50-300	+	+†
Rhabdoviridae	4-7	ss, −	Bullet-shaped	180 × 75	+	+
Filoviridae	4-7	ss, −	Filamentous	800 × 80	+	+
Bunyaviridae	4-7	ss, −	Spherical	90-100	+	+†
Retroviridae	2 × (2-3)‡	ss, +	Spherical	80-110	+§	+
Reoviridae	11-15	ds, seg	Icosahedral	60-80	+	−
Picornaviridae	2.5	ss, +	Icosahedral	25-30	−	−
Togaviridae	4-5	ss, +	Icosahedral	60-70	−	+
Flaviviridae	4-7	ss, +	Spherical	40-50	−	+
Caliciviridae	2.6	ss, +	Icosahedral	35-40	−	−

ds, Double-stranded; seg, segmented; ss, single-stranded; + or −, polarity of single-stranded nucleic acid.
*Some enveloped viruses are very pleomorphic (sometimes filamentous).
†No matrix protein.
‡Genome has two identical single-stranded RNA molecules.
§Reverse transcriptase.

Figure 4—4. Relative sizes of viruses and bacteria. (*Courtesy the Upjohn Company, Kalamazoo, Mich.*)

genes. Just as there are many different types of computer memory devices, all of these forms of nucleic acid can maintain and transmit the genetic information of the virus. Similarly, the larger the genome, the more information (genes) it can carry and the larger the capsid or envelope structure required to contain the genome.

The outer layer of the virion is the **capsid** or **envelope**. These structures are the package, protection, and delivery vehicle during transmission of the virus from one host to another and for spread within the host to the target cell. The surface structures of the capsid and envelope mediate the interaction of the virus with the target cell through a **viral attachment protein (VAP)** or structure. Removal or disruption of the outer package inactivates the virus. Antibodies generated against the components of these structures prevent virus infection.

The **capsid** is a rigid structure able to withstand harsh environmental conditions. Viruses with naked capsids are generally resistant to drying, acid, and detergents, including the acid and bile of the enteric tract. Many of these viruses are transmitted by the fecal-oral route and can endure transmission even in sewage.

42

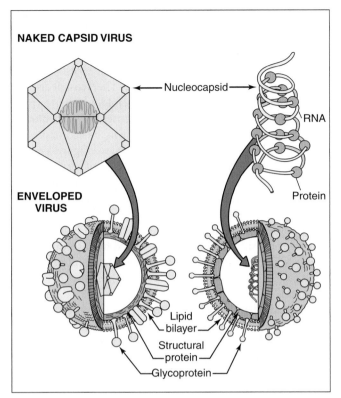

Figure 4—5. The structures of a naked capsid virus (*top left*) and enveloped viruses with an icosahedral (*left*) nucleocapsid or a helical (*right*) ribonucleocapsid. The helical ribonucleocapsid is formed by viral proteins associated with an RNA genome.

The **envelope** is a membrane composed of lipids, proteins, and glycoproteins. The membranous structure of the envelope can be maintained only in aqueous solutions. It is readily disrupted by drying, acidic conditions, detergents, and solvents such as ether, which results in inactivation of the virus. As a result, enveloped viruses must remain wet and are generally transmitted in fluids, respiratory droplets, blood, and tissue. Most cannot survive the harsh conditions of the gastrointestinal tract. The influence of virion structure on viral properties is summarized in Boxes 4-4 and 4-5.

Capsid Viruses

The viral capsid is assembled from individual proteins associated into progressively larger units. All of the components of the capsid have chemical features that allow them to fit together and to assemble into a larger unit. Individual structural proteins associate into **subunits**, which associate into **protomers, capsomeres** (distinguishable in electron micrographs), and finally, a recognizable **procapsid** or **capsid** (Figure 4-6). A procapsid requires further processing to the final, transmissible capsid. For some viruses the capsid forms around the genome; for others the capsid forms as an empty shell (procapsid) to be filled by the genome.

The simplest viral structures that can be built stepwise are symmetrical and include **helical** and **icosahedral** structures. Helical structures appear as rods, whereas the

Box 4—4. Virion Structure: Naked Capsid

Component

Protein

Properties*

Is environmentally stable to the following:
   Temperature
   Acid
   Proteases
   Detergents
   Drying
Is released from cell by lysis

Consequences*

Can be spread easily (on fomites, from hand to hand, by dust, by small droplets)
Can dry out and retain infectivity
Can survive the adverse conditions of the gut
Can be resistant to detergents and poor sewage treatment
Antibody may be sufficient for immunoprotection

Exceptions exist.

icosahedron is an approximation of a sphere assembled from symmetrical subunits (Figure 4-7). Nonsymmetrical capsids are complex forms and are associated with certain bacterial viruses (phages).

The classic example of a virus with helical symmetry is the tobacco mosaic plant virus. Its capsomeres self-assemble on the RNA genome into rods that extend the length of

Box 4—5. Virion Structure: Envelope

Components

Membrane
Lipids
Proteins
Glycoproteins

Properties*

Is environmentally labile—is disrupted by the following:
   Acid
   Detergents
   Drying
   Heat
Modifies cell membrane during replication
Is released by budding and cell lysis

Consequences*

Must stay wet
Cannot survive the gastrointestinal tract
Spreads in large droplets, secretions, organ transplants, and blood transfusions
Does not need to kill the cell to spread
May need antibody and cell-mediated immune response for protection and control
Elicits hypersensitivity and inflammation to cause immunopathogenesis

Exceptions exist.

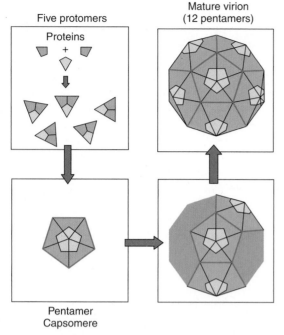

Five protomers

Proteins

Mature virion
(12 pentamers)

Pentamer
Capsomere

Figure 4—6. Capsid assembly of the icosahedral capsid of a picornavirus. Individual proteins associate into subunits, which associate into protomers, capsomeres, and an empty procapsid. Inclusion of the (+) RNA genome triggers its conversion to the final capsid form.

the genome. The capsomeres cover and protect the RNA. Helical nucleocapsids are observed within the envelope of most negative-strand RNA viruses (see Figure 58-1).

Simple **icosahedrons** are used by small viruses such as the picornaviruses and parvoviruses. The icosahedron is made of 12 capsomeres, each with fivefold symmetry (**pentamer** or **penton**). For the picornaviruses, every pentamer is made up of five protomers, each of which is composed of three subunits of four separate proteins (see Figure 4-6). X-ray crystallography and image analysis of cryoelectron microscopy have defined the structure of the picornavirus capsid to the molecular level. These studies have depicted a canyon-like cleft, which is a "docking site" to bind to the receptor on the surface of the target cell (see Figure 56-2).

Larger capsid virions are constructed by inserting structurally distinct capsomeres between the pentons at the vertices. These capsomeres have six nearest neighbors (**hexons**). This extends the icosahedron and is called an **icosadeltahedron**, and its size is determined by the number of hexons inserted along the edges and within the surfaces between the pentons. *A soccer ball is an icosadeltahedron.* For example, the herpesvirus nucleocapsid has 12 pentons and 150 hexons. The herpesvirus nucleocapsid is also surrounded by an envelope. The adenovirus capsid is composed of 252 capsomeres, with 12 pentons and 240 hexons. A long fiber is attached to each penton of

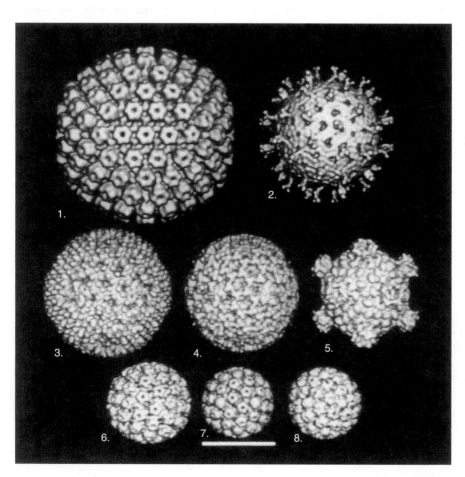

Figure 4—7. Cryoelectron microscopy and computer-generated three-dimensional image reconstructions of several icosahedral capsids. These images show the symmetry of capsids and the individual capsomeres. During assembly, the genome may fill the capsid through the holes in the herpesvirus and papovavirus capsomeres. *1*, Equine herpesvirus nucleocapsid; *2*, simian rotavirus; *3*, reovirus type 1 (Lang) virion; *4*, intermediate subviral particle (reovirus); *5*, core (inner capsid) particle (reovirus); *6*, human papillomavirus type 19; *7*, mouse polyomavirus; *8*, cauliflower mosaic virus. Bar = 50 nm. *(Courtesy Dr. Tim Baker, Purdue University, West Lafayette, Ind.)*

adenovirus to serve as the viral attachment protein (VAP) to bind to target cells, and it also contains the type-specific antigen (see Figure 52-1). The reoviruses have an icosahedral double capsid with fiberlike proteins partially extended from each vertex. The outer capsid protects the virus and promotes its uptake across the gastrointestinal tract and into target cells, whereas the inner capsid contains enzymes for the synthesis of RNA (see Figures 4-7 and 61-2).

Enveloped Viruses

The virion envelope is composed of lipids, proteins, and glycoproteins (see Figure 4-5 and Box 4-5). It has a membrane structure similar to cellular membranes. Cellular proteins are rarely found in the viral envelope, even though the envelope is obtained from cellular membranes. Most enveloped viruses are round or pleomorphic. (See Figures 4-2 and 4-3 for the complete listing of enveloped viruses.) Two exceptions are the poxvirus, which has a complex internal and a bricklike external structure, and the rhabdovirus, which is bullet shaped.

Most viral glycoproteins have asparagine-linked (*N*-linked) carbohydrate and extend through the envelope and away from the surface of the virion. For many viruses, these can be observed as spikes (Figure 4-8). Most glycoproteins act as **VAPs**, capable of binding to structures on target cells. VAPs that also bind to erythrocytes are termed **hemagglutinins (HAs)**. Some glycoproteins have other functions, such as the neuraminidase of orthomyxoviruses (influenza) and the Fc receptor and the C3b receptor associated with

Figure 4—8. Diagram of the hemagglutinin glycoprotein trimer of influenza A virus, a representative spike protein. The region for attachment to the cellular receptor is exposed on the spike protein's surface. Under mild acidic conditions the hemagglutinin changes conformation to expose a hydrophobic sequence at the "fusion region." CHO, *N*-linked carbohydrate attachment sites. *(Modified from Schlesinger MJ, Schlesinger S: Domains of virus glycoproteins. Adv Virus Res 33:1-44, 1987.)*

herpes simplex virus glycoproteins, or the fusion glycoproteins of paramyxoviruses. Glycoproteins, especially the VAP, are also major antigens that elicit protective immunity.

The envelope of the togaviruses surrounds an icosahedral nucleocapsid containing a positive-strand RNA genome. The envelope contains spikes consisting of two or three glycoprotein subunits anchored to the virion's icosahedral capsid. This causes the envelope to adhere tightly and conform (shrink-wrap) to an icosahedral structure discernible by cryoelectron microscopy.

All of the negative-strand RNA viruses are enveloped. Components of the viral RNA-dependent RNA polymerase associate with the (−) RNA genome of the orthomyxoviruses, paramyxoviruses, and rhabdoviruses to form helical nucleocapsids (see Figure 4-5). These enzymes are required to initiate virus replication, and their association with the genome ensures their delivery into the cell. Matrix proteins lining the inside of the envelope facilitate the assembly of the ribonucleocapsid into the virion. Influenza A (orthomyxovirus) is an example of a (−) RNA virus with a segmented genome. Its envelope is lined with matrix proteins and has two glycoproteins: the hemagglutinin, which is the VAP, and a neuraminidase (NA) (see Figure 59-1). Bunyaviruses do not have matrix proteins.

The herpesvirus envelope is a baglike structure that encloses the icosadeltahedral nucleocapsid (see Figure 59-1). Depending on the specific herpesvirus, the envelope may contain as many as 11 glycoproteins. The interstitial space between the nucleocapsid and the envelope is called the **tegument**, and it contains enzymes, other proteins, and even mRNA that facilitate the viral infection.

The poxviruses are enveloped viruses with large, complex, bricklike shapes (see Figure 54-1). The envelope encloses a dumbbell-shaped, DNA-containing nucleoid structure; lateral bodies; fibrils; and many enzymes and proteins, including the enzymes and transcriptional factors required for mRNA synthesis.

Viral Replication

The major steps in viral replication are the same for all viruses (Figure 4-9 and Box 4-6). The cell acts as a factory, providing the substrates, energy, and machinery necessary for the synthesis of viral proteins and replication of the genome. Processes not provided by the cell must be encoded in the genome of the virus. The manner in which each virus accomplishes these steps and overcomes the cell's biochemical limitations is determined by the structure of the genome and of the virion (whether it is enveloped or has a naked capsid). This is illustrated in the examples in Figures 4-12 to 4-14.

A single round of the viral replication cycle can be separated into several phases. During the **early phase** of infection, the virus must recognize an appropriate target cell, attach to the cell, penetrate the plasma membrane and

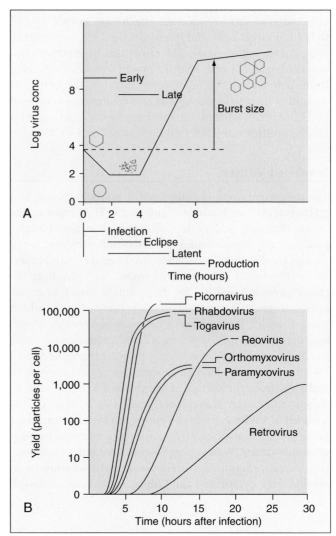

Figure 4—9. A general scheme of viral replication. Enveloped viruses have alternative means of entry (3) assembly, and exit from the cell (8′ and 9′). The antiviral drugs for susceptible steps in viral replication are listed in magenta.

Figure 4—10. A, Single-cycle growth curve of a virus that is released on cell lysis. The different stages are defined by the presence or absence of visible viral components (eclipse period), infectious virus in the media (latent period), or macromolecular synthesis (early/late phases). **B,** Growth curve and burst size of representative viruses. (*A modified from Davis BD, et al: Microbiology, 4th ed. Philadelphia, Lippincott, 1990; B modified from White DO, Fenner F: Medical Virology, 3rd ed. New York, Academic, 1986.*)

be taken up by the cell, release (uncoat) its genome into the cytoplasm, and if necessary, deliver the genome to the nucleus. The **late phase** begins with the start of genome replication and viral macromolecular synthesis and proceeds through viral assembly and release. Uncoating of the genome from the capsid or envelope during the early phase abolishes its infectivity and identifiable structure, thus initiating the eclipse period. The **eclipse period**, like a solar eclipse, ends with the appearance of new virions after virus assembly. The **latent period**, during which extracellular infectious virus is not detected, includes the eclipse period and ends with the release of new

viruses (Figure 4-10). Each infected cell may produce as many as 100,000 particles; however, only 1% to 10% of these particles may be infectious. The noninfectious particles (**defective particles**) result from mutations and errors in the manufacture and assembly of the virion. The yield of infectious virus per cell, or **burst size**, and the time required for a single cycle of virus reproduction are determined by the properties of the virus and the target cell.

Recognition of and Attachment to the Target Cell

The binding of the **VAPs** or structures on the surface of the virion capsid (Table 4-5) to **receptors on the cell** (Table 4-6) initially determines which cells can be infected by a virus. *The receptors for the virus on the cell may be*

Box 4—6. Steps in Viral Replication

1. Recognition of the target cell
2. Attachment
3. Penetration
4. Uncoating
5. Macromolecular synthesis
   a. Early messenger RNA (mRNA) and nonstructural protein synthesis: genes for enzymes and nucleic acid—binding proteins
   b. Replication of genome
   c. Late mRNA and structural protein synthesis
   d. Post-translational modification of protein
6. Assembly of virus
7. Budding of enveloped viruses
8. Release of virus

Table 4–5. Examples of Viral Attachment Proteins

Virus Family	Virus	VAP
Picornaviridae	Rhinovirus	VP1-VP2-VP3 complex
Adenoviridae	Adenovirus	Fiber protein
Reoviridae	Reovirus	σ-1
	Rotavirus	VP7
Togaviridae	Semliki Forest virus	E1-E2-E3 complex gp
Rhabdoviridae	Rabies virus	G protein gp
Orthomyxoviridae	Influenza A virus	HA gp
Paramyxoviridae	Measles virus	HA gp
Herpesviridae	Epstein-Barr virus	gp350 and gp220
Retroviridae	Murine leukemia virus	gp70
	Human immunodeficiency virus	gp120

gp, glycoprotein; HA, hemagglutinin; VAP, viral attachment protein.

proteins or carbohydrates on glycoproteins or glycolipids. Viruses that bind to receptors expressed on specific cell types may be restricted to certain species (**host range**) (e.g., human, mouse) or specific cell types. The susceptible target cell defines the **tissue tropism** (e.g., neurotropic, lymphotropic). Epstein-Barr virus, a herpesvirus, has a very limited host range and tropism because it binds to the C3d receptor (CR2) expressed on human B cells. The B19 parvovirus binds to globoside (blood group P antigen) expressed on erythroid precursor cells.

The viral attachment structure for a capsid virus may be part of the capsid or a protein that extends from the capsid. A canyon on the surface of picornaviruses, such as the rhinovirus 14, serves as a "keyhole" for the insertion of a portion of the intercellular adhesion molecule (ICAM-1) from the cell surface. The fibers of the adenoviruses and the σ-1 proteins of the reoviruses at the vertices of the capsid interact with receptors expressed on specific target cells.

VAPs are specific glycoproteins of enveloped viruses. The HA of influenza A virus binds to sialic acid expressed on many different cells and has a broad host range and tissue tropism. Similarly, the α-togaviruses and the flaviviruses are able to bind to receptors expressed on cells of many animal species, including arthropods, reptiles, amphibians, birds, and mammals. This allows them to infect animals, mosquitoes, and other insects and to be spread by them.

Penetration

Many interactions between the VAPs and the cellular receptors initiate the internalization of the virus into the cell. The mechanism of internalization depends on the virion structure and cell type. Most nonenveloped viruses enter the cell by receptor-mediated endocytosis or by viropexis. **Endocytosis** is a normal process used by the cell for the uptake of receptor-bound molecules such as hormones, low-density lipoproteins, and transferrin. Picornaviruses and papovaviruses may enter by **viropexis**. Hydrophobic structures of capsid proteins may be exposed after viral binding to the cells, and these structures help the virus or the viral genome slip through (direct penetration) the membrane.

Enveloped viruses fuse their membranes with cellular membranes to deliver the nucleocapsid or genome directly into the cytoplasm. The optimum pH for fusion determines

Table 4–6. Examples of Viral Receptors

Virus	Target Cell	Receptor*
Epstein-Barr virus	B cell	C3d complement receptor CR2 (CD21)
Human immunodeficiency virus	Helper T cell	CD4 molecule and chemokine coreceptor
Rhinovirus	Epithelial cells	ICAM-1 (immunoglobulin superfamily protein)
Poliovirus	Epithelial cells	Immunoglobulin superfamily protein
Herpes simplex virus	Many cells	Herpesvirus entry mediator (HᴠᴇA), nectin-1
Rabies virus	Neuron	Acetylcholine receptor, NCAM (neural cell adhesion molecule)
Influenza A virus	Epithelial cells	Sialic acid
B19 parvovirus	Erythroid precursors	Erythrocyte P antigen (globoside)

ICAM-1, Intercellular adhesion molecule.
*Other receptors for these viruses may also exist.

whether penetration occurs at the cell surface at neutral pH or whether the virus must be internalized by endocytosis, and fusion occurs in an endosome at acidic pH. The fusion activity may be provided by the VAP or another protein. The HA of influenza A (see Figure 4-8) binds to sialic acid receptors on the target cell. Under the mild acidic conditions of the endosome, the HA undergoes a dramatic conformational change to expose hydrophobic portions capable of promoting membrane fusion. Paramyxoviruses have a fusion protein that is active at neutral pH to promote virus-cell fusion. Paramyxoviruses can also promote cell–cell fusion to form multinucleated giant cells (**syncytia**). Some herpesviruses and retroviruses fuse with cells at a neutral pH and induce syncytia after replication.

Uncoating

Once internalized, the nucleocapsid must be delivered to the site of replication within the cell and the capsid or envelope removed. The genome of DNA viruses, except for poxviruses, must be delivered to the nucleus, whereas most RNA viruses remain in the cytoplasm. The uncoating process may be initiated by attachment to the receptor or promoted by the acidic environment or proteases found in an endosome or lysosome. Picornavirus capsids are weakened by the release of the VP4 capsid protein to allow uncoating. VP4 is released by insertion of the receptor into the keyhole-like canyon attachment site of the capsid. Enveloped viruses are uncoated on fusion with cell membranes. Fusion of the herpesvirus envelope with the plasma membrane releases its nucleocapsid, which then "docks" with the nuclear membrane to deliver its DNA genome directly to the site of replication. The release of the influenza nucleocapsid from its matrix and envelope is facilitated by the passage of protons from inside the endosome through the ion pore formed by the influenza M2 matrix protein to acidify the virion.

The reovirus and poxvirus are only partially uncoated on entry. The outer capsid of reovirus is removed, but the genome remains in an inner capsid which contains the polymerases necessary for RNA synthesis. The initial uncoating of the poxviruses exposes a subviral particle to the cytoplasm, allowing synthesis of mRNA by virion-contained enzymes. An uncoating enzyme can then be synthesized to release the DNA-containing core into the cytoplasm.

Macromolecular Synthesis

Once inside the cell the genome must direct the synthesis of viral mRNA and protein and generate identical copies of itself. The genome is useless unless it can be transcribed into functional mRNAs capable of binding to ribosomes and being translated into proteins. The means by which each virus accomplishes these steps depends on the structure of the genome (Figure 4-11) and the site of replication.

Figure 4–11. Viral macromolecular synthesis steps: The mechanism of viral mRNA and protein synthesis and genome replication are determined by the structure of the genome. *1.* Double-stranded DNA (DS DNA) uses host machinery in the nucleus (except poxviruses) to make mRNA, which is translated by host cell ribosomes into proteins. Replication of viral DNA occurs by semiconservative means, by rolling circle, linear, and in other ways. *2.* Single-stranded DNA (SS DNA) is converted into DS DNA and replicates like DS DNA. *3.* (+) RNA resembles an mRNA that binds to ribosomes to make a polyprotein that is cleaved into individual proteins. One of the viral proteins is an RNA polymerase that makes a (−) RNA template and then more (+) RNA genome progeny and mRNAs. *4.* (−) RNA is transcribed into mRNAs and a full-length (+) RNA template by the RNA polymerase carried in the virion. The (+) RNA template is used to make (−) RNA genome progeny. *5.* DS RNA acts like (−) RNA. The (−) strands are transcribed into mRNAs by an RNA polymerase in the capsid. (+) RNAs get encapsidated and (−) RNAs are made in the capsid. *6.* Retroviruses are (+) RNA that are converted to complementary DNA (cDNA) by reverse transcriptase carried in the virion. cDNA integrates into the host chromosome, and the host makes mRNAs, proteins, and full-length RNA genome copies.

The cell's machinery for transcription and mRNA processing is found in the nucleus. *Most DNA viruses use the cell's DNA-dependent RNA polymerase II and other enzymes to make mRNA.* For example, eukaryotic mRNAs acquire a 3' polyadenylated (poly A) tail and a 5' methylated cap (for binding to the ribosome) and are processed to remove introns before being exported to the cytoplasm. Viruses that replicate in the cytoplasm must provide these functions or an alternative. Although poxviruses are DNA viruses, they replicate in the cytoplasm and therefore must encode enzymes for all these functions. *Most RNA viruses replicate and produce mRNA in the cytoplasm,* except for orthomyxoviruses and retroviruses. *RNA viruses must encode the necessary enzymes for transcription and replication, because the cell has no means of replicating RNA.* The mRNAs for RNA viruses may or may not acquire a 5' cap or poly A tail.

The naked genome of DNA viruses (except poxviruses) and the positive-sense RNA viruses (except retroviruses) are sometimes referred to as **infectious nucleic acids**, because they are sufficient for initiating replication on injection into a cell. These genomes can interact directly with host machinery to promote mRNA or protein synthesis, or both.

In general, mRNA for nonstructural proteins is transcribed first (see Figure 4-12). **Early gene products** (nonstructural proteins) are often DNA-binding proteins and enzymes, including virus-encoded polymerases. These proteins are catalytic, and only a few are required. *Replication of the genome usually initiates the transition to transcription of late gene products.* **Late viral genes** encode structural proteins. Many copies of these proteins are required to package the virus, but are generally not required before the genome is replicated. Newly replicated genomes also provide new templates for more late gene mRNA synthesis. Different DNA and RNA viruses control the time and amount of viral gene and protein synthesis in different ways.

DNA Viruses

Replication of the DNA genome requires a DNA-dependent DNA polymerase, other enzymes, and deoxyribonucleotide

Figure 4–12. Replication of herpes simplex virus, a complex enveloped DNA virus. The virus binds to specific receptors and fuses with the plasma membrane. The nucleocapsid then delivers the DNA genome to the nucleus. Transcription and translation occur in three phases: immediate early, early, and late. Immediate early proteins promote the takeover of the cell; early proteins consist of enzymes, including the DNA-dependent DNA polymerase; and the late proteins are structural proteins, including the viral capsid and glycoproteins. The genome is replicated before transcription of the late genes. Capsid proteins migrate into the nucleus, assemble into icosadeltahedral capsids, and are filled with the DNA genome. The capsids filled with genomes bud through the nuclear and endoplasmic reticulum membranes into the cytoplasm, acquire tegument proteins, and then acquire their envelope as they bud through the viral glycoprotein modified membranes of the trans-Golgi network. The virus is released by exocytosis or cell lysis.

Box 4—7. Properties of DNA Viruses

DNA is not transient or labile.

Many DNA viruses establish persistent infections (e.g., latent, immortalizing).

DNA genomes reside in the nucleus (except for poxviruses).

Viral DNA resembles host DNA for transcription and replication.

Viral genes must interact with host transcriptional machinery (except for poxviruses).

Viral gene transcription is temporally regulated.

Early genes encode DNA-binding proteins and enzymes.

Late genes encode structural and other proteins.

DNA polymerases require a primer to replicate the viral genome.

The larger DNA viruses encode means to promote efficient replication of their genome.

Parvovirus: requires cells undergoing DNA synthesis to replicate.

Papovavirus: stimulates cell growth and DNA synthesis.

Hepadnavirus: stimulates cell growth and encodes its own polymerase.

Adenovirus: stimulates cellular DNA synthesis and encodes its own polymerase.

Herpesvirus: stimulates cell growth, encodes its own polymerase and enzymes to provide deoxyribonucleotides for DNA synthesis, establishes latent infection in host.

Poxvirus: encodes its own polymerase and enzymes to provide deoxyribonucleotides for DNA synthesis, replication machinery, and transcription machinery in the cytoplasm.

triphosphates, especially thymidine (Box 4-7). Transcription of the DNA virus genome (except for poxviruses) occurs in the nucleus, using host cell polymerases and other enzymes for viral mRNA synthesis. Transcription of the viral genes is regulated by the interaction of specific DNA-binding proteins with promoter and enhancer elements in the viral genome. The viral promoter and enhancer elements are similar in sequence to those of the host cell to allow binding of the cell's transcriptional activation factors and DNA-dependent RNA polymerase. Cells from some tissues do not express the DNA-binding proteins necessary for activating the transcription of viral genes, and replication of the virus in that cell is thus prevented or limited.

Different DNA viruses control the duration, timing, and quantity of viral gene and protein synthesis in different ways. The more complex viruses encode their own transcriptional activators, which enhance or regulate the expression of viral genes. For example, the herpes simplex virus encodes many proteins that regulate the kinetics of viral gene expression, including the VMW 65 (α-TIF protein, VP16). VMW 65 is carried in the virion, binds to the host cell transcription-activating complex (Oct-1), and enhances its ability to stimulate transcription of the immediate early genes of the virus.

Genes may be transcribed from either DNA strand of the genome and in opposite directions. For example, the early and late genes of the SV40 papovavirus are on opposite, non-overlapping DNA strands. Viral genes may have introns requiring post-transcriptional processing of the mRNA by the cell's nuclear machinery (splicing). The

late genes of papovaviruses and adenoviruses are initially transcribed as a large RNA from a single promoter and then processed to produce several different mRNAs after removal of different intervening sequences (introns).

Replication of viral DNA follows the same biochemical rules as for cellular DNA. Replication is initiated at a unique DNA sequence of the genome called the **origin (ori)**. This is a site recognized by cellular or viral nuclear factors and the **DNA-dependent DNA polymerase**. Viral DNA synthesis is semiconservative, and viral and cellular *DNA polymerases require a primer* to initiate synthesis of the DNA chain. The parvoviruses have DNA sequences that are inverted and repeated to allow the DNA to fold back and hybridize with itself to provide a primer. Replication of the adenovirus genome is primed by deoxycytidine monophosphate attached to a terminal protein. A cellular enzyme (primase) synthesizes an RNA primer to start the replication of the papovavirus genome, whereas the herpesviruses encode a primase.

Replication of the genome of the simple DNA viruses (e.g., parvoviruses, papovaviruses) uses the host DNA-dependent DNA polymerases, whereas the larger, more complex viruses (e.g., adenoviruses, herpesviruses, poxviruses) encode their own polymerases. Viral polymerases are usually faster but less precise than host cell polymerases, causing a higher mutation rate in viruses and providing a target for nucleotide analogues as antiviral drugs.

Hepadnavirus replication is unique in that a circular, positive-strand RNA intermediate is first synthesized by the cell's DNA-dependent RNA polymerase. Viral proteins surround the RNA, an RNA-dependent DNA polymerase (reverse transcriptase) in this virion core makes a negative-strand DNA, and then the RNA is degraded. Positive-strand DNA synthesis is initiated but stops when the genome and core are enveloped, yielding a partially double-stranded circular DNA genome.

Major limitations for replication of a DNA virus include availability of the DNA polymerase and deoxyribonucleotide substrates. Most cells in the resting phase of growth are not undergoing DNA synthesis, because the necessary enzymes are not present, and deoxythymidine pools are limited. *The smaller the DNA virus, the more dependent the virus is on the host cell* to provide these functions (see Box 4-7). The parvoviruses are the smallest DNA viruses and replicate only in growing cells, such as erythroid precursor cells or fetal tissue. Speeding up the growth of the cell can enhance viral DNA and mRNA synthesis. The T antigen of SV40, the E6 and E7 of papillomavirus, and the E1a and E1b proteins of adenovirus bind to and prevent the function of growth-inhibitory proteins (p53 and the retinoblastoma gene product), resulting in cell growth, which also promotes virus replication. The larger DNA viruses may encode a DNA polymerase and other proteins to facilitate DNA synthesis and are more independent. Herpes simplex virus encodes a DNA polymerase and scavenging enzymes, such as deoxyribonuclease, ribonucleotide reductase, and thymidine kinase, to generate the necessary deoxyribonucleotide substrates for replication of its genome.

RNA Viruses

Replication and transcription of RNA viruses are similar processes, because the viral genomes are usually either an mRNA (positive-strand RNA) (see Figure 4-13) or a template for mRNA (negative-strand RNA) (Box 4-8; see Figure 4-14). During replication and transcription, a double-stranded RNA replicative intermediate, a structure not normally found in uninfected cells, is formed.

The RNA virus genome must code for **RNA-dependent RNA polymerases (replicases and transcriptases)**, because the cell has no means of replicating RNA. Because RNA is degraded relatively quickly, the RNA-dependent RNA polymerase must be provided or synthesized soon after uncoating to generate more viral RNA, or the infection will be aborted. Most viral RNA polymerases work at a fast pace but are also error prone, causing mutations. Replication of the genome provides new templates for production of more mRNA, which amplifies and accelerates virus replication.

Figure 4–13. Replication of picornaviruses: a simple (+) RNA virus. *1*, Interaction of the picornaviruses with receptors on the cell surface defines the target cell and weakens the capsid. *2*, The genome is injected through the virion and across the cell membrane. *2′*, The virion is endocytosed, and then the genome is released. *3*, Alternatively, the genome is used as mRNA for protein synthesis. One large polyprotein is translated from the virion genome. *4*, Then the polyprotein is proteolytically cleaved into individual proteins, including an RNA-dependent RNA polymerase. *5*, The polymerase makes a (−) strand template from the genome and replicates the genome. A protein (VPg) is covalently attached to the 5′ end of the viral genome. *6*, The structural proteins associate into the capsid structure, the genome is inserted, and the virions are released on cell lysis.

Box 4—8. Properties of RNA Viruses

RNA is labile and transient.
Most RNA viruses replicate in the cytoplasm.
Cells cannot replicate RNA. RNA viruses must encode an RNA-dependent RNA polymerase.
The genome structure determines the mechanism of transcription and replication.
RNA viruses are prone to mutation.
The genome structure and polarity determine how viral messenger RNA (mRNA) is generated and proteins are processed.
RNA viruses, except (+) RNA genome, must carry polymerases.
All (−) RNA viruses are enveloped.
Picornaviruses, togaviruses, flaviviruses, caliciviruses, and coronaviruses
(+) RNA genome resembles mRNA and is translated into a polyprotein, which is proteolyzed. A (−) RNA template is used for replication. Togaviruses, coronaviruses, and noroviruses have early and late genes.
Orthomyxoviruses, paramyxoviruses, rhabdoviruses, filoviruses, and bunyaviruses
(−) RNA genome is a template for individual mRNAs, but full-length (+) RNA template is required for replication. Orthomyxoviruses replicate and transcribe in nucleus, and each segment of the genome encodes one mRNA and template.
Reoviruses
(+/−) Segmented RNA genome is a template for mRNA. (+) RNA may also be encapsulated to generate the (+/−) RNA and then more mRNA.
Retroviruses
(+) Retrovirus RNA genome is converted into DNA, which is integrated into the host chromatin and transcribed as a cellular gene.

The **positive-strand RNA viral genomes** of the picornaviruses, caliciviruses, coronaviruses, flaviviruses, and togaviruses act as mRNA, bind to ribosomes, and direct protein synthesis. *The naked positive-strand RNA viral genome is sufficient to initiate infection by itself.* After the virus-encoded, RNA-dependent RNA polymerase is produced, a negative-strand RNA template is synthesized. The template can then be used to generate more mRNA and to replicate the genome. For the togaviruses and caliciviruses, the negative-sense RNA template is also used to produce a smaller RNA for the structural proteins (late genes). The mRNAs for these viruses are not capped at the 5′ end, but the genome encodes a short poly A sequence. Transcription and replication of coronaviruses share many of these aspects but are more complex.

The **negative-strand RNA virus genomes** of the rhabdoviruses, orthomyxoviruses, paramyxoviruses, filoviruses, and bunyaviruses are the templates for production of mRNA. The negative-strand RNA genome is not infectious by itself, and *a polymerase must be carried into the cell with the genome* (associated with the genome as part of the nucleocapsid) to make individual mRNA for the different viral proteins. As a result, a full-length positive-strand RNA must also be produced by the viral polymerase to act as a template to generate more copies of the genome.

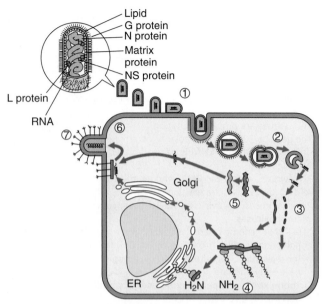

Figure 4–14. Replication of rhabdoviruses: a simple enveloped (−) RNA virus. *1*, Rhabdoviruses bind to the cell surface and are *(2)* endocytosed. The envelope fuses with the endosome vesicle membrane to deliver the nucleocapsid to the cytoplasm. The virion must carry a polymerase, which *(3)* produces five individual messenger RNAs (mRNAs) and a full-length (+) RNA template. *4*, Proteins are translated from the mRNAs, including one glycoprotein (G) which is co-translationally glycosylated in the endoplasmic reticulum (ER), processed in the Golgi apparatus, and delivered to the cell membrane. *5*, The genome is replicated from the (+) RNA template, and N, L, and NS proteins associate with the genome to form the nucleocapsid. *6*, The matrix protein associates with the G protein—modified membrane, which is followed by assembly of the nucleocapsid. *7*, The virus buds from the cell in a bullet-shaped virion.

The (−) RNA genome is like the negatives from a roll of 35-mm film: Each frame encodes a photo/mRNA, but a full-length positive is required for replicating the roll. *Except for influenza viruses, transcription and replication of negative-strand RNA viruses occur in the cytoplasm.* The influenza transcriptase requires a primer to produce mRNA. It uses the 5′ ends of cellular mRNA in the nucleus as primers for its polymerase and in the process steals the 5′ cap from the cellular mRNA. The influenza genome is also replicated in the nucleus.

The reoviruses have a **segmented, double-stranded RNA genome** and undergo a more complex means of replication and transcription. The reovirus RNA polymerase is part of the inner capsid core; mRNA units are transcribed from each of the 10 or more segments of the genome while they are still in the core. The negative strands of the genome segments are used as templates for mRNA in a manner similar to that of the negative-strand RNA viruses. Reovirus-encoded enzymes contained in the inner capsid core add the 5′ cap to viral mRNA. The mRNA does not have poly A. The mRNAs are released into the cytoplasm, where they direct protein synthesis or are sequestered into new cores. The positive-strand RNA in the new cores acts as a template for negative-strand RNA, and the core polymerase produces the progeny double-stranded RNA.

The arenaviruses have an **ambisense circular genome** with (+) sequences adjacent to (−) sequences. The early genes of the virus are transcribed from the negative-sense portion of the genome, and the late genes of the virus are transcribed from the full-length replicative intermediate.

Although the **retroviruses** have a positive-strand RNA genome, the virus provides no means for replication of the RNA in the cytoplasm. Instead, the retroviruses carry two copies of the genome, two transfer RNA (tRNA) molecules, and an RNA-dependent DNA polymerase (**reverse transcriptase**) in the virion. The tRNA is used as a primer for synthesis of a circular complementary DNA copy (**cDNA**) of the genome. The cDNA is synthesized in the cytoplasm, travels to the nucleus, and is then integrated into the host chromatin. The viral genome becomes a cellular gene. Promoters at the end of the integrated viral genome enhance the transcription of the viral DNA sequences by the cell. Full-length RNA transcripts are used as new genomes, and individual mRNAs are generated by differential splicing of this RNA.

The most unusual mode of replication is reserved for the **deltavirus**. The deltavirus resembles a viroid. The genome is a circular, rod-shaped, single-stranded RNA, which is extensively hybridized to itself. As the exception, the deltavirus RNA genome is replicated by the host cell DNA-dependent RNA polymerase II in the nucleus. A portion of the genome forms an RNA structure called a ribozyme, which cleaves the RNA circle to produce an mRNA.

Viral Protein Synthesis

All viruses depend on the host cell ribosomes, tRNA, and mechanisms for post-translational modification to produce their proteins. The binding of mRNA to the ribosome is mediated by a 5′ cap structure of methylated guanosine or a special RNA loop structure (internal ribosome entry sequence [IRES]), which binds within the ribosome to initiate protein synthesis. The cap structure, if used, is attached to mRNA in different ways by different viruses. The IRES structure was discovered first in the picornavirus genome and then in selected cellular mRNAs. Most but not all viral mRNA have a polyadenosine (polyA) tail, like eukaryotic mRNAs.

Unlike bacterial ribosomes, which can bind to a polycistronic mRNA and translate several gene sequences into separate proteins, the eukaryotic ribosome binds to mRNA and can make only one continuous protein, and then it falls off the mRNA. Each virus deals with this limitation differently, depending on the structure of the genome. For example, the entire genome of a positive-strand RNA virus is read by the ribosome and translated into one giant **polyprotein**. The polyprotein is subsequently cleaved by cellular and viral proteases into functional proteins. DNA viruses, retroviruses, and most negative-strand RNA viruses transcribe separate mRNA for smaller polyproteins or individual proteins. The orthomyxovirus and reovirus genomes are segmented, and most of the segments code for single proteins for this reason.

Viruses use different tactics to promote preferential translation of their viral mRNA instead of cellular mRNA. In many cases, the concentration of viral mRNA in the cell is so large that it occupies most of the ribosomes, preventing translation of cellular mRNA. Adenovirus infection blocks the egress of cellular mRNA from the nucleus. Herpes simplex virus and other viruses inhibit cellular macromolecular synthesis and induce degradation of the cell's DNA and mRNA. To promote selective translation of its mRNA, poliovirus uses a virus-encoded protease to inactivate the 200,000-Da cap-binding protein of the ribosome to prevent binding and translation of 5′ capped cellular mRNA. Togaviruses and many other viruses increase the permeability of the cell's membrane; thus the ribosomal affinity for most cellular mRNA is decreased. All these actions also contribute to the cytopathology of the virus infection. The pathogenic consequences of these actions are discussed further in Chapter 48.

Some viral proteins require **post-translational modifications**, such as phosphorylation, glycosylation, acylation, or sulfation. Protein phosphorylation is accomplished by cellular or viral protein kinases and is a means of modulating, activating, or inactivating proteins. Several herpesviruses and other viruses encode their own protein kinase. *Viral glycoproteins are synthesized on membrane-bound ribosomes and have the amino acid sequences to allow insertion into the rough endoplasmic reticulum and N-linked glycosylation.* The high-mannose precursor form of the glycoproteins progresses from the endoplasmic reticulum through the vesicular transport system of the cell and is processed through the Golgi apparatus. The sialic acid–containing mature glycoprotein is expressed on the plasma membrane of the cell unless the glycoprotein expresses protein sequences for retention in an intracellular organelle. The presence of the glycoproteins determines where the virion will assemble. Other modifications, such as O-glycosylation, acylation, and sulfation of the proteins, can also occur during progression through the Golgi apparatus.

Assembly

Virion assembly is analogous to a three-dimensional interlocking puzzle that puts itself together in the box. The virion is built from small, easily manufactured parts that enclose the genome in a functional package. Each part of the virion has recognition structures that allow the virus to form the appropriate protein–protein, protein–nucleic acid, and (for enveloped viruses) protein–membrane interactions needed to assemble into the final structure. The assembly process begins when the necessary pieces are synthesized and the concentration of structural proteins in the cell is sufficient to drive the process thermodynamically, much like a crystallization reaction. The assembly

process may be facilitated by scaffolding proteins or other proteins that are activated or release energy on proteolysis. For example, cleavage of the VP0 protein of poliovirus releases the VP4 peptide, which solidifies the capsid.

The site and mechanism of virion assembly in the cell depend on where genome replication occurs and whether the final structure is a naked capsid or an enveloped virus. Assembly of the DNA viruses, other than poxviruses, occurs in the nucleus and requires transport of the virion proteins into the nucleus. RNA virus and poxvirus assembly occurs in the cytoplasm.

Capsid viruses may be assembled as empty structures (procapsids) to be filled with the genome (e.g., picornaviruses), or they may be assembled around the genome. Nucleocapsids of the retroviruses, togaviruses, and the negative-strand RNA viruses assemble around the genome and are subsequently enclosed in an envelope. The helical nucleocapsid of negative-strand RNA viruses includes the RNA-dependent RNA polymerase necessary for mRNA synthesis in the target cell.

For enveloped viruses, newly synthesized and processed viral glycoproteins are delivered to cellular membranes by vesicular transport. Acquisition of an envelope occurs after association of the nucleocapsid with the viral glycoprotein-containing regions of host cell membranes in a process called **budding**. Matrix proteins for negative-strand RNA viruses line and promote the adhesion of nucleocapsids with the glycoprotein-modified membrane. As more interactions occur, the membrane surrounds the nucleocapsid, and the virus buds from the membrane.

The type of genome and the protein sequence of the glycoproteins determine the site of budding. Most RNA viruses bud from the plasma membrane, and the virus is released from the cell at the same time. The flaviviruses, coronaviruses, and bunyaviruses acquire their envelope by budding into the endoplasmic reticulum and Golgi membranes and may remain cell-associated in these organelles. The herpes simplex virus nucleocapsid assembles in the nucleus and buds into and then out of the endoplasmic reticulum. The nucleocapsid is dumped into the cytoplasm, viral proteins associate with the capsid, and then the envelope is acquired by budding into a trans-Golgi network membrane decorated with the 10 viral glycoproteins. The virion is transported to the cell surface and released by exocytosis, on cell lysis, or transmitted through cell–cell bridges.

Viruses use different tricks to ensure that all the parts of the virus are assembled into complete virions. The RNA polymerase required for infection by negative-strand RNA viruses is carried on the genome as a helical nucleocapsid. The human immunodeficiency virus and other retrovirus genomes are packaged in a procapsid consisting of a polyprotein containing the protease, polymerase, integrase, and structural proteins. This procapsid binds to viral glycoprotein-modified membranes, and the virion buds from the membrane. The virus-encoded protease is activated within the virion and cleaves the polyprotein to produce the final infectious nucleocapsid and the required proteins within the envelope.

Assembly of viruses with segmented genomes, such as influenza or reovirus, requires accumulation of at least one copy of each gene segment. This can be accomplished if the segments assemble together like capsid subunits or randomly package more segments per virion than necessary. This will statistically generate a small but acceptable percentage of functional viruses. Errors are made by the viral polymerase and during viral assembly. Empty virions and virions containing defective genomes are produced. As a result, the particle to infectious virus ratio, also called *particle to plaque-forming unit ratio*, is high, usually greater than 10, and during rapid viral replication can even be 10^4. Defective viruses can occupy the machinery required for normal virus replication to prevent (interfere with) virus production (**defective interfering particles**).

Release

Viruses can be released from cells after lysis of the cell, by exocytosis, or by budding from the plasma membrane. Naked capsid viruses are generally released after lysis of the cell. Release of most enveloped viruses occurs after budding from the plasma membrane without killing the cell. Lysis and plasma membrane budding are efficient means of release. Viruses that bud or acquire their membrane in the cytoplasm (e.g., flaviviruses, poxviruses) remain cell-associated and are released by exocytosis or cell lysis. Viruses that bind to sialic acid receptors (e.g., orthomyxoviruses, certain paramyxoviruses) may also have a neuraminidase. The neuraminidase removes potential sialic acid receptors on the glycoproteins of the virion and the host cell to prevent clumping and facilitate release.

Reinitiation of the Replication

The virus released to the extracellular medium is usually responsible for initiating new infections; however, *traversal of cell–cell bridges, virus-induced cell–cell fusion, or vertical transmission* of the genome to daughter cells can also spread the infection. These allow the virus to escape antibody detection. Some herpesviruses, retroviruses, and paramyxoviruses can induce cell–cell fusion to merge the cells into multinucleated giant cells (**syncytia**), which become huge virus factories. The retroviruses and some DNA viruses can transmit their integrated copy of the genome vertically to daughter cells on cell division.

Viral Genetics

Mutations spontaneously and readily occur in viral genomes, creating new virus strains with properties differing from the **parental**, or **wild-type, virus**. These variants can be identified by their nucleotide sequences, antigenic differences (serotypes), or differences in functional or structural properties. Most mutations have no effect or are detrimental to the virus. Mutations in essential genes inactivate the virus, but mutations in other genes can produce antiviral drug resistance or alter the antigenicity or pathogenicity of the virus.

Errors in copying the viral genome during virus replication produce many mutations. This is because of the poor fidelity of the viral polymerase and the rapid rate of genome replication. In addition, RNA viruses do not have a genetic error-checking mechanism. As a result, the rates of mutation for RNA viruses are usually greater than for DNA viruses.

Mutations in essential genes are termed **lethal mutations**. These mutants are difficult to isolate, because the virus cannot replicate. A **deletion mutant** results from the loss or selective removal of a portion of the genome and the function that it encodes. Other mutations may produce **plaque mutants**, which differ from the wild type in the size or appearance of the infected cells; **host range mutants**, which differ in the tissue type or species of target cell that can be infected; or **attenuated mutants**, which are variants that cause less serious disease in animals or humans. **Conditional mutants**, such as **temperature-sensitive (ts)** or **cold-sensitive mutants**, have a mutation in a gene for an essential protein that allows virus production only at certain temperatures. Whereas ts mutants generally grow well or relatively better at 30° C to 35° C, the encoded protein is inactive at elevated temperatures of 38° C to 40° C, preventing virus production.

New virus strains can also arise by genetic interactions between viruses or between the virus and the cell (Figure 4-15). Intramolecular genetic exchange between

Figure 4–15. Genetic exchange between viral particles can give rise to new viral types, as illustrated. Representative viruses include the following: *1*, intertypic recombination of herpes simplex virus type 1 (HSV1) and type 2 (HSV2); *2*, reassortment of two strains of influenza virus; *3*, rescue of a papovavirus defective in assembly by a complementary defective virus (transcapsidation); and *4*, marker rescue of a lethal or conditional mutation.

viruses or the virus and the host is termed **recombination**. Recombination can occur readily between two related DNA viruses. For example, coinfection of a cell with the two closely related herpesviruses (herpes simplex virus types 1 and 2) yields intertypic recombinant strains. These new hybrid strains have genes from types 1 and 2. Integration of retroviruses into host cell chromatin is a form of recombination. Recombination of two related RNA viruses, Sindbis and eastern equine encephalitis virus, resulted in creation of another togavirus, western equine encephalitis virus.

Viruses with segmented genomes (e.g., influenza viruses and reoviruses) form hybrid strains on infection of one cell with more than one virus strain. This process, termed **reassortment**, is analogous to picking 10 marbles out of a box containing 10 black and 10 white marbles. Very different strains of influenza A virus are created on coinfection with a virus from different species (see Figure 59-5).

In some cases, a defective viral strain can be rescued by the replication of another mutant, by the wild-type virus, or by a cell line bearing a replacement viral gene. Replication of the other virus or expression of the gene in the cell provides the missing function required by the mutant (**complementation**), allowing replication to occur. A disabled infectious single-cycle herpes simplex virus (DISC-HSV) vaccine lacks an essential gene and is grown in a cell line that expresses that gene product to "complement" the virus. The virus that is produced can infect the normal cells of the vaccinated individual, but the virions that are produced lack the function necessary for replication in that person's cells. Rescue of a lethal or conditional-lethal mutant with a defined genetic sequence, such as a restriction endonuclease DNA fragment, is called **marker rescue**. Marker rescue is used to map the genomes of viruses such as herpes simplex virus. Virus produced from cells infected with different virus strains may be phenotypically mixed and have the proteins of one strain but the genome of the other (**transcapsidation**). **Pseudotypes** are generated when transcapsidation occurs between different types of virus, but this is rare.

Individual virus strains or mutants are **selected** by their ability to use the host cell machinery and to withstand the conditions of the body and the environment. Cellular properties that can act as selection pressures include the growth rate of the cell and tissue-specific expression of certain proteins required by the virus (e.g., enzymes, glycoproteins, transcription factors). The conditions of the body, its elevated temperature, innate and immune defenses, and tissue structure are also selection pressures for viruses. The viruses that cannot endure these conditions or evade the host defenses are eliminated. A small selective advantage in a mutant virus can shortly lead to its becoming the predominant viral strain. The high mutation rate of the human immunodeficiency virus promotes a switch in target cell tropism from macrophage to T cell, the development of antiviral drug-resistant strains after treatment, and the generation of antigenic variants during a patient's course of infection.

The growth of virus under benign laboratory conditions allows weaker strains to survive because of the absence of the selective pressures of the body. This process is used to select attenuated virus strains for use in vaccines.

Viral Vectors for Therapy

Genetically manipulated viruses can be excellent delivery systems for foreign genes. Viruses can provide gene replacement therapy, can be used as vaccines to promote immunity to other agents or tumors, and can act as targeted killers of tumors. The advantages of using viruses are that they can be readily amplified by replication in appropriate cells, and they target specific tissues and deliver the DNA or RNA into the cell. Viruses that are being developed as vectors include retroviruses, adenoviruses, herpes simplex virus, adeno-associated virus (parvovirus), poxviruses (e.g., vaccinia and canarypox) (see Figure 54-3), and even some togaviruses. The viral vectors are usually defective or attenuated viruses, in which the foreign DNA replaces a virulence or unessential gene. The foreign gene may be under the control of a viral promoter or even a tissue-specific promoter. Defective virus vectors are grown in cell lines that express the missing viral functions "complementing" the virus. The progeny can deliver their nucleic acid but not produce infectious virus. Retroviruses and adeno-associated viruses can integrate into cells and permanently deliver a gene into the cell's chromosome. Adenovirus and herpes simplex virus promote targeted delivery of the foreign gene to receptor-bearing cells. Genetically attenuated herpes simplex viruses are being developed to specifically kill the growing cells of glioblastomas while sparing the surrounding neurons. Vaccinia virus carrying a gene for the rabies glycoprotein is already being used successfully to immunize raccoons, foxes, and skunks in the wild. Some day, virus vectors may be routinely used to treat cystic fibrosis, Duchenne muscular dystrophy, lysosomal storage diseases, and immunologic disorders.

Questions

1. Describe the features of these viruses that are similar, and those that are different.

   a. Poliovirus and rhinovirus
   b. Poliovirus and rotavirus
   c. Poliovirus and western equine encephalitis virus
   d. Yellow fever virus and dengue virus
   e. Epstein-Barr virus and cytomegalovirus

Continued

Questions—cont'd

2. Match the characteristics from column A with the appropriate viral families in column B, based on your knowledge of their physical and genome structure and their implications.

A	B
1. Are resistant to detergents	Picornaviruses
2. Are resistant to drying	Togaviruses
3. Replication in the nucleus	Orthomyxoviruses
4. Replication in the cytoplasm	Paramyxoviruses
5. Can be released from the cell without cell lysis	Rhabdoviruses
6. Provide a good target for antiviral drug action	Reoviruses
7. Undergo reassortment on coinfection with two strains	Retroviruses
8. Make DNA from an RNA template	Herpesviruses
9. Use a (+) RNA template to replicate the genome	Papovaviruses
10. Genome translated into a polyprotein	Adenoviruses
	Poxviruses
	Hepadnaviruses

3. Based on structural considerations, which of the virus families listed in question 2 should be able to endure fecal-oral transmission?

4. List the essential enzymes encoded by the virus families listed in question 2.

5. A mutant defective in the herpes simplex virus type 1 DNA polymerase gene replicates in the presence of herpes simplex virus type 2. The progeny virus contains the herpes simplex virus type 1 genome, but is recognized by antibodies to herpes simplex virus type 2. Which genetic mechanisms may be occurring?

6. How are the early and late genes of the togaviruses, papovaviruses, and herpesviruses distinguished, and how is the time of their expression regulated?

7. What are the consequences (no effect, decreased efficiency, or inhibition of replication) of a deletion mutation in the following viral enzymes?

   a. Epstein-Barr virus polymerase

   b. Herpes simplex virus thymidine kinase

   c. Human immunodeficiency virus reverse transcriptase

   d. Influenza B virus neuraminidase

   e. Rabies virus (rhabdovirus) G protein

Bibliography

Big Picture Book of Viruses online: Available at http://www.virology.net/Big_Virology/BVHomePage.html

Cann AJ: Principles of Molecular Virology. San Diego, Academic, 2001.

Cohen J, Powderly WG: Infectious Diseases, 2nd ed. St Louis, Mosby, 2004.

Electron microscopic images of viruses, by Linda Stannard, University of Capetown, South Africa, online: Available at www.uct.ac.za/depts/mmi/stannard/linda.html.

Flint SJ, et al: Principles of Virology: Molecular Biology, Pathogenesis and Control of Animal Viruses, 2nd ed. Washington, DC, ASM Press, 2003.

Knipe DM, Howley PM: Fields Virology, 4th ed. New York, Lippincott Williams & Wilkins, 2001.

Richman DD, Whitley RJ, Hayden FG: Clinical Virology. New York, Churchill Livingstone, 1997.

Rosenthal KS: Viruses: Microbial spies and saboteurs. Infect Dis Clin Practice 14:97-106, 2006.

Specter S, Hodinka RL, Young SA: Clinical Virology Manual, 3rd ed. Washington, DC, ASM Press, 2000.

Strauss JM, Strauss EG: Viruses and Human Disease, 2nd ed. San Diego, Academic, 2007.

Virology on the web: Available at http://www.virology.net/garryfavweb.html

Viruses in cell culture: Available at www.uct.ac.za/depts/mmi/stannard/linda.html

Fungal Classification, Structure, and Replication

This chapter provides an overview of fungal classification, structure, and reproduction. The very basic aspects of fungal cell organization and morphology are discussed, as well as the broad categories of human mycoses. We have purposely simplified the fungal taxonomy and use it to highlight the major classes of fungi causing disease in humans: the Zygomycetes, the Basidiomycetes, the Archiascomycetes, the Hemiascomycetes, and the Euascomycetes.

The Importance of Fungi

The fungi represent a ubiquitous and diverse group of organisms, the main purpose of which is to degrade organic matter. All fungi lead a heterotrophic existence as **saprobes** (organisms that live on dead or decaying matter), **symbionts** (organisms that live together and in which the association is of mutual advantage), **commensals** (organisms living in a close relationship in which one benefits from the relationship, and the other neither benefits nor is harmed), or as **parasites** (organisms that live on or within a host from which they derive benefits without making any useful contribution in return; in the case of pathogens, the relationship is harmful to the host).

Fungi have emerged in the past two decades as major causes of human disease (Table 5-1), especially among those individuals who are immunocompromised or hospitalized with serious underlying diseases. Among these patient groups, fungi serve as opportunistic pathogens, causing considerable morbidity and mortality. The overall incidence of specific invasive mycoses continues to increase with time (Table 5-2), and the list of opportunistic fungal pathogens likewise increases each year. In short, *there are no nonpathogenic fungi!* This increase in fungal infections can be attributed to the ever-growing number of immunocompromised patients, including transplant patients, individuals with AIDS, patients with cancer and undergoing chemotherapy, and those individuals who are hospitalized with other serious underlying conditions and who undergo a variety of invasive procedures.

Fungal Taxonomy, Structure, and Replication

The fungi are classified in their own separate kingdom, Kingdom Fungi. They are eukaryotic organisms that are distinguished from other eukaryotes by a rigid cell wall composed of chitin and glucan and a cell membrane in which ergosterol is substituted for cholesterol as the major sterol component (Figure 5-1).

Classic fungal taxonomy relies heavily on morphology and mode of spore production. Increasingly, however, ultrastructural features, biochemical, and molecular characteristics are brought to bear, often resulting in changes in the original taxonomic designation. Fungi may be unicellular or multicellular. The most simple grouping, based on morphology, lumps fungi into either **yeasts** or **molds**. A yeast can be defined morphologically as a cell that reproduces by budding or by fission (Figure 5-2), where a progenitor or "mother" cell pinches off a portion of itself to produce a progeny or "daughter" cell. The daughter cells may elongate to form sausage-like **pseudohyphae**. Yeasts are usually unicellular and produce round, pasty, or mucoid colonies on agar. Molds, on the other hand, are multicellular organisms consisting of threadlike tubular structures called **hyphae** (see Figure 5-2) that elongate at their tips by a process known as **apical extension**. Hyphae are either **coenocytic** (hollow and multinucleate) or **septate** (divided by partitions or cross-walls) (see Figure 5-2). The hyphae form together to produce a matlike structure called a **mycelium**. The colonies formed by molds are often described as **filamentous, hairy,** or **woolly.**

Table 5—1. Incidence and Case-Fatality Ratios of Selected Invasive Fungal Infections

Pathogen	No. of Cases per Million per Year Incidence	Case-Fatality Ratio (%) for First Episode
Candida species	72.8	33.9
Cryptococcus neoformans	65.5	12.7
Coccidioides immitis	15.3	11.1
Aspergillus species	12.4	23.3
Histoplasma capsulatum	7.1	21.4
Agents of zygomycosis	1.7	30.0
Agents of hyalohyphomycosis	1.2	14.3
Agents of phaeohyphomycosis	1.0	0
Sporothrix schenckii	<1	20.0
Malassezia furfur	<1	0
Total	178.3	22.4

Adapted from Rees JR, et al: The epidemiological features of invasive mycotic infections in the San Francisco Bay Area, 1992-1993: Results of population-based laboratory active surveillance. Clin Infect Dis 27:1138-1147, 1998.

When growing on agar or other solid surfaces, molds produce hyphae, termed **vegetative hyphae**, that grow on or beneath the surface of the culture medium, and also hyphae that project above the surface of the medium, so-called **aerial hyphae**. The aerial hyphae may produce specialized structures known as **conidia** (asexual reproductive

Table 5—2. Cumulative Incidences of Selected Invasive Mycoses

Mycosis	Incidence per Million per Year			
	CPHA[a]	CDC[b]	NHDS[c]	NHDS[d]
	1980-82	1992-93	1996	2003
Candidiasis	2.6	72.8	228.2	290.0
Histoplasmosis	13.9	7.1	13.6	NA
Aspergillosis	8.4	12.4	34.3	22.0
Cryptococcosis	4.0	65.5	29.6	NA

[a]CPHA, Commission on Hospital and Professional Activities (Reingold et al, 1986).
[b]CDC, Centers for Disease Control (Rees et al, 1998).
[c]NHDS, National Hospital Discharge Survey (Wilson et al, 2002).
[d]NHDS, National Hospital Discharge Survey (Pfaller and Diekema, 2007)
NA, data not available

elements) (Figure 5-3). The conidia may be produced by either a blastic (budding) process or a thallic process, where hyphal segments fragment into individual cells or **arthroconidia**. The conidia are easily airborne and serve to disseminate the fungus. The size, shape, and certain developmental features of conidia are used as a means of identifying fungi to genus and species. Many fungi of medical importance are termed **dimorphic**, because they may exist in both a yeast form and a mold form.

Most fungi exhibit aerobic respiration, although some are facultatively anaerobic (fermentative), and others are strict anaerobes. Metabolically fungi are heterotrophic and biochemically versatile, producing both primary (e.g., citric acid, ethanol, glycerol) and secondary (e.g., antibiotics [penicillin], amanitens, aflatoxins) metabolites. Relative to the bacteria, fungi are slow growing, with cell doubling times in terms of hours rather than minutes.

A simplified taxonomic scheme listing the five major classes of fungi of medical importance is shown in Table 5-3. Of the estimated several hundred thousand different fungi, only about 200 are known to cause human disease, although this number appears to be increasing.

Fungi reproduce by the formation of spores which may be sexual (involving meiosis, preceded by fusion of the protoplasm and nuclei of two compatible mating types) or asexual (involving mitosis only). The fungi in the classes Zygomycetes, Archiascomycetes, Basidiomycetes, Hemiascomycetes, and Euascomycetes produce both sexual and asexual spores (Table 5-4). The form of the fungus producing sexual spores is termed the **teleomorph**, and the form producing asexual spores is termed the **anamorph**. The fact that the teleomorph and anamorph of the same fungus have different names (e.g., *Ajellomyces capsulatum* [teleomorph] and *Histoplasma capsulatum* [anamorph]) is a source of confusion for nonmycologists.

In some fungi the asexual stage, or anamorph, has proved so successful as a means of rapid dispersal and adaptation to new habitats that the sexual stage, or teleomorph, has disappeared or has not yet been discovered. Even in the absence of the teleomorph, it is often possible to assign these fungi to the Basidiomycetes, Archiascomycetes, or Hemiascomycetes on the basis of DNA sequences of their anamorphs. In the past these asexual fungi were classified in an artificial group, the "Fungi Imperfecti" (form-division Deuteromycota).

Irrespective of the ability of a given fungus to produce sexual spores, in clinical situations it is common to refer to the organisms by their asexual designations. This is because the anamorphic (asexual) state is isolated from clinical specimens, and the sexual or teleomorphic phase occurs only under very specialized conditions in the laboratory.

Asexual spores consist of two general types: **sporangiospores** and **conidia**. Sporangiospores are asexual spores produced in a containing structure or **sporangia** (see Figure 5-3) and are characteristic of genera belonging

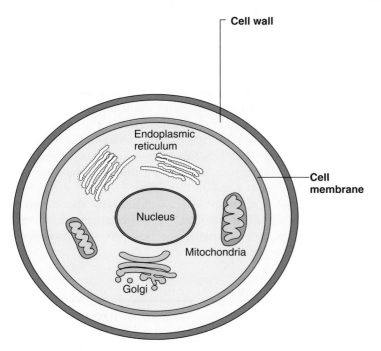

Figure 5—1. Diagram of a fungal cell.

to the class Zygomycetes, such as *Rhizopus* and *Mucor* spp. Conidia are asexual spores that are borne naked on specialized structures as seen in *Aspergillus* spp. (see Figure 5-3), *Penicillium* spp., and the dermatophytes.

Figure 5—2. Fungal cell morphology. **A,** Yeast cells reproducing by nuclear fission and by blastoconidia formation. The elongation of budding yeast cells to form pseudohyphae is shown, as is the formation of a germ tube. **B,** Types of hyphae seen with various molds.

Zygomycetes

The Zygomycetes are molds with broad, sparsely septate, coenocytic hyphae. The Zygomycetes produce sexual zygospores following the fusion of two compatible mating types. The asexual spores of the order Mucorales (see Table 5-3) are contained within a sporangium (sporangiospores). The sporangia are borne at the tips of stalklike **sporangiophores** that terminate in a bulbous swelling called the **columella** (see Figure 5-3). The presence of rootlike structures, called **rhizoids**, is helpful in identifying specific genera within the Mucorales. Most Zygomycetes encountered clinically belong to the order Mucorales. The other order, the Entomophthorales, are less common and include the genera *Basidiobolus* and *Conidiobolus*. These organisms cause tropical subcutaneous zygomycosis. The asexual spores are borne singly on short sporophores and are forcibly ejected when mature.

Basidiomycetes

Most members of the Basidiomycetes have a separate filamentous form, but some are typical yeasts. Sexual reproduction leads to the formation of haploid basidiospores on the outside of a generative cell termed a **basidium**. The most prominent human pathogens in the class Basidiomycetes are the basidiomycetous yeasts with anamorphic stages belonging to the genera *Cryptococcus*, *Malassezia*, and *Trichosporon*. The genus *Cryptococcus*, which contains more than 30 different species, has teleomorphs (sexual stages) that have been assigned to the genera *Filobasidium* and *Filobasidiella*.

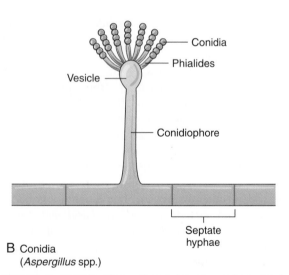

Figure 5–3. Examples of asexual spore formation and associated structures seen with a Zygomycete (**A**) and an *Aspergillus* spp. (**B**).

Archiascomycetes

Archiascomycetes is a new class that was recently described to include an organism, *Pneumocystis carinii*, which had formerly been considered a protozoan. The reclassification of *Pneumocystis* was based on molecular evidence that it was most closely related to the ascomycete *Schizosaccharomyces pombe*. Further molecular studies resulted in the naming of human-derived strains as *Pneumocystis jirovecii*. The organism exists in a vegetative trophic form that reproduces asexually by binary fission.

Fusion of compatible mating types results in a spherical cyst or spore case, which on maturity contains eight spores.

Hemiascomycetes

The class Hemiascomycetes contains the ascomycetous yeasts (order Saccharomycetales) which are characterized by vegetative yeast cells that proliferate by budding or fission (see Figure 5-2A). Many members of the order Saccharomycetales have an anamorphic stage belonging to the genus *Candida* (see Table 5-3). This genus, which consists of approximately 200 anamorphic species, has teleomorphs in more than 10 different genera, including *Clavispora*, *Debaromyces*, *Issatchenkia*, *Kluyveromyces*, and *Pichia*.

Euascomycetes

In the class Euascomycetes, sexual reproduction leads to the formation of a thin-walled sac, or ascus, which contains the haploid ascospores. Although most of the septate molds that are isolated in the clinical laboratory belong to the class Euascomycetes, it is unusual to encounter their sexual reproductive structures in routine cultures.

This class has 12 orders that include species pathogenic to humans. Among the more important are the order Onygenales, which contains the dermatophytes and a number of dimorphic systemic pathogens (including *Histoplasma capsulatum* and *Blastomyces dermatitidis*); the order Eurotiales, which contains the teleomorphs of the anamorphic genera *Aspergillus* and *Penicillium*; the order Hypocreales, which contains the teleomorphs of the anamorphic genus *Fusarium*; and the order Microascales, which contains the teleomorphs (*Pseudallescheria*) of the anamorphic genus *Scedosporium* (see Table 5-3). In addition, the teleomorphs of numerous melanized (dematiaceous) fungi of medical importance belong to orders in this class.

Classification of Human Mycoses

In addition to the formal taxonomic classification of fungi, fungal infections may be classified according to the tissues infected, as well as by specific characteristics of organism groups. These classifications include the superficial, cutaneous, and subcutaneous mycoses, the endemic mycoses, and the opportunistic mycoses (Table 5-5).

Superficial Mycoses

The superficial mycoses are those infections that are limited to the very superficial surfaces of the skin and hair. They are nondestructive and of cosmetic importance only. The clinical infection termed *pityriasis versicolor* is characterized by discoloration or depigmentation

Table 5–3. Medically Important Fungi (Kingdom Fungi)

Taxonomic Designation	Representative Genera	Human Disease
Class: Zygomycetes		
Order: Mucorales	*Rhizopus, Mucor, Absidia, Saksenaea*	Zygomycosis: opportunistic in patients with diabetes, leukemia, severe burns, or malnutrition; rhinocerebral infections.
Order: Entomophthorales	*Basidiobolus, Conidiobolus*	Zygomycosis: subcutaneous and gastrointestinal infections
Class: Basidiomycetes	Teleomorphs of *Cryptococcus, Malassezia*, and *Trichosporon* species.	Cryptococcosis and numerous mycoses
Class: Archiascomycetes	*Pneumocystis jirovecii*	*Pneumocystis* pneumonia
Class: Hemiascomycetes	Teleomorphs of *Candida* species; *Saccharomyces*	Numerous mycoses
Class: Euascomycetes		
Order: Onygenales	*Arthroderma* (teleomorphs of *Trichophyton* and *Microsporum*); *Ajellomyces* (teleomorphs of *Blastomyces* and *Histoplasma* species)	Dermatophytoses; systemic mycoses
Order: Eurotiales	Teleomorphs of *Aspergillus* species	Aspergillosis
Order: Hypocreales	Teleomorphs of *Fusarium* species	Keratitis and other invasive mycoses
Order: Microascales	*Pseudallescheria* (teleomorph of *Scedosporium* species)	Pneumonia, mycetoma, and invasive mycoses

Adapted from Warnock DW: Taxonomy and classification of fungi. In Murray PR, et al (eds): Manual of Clinical Microbiology, 9th ed. Washington, DC, ASM Press, 2007.

Table 5–4. Biologic, Morphologic, and Reproductive Characteristics of Pathogenic Fungi

Organism Class	Representative Genera	Morphology	Reproduction
Zygomycetes	*Rhizopus, Mucor, Absidia, Basidiobolus*	Broad, thin-walled, coenocytic hyphae, 6-25 μm with nonparallel sides; spores contained within sporangium; rootlike structures called *rhizoids* characteristic of some genera	Asexual: production of sporangiospores within sporangium. Sexual: production of zygospores formed by fusion of compatible mating types
Basidiomycetes	Anamorphic basidiomycetous yeasts (*Cryptococcus, Malassezia, Trichosporon*)	Budding yeasts, hyphae, and arthroconidia. Hyphae that produce basidiospores (not seen in nature or in patients). Hyphae with clamp connections.	Asexual: production of conidia by budding from a mother cell or within a hyphal fragment. Sexual: fusion of compatible nuclei followed by meiosis to form basidiospores or not identified
Archiascomycetes	*Pneumocystis jirovecii*	Trophic forms and cystlike structures	Asexual: binary fission. Sexual: fusion of compatible mating types to form zygote; compartmentalization of spores within cyst
Hemiascomycetes	*Candida* and *Saccharomyces*	Budding yeasts and hyphae, pseudohyphae	Asexual: production of conidia by budding from a mother cell. Sexual: either not seen or by conjugation between two single cells or by "mother-bud" conjugation
Euascomycetes	Dermatophytes, *Blastomyces, Histoplasma, Aspergillus, Fusarium, Scedosporium* species	Budding yeasts, septate hyphae, asexual conidia borne on specialized structures.	Asexual: production of conidia by budding from a mother cell. Sexual: ascospores produced in a specialized structure called an *ascus* or not seen

Table 5—5. Classification of Human Mycoses and Representative Etiologic Agents

Superficial Mycoses	Cutaneous and Subcutaneous Mycoses	Endemic Mycoses	Opportunistic Mycoses
Black piedra	Dermatophytoses	Blastomycosis	Aspergillosis
Piedraia hortae	*Microsporum* spp.	*Blastomyces dermatitidis*	*Aspergillus fumigatus*
Tinea nigra	*Trichophyton* spp.	Histoplasmosis	*A. flavus*
Hortae werneckii	*Epidermophyton floccosum*	*Histoplasma capsulatum*	*A. niger*
Pityriasis versicolor	Tinea unguium	Coccidioidomycosis	*A. terreus*
Malassezia furfur	*Trichophyton* spp.	*Coccidioides immitis/*	Candidiasis
White piedra	*E. floccosum*	*posadasii*	*Candida albicans*
Trichosporon spp.	Onychomycosis	Penicilliosis	*C. glabrata*
	Candida spp.	*Penicillium marneffei*	*C. parapsilosis*
	Aspergillus spp.	Paracoccidioidomycosis	*C. tropicalis*
	Trichosporon spp.	*Paracoccidioides brasiliensis*	Cryptococcosis
	Geotrichum spp.		*Cryptococcus neoformans*
	Mycotic keratitis		Trichosporonosis
	Fusarium spp.		*Trichosporon* spp.
	Aspergillus spp.		Hyalohyphomycosis
	Candida spp.		*Acremonium* spp.
	Chromoblastomycosis		*Fusarium* spp.
	Fonsecaea spp.		*Paecilomyces* spp.
	Phialophora spp.		*Scedosporium* spp.
			Zygomycosis
			Rhizopus spp.
			Mucor spp.
			Absidia spp.
			Phaeohyphomycosis
			Alternaria spp.
			Curvularia spp.
			Bipolaris spp.
			Wangiella spp.
			Pneumocystosis
			Pneumocystis jirovecii

and scaling of the skin. *Tinea nigra* refers to brown or black pigmented macular patches localized primarily to the palms. The clinical entities of black and white piedra involve the hair and are characterized by nodules composed of hyphae that encompass the hair shaft. The fungi associated with these superficial infections include *Malassezia furfur, Hortae werneckii, Piedraia hortae* and *Trichosporon* spp.

Cutaneous Mycoses

Cutaneous mycoses are infections of the keratinized layer of skin, hair, and nails. These infections may elicit a host response and become symptomatic. Signs and symptoms include itching, scaling, broken hairs, ringlike patches of the skin, and thickened, discolored nails. The Dermatophytes are fungi classified in the genera *Trichophyton, Epidermophyton,* and *Microsporum.* Infections of the skin involving these organisms are called **dermatophytoses. Tinea unguium** refers to infections of the toes involving these agents. Onychomycoses includes infections of the nails caused by the dermatophytes, as well as nondermatophytic fungi such as *Candida* spp. and *Aspergillus* spp.

Subcutaneous Mycoses

Subcutaneous mycoses involve the deeper layers of the skin, including the cornea, muscle, and connective tissue and are caused by a broad spectrum of taxonomically diverse fungi. The fungi gain access to the deeper tissues usually by traumatic inoculation and remain localized, causing abscess formation, nonhealing ulcers, and draining sinus tracts. The host immune system recognizes the fungi, resulting in variable tissue destruction and frequently epitheliomatous hyperplasia. Infections may be caused by hyaline molds such as *Acremonium* spp. and *Fusarium* spp. and by pigmented or dematiaceous fungi such as *Alternaria* spp., *Cladosporium* spp., and *Exophiala* spp. (Phaeohyphomycoses, Chromoblastomycoses). Subcutaneous mycoses tend to remain localized and rarely disseminate systemically.

Endemic Mycoses

The endemic mycoses are fungal infections caused by the classic dimorphic fungal pathogens *Histoplasma capsulatum, Blastomyces dermatitidis, Coccidioides immitis, Coccidioides posadasii,* and *Paracoccidioides brasiliensis.*

These fungi exhibit thermal dimorphism (exist as yeasts or spherules at 37° C and molds at 25° C) and are generally confined to geographic regions where they occupy specific environmental or ecological niches. The endemic mycoses are often referred to as **systemic mycoses**, because these organisms are true pathogens and can cause infection in healthy individuals. Recently the dimorphic fungus *Penicillium marneffei* has been added to the list of agents causing endemic mycoses. All of these agents produce a primary infection in the lung, with subsequent dissemination to other organs and tissues.

Opportunistic Mycoses

The opportunistic mycoses are infections attributable to fungi that are normally found as human commensals or in the environment. With the exception of *Cryptococcus neoformans*, these organisms exhibit inherently low or limited virulence and cause infection in individuals who are debilitated, immunosuppressed, or who carry implanted prosthetic devices or vascular catheters. Virtually any fungus can serve as an opportunistic pathogen, and the list of those identified as such becomes longer each year. The most common opportunistic fungal pathogens are the yeasts *Candida* spp. and *Cryptococcus neoformans*, the mold *Aspergillus* spp., and *Pneumocystis jirovecii*. Due to its inherent virulence, *Cryptococcus neoformans* is often considered a "systemic" pathogen. Although this fungus may cause infection in immunologically normal individuals, it clearly is seen more frequently as an opportunistic pathogen in the immunocompromised population.

Summary

With the ever-increasing number of individuals at risk for fungal infection, it is imperative that physicians "think fungus" when confronting a suspected infection. The list of documented fungal pathogens is extensive, and one can no longer ignore or dismiss fungi as "contaminants" or clinically insignificant when isolated from clinical material. It is also apparent that the prognosis and response to therapy may vary with the type of fungus causing infection, as well as with the immunological status of the host. Thus physicians must become familiar with the various fungi, their epidemiologic and pathogenic features, as well as the optimal approaches to diagnosis and therapy. These issues will be discussed in detail in subsequent chapters according to the classification scheme shown in Table 5-5.

Questions

1. How do fungi differ from bacteria (size, nucleus, cytosol, plasma membrane, cell wall, physiology, generation time)?
2. How does the plasma membrane of fungi differ from that of other eukaryotic (e.g., mammalian) cells?
3. What is the difference between a yeast and a mold?
4. What do the terms *anamorph* and *teleomorph* mean and why are they important?

Bibliography

Pfaller MA, Diekema DJ: The epidemiology of invasive candidiasis: A persistent public health problem. Clin Microbiol Rev 20:133-163, 2007.

Rees JR, et al: The epidemiological features of invasive mycotic infections in the San Francisco Bay Area, 1992-1993: Results of population-based laboratory active surveillance. Clin Infect Dis 27:1138-1147, 1998.

Rheingold AL, et al: Systemic mycoses in the United States, 1980-1982. J Med Vet Mycol 24:433-436, 1986.

Warnock DW: Taxonomy and classification of fungi. In Murray PR, et al (eds): Manual of Clinical Microbiology, 9th ed. Washington, DC, ASM Press, 2007.

Wilson LS, et al: The direct cost and incidence of systemic fungal infections. Value Health 5:26-34, 2002.

Parasitic Classification, Structure, and Replication

This chapter provides an introduction to parasite classification and physiology. This brief review is intended to enhance the reader's comprehension of the interrelationships among parasitic organisms, their epidemiology and transmission of disease, the specific disease processes involved, and the possibilities for prevention and control of maladies. We have deliberately attempted to simplify the taxonomy by using it to address the major divisions involved in medical parasitology—specifically, intestinal and urogenital protozoa, blood and tissue protozoa, nematodes, trematodes, cestodes, and arthropods.

Importance of Parasites

Medical parasitology is the study of invertebrate animals capable of causing disease in humans and other animals. Although parasitic diseases are frequently considered "tropical" and thus of little importance to physicians practicing in the more temperate, developed countries of the world, it is clear that the world has become a very small place and that physicians' knowledge of parasitic diseases is essential. The global impact of parasitic infections and the number of parasite-associated deaths is staggering and must be of concern to all health care workers (Table 6-1). Increasingly tourists, missionaries, Peace Corps volunteers, and others are visiting and working for extended periods of time in exotic, remote parts of the world. Thus they are at risk for parasitic and other infections that are rare in the United States and other more developed countries. Another source of infected patients is the ever-increasing number of refugees from developing countries. Finally, the profound immunosuppression problems that accompany advances in medical therapy (e.g., organ transplantation), as well as those associated with persons infected with the human immunodeficiency virus (HIV), place a growing number of individuals at risk for developing infections caused by

certain parasites. Given these considerations, clinicians and laboratory workers should be aware of the possibility of parasitic disease and should be trained in ordering, performing, and interpreting the appropriate laboratory tests to aid in the diagnosis and therapy.

Classification and Structure

The parasites of humans are classified within the four eukaryotic kingdoms: Protozoa, Animalia (Metazoa), Fungi, and Chromista (Table 6-2). Traditionally parasite classification has taken into account the morphology of intracytoplasmic structures, such as the nucleus, the type of locomotive organelles, and the mode of reproduction (Table 6-3). More recently the new taxonomic consensus has emerged based mainly on advances in our understanding of the biochemistry and molecular biology of lower organisms (e.g., Protozoa, Fungi, and Chromista). Comparisons of small subunit ribosomal RNA (SSU rRNA) and protein sequences have made it possible to arrange organisms within groups based on evolutionary distances. Furthermore, the identification of certain organelles found in eukaryotic cells, with their prokaryote origins, has made it possible to organize all living organisms within a realistic and evolutionarily sound overall taxonomic scheme. The Protozoa and Chromista are animals whose life functions occur in a single cell. The microsporidians are also single-celled organisms and were previously classified among the protozoans; however, they are now thought to be more closely related to fungi than to protozoa and have been reclassified with the Fungi. Despite this reclassification, there has been reluctance among parasitologists to part with this group, whereas mycologists have been reluctant to accept it. Thus for historical, as well as established diagnostic, epidemiologic, and therapeutic reasons, we will retain discussion of microsporidians

Table 6—1. Estimated Worldwide Disease Burden of Parasitic Infections

Infection	Disease Burden in DALYs (thousands)*	Deaths (thousands)†
Malaria	42,280	1124
Lymphatic filariasis	5644	0
Leishmaniasis	2357	59
Hookworm	1825	—
Schistosomiasis	1760	15
Trichuriasis	1649	—
African trypanosomiasis	1598	50
Ascariasis	1181	—
Onchocerciasis	987	0
Chagas disease	649	13

Adapted from Edwards G, Krishna S: Pharmacokinetic and pharmacodynamic issues in the treatment of parasite infections. Eur J Clin Microbiol Infect Dis 23:233-242, 2004; and Hoetz PJ, et al: Control of neglected tropical diseases. N Engl J Med 357:1018-1027, 2007.
*DALYs, disability-adjusted life years (the number of healthy years of life lost due to premature death and disability).
†Mortality data included where available.

alongside the Protozoa with the understanding that they are most likely fungi. The members of the kingdom Animalia, also known as **metazoans**, are multicellular animals in which life functions occur in cellular structures organized as tissue and organ systems.

Protozoa

Protozoa are simple microorganisms that range in size from 2 to 100 μm. Their protoplasm is enclosed by a cell membrane and contains numerous organelles, including a membrane-bound nucleus, an endoplasmic reticulum, food-storage granules, and contractile and digestive vacuoles. The nucleus contains clumped or dispersed chromatin and a central karyosome. Organs of motility vary from simple cytoplasmic extrusions or pseudopods to more complex structures, such as flagella or cilia. The kingdom Protozoa comprises 13 major subgroups, or phyla, seven of which are the concern of medical parasitology.

The Flagellates: Metamonada, Parabasala, Percolozoa, and Euglenozoa

Previously grouped under the former subphylum Mastigophora, the flagellates are now distributed under four phyla, Metamonada, Parabasala, Percolozoa, and Euglenozoa. The flagellates move by the lashing of their whiplike flagella. The number and position of the flagella vary a great deal in different species. In addition, specialized structures associated with the flagella may produce a characteristic morphologic appearance that may be useful in species identification.

Table 6—2. Medically Important Parasites

Kingdom	Phylum	Organisms
Protozoa	Metamonada (flagellates)	*Giardia, Chilomastix*
	Parabasala (flagellates)	*Dientamoeba, Trichomonas*
	Percolozoa (flagellates)	*Naegleria*
	Euglenozoa (flagellates)	*Leishmania, Trypanosoma*
	Amoebozoa (amebae)	*Acanthamoeba, Balamuthia, Entamoeba*
	Sporozoa (sporozoans)	*Cryptosporidium, Cyclospora, Toxoplasma, Babesia, Plasmodium*
	Ciliophora (ciliates)	*Balantidium coli*
Chromista	Bigyra	*Blastocystis hominis*
Fungi	Microspora (microsporidians)	*Encephalitozoon, Enterocytozoon, Brachiola, Microsporidium, Nosema*
Animalia	Nemathelminthes (Nematoda, roundworms)	*Trichinella, Trichuris, Ancylostoma, Necator, Ascaris, Dracunculus filaria, Enterobius, Strongyloides*
	Platyhelminthes	Trematodes, Cestodes
	Arthropoda	Crustaceans, spiders, insects, true bugs

Table 6—3. Biologic, Morphologic, and Physiologic Characteristics of Pathogenic Parasites

Organism Class	Morphology	Reproduction	Organelles of Locomotion	Respiration	Nutrition
Protozoa					
Ameba	Unicellular; cyst and trophocyte forms	Binary fission	Pseudopods	Facultative anaerobe	Assimilation by pinocytosis or phagocytosis
Flagellates	Unicellular; cyst and trophozoite forms; possibly intracellular	Binary fission	Flagella	Facultative anaerobe	Simple diffusion or ingestion via cytostome, pinocytosis, or phagocytosis
Ciliates	Unicellular; cysts and trophozoite	Binary fission or conjugation	Cilia	Facultative anaerobe	Ingestion via cytostome, food vacuole
Sporozoa	Unicellular, frequently intracellular; multiple forms, including trophozoites, sporozoites, cysts (oocysts), gametes	Schizogony and sporogony	None	Facultative anaerobe	Simple diffusion
Fungi					
Microsporidia	Obligate intracellular forms; small, simple cells and spores	Binary fission, schizogony, and sporogony	None	Facultative anaerobe	Simple diffusion
Helminths					
Nematodes	Multicellular; round, smooth, spindle-shaped, tubular alimentary tract; possibility of teeth or plates for attachment	Separate sexes	No single organelle; active muscular motility	Adults: usually anaerobic; larvae: possibly aerobic	Ingestion or absorption of body fluids, tissue, or digestive contents
Trematodes	Multicellular; leaf-shaped with oral and ventral suckers, blind alimentary tract	Hermaphroditic (*Schistosoma* group has separate sexes)	No single organelle; muscle-directed motility	Adults: usually anaerobic	Ingestion or absorption of body fluids, tissue, or digestive contents
Cestodes	Multicellular; head with segmented body (proglottids); lack of alimentary tract; head equipped with hooks and/or suckers for attachment	Hermaphroditic	No single organelle; usually attachment to mucosa; possible muscular motility (proglottids)	Adults: usually anaerobic	Absorption of nutrients from intestine
Arthropods					
Myriapoda	Elongated; many legs; distinctive head and trunk; poison claws on first segment	Separate sexes	Legs	Aerobic	Carnivore
Pentastomida	Wormlike; cylindrical or flattened; two distinct body regions; digestive and reproductive organs; lack of circulatory and respiratory systems	Separate sexes	Muscle-directed motility	Aerobic	Ingestion of body fluids and tissue
Crustacea	Hard external carapace; one pair of maxillae; five pairs of biramous legs	Separate sexes	Legs	Aerobic	Ingestion of body fluids and tissue, carnivorous

Continued

Table 6—3. Biologic, Morphologic, and Physiologic Characteristics of Pathogenic Parasites—cont'd

Organism Class	Morphology	Reproduction	Organelles of Locomotion	Respiration	Nutrition
Chelicerata (Arachnida)	Body divided into cephalothorax and abdomen; eight legs and poisoning fangs	Separate sexes	Legs	Aerobic	Carnivore
Insecta	Body: head, thorax, and abdomen; one pair of antennae; three pairs of appendages, up to two pairs of wings	Separate sexes	Legs, wings	Aerobic	Ingestion of fluids and tissues

Amoebozoa

The phylum Amoebozoa, containing the amebae, is equivalent to the old subphylum Sarcodina. Locomotion of amebae is accomplished by the extrusion of pseudopodia ("false feet"). Amebae are phagocytic and contain mitochondria with tubular cristae.

Sporozoa

Phylum Sporozoa organisms are often referred to as **Apicomplexa** or **Coccidia**. The Sporozoa include a large group of sexually reproducing, spore-forming protozoans with comparable life cycles and similar morphology at the electron microscopic level. These organisms have a system of organelles at their apical end that produces substances to help the organism penetrate host cells and thus become an intracellular parasite.

Ciliophora

Phylum Ciliophora consists of the ciliates, which include a variety of free-living and symbiotic species. Ciliate locomotion involves the coordinated movement of rows of hairlike structures, or cilia. Cilia are structurally similar to flagella but are usually shorter and more numerous. Some ciliates are multinucleate. The only ciliate parasite of humans, *Balantidium coli*, contains two nuclei: a large macronucleus and a small micronucleus.

Chromista

The kingdom Chromista was created in 1989 to accommodate a number of plantlike organisms, mainly algae, that were originally chimeras between eukaryotic biflagellate hosts and symbiotic red algae that had lost their chloroplasts over evolutionary time, yet still retain elements of their red algae ancestry. Although previously shuffled between the Fungi and Protozoa, *Blastocystis hominis* is now placed within the Chromista (phylum Bigyra, class Blastocystea) based on analysis of 18S rRNA and other molecular evidence. *B. hominis* is the first chromist known to parasitize humans.

Fungi

Microspora (Microsporidians)

Previously classified with the Protozoa, Microsporidia are now considered to be degenerate fungi based on sequences of α- and β-tubulin and sequence trees for the molecular chaperone hsp70. Further evidence for the fungal nature of microsporidia includes spores with walls of chitin, a lack of Golgi stacks, and a mitotic mechanism that is indistinguishable from that of fungal ascomycetes. The Microspora are small intracellular parasites that lack both mitochondria and peroxisomes. They are further characterized by the structure of their spores, which have a complex tubular extrusion mechanism (polar tube) used to inject the infective material (sporoplasm) into host cells. The origin of the polar tube and the unique method of infection are considered both necessary and sufficient for the origin of intracellular parasitism.

Animalia (Metazoa)

The kingdom Animalia (Metazoa) includes all eukaryotic organisms that are not Protozoa, Chromista, or Fungi. This chapter discusses two broad groups of organisms of major importance: the helminths ("worms") and the arthropods (crabs, insects, ticks, and the like).

Helminths

The helminths are complex multicellular organisms that are elongated and bilaterally symmetrical. They are considerably larger than the protozoan parasites and generally are macroscopic, ranging in size from less than 1 mm to 1 m or larger. The external surface of some worms is covered with a protective cuticle, which is acellular and may be smooth or possess ridges, spines, or tubercles. The protective covering of flatworms is known as a **tegument**. Often helminths possess elaborate attachment structures such as hooks, suckers, teeth, or plates. These structures are usually located anteriorly and may be useful in classifying and identifying the organisms (see Table 6-3). Helminths typically have primitive nervous and excretory systems. Some have alimentary tracts; however, none have a circulatory system. The helminths are separated into two phyla, the Nemathelminthes and the Platyhelminthes.

NEMATHELMINTHES

Phylum Nemathelminthes consists of the roundworms, which have cylindrical bodies. The sexes of roundworms are separate, and these organisms have a complete digestive system. The Nemathelminths may be intestinal parasites or may infect the blood and tissue.

PLATYHELMINTHES

Phylum Platyhelminthes consists of the flatworms, which have flattened bodies that are leaflike or resemble ribbon segments. Platyhelminthes can be further divided into trematodes and cestodes.

Trematodes, or flukes, have leaf-shaped bodies. Most are hermaphroditic, with male and female sex organs in a single body. Their digestive systems are incomplete and only have saclike tubes. Their life cycle is complex; snails serve as first intermediate hosts, and other aquatic animals or plants serve as second intermediate hosts.

Cestodes, or tapeworms, have bodies composed of ribbons of proglottids, or segments. All are hermaphroditic, and all lack digestive systems, with nutrition being absorbed through the body walls. The life cycles of some cestodes are simple and direct, whereas those of others are complex and require one or more intermediate hosts.

Arthropods

Phylum Arthropoda is the largest group of animals in the kingdom Animalia. Arthropods are complex multicellular organisms that may be involved directly in causing invasive or superficial (infestation) disease processes or indirectly as intermediate hosts and vectors of many infectious agents, including protozoan and helminthic parasites (Table 6-4). In addition, envenomization by biting and stinging arthropods can result in adverse reactions in humans that range from local allergic and hypersensitivity reactions to severe anaphylactic shock and death. There are five major categories of arthropods.

MYRIAPODA

The Myriapoda (formerly Chilopoda) consist of terrestrial forms, such as centipedes. These organisms are of medical importance because of their poisoning claws, which may produce a painful "bite."

PENTASTOMIDA

The pentastomids, or tongue worms, are bloodsucking endoparasites of reptiles, birds, and mammals. Adult pentastomids are white and cylindrical or flattened parasites that possess two distinct body regions: an anterior cephalothorax and an abdomen. Humans may serve as intermediate hosts for these parasites.

CRUSTACEA

The crustaceans include familiar aquatic forms such as crabs, crayfish, shrimp, and copepods. Several are involved as intermediate hosts in life cycles of various intestinal or blood and tissue helminths.

CHELICERATA

The Chelicerata (formerly Arachnida) consists of familiar terrestrial forms, such as mites, ticks, spiders, and scorpions. Unlike insects, these animals have no wings or antennae, and adults have four pairs of legs, as opposed to three pairs for insects. Of medical importance are those serving as vectors for microbial diseases (mites and ticks) or as venomous animals that bite (spiders) or sting (scorpions).

INSECTA

Insecta consist of familiar aquatic and terrestrial forms, such as mosquitoes, flies, midges, fleas, lice bugs, wasps, and ants. Wings and antennae are present, and adult forms have three pairs of legs. Of medical importance are the many insects that serve as vectors for microbial diseases (mosquitoes, fleas, lice, and bugs) or as venomous animals that sting (bees, wasps, and ants).

Physiology and Replication

Protozoa

The nutritional requirements of the parasitic protozoa are generally simple and require the assimilation of organic nutrients. The amebae, ameboflagellates, and certain other protozoa accomplish this assimilation by the rather primitive process of pinocytosis or phagocytosis of soluble or particulate matter (see Table 6-3). The engulfed material is enclosed in digestive vacuoles. The flagellates and ciliates generally ingest food at a definitive site or structure, the peristome or cytostome. Other unicellular parasites, such as the intracellular microsporidia, assimilate nutrients by simple diffusion. The ingested food material may be retained in intracytoplasmic granules or in vacuoles. The undigested particles and waste may be eliminated from the cell by extrusion of the material at the cell surface. Respiration in most parasitic protozoa is accomplished by facultatively anaerobic processes.

To ensure survival under harsh or unfavorable environmental conditions, many parasitic protozoa develop into a cyst form that is less metabolically active. This cyst is surrounded by a thick external cell wall capable of protecting the organism from otherwise lethal physical and chemical insults. The cyst form is an integral part of the life cycle of many protozoan parasites and facilitates the transmission of the organism from host to host in the external environment (see Table 6-4). Parasites that cannot form cysts must rely on direct transmission from host to host or require an arthropod vector to complete their life cycles (see Table 6-4).

Table 6—4. Transmission and Distribution of Pathogenic Parasites

Organism	Infective Form	Mechanism of Spread	Distribution
Intestinal Protozoa			
Entamoeba histolytica	Cyst/trophozoite	Indirect (fecal-oral) Direct (venereal)	Worldwide
Giardia lamblia	Cyst	Fecal-oral route	Worldwide
Dientamoeba fragilis	Trophozoite	Fecal-oral route	Worldwide
Balantidium coli	Cyst	Fecal-oral route	Worldwide
Isospora belli	Oocyst	Fecal-oral route	Worldwide
Cryptosporidium species	Oocyst	Fecal-oral route	Worldwide
Enterocytozoon bieneusi	Spore	Fecal-oral route	North America, Europe
Urogenital Protozoa			
Trichomonas vaginalis	Trophozoite	Direct (venereal) route	Worldwide
Blood and Tissue Protozoa			
Naegleria and *Acanthamoeba* species	Cyst/trophozoite	Direct inoculation, inhalation	Worldwide
Plasmodium species	Sporozoite	*Anopheles* mosquito	Tropical and subtropical areas
Babesia species	Pyriform body	Ixodes tick	North America, Europe
Toxoplasma gondii	Oocysts and tissue cysts	Fecal-oral route, carnivorism	Worldwide
Leishmania species	Promastigote	Phlebotomus sandfly	Tropical and subtropical areas
Trypanosoma cruzi	Trypomastigote	Reduviid bug	North, Central, and South America
Trypanosoma brucei	Trypomastigote	Tsetse fly	Africa
Nematodes			
Enterobius vermicularis	Egg	Fecal-oral route	Worldwide
Ascaris lumbricoides	Egg	Fecal-oral route	Areas of poor sanitation
Toxocara species	Egg	Fecal-oral route	Worldwide
Trichuris trichiura	Egg	Fecal-oral route	Worldwide
Ancylostoma duodenale	Filariform lava	Direct skin penetration from contaminated soil	Tropical and subtropical areas
Necator americanus	Filariform larva	Direct skin penetration, autoinfection	Tropical and subtropical areas
Strongyloides stercoralis	Filariform larva	Direct skin penetration, autoinfection	Tropical and subtropical areas
Trichinella spiralis	Encysted larva in tissue	Carnivorism	Worldwide
Wuchereria bancrofti	Third-stage larva	Mosquito	Tropical and subtropical areas
Brugia malayi	Third-stage larva	Mosquito	Tropical and subtropical areas
Loa loa	Filariform larva	Chrysops fly	Africa
Mansonella species	Third-stage larva	Biting midges or black flies	Africa, Central and South America
Onchocerca volvulus	Third-stage larva	Simulium black fly	Africa, Central and South America

Table 6—4. Transmission and Distribution of Pathogenic Parasites—cont'd

Organism	Infective Form	Mechanism of Spread	Distribution
Dracunculus medinensis	Third-stage larva	Ingestion of infected Cyclops	Africa, Asia
Dirofilaria immitis	Third-stage larva	Mosquito	Japan, Australia, United States
Trematodes			
Fasciolopsis buski	Metacercaria	Ingestion of metacercaria encysted on aquatic plants	China, Southeast Asia, India
Fasciola hepatica	Metacercaria	Metacercaria on water plants	Worldwide
Opisthorchis (Clonorchis) sinensis	Metacercaria	Metacercaria encysted in freshwater fish	China, Japan, Korea, Vietnam
Paragonimus westermani	Metacercaria	Metacercaria encysted in freshwater crustaceans	Asia, Africa, India, Latin America
Schistosoma species	Cercaria	Direct penetration of skin by free-swimming cercaria	Africa, Asia, India, Latin America
Cestodes			
Taenia solium	Cysticercus, embryonated egg or proglottid	Ingestion of infected pork; ingestion of egg (cysticercosis)	Pork-eating countries: Africa, Southeast Asia, China, Latin America
Taenia saginata	Cysticercus	Ingestion of cysticercus in meat	Worldwide
Diphyllobothrium latum	Sparganum	Ingestion of sparganum in fish	Worldwide
Echinococcus granulosus	Embryonated egg	Ingestion of eggs from infected canines	Sheep-raising countries: Europe, Asia, Africa, Australia, United States
Echinococcus multilocularis	Embryonated egg	Ingestion of eggs from infected animals, fecal-oral route	Canada, Northern United States, Central Europe
Hymenolepsis nana	Embryonated egg	Ingestion of eggs, fecal-oral route	Worldwide
Hymenolepsis diminuta	Cysticercus	Ingestion of infected beetle larvae in contaminated grain products	Worldwide
Dipylidium caninum	Cysticercoid	Ingestion of infected fleas	Worldwide

In addition to cyst formation, many protozoan parasites have developed elaborate immunoevasive mechanisms that allow them to respond to attack by the host immune system by continuously changing their surface antigens, thus ensuring continued survival within the host. Reproduction among the protozoa is generally by simple binary fission (merogony), although the life cycle of some protozoa, such as the sporozoans, includes cycles of multiple fission (schizogony) alternating with a period of sexual reproduction (sporogony or gametogony).

Animalia (Metazoa)

Helminths

The nutritional requirements of helminthic parasites are met by active ingestion of host tissue, fluids, or both, with resultant tissue destruction, or by more passive absorption of nutrients from the surrounding fluids and intestinal contents (see Table 6-3). The muscular motility of many helminths expends considerable energy, and the worms rapidly metabolize carbohydrates. Nutrients are stored in the form of glycogen, the content of which is high in most helminths. Similar to respiration in protozoa, respiration in helminths is primarily anaerobic, although the larval forms may require oxygen.

A significant proportion of the energy requirement of helminths is dedicated to supporting the reproductive process. Many worms are quite prolific, producing as many as 200,000 offspring each day. In general, helminthic parasites are egg laying (oviparous), although a few species may bear live young (viviparous). The resulting larvae are always morphologically distinct from the adult parasites and must undergo several developmental stages or molts before attaining adulthood.

The major protective barrier for most helminths is the tough external layer (cuticle or tegument). Worms may also secrete enzymes that destroy host cells and neutralize immunological and cellular defense mechanisms. Similar to protozoan parasites, some helminths possess the ability to alter the antigenic properties of their external surfaces and thus evade the host immune response. This is accomplished in part by incorporating host antigens into their external cuticular layer. In this way the worm avoids immunological recognition, and in some diseases (e.g., schistosomiasis), it allows the parasite to survive within the host for decades.

Arthropods

Arthropods have segmented bodies, paired jointed appendages, and well-developed digestive and nervous systems. Sexes are separate. Respiration by aquatic forms is via gills and by terrestrial forms is via tubular body structures. All have a hard chitin covering as an exoskeleton.

Proper education regarding parasitic diseases in medical curricula cannot be overemphasized as a requirement for physicians whose practice includes travelers to foreign countries and refugee populations. Many of the important parasites responsible for human diseases are transmitted by arthropod vectors or are acquired by the consumption of contaminated food or water. The various modes of transmission and distribution of parasitic diseases are presented in appropriate detail in the following chapters; however, the data in Table 6-4 are provided as an outline.

Questions

1. How do protozoa adapt to harsh environmental conditions?
2. Which morphologic form is important in the transmission of protozoa from host to host?
3. How do helminths, such as schistosomes, avoid the host immune response?
4. How do arthropods cause human disease?

Summary

Physician awareness of parasitic diseases is undoubtedly more critical now than at any time in the history of medical practice. Physicians today must be prepared to answer questions from patients about protection from malaria and the risks of drinking water and eating fresh fruits and vegetables in remote areas where they may be traveling. With this knowledge of parasitic diseases, the physician can also evaluate signs, symptoms, and incubation periods in returning travelers, make a diagnosis, and begin treatment for a patient with a possible parasitic disease. The risks of parasitic diseases in immunosuppressed individuals and those with acquired immunodeficiency syndrome must also be understood and taken into account.

Bibliography

Cavalier-Smith T: A revised six-kingdom system of life. Biol Rev 73:203-266, 1998.
Cox FEG: History of human parasitology. Clin Microbiol Rev 15:595-612, 2002.
Cox FEG: Taxonomy and classification of human parasites. In Murray PR, et al (eds): Manual of Clinical Microbiology, 9th ed. Washington, DC, ASM Press, 2007.
Edwards G, Krishna S: Pharmacokinetic and pharmacodynamic issues in the treatment of parasite infections. Eur J Clin Microbiol Infect Dis 23:233-242, 2004.
Garcia LS: Diagnostic Medical Parasitology, 5th ed. Washington, DC, ASM Press, 2006.
Hoetz PJ, Molyneux DH, Fenwick A, et al: Control of neglected tropical diseases. N Engl J Med 357:1018-1027, 2007.
Markell EK, John DT, Krotoski WA: Markell and Voge's Medical Parasitology, 8th ed. Philadelphia, WB Saunders, 1999.
Murray PR, et al: Manual of Clinical Microbiology, 9th ed. Washington, DC, ASM Press, 2007.

Commensal and Pathogenic Microbial Flora in Humans

Medical microbiology is the study of the interactions between animals (primarily humans) and microorganisms, such as bacteria, viruses, fungi, and parasites. Although the primary interest is in diseases caused by these interactions, it must also be appreciated that microorganisms play a critical role in human survival. The normal commensal population of microbes participates in the metabolism of food products, provides essential growth factors, protects against infections with highly virulent microorganisms, and stimulates the immune response. In the absence of these organisms, life as we know it would be impossible.

The microbial flora in and on the human body is in a continual state of flux determined by a variety of factors, such as age, diet, hormonal state, health, and personal hygiene. Whereas the human fetus lives in a protected, sterile environment, the newborn human is exposed to microbes from the mother and the environment. The infant's skin is colonized first, followed by the oropharynx, gastrointestinal tract, and other mucosal surfaces. Throughout the life of a human being, this microbial population continues to change. Changes in health can drastically disrupt the delicate balance that is maintained among the heterogeneous organisms coexisting within us. For example, hospitalization can lead to the replacement of normally avirulent organisms in the oropharynx with gram-negative rods (e.g., *Klebsiella*, *Pseudomonas*) that can invade the lungs and cause pneumonia. Likewise, the indigenous bacteria present in the intestines restrict the growth of *Clostridium difficile* in the gastrointestinal tract. In the presence of antibiotics, however, this indigenous flora is eliminated, and *C. difficile* is able to proliferate and produce diarrheal disease and colitis.

Exposure of an individual to an organism can lead to one of three outcomes. The organism can: (1) transiently colonize the person, (2) permanently colonize the person, or (3) produce disease. It is important to understand the distinction between **colonization** and **disease**. (Note: many

people use the term *infection* inappropriately as a synonym for both terms.) Organisms that colonize humans (whether for a short period such as hours or days [transient] or permanently) do not interfere with normal body functions. In contrast, disease occurs when the interaction between microbe and human leads to a pathologic process characterized by damage to the human host. This process can result from microbial factors (e.g., damage to organs caused by the proliferation of the microbe or the production of toxins or cytotoxic enzymes) or the host's immune response to the organism (e.g., the pathology of severe acute respiratory syndrome [SARS] coronavirus infections is primarily caused by the patient's immune response to the virus).

An understanding of medical microbiology requires knowledge not only of the different classes of microbes but also of their propensity for causing disease. A few infections are caused by **strict pathogens** (i.e., organisms always associated with human disease). A few examples of strict pathogens and the diseases they cause include *Mycobacterium tuberculosis* (tuberculosis), *Neisseria gonorrhoeae* (gonorrhea), *Francisella tularensis* (tularemia), *Plasmodium* spp. (malaria), and rabies virus (rabies). Most human infections are caused by **opportunistic pathogens**, organisms that are typically members of the patient's normal microbial flora (e.g., *Staphylococcus aureus*, *Escherichia coli*, *Candida albicans*). These organisms do not produce disease in their normal setting but establish disease when they are introduced into unprotected sites (e.g., blood, tissues). The specific factors responsible for the virulence of strict and opportunistic pathogens are discussed in later chapters. If a patient's immune system is defective, that patient is more susceptible to disease caused by opportunistic pathogens.

The microbial population that colonizes the human body is numerous and diverse. Our knowledge of the composition of this population is currently based on comprehensive culture methods; however, it is estimated that only a small proportion of the microbes can be cultivated. To better understand the microbial population, a large-scale project has been initiated to characterize comprehensively the human microbiota and analyze its role in human health and disease. The skin and all mucosal surfaces of the human body will be systematically analyzed by genomic techniques. Because the project (**Human Microbiome Project, HMP**) will be initiated in 2008, the results of this work are not available at the time this chapter is written. However, I would refer you to the HMP website for the most current information: http://nihroadmap.nih.gov/hmp/. Thus, the information discussed in this chapter will be based on data collected from systematic cultures, with the understanding that much of what we currently know may be very different from what we will learn in the next 5 years.

Respiratory Tract and Head

Mouth, Oropharynx, and Nasopharynx

The upper respiratory tract is colonized with numerous organisms, with 10 to 100 anaerobes for every aerobic bacterium (Box 7-1). The most common anaerobic bacteria are *Peptostreptococcus* and related anaerobic cocci, *Veillonella*, *Actinomyces*, and *Fusobacterium* spp. The most common aerobic bacteria are *Streptococcus*, *Haemophilus*, and *Neisseria* spp. The relative proportion of these organisms varies at different anatomic sites; for example, the

microbial flora on the surface of a tooth is quite different from the flora in saliva or in the subgingival spaces. Most of the common organisms in the upper respiratory tract are relatively avirulent and are rarely associated with disease unless they are introduced into normally sterile sites (e.g., sinuses, middle ear, and brain). Potentially pathogenic organisms, including *Streptococcus pyogenes*, *Streptococcus pneumoniae*, *S. aureus*, *Neisseria meningitidis*, *Haemophilus influenzae*, *Moraxella catarrhalis*, and Enterobacteriaceae, can also be found in the upper airways. Isolation of these organisms from an upper respiratory tract specimen does not define their pathogenicity (remember the concept of colonization vs. disease). Their involvement with a disease process must be demonstrated by the exclusion of other pathogens. For example, with the exception of *Streptococcus pyogenes*, these organisms are rarely responsible for pharyngitis, even though they can be isolated from patients with this disease. *S. pneumoniae*, *S. aureus*, *H. influenzae*, and *M. catarrhalis* are organisms commonly associated with infections of the sinuses.

Ear

The most common organism colonizing the outer ear is coagulase-negative *Staphylococcus*. Other organisms colonizing the skin have been isolated from this site, as well as potential pathogens such as *S. pneumoniae*, *Pseudomonas aeruginosa*, and members of the Enterobacteriaceae family.

Eye

The surface of the eye is colonized with coagulase-negative staphylococci, as well as rare numbers of organisms found in the nasopharynx (e.g., *Haemophilus* spp., *Neisseria* spp., viridans streptococci). Disease is typically associated with *S. pneumoniae*, *S. aureus*, *H. influenzae*, *N. gonorrhoeae*, *Chlamydia trachomatis*, *P. aeruginosa*, and *Bacillus cereus*.

Lower Respiratory Tract

The larynx, trachea, bronchioles, and lower airways are generally sterile, although transient colonization with secretions of the upper respiratory tract may occur. More virulent bacteria present in the mouth (e.g., *S. pneumoniae*, *S. aureus*, members of the family Enterobacteriaceae such as *Klebsiella*) cause acute disease of the lower airway. Chronic aspiration may lead to a polymicrobial disease in which anaerobes are the predominant pathogens, particularly *Peptostreptococcus*, related anaerobic cocci, and anaerobic gram-negative rods. Fungi such as *Candida albicans* are a rare cause of disease in the lower airway, and invasion of these organisms into tissue must be demonstrated to exclude simple colonization. In contrast, the presence of the dimorphic fungi (e.g., *Histoplasma*,

---

Box 7—1. Most Common Microbes That Colonize the Upper Respiratory Tract

Bacteria

Acinetobacter	Mycoplasma
Actinobacillus	Neisseria
Actinomyces	Peptostreptococcus
Cardiobacterium	Porphyromonas
Corynebacterium	Prevotella
Eikenella	Propionibacterium
Enterobacteriaceae	Staphylococcus
Eubacterium	Streptococcus
Fusobacterium	Stomatococcus
Haemophilus	Treponema
Kingella	Veillonella
Moraxella	

Fungi

Candida

Parasites

Entamoeba	Trichomonas

Box 7–2. Most Common Microbes That Colonize the Gastrointestinal Tract

Bacteria

Acinetobacter	Helicobacter
Actinomyces	Lactobacillus
Bacteroides	Mobiluncus
Bifidobacterium	Peptostreptococcus
Campylobacter	Porphyromonas
Clostridium	Prevotella
Corynebacterium	Propionibacterium
Eubacterium	Pseudomonas
Enterobacteriaceae	Staphylococcus
Enterococcus	Streptococcus
Fusobacterium	Veillonella
Haemophilus	

Fungi

Candida

Parasites

Blastocystis	Entamoeba
Chilomastix	Iodamoeba
Endolimax	Trichomonas

Coccidioides, and *Blastomyces* spp.) is diagnostic because asymptomatic colonization with these organisms never occurs.

Gastrointestinal Tract

The gastrointestinal tract is colonized with microbes at birth and remains the home for a diverse population of organisms throughout the life of the host (Box 7-2). Although the opportunity for colonization with new organisms occurs daily with the ingestion of food and water, the population remains relatively constant, unless exogenous factors such as antibiotic treatment disrupt the balanced flora.

Esophagus

Oropharyngeal bacteria and yeast, as well as the bacteria that colonize the stomach, can be isolated from the esophagus; however, most organisms are believed to be transient colonizers that do not establish permanent residence. Bacteria rarely cause disease of the esophagus (esophagitis); *Candida* spp. and viruses such as herpes simplex virus and cytomegalovirus cause most infections.

Stomach

Because the stomach contains hydrochloric acid and pepsinogen (secreted by the parietal and chief cells lining the gastric mucosa), the only organisms present are small numbers of acid-tolerant bacteria, such as the lactic acid–producing bacteria (*Lactobacillus* and *Streptococcus* spp.) and *Helicobacter pylori*. *H. pylori* is a cause of gastritis and ulcerative disease. The microbial population can dramatically change in numbers and diversity in patients receiving drugs that neutralize or reduce the production of gastric acids.

Small Intestine

In contrast with the anterior portion of the digestive tract, the small intestine is colonized with many different bacteria, fungi, and parasites. Most of these organisms are anaerobes, such as *Peptostreptococcus*, *Porphyromonas*, and *Prevotella*. Common causes of gastroenteritis (e.g., *Salmonella* and *Campylobacter* spp.) can be present in small numbers as asymptomatic residents; however, their detection in the clinical laboratory generally indicates disease. If the small intestine is obstructed, such as after abdominal surgery, then a condition called **blind loop syndrome** can occur. In this case, stasis of the intestinal contents leads to the colonization and proliferation of the organisms typically present in the large intestine, with a subsequent malabsorption syndrome.

Large Intestine

More microbes are present in the large intestine than anywhere else in the human body. It is estimated that more than 10^{11} bacteria per gram of feces can be found, with anaerobic bacteria in excess by more than 1000-fold. Various yeasts and nonpathogenic parasites can also establish residence in the large intestine. The most common bacteria include *Bifidobacterium*, *Eubacterium*, *Bacteroides*, *Enterococcus*, and the Enterobacteriaceae. *E. coli* is present in virtually all humans from birth until death. Although this organism represents less than 1% of the intestinal population, it is the most common aerobic organism responsible for intraabdominal disease. Likewise, *Bacteroides fragilis* is a minor member of the intestinal flora, but it is the most common anaerobe responsible for intraabdominal disease. In contrast, *Eubacterium* and *Bifidobacterium* are the most common bacteria in the large intestine but are rarely responsible for disease. These organisms simply lack the diverse virulence factors found in *B. fragilis*.

Antibiotic treatment can rapidly alter the population, causing the proliferation of antibiotic-resistant organisms, such as *Enterococcus*, *Pseudomonas*, and fungi. *C. difficile* can also grow rapidly in this situation, leading to diseases ranging from diarrhea to pseudomembranous colitis. Exposure to other enteric pathogens, such as *Shigella*, enterohemorrhagic *E. coli*, and *Entamoeba histolytica*, can also disrupt the colonic flora and produce significant intestinal disease.

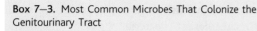

Box 7–3. Most Common Microbes That Colonize the Genitourinary Tract

Bacteria

Actinomyces	*Lactobacillus*
Bacteroides	*Mobiluncus*
Bifidobacterium	*Mycoplasma*
Clostridium	*Peptostreptococcus*
Corynebacterium	*Porphyromonas*
Enterococcus	*Prevotella*
Enterobacteriaceae	*Propionibacterium*
Eubacterium	*Staphylococcus*
Fusobacterium	*Streptococcus*
Gardnerella	*Treponema*
Haemophilus	*Ureaplasma*

Fungi

Candida

Genitourinary System

In general the anterior urethra and vagina are the only anatomic areas of the genitourinary system permanently colonized with microbes (Box 7-3). Although the urinary bladder can be transiently colonized with bacteria migrating upstream from the urethra, these should be cleared rapidly by the bactericidal activity of the uroepithelial cells and the flushing action of voided urine. The other structures of the urinary system should be sterile, except when disease or an anatomic abnormality is present. Likewise the uterus should also remain free of organisms.

Anterior Urethra

The commensal population of the urethra consists of a variety of organisms, with lactobacilli, streptococci, and coagulase-negative staphylococci the most numerous. These organisms are relatively avirulent and are rarely associated with human disease. In contrast, the urethra can be colonized transiently with fecal organisms such as *Enterococcus*, Enterobacteriaceae, and *Candida*—all of which can invade the urinary tract, multiply in urine, and lead to significant disease. Pathogens such as *N. gonorrhoeae* and *C. trachomatis* are common causes of urethritis and can persist as asymptomatic colonizers of the urethra. The isolation of these two organisms in clinical specimens should always be considered significant, regardless of the presence or absence of clinical symptoms.

Vagina

The microbial population of the vagina is more diverse and is dramatically influenced by hormonal factors. Newborn girls are colonized with lactobacilli at birth, and these bacteria predominate for approximately 6 weeks. After that time, the levels of maternal estrogen have declined, and the vaginal flora changes to include staphylococci, streptococci, and Enterobacteriaceae. When estrogen production is initiated at puberty, the microbial flora again changes. Lactobacilli reemerge as the predominant organisms, and many other organisms are also isolated, including staphylococci (*S. aureus* less commonly than the coagulase-negative species), streptococci (including group B *Streptococcus*), *Enterococcus*, *Gardnerella*, *Mycoplasma*, *Ureaplasma*, Enterobacteriaceae, and a variety of anaerobic bacteria. *N. gonorrhoeae* is a common cause of vaginitis. In the absence of this organism, significant numbers of cases develop when the balance of vaginal bacteria is disrupted, resulting in decreases in the number of lactobacilli and increases in the number of *Mobiluncus* and *Gardnerella*. *Trichomonas vaginalis*, *C. albicans*, and *Candida glabrata* are also important causes of vaginitis. Although herpes simplex virus and papillomavirus would not be considered normal flora of the genitourinary tract, these viruses can establish persistent infections.

Cervix

Although the cervix is not normally colonized with bacteria, *N. gonorrhoeae* and *C. trachomatis* are important causes of cervicitis. *Actinomyces* can also produce disease at this site.

Skin

Although many organisms come into contact with the skin surface, this relatively hostile environment does not support the survival of most organisms (Box 7-4). Gram-positive bacteria (e.g., coagulase-negative *Staphylococcus* and less commonly *S. aureus*, corynebacteria, and propionibacteria) are the most common organisms found on the skin surface. *Clostridium perfringens* is isolated on the skin of approximately 20% of healthy individuals, and the fungi *Candida* and *Malassezia* are also found on skin surfaces, particularly in moist sites. Streptococci can colonize the skin transiently,

Box 7–4. Most Common Microbes That Colonize the Skin

Bacteria

Acinetobacter	*Micrococcus*
Aerococcus	*Peptostreptococcus*
Bacillus	*Propionibacterium*
Clostridium	*Staphylococcus*
Corynebacterium	*Streptococcus*

Fungi

Candida	*Malassezia*

but the volatile fatty acids produced by the anaerobe propionibacteria are toxic for these organisms. Gram-negative rods do not permanently colonize the skin surface (with the exception of *Acinetobacter* and a few other less common genera), because the skin is too dry.

Questions

1. What is the distinction between *colonization* and *disease*?
2. Give examples of strict pathogens and opportunistic pathogens.
3. What factors regulate the microbial populations of organisms that colonize humans?

Bibliography

Balows A, Truper H: The Prokaryotes, 2nd ed. New York, Springer-Verlag, 1992.

Murray P: Human microbiota. In Balows A, et al: Topley and Wilson's Microbiology and Microbial Infections, 10th ed. London, Edward Arnold, 2005.

Murray P, Shea Y: Pocket Guide to Clinical Microbiology, 3rd ed. Washington, DC, ASM Press, 2004.

Sterilization, Disinfection, and Antisepsis

An important aspect of the control of infections is an understanding of the principles of sterilization, disinfection, and antisepsis (Box 8-1).

Sterilization

Sterilization is the total destruction of all microbes, including the more resilient forms such as bacterial spores, mycobacteria, nonenveloped (nonlipid) viruses, and fungi. This can be accomplished using physical, gas vapor, or chemical sterilants (Table 8-1).

Physical sterilants such as **moist** and **dry heat** are the most common sterilizing methods used in hospitals and are indicated for most materials, except those that are heat sensitive or consist of toxic or volatile chemicals. **Filtration** is useful for removing bacteria and fungi from air (with high-efficiency particulate air [HEPA] filters) or from solutions. However, these filters are unable to remove viruses and some small bacteria. Sterilization by **ultraviolet** or **ionizing radiation** (e.g., microwave or gamma rays) is also commonly used. The limitation of ultraviolet radiation is that direct exposure is required.

Ethylene oxide is the most commonly used **gas vapor sterilant**. Although it is highly efficient, strict regulations limit its use because ethylene oxide is flammable, explosive, and carcinogenic to lab animals. Sterilization with **formaldehyde gas** is also limited because the chemical is carcinogenic. Its use is restricted primarily to sterilization of HEPA filters. **Hydrogen peroxide** vapors are effective sterilants because of the oxidizing nature of the gas. This sterilant is used for the sterilization of instruments. A variation is **plasma gas sterilization**, in which hydrogen peroxide is vaporized, and then reactive free radicals are produced with either microwave-frequency or radiofrequency energy. Because this is an efficient sterilizing method that does not produce toxic byproducts, it is anticipated that plasma gas sterilization will replace many of the applications for ethylene oxide. However, it cannot be used with materials that absorb hydrogen peroxide or react with it.

Two **chemical sterilants** have also been used: **peracetic acid** and **glutaraldehyde**. Peracetic acid, an oxidizing agent, has excellent activity, and the end products (i.e., acetic acid and oxygen) are nontoxic. In contrast, safety is a concern with glutaraldehyde, and care must be used when handling this chemical.

Disinfection

Microbes are also destroyed by disinfection procedures, although more resilient organisms can survive. Unfortunately the terms **disinfection** and **sterilization** are casually interchanged, which can result in some confusion. This occurs because disinfection processes have been categorized as high level, intermediate level, and low level. High-level disinfection can generally approach sterilization in effectiveness, whereas spore forms can survive intermediate-level disinfection, and many microbes can remain viable when exposed to low-level disinfection.

Even the classification of disinfectants (Table 8-2) by their level of activity is misleading. The effectiveness of these procedures is influenced by the nature of the item to be disinfected, number and resilience of the contaminating organisms, amount of organic material present (which can inactivate the disinfectant), type and concentration of disinfectant, and duration and temperature of exposure.

High-level disinfectants are used for items involved with invasive procedures that cannot withstand sterilization procedures (e.g., certain types of endoscopes, surgical instruments with plastic or other components that cannot be autoclaved). Disinfection of these and other items is most effective if cleaning the surface to remove organic matter precedes treatment. Examples of high-level disinfectants include treatment with moist heat and use of liquids such as glutaraldehyde, hydrogen peroxide, peracetic acid, and chlorine compounds.

Table 8–2. Methods of Disinfection

Method	Concentration (Level of Activity)
Heat	
Moist heat	75° C to 100° C for 30 min (high)
Liquid	
Glutaraldehyde	2%-3.5% (high)
Hydrogen peroxide	3%-25% (high)
Formaldehyde	3%-8% (high/intermediate)
Chlorine dioxide	Variable (high)
Peracetic acid	Variable (high)
Chlorine compounds	100-1000 ppm of free chlorine (high)
Alcohol (ethyl, isopropyl)	70%-95% (intermediate)
Phenolic compounds	0.4%-5.0% (intermediate/low)
Iodophor compounds	30-50 ppm of free iodine/L (intermediate)
Quaternary ammonium compounds	0.4%-1.6% (low)

Table 8–3. Antiseptic Agents

Antiseptic Agent	Concentration
Alcohol (ethyl, isopropyl)	70%-90%
Iodophors	1-2 mg of free iodine/L; 1%-2% available iodine
Chlorhexidine	0.5%-4.0%
Parachlorometaxylenol	0.50%-3.75%
Triclosan	0.3%-2.0%

preparations are frequently used with alcohols for disinfecting the skin surface. **Chlorhexidine** has broad antimicrobial activity, although it kills organisms at a much slower rate than alcohol. Its activity persists, although organic material and high pH levels decrease its effectiveness. The activity of **parachlorometaxylenol** (PCMX) is limited primarily to gram-positive bacteria. Because it is nontoxic and has residual activity, it has been used in handwashing products. **Triclosan** is active against bacteria but not against many other organisms. It is a common antiseptic agent in deodorant soaps and some toothpaste products.

Mechanisms of Action

The following section briefly reviews the mechanisms by which the most common sterilants, disinfectants, and antiseptics work.

Moist Heat

Attempts to sterilize items using boiling water are inefficient because only a relatively low temperature (100° C) can be maintained. Indeed, spore formation by a bacterium is commonly demonstrated by boiling a solution of organisms and then subculturing the solution. Boiling vegetative organisms kills them, but the spores remain viable. If organisms grow on the subculture plate, the bacteria are capable of sporulating. In contrast, steam under pressure in

an autoclave is a very effective form of sterilization; the higher temperature causes denaturation of microbial proteins. The rate of killing organisms during the autoclave process is rapid but is influenced by the temperature and duration of autoclaving, size of the autoclave, flow rate of the steam, density and size of the load, and placement of the load in the chamber. Care must be taken to avoid creating air pockets, which inhibit penetration of the steam into the load. In general, most autoclaves are operated at 121° C to 132° C for 15 minutes or longer. Including commercial preparations of *Bacillus stearothermophilus* spores can help monitor the effectiveness of sterilization. An ampule of these spores is placed in the center of the load, removed at the end of the autoclave process, and incubated at 37° C. If the sterilization process is successful, the organisms fail to sporulate and do not grow.

Ethylene Oxide

Ethylene oxide is a colorless gas, soluble in water and common organic solvents, that is used to sterilize heat-sensitive items. The sterilization process is relatively slow and is influenced by the concentration of gas, relative humidity and moisture content of the item to be sterilized, exposure time, and temperature. The exposure time is reduced by 50% for each doubling of ethylene oxide concentration. Likewise the activity of ethylene oxide approximately doubles with each temperature increase of 10° C. Sterilization with ethylene oxide is optimal in a relative humidity of approximately 30%, with decreased activity at higher or lower humidity. This is particularly problematic if the contaminated organisms are dried onto a surface or lyophilized. Ethylene oxide exerts its sporicidal activity through the alkylation of terminal hydroxyl, carboxyl, amino, and sulfhydryl groups. This process blocks the reactive groups required for many essential metabolic processes. Examples of other strong alkylating gases used as sterilants are formaldehyde and β-propiolactone. Because ethylene oxide can damage viable tissues, the gas must be dissipated before the item can be used. This aeration period is generally 16 hours or longer. The effectiveness of sterilization is monitored with the *B. subtilis* spore test.

Table 8—4. Germicidal Properties of Disinfectants and Antiseptic Agents

Agents	Bacteria	Mycobacteria	Bacterial Spores	Fungi	Viruses
Disinfectants					
Alcohol	+	+	−	+	+/−
Hydrogen peroxide	+	+	+/−	+	+
Formaldehyde	+	+	+	+	+
Phenolics	+	+	−	+	+/−
Chlorine	+	+	+/−	+	+
Iodophors	+	+/−	−	+	+
Glutaraldehyde	+	+	+	+	+
Quaternary ammonium compounds	+/−	−	−	+/−	+/−
Antiseptic Agents					
Alcohol	+	+	−	+	+
Iodophors	+	+	−	+	+
Chlorhexidine	+	+	−	+	+
Parachlorometaxylenol	+/−	+/−	−	+	+/−
Triclosan	+	+/−	−	+/−	+

Aldehydes

As with ethylene oxide, aldehydes exert their effect through alkylation. The two best-known aldehydes are **formaldehyde** and **glutaraldehyde**, both of which can be used as sterilants or high-level disinfectants. Formaldehyde gas can be dissolved in water (creating a solution called **formalin**) at a final concentration of 37%. Stabilizers such as methanol are added to formalin. Low concentrations of formalin are bacteriostatic (i.e., they inhibit but do not kill organisms), whereas higher concentrations (e.g., 20%) can kill all organisms. Combining formaldehyde with alcohol (e.g., 20% formalin in 70% alcohol) can enhance this microbicidal activity. Exposure of skin or mucous membranes to formaldehyde can be toxic. Glutaraldehyde is less toxic for viable tissues, but it can still cause burns on the skin or mucous membranes. Glutaraldehyde is more active at alkaline pH levels ("activated" by sodium hydroxide) but is less stable. Glutaraldehyde is also inactivated by organic material, so items to be treated must first be cleaned.

Oxidizing Agents

Examples of oxidants include ozone, peracetic acid, and hydrogen peroxide, the last used most commonly. **Hydrogen peroxide** effectively kills most bacteria at a concentration of 3% to 6% and kills all organisms, including spores, at higher concentrations (10% to 25%). The active oxidant form is not hydrogen peroxide but rather the free hydroxyl radical formed by the decomposition of hydrogen peroxide. Hydrogen peroxide is used to disinfect plastic implants, contact lenses, and surgical prostheses.

Halogens

Halogens, such as compounds containing iodine or chlorine, are used extensively as disinfectants. **Iodine compounds** are the most effective halogens available for disinfection. Iodine is a highly reactive element that precipitates proteins and oxidizes essential enzymes. It is microbicidal against virtually all organisms, including spore-forming bacteria and mycobacteria. Neither the concentration nor the pH of the iodine solution affects the microbicidal activity, although the efficiency of iodine solutions is increased in acid solutions because more free iodine is liberated. Iodine acts more rapidly than do other halogen compounds or quaternary ammonium compounds. However, the activity of iodine can be reduced in the presence of some organic and inorganic compounds, including serum, feces, ascitic fluid, sputum, urine, sodium thiosulfate, and ammonia. Elemental iodine can be dissolved in aqueous potassium iodide or alcohol, or it can be complexed with a carrier. The latter compound is referred to as an *iodophor* (*iodo*, "iodine"; *phor*, "carrier"). Povidone iodine (iodine complexed with polyvinylpyrrolidone) is used most commonly and is relatively stable and nontoxic to tissues and metal surfaces, but it is expensive compared with other iodine solutions.

Chlorine compounds are also used extensively as disinfectants. Aqueous solutions of chlorine are rapidly bactericidal, although their mechanisms of action are not defined. Three forms of chlorine may be present in water: elemental chlorine (Cl_2), which is a very strong oxidizing agent; hypochlorous acid (HOCl); and hypochlorite ion (OCl_2). Chlorine also combines with ammonia and other nitrogenous compounds to form chloramines, or *N*-chloro compounds. Chlorine can exert its effect by the irreversible oxidation of sulfhydryl (SH) groups of essential enzymes. Hypochlorites are believed to interact with cytoplasmic components to form toxic *N*-chloro compounds, which interfere with cellular metabolism. The efficacy of chlorine is inversely proportional to the pH, with greater activity observed at acid pH levels. This is consistent with greater activity associated with hypochlorous acid rather than with hypochlorite ion concentration. The activity of chlorine compounds also increases with concentration (e.g., a twofold increase in concentration results in a 30% decrease in time required for killing) and temperature (e.g., a 50% to 65% reduction in killing time with a $10°$ C increase in temperature). Organic matter and alkaline detergents can reduce the effectiveness of chlorine compounds. These compounds demonstrate good germicidal activity, although spore-forming organisms are tenfold to 1000-fold more resistant to chlorine than are vegetative bacteria.

Phenolic Compounds

Phenolic compounds (germicides) are rarely used as disinfectants. However, they are of historical interest because they were used as a comparative standard for assessing the activity of other germicidal compounds. The ratio of germicidal activity by a test compound to that by a specified concentration of phenol yielded the phenol coefficient. A value of 1 indicated equivalent activity, greater than 1 indicated activity less than phenol, and less than 1 indicated activity greater than phenol. These tests are limited because phenol is not sporicidal at room temperature (but is sporicidal at temperatures approaching $100°$ C) and has poor activity against non-lipid-containing viruses. This is understandable, because phenol is believed to act by disrupting lipid-containing membranes, resulting in leakage of cellular contents. Phenolic compounds are active against the normally resilient mycobacteria because the cell wall of these organisms has a very high concentration of lipids. Exposure of phenolics to alkaline compounds significantly reduces their activity, whereas halogenation of the phenolics enhances their activity. The introduction of aliphatic or aromatic groups into the nucleus of halogen phenols also increases their activity. Bisphenols are two phenol compounds linked together. The activity of these compounds can also be potentiated by halogenation. One example of a halogenated bisphenol is **hexachlorophene**, an antiseptic with activity against gram-positive bacteria.

Quaternary Ammonium Compounds

Quaternary ammonium compounds consist of four organic groups covalently linked to nitrogen. The germicidal activity of these cationic compounds is determined by the nature of the organic groups, with the greatest activity observed with compounds with 8- to 18-carbon–long groups. Examples of quaternary ammonium compounds include **benzalkonium chloride** and **cetylpyridinium chloride**. These compounds act by denaturing cell membranes to release the intracellular components. Quaternary ammonium compounds are bacteriostatic at low concentrations and bactericidal at high concentrations. However, organisms such as *Pseudomonas, Mycobacterium*, and the fungus *Trichophyton*, among others, are resistant to these compounds. Indeed, some *Pseudomonas* strains can grow readily in quaternary ammonium solutions. Many viruses and all bacterial spores are also resistant. Ionic detergents, organic matter, and dilution neutralize quaternary ammonium compounds.

Alcohols

The germicidal activity of alcohols increases with increasing chain length (maximum of five to eight carbons). The two most commonly used alcohols are **ethanol** and **isopropanol**. These alcohols are rapidly bactericidal against vegetative bacteria, mycobacteria, some fungi, and lipid-containing viruses. Unfortunately alcohols have no activity against bacterial spores and have poor activity against some fungi and non-lipid-containing viruses. Activity is greater in the presence of water. Thus 70% alcohol is more active than is 95% alcohol. Alcohol is a common disinfectant for skin surfaces and is extremely effective for this purpose when followed by treatment with an iodophor. Alcohols are also used to disinfect items such as thermometers.

Questions

1. Define the following terms and give three examples of each: *sterilization, disinfection*, and *antisepsis*.
2. Define the three levels of disinfection, and give examples of each. When would each type of disinfectant be used?
3. What factors influence the effectiveness of sterilization with moist heat, dry heat, and ethylene oxide?
4. Give examples of each of the following disinfectants and their mode of action: iodine compounds, chlorine compounds, phenolic compounds, and quaternary ammonium compounds.

Bibliography

Block SS: Disinfection, Sterilization, and Preservation, 2nd ed. Philadelphia, Lea and Febiger, 1977.
Brody TM, Larner J, Minneman KP: Human Pharmacology: Molecular to Clinical, 3rd ed. St Louis, Mosby, 1998.
Widmer A, Frei R: Decontamination, disinfection, and sterilization. In Murray P, et al (eds): Manual of Clinical Microbiology, 9th ed. Washington, DC, ASM Press, 2007.

Basic Concepts in the Immune Response

Elements of Host Protective Responses

We live in a microbial world, and our bodies are constantly being exposed to bacteria, fungi, parasites, and viruses. Our bodies' defenses to this onslaught are similar to a military defense. The initial defense mechanisms are **barriers**, such as the skin, acid and bile of the gastrointestinal tract, and mucus that inactivate and prevent entry of the foreign agents. If these barriers are compromised or the agent gains entry in another way, the local militia of **innate responses** (e.g., complement, interferon, cytokines, natural killer cells, neutrophils, macrophages) must quickly rally to the challenge and prevent expansion of the invasion. Once activated, these responses send an alarm (complement, cytokines, and chemokines) and open the vasculature (complement) to provide access to the site. Finally, if these steps are not effective, the innate responses activate a major campaign specifically directed against the invader by **antigen-specific immune responses** (B cells, antibody and T cells) at whatever cost (immunopathogenesis). Similarly, knowledge of the characteristics (antigens) of the enemy through immunization enables the body to mount a faster, more effective response (activation of memory B and T cells) on rechallenge.

The different elements of the immune system interact and communicate using soluble molecules and by direct cell-to-cell interaction. These interactions provide the mechanisms for activation and control of the protective responses. Unfortunately the protective responses to some infectious agents are insufficient; in other cases, the response to the challenge is excessive. In either case, disease occurs.

Soluble Activators and Stimulators of Immune Function

Innate and immune cells communicate by interactions of specific cell surface receptors and with soluble molecules, including cytokines, interferons, and chemokines. **Cytokines** are proteins that are produced by specific lymphoid and other cell types to stimulate and regulate other cells to activate and regulate the immune response (Table 9-1 and Box 9-1).

Interferons are proteins produced in response to viral and other infections (interferon-α and interferon-β) or on activation of the immune response (interferon-γ); they promote antiviral and antitumor responses and stimulate immune responses (see Chapter 12). **Chemokines** are small proteins (approximately 8000 Da) that are associated with inflammatory responses. Neutrophils, basophils, monocytes, and T cells express receptors and can be activated by specific chemokines. The chemokines and other proteins (e.g., the C3a and C5a products of the complement cascade) are chemotactic factors that establish a chemical path to attract phagocytic and inflammatory cells to the site of infection. The triggers that stimulate the production of these molecules and the consequences of the interactions with their receptors on specific cells determine the nature of the innate and immune response.

Cells of the Immune Response

Immune responses are mediated by specific cells with defined functions. The characteristics of the most important cells of the immune system and their appearances are presented in Figure 9-1 and in Tables 9-2 and 9-3.

The white blood cells can be distinguished on the basis of (1) morphology, (2) histologic staining, (3) immunologic functions, and (4) intracellular and cell surface markers. Monoclonal antibodies are used to distinguish subsets of the different types of cells according to their cell surface markers. These markers have been defined within clusters of differentiation, and the markers indicated by **"CD"** (cluster of differentiation) numbers (Table 9-4). In addition, **all nucleated cells express class I MHC (MHC I) antigens** (HLA-A, HLA-B, HLA-C).

A special class of cells that are **antigen-presenting cells (APCs)** express class II major histocompatibility complex (MHC) antigens (HLA-DR, HLA-DP, HLA-DQ). APCs include dendritic cells, macrophage family cells, B lymphocytes, and a limited number of other cell types.

Table 9–1. Cytokines and Chemokines

Factor	Source	Major Target	Function
Innate and Acute Phase Responses			
Interferon-α, interferon-β	Leukocytes, fibroblasts, and other cells	Virally infected cells, tumor cells, NK cells	Induction of antiviral state; activation of NK cells, enhancement of cell-mediated immunity
IL-1α, IL-1β	Macrophage, fibroblasts, epithelial cells, endothelial cells	T cells, B cells, PMN, tissue, central nervous system, liver, etc.	Many actions: promotion of inflammatory and acute phase responses, fever, activation of T cells and macrophages
TNF-α (cachectin)	Similar to IL-1	Macrophages, T cells, NK cells	Similar to IL-1, antitumor and wasting (cachexia, weight loss) functions, sepsis, endothelial activation
IL-6	DCs, Macrophages, T and B cells, fibroblasts, epithelial cells, endothelial cells	T and B cells, hepatocytes	Stimulation of acute-phase and inflammatory responses, fever, Ig secretion, T and B cell growth and development
IL-12, IL-23	DC, macrophage	NK cells, CD4 TH1 cells	Activation of T cell mediated and inflammatory responses, IFN-gamma production
Growth and Differentiation			
Colony-stimulating factors (e.g., GM-CSF)	T cells, stromal cells	Stem cells	Growth and differentiation of specific cell types, hematopoiesis
IL-3	CD4 T cells, keratinocytes	Stem cells	Hematopoiesis
IL-7	Bone marrow, stroma	Precursor cells and stem cells	Growth of pre-B cell, thymocyte, T cell, and cytotoxic lymphocyte
TH1 and TH17 Responses			
IL-2	CD4 T cells (TH0, TH1)	T cells, B cells, NK cells	T and B cell growth, NK activation
Interferon-γ	CD4 TH1 cells, NK cells	Macrophages,* T cells, B cells	Activation of macrophage, promotion of IgG class switch, inflammation and TH1 but inhibition of TH2 responses
TNF-β	T cells	PMN, tumors	Lymphotoxin: tumor killing, activation of PMN, endothelial activation
IL-17	T cells (TH17)	Epithelial, endothelial, and fibroblast cells	Activate tissue to promote inflammation, even in the presence of TGF-beta.
TH2 Responses			
IL-4	CD4 (TH0, TH2), T cells	B and T cells	T and B cell growth; IgG, IgA, IgE production; TH2 responses
IL-5	CD4 TH2 cells	B cells, eosinophils	B cell growth and differentiation, IgG, IgA, and IgE production, eosinophil production, allergic responses
IL-7	Bone marrow, stroma	Precursor cells and stem cells	Growth of pre-B cell, thymocyte, T cell, and cytotoxic lymphocyte
IL-10	CD4 TH2 cells	B cells, CD4 TH1 cells	B cell growth, inhibition of TH1 response
Regulatory Response			
TGF-β	CD4 Treg cells	B cells, T cells, macrophages	Immunosuppression of B, T, NK cells and macrophages; promotion of oral tolerance, wound healing, IgA production

Table 9—1. Cytokines and Chemokines—cont'd

Factor	Source	Major Target	Function
Chemokines			
α-chemokines: C-X- C chemokines—two cysteines separated by one amino acid (IL-8; IP-10; GRO-α, GRO-β, GRO-γ)	Many cells	Neutrophils, T cells, macrophages	Chemotaxis, activation
β-chemokines: C-C chemokines—two adjacent cysteines (MCP-1; MIP-α; MIP-β; RANTES)	Many cells	T cells, macrophages, basophils	Chemotaxis, activation

GM-CSF, Granulocyte-macrophage colony-stimulating factor; GRO, growth-related oncogene; Ig, immunoglobulin; IL, interleukin; IP, interferon-α protein; MCP, monocyte chemoattractant protein; MIP, macrophage inflammatory protein; NK, natural killer; PMN, polymorphonuclear leukocyte; RANTES, regulated on activation, normal T expressed and secreted; TNF, tumor necrosis factor.
*Applies to one or more cells of the monocyte-macrophage lineage.

Hematopoietic Cell Differentiation

Differentiation of a common progenitor cell, termed the **pluripotent stem cell**, gives rise to all blood cells. Differentiation of these cells begins during development of the fetus and continues throughout life. The pluripotent stem cell differentiates into stem cells (sometimes referred to as colony-forming units) for different lineages of blood cells, including the lymphoid (T and B cells), myeloid, erythrocytic, and megakaryoblastic (source of platelets) lineages (see Fig. 9-1). The stem cells reside primarily in the bone marrow, but can also be isolated from the fetal blood in umbilical cords and as rare cells in adult blood. Differentiation of stem cells into the functional blood cells is triggered by specific cell surface interactions with the stromal cells of the marrow and specific cytokines produced by these and other cells. The **thymus and the "bursal equivalent" in the Peyer patches promote development of T cells and B cells, respectively.** Specific cytokines that promote hematopoietic cell growth and terminal differentiation are released by helper T cells, dendritic cells, macrophages, and other cells in response to infections and on activation.

The bone marrow and thymus are considered **primary lymphoid organs** (Figure 9-2). These sites of initial lymphocyte differentiation are essential to the development of the immune system. **Secondary lymphoid organs** include the **lymph nodes, spleen,** and **mucosa-associated lymphoid tissue (MALT)**, the latter also includes gut-associated lymphoid tissue (GALT) (e.g., Peyer patches) and bronchus-associated lymphoid tissue (BALT) (e.g., tonsils, appendix). These sites are where dendritic cells and B and T lymphocytes reside and respond to antigenic challenges. Proliferation of the lymphocytes in response to infectious challenge causes these tissues to swell (i.e., "swollen glands"). The cells of the primary and secondary lymphoid organs express cell surface adhesion molecules (**addressins**) that interact with homing receptors (**cell adhesion molecules**) expressed on B and T cells.

The spleen and lymph nodes are encapsulated organs in which the macrophages and B and T cells reside in defined regions. Their location facilitates interactions that promote immune responses to antigen (Figure 9-3). The **lymph nodes** are kidney-shaped organs 2 to 10 mm in diameter that filter the fluid that passes from intercellular spaces into the lymphatic system, almost like a sewage processing plant. The lymph node is constructed to optimize the meeting of the innate (dendritic cells and macrophages) and the immune response (B and T) cells to initiate and expand specific immune responses. A lymph node consists of the following three layers:

1. The cortex, the outer layer that contains mainly B cells, follicular dendritic cells, and macrophages arranged in clusters called *follicles*.

Box 9—1. Major Cytokine-Producing Cells

Innate (Acute Phase Responses)

Dendritic cells and macrophages: IL-1, TNF-α, TNF-β, IL-6, IL-12, IL-18, IL-23, GM-CSF, chemokines, interferons α, β

Immune: T cells (CD4 and CD8)

TH1 cells: IL-2, IL-3, GM-CSF, interferon-γ, TNF-α, TNF-β
TH2 cells: IL-4, IL-5, IL-6, IL-10, IL-3, IL-9, IL-13, GM-CSF, TNF-α TH17 cells: IL-17
Treg cells: TGF-beta and IL-10
GM-CSF, granulocyte-macrophage colony-stimulating factor; IL, interleukin; TNF, tumor necrosis factor

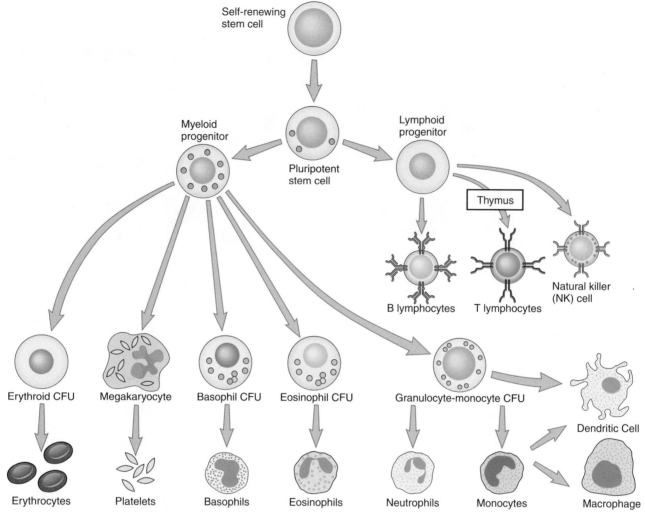

Figure 9–1. Morphology and lineage of cells involved in the immune response. Pluripotent stem cells and colony-forming units (CFU) are long-lived cells capable of replenishing the more differentiated functional and terminally differentiated cells. *(From Abbas K, et al: Cellular and Molecular Immunology, 5th ed. Philadelphia, WB Saunders, 2003.)*

2. The paracortex, which contains dendritic cells that bring antigens from the tissues to be presented to the T cells to initiate immune responses.
3. The medulla, which contains B and T cells and antibody-producing plasma cells.

The **spleen** is a large organ that acts like a lymph node and also filters antigens, encapsulated bacteria, and viruses from blood and removes aged blood cells and platelets (Figure 9-4). The spleen consists of two types of tissue, the white pulp and the red pulp. The white pulp consists of arterioles surrounded by lymphoid cells (periarteriolar lymphoid sheath), in which the T cells surround the central arteriole. B cells are organized into primary unstimulated or secondary stimulated follicles that have a germinal center. The germinal center contains memory cells, macrophages, and follicular dendritic cells. The red pulp is a storage site for blood cells and the site of turnover of aged platelets and erythrocytes.

MALT contains less structured aggregates of lymphoid cells (Figure 9-5). For example, the **Peyer patches** along the intestinal wall have special cells in the epithelium (M cells) that deliver antigens to the lymphocytes contained in defined regions (T [interfollicular] and B [germinal]). Once thought to be expendable, the **tonsils** are an important part of the MALT. These lymphoepithelial organs sample the microbes in the oral and nasal area. The tonsils contain a large number of mature and memory B cells (50% to 90% of the lymphocytes) that use their antibodies to sense specific pathogens and, with dendritic cells and T cells, can initiate immune responses. Swelling of the tonsils may be caused by infection or a response to infection.

Polymorphonuclear Leukocytes

Polymorphonuclear leukocytes (neutrophils) are short-lived cells that constitute 50% to 70% of circulating white

Table 9—2. Cells of the Immune Response

Cells	Characteristics and Functions
Natural Cytolytic Cells	
Natural killer cells	Large, granular lymphocytes Markers: Fc receptors for antibody Kill antibody-decorated cells and virus-infected or tumor cell (no MHC restriction)
Phagocytic Cells	
Neutrophils	Granulocytes with short life span, multilobed nucleus and granules, segmented band forms (more immature) **Phagocytose** and **kill bacteria** (polymorphonuclear leukocytes)
Eosinophils	Bilobed nucleus, heavily granulated cytoplasm Marker: staining with eosin Involved in parasite defense and allergic response
Antigen-Presenting Cells (APCs)	Marker: Class II MHC—expressing cells Present antigen to CD4 T cells
Monocytes*	Found in lymphocytes, blood, lungs, and other organs Horseshoe-shaped nucleus, lysosomes, granules *Precursors to macrophage-lineage and dendritic cells*, cytokine release
Immature dendritic cells	Blood and tissue Cytokine response to infection, process antigen
Dendritic cells*	Lymph nodes, tissue Most efficient antigen presenters, determines nature of T cell response
Langerhans cells*	Presence in skin Transport antigen to lymph nodes
Macrophages*	Possible residence in tissue, spleen, lymph nodes, and other organs; activated by IFN-γ and TNF Markers: large, granular cells; Fc and C3 receptors Initiate inflammatory and acute phase response; activated cells are antibacterial and have antiviral and antitumor activities
Microglial cells*	Presence in CNS and brain Produce cytokines
Kupffer cells*	Presence in liver Filter particles from blood (e.g., viruses)
Antigen-Responsive Cells	
T cells (all)	Mature in thymus; large nucleus, small cytoplasm Markers: CD2, CD3, T cell receptor (TCR)
αβTCR CD4 T cells	Helper/DTH cells; **activation** by APCs through **class II MHC antigen presentation** Produce IL-2, other cytokines; stimulate T and B cell growth; promote B-cell differentiation (class switching, antibody production) **TH1 subtype** (IL-2, IFN-γ, LT production): promote initial defenses (local), DTH, T killer cells, and antibody **TH2 subtype** (IL-4, IL-5, IL-6, IL-10 production): promote later humoral responses **TH17 subtype** (IL-17, TNF-α, IL-6): stimulate inflammation in presence of TGFβ **T regulator (Treg) cells** (TGFβ): control CD4 and CD8 T cell activation, important for immunotolerance
αβTCR CD8 T-killer cells	**Recognition** of antigen presented by **class I MHC antigens** Kill viral, tumor, nonself (transplant) cells; secrete TH1 cytokines
αβTCR CD8 T cells (suppressor cells)	**Recognition** of antigen presented by **class I MHC antigens** Suppress T- and B-cell response
γδ TCR T cells	CD2, CD3, γδ T-cell receptor Marker: early sensor of some bacterial infections in tissue and blood

Continued

Table 9–2. Cells of the Immune Response—cont'd

Cells	Characteristics and Functions
NKT cells	Express NK cell receptors Rapid response to infection, cytokine release
Antibody-Producing Cells	
B cells	Mature in bone marrow, bursal equivalent, Peyer patches Large nucleus, small cytoplasm; activation by antigens and T-cell factors Markers: surface antibody, **class II MHC antigens** Produce antibody and present antigen
Plasma cells	Small nucleus, large cytoplasm Terminally differentiated, antibody factories
Other Cells	
Basophils/mast cells	Granulocytic Marker: Fc receptors for IgE Release histamine, provide allergic response, are antiparasitic

APCs, antigen-presenting cells; CNS, central nervous system; DTH, delayed-type hypersensitivity; IFN, interferon; Ig, immunoglobulin; IL, interleukin; LT, lymphotoxin; MHC, major histocompatibility complex; TNF, tumor necrosis factor.
*Monocyte/macrophage lineage.

blood cells (see Figure 9-1) and are a primary **phagocytic defense** against bacterial infection and major component of the **inflammatory response. Neutrophils** are 9 to 14 μm in diameter, lack mitochondria, have a granulated cytoplasm in which granules stain with both acidic and basic stains, and have a multilobed nucleus. Neutrophils leave the blood and concentrate at the site of infection in response to chemotactic factors. During infection, the neutrophils in the blood increase in number and include precursor forms. These precursors are termed **band forms**, in contrast to the terminally differentiated and **segmented neutrophils**. The finding of such an increase and change in neutrophils by a blood count is sometimes termed *a left shift with an increase in bands versus segs*. Neutrophils ingest bacteria by phagocytosis and expose the bacteria to antibacterial substances and enzymes contained in **primary (azurophilic)** and **secondary (specific) granules**. Azurophilic granules are reservoirs for enzymes such as myeloperoxidase, β-glucuronidase, elastase, and cathepsin G. Specific granules serve as reservoirs for lysozyme and lactoferrin. Dead neutrophils are the major component of pus.

Eosinophils are heavily granulated cells (11 to 15 μm in diameter) with a bilobed nucleus that stain with the acid dye eosin Y. They are also phagocytic, motile, and granulated. The granules contain acid phosphatase, peroxidase, and eosinophilic basic proteins. Eosinophils play a role in the defense against **parasitic infections**. The eosinophilic basic proteins are toxic to many parasites. **Basophils**, another type of granulocyte, are not phagocytic but release the contents of their granules during allergic responses (type 1 hypersensitivity).

Table 9–3. Normal Blood Cell Counts

	Mean Number per Microliter	Normal Range
White blood cells (leukocytes)	7400	4500-11,000
Neutrophils	4400	1800-7700
Eosinophils	200	0-450
Basophils	40	0-200
Lymphocytes	2500	1000-4800
Monocytes	300	0-800

From Abbas AK, Lichtman AH, Pober JS: Cellular and Molecular Immunology, 4th ed. Philadelphia, WB Saunders, 2000.

Mononuclear Phagocyte System

The **mononuclear phagocyte system** are myeloid cells and consist of monocytes (see Fig. 9-1) in the blood and cells derived from **monocytes**. Different cytokines or tissue environments promote myeloid stem cells and monocytes to differentiate into the various macrophages and dendritic cells. These cells include *macrophages, alveolar macrophages in the lungs, Kupffer cells in the liver, intraglomerular mesangial cells in the kidney,*

Table 9—4. Selected CD Markers of Importance

CD Markers	Identity and Function	Cell
CD1	MHC I-like, nonpeptide antigen presentation	DC, macrophage
CD2 (LFA-3R)	Erythrocyte receptor	T
CD3	TCR subunit (γ, δ, ϵ, ζ, η); activation	T
CD4	Class II MHC receptor	T-cell subset, monocytes, some DCs
CD8	Class I MHC receptor	T-cell subset, some DCs
CD11b (CR3)	C3b complement receptor 3 (α chain)	NK, myeloid cells
CD14	LPS-binding protein receptor	Myeloid cells (monocytes, macrophages)
CD16 (Fc-γ RIII)	Phagocytosis and ADCC	NK cell marker, macrophages, neutrophils
CD21 (CR2)	C3d complement receptor, EBV receptor, B cell activation	B cells
CD25	IL-2 receptor (α chain), early activation marker, marker for regulatory cells	Activated T cells, regulatory T cells
CD28	Receptor for B-7 co-stimulation: activation	T cells*
CD40	Stimulation of B cell, DC, and macrophage	B cell, macrophage
CD40 L	Ligand for CD40	T cell
CD45RO	Isoform (on memory cells)	T cell, B cell
CD56 (NKH1)	Adhesion molecule	NK cell
CD69	Marker of cell activation	Activated T, B, NK cells and macrophages
CD80 (B7-1)	Co-stimulation of T cells on APCs	DC, macrophages, B cell
CD86(B7-2)	Co-stimulation of T cells on APCs	DC, macrophages, B cell
CD95(Fas)	Apoptosis inducer	Many cells
CD152 (CTLA-4)	Receptor for B-7; tolerance	T cell
CD178 (FasL)	Fas Ligand: apoptosis inducer	Killer T and NK cells
Adhesion Molecules		
CD11a	LFA-1 (α chain)	
CD29	VLA (β chain)	
VLA-1, VLA-2, VLA-3	α integrins	T cells
VLA-4	α_4 integrin homing receptor	T cell, B cell, monocyte
CD50	ICAM-3	Lymphocytes and leukocytes
CD54	ICAM-1	
CD58	LFA-3	

ADCC, antibody-dependent cellular cytotoxicity; APCs, antigen-presenting cells; CTLA, cytotoxic T-lymphocyte—associated protein; EBV, Epstein Barr virus; ICAM, intercellular adhesion molecule; Ig, immunoglobulin; IL, interleukin; LCA, leukocyte common antigen; LFA, leukocyte function—associated antigen; LPS, lipopolysaccharide; MHC, major histocompatibility complex; TAC, T-cell activation complex; TCR, T-cell antigen receptor; VLA, very late activation (antigen).
*Activated cells only.
Modified from Male D, et al: Advanced Immunology, 3rd ed. St Louis, Mosby, 1996.

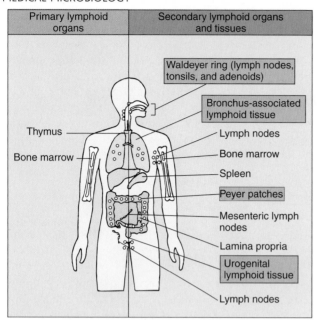

Figure 9—2. Organs of the immune system. Thymus and bone marrow are primary lymphoid organs. They are sites of maturation for T and B cells, respectively. Cellular and humoral immune responses develop in the secondary (peripheral) lymphoid organs and tissues; effector and memory cells are generated in these organs. The spleen responds predominantly to blood-borne antigens. Lymph nodes mount immune responses to antigens in intercellular fluid and in the lymph, absorbed either through the skin (superficial nodes) or from internal viscera (deep nodes). Tonsils, Peyer patches, and other mucosa-associated lymphoid tissues (blue boxes) respond to antigens that have penetrated the surface mucosal barriers. *(From Roitt I, et al: Immunology, 4th ed. St Louis, Mosby, 1996.)*

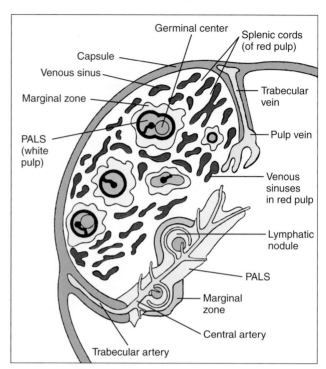

Figure 9—4. Organization of lymphoid tissue in the spleen. The white pulp contains germinal centers and is surrounded by the marginal zone, which contains numerous macrophages, antigen-presenting cells, slowly recirculating B cells, and natural killer cells. The red pulp contains venous sinuses separated by splenic cords. Blood enters the tissues via the trabecular arteries, which give rise to the many-branched central arteries. Some end in the white pulp, supplying the germinal centers and mantle zones, but most empty into or near the marginal zones. PALS, periarteriolar lymphoid sheath. *(From Roitt I, et al: Immunology, 4th ed. St Louis, Mosby, 1996.)*

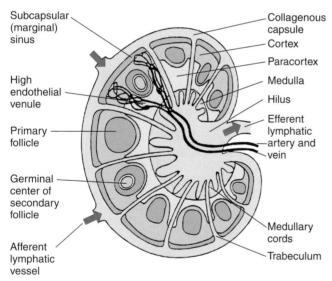

Figure 9—3. Organization of the lymph node. Beneath the collagenous capsule is the subcapsular sinus, which is lined with phagocytic cells. Lymphocytes and antigens from surrounding tissue spaces or adjacent nodes pass into the sinus via the afferent lymphatic system. The cortex contains B cells grouped in primary follicles and stimulated B cells in secondary follicles (germinal centers). The paracortex contains mainly T cells and dendritic cells (antigen-presenting cells). Each lymph node has its own arterial and venous supplies. Lymphocytes enter the node from the circulation through the specialized high endothelial venules in the paracortex. The medulla contains both T and B cells, as well as most of the lymph node plasma cells organized into cords of lymphoid tissue. Lymphocytes can leave the node only through the efferent lymphatic vessel. *(From Roitt I, et al: Immunology, 4th ed. St Louis, Mosby, 1996.)*

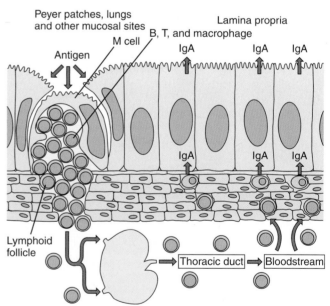

Figure 9—5. Lymphoid cells stimulated with antigen in Peyer patches (or the lungs or another mucosal site) migrate via the regional lymph nodes and thoracic duct into the bloodstream, then to the lamina propria of the gut and probably other mucosal surfaces. Thus lymphocytes stimulated at one mucosal surface may become distributed throughout the MALT (mucosa-associated lymphoid tissue) system. IgA, immunoglobulin A. *(From Roitt I, et al: Immunology, 4th ed. St Louis, Mosby, 1996.)*

histiocytes in connective tissue, osteoclasts, synovial cells, and microglial cells in the brain. Alveolar and serosal (e.g., peritoneal) macrophages are examples of "wandering" macrophages. Brain microglia are cells that enter the brain around the time of birth and differentiate into fixed cells. Some dendritic cells are myeloid cells and may be derived from monocytes. These mature forms have different morphologies corresponding to their ultimate tissue location and function and may express a subset of macrophage activities or cell surface markers.

Monocytes are 10 to 18 μm in diameter, with a single-lobed, kidney bean–shaped nucleus. They represent 3% to 8% of peripheral blood leukocytes. Monocytes follow neutrophils as an early cellular component of inflammation.

Macrophages are long-lived cells that are phagocytic, contain lysosomes, and unlike neutrophils, have mitochondria. Macrophages have the following basic functions: (1) phagocytosis, (2) antigen presentation to T cells to initiate specific immune responses, and (3) secretion of cytokines to activate and promote innate and immune responses (Figure 9-6). Macrophages express cell surface receptors for the Fc portion of immunoglobulin (Ig) G (Fc-γ RI, Fc-γ RII, Fc-γ RIII) and for the C3b product of the complement cascade (CR1, CR3). These receptors facilitate the phagocytosis of antigen, bacteria, or viruses coated with these proteins. Toll-like and other pattern-recognition receptors recognize pathogen-associated molecular patterns and activate protective responses.

Macrophages also express the class II MHC antigen, which allows these cells to present antigen to CD4 helper T cells to expand the immune response. Macrophages secrete interleukin-1, interleukin-6, tumor necrosis factor, interleukin-12, and other molecules upon sensing bacteria, which stimulates immune and inflammatory responses, including fever. A T-cell–derived lymphokine, interferon-γ, activates macrophages. Activated macrophages have enhanced phagocytic, killing, and antigen-presenting capabilities.

Dendritic Cells

Dendritic cells (DCs) of myeloid and lymphoid origins have octopus-like tendrils and are professional APCs that can also produce cytokines. Different types of immature and mature dendritic cells are found in tissue and blood; they include Langerhans cells in the skin, dermal interstitial cells, splenic marginal dendritic cells, and dendritic cells in the liver, thymus, germinal centers of the lymph nodes, and blood. Plasmacytoid dendritic cells are present in blood and produce large amounts of interferon alpha and cytokines in response to viral and other infections. Follicular dendritic cells present in lymph nodes and spleen are not hematopoietic in origin but have tendrils and a "sticky" surface to concentrate and present antigens to B cells. Immature DCs capture and phagocytose antigen efficiently, release cytokines to activate and steer the subsequent immune response, and then

Figure 9—6. Macrophage surface structures mediate cell function. Receptors for bacterial components, antibody, and complement (for opsonization) promote activation and phagocytosis of antigen; other receptors promote antigen presentation and activation of T cells. The dendritic cell shares many of these characteristics. *MHC*, major histocompatibility antigen I or II; *LFA*, leukocyte function associated antigen; *ICAM*, intercellular adhesion molecule; *LPS*, lipopolysaccharide; *Ig*, immunoglobulin; *TNF*, tumor necrosis factor.

mature into dendritic cells. These cells move to lymph node regions rich in T cells to present antigen on class I and class II MHC antigens. Dendritic cells are the only antigen-presenting cell that can initiate an immune response with a naïve T lymphocyte and also determine the type of response (TH1, TH2, Treg).

Lymphocytes

The lymphocytes are 6 to 10 μm in diameter, which is smaller than leukocytes. The two major classes of lymphocytes, **B cells** and **T cells**, have a large nucleus and smaller, agranular cytoplasm. Although B and T cells are indistinguishable by their morphologic features, they can be distinguished on the basis of function and surface markers (Table 9-5). Lymphoid cells that are not B or T cells (non-B/non-T cells, or null cells) are large, granular lymphocytes (LGLs), also known as **natural killer (NK) cells**.

The primary function of **B cells** is to **make antibody**, but they also internalize antigen, process the antigen, and present the antigen to T cells to expand the immune response. B cells can be identified by the presence of immunoglobulins, class II MHC molecules, and receptors for the C3b and C3d products of the complement cascade (CR1, CR2) on their cell surfaces (Figure 9-7). The B-cell name is derived from its site of differentiation in birds, the *b*ursa of Fabricius and the *b*one marrow of mammals. B-cell differentiation also takes place in the fetal liver and fetal spleen. Activated B cells either develop into **memory cells**, which express the CD45RO cell surface marker and circulate until activated by specific antigen, or terminally differentiate into plasma cells. **Plasma cells** have small nuclei and a large cytoplasm for their job as producers of antibody.

T cells acquired their name because they develop in the *t*hymus. T cells have the following two major functions in response to foreign antigen:

1. Control, suppress (when necessary), and activate immune and inflammatory responses by cell-cell interactions and by releasing cytokines.
2. Directly kill virally infected cells, foreign cells (e.g., tissue grafts), and tumors.

T cells make up 60% to 80% of peripheral blood lymphocytes.

Table 9—5. Comparison of B and T Cells

Property	T Cells	B Cells
Origin	Bone marrow	Bone marrow
Maturation	Thymus	Bursal equivalent: bone marrow, Peyer patches
Functions	Helper: cytokine production for initiation and promotion of immune response DTH: promotion and amplification of inflammatory response CTL: class I MHC—restricted cytolysis NKT: rapid response to infection Treg: control and suppress T cell and other responses	**Antibody production** Antigen presentation to T cells
Protective response	Resolution of intracellular and fungal infections	Antibody protects against rechallenge, block spread of agent in blood, opsonize, etc.
Products*	Cytokines, interferon-γ, growth factors, cytolytic substances (perforin, granzymes)	IgM, IgD, IgG, IgA, or IgE
Distinguishing surface markers	CD2 (sheep red blood cell receptor), TCR, CD3, CD4, or CD8	Surface antibody, complement receptors, class II MHC antigens
Subsets	CD4 TH0: helper precursor CD4 TH1: activates B, T, and NK cell growth, activates macrophages, CTLs and DTH responses, and IgG production CD4 TH2: activates B and T cell growth, IgG, IgE, and IgA production CD4 TH17: inflammation CD4 CD25 Treg: suppression CD8: cytotoxic T cells (CTL) CD8: suppressor cells NKT: rapid response to infection Memory cells: long-lived, anamnestic response	B cells: antibody, antigen presentation Plasma cell: terminally differentiated antibody factories Memory cells: long-lived, anamnestic response

CTL, Cytotoxic lymphocyte; DTH, delayed-type hypersensitivity; Ig, immunoglobulin; MHC, major histocompatibility complex; TCR, T-cell receptor.
*Depending on subset.

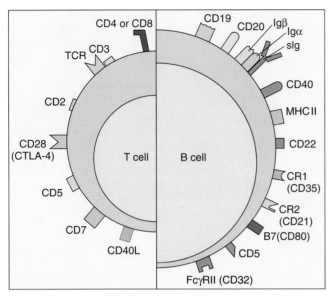

Figure 9–7. Surface markers of human B and T cells.

T cells were initially distinguished from B cells on the basis of their ability to bind and surround themselves (forming rosettes) with sheep erythrocytes through the CD2 molecule. All T cells express an antigen-binding **T-cell receptor (TCR)**, which resembles but differs from antibody, and **CD2**- and **CD3**-associated proteins on their cell surface (see Figure 9-7). T cells are divided into three major groups on the basis of the type of TCR and the cell surface expression of two proteins, CD4 and CD8. Most lymphocytes express the $\alpha\beta$ TCR. **CD4-expressing T cells** are primarily cytokine-producing cells which help initiate and mature immune responses, activate macrophages to induce delayed-type hypersensitivity responses (DTH), and a subset of these cells suppress responses. The CD4 T cells can be further divided into TH0, TH1, TH2, TH17, and Treg subgroups according to the spectrum of cytokines they secrete and the type of immune response that they promote. TH1 cells promote local, antibody and cellular inflammatory, and DTH responses, whereas TH2 cells promote antibody production. TH17 cells activate neutrophil responses and Treg cells promote T-cell tolerance. The **CD8 T cells** also release cytokines but are better known for their ability to recognize and kill virally infected cells, foreign tissue transplants (nonself-grafts), and tumor cells as cytotoxic killer T cells. CD8 T cells are also responsible for suppressing immune responses. T cells also produce **memory cells** that express CD45RO. Terminally differentiated effector CD4 and CD8 T cells express the class II MHC antigen. A variable number of T cells express the $\gamma\delta$ TCR but do not express CD4 or CD8. These cells

generally reside in skin and mucosa and are important for innate immunity. **NKT** cells are T cells, which share characteristics with NK cells.

The **large, granular lymphocyte NK cells** resemble the CD8 T cells in cytolytic function toward virally infected and tumor cells, but they differ in the mechanism for identifying the target cell. NK cells also have Fc receptors, which are used in antibody-dependent killing and hence are also called **antibody-dependent cellular cytotoxicity (ADCC or K) cells**. The cytoplasmic granules contain cytolytic proteins to mediate the killing.

Questions

A professor was teaching an introductory course and described the different immune cells with the following nicknames. Explain why the nicknames are appropriate or why they are not.

1. Macrophage: Pac-Man (a computer game character who normally eats dots but eats bad guys when activated)
2. Lymph node: police department
3. CD4 T cell: desk sergeant/dispatch officer
4. CD8 T cell: "cop on the beat"/patrol officer
5. B cell: product design and building company
6. Plasma cell: factory
7. Mast cell: activatable chemical warfare unit
8. Neutrophil: trash collector and disinfector
9. Dendritic cell: billboard display

Bibliography

Abbas AK, et al: Cellular and Molecular Immunology, 6th ed. Philadelphia, WB Saunders, 2007.

DeFranco AL, Locksley RM, Robertson M: Immunity: The Immune Response in Infectious and Inflammatory Disease. Sunderland, Mass, Sinauer Associates, 2007.

Janeway CA, et al: Immunobiology: The Immune System in Health and Disease, 6th ed. New York, Current Biology and Garland, 2004.

Kindt TJ, Goldsby RA, Osborne BA: Kuby Immunology, 6th ed. New York, WH Freeman, 2007.

Kumar V, Abbas AK, Fausto N: Robbins and Cotran Pathologic Basis of Disease, 7th ed. Philadelphia, Elsevier, 2005.

Rosenthal KS, Wilkinson JG: Flow cytometry and immunospeak. Infect Dis Clin Pract 15:183-191, 2007.

Rosenthal KS: Vaccines make good immune theater: Immunization as described in a three-act play. Infect Dis Clin Pract 14:35-45, 2006.

Rosenthal KS: Are microbial symptoms "self-inflicted"?: The consequences of immunopathology. Infect Dis Clin Pract 13:306-310, 2005.

Sompayrac L: How the Immune System Works, 2nd ed. Malden, Mass, Blackwell Scientific, 2003.

Trends in Immunology: Issues contain understandable reviews on current topics in immunology.

Humoral Immune Responses

The primary molecular component of the humoral immune response is antibody. B cells and plasma cells synthesize antibody molecules in response to challenge by antigen. Antibodies provide protection from rechallenge by an infectious agent, block spread of the agent in the blood, and facilitate elimination of the infectious agent. To accomplish these tasks, an incredibly large repertoire of antibody molecules must be available to recognize the tremendous number of infectious agents and molecules that challenge our bodies. In addition to interacting specifically with foreign structures, the antibody molecules must interact with host systems and cells (e.g., complement, macrophages) to promote clearance of antigen and activation of subsequent immune responses (Box 10-1). Antibody molecules also serve as the cell surface receptors that stimulate the appropriate B cell antibody factories to grow and produce more antibody in response to antigenic challenge.

Immunogens, Antigens, and Epitopes

Almost all of the proteins and carbohydrates associated with an infectious agent, whether a bacterium, fungus, virus, or parasite, are considered foreign to the human host and have the potential to induce an immune response. A protein or carbohydrate that challenges the immune system and can initiate an immune response is called an **immunogen** (Box 10-2). Immunogens may contain more than one antigen (e.g., bacteria). An **antigen** is a molecule that is recognized by specific antibody or T cells. An **epitope (antigenic determinant)** is the actual molecular structure that interacts with a single antibody molecule or T-cell receptor. Within a protein, an epitope may be formed by a specific sequence (**linear epitope**) or a three-dimensional structure (**conformational epitope**). Antigens and immunogens usually contain several epitopes, each capable of binding to a different antibody molecule. As described later in this chapter, a **monoclonal antibody** recognizes a single epitope.

Not all molecules are immunogens. In general, *proteins are the best immunogens, carbohydrates are weaker immunogens, and lipids and nucleic acids are poor immunogens.* **Haptens (incomplete immunogens)** are often too small to immunize (i.e., initiate a response) an individual but can be recognized by antibody. Haptens can be made immunogenic by attachment to a **carrier molecule**, such as a protein. For example, dinitrophenol conjugated to bovine serum albumin is an immunogen for the dinitrophenol hapten.

During artificial immunization (e.g., vaccines), an adjuvant is used to enhance the response to antigen. **Adjuvants** usually prolong the presence of antigen in the tissue, promote uptake of the immunogen or activate dendritic cells (DCs), macrophages, and lymphocytes. Some adjuvants mimic the activators (e.g., microbial ligands for Toll-like receptors) present in a natural immunization.

Some molecules will not elicit an immune response in an individual. During growth of the fetus, the body develops **central immune tolerance** toward self-antigens and any foreign antigens that may be introduced before maturation of the immune system. Later in life, **peripheral tolerance** develops to other proteins to prevent uncontrolled or autoimmune responses. For example, our immune response is tolerant of the food we eat; alternatively, eating steak would induce an anti-muscle response.

The type of immune response initiated by an immunogen depends on its molecular structure. A primitive but rapid antibody response can be initiated toward *bacterial polysaccharides (capsule), peptidoglycan, or flagellin.* Termed **T-independent antigens**, these molecules have a large, repetitive structure, which is sufficient to activate B cells directly to make antibody without the participation of T-cell help. In these cases, the response is limited to production of **IgM** antibody and fails to stimulate an **anamnestic (booster) response**. The transition from an IgM response to an IgG, IgE, or IgA response results from a big change in the B cell and is equivalent to differentiation of the cell. This requires help provided by T-cell interactions

Box 10—1. Antimicrobial Action of Antibodies

Are opsonic: promote ingestion and killing by phagocytic cells (IgG)

Neutralize (block attachment) toxins and virus

Agglutinate bacteria: may aid in clearing

Render motile organisms nonmotile

Combine with antigens on the microbial surface and activate the complement cascade, thus inducing an inflammatory response, bringing fresh phagocytes and serum antibodies into the site

Combine with antigens on the microbial surface, activate the complement cascade, and anchor the membrane attack complex involving C5b to C9

Box 10—2. Definitions

Adjuvant: substance that promotes immune response to immunogen

Antigen: substance recognized by immune response

Carrier: protein modified by hapten to elicit response

Epitope: molecular structure recognized by immune response

Hapten: incomplete immunogen that cannot initiate response but can be recognized by antibody

Immunogen: substance capable of eliciting an immune response

T-dependent antigens: antigens that must be presented to T and B cells for antibody production

T-independent antigens: antigens with large, repetitive structures (e.g., bacteria, flagellin, lipopolysaccharide, polysaccharide)

and cytokines. The antigen must therefore be recognized and stimulate both T and B cells. **T-dependent antigens** are proteins; they stimulate all five classes of immunoglobulins and can elicit an anamnestic (secondary-booster) response.

In addition to the structure of the antigen, the amount, route of administration, and other factors influence the type of immune response, including the types of antibody produced. For example, oral or nasal administration of a vaccine across mucosal membranes promotes production of a secretory form of **IgA** (sIgA) that would not be produced on intramuscular challenge.

Immunoglobulin Types and Structures

Immunoglobulins are composed of at least two heavy chains and two light chains, a dimer of dimers. They are subdivided into classes and subclasses based on the structure and antigenic distinction of their heavy chains. IgG, IgM, and IgA are the major antibody forms, whereas IgD

and IgE make up less than 1% of the total immunoglobulins. The IgA and IgG classes of immunoglobulin are divided further into subclasses based on differences in the Fc portion. There are four subclasses of IgG, designated as IgG1 through IgG4, and two IgA subclasses (IgA1 and IgA2) (Figure 10-1).

Antibody molecules are Y-shaped molecules with two major structural regions that mediate the two major functions of the molecule (see Figure 10-1; Table 10-1). The **variable-region/antigen-combining site** must be able to identify and specifically interact with an epitope on an antigen. A large number of different antibody molecules, each with a different variable region, are produced in every individual to recognize the seemingly infinite number of different antigens in nature. The **Fc portion** (stem of the antibody Y) interacts with host systems and cells to promote clearance of antigen and activation of subsequent immune responses. The Fc portion is responsible for fixation of complement and binding of the molecule to cell surface immunoglobulin receptors (**FcR**) on macrophages, natural killer cells, and T cells. For IgG and IgA, the

Figure 10—1. Comparative structures of the immunoglobulin (Ig) classes and subclasses in humans. IgA and IgM are held together in multimers by the J chain. IgA can acquire the secretory component for the traversal of epithelial cells.

Table 10–1. Immunoglobulins

Ig	IgM	IgD	IgG	IgE	IgA
CD4 T-helper subclass association	T independent and TH1	—	TH1, TH2	TH2	TH2
Total Ig (%)	5-10	<1	85	<1	5-15
Molecular mass (kDa)	900	185	154	190	160 (+ dimer)
H-chain class	μ	δ	γ	ε	α
Subclass	—	—	γ-1, γ-2, γ-3, γ-4	—	α-1, α-2
Serum half-life (days)	5	2-3	23	2-3	6
Principal site of action	Serum	Receptor for B cells	Serum and tissue	Mast cells	Secretions
Principal biologic effect	Resistance: precipitin, primary response	B-cell activation	Resistance: opsonin, secondary response	Anaphylaxis	Resistance: protection of mucous membranes
Complement fixation	++++	—	+++	—	+
Opsonin for macrophage, PMN			+		
Mucosal secretion	—	—	—	—	+
Crossing of placenta	—	—	+	—	—

PMN, polymorphonuclear neutrophil (leukocyte); +/−, relative activity.

10

Fc portion interacts with other proteins to promote transfer across the placenta and the mucosa, respectively (Table 10-2). In addition, each of the different types of antibody can be synthesized with a **membrane-spanning portion** to make it a cell surface antigen receptor.

IgG and IgA have a flexible **hinge region** rich in proline and susceptible to cleavage by proteolytic enzymes. Digestion of IgG molecules with **papain** yields two **Fab** fragments and one **Fc** fragment (Figure 10-2). Each Fab fragment has one antigen-binding site. **Pepsin** cleaves the molecule, producing an **F(ab′)₂** fragment with two antigen-binding sites and a **pFc′** fragment.

The different types and parts of immunoglobulin can also be distinguished using antibodies directed against different portions of the molecule. **Isotypes (IgM, IgD, IgG, IgA, IgE)** are determined by antibodies directed against the Fc portion of the molecule (*iso* meaning the same for all people.) **Allotypic** differences occur for antibody molecules with the same isotype but contain protein sequences that differ from one person to another (in addition to the antigen-binding region). (*Every one ["allo"] of them cannot have the same IgG.*) The **idiotype** refers to the protein sequences in the variable region that generate the large number of antigen-binding regions. (*There are many different idiots in the world.*)

On a molecular basis, each antibody molecule is made up of heavy and light chains encoded by separate genes. The basic

immunoglobulin unit consists of **two heavy (H)** and **two light (L) chains**. IgM and IgA consist of multimers of this basic structure. The heavy and light chains of immunoglobulin are fastened together by **interchain disulfide bonds**. Two types of light chains—κ and λ—are present in all five immunoglobulin classes, although only one type is present in an individual molecule. Approximately 60% of human immunoglobulin molecules have κ light chains, and 40% have λ light chains.

Table 10–2. Fc Interactions with Immune Components

Immune Component	Interaction	Function
Fc receptor	Macrophages	Opsonization
	PMNs	Opsonization
	T cells	Activation
	NK cells (antibody-dependent cellular cytotoxicity)	Killing
		Allergic reactions, antiparasitic
	Mast cells for immunoglobulin E	
Complement	Complement system	Opsonization, killing (especially bacteria)

NK, natural killer; PMN, polymorphonuclear neutrophils.

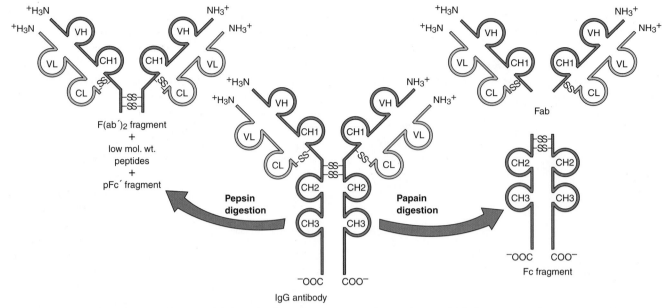

Figure 10–2. Proteolytic digestion of immunoglobulin G (IgG). Pepsin treatment produces a dimeric F(ab′)$_2$ fragment. Papain treatment produces monovalent Fab fragments and an Fc fragment. The F(ab′)$_2$ and the Fab fragments bind antigen but lack a functional Fc region. The heavy chain is depicted in *blue*; the light chain in *orange*.

There are **five types of heavy chains**, one for each isotype of antibody (**IgM, μ; IgG, γ; IgD, δ; IgA, α; and IgE, ε**). Intrachain disulfide bonds define molecular domains within each chain. Light chains have a variable and a constant domain. The heavy chains have a variable and three (IgG, IgA) or four (IgM, IgE) constant domains. The variable domains on the heavy and light chains interact to form the antigen-binding site. The constant domains from each chain make up the Fc portion, provide the molecular structure to the immunoglobulin and define the interaction of the antibody molecule with host systems, hence its ultimate function. The heavy chain of the different antibody molecules can also be synthesized with a membrane-spanning region to make the antibody an antigen-specific cell surface receptor for the B cell.

Immunoglobulin D

IgD, which has a molecular mass of 185 kDa, accounts for less than 1% of serum immunoglobulins. IgD exists primarily as membrane IgD, which serves with IgM as an antigen receptor on early B-cell membranes to help initiate antibody responses by activating B cell growth. IgD and IgM are the only isotypes that can be expressed together by the same cell.

Immunoglobulin M

IgM is the first antibody produced in response to antigenic challenge and can be produced in a T-cell–independent manner. IgM makes up 5% to 10% of the total immunoglobulins in adults and has a half-life of 5 days. It is a **pentameric molecule** with five immunoglobulin units joined by disulfide bonds and the **J chain**, with a total molecular mass of 900 kDa.

Theoretically, this immunoglobulin has 10 antigen-binding sites. IgM is the most efficient immunoglobulin for fixing (binding) complement. A single IgM pentamer can activate the classical complement pathway. Monomeric IgM is found with IgD on the B-cell surface, where it serves as the receptor for antigen. Because IgM is relatively large, it remains in the blood and spreads inefficiently from the blood into tissue. IgM is particularly important for immunity against polysaccharide antigens on the exterior of pathogenic microorganisms. It also promotes phagocytosis and promotes bacteriolysis by activating complement through its Fc portion. IgM is also a major component of rheumatoid factors (autoantibodies).

Immunoglobulin G

IgG comprises approximately 85% of the immunoglobulins in adults. It has a molecular mass of 154 kDa, based on two L chains of 22,000 Da each and two H chains of 55,000 Da each. The four subclasses of IgG differ in structure (see Figure 10-1), relative concentration, and function. Production of IgG requires T-cell help. IgG, as a class of antibody molecules, has the longest half-life (23 days) of the five immunoglobulin classes, crosses the placenta, and is the principal antibody in the **anamnestic or booster response**. IgG shows high avidity (binding capacity) for antigens, fixes complement, stimulates chemotaxis, and acts as an opsonin to facilitate phagocytosis.

Immunoglobulin A

IgA comprises 5% to 15% of the serum immunoglobulins and has a half-life of 6 days. It has a molecular mass of

160 kDa and a basic four-chain monomeric structure. However, it can occur as monomers, dimers, trimers, and multimers combined by the J chain (similar to IgM). In addition to serum IgA, a **secretory IgA** appears in body secretions and provides localized immunity. IgA production requires specialized T-cell help and mucosal stimulation. Adjuvants, such as cholera toxin and attenuated *Salmonella* bacteria, can promote an IgA response. IgA binds to a **poly-Ig receptor** on epithelial cells for transport across the cell. The poly-Ig receptor remains bound to IgA and is then cleaved to become the **secretory component** when secretory IgA is secreted from the cell. An adult secretes approximately 2 gm of IgA per day. Secretory IgA appears in colostrum, intestinal and respiratory secretions, saliva, tears, and other secretions. IgA-deficient individuals have an increased incidence of respiratory tract infections.

Immunoglobulin E

IgE accounts for less than 1% of the total immunoglobulins and has a half-life of approximately 2.5 days. Most IgE is bound to Fc receptors on **mast cells**, on which it serves as a receptor for allergens and parasite antigens. When sufficient antigen binds to the IgE on the mast cell, the mast cell releases histamine, prostaglandin, platelet-activating factor, and cytokines. IgE is important for protection against parasitic infection and is responsible for **anaphylactic hypersensitivity** (Type 1) (rapid allergic reactions).

Immunogenetics

The antibody response can recognize as many as 10^8 structures but can still specifically amplify and focus a response directed to a specific challenge. The mechanisms for generating this antibody repertoire and the different immunoglobulin subclasses are tied to random genetic events that accompany the development (differentiation) of the B cell (Figure 10-3).

Human chromosomes 2, 22, and 14 contain immunoglobulin genes for κ, λ, and H chains, respectively. The **germline forms** of these genes consist of different and separate sets of genetic building blocks for the light (**V and J gene segments**) and heavy chains (**V, D, and J gene segments**), which are genetically recombined to produce the immunoglobulin variable regions. These variable regions are then associated with the constant-region C gene segments. For the κ light chain, there are 300 V gene segments, 5 J gene segments, and 1 C gene segment. The number of λ gene segments for V and J is more limited. For the heavy chain, there are 300 to 1000 V genes, 12 D genes, and 6 (heavy-chain) J genes, but only 9 C genes (one for each class and subclass of antibody [μ; δ; γ_3, γ_1, γ_2, and γ_4; ϵ; α_1 and α_2]). In addition, gene segments for membrane-spanning peptides can be attached to the heavy-chain genes

to allow the antibody molecule to insert into the B-cell membrane as an antigen-activation receptor.

Production of the final antibody molecule in the pre-B and B cell requires genetic recombination at the deoxyribonucleic acid (DNA) level and post-transcriptional processing at the ribonucleic acid (RNA) level to assemble the immunoglobulin gene and produce the functional messenger RNA (mRNA) (see Figure 10-3). Each of the V, D, and J segments is surrounded by DNA sequences that promote **directional recombination and loss of the intervening DNA sequences**. Each of the recombination sites are joined by randomly inserted nucleotides, which can enhance the diversity of sequences or disrupt the gene depending upon the number of inserted nucleotides. Juxtaposition of randomly chosen V and J gene segments of the light chains and the V, D, and J gene segments of the heavy chains produces the variable region of the immunoglobulin chains. These recombination reactions are analogous to matching and sewing together similar patterns from a long swatch of cloth, then cutting out the intervening loops of extra cloth. **Somatic mutation** of the immunoglobulin gene can also occur later in activated, growing B cells to add to the enormous number of possible coding sequences for the variable region and to fine-tune a specific immune response. The variable-region sequences (VDJ) are attached by recombination to the μ; δ; γ_3, γ_1, γ_2, and γ_4; ϵ; or α_1 and α_2 sequences of the C gene segments to produce a heavy-chain gene. In the pre-B and immature B cells, mRNAs are produced and contain the variable-region gene segments connected to the C gene sequences for μ and δ. Processing of the mRNA removes either the μ or δ, as if it were an intron, to produce the final immunoglobulin. The pre-B cell expresses cytoplasmic IgM, whereas the B cell expresses cytoplasmic and cell surface IgM and cell surface IgD. IgM and IgD are the only pair of isotypes that can be expressed on the same cell.

Class switching (IgM to IgG, IgE, or IgA) occurs in mature B cells in response to different cytokines produced by TH1 or TH2 CD4 helper T cells (see Figure 10-3). Each of the C gene segments, except for δ, is preceded by a DNA sequence called the **switch site**. After the appropriate cytokine signal, the switch in front of the μ sequence recombines with the switch in front of the γ_3, γ_1, γ_2, or γ_4; ϵ; or α_1, or α_2 sequences, creating a DNA loop that is subsequently removed. Processing of the RNA transcript yields the final mRNA for the immunoglobulin heavy-chain protein. For example, IgG1 production would result from excision of DNA containing the C gene segments C_μ, C_δ, and $C\gamma_3$ to attach the variable region to the γ_1 C gene segment. **Class switching does not change the variable region**.

The final steps in B-cell differentiation to memory cells or plasma cells do not change the antibody gene. **Memory cells** are long-lived, antigen-responsive B cells expressing the CD45RO surface marker. Memory cells can be

Figure 10—3. T-cell help induces differentiation of the B cell and promotes genetic recombination and Ig class switching. Switch regions in front of the constant-region genes (including immunoglobulin [Ig] G subclasses) allow attachment of the preformed VDJ region with different heavy-chain constant-region genes, genetically removing the μ, δ, and other intervening genes. This produces an immunoglobulin gene with the same VDJ region (except for somatic mutation) but different heavy-chain genes. Splicing of messenger RNA (mRNA) produces the final IgM and IgD mRNA. *(Redrawn from Abbas AK, Lichtman AH, Pillai S: Cellular and Molecular Immunology, 6th ed. Philadelphia: WB Saunders, 2007.)*

activated in response to antigen later in life to divide and then produce its specific antibody. **Plasma cells** are terminally differentiated B cells with a small nucleus but a large cytoplasm filled with endoplasmic reticulum. Plasma cells are antibody factories.

Antibody Response

An initial repertoire of IgM and IgD immunoglobulins is generated in pre-B cells by the genetic events previously described (Figure 10-4). Expression of cell surface IgM and

Figure 10—4. B-cell activation. IgM production is activated by binding of antigen, cross-linking of cell surface receptors, and the C3d product of complement, endotoxin, and cytokines. Binding of T cells and cytokines associated with TH1, TH2, or TH3 responses activate the growth and differentiation of B cells to produce different antibody isotypes. APC, antigen-presenting cell; IFNγ, interferon-γ; Ig, immunoglobulin; IL, interleukin; TGF-β, transforming growth factor-β.

IgD accompany differentiation of the pre-B cell to the B cell. The cell surface antibody acts as an antigen receptor to trigger activation of the B cell through its associated signal transduction receptors, Ig-α (CD79a) and Ig-β (CD79b). A cascade of protein tyrosine kinases, phospholipase C, and calcium fluxes activate transcription and cell growth to mediate the activation signal. Other surface molecules, including the CR2 (CD21) complement (C3d) receptor, amplify the activation signal. The combination of these signals triggers the growth and increases the number of cells making antibodies to that antigen. In this manner, the B cells that best recognize the different epitopes of the

antigen are selected to increase in number in a process termed **clonal expansion**.

Clonal expansion of the antigen-specific B cells increases the number of antibody factories making the relevant antibody, and the strength of the antibody response is thus increased. Activation of the B cells also promotes *somatic mutation of the variable region, increasing the diversity of antibody molecules* directed at the specific antigen. The B-cell clones that express antibody with the strongest antigen binding are preferentially stimulated. This selects a better antibody response.

T-independent antigens cross-link sufficient numbers of surface antibody to stimulate growth of the antigen-specific B cells. In contrast, production of antibody to **T-dependent antigens** requires receptor interactions of the B cell with the helper T cell through CD40 (on the B cell), CD40L (T cell), and the action of cytokines. Different combinations of cytokines produced by helper T cells induce class switching. *TH1-helper responses (interferon-γ) promote production of IgG. TH2-helper responses (IL-4, IL-5, IL-6) promote production of IgG, IgE, and IgA. IgA production is especially promoted by IL-5 and transforming growth factor-β (TGF-β)* (TH3). Memory cells are developed with T-cell help. Terminal differentiation produces the ultimate antibody factory, the plasma cell.

During an immune response, antibodies are made against different epitopes of the foreign object, protein, or infectious agent. *Specific antibody is a mixture of many different immunoglobulin molecules made by many different B cells* (**polyclonal antibody**), each immunoglobulin molecule differing in the epitope it recognizes and the strength of the interaction. Different antibody molecules are made against different epitopes on the antigen, and each binds with different strengths (**affinity**, monovalent binding to an epitope; **avidity**, multivalent binding of antibody to antigen) for the same antigen.

Monoclonal antibodies are identical antibodies produced by a single clone of cells or by myelomas (cancers of plasma cells) or hybridomas. Hybridomas are cloned, laboratory-derived cells obtained by the fusion of antibody-producing spleen cells and a myeloma cell. In 1975, Kohler and Millstein developed the technique for producing monoclonal antibodies from B-cell hybridomas. The hybridoma is immortal and produces a single (monoclonal) antibody. This technique has revolutionized the study of immunology because it allows selection (cloning) of individual antibody-producing cells and their development into cellular factories for production of large quantities of that antibody. Monoclonal antibodies have been commercially produced for both diagnostic reagents and therapeutic purposes.

The primary antibody response is characterized by the initial production of IgM. As the response matures, IgG antibodies rapidly increase in concentration (Figure 10-5). IgM antibodies appear in the blood within 3 days to 2 weeks after

Figure 10–5. Time course of immune responses. The primary response occurs after a lag period. The immunoglobulin (Ig) M response is the earliest response. The secondary immune response (anamnestic response) reaches a higher titer, lasts longer, and consists predominantly of IgG.

exposure to a novel immunogen. The first antibodies that are produced react with residual antigen and therefore are rapidly cleared. After the initial lag phase, however, the antibody titer increases logarithmically to reach a plateau.

Reexposure to an immunogen, a **secondary response**, induces a heightened antibody response (also termed **anamnestic response**). The antibodies develop more rapidly, last longer, and reach a higher titer. The antibodies in a secondary response are principally of the IgG class.

Complement

The complement system is an alarm and a weapon against infection, especially bacterial infection. The complement system is activated directly by bacteria and bacterial products (**alternate or properdin pathway**), by lectin binding to sugars on the bacterial cell surface (**mannose-binding protein**), or by complexes of antibody and antigen (**classical pathway**) (Figure 10-6). Activation by either pathway initiates a cascade of proteolytic events that produce chemotactic factors to attract phagocytic and inflammatory cells to the site, increase vascular permeability to allow access to the site of infection, bind to the agent to promote their phagocytosis (**opsonization**) and elimination, and directly kill the infecting agent. The three activation pathways of complement coalesce at a common junction point, the activation of the **C3 component**.

Alternate Pathway

The alternate pathway is activated directly by bacterial cell surfaces and their components (e.g., endotoxin, microbial polysaccharides), as well as other factors. This pathway can be activated before the establishment of an immune response to the infecting bacteria because

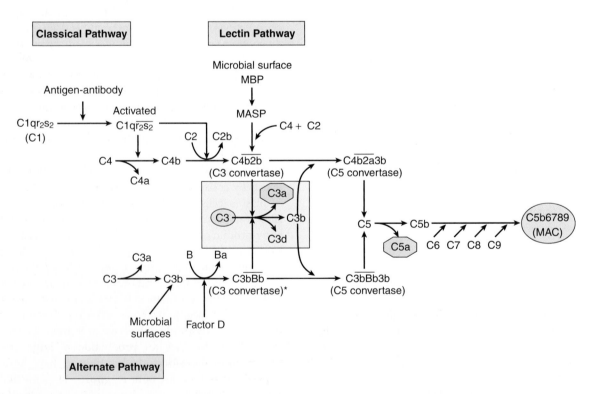

* Stabilized by properdin.

Figure 10–6. The classical, lectin, and alternate complement pathways. Despite different activators, the goal of these pathways is cleavage of C3 and C5 to provide chemoattractants and anaphylotoxins (C3a, C5a), an opsonin (C3b) that adheres to membranes, and to initiate the membrane attack complex to kill cells. MASP, MBP-associated serine protease; MBP, mannose-binding protein. *(Redrawn from Rosenthal KS, Tan JS: Rapid Review Microbiology and Immunology. St Louis, Mosby, 2002.)*

it does not depend on antibody and does not involve the early complement components (C1, C2, and C4). The initial activation of the alternate pathway is mediated by *properdin factor B* binding to C3b and then with *properdin factor D*, which splits *factor B* in the complex to yield the *Bb active fragment* that remains linked to *C3b (activation unit)*. The C3b sticks to the cell surface and anchors the complex. Inactive *Ba* is split from this complex, leading to cleavage and activation of many C3 molecules (amplification). The complement cascade continues in a manner analogous to the classical pathway.

Classical Pathway

The classical complement cascade is initiated by *binding to the Fc portion of antibody that is bound to cell surface antigens, or in an immune complex with soluble antigens.* Aggregation of antibody (**IgG or IgM, not IgA or IgE**) changes the structure of the heavy chain to allow binding to complement (see Figure 10-6).

The first complement component, designated *C1*, consists of a complex of three separate proteins designated *C1q, C1r, and C1s* (see Figure 10-6). One molecule each of C1q and C1s with two molecules of C1r constitutes the C1 complex or **recognition unit**. C1q facilitates binding of the recognition unit to cell surface antigen-antibody complexes. Activation of the classical complement cascade requires linkage of C1q to two IgG antibodies through their Fc regions. In contrast, one pentameric IgM molecule attached to a cell surface may interact with C1q to initiate the classical pathway. Binding of C1q activates C1r (referred to now as *C1r**) and in turn C1s (C1s*). C1s* then cleaves *C4* to C4a and C4b, and *C2* to C2a and C2b. The convention is that the b fragment is bigger and bound to something. The ability of a single recognition unit to split numerous C2 and C4 molecules represents an amplification mechanism in the complement cascade. The union of *C4b* and *C2b* produces **C4b2b**, which is known as **C3 convertase**. This complex binds to the cell membrane and cleaves *C3* into *C3a* and *C3b* fragments. The C3b protein has a unique thioester bond that will covalently attach C3b to a cell surface or be hydrolyzed. The C3 convertase amplifies the response by splitting many C3 molecules. The interaction of C3b with C4b2a bound to the cell membrane produces **C4b3b2b**, which is termed **C5 convertase**. This activation unit splits *C5* into *C5a* and *C5b* fragments and represents yet another amplification step.

Lectin Pathway

The lectin pathway is also a bacterial and fungal defense mechanism. **Mannose-binding protein** (previously known as *RaRF*) is a large serum protein that binds to nonreduced mannose, fucose, and glucosamine on bacterial, fungal, and other cell surfaces. Mannose-binding protein resembles and replaces the C1q component and on binding to bacterial surfaces, activates the cleavage of mannose-binding protein–associated serine protease. Mannose-binding protein–associated serine protease cleaves the C4 and C2 components to produce the C3 convertase, the junction point of the complement cascade.

Biologic Activities of Complement Components

Cleavage of the C3 and C5 components produces important factors that enhance clearance of the infectious agent by promoting access to the infection site and attracting the cells that mediate protective inflammatory reactions. **C3b** is an **opsonin** that promotes clearance of bacteria by binding directly to the cell membrane to make the cell more attractive to phagocytic cells such as neutrophils and macrophages, which have receptors for C3b. C3b can be cleaved further to generate **C3d**, which is an activator of B lymphocytes. Complement fragments **C3a** and **C5a** serve as powerful **anaphylatoxins** that stimulate mast cells to release histamine, which *enhances vascular permeability and smooth muscle contraction*. **C3a** and **C5a** also act as attractants (**chemotactic factors**) for neutrophils and macrophages. These cells also express receptors for C3b, are phagocytic, and promote inflammatory reactions.

Membrane Attack Complex

The terminal stage of the classical pathway involves creation of the **membrane attack complex**, which is also called **the lytic unit** (Figure 10-7). The five terminal complement proteins (C5 through C9) associate into a membrane attack complex on target cell membranes to mediate injury. Initiation of the membrane attack complex assembly begins with C5 cleavage into C5a and C5b fragments. A $(C5b,6,7,8)_1(C9)_n$ complex forms and drills a hole in the membrane, leading to the hypotonic lysis of cells. The C9 component is similar to perforin, which is produced by cytolytic T cells and natural killer cells.

Regulation of Complement Activation

Humans have several mechanisms for preventing generation of the C3 convertase to protect against inappropriate complement activation. These include C1 inhibitor, C4 binding protein, Factor H, Factor I, and the cell surface proteins, which are decay-accelerating factor (DAF) and membrane cofactor protein. In addition, CD59 (protectin) prevents formation of the membrane attack complex. Most infectious agents lack these protective mechanisms and remain susceptible to complement. A genetic deficiency in these protection systems can result in disease.

Figure 10–7. Cell lysis by complement. Activation of C5 initiates the molecular construction of an oil-well–like membrane attack complex (MAC).

C5b

C6

C7

C5b67

C7 C6

C5b

1

C5b678

C7 C6

C8

C5b

C8

2

C5b6789n
MAC

C7 C6

C8

C5b

C9

3

Questions

What is wrong with each of the following statements, and why?

1. The laboratory tested a baby for IgM maternal antibodies.

2. An investigator attempted to use fluorescent-labeled $F(ab')_2$ fragments to locate class II major histocompatibility complex molecules on the cell surface of antigen-presenting cells without cross-linking (binding two molecules together) these cell surface molecules.

3. A patient is diagnosed as having been infected with a specific strain of influenza A (A/Bangkok/1/79/H3N2) on the basis of the presence of anti-influenza IgG in serum taken from the patient at the initial visit (within 2 days of symptoms).

4. A patient was considered unable to use the complement systems because of a T-cell deficiency, which precluded the ability to promote class switching of B cells.

5. Analysis of immunoglobulin genes from B cells taken from the patient described in statement 4 did not contain recombined VDJ variable-region gene sequences.

6. A patient was considered to have a B-cell deficiency because serum levels of IgE and IgD were undetectable despite proper concentrations of IgG and IgM.

Bibliography

Abbas AK, et al: Cellular and Molecular Immunology, 6th ed. Philadelphia, Saunders, 2007.

DeFranco AL, Locksley RM, Robertson M: Immunity: The Immune Response in Infectious and Inflammatory Disease. Sunderland, Mass, Sinauer, 2007.

Janeway CA, et al: Immunobiology: The Immune System in Health and Disease, 6th ed. New York, Current Biology and Garland, 2004.

Kindt TJ, Goldsby RA, Osborne BA: Kuby Immunology, 6th ed. New York, WH Freeman, 2007.

Kumar V, Abbas AK, Fausto N: Robbins and Cotran Pathologic Basis of Disease, 7th ed. Philadelphia, Saunders, 2005.

Sompayrac L: How the Immune System Works, 2nd ed. Malden, Mass, Blackwell Scientific, 2003.

Trends in Immunology: Issues contain understandable reviews on current topics in immunology.

Cellular Immune Responses

The drama of the immune response unfolds in several acts after an antigenic challenge. The actors include cells of the innate response, including neutrophils, monocyte-macrophage lineage cells, immature dendritic (iDCs) and dendritic cells (DCs), natural killer (NK) cells, the T and B lymphocytes of the antigen-specific response, and other cells. These cells are distinguished by their outer structures, their costumes, which also define their roles in the immune response. Act 1 starts at the site of infection and involves innate responses. Neutrophils and activated macrophages act directly on bacteria and infection. The NK cells provide early responses to infection and kill virally infected and tumor cells. The NK cells return in Act 2 to kill cells decorated with antibody (antibody-dependent cellular cytotoxicity [ADCC]). Immature dendritic cells bridge the gap between the innate and the antigen-specific protective responses by first producing cytokines to enhance the action and then taking their phagocytosed and pinocytosed cargo to the lymph node as the only antigen-presenting cell (APC) that can **initiate** an immune response. Act 2 includes the adaptive immune responses and commences in the lymph node, where the mature DCs present antigen to the T lymphocytes. The plot of this story may proceed to reinforce local site inflammatory responses (TH1) or initiate systemic, humoral responses (TH2), depending on the cytokine dialogue of the DC and the T cell. The T cells play a central role in activating and controlling (helping) immune and inflammatory responses through the release of cytokines. In Act 3, the cast of T cells and B lymphocytes responding to the infection expands to deliver antigen-specific cellular and antibody immune responses and then terminally differentiates into effector and plasma cells. Macrophages and B cells refine and strengthen the direction of the response as APCs. Certain members of the B- and T-cell cast maintain a low profile and become memory cells to be able to replay the drama more quickly and efficiently in the future. This chapter will introduce the cast of cellular actors, their costumes, the cytokine dialogue, and the roles they play in the immune response drama.

Immature Dendritic and Dendritic Cells

Dendritic cells provide the bridge between the innate and the immune responses, and the cytokines they produce determine the nature of the T cell response. **Immature dendritic cells (iDCs)** provide an early cytokine-mediated warning system and then mature into **dendritic cells,** which are the ultimate antigen-presenting cell, the only antigen-presenting cell that can initiate an antigen-specific T cell response (Box 11-1). DCs have octopus-like arms (dendrites), an antigen-sticky cell surface, produce cytokines, and present antigen to T and B cells.

Precursor DCs of myeloid (including monocytes) or lymphoid origin circulate in the blood and then differentiate into immature DCs in tissue. Some of the various immature DCs found in tissue and blood are specialized and include: (1) **Langerhans cells** in the skin, (2) **dermal interstitial cells**, (3) **interdigitating cells** (lymph node and spleen), and (4) **splenic marginal DCs**; but DCs are also present in the **liver, thymus, germinal centers of the lymph nodes**, and **blood. These cells present antigen to T cells** on major histocompatibility complex (MHC) I and MHC II molecules. **Follicular DCs** (FDC) present in the lymph node and spleen are different. FDCs lack MHC II molecules but have sticky cell surfaces, which capture antigen (through lectins and other molecules) to present to B cells.

Immature DCs sense the presence of microbes and release cytokines, which determine whether the subsequent immune response will develop into a TH1 or a TH2 type of immune response, depending on the nature of the activation signals. These cells express different combinations of microbial sensors from the **Toll-like receptors (TLRs)** family of proteins, as well as other receptors. The TLRs include 10 different cell surface and intracellular proteins that sense the presence of microbial infection by binding to the characteristic patterns within molecules on the outside of bacteria, fungi, and viruses, and even to forms of the deoxyribonucleic acid (DNA) and ribonucleic acid (RNA)

Box 11–1. Dendritic Cells

Myeloid and lymphoid
Morphology: octopus-like with tendrils
Activities:

Immature DC:
In blood and tissue
Phagocytosis and cytokine production directs TH1 or TH2 responses

Mature DC:
In lymphoid tissues (up-regulated MHC II and B7-1 and B7-2 molecules)
In T-cell areas of lymph node, process and present antigen to initiate T-cell response
MHC I-peptide: CD8 T cells
CD1-glycolipids: CD8 T cells
MHC II-peptide: CD4 T cells
Activate naïve T-cells and determine response through specific cytokines

Follicular DC:
In B-cell areas of lymphoid tissues (Fc and CR1, CR2, and CR3 complement receptors, lack MHC II)
Presentation of antigen stuck to membrane to B cells

defenses (TH1 responses). DCs present antigenic material attached to MHC class I and CD1 molecules to CD8 T and NKT cells, and on MHC class II molecules to CD4 T cells. DCs are so effective at presenting antigen that 10 cells loaded with antigen are sufficient to initiate protective immunity to a lethal bacterial challenge in a mouse.

Cells of the Monocyte-Macrophage Lineage

Monocytes are myeloid cells that develop from the same lineage as polymorphonuclear granulocytes. Monocytes mature into different types of **macrophages**, other cells of the macrophage lineage, and dendritic cells that differ in function and tissue location. The surface markers on monocyte/macrophages correspond to the cells' functions. These cells express the following proteins:

1. **Receptors for opsonins** (e.g., immunoglobulin Fc receptors [Fc-γ RI, Fc-γ RII, Fc-γ RIII] and **complement receptors** [CR1, CR3])
2. **Lectins** (specific sugar-binding proteins, such as mannosyl-fucosyl receptors)
3. **Toll-like receptors**, which recognize **pathogen-associated molecular patterns** and provide signals for cell activation
4. A **receptor (CD14) for the lipopolysaccharide-binding protein** to facilitate bacterial uptake and promote activation
5. Adhesion molecules to promote cell-to-cell interactions; for example, leukocyte function–associated antigen-1 (LFA-1)
6. The class II MHC proteins to allow **antigen presentation** to T cells and the B7 and CD40 co-receptors for activation

Binding and ingestion of microbes by monocytes and macrophages promote the release of interleukin-1 (IL-1), IL-12, and tumor necrosis factor (TNF), which initiate inflammatory reactions. Interferon-γ (IFN-γ) made by NK or T cells activates killing mechanisms in the macrophage (activated/angry macrophage) and the production of more IL-12, which reinforces CD4 TH1 immune responses. Macrophage presentation of antigenic peptides on MHC II molecules and binding of their CD40 molecules to the CD40L on the CD4 TH1 cells promotes the production of IFN-γ to continue the activation of the macrophage. The **activated macrophages** reinforce local inflammatory reactions by producing various chemokines to attract neutrophils, immature DCs, NK cells, and activated T cells. Activation of the macrophages makes them more efficient killers of phagocytosed microbes, virally infected cells, and tumor cells. Macrophages activated by IL-4 and IL-13 support TH2 antiparasitic responses. Continuous stimulation of macrophages by T cells, as in the case of an unresolved mycobacterial infection, promotes the fusion of macrophages into **multinucleate giant cells** and large

of these microbes, termed **pathogen-associated molecular patterns (PAMPs)** (Table 11-1). These patterns are present within the endotoxin component of lipopolysaccharide (LPS) and in teichoic acid, fungal glycans, unmethylated cytosine-guanosine units of DNA (CpG ODN) commonly found in bacteria, double-stranded RNA produced during the replication of some viruses, and other molecules. Activation of the TLR triggers either of two cascades of protein kinases and other responses that result in the activation of the cell and production of specific cytokines. Cytoplasmic sensors of bacterial peptidoglycan include NOD1, NOD2 and cryopyrin.

The iDCs are constantly acquiring antigenic material by macropinocytosis, pinocytosis, or phagocytosis of apoptotic cells, debris, and proteins in normal tissue and at the site of infection or tumor. However, on activation of the iDC by a TLR cascade in response to infection, the iDC matures into a DC, and its role changes. The DC loses its ability to phagocytize, preventing it from acquiring irrelevant antigenic material other than the microbial debris, and progresses to the lymph node. As an analogy, the immature DC is like a clam, constantly surveying its environment by filter feeding the cellular and microbial debris (if present), but when triggered by a TLR signal that microbes are present, it releases a local cytokine alarm, closes its shell, and moves to the lymph node to trigger a response to the challenge. The mature DC moves to T-cell areas of lymph nodes and up-regulates its cell surface molecules for antigen presentation (class II MHC and B7-1 and B7-2 [co-stimulatory] molecules). Microbe-activated mature DCs release cytokines (e.g., IL-12), which activate responses to reinforce local host

Table 11—1. Pathogen Pattern Receptors

Toll-Like Receptor*	Cell Types†	Microbial Activators	Ligand
TLR 1	MDTBcG	Bacteria, mycobacteria *Neisseria meningitidis*	Lipopeptides Soluble factors
TLR2	MDG	Bacteria Fungi Cells	LPS, LTA, PGN, etc. Zymosan Necrotic cells
TLR3	MDT	Viruses	Double-stranded RNA
TLR4	MDTGBc	Bacteria Viruses	**LPS**, LTA RSV, HCV glycoproteins
TLR5	MDG	Bacteria	Flagellin
TLR6	MDBc	Bacteria Fungi	LTA, lipopeptides, zymosan
TLR7	MDBc	Viruses	Single-stranded RNA Imidazoquinolines
TLR8	MD	Viruses	Single-stranded RNA Imidazoquinolines
TLR9	MDBc	Bacteria Viruses	Unmethylated DNA (CpG)
NOD1	MD	Bacteria	Peptidoglycan
NOD2	MD	Bacteria	Peptidoglycan
Cryopyrin	MD	Bacteria	Peptidoglycan

Activators: CMV, cytomegalovirus; dsRNA, double-stranded RNA; gram +/−, gram-positive and gram-negative bacteria; HCV, hepatitis C virus; LPS, lipopolysaccharide; LTA, lipoteichoic acid; PGN, peptidoglycan; RSV, respiratory syncytial virus, NOD, nucleotide-binding oligomerization domain
*Information about Toll-like receptors from Takeda A, Kaisho T, Akira S: Annu Rev Immunol 21:335-376, 2003; Akira S, Takeda K: Nat Rev Immunol 4:499-511, 2003.
†Cell types: Bc, B cell; D, dendritic cell; G, granulocyte; M, macrophage; T, T cell.

macrophages called **epithelioid cells** that surround the infection and form a **granuloma**.

Natural Killer Cells

NK cells are an important part of the natural immune (innate) system. NK cells provide an early cellular response to a viral infection, have antitumor activity, and amplify inflammatory reactions after bacterial infection. NK cells are also responsible for **ADCC**, in which they bind and kill antibody-coated cells.

NK cells are large granular lymphocytes (LGLs) that share many characteristics with T cells, except the mechanism for target cell recognition. NK cells are stimulated by (1) IFN-α and IFN-β (produced early in response to viral and other infections), (2) TNF-α, (3) IL-12, IL-15, and

IL-18 (produced by pre-DCs and activated macrophages), and (4) IL-2 (produced by CD4 TH1 cells). The NK cells express many of the same cell surface markers as T cells (e.g., CD2, CD7, IL-2 receptor [IL-2R], and **FasL** [Fas ligand]) but also the **Fc receptor for IgG (CD16)**, complement receptors for ADCC, and NK-specific inhibitory receptors and activating receptors (including NK immunoglobulin-like receptors (KIR)). Activated NK cells produce IFN-γ, IL-1, and granulocyte-macrophage colony-stimulating factor (GM-CSF). These cytokines reinforce local initial protective responses (TH1) by encouraging the production of IL-12 by pre-DCs and activated macrophages. The granules in an NK cell contain **perforin**, a pore-forming protein, and **granzymes** (esterases), which are similar to the contents of the granules of a CD8 cytotoxic T lymphocyte (CTL). These molecules promote the death of the target cell.

Unlike T cells, NK cells do not express a TCR or CD3 and cannot make IL2. They neither recognize a specific antigen nor require presentation of antigen by MHC molecules. The NK system does not involve memory or require sensitization and cannot be enhanced by specific immunization.

The NK cell sees every cell as a potential victim, especially those that appear in distress, unless it receives an inhibitory signal from the target cell. NK cells interact closely with the target cell by binding to carbohydrates and surface proteins on the cell surface. The interaction of a class I MHC molecule on the target cell with a KIR **inhibitory receptor** is like communicating a secret password, indicating that all is normal, and then providing an inhibitory signal to prevent NK killing of the target cell. Virus-infected and tumor cells express "stress-related receptors" and are often deficient in MHC I molecules and become NK cell targets. Binding of the NK cell to antibody-coated target cells (ADCC) also initiates killing, but this is not controlled by an inhibitory signal. The **killing mechanisms** are similar to those of CTLs. A synapse (pocket) is formed between the NK and target cell, and **perforin and granzymes** are released to disrupt the target cell and induce apoptosis. In addition, the interaction of the **FasL** on the NK cell with **Fas** protein on the target cell can also induce apoptosis. (See the discussion of CD8 T cells later in this chapter.)

T Cells

The T cells are the directors and also play a starring role in the immune response drama. T cells were initially distinguished from B cells on the basis of their ability to bind sheep red blood cells through the CD2 molecule and form rosettes. These cells communicate through direct cell-to-cell interactions and with cytokines. T cells are defined through the use of antibodies that distinguish their cell surface molecules. The T-cell surface proteins include: (1) the **T-cell receptor (TCR)**, (2) the CD4 and CD8 co-receptors, (3) accessory proteins that promote recognition and activation, (4) cytokine receptors, and (5) adhesion proteins. All of these proteins determine the types of cell-to-cell interactions for the T cell and therefore the functions of the cell.

Development of T Cells

T-cell precursors develop into T cells in the thymus (Figure 11-1; Box 11-2). Contact with the thymic epithelium and hormones such as thymosin, thymulin, and thymopoietin II in the thymus promote extensive proliferation and differentiation of the individual's T-cell population during fetal development. While T-cell precursors are in the thymus, genetic events similar to those for

Figure 11–1. Human T-cell development. T-cell markers are useful for the identification of the differentiation stages of the T cell and for characterizing T-cell leukemias and lymphomas. TdT, cytoplasmic terminal deoxynucleotidyl transferase.

immunoglobulin generate numerous TCRs, each expressed on a different T-cell clone. T cells that cannot interact with MHC molecules do not grow, and those that react with the host (self-reactive) are forced into committing suicide (apoptosis). The remaining T cells differentiate into the

---

Box 11–2. T Cells

γ/δ T cells:
γ/δ TCR reactive to microbial metabolites
Local responses: resident in blood and tissue
Quicker responses than α/β T cells
Produce IFN-γ; activate DCs and macrophages

α/β T cells:
CD4: α/β TCR reactive with APC presented peptides on MHC II
Activated in lymph nodes then progresses to tissue
Cytokines activate and direct immune response (TH1, TH2, TH17)
Cytotoxic through Fas-Fas ligand interactions
CD4 CD25 Treg cells:
Control and limit expansion of immune response; promote tolerance and memory cell development
CD4 TH17 cells: IL-17-producing cells that reinforce inflammatory responses especially for immunosuppressive environments, like the eye
CD8: α/β TCR reactive with peptides presented on MHC I
Activated in lymph nodes, then progress to tissue
Produce similar cytokines as CD4 cells
Cytotoxic through perforin and granzymes and Fas-Fas ligand induction of apoptosis
NKT cells: α/β TCR reactive with glycolipids (mycobacteria) on CD1 molecules
Kill tumor and viral infected cells similar to NK cells
Provide early support to antibacterial responses

subpopulations of T cells. T cells can be distinguished by the type of T-cell antigen receptor, either consisting of **γ and δ chains** or **α and β chains**; and for α/β T cells, the presence of **CD4** or **CD8 co-receptors**. T cells can be further distinguished by the cytokines they produce.

T cells expressing the **γ/δ TCR** are present in blood, mucosal epithelium, and other tissue locations and are important for stimulating innate and mucosal immunity. These cells make up 5% of circulating lymphocytes but expand to between 20% and 60% of T cells during certain bacterial and other types of infections. The γ/δ TCR senses unusual microbial metabolites and initiates cytokine-mediated immune responses.

The **α/β TCR** is expressed on most T cells, and these cells are primarily responsible for antigen-activated immune responses. T cells with the α/β TCR are distinguished further by the expression of either a CD4 or a CD8 molecule.

The helper T cells (**CD4**) activate and control immune and inflammatory responses by specific cell—cell interactions and by releasing cytokines (soluble messengers). Helper T cells interact with peptide antigens presented on class II MHC molecules expressed on APCs (DCs, macrophages, and B cells) (Figure 11-2). The vocabulary of cytokines secreted by a specific CD4 T cell in response to antigenic challenge defines the type of CD4 T cell. **TH0** cells respond to antigen and can be converted to either TH1 or TH2 cells, depending on the cytokines produced by the antigen-presenting cells. **TH1 cells** promote inflammatory responses, which are especially important for controlling intracellular (mycobacterial and viral) and fungal infections and promoting certain subtypes of IgG antibody production. **TH2 cells** promote antibody responses. A **TH3**

subtype has also been described; it helps promote production of immunoglobulin (Ig) A. **TH17** cells secrete IL-17 and IL-23 in response to bacterial infection to promote inflammation. T-regulator cells (**Treg**) express CD4 and CD25, prevent spurious activation of T cells, and control the immune response. The TH1 and TH2 responses are antagonistic, and TH3 responses suppress TH1 and TH2 responses.

CD8 T cells are categorized as cytolytic and suppressor T cells but can also make cytokines similar to CD4 cells. Activated CD8 T cells "patrol" the body for virus-infected or tumor cells, which are identified by antigenic peptides presented by class I MHC molecules. Class I MHC molecules are found on all nucleated cells.

Cell Surface Receptors of T cells

The **TCR complex** is a combination of the antigen recognition structure (TCR) and cell-activation machinery (**CD3**) (Figure 11-3). The specificity of the TCR determines the antigenic response of the T cell. Each TCR molecule is made up of two different polypeptide chains. As with antibody (as described in Chapter 12), each TCR chain has a constant region and a variable region. The repertoire of TCRs is very large and can identify a tremendous number of antigenic specificities (estimated to be able to recognize 10^{15} separate epitopes). The genetic mechanisms for the development of this diversity are also similar to those for antibody (Figure 11-4). The TCR gene is made up of multiple V ($V_1V_2V_3 \ldots V_n$), D, and J segments. In the early stages of T cell development, a particular V segment genetically recombines with one or more D segments,

Figure 11—2. MHC restriction and antigen presentation to T cells. *Left,* Antigenic peptides bound to class I MHC molecules are presented to the T-cell receptor (TCR) on CD8 T killer/suppressor cells. *Right,* Antigenic peptides bound to class II MHC molecules on the antigen-presenting cell (APC) (B cell, dendritic cell, or macrophage) are presented to CD4 helper cells and delayed-type hypersensitivity T cells.

Figure 11—3. T-cell receptor (TCR). The TCR consists of different subunits. Antigen recognition occurs through the α/β or γ/δ subunits. The CD3 complex of γ, δ, ϵ, and ζ subunits promotes T-cell activation. C, constant region; V, variable region.

Figure 11–4. Structure of the embryonic T-cell receptor (TCR) gene. Note the similarity in structure to the immunoglobulin genes. Recombination of these segments also generates a diverse recognition repertoire.

deleting intervening V and D segments, and then recombines with a J segment to form a unique TCR gene. Like antibody, random insertion of nucleotides at the recombination junctions increases the potential for diversity and the possibility of producing inactive TCRs. Only cells with functional TCRs will survive. Each T-cell clone expresses a unique TCR.

The **CD3 complex** is found on all T cells and consists of the γ-, δ-, ε-, and ζ-polypeptide chains. The CD3 complex is the **signal transduction unit** for the TCR. **Tyrosine protein kinases** (ZAP70, Lck) associate with the CD3 complex when antigen is bound to the TCR complex, promote a cascade of protein phosphorylations, activation of phospholipase C (PLC), and other events. The products of cleavage of inositol triphosphate by PLC cause the release of calcium and activate protein kinase C and **calcineurin**, a protein phosphatase. Calcineurin is a target for the immunosuppressive drugs cyclosporine and tacrolimus. Activation of membrane G-proteins such as Ras and the consequences of the previously described cascades result in the activation of specific transcription factors in the nucleus, the activation of the T cell, and production of IL-2 and its receptor, IL-2R. These steps are depicted in Figure 11-5.

The **CD4 and CD8 proteins** are co-receptors for the TCR because they facilitate the interaction of the TCR with the antigen-presenting MHC molecule and can enhance the activation response. CD4 binds to class II MHC molecules on the surface of APCs. CD8 binds to class I MHC molecules on the surface of the target cell. Class I MHC molecules are expressed on all nucleated cells (see more on MHC later in this chapter). The cytoplasmic tails of CD4 and CD8 associate with a protein tyrosine kinase (p56^{Lck}), which enhances the TCR-induced activation of the cell on binding to the APC or target cell. CD4 or CD8 is found on α/β T cells but not on γ/δ T cells.

Accessory molecules expressed on the T cell include several protein receptors on the cell surface that interact with proteins on APCs and target cells, leading to activation of the T cell, promoting tighter interactions between the cells, or facilitating the killing of the target cell. These accessory molecules are as follows:

1. **CD45RA (native T cells)** or **CD45RO (memory T cells)**, a transmembrane protein tyrosine phosphatase (PTP).
2. **CD28** or cytotoxic T-lymphocyte–associated protein 4 (**CTLA-4**) (on activated T cells), which binds to the B7 protein on APCs to deliver a co-stimulation or inhibitory signal to the T cell.
3. **CD154 (CD40L)**, which is present on all T cells and promotes activation on binding to CD40 on DCs, macrophages, and B cells.
4. **FasL**, which initiates apoptosis in a target cell that expresses **Fas** on its cell surface.

Adhesion molecules tighten the interaction of the T cell with the APC or target cell and may also promote activation. Adhesion molecules include **LFA-1**, which interacts with the **intercellular adhesion molecules (ICAM-1, ICAM-2, and ICAM-3)** on the target cell. **CD2** was originally identified by its ability to bind to sheep red blood cells (**erythrocyte receptors**). CD2 binds to LFA-3 on the target cell and promotes cell-to-cell adhesion and T-cell activation. **Very late antigens (VLA-4 and VLA-5)** are expressed on activated cells later in the response and bind to fibronectin on target cells to enhance the interaction.

T cells express receptors for many cytokines that activate and regulate T-cell function (Table 11-2). The **cytokine receptors** activate protein kinase cascades on binding of cytokine to deliver their signal to the nucleus. **The IL-2 receptor (IL-2R)** is composed of three subunits. β/γ subunits are on most T cells (also NK cells) and have intermediate affinity for IL-2. The α subunit (**CD25**) is induced by cell activation (a marker of activation) to form a high-affinity α/β/γ IL-2R. Binding of IL-2 to the IL-2R initiates a growth-stimulating signal to the T cell, which also promotes the production of more IL-2 and IL-2R. CD25 is also expressed on the Treg subset of CD4 T cells (CD4+CD25+), which regulate and suppress the immune response.

Antigen Presentation to T Cells

Activation of an antigen-specific T-cell response requires a combination of cytokine and cell–cell receptor interactions (Table 11-3). Unlike cell surface immunoglobulin on the B cell, which senses ("tastes" or "sniffs") the presence of soluble foreign molecules floating past the cell, the TCR on the T cell must be presented with the relevant epitope, which is cleaved from the protein and cradled in a molecular holder on the surface of an APC, allowing the T cell to "touch" and respond to it. **Class I and II MHC** molecules provide the molecular cradle for the peptide. The **CD8** molecule on cytolytic/suppressor T cells binds to and promotes the interaction with class I MHC molecules on target cells. The **CD4** molecule on helper/DTH T cells binds to and promotes interactions with class II MHC molecules

Figure 11—5. Activation pathways for T cells. Binding of MHC II-peptide to CD4 and the TCR activate kinase cascades and phospholipase C to activate the NF-AT, NF-κβ, AP-1, and other transcription factors. DAG, diacylglycerol; PIP2, phosphatidylinositol 4,5-bisphosphate; IP3, inositol 1,4,5-triphosphate; PLC-γ, MAP kinase, mitogen-activated protein kinase; NF-AT, nuclear factor of activated T cells; NF-κB, nuclear factor-kappa B; AP-1, activation protein 1. (*Modified from Nairn R, Helbert M: Immunology for Medical Students, 2nd ed. Philadelphia, Mosby, 2007.*)

Table 11—2. Cytokines That Modulate T-cell Function

Cytokine	Source	Action
IL-1	APC	Activation
IL-2	CD4 TH1	Growth
IL-4	CD4 TH2	Growth and TH2 focus
IL-6	DC, etc.	Overturns Treg suppression
IL-10	TH2, Treg	Suppress TH1
IL-12	DC, macrophage	Promotes TH1
IL-23	DC	Promotes TH17
TGF-β	Treg, etc.	Suppress TH1, TH2, promote TH17

on APCs. The MHC molecules are encoded within the major histocompatibility complex (MHC) gene locus (Figure 11-6). The MHC contains a cluster of genes important to the immune response.

Class I MHC molecules are found on all nucleated cells and are the major determinant of "self." The class I MHC molecule, also known as **HLA** for human and H-2 for mouse, consists of two chains, a **variable heavy chain** and a **light chain (β₂-microglobulin)** (Figure 11-7). Differences in the heavy chain of the HLA molecule between individuals (*allotypic differences*) elicit the T-cell response that prevents graft (tissue) transplantation. There are three major HLA genes: HLA-A, HLA-B, and HLA-C and other minor HLA genes. Each cell expresses a pair of different **HLA-A, HLA-B**, and **HLA-C** proteins, one from each parent. *The heavy chain of the class I MHC molecule forms a closed-ended cleft, like a pita bread pocket, that holds a peptide of eight to nine amino acids.*

Table 11–3. Antigen-Specific T-Cell Responses

APC Activation of Naïve T Cells

Activation of the T Cell Requires Antigen, Co-Receptor, and Cytokine Interactions

DC	CD4 T cell	Function
MHCII-peptide complex	TCR/CD4	Antigen specificity
B-7	CD28 or CTLA4	Activation or suppression
IL-1	IL-1R	Activation
IL-6	IL-6R	Overcomes Treg-induced tolerance

T-Cell Activation of APC

Enhanced Antigen Presentation of APCs, Enhanced Antimicrobial Activity of Macrophages, and Class Switch of Immunoglobulin Production by the B Cell Requires Antigen, Co-Receptor, and Cytokine Interactions

DC, macrophage, or B cell	CD4 T cell	Function
MHCII-peptide complex	CD4T cell: TCR/CD4	Antigen specificity
B7-1, B7-2	CD28	Activation of T cell
CD40	CD40L	Activation of other functions in APC
IL-12		Activation/reinforcement of TH1 responses
IFN-γ		Activation of macrophages and B-cell class switch
IL-4		TH2 functions: growth and B-cell class switch
IL-5		TH2 functions: B-cell class switch

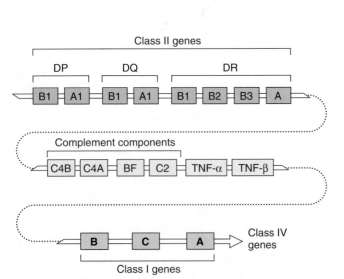

Figure 11–6. Genetic map of the major histocompatibility complex (MHC). Genes for class I and class II molecules, as well as complement components and tumor necrosis factor (TNF), are within the MHC gene complex.

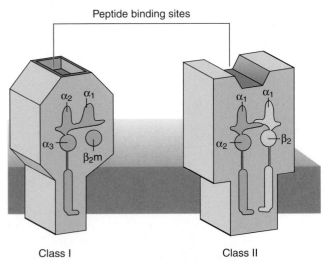

Figure 11–7. Structure of class I and class II major histocompatibility complex (MHC) molecules. The class I MHC molecules consist of two subunits, the heavy chain, and β₂-microglobulin. The binding pocket is closed at each end and can only hold peptides of 8 to 9 amino acids. Class II MHC molecules consist of two subunits, α and β, and hold peptides of 11 or more amino acids.

The class I MHC molecule presents antigenic peptides from within the cell (**endogenous**) to CD8-expressing T cells. Up-regulation of class I MHC molecules makes the cell a better target for T cell action. Some cells (brain) and some virus infections (herpes simplex virus, cytomegalovirus) down-regulate the expression of MHC I antigens to reduce their potential as targets for T cells.

Class II MHC molecules are normally expressed on antigen-presenting cells, cells that interact with CD4 T cells (e.g., macrophages, dendritic cells, B cells). The class II MHC molecules are encoded by the **DP, DQ,** and **DR** loci. The class II MHC molecules are a dimer of α and β subunits (see Figure 11-7). *Both chains of the class II MHC molecule form an open-ended peptide-binding cleft that resembles a hot dog bun and holds a peptide of 11 to 12 amino acids.* The class II MHC molecule presents ingested (**exogenous**) antigenic peptides to CD4-expressing T cells.

CD1 MHC molecules resemble MHC I molecules, have a heavy chain and a light chain (β₂-microglobulin), but bind glycolipids rather than peptides. CD1 molecules are primarily expressed on DC and present antigen to the TCR on CD8T or NKT (CD4⁻CD8⁻) cells. CD1 molecules are especially important for defense against mycobacterial infections.

Peptide Presentation by Class I and Class II MHC Molecules

Unlike antibodies that can recognize conformational epitopes, T-cell antigenic peptides must be linear epitopes. A T-cell antigen must be a peptide of 8 to 12 amino acids with a hydrophobic backbone that binds to the molecular cleft of the class I or class II MHC molecule and exposes a T-cell epitope to the TCR. Because of these constraints, there may be only one T-cell antigenic peptide in a protein. All nucleated cells proteolytically process a set of intracellular proteins and display the peptides to CD8 T cells (**endogenous route of antigen presentation**) to distinguish "self," "nonself," and the presence of intracellular infections, whereas APCs process and present phagocytized proteins to CD4 T cells (**exogenous route of antigen presentation**) (Figure 11-8). Dendritic cells can cross these routes (**cross-presentation**) to present exogenous antigen to CD8 T cells to initiate antiviral and antitumor responses.

Class I MHC molecules bind and present peptides that are degraded from cellular proteins by the **proteosome** (a protease machine) and then shuttled into the endoplasmic reticulum (ER) through the **TAP** (transporter associated with antigen processing). Most of these peptides come from misfolded or excess proteins (trash) marked by attachment of the **ubiquitin** protein. The antigenic peptide binds to the heavy chain of the class I MHC molecule. Then the MHC heavy chain can assemble properly with β₂-microglobulin, exit the ER, and proceed to the cell membrane.

During a **viral infection**, large quantities of viral proteins are produced and degraded into peptides and become the predominant source of peptides occupying the class I MHC molecules to be presented to CD8 T cells. **Transplanted cells (grafts)** express peptides on their MHC molecules, which differ from those of the host and therefore may be recognized as foreign. **Tumor cells** often express peptides derived from abnormal or embryonic proteins, which may elicit responses in the host because the host was not tolerized to these proteins. Expression of these "foreign" peptides on MHC I at the cell surface allows the T cell to "see" what is going on within the cell.

Class II MHC molecules present peptides from exogenous proteins that were acquired by macropinocytosis, pinocytosis, or phagocytosis and then degraded in lysosomes by APCs. The class II MHC protein is also synthesized in the ER but unlike MHC I, the invariant chain associates with MHC II to prevent acquisition of a peptide. MHC II acquires its antigenic peptide as a result of a merging of the vesicular transport pathway (carrying newly synthesized class II MHC molecules) and the lysosomal degradation pathway (carrying phagocytosed and proteolyzed proteins). The antigenic peptides displace a peptide from the invariant chain and associate with the cleft formed in the class II MHC protein; the complex is then delivered to the cell surface.

Cross-presentation of antigen is used by dendritic cells to present antigen to naïve CD8 T cells to initiate the response to viruses and tumor cells. After picking up antigen (including debris from apoptotic cells) in the periphery, the protein is degraded or its peptides enter the cytoplasm and are then shuttled through the TAP into the ER to bind to MHC I molecules. The DCs present the antigenic peptide to CD8 T cells in the lymph node to initiate the response.

The following analogy might aid in the understanding of antigen presentation: All cells degrade their protein "trash" and then display it on the cell surface on class I MHC trash cans. CD8 T cells "policing" the neighborhood are not alarmed by the normal, everyday peptide trash. A viral intruder would produce large amounts of viral peptide trash (e.g., beer cans, pizza boxes) displayed on class I MHC molecular garbage cans, which would alert the policing CD8 T cells. APCs (dendritic cells, macrophages, and B cells) are similar to garbage collectors or sewage workers; they gobble up the neighborhood trash or lymphatic sewage, degrade it, display it on class II MHC molecules, and then move to a lymph node to present the antigenic peptides to the CD4 T cells in the "police station." Foreign antigens would alert the CD4 T cells to release cytokines and activate an immune response.

Activation of CD4 T Cells and Their Response to Antigen

Activation of naïve T cell responses is initiated by DCs and then expanded by other APCs. CD4 helper T cells are activated by the interaction of the TCR with antigenic peptide presented by class II MHC molecules on the APC (Figures 11-9

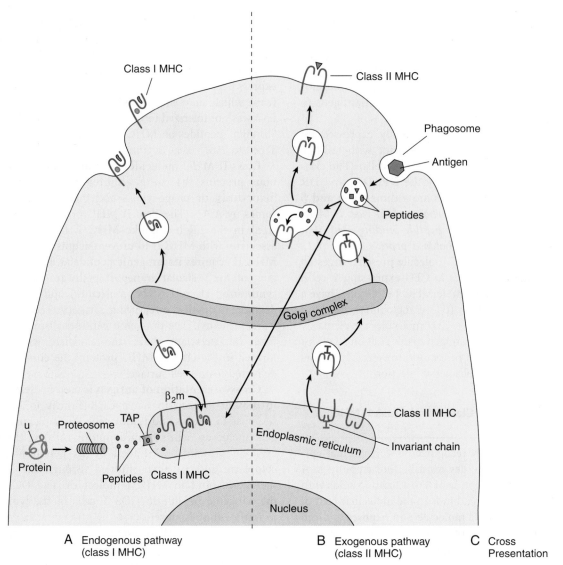

Figure 11–8. Antigen presentation. **A, Endogenous**: Endogenous antigen (produced by the cell and analogous to cell trash) is targeted by attachment of ubiquitin (u) for digestion in the proteosome. Peptides of eight to nine amino acids are transported through the TAP (transporter associated with antigen processing) into the endoplasmic reticulum (ER). The peptide binds to a groove in the heavy chain of the class I MHC molecule, and the β_2 microglobulin (β_2m) binds to the heavy chain β_2 microglobulin (β_2m). The complex is processed through the Golgi apparatus and delivered to the cell surface for presentation to CD8 T cells. **B, Exogenous**: Class II MHC molecules assemble in the ER with an invariant chain protein to prevent acquisition of a peptide in the ER. They are transported in a vesicle through the Golgi apparatus. Exogenous antigen (phagocytosed) is degraded in lysosomes, which then fuse with a vesicle containing the class II MHC molecules. The invariant chain is degraded and displaced by peptides of 11 to 13 amino acids, which bind to the class II MHC molecule. The complex is then delivered to the cell surface for presentation to CD4 T cells. **C, Cross presentation**: Exogenous antigen enters the ER of dendritic cells and is presented on MHC I molecules to CD8 T cells.

and 11-10; see also Fig 11-5). The interaction is strengthened by the binding of CD4 to the class II MHC molecule and the linkage of adhesion proteins on the T cell and the APC. A **co-stimulatory signal** is required to induce growth of the T cell as a fail-safe mechanism to ensure legitimate activation. Co-stimulatory signals are generated by the interaction of CD28 on the T cell with the B7 molecules on the macrophage, dendritic, or B cell APC and by cytokines binding to their receptors. Resting T cells require cytokine signals (e.g., IL-1, IL-2, IL-6) to initiate growth and overcome regulatory suppression of the cell. Proper activation of the helper T cell promotes production of IL-2 to promote growth of other

T cells and B cells and increase expression of IL-2Rs on the cell surface, enhancing the cell's own ability to bind and maintain activation by IL-2. Once activated, the IL-2 sustains the growth of the cell, and other cytokines influence whether the helper T cell matures into a TH1 or TH2 helper cell (see following section).

Partial activation (T-cell receptor interaction with MHC peptide) without appropriate cytokine or CD28-B7 co-stimulation leads to **anergy** (unresponsiveness) or apoptotic death (cell suicide) of the T cell. This is a mechanism for (1) eliminating self-reactive T cells in the thymus and (2) promoting the development of **tolerance** to self proteins.

11

Figure 11–9. The molecules involved in the interaction between CD4 T cells and antigen-presenting cells (APCs). The various cytokines and their direction of action are also shown. GM-CSF, granulocyte-macrophage colony-stimulating factor; ICAM-1, intercellular adhesion molecule 1, IFN-γ, interferon-γ; TNF, tumor necrosis factor. *(From Roitt I, et al: Immunology, 4th ed. St Louis, Mosby, 1996.)*

In addition, binding of the CTLA-4 co-stimulator molecule instead of CD28 on T cells with B7 on target or APC cells can result in anergy toward the antigen.

Once activated, the CD4 T cells can move into the body or to B-cell zones of the lymph nodes and spleen. Antigen presentation initiates close interactions between the T cell and APC that allow the CD40L and CD28 molecules on the T cell to bind CD40 and B7 molecules on the APC. These interactions stimulate the activation of the T cell and the APC. This interaction and the cytokines produced by the T cell will determine the function of the macrophages and DC and which immunoglobulin the B cell will produce.

CD4 T-Helper Cell Functions

The CD4 T cells start as a TH0 cell that can develop into TH0, TH1, TH2, and other TH cells with different functions, as determined by the initial dendritic cell and cytokine interactions. The different types of TH cells are defined by the cytokines they secrete and thus the responses that they induce (Figure 11-11; see Table 11-2; Table 11-4). Understanding the TH0, TH1, and TH2 division of cytokine production is the basis for understanding the generation of immune responses. All three types of T cells produce GM-CSF, IL-3, TNF-α, and some chemokines.

Figure 11–10. Dendritic cells initiate immune responses. Immature dendritic cells constantly internalize and process proteins, debris, and microbes, when present. Binding of microbial components to Toll-like receptors (TLRs) activates the maturation of the DC so that it ceases to internalize any new material, moves to the lymph node, up-regulates MHC II, B7 and B7.1 molecules for antigen presentation, and produces cytokines to activate T cells. Release of IL-6 inhibits release of TGF-β and IL-10 by T-regulatory cells. The cytokines produced by DC and its interaction with TH0 cells initiate immune responses. IL-12 and IL-2 promote TH1 responses while IL-4 promotes TH2 responses. Most of the T cells divide to enlarge the response, but some remain as memory cells. Memory cells can be activated by DC-, macrophage-, or B-cell presentation of antigen for a secondary response.

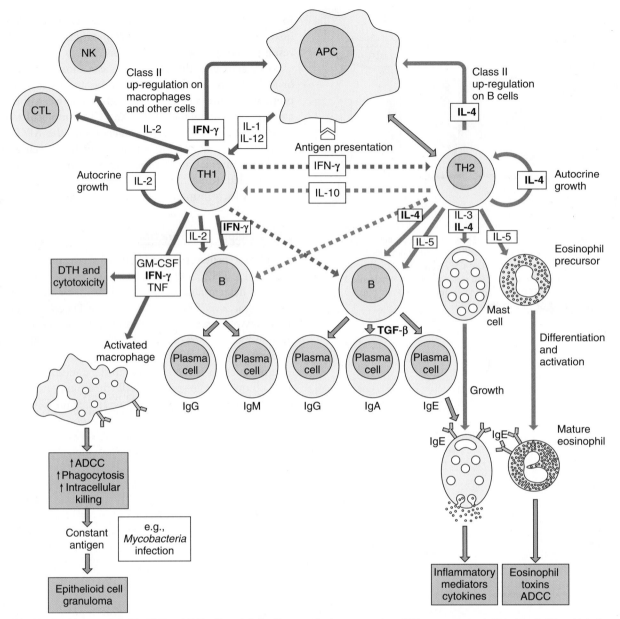

Figure 11–11. Cytokines produced by TH1 and TH2 cells and their effects on the immune system. TH1 responses are initiated by IL-12 and interferon-γ and TH2 responses by IL-4. TH1 cells promote inflammation and production of complement and macrophage-binding antibody *(solid blue lines)* and inhibit TH2 responses *(dotted blue lines)*. TH2 cells promote humoral responses *(solid red lines)* and inhibit TH1 responses *(dotted red lines)*. Colored square denotes end result. ADCC, antibody-dependent cellular cytotoxicity; APC, antigen-presenting cell; CTL, cytotoxic T cell; DTH, delayed-type hypersensitivity; GM-CSF, granulocyte-macrophage colony-stimulating factor; TNF, tumor necrosis factor.

TH0 cells have not committed to TH1 or TH2 and produce cytokines of both responses, including IL-2, IFN-γ, and IL-4. TH0 cells mature into either TH1 or TH2 cells, depending on the antigen, how it is presented, the type of APC, the concentration of antigen, and most importantly, the cytokine environment. Once activated, the TH1 and TH2 cells produce cytokines that stimulate their own growth and development (autocrine) but inhibit the development of the other type of CD4 T cell.

TH1 cells are activated by dendritic cells and the response reinforced by macrophages which produce **IL-12** and present antigen to the CD4 T cell. TH1 cells are characterized by secretion of **IL-2, IFN-γ, and TNF-β**

(lymphotoxin). These cytokines stimulate inflammatory responses and the production of IgM and specific subclasses of IgG that bind to Fc receptors on neutrophils and NK cells and can fix complement. **IFN-γ**, also known as **macrophage activation factor**, reinforces TH1 responses by promoting more IL-12 production, creating a self-sustaining cycle. TH1 cells are inhibited by IL-10, which is produced by TH2 cells. Activated TH1 cells also express the **FasL**, which can interact with **Fas** on target cells to promote apoptosis (killing) of the target cell.

The **TH1 response (1 meaning *first*)** *usually occurs first and reinforces local responses.* It often occurs early in an infection. The TH1 responses amplify local inflammatory

Table 11—4. Cytokines Produced by TH0, TH1, and TH2 Cells*

Cytokine	TH0	TH1	TH2
IFN-γ	+	++	−
IL-2	+	++	−
TNF-β (LT)	+	++	−
Chemokines	+	+	−
GM-CSF	+	++	+
TNF-α	+	++	+
IL-3	+	++	++
IL-4	+	−	++
IL-5	+	−	++
IL-6		−	++
IL-10	+	−	++

GM-CSF, granulocyte-macrophage colony-stimulating factor; IFN, interferon; IL, interleukin; LT, lymphotoxin; TNF, tumor necrosis factor; +, minor product; ++, major product; −, no product.
*The relative ability of TH0, TH1, and TH2 cells to produce different cytokines after activation.

reactions and DTH reactions by activating macrophages, NK cells, and CD8 cytotoxic T cells and also expand the immune response by stimulating growth of B and T cells with IL-2. The inflammatory responses and antibody stimulated by TH1 responses are important for eliminating intracellular infections (e.g., viruses, bacteria, and parasites) and fungi but are also associated with cell-mediated autoimmune inflammatory diseases (e.g., multiple sclerosis, Crohn disease, rheumatoid arthritis).

Reinforcement of antibacterial responses is also mediated by the TH17 cells. These are CD4 T-helper cells stimulated by IL-23 or IL-6 plus TGF-β instead of IL-12. IL-23 is in the IL-12 family of cytokines. TH17 cells make cytokines such as IL-17, IL-6, and TNF-α, associated with chronic inflammation, and proinflammatory chemokines instead of IFN-γ to promote inflammatory responses. TH17 responses would also provide protection in immunoprivileged sites, like the eye, which protect themselves against detrimental TH1 responses with TGF-β.

The **TH2 response (2 meaning *second*)** *occurs later and acts systemically.* The TH2 response occurs in the absence of an IL-12/IFN-γ signal from innate responses, and then IL-4 reinforces the continuation of TH2 responses. TH2 cell development is inhibited by IFN-γ. The TH2 response may be stimulated later in an infection, when antigen reaches the lymph nodes and is presented by DCs, macrophages, and B cells. B cells expressing specific cell surface antibody can capture, process, and present antigen to TH2 cells to initiate an antigen-specific circuit, stimulating the growth of and clonally expanding the helper T cells and B cells, which are specific for the same antigen. TH2 cells release IL-4, IL-5, IL-6, and IL-10 cytokines that promote humoral (systemic) responses. These cytokines stimulate B-cell differentiation, resulting in deletions in the immunoglobulin gene to switch from production of IgM and IgD to production of specific subtypes of IgG, IgE, or IgA. TH2 responses can limit the development of inflammatory and autoimmune diseases but can exacerbate an intracellular infection (e.g., *Mycobacterium leprae*) by prematurely shutting off protective TH1 responses.

TH3 cells are characterized by their production of IL-5 and transforming growth factor β (TGF-β), which are important for promoting B-cell differentiation to produce IgA. TH3 cells are also important for promoting immunotolerance to proteins in food. TGF-β inhibits TH1 and TH2 cell action to promote tolerance.

Treg cells expressing CD4$^+$CD25$^+$ are antigen-specific suppressor cells. These cells prevent the development of autoimmune responses by producing TGF-β and IL-10, help to keep T-cell responses under control, and promote memory cell development.

CD8 T Cells

CD8 T cells include **CTLs** and **suppressor cells**. CTLs are part of the TH1 response and are important for eliminating virally infected cells and tumor cells. CD8 T cells can also secrete TH1-like cytokines. Less is known about suppressor cells.

The CTL response is initiated when naïve CD8 cells in the lymph node are stimulated to grow by IL-2 produced by CD4 T cells and by antigen-specific activation by DCs that may be reinforced by macrophages (Figure 11-12). Presentation of the antigen may be the result of a virus infection of the APC or caused by cross-presentation of

Figure 11—12. Interactions between CD8 cytotoxic T lymphocyte (CTL) and target cells. The Fas-FasL interaction promotes apoptosis. ICAM-1, Intercellular adhesion molecule 1. (*From Roitt I, et al: Immunology, 4th ed. St Louis, Mosby, 1996.*)

an antigen acquired at the site of infection or tumor by a DC. The activated CD8 T cells divide and differentiate into mature CTLs. During a viral challenge of mice, the numbers of specific CTLs will increase up to 100,000 times. When the activated CTL finds a target cell, it binds tightly through interactions of the TCR with antigen-bearing class I MHC proteins and adhesion molecules on both cells (similar to the closing of a zipper). **Granules** containing toxic molecules, **granzymes** (**esterases**), and a pore-forming protein (**perforin**) move to the site of interaction and release their contents into the pocket (**immune synapse**) formed between the T cell and target cell. **Perforin** generates holes in the target cell membrane to allow the granule contents to enter and induce **apoptosis (programmed cell death)** in the target cell. CD8 T cells can also initiate apoptosis in target cells through the interaction of the **FasL on the T cell with the Fas protein on the target cell surface**. FasL is a member of the TNF family of proteins, and Fas is a member of the TNF receptor family of proteins. Apoptosis is characterized by degradation of the target cell DNA into discrete fragments of approximately 200 base pairs and disruption of internal membranes. The cells shrink into apoptotic bodies, which are readily phagocytosed by macrophages and dendritic cells. Apoptosis is a clean method of cell death, unlike necrosis, which signals neutrophil action and further tissue damage. TH1 CD4 T cells and NK cells also express FasL and can initiate apoptosis in target cells.

Suppressor T cells provide antigen-specific regulation of helper T cell function through inhibitory cytokines and other means. Like CTLs, suppressor T cells interact with class I MHC molecules.

NKT Cells

NKT cells are like a hybrid between NK cells and T cells. They express a natural killer cell marker, NK1.1 and an α/β TCR. Unlike other T cells, the TCR repertoire is very limited. They may express CD4, but most lack CD4 and CD8 molecules ($CD4^-CD8^-$). Like the $\gamma\delta$ TCR, the TCR of most NK T cells react with CD1 molecules, which present microbial glycolipids and glycopeptides. Upon activation, NKT cells release large amounts of IL-4 and IFN-γ. NK T cells help in the initial responses to infection and are very important for defense against mycobacterial infections.

Bibliography

Abbas AK, et al: Cellular and Molecular Immunology, 6th ed. Philadelphia, WB Saunders, 2007.

Akira S, Takeda K: Toll-like receptor signaling. Nat Rev Immunol 4:499-511, 2004.

DeFranco AL, Locksley RM, Robertson M: Immunity: The Immune Response in Infectious and Inflammatory Disease. Sunderland, Mass, Sinauer, 2007.

Janeway CA, et al: Immunobiology: The Immune System in Health and Disease, 6th ed. New York, Current Biology and Garland, 2004.

Kindt TJ, Goldsby RA, Osborne BA: Kuby Immunology, 6th ed. New York, WH Freeman, 2007.

Kumar V, Abbas AK, Fausto N: Robbins and Cotran Pathologic Basis of Disease, 7th ed. Philadelphia, Elsevier, 2005.

Sompayrac L: How the Immune System Works, 2nd ed. Malden, Mass, Blackwell Scientific, 2003.

Takeda K, Kaisho T, Akira S: Toll-like receptors. Annu Rev Immunol 21:335-376, 2003.

Trends in Immunology: Issues contain understandable reviews on current topics in immunology.

Questions

1. The importance of specific molecules can be determined through development of genetically deficient strains of mice (knockout mice) or study of human genetic deficiency diseases. Describe the immune functions that should be missing and the cell types that should be affected for the mice deficient in the following molecules:
   a. Class I MHC
   b. Class II MHC
   c. TCR-γ/δ
   d. IL-2 receptor
   e. CD4
   f. B7-1 and B7-2
   g. IFN-γ
   h. IL-1
   i. CD40L

2. The division of helper T cell responses into TH1 and TH2 subsets provides one of the most useful approaches to understanding immune responses to challenge. What would be the consequence of each of the following?
   a. Initiation of TH2 response to an intracellular infection (e.g., *Mycobacterium leprae*) before a TH1 response
   b. Uncontrolled TH1 response to a vaginal yeast infection (e.g., *Candida albicans*)
   c. Insufficient TH1 response to viral infection of a neonate as a result of low levels of IFN-γ (e.g., herpes simplex virus)
   d. Immunization with a mixture of IL-2, GM-CSF, and IFN-γ and human immunodeficiency virus glycoprotein 120 antigen, rather than the antigen alone

3. Manipulation of antigen presentation can change the subsequent immune response in ways that may enhance or inhibit the response. What would be the consequences of the following blocks to the subsequent response?
   a. Blockage of the TAP
   b. Inhibition of expression of the invariant chain
   c. Lack of β_2-microglobulin
   d. Inhibition of lysosomal proteases

Immune Responses to Infectious Agents

The previous chapters in this section introduced the different immunologic actors and their characteristics. This chapter describes the different roles they play in host protection from infection, their interactions, and the immunopathogenic consequences that may arise as a result of the response. The importance of each of the components of the host response differs for different infectious agents (Table 12-1), and their importance becomes obvious when it is genetically deficient or is blocked by chemotherapy, disease, or infection (e.g., acquired immune deficiency syndrome [AIDS]).

Human beings have three basic lines of protection against invasion by infectious agents, which are as follows:

1. **Natural barriers**, such as skin, mucus, ciliated epithelium, gastric acid, and bile, which restrict entry of the agent
2. **Innate, antigen-nonspecific immune defenses**, such as fever, interferon, complement, neutrophils, macrophages, dendritic cells, and natural killer (NK) cells, which provide rapid, local responses to challenge by an invader
3. **Adaptive, antigen-specific immune responses**, such as antibody and T cells, which specifically target, attack, and eliminate the invaders that succeed in passing the first two defenses

Barriers to Infection

The **skin** and **mucous membranes** serve as barriers to most infectious agents (Figure 12-1 and Table 12-2), with few exceptions (e.g., papillomavirus, dermatophytes ["skin-loving" fungi]). Free fatty acids produced in sebaceous glands and by organisms on the skin surface, lactic acid in perspiration, and the low pH and relatively dry environment of the skin all form unfavorable conditions for the survival of most organisms.

The mucosal epithelium covering the orifices of the body is protected by mucus secretions and cilia. For example, pulmonary airways are coated with mucus, which is continuously transported toward the mouth by ciliated epithelial cells. Large, airborne particles get caught in the mucus, whereas small particles (0.05 to 3 microns [μm]), the size of viruses or bacteria) that reach the alveoli are phagocytosed by macrophages and transported out of the airspaces. Some bacteria and viruses (e.g., *Bordetella pertussis*, influenza virus), cigarette smoke, or other pollutants can interfere with this clearance mechanism by damaging the ciliated epithelial cells, thus rendering the patient susceptible to secondary bacterial pneumonia. Antimicrobial substances (cationic peptides [**defensins**], lysozyme, lactoferrin, and secretory [IgA]) found in secretions at mucosal surfaces (e.g., tears, mucus, and saliva) also provide protection. Different defensins can disrupt bacterial, viral, and fungal membranes. Lysozyme induces lysis of bacteria by cleaving the polysaccharide backbone of the peptidoglycan of gram-positive bacteria. Lactoferrin, an iron-binding protein, deprives microbes of the free iron they need for growth.

The **acidic environment** of the stomach, bladder, and kidneys and the **bile** of the intestines inactivate many viruses and bacteria. **Urinary flow** also limits the establishment of infection.

Body temperature, and especially **fever**, limits or prevents the growth of many microbes. In addition, the immune response is more efficient at elevated temperatures.

Antibacterial Responses

Figure 12-2 illustrates the progression of protective responses to a bacterial challenge. Protection is initiated by activation of innate and inflammatory responses on a local basis and progresses to acute-phase and antigen-specific responses on a systemic scale. A summary of antibacterial responses is presented in Box 12-1.

Activation of Response

Bacterial components are excellent activators of the innate antigen-nonspecific protective and inflammatory responses

Table 12–1. Importance of Antimicrobial Defenses for Infectious Agents

	Bacteria	Intracellular Bacteria	Viruses	Fungi	Parasites
Complement	+	–	–	–	–
Interferon-α/β	–	–	++++	–	–
Neutrophils	++++	–	–	+	+
Macrophages	++	+++	++	++	+
NK cells	–	–	+++	–	–
CD4 TH1, DTH	–	++	+++	+*	+
CD8 CTL	–	++	++++	–	–
Antibody	++	+	+	+	++ (IgE)†

CTL, cytotoxic T lymphocytes; NK, natural killer.
*By activation of macrophages.
†Immunoglobulin E and mast cells are especially important for worm infections.

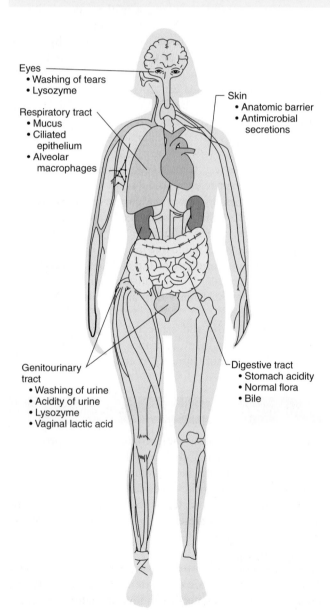

Eyes
• Washing of tears
• Lysozyme

Respiratory tract
• Mucus
• Ciliated epithelium
• Alveolar macrophages

Skin
• Anatomic barrier
• Antimicrobial secretions

Genitourinary tract
• Washing of urine
• Acidity of urine
• Lysozyme
• Vaginal lactic acid

Digestive tract
• Stomach acidity
• Normal flora
• Bile

Figure 12–1. Barrier defenses of the human body.

Table 12–2. Nonspecific Humoral Defense Mechanisms

Factor	Function	Source
Lysozyme	Catalyzes hydrolysis of bacterial peptidoglycan	Tears, saliva, nasal secretions, body fluids, lysosomal granules
Lactoferrin, transferrin	Bind iron and compete with microorganisms for it	Specific granules of PMNs
Lactoperoxidase	May be inhibitory to many microorganisms	Milk and saliva
β-Lysin	Is effective mainly against gram-positive bacteria	Thrombocytes, normal serum
Chemotactic factors	Induce directed migration of PMNs, monocytes, and other cells	Bacterial substances, products of cell injury, denatured proteins, complement, and chemokines
Properdin	Activates complement in the absence of antibody-antigen complex	Normal plasma
Cationic peptides	Disrupt membranes, block cell transport activities	Polymorphonuclear granules (defensins, etc.)

PMNs, Polymorphonuclear neutrophils (leukocytes).

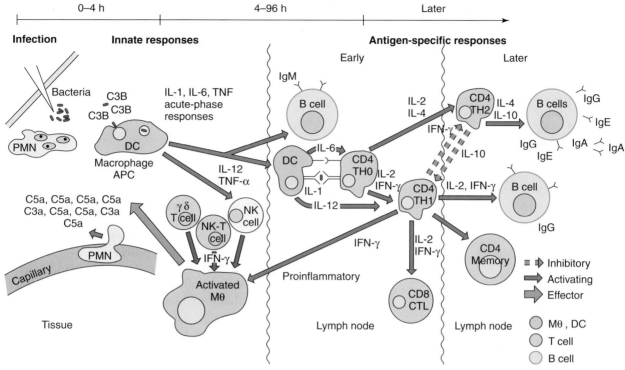

Figure 12–2. Antibacterial responses. First, innate antigen-nonspecific responses attract and promote polymorphonuclear neutrophil (PMN) and macrophage (Mθ) responses. Dendritic cells (DC) and antigen reach the lymph node to activate early immune responses (TH1 and immunoglobulin M[IgM]). Later, TH2 systemic antibody responses and memory cells are developed. The time course of events is indicated at the top of the figure. CTL, cytotoxic T lymphocyte; IFN, interferon; IL, interleukin, TNF, tumor necrosis factor.

(Box 12-2). The bacterial cell walls (teichoic acid and peptidoglycan fragments of gram-positive bacteria), and especially the lipopolysaccharide (LPS) of gram-negative bacterial cell walls contain repetitive structures that can be recognized by **pathogen-associated molecular pattern recognition (PAMP) receptors**, including the cell surface **Toll-like receptors (TLRs)** (see Table 11-1) and the cytoplasmic peptidoglycan receptors NOD1, NOD2, and cryopyrin. Binding of these PAMPs to receptors on macrophages, Langerhans cells, and dendritic cells activate kinase cascades that promote cytokine production (including IL-1, IL-6, and TNF), protective responses, and maturation of dendritic cells. **LPS (endotoxin)** binds to TLR4 and other PAMP receptors and is a very strong activator of dendritic cells, macrophages, B cells, and selected other cells (e.g., endothelial cells). NK cells, NKT, and γ/δ T cells residing in tissue also respond, produce cytokines, and reinforce cellular responses.

The **alternative complement pathway (properdin)** can be activated by teichoic acid, peptidoglycan, and LPS in the absence of antibody and, with **mannose-binding protein**, can activate the classic complement pathway. Activation of the **complement system** (see Chapter 10) is a very early and important antibacterial defense. Complement activates inflammatory responses and can also directly kill gram-negative bacteria and, to a much lesser extent, gram-positive

bacteria (the thick peptidoglycan of gram-positive bacteria shields them from lysis). Activation of the complement cascade by gram-positive or gram-negative bacteria provides the following protective factors:

1. **Chemotactic factors (C5a)** to attract neutrophils and macrophages to the site of infection
2. **Anaphylotoxins (C3a and C5a)** to stimulate mast cell release of histamine and thereby increase vascular permeability, allowing access to the infection site
3. **Opsonins (C3b)**, which bind to bacteria and promote their phagocytosis
4. A B-cell activator (C3d)

Antibody (**IgM** or **IgG**), which is present later in an infection, enhances the complement response through activation of the **classical complement cascade**.

Chemotaxis and Leukocyte Migration

Chemotactic factors produced in response to infection and inflammatory responses, such as complement components (C3a, C5a), bacterial products (e.g., formyl-methionyl-leucyl-phenylalanine [f-met-leu-phe]), and chemokines, are powerful chemoattractants for neutrophils, macrophages, and later in the response, lymphocytes. **Chemokines** are sticky proteins that establish a chemically lighted "runway"

Box 12–1. Summary of Antibacterial Responses

Complement

Alternative and lectin pathways activated by bacterial surfaces
Classic pathway activated later by antibody-antigen complexes
Production of chemotactic and anaphylotoxic proteins (C3a, C5a)
Opsonization of bacteria (C3b)
Promotion of killing of gram-negative bacteria
Activation of B cells (C3d)

Neutrophils

Important antibacterial phagocytic cell
Killing by oxygen-dependent and oxygen-independent mechanisms

Dendritic Cells

Production of cytokines and interferon (IFN)-α
Initiation of immune responses

Macrophages

Important antibacterial phagocytic cell
Killing by oxygen-dependent mechanisms
Production of interleukins IL-1, IL-6, and IL-12; tumor necrosis
   factor (TNF)-α and TNF-β, and IFN-α
Activation of acute-phase and inflammatory responses
Presentation of antigen to CD4 T cell

T Cells

γ/λ T-cell response to bacterial metabolites
Natural killer (NK)-1 T-cell response to CD1 presentation
   of mycobacterial glycolipids
TH1 CD4 responses important for bacterial, especially
   intracellular, infections
TH2 CD4 response important for antibody protections
TH17 CD4 response activates neutrophils

Antibody

Binding to surface structures of bacteria (fimbriae, lipoteichoic
   acid, capsule)
Blocking of attachment
Opsonization of bacteria for phagocytosis
Promotion of complement action
Promotion of clearance of bacteria
Neutralization of toxins and toxic enzymes

Box 12–2. Bacterial Components That Activate Protective
Responses

Direct Activation through TLRs and Other Receptors:

Lipopolysaccharide (endotoxin)
Lipoteichoic acid
Lipoarabinomannan
Glycolipids and glycopeptides
Polyanions
N-Formyl peptides (formyl-methionyl-leucyl-phenylalanine)
Peptidoglycan fragments

Chemotaxis via C3a, C5a, and Other Mechanisms:

Peptidoglycan fragments
Cell surface activation of alternative pathways of complement

---

to guide these cells to the site of an infection and also activate them. The chemokines and **tumor necrosis factor-α (TNF-α)** cause the endothelial cells lining the capillaries (near the inflammation) and the leukocytes passing by to express complementary adhesion molecules (molecular "Velcro"). The leukocytes slow, roll, attach to the lining, and then extravasate across (i.e., pass through) the capillary wall to the site of inflammation (in a process called **diapedesis**) (Figure 12-3).

Phagocytic Responses

Polymorphonuclear neutrophils (PMNs), monocytes, and occasionally eosinophils are the first cells to arrive at the site in response to infection; they are followed later by macrophages. **Neutrophils** provide a major antibacterial response and contribution to inflammation. An increased number of neutrophils in the blood, body fluids (e.g., cerebrospinal fluid), or tissue indicates a bacterial infection. The mobilization of neutrophils is accompanied by a "left shift," an increase in the number of immature **band forms** released from the bone marrow (*left* refers to the beginning of a chart of neutrophil development).

Phagocytosis of bacteria by macrophages and neutrophils involves three steps: attachment, internalization, and digestion. **Attachment of the bacteria** to the macrophage is mediated by receptors for bacterial carbohydrates (**lectins** [specific sugar-binding proteins]), fibronectin receptors (especially for *Staphylococcus aureus*), and **receptors for opsonins**, including complement (C3b), mannose-binding protein, and the Fc portion of antibody. After attachment, a section of plasma membrane surrounds the particle, which forms a **phagocytic vacuole** around the microbe. This vacuole fuses with the **primary lysosomes** (macrophages) or **granules** (PMNs) to allow inactivation and digestion of the vacuole contents.

Phagocytic killing may be oxygen dependent or oxygen independent, depending on the antimicrobial chemicals produced by the granules (Figure 12-4). Activation of macrophages is promoted by interferon-γ (IFN-γ) (best), granulocyte-macrophage colony-stimulating factor (GM-CSF), TNF-α, and lymphotoxin (TNF-β), which are produced early in the infection by NK and NKT cells or later by CD4 T cells. Activation of macrophages is required for macrophages to kill internalized microbes.

Oxygen-dependent killing is activated by a powerful oxidative burst that culminates in the formation of hydrogen peroxide and other antimicrobial substances (Box 12-3). In the neutrophil, but not the macrophage, hydrogen peroxide with **myeloperoxidase** (released by primary granules during fusion to the phagolysosome) transforms chloride ions into hypochlorous ions that kill the microorganisms. **Nitric oxide** produced by neutrophils and activated macrophages has antimicrobial activity and is also a major second messenger molecule (like cyclic adenosine monophosphate

Figure 12—3. Neutrophil diapedesis in response to inflammatory signals. Tumor necrosis factor-α (TNF-α) and chemokines activate the expression of selectins and intercellular adhesion molecules (ICAM-1) on the endothelium near the inflammation and their ligands on the neutrophil: integrins, L-selectin, and LFA-1 (leukocyte function—associated antigen). The neutrophil binds progressively tighter to the endothelium until it finds its way through the endothelium.

[cAMP]) which enhances the inflammatory and other responses.

The **neutrophil** can also mediate **oxygen-independent killing** upon fusion of the phagosome with azurophilic granules containing cationic proteins (e.g., cathepsin G) and specific granules containing lysozyme and lactoferrin. These proteins kill gram-negative bacteria by disrupting their cell membrane integrity, but they are far less effective against gram-positive bacteria, which are killed principally through the oxygen-dependent mechanism.

The neutrophils contribute to the inflammation in several ways. Prostaglandins and leukotrienes, which increase vascular permeability, are released, causing swelling (edema) and stimulating pain receptors. In addition, during phagocytosis the granules may leak their contents to cause tissue damage. The neutrophils have short lives, and dead neutrophils produce **pus**.

In addition to the tissue macrophages, **splenic macrophages** are important for clearing bacteria, especially encapsulated bacteria, from blood. Asplenic (congenitally or surgically) individuals are highly susceptible to pneumonia, meningitis, and other manifestations of *Streptococcus pneumoniae, Neisseria meningitidis,* and other encapsulated bacteria.

Cytokine-Induced Responses

LPS and other bacterial cell wall components stimulate immature dendritic cells and macrophages to release interleukins IL-1, IL-6, TNF-α, and chemokines. These cytokines are **endogenous pyrogens** because they promote **fever** production and enhance the inflammatory response by further activating macrophages and promoting the acute-phase response. The **acute-phase response** (Box 12-4) is triggered by IL-1, IL-6, TNF-α, inflammation, tissue injury,

Figure 12—4. Phagocytosis and killing of bacteria. Bacteria are bound directly or are opsonized by mannose-binding protein, immunoglobulin G (IgG) and/or C3b receptors promoting their adherence and uptake by phagocytes. Within the phagosome, oxygen-dependent and oxygen-independent mechanisms kill and degrade the bacteria. NADPH, reduced form of nicotinamide-adenine dinucleotide phosphate.

Box 12—3. Antibacterial Compounds of the Phagolysosome

Oxygen-Dependent Compounds

Hydrogen peroxide: NADPH oxidase and NADH oxidase
Superoxide
Hydroxyl radicals (•OH⁻)
Activated halides (Cl⁻, I⁻, Br⁻): myeloperoxidase (neutrophil)
Nitrous oxide

Oxygen-Independent Compounds

Acids
Lysosome (degrades bacterial peptidoglycan)
Lactoferrin (chelates iron)
Defensins and other cationic proteins (damage membranes)
Proteases, elastase, cathepsin G

prostaglandin E_2, and interferons associated with infection (Box 12-5). The acute-phase response promotes changes that support host defenses and include fever, anorexia, sleepiness, metabolic changes, and production of proteins. Acute-phase proteins that are produced and released into the serum include C-reactive protein, complement components, coagulation proteins, LPS-binding proteins, transport proteins, protease inhibitors, and adherence proteins. **C-reactive protein** complexes with the polysaccharides of numerous bacteria and fungi and activates the complement pathway, facilitating removal of these organisms from the body through greater phagocytosis. The acute-phase

proteins reinforce the innate defenses against infection, but their excessive production during sepsis (induced by endotoxin) can cause serious problems, such as shock.

Immature dendritic cells, macrophages, and other cells of the macrophage lineage play many roles in addition to the phagocytosis of bacteria and antigen (Figure 12-5), including a major role in the transition between the antigen-nonspecific and antigen-specific responses. The immature dendritic cells and macrophages produce IL-12, which activates NK cells at the site of infection and initiates the TH1 response.

γ/δ T cells in tissue and in the blood sense phosphorylated amine metabolites from some bacteria (*Escherichia coli*, mycobacteria) but not others (streptococci, staphylococci). Dendritic cells can present bacterial glycolipids to activate **NK1-T** cells. These T cells and NK cells produce IFN-γ, which activate macrophages and dendritic cells to enforce a protective TH1 cycle of cytokines and local cellular inflammatory reactions.

Acute Inflammation

Acute inflammation is an early defense mechanism to contain an infection, prevent its spread from the initial focus, and signal subsequent specific immune responses. The three major events in acute inflammation are (1) expansion of capillaries to increase blood flow (causing redness or a rash and releasing heat); (2) increase in permeability of the

Figure 12—5. The many functions of macrophages and members of the macrophage family. IL, Interleukin; TNF, tumor necrosis factor. (*From Roitt, et al: Immunology, 4th ed. St Louis, Mosby, 1996.*)

microvasculature structure to allow escape of fluid, plasma proteins, and leukocytes from the circulation (swelling or edema); and (3) recruitment of neutrophils and their accumulation and response to infection at the site of injury.

Inflammatory responses are beneficial but are associated with pain, redness, heat, and swelling and can also cause tissue damage. The mediators of inflammation are listed in Table 12-3. Tissue damage is caused to some extent by complement and macrophages but mostly by neutrophils. Dead neutrophils are a major component of **pus**. Kinins and clotting factors induced by tissue damage (e.g., factor XII [Hageman factor], bradykinin, fibrinopeptides) are also involved in inflammation. These factors increase vascular permeability and are chemotactic for leukocytes. Products of arachidonic acid metabolism also affect inflammation. Cyclooxygenase-2 (COX-2) and 5-lipooxygenase convert arachidonic acid to **prostaglandins and leukotrienes**, respectively, which can mediate essentially every aspect of acute inflammation. The course of inflammation can be followed by rapid increases in acute phase proteins, especially C-reactive protein (which can increase a thousand fold within 24 to 48 hours) and serum amyloid A.

Antigen-Specific Response to Bacterial Challenge

On ingestion of bacteria and stimulation of TLRs by bacterial components, the immature dendritic cell (iDC)

Table 12—3. Mediators of Acute and Chronic Inflammation

Action	Mediators
Acute Inflammation	
Increased vascular permeability	Histamine, bradykinin, C3a, C5a, leukotrienes, PAF, Substance P
Vasodilation	Histamine, prostaglandins, PAF, Nitric oxide
Pain	Bradykinin, prostaglandins
Leukocyte adhesion	LTB4, IL-1, TNF-α, C5a
Leukocyte chemotaxis	C5a, C3a, IL-8, Chemokines, PAF, Leukotriene B4
Acute phase response	IL-1, IL-6, TNF-α
Tissue damage	Proteases, free radicals, NO, neutrophil granule contents
Fever	IL-1, TNF, prostaglandins
Chronic Inflammation	
Activation of T cells and macrophages, and acute phase processes	T cell (IFN-γ, TNF) and macrophages (IL-1, TNF-α, IL-12) cytokines

From Novak R: Crash Course Immunology. Philadelphia, Mosby, 2006.

matures to a dendritic cell (DC), ceases to phagocytize, and moves to the lymph nodes to process and deliver their internalized antigen for presentation to T cells (see Figure 12-2; Figure 12-6). Antigenic peptides (having more than 11 amino acids) produced from phagocytosed proteins (exogenous route) are bound to class II major histocompatibility complex (MHC) molecules and presented by these antigen-presenting cells (APCs) to naïve CD4 TH0 cells. The CD4 T cells are activated by a combination of (1) antigenic peptide in the MHC II complex with the T-cell antigen receptor and CD4, (2) co-stimulatory signals provided by the interaction of CD28 molecules on the T cells with the B7 molecule on the DC, and (3) IL-1, IL-12, and other cytokines produced by the DC. In addition, IL-6 produced by the DC inhibits the production of suppressive cytokines (transforming growth factor-β [TGF-β] and IL-10) by $CD4^+CD25^+$ regulatory T cells to allow the activation of the naïve T cells. The TH0 cells produce IL-2, IFN-γ, and IL-4. Simultaneously, bacterial antigens stuck to the surface of the DC or free antigen interacts with B cells expressing surface IgM and IgD specific for the antigen and activates the cell to grow and produce IgM. Microbial cell-wall polysaccharides, especially LPS and also the C3d component of complement, activate B cells and promote the specific IgM antibody responses. Swollen lymph nodes are an indication of lymphocyte activation in response to antigenic challenge.

The conversion of TH0 cells to TH1 cells is promoted by IL-12 and reinforced by IFN-γ. **CD4 TH1 T cells** (1) promote and reinforce inflammatory responses (e.g., IFN-γ activation of macrophage) and growth of T and B cells (IL-2) to expand the immune response; and (2) promote B cells to produce complement-binding antibodies (IgM, IgG upon class-switching). These responses are important for the early phases of an antibacterial defense. TH1 responses are also essential for combating intracellular bacterial infections and mycobacteria, which are hidden from antibody. IFN-γ activates macrophage and other inflammatory processes (DTH) to kill the infected cell. Chronic stimulation of CD4 TH1 T cells by macrophages expressing microbial (mycobacterial or histoplasmic) antigen and production of IFN-γ may cause the transformation of other macrophages into epithelioid cells and giant cells, which can surround the infection and produce a granuloma. *CD8 T cells are not very important for antibacterial immunity.*

CD4 TH2 T-cell responses occur in the absence of IL-12 at more distant lymph nodes. These responses are also initiated by dendritic cells and later by the B-cell presentation of antigen. Binding of antigen to the cell surface antibody on B cells activates the B cells and also promotes uptake, processing of the antigen, and presentation of antigenic peptides on class II MHC molecules to the CD4 TH2 cell. The TH2 cell produces IL-4, IL-5, IL-6, IL-10, and IL-13, which enhance IgG production and, depending on other factors, the production of IgE or IgA. The TH2

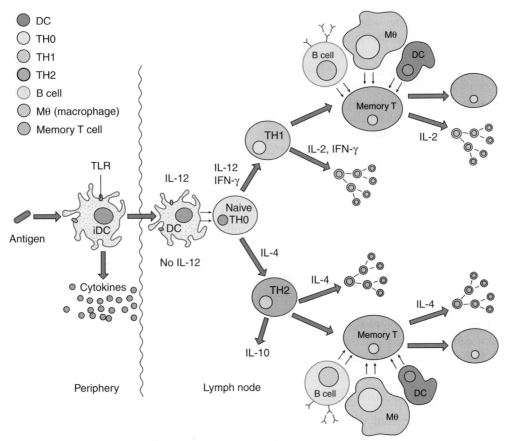

DC
TH0
TH1
TH2
B cell
Mθ (macrophage)
Memory T cell

Figure 12—6. Initiation and expansion of specific immune responses. Immature dendritic cells at the site of infection acquire bacteria and debris, bacterial components activate the cell through Toll-like receptors, and DCs mature, move to the lymph node, and present antigen to naïve T cells to initiate the antigen-specific response. During a secondary or memory response, B cells, macrophages, and DCs can present antigen to initiate the response.

response also promotes terminal differentiation of B cells to plasma-cell antibody factories. **CD4$^+$CD25$^+$ regulatory T cells** curtail both TH1 and TH2 responses and promote the development of some of the antigen-specific cells into memory T cells.

Antibodies are the primary protection against extracellular bacteria and reinfection. Antibody is important for promoting complement activation, opsonizing the bacteria for phagocytosis, blocking bacterial adhesion, and neutralizing (inactivating) exotoxins (e.g., tetanospasmin, botulinum toxin) and other cytotoxic proteins produced by bacteria (e.g., degradative enzymes). Vaccine immunization with inactivated exotoxins (toxoids) is the primary means of protection against the potentially lethal effects of exotoxins.

IgM antibodies are produced early in the antibacterial response. IgM bound to bacteria activates the classical complement cascade, promoting both the direct killing of gram-negative bacteria and the inflammatory responses. The large size of IgM limits its ability to spread into the tissue. Later in the immune response, T-cell help promotes differentiation of the B cell and immunoglobulin class switching to produce IgG. **IgG** antibodies are the predominant antibody, especially on rechallenge. IgG antibodies, except IgG4, fix complement and promote phagocytic

uptake of the bacteria through Fc receptors on macrophages. The production of **IgA** requires TH2 cytokines and other factors. IgA is the primary secretory antibody and is important for protecting mucosal membranes. Secretory IgA acquires the secretory component that promotes interaction and passage of IgA through mucosal epithelial cells. IgA neutralizes the binding of bacteria and their toxins at epithelial cell surfaces.

A primary antigen-specific response to bacterial infection takes at least 5 to 7 days. Movement of the DC to the lymph node may take 1 to 3 days, followed by activation, expansion, and maturation of the response. On rechallenge to infection, memory T cells can respond quickly to antigen presentation by DC, macrophage, or B cells, not just DC; memory B cells can respond to antigen; and the secondary response occurs within 2 to 3 days.

Bacterial Immunopathogenesis

Activation of the inflammatory and acute-phase responses can initiate significant tissue and systemic damage. Although IL-1, IL-6, and TNF-α promote protective responses to a local infection, these same responses can be life threatening when activated by systemic infection.

Activation of macrophages in the liver and spleen by endotoxin can promote release of TNF-α into the blood, causing many of the symptoms of **sepsis**, including hemodynamic failure, shock, and death (see Chapter 18). Antibodies produced against bacterial antigens that share determinants with human proteins can initiate tissue destruction (e.g., antibodies produced in poststreptococcal glomerulonephritis and rheumatic fever). Nonspecific activation of CD4 T cells by **superantigens** (e.g., toxic shock syndrome toxin of *S. aureus*) promotes the production of large amounts of cytokines and eventually the death of large numbers of T cells. The sudden, massive release of cytokines ("cytokine storm") can cause shock and severe tissue damage (e.g., toxic shock syndrome) (see Chapter 18).

Bacterial Evasion of Protective Responses

The mechanisms used by bacteria to evade host-protective responses are discussed in Chapter 18 as virulence factors. These mechanisms include: (1) the inhibition of phagocytosis and intracellular killing in the phagocyte, (2) inactivation of complement function, (3) cleavage of IgA, (4) intracellular growth (avoidance of antibody), and (5) change in bacterial antigenic appearance. Some microorganisms, including but not limited to mycobacteria (also *Listeria* and *Brucella* species), survive and multiply within macrophages and use the macrophages as a protective

reservoir or transport system to help spread the organisms throughout the body. However, cytokine-activated macrophages can kill the intracellular pathogens.

Antiviral Responses

Host Defenses against Viral Infection

The immune response is the best and in most cases the only means of controlling a viral infection (Figure 12-7). Unfortunately it is also the source of pathogenesis for many viral diseases. The humoral and cellular immune responses are important for antiviral immunity. Unlike for a bacterial infection, the ultimate goal of the immune response in a viral infection is to eliminate both the virus and the host cells harboring or replicating the virus. Interferons, NK cells, CD4 TH1 responses, and CD8 cytotoxic killer T cells are more important for viral infections than for bacterial infections. Failure to resolve the infection may lead to persistent or chronic infection or death.

Innate Defenses

Body temperature, fever, interferons, other cytokines, the mononuclear phagocyte system, and NK cells provide a local rapid response to viral infection and also activate the specific immune defenses. Often the nonspecific defenses

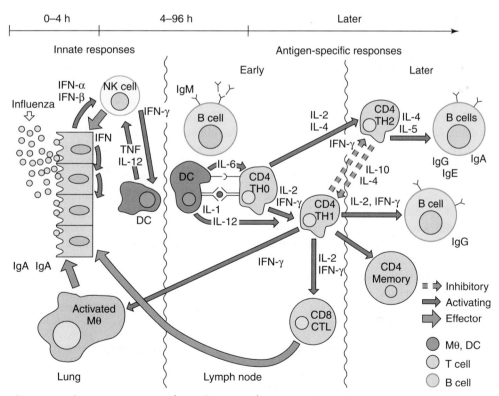

Figure 12–7. Antiviral responses. The response to a virus (e.g., influenza virus) initiates with interferon production and action and NK cells. Activation of antigen-specific immunity resembles the antibacterial response, except that CD8 cytotoxic T lymphocytes (CTLs) are important antiviral responses. The time course of events is indicated at the top of the figure. APC, antigen-presenting cell; HLA, human leukocyte antigen; IFN, interferon, Mθ, macrophage; NK, natural killer, TNF, tumor necrosis factor.

are sufficient to control a viral infection, thus preventing the occurrence of symptoms.

Viral infection can induce the release of cytokines (e.g., TNF, IL-1) and interferon from infected cells, immature dendritic cells, and macrophages. Viral RNA (especially double-stranded RNA), DNA, and some viral glycoproteins are potent activators of membrane-bound TLRs, and viral nucleic acids can also trigger cytoplasmic pathogen pattern receptors to promote these interferon and cytokine responses. These soluble protein factors trigger early local and systemic responses. Induction of fever and stimulation of the immune system are two of these systemic effects.

Body temperature and fever can limit the replication of or destabilize some viruses. Many viruses are less stable (e.g., herpes simplex virus) or cannot replicate (rhinoviruses) at 37° C or higher.

Cells of the **dendritic and mononuclear phagocyte system** phagocytose the viral and cell debris from virally infected cells. Macrophages in the liver (Kupffer cells) and spleen rapidly filter many viruses from the blood. Antibody and complement bound to a virus facilitate its uptake by macrophages (opsonization). Dendritic cells and macrophages also present antigen to T cells and release IL-1, IL-12, and IFN-α to expand the innate and initiate the antigen-specific immune responses. Activated macrophages can also distinguish and kill infected target cells.

NK cells are activated by interferon and IL-12 to kill virally infected cells. Viral infection may reduce the expression of MHC antigens or may alter the carbohydrates on cell surface proteins to provide cytolytic signals to the NK cell.

Interferon

Interferon was first described by Isaacs and Lindemann as a factor that "interferes with" the replication of many different viruses. Interferon is the body's *first* active defense against a viral infection, an "early warning system" at the local and systemic levels. *In addition to activating a target-cell antiviral defense to block viral replication, interferons activate the immune response and enhance T-cell recognition of the infected cell.* Interferon is a very important defense against infection, but it is also a cause of the systemic symptoms associated with many viral infections, such as malaise, myalgia, chills, and fever (nonspecific flulike symptoms), especially during viremia.

IFN comprises a family of proteins that can be subdivided according to several properties, including size, stability, cell of origin, and mode of action (Table 12-4). **IFN-α** and **IFN-β** are type 1 interferons that share many properties, including structural homology and mode of action. B cells, epithelial cells, monocytes, macrophages, and immature dendritic cells make **IFN-α**. Fibroblasts and other cells make **IFN-β** in response to viral infection and other stimuli. **IFN-γ** is a type 2 interferon, a cytokine produced by activated T and NK cells later in the infection. Although IFN-γ inhibits viral replication, its structure and mode of

Table 12—4. Basic Properties of Human Interferons (IFNs)

Property	IFN-α	IFN-β	IFN-γ
Previous designations	Leukocyte IFN Type I	Fibroblast IFN Type I	Immune IFN Type II
Genes	> 20	1	1
Molecular mass (Da)*			
Major subtypes	16,000-23,000	23,000	20,000-25,000
Cloned†	19,000	19,000	16,000
Glycosylation	No‡	Yes	Yes
pH 2 stability	Stable‡	Stable	Labile
Induction	Viruses	Viruses	Immune activation
Principal source	Epithelium, leukocytes	Fibroblast	Lymphocyte
Introns in gene	No	No	Yes
Homology with human IFN-α	100%	30%-50%	<10%

Data from White DO: Antiviral Chemotherapy, Interferons and Vaccines. Basel, Switzerland, Karger, 1984; Samuel CE: Virology 183:1-11, 1991.
*Molecular mass of monomeric form.
†Nonglycosylated form, as produced in bacteria by recombinant DNA technology.
‡Most subtypes but not all.

action differ from those of the other interferons. IFN-γ is also known as **macrophage activation factor** and is the defining component of the TH1 response.

The best inducer of IFN-α and IFN-β production is **double-stranded RNA (dsRNA),** *produced as the replicative intermediates of RNA viruses* or from the interaction of sense/antisense messenger RNAs (mRNAs) for some DNA viruses (Box 12-6). One dsRNA molecule per cell is sufficient to induce the production of interferon. Interaction of some enveloped viruses (e.g., herpes simplex virus and human immunodeficiency virus [HIV]) with immature dendritic cells can promote production of IFN-α. Alternatively, inhibition of protein synthesis in a virally infected cell can decrease the production of a repressor protein of the interferon gene, allowing expression of the interferon gene. Nonviral interferon inducers include the following:

1. Intracellular microorganisms (e.g., mycobacteria, fungi, protozoa)
2. Activators of certain TLRs or mitogens (e.g., endotoxins, phytohemagglutinin)
3. Double-stranded polynucleotides (e.g., poly I:C, poly dA:dT)

Box 12–6. Interferons

Induction

Double-stranded ribonucleic acid (dsRNA) (e.g., RNA virus
   intermediate)
Viral inhibition of cellular protein synthesis
Enveloped virus interaction with immature dendritic cell

Mechanism of Action

Initial infected cell releases interferon
Interferon binds to a specific cell surface receptor on another cell
Interferon induces the "antiviral state":

   Synthesis of protein kinase R (PKR), 2′,5′-oligoadenylate
      synthetase, and ribonuclease L
Viral infection of the cell activates these enzymes
Protein synthesis inhibited to block viral replication
   Degradation of mRNA (2′,5′-oligoadenylate synthase
      and RNAase L)
   Inhibition of ribosome assembly (PKR)
Initiation of innate and immune antiviral responses

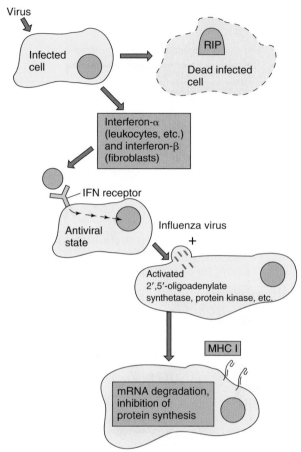

Figure 12–8. Induction of the antiviral state by interferon-α or
interferon-β. Interferon is produced in response to viral infection but
does not affect the initially infected cell. The interferon binds to a cell
surface receptor on other cells and induces production of antiviral
enzymes (antiviral state). The infection and production of double-
stranded RNA activates the antiviral activity. MHC I, major
histocompatibility antigen type 1.

4. Synthetic polyanion polymers (e.g., polysulfates,
   polyphosphates, pyran)
5. Antibiotics (e.g., kanamycin, cycloheximide)
6. Low-molecular-weight synthetic compounds (e.g.,
   tilorone, acridine dyes)

IFN-α and IFN-β can be induced and released within
hours of infection (Figure 12-8). The interferon binds to
specific receptors on the neighboring cells and induces the
production of antiviral proteins—**the antiviral state.**
However, these antiviral proteins are not activated until
they bind dsRNA. The major antiviral effects of interferon
are produced by two enzymes, **2′,5′-oligoadenylate synthetase** (an unusual polymerase) and **protein kinase R (PKR)**
(Figure 12-9), and for influenza, the **mx protein** is also
important. Viral infection of the cell and production of
dsRNA activate these enzymes and trigger a cascade of
biochemical events that leads to (1) the inhibition of protein synthesis by PKR phosphorylation of an important
ribosomal initiation factor (elongation initiation factor
2-alpha [eIF-2α]) and (2) the degradation of mRNA (preferentially, viral mRNA) by ribonuclease L, activated by
2′,5′-oligoadenosine. This process essentially puts the cellular protein synthesis factory "on strike" and prevents
viral replication. It must be stressed that interferon does
not directly block viral replication. The antiviral state lasts
for 2 to 3 days, which may be sufficient for the cell to
degrade and eliminate the virus without being killed.

Interferons stimulate cell-mediated immunity by activating effector cells and enhancing recognition of the virally
infected target cell. Interferons stimulate pre-NK cells to
differentiate to NK cells to *activate an early, local, natural
defense against infection.* Activation of macrophages by

IFN-γ promotes production of more IFN-α and IFN-β,
secretion of other biologic response modifiers, phagocytosis, recruitment, and inflammatory responses. IFN-γ
increases the expression of class II MHC antigens on the
macrophage to help promote antigen presentation to T cells.
IFN-α and IFN-β increase the expression of class I MHC
antigens, enhancing the cell's ability to present antigen and
making the cell a better target for cytotoxic T cells (CTLs).

Interferon also has widespread regulatory effects on cell
growth, protein synthesis, and the immune response. All
three interferon types block cell proliferation at appropriate
doses.

Genetically engineered recombinant interferon is being
used as an antiviral therapy for some viral infections (e.g.,
human papilloma and hepatitis C viruses). Effective treatment requires the use of the correct interferon subtype(s)
and its prompt delivery at the appropriate concentration.
The use of IFN-β for treatment of multiple sclerosis is based
on prevention of myelin basic protein presentation by DCs.
Interferons have also been used in clinical trials for the

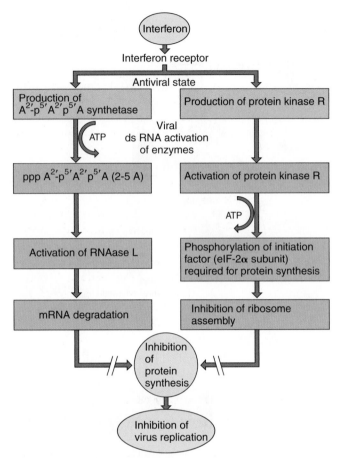

Figure 12—9. The two major routes for interferon inhibition of viral protein synthesis. One mechanism involves the induction of an unusual polymerase (2′,5′-oligoadenylate synthetase [2-5A]) that is activated by double-stranded RNA (dsRNA). The activated enzyme synthesizes an unusual adenine chain with a 2′,5′-phosphodiester linkage. The oligomer activates RNAase L that degrades messenger RNA (mRNA). The other mechanism involves the induction of protein kinase R (PKR), which prevents assembly of the ribosome by phosphorylation of the elongation initiation factor (eIF-2α) to prevent initiation of protein synthesis. ATP, adenosine triphosphate.

treatment of certain cancers. However, interferon treatment has flulike side effects, such as chills, fever, and fatigue.

Antigen-Specific Immunity

Humoral immunity and cell-mediated immunity play different roles in resolving viral infections (i.e., eliminating the virus from the body). Humoral immunity (antibody) acts mainly on extracellular virions, whereas cell-mediated immunity (T cells) is directed at the virus-producing cell (see Figure 12-7).

Humoral Immunity

Practically all viral proteins are foreign to the host and are immunogenic (i.e., capable of eliciting an antibody response). However, not all immunogens elicit protective immunity.

Antibody blocks the progression of disease through the **neutralization and opsonization** of cell-free virus. Protective antibody responses are generated toward the viral capsid proteins of naked viruses and the glycoproteins of enveloped viruses that interact with cell surface receptors (viral attachment proteins). These antibodies can neutralize the virus by preventing viral interaction with target cells or by destabilizing the virus, thus initiating its degradation. Binding of antibody to these proteins also opsonizes the virus, promoting its uptake and clearance by macrophages. Antibody recognition of infected cells can also promote antibody-dependent cellular cytotoxicity (ADCC) by NK cells. Antibodies to other viral antigens may be useful for serologic analysis of the viral infection (Box 12-7).

The major antiviral role of antibody is to prevent the spread of extracellular virus to other cells. Antibody is especially important in limiting the spread of the virus by **viremia**, preventing the virus from reaching the target tissue for disease production. Antibody is most effective at resolving cytolytic infections. Resolution occurs because the virus kills the cell factory and the antibody eliminates the extracellular virus. Antibody is the primary defense initiated by vaccination.

T-Cell Immunity

T cell-mediated immunity promotes antibody and inflammatory responses (CD4 helper T cells) and kills infected cells (cytotoxic T cells [CD4 and CD8]) (see Box 12-7). The **CD4 TH1** response is generally more important than TH2 responses for controlling a viral infection, especially noncytolytic and enveloped viruses. **CTLs** induce apoptosis on interaction of their Fas ligand protein with the Fas protein on the target cell. **CD8** killer T cells can also kill cells after their T-cell receptor binds to a viral peptide presented by a class I MHC protein. The peptides expressed on class I MHC antigens are obtained from viral proteins synthesized within the infected cell (endogenous route). *The viral protein from which these peptides are derived may not elicit protective antibody* (e.g., intracellular or internal virion proteins, nuclear proteins, improperly folded or processed proteins [cell trash]), in addition to viral glycoproteins. For example, the matrix and nucleoproteins of the influenza virus and the ICP4 (nuclear) protein of herpes simplex virus are targets for CTL lysis but do not elicit protective antibody. An **immune synapse** formed by interactions of the TCR and MHC I, the co-receptors, and adhesion molecules is formed, and **perforin**, a complement-like membrane pore-former, and granzymes (degradative enzymes) are released into this space between the CTL and target cell and induce apoptosis in the target cell.

The CD8 CTL response probably evolved as a defense against virus infection. Cell-mediated immunity is especially important for resolving infections by syncytia-forming viruses (e.g., measles, herpes simplex, and varicella-zoster viruses), which can spread from cell to cell without exposure

Immune Response to Viral Challenge

Primary Viral Challenge

12

The innate host responses are the earliest responses to viral challenge and are often sufficient to limit viral spread (see Figure 12-7). The **interferon** produced in response to most viral infections initiates the protection of adjacent cells, enhances antigen presentation by increasing the expression of MHC antigens, and initiates the clearance of infected cells by activating NK cells and antigen-specific responses. Virus and viral components released from the infected cells are phagocytosed by and activate **immature dendritic cells** to produce cytokines and then move to the lymph nodes. Macrophages in the liver and spleen are especially important for clearing virus from the bloodstream (filters). These phagocytic cells degrade and process the viral antigens. Dendritic cells present the appropriate peptide fragments bound to class II MHC antigens to CD4 T cells and can also cross-present these antigens on MHC I molecules to CD8 T cells to initiate the response. The APCs also release IL-1, IL-6, and TNF to induce fever and, with IL-12, promote activation of helper T cells and specific cytokine production (TH1 response). The activated T cells move to the site of infection and B-cell areas of the lymph node, and macrophages and B cells present antigen and become stimulated by the T cells.

Antiviral antigen-specific responses are similar to antibacterial antigen-specific responses, except that the CD8 T cell plays a more important role. **IgM** is produced approximately 3 days after infection. Its production indicates a primary infection. **IgG** and **IgA** are produced 2 to 3 days after IgM. Secretory IgA is made in response to a viral challenge of mucosal surfaces at the natural openings of the body (i.e., eyes, mouth, and respiratory and gastrointestinal systems). Activated **CD4** and **CD8** T cells are present at approximately the same time as serum IgG. During infection, the number of CD8 T cells specific for antigen may increase 50,000 to 100,000 times. The antigen-specific CD8 T cells move to the site of infection and kill virally infected cells. Recognition and binding to class I MHC viral-peptide-expressing target cells promotes apoptotic killing of the target cells, either through the release of perforin and granzymes (to disrupt the cell membrane) or through the binding of the Fas ligand with Fas on the target cell. Resolution of the infection occurs later, when sufficient antibody is available to neutralize all virus progeny or when cellular immunity has been able to reach and eliminate the infected cells. For the resolution of most enveloped and noncytolytic viral infections, TH1-mediated responses are required (in addition to antibody) to kill the viral factory.

Viral infections of the brain and the eye can cause serious damage because these tissues cannot repair tissue damage and are **immunologically privileged sites** of the body. T-cell responses are suppressed to prevent the serious

---

Box 12–7. Summary of Antiviral Responses

Interferon

Interferon is induced by double-stranded RNA, inhibition of cellular protein synthesis, or enveloped virus.
Interferon initiates the antiviral state in surrounding cells.
Interferon blocks local viral replication.
Interferon initiates systemic antiviral responses.

Natural Killer (NK) Cells

NK cells are activated by interferon-α (IFN-α) and IL-12 and activate macrophages (IFN-γ).
NK cells target and kill virus-infected cells (especially enveloped viruses).

Macrophage and Dendritic Cells

Macrophages filter viral particles from blood.
Macrophages inactivate opsonized virus particles.
Immature dendritic cells (iDCs) produce IFN-α and other cytokines.
DC initiate CD4 and CD8 T-cell response.
DC and macrophage present antigen to CD4 T cells.

T Cells

T cells are essential for controlling enveloped and noncytolytic viral infections.
T cells recognize viral peptides presented by major histocompatibility complex (MHC) molecules on cell surfaces.
Antigenic viral peptides (linear epitopes) can come from any viral protein (e.g., glycoproteins, nucleoproteins).
CD4 TH1 responses are more important than TH2 responses.
CD8 cytotoxic T cells respond to viral peptide class I MHC protein complexes on the cell surface.
CD4 TH2 responses are important for the maturation of the antibody response.
CD4 TH2 responses may be detrimental if they prematurely limit the TH1 inflammatory and cytolytic responses.

Antibody

Antibody neutralizes extracellular virus:
  It blocks viral attachment proteins (e.g., glycoproteins, capsid proteins).
  It destabilizes viral structure.
Antibody opsonizes virus for phagocytosis.
Antibody promotes killing of target cell by the complement cascade and antibody-dependent cellular cytotoxicity.
Antibody resolves lytic viral infections.
Antibody blocks viremic spread to target tissue.
IgM is an indicator of recent or current infection.
IgG is a more effective antiviral than IgM.
Secretory IgA is important for protecting mucosal surfaces.

---

to antibody; by noncytolytic viruses (e.g., hepatitis A and measles viruses); and for controlling latent viruses (herpes viruses and papillomaviruses). *CTLs kill infected cells and, as a result, eliminate the source of new virus.*

tissue destruction that accompanies inflammation. These sites depend on innate, cytokine, and antibody control of infection. If cell-mediated responses become necessary, permanent tissue damage often results.

Cell-mediated and IgG immune responses do not arise until 6 to 8 days after viral challenge. For many viral infections, this is after innate responses have controlled viral replication. However, for other viral infections, this period allows the virus to expand the infection, spread through the body and infect the target tissue, and cause disease (e.g., brain: encephalitis, liver: hepatitis). The response to the expanded infection may require a larger and more intense immune response, which often includes the immunopathogenesis and tissue damage that cause disease symptoms.

Secondary Viral Challenge

In any war, it is easier to eliminate an enemy if its identity and origin are known and if establishment of its foothold can be prevented. Similarly in the human body, prior immunity, established by prior infection or vaccination, allows rapid, specific mobilization of defenses to prevent disease symptoms, promote rapid clearance of the virus, and block viremic spread from the primary site of infection to the target tissue to prevent disease. As a result, most secondary viral challenges are asymptomatic. Antibody and memory B and T cells are present in an immune host to generate a more rapid and extensive anamnestic (booster) response to the virus. Secretory IgA is produced quickly to provide an important defense to reinfection through the natural openings of the body, but it is produced only transiently.

Host, viral, and other factors determine the outcome of the immune response to a viral infection. Host factors include genetic background, immune status, age, and the general health of the individual. Viral factors include viral strain, infectious dose, and route of entry. The time required to initiate immune protection, the extent of the response, the level of control of the infection, and the potential for immunopathology (see Chapter 48) resulting from the infection differ after a primary infection and a rechallenge.

Viral Mechanisms for Escaping the Immune Response

A major factor in the virulence of a virus is its ability to escape immune resolution. Viruses may escape immune resolution by evading detection, preventing activation, or blocking the delivery of the immune response. Specific examples are presented in Table 12-5. Some viruses even encode special proteins that suppress the immune response.

Viral Immunopathogenesis

The symptoms of many viral diseases are the consequence of cytokine action or overzealous immune responses. The flulike symptoms of influenza and any virus that establishes a viremia (e.g., arboviruses) are a result of the interferon and other cytokine responses induced by the virus. Antibody interactions with large amounts of viral antigen in blood, such as occurs with hepatitis B virus infection, can lead to immune complex diseases. The measles rash, the extensive tissue damage to the brain associated with herpes simplex virus encephalitis (-itis means "inflammation"), and the tissue damage and symptoms of hepatitis are a result of cell-mediated immune responses. The more aggressive NK-cell and T-cell responses of adults exacerbate some diseases that are benign in children, such as varicella-zoster virus, Epstein-Barr virus infectious mononucleosis, and hepatitis B infection. Yet the lack of such a response in children makes them prone to chronic hepatitis B infection because the response is insufficient to kill the infected cells and resolve the infection.

Specific Immune Responses to Fungi

The primary protective responses to fungal infection are promoted by **TH1-mediated inflammatory reactions**. Patients deficient in these responses (e.g., patients with AIDS) are most susceptible to fungal (opportunistic) infections. **Macrophages activated by IFN-γ** are important for killing the fungi. Neutrophil production of cationic proteins may be important for some fungal infections (e.g., mucormycosis), and nitric oxide may be important against *Cryptococcus* and other fungi. Antibody, as an opsonin, may facilitate clearance of the fungi.

Specific Immune Responses to Parasites

It is difficult to generalize about the mechanisms of antiparasitic immunity, because there are many different parasites that have different forms and reside in different tissue locations during their life cycles (Table 12-6). Stimulation of *CD4 TH1, CD8 T-cell, and macrophage responses are important for intracellular infections, and TH2 antibody responses are important for extracellular parasites in blood and fluids.* **IgE, eosinophil**, and **mast cell** action are especially important for eliminating worm (cestode and nematode) infections. The efficiency of control of the infection may depend on which response is initiated in the host. Initiation of a TH2 response to *Leishmania* infection results in the inhibition of protective inflammatory responses and a poor outcome. This observation provided the basis for the discovery that TH1 and TH2 responses are separate and antagonistic. Parasites have developed sophisticated mechanisms for avoiding immune clearance and often establish chronic infections.

Extracellular parasites, such as *Trypanosoma cruzi, Toxoplasma gondii*, and *Leishmania* species, are phagocytosed by **macrophage**. **Antibody** may facilitate the uptake of (opsonize) the parasites. Killing of the parasites follows

Table 12—5. Examples of Viral Evasion of Immune Responses

Mechanism	Viral Examples	Action
Humoral Response		
Hidden from antibody	Herpesviruses, retroviruses	Latent infection
	Herpes simplex virus, varicella-zoster virus, paramyxoviruses, human immunodeficiency virus	Cell-to-cell infection (syncytia formation)
Antigenic variation	Lentiviruses (human immunodeficiency virus)	Genetic change after infection
	Influenza virus	Annual genetic changes
Secretion of blocking antigen	Hepatitis B virus	Hepatitis B surface antigen
Decay of complement	Herpes simplex virus	Glycoprotein C, which binds and promotes C3 decay
Interferon		
Block production	Hepatitis B virus	Inhibition of IFN transcription
	Epstein-Barr virus	IL-10 analogue (BCRF-1) blocks IFN-γ production
Block action	Adenovirus	Inhibits up-regulation of MHC expression, VA1 blocks double-stranded RNA activation of interferon- induced protein kinase (PKR)
	Herpes simplex virus	Inactivates PKR and activates phosphatase (PP1) to reverse inactivation of initiation factor for protein synthesis
Immune Cell Function		
Impairment of dendritic cell (DC) function	Measles, hepatitis C	Induction of IFN-β, which inhibits DC function
Impairment of lymphocyte function	Herpes simplex virus	Prevention of CD8 T-cell killing
	Human immunodeficiency virus	Kills CD4 T cells and alteration of macrophages
	Measles virus	Suppression of NK, T, and B cells
Immunosuppressive factors	Epstein-Barr virus	BCRF-1 (similar to IL-10) suppression of CD4 TH1 helper T-cell responses
Decreased Antigen Presentation		
Reduced class I MHC expression	Adenovirus 12	Inhibition of class I MHC transcription 19-kDa protein (E3 gene) binds class I MHC heavy chain, blocking translocation to surface
	Cytomegalovirus	H301 protein blocks surface expression of β_2-microglobulin and class I MHC molecules
	Herpes simplex virus	ICP47 blocks TAP, preventing peptide entry into ER and binding to class I MHC molecules
Inhibition of Inflammation		
	Poxvirus, adenovirus	Blocking of action of IL-1 or tumor necrosis factor

IFN, interferon; IL, interleukin; MHC I, major histocompatibility complex, antigen type 1; NK, natural killer; PMN, polymorphonuclear neutrophil; TAP, transporter associated with antigen production.

Table 12—6. Examples of Antiparasitic Immune Responses

Parasite	Habitat	Main Host Effector Mechanism*	Method of Avoidance
Trypanosoma brucei	Bloodstream	Antibody + complement	Antigenic variation
Plasmodium species	Hepatocyte, blood cell	Antibody, cytokines (TH1)	Intracellular, antigenic variation
Toxoplasma gondii	Macrophage	O_2 metabolites, NO, lysosomal enzymes (TH1)	Inhibition of fusion with lysosomes
Trypanosoma cruzi	Many cells	O_2 metabolites, NO, lysosomal enzymes (TH1)	Escape into cytoplasm, thus avoiding digestion in lysosome
Leishmania species	Macrophage	O_2 metabolites, NO, lysosomal enzymes (TH1)	Impairment of O_2 burst and scavenging of products; avoidance of digestion
Trichinella spiralis	Gut, blood, muscle	Myeloid cells, antibody + complement (TH2)	Encystment in muscle
Schistosoma mansoni	Skin, blood, lungs, portal vein	Myeloid cells, antibody + complement (TH2)	Acquisition of host antigens, blockade by antibody; soluble antigens and immune complexes; antioxidants
Wuchereria bancrofti	Lymphatic system	Myeloid cells, antibody + complement (TH2)	Thick, extracellular cuticle; antioxidants
Helminths	Gut	IgE	Extracellular cuticle

From Roitt, et al: Immunology, 4th ed. St Louis, Mosby, 1996.
*Antibody is most important for extracellular pathogens. Cell-mediated immunity (TH1 response) is most important for intracellular pathogens.

activation of the macrophage by IFN-γ (produced by NK, γ/δ T, or CD4 TH1 cells) or TNF-α (produced by other macrophages) and induction of **oxygen-dependent killing mechanisms** (peroxide, superoxide, nitric oxide). The parasites may replicate in the macrophage and hide from subsequent immune detection unless the macrophage is activated by TH1 responses.

TH1 production of IFN-γ and activation of macrophages are also essential for defense against intracellular protozoa and for the development of **granulomas** around *Schistosoma mansoni* eggs and worms in the liver. The granuloma, formed by layers of inflammatory cells, protects the liver from toxins produced by the eggs. However, the granuloma also causes fibrosis, which interrupts the venous blood supply to the liver, leading to hypertension and cirrhosis.

Neutrophils phagocytose and kill extracellular parasites through both oxygen-dependent and oxygen-independent mechanisms. **Eosinophils** localize near parasites, bind to IgG or IgE on the surface of larvae or worms (e.g., helminths, *S. mansoni, and Trichinella spiralis*), degranulate by fusing their intracellular granules with the plasma membrane, and release the **major basic protein** into the intercellular space. The major basic protein is toxic to the parasite.

For parasitic worm infections, cytokines produced by CD4 TH2 T cells are very important for stimulating the production of IgE and the activation of mast cells (Figure 12-10). IgE bound to Fc receptors on mast cells targets the

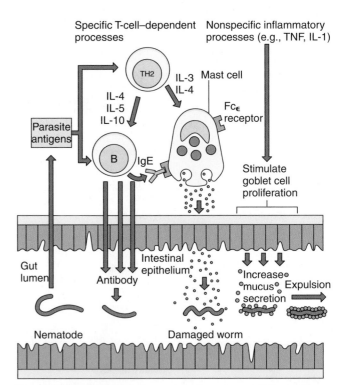

Figure 12—10. Elimination of nematodes from the gut. TH2 responses are important for stimulating the production of antibody. Antibody can damage the worm. Immunoglobulin E (IgE) is associated with mast cells, the release of histamine, and toxic substances. Increased mucus secretion also promotes expulsion. IL, interleukin; TNF, tumor necrosis factor. *(From Roitt I, et al: Immunology, 4th ed. St Louis, Mosby, 1996.)*

cells to antigens of the infecting parasite. In the lumen of the intestine, antigen binding and cross-linking of the IgE on the mast cell surface stimulate the release of histamine and substances toxic to the parasite and promote mucus secretion to coat and promote expulsion of the worm.

IgG antibody also plays an important role in antiparasitic immunity, as an opsonin and by activating complement on the surface of the parasite.

Evasion of Immune Mechanisms by Parasites

Animal parasites have developed remarkable mechanisms for establishing chronic infections in the vertebrate host (see Table 12-6). These mechanisms include intracellular growth, inactivation of phagocytic killing, release of blocking antigen (e.g., *Trypanosoma brucei*, *Plasmodium falciparum*), and development of cysts (e.g., protozoa: *Entamoeba histolytica*; helminths: *T. spiralis*) to limit access by the immune response. The African trypanosomes can reengineer the genes for their surface antigen (variable surface glycoprotein) and therefore change their antigenic appearance. Schistosomes can coat themselves with host antigens, including MHC molecules.

Other Immune Responses

Antitumor responses and **rejection of tissue transplants** are primarily mediated by T cells. CD8 cytolytic T cells recognize and kill tumors expressing peptides from embryologic proteins, mutated proteins, or other proteins on class I MHC molecules (endogenous route of peptide presentation). These proteins may be expressed inappropriately by the tumor cell, and the host immune response may not be tolerized to them. In addition, IL-2 treatment in vitro generates lymphokine-activated killer (LAK) cells and NK cells that target tumor cells, and IFN-γ-activated ("angry") macrophages can also distinguish and kill tumor cells.

T cell rejection of **allografts** used for tissue transplants is triggered by recognition of foreign peptides expressed on foreign class I MHC antigens. In addition to host rejection of the transplanted tissue, cells from the donor of a blood transfusion or a tissue transplant can react against the new host in a **graft versus host (GVH) response**. An in vitro test of T-cell activation and growth in a GVH-like response is the **mixed lymphocyte reaction**. Activation is usually measured as DNA synthesis (radioactive thymidine uptake).

Immunopathogenesis

Hypersensitivity Responses

Once activated, the immune response is sometimes difficult to control and causes tissue damage. Hypersensitivity reactions are responsible for many of the symptoms associated with microbial infections, especially viral infections. *The mediator and the time course* primarily distinguish the four types of hypersensitivity responses (Table 12-7).

Type I hypersensitivity is caused by **IgE** and is associated with **allergic, atopic**, and **anaphylactic reactions** (Figure 12-11). IgE allergic reactions are rapid-onset reactions. IgE binds to Fc receptors on mast cells and becomes the cell surface receptor for antigens (**allergens**). Cross-linking of several cell surface IgE molecules by an allergen (e.g., pollen) triggers degranulation, releasing **chemoattractants** (cytokines, leukotrienes) to attract eosinophils,

Table 12—7. Hypersensitivity Reactions

Reaction Type	Onset Time	Key Features	Beneficial Effects	Pathologic Effects
Type I	< 30 min	Soluble antigen-triggered, immunoglobulin E-dependent release of vasoactive mediators	Antiparasitic responses and toxin neutralization	Localized allergies (e.g., hay fever, asthma) Systemic anaphylaxis
Type II	< 8 h	Cell-bound antibody promoting C'-mediated cytotoxicity and ADCC	Direct lysis and phagocytosis of extracellular bacteria and other susceptible microbes	Destruction of red blood cells (e.g., transfusion reactions, Rh disease) Organ-specific tissue damage in some autoimmune diseases (e.g., Goodpasture syndrome)
Type III	< 8 h	Soluble antigen-antibody complexes activate C'	Acute inflammatory reaction at site of extracellular microbes and their clearance	Arthus reaction (localized) Serum sickness and drug reactions (generalized) Systemic autoimmune diseases
Type IV	24-72 h (acute) >1 week (chronic)	Soluble antigen presented to CD4 T cells by MHC II leads to release of TH1 cytokines, activating macrophages and cytotoxic T lymphocytes	Protection against infection by fungi, intracellular bacteria, and viruses	Acute: contact dermatitis, tuberculosis skin test Chronic: granuloma formation, graft rejection

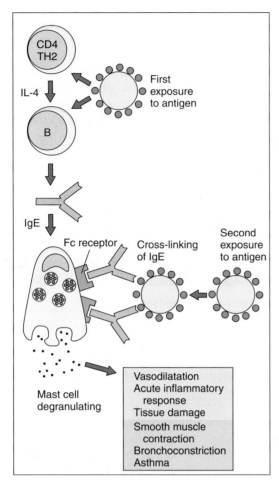

Figure 12—11. Type I hypersensitivity: immunoglobulin E (IgE)-mediated atopic and anaphylactic reactions. IgE produced in response to the initial challenge binds to Fc receptors on mast cells and basophils. Allergen binding to the cell surface IgE promotes the release of histamine and prostaglandins from granules to produce symptoms. Examples are hay fever, asthma, penicillin allergy, and reaction to bee stings. IL, interleukin.

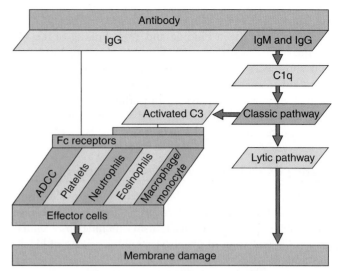

Figure 12—12. Type II hypersensitivity: mediated by antibody and complement. Complement activation promotes direct cell damage through the complement cascade and by the activation of effector cells. Examples are Goodpasture syndrome, the response to Rh factor in newborns, and autoimmune endocrinopathies. ADCC, antibody-dependent cellular cytotoxicity; Ig, immunoglobulin.

neutrophils, and mononuclear cells; **activators** (histamine, platelet-activating factor, tryptase, kininogenase) to promote vasodilation and edema; and **spasmogens** (histamine, prostaglandin D_2, leukotrienes) to directly affect bronchial smooth muscle and promote mucus secretion. Desensitization (allergy shots) produces IgG to bind the allergen and prevent allergen binding to IgE. After 8 to 12 hours, a late phase reaction develops because of the infiltration of eosinophils and CD4 TH2 cells and cytokine reinforcement of inflammation.

Type II hypersensitivity is caused by **antibody binding** to cell surface molecules and the subsequent activation of *cytolytic responses by the* **classic complement cascade** *or by cellular mechanisms* (Figure 12-12). These reactions occur as early as 8 hours following a tissue or blood transplant or as part of a chronic disease. Examples of these reactions are (1) myasthenia gravis (due to antibodies to acetylcholine receptors on neurons), (2) autoimmune hemolytic anemia, and (3) Goodpasture syndrome (lung and kidney basement membrane damage). Another example is hemolytic disease

of newborns (blue babies), which is caused by the reaction of maternal antibody generated during the first pregnancy to Rh factors on fetal erythrocytes of a second baby (Rh incompatibility).

Type III hypersensitivity responses result from activation of **complement** by **immune complexes** (Figure 12-13).

Figure 12—13. Type III hypersensitivity: immune complex deposition. Immune complexes can be trapped in the kidney and elsewhere in the body, can activate complement, and can cause other damaging responses. Examples are serum sickness, nephritis associated with chronic hepatitis B infection, and Arthus reaction.

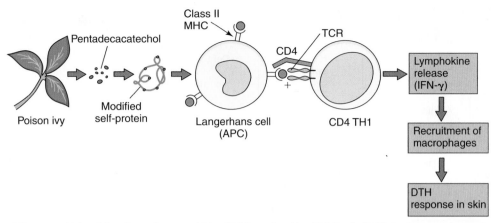

Figure 12—14. Type IV hypersensitivity: delayed-type hypersensitivity (DTH) mediated by CD4 T cells (TH1). In this case, chemically modified self-proteins are processed and presented to CD4 T cells, which release cytokines (including interferon-γ [IFN-γ]) that promote inflammation. Other examples of DTH are the tuberculin response (purified protein derivative [PPD] test) and reaction to metals such as nickel. APC, antigen-presenting cell; TCR, T-cell receptor.

In the presence of an abundance of soluble antigen in the bloodstream, large antigen-antibody complexes form, become trapped in capillaries (especially in the kidney), and then initiate the classic complement cascade. Activation of the complement cascade initiates inflammatory reactions. Immune complex disease may be caused by persistent infections (e.g., hepatitis B, malaria, staphylococcal infective endocarditis), autoimmunity (e.g., rheumatoid arthritis, systemic lupus erythematosus), or consistent inhalation of antigen (e.g., mold, plant, or animal antigens). For example, hepatitis B infection produces large amounts of hepatitis B surface antigen, which may promote formation of immune complexes that lead to glomerulonephritis. Type III hypersensitivity reactions can be induced in presensitized people by the intradermal injection of antigen to cause an **Arthus reaction**, a skin reaction characterized by redness and swelling. Serum sickness, extrinsic allergic alveolitis (a reaction to inhaled fungal antigen), and glomerulonephritis result from type III hypersensitivity reactions.

Type IV hypersensitivity responses are **TH1-mediated delayed-type hypersensitivity (DTH)** inflammatory responses (Figure 12-14 and Table 12-8). It usually takes 24 to 48 hours for antigen to be presented to **CD4 T cells** and for them to **activate macrophages** to induce the response. Although essential for the control of fungal infections and intracellular bacteria (e.g., mycobacteria), DTH is also responsible for **contact dermatitis** (e.g., cosmetics, nickel) and the response to poison ivy. Intradermal injection of **tuberculin antigen** (purified protein derivative [PPD]) elicits firm swelling that is maximal 48 to 72 hours after injection and indicative of prior exposure to *Mycobacterium tuberculosis* (Figure 12-15). **Granulomas** form in response to continued stimulation by the intracellular growth of *M. tuberculosis*. These structures consist of epithelioid cells created from chronically activated macrophages, fused epithelioid cells (multinucleated giant cells) surrounded by lymphocytes, and fibrosis caused by the deposition of collagen from fibroblasts. The granulomas restrict the spread of *M. tuberculosis* as long as CD4 T cells can provide IFN-γ. Granulomatous hypersensitivity occurs with tuberculosis, leprosy, schistosomiasis, sarcoidosis, and Crohn disease.

Table 12—8. Important Characteristics of Four Types of Delayed-Type Hypersensitivity Reactions

Type	Reaction Time	Clinical Appearance	Histologic Appearance	Antigen
Jones-Mote	24 h	Skin swelling	Basophils, lymphocytes, mononuclear cells	Intradermal antigen: ovalbumin
Contact	48 h	Eczema	Mononuclear cells, edema, raised epidermis	Epidermal: nickel, rubber, poison ivy
Tuberculin	48 h	Local induration and swelling with or without fever	Mononuclear cells, lymphocytes and monocytes, reduced macrophages	Dermal: tuberculin, mycobacterial, and leishmanial
Granulomatous	4 wk	Skin induration	Epithelioid cell granuloma, giant cells, macrophages, fibrosis with or without necrosis	Persistent antigen or antigen-antibody complexes in macrophages or "nonimmunologic" (e.g., talcum powder)

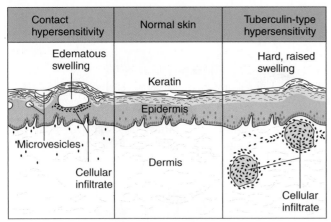

Figure 12—15. Contact and tuberculin hypersensitivity responses. These type IV responses are cell mediated but differ in the site of cell infiltration and in the symptoms. Contact hypersensitivity occurs in the epidermis and leads to the formation of blisters; tuberculin-type hypersensitivity occurs in the dermis and is characterized by swelling.

Autoimmune Responses

Normally a person is tolerized to self-antigens during the development of the immune system as a fetus and later in life by other mechanisms (e.g., oral tolerization). However, deregulation of the immune response may be initiated by cross-reactivity with microbial antigens (e.g., group A streptococcal infection, rheumatic fever), polyclonal activation of lymphocytes induced by tumors or infection (e.g., malaria, Epstein-Barr virus infection), or a genetic predisposition caused by lack of tolerization to specific antigens.

Autoimmune reactions result from the presence of autoantibodies, activated T cells, and hypersensitivity reactions. People with certain MHC antigens are at higher risk for autoimmune responses (e.g., HLA-B27 [human leukocyte antigen]: juvenile rheumatoid arthritis, ankylosing spondylitis). Evidence suggests that multiple sclerosis, an inflammatory response directed against myelin basic protein, may be triggered by immune responses to one or more viruses, such as human herpesvirus 6 or measles.

Immunodeficiency

Immunodeficiency may result from genetic deficiencies, starvation, drug-induced immunosuppression (e.g., steroid treatment, cancer chemotherapy, chemotherapeutic suppression of tissue graft rejection), cancer (especially of immune cells), or disease (e.g., AIDS) and naturally occurs in neonates and pregnant women. Deficiencies in specific protective responses put a patient at high risk for serious disease caused by infectious agents that should be controlled by that response (Table 12-9). These "natural experiments" illustrate the importance of specific responses in controlling specific infections.

Table 12—9. Infections Associated with Defects in Immune Responses

Defect	Pathogen
Induction by physical means (e.g., burns, trauma)	*Pseudomonas aeruginosa*
	Staphylococcus aureus
	Staphylococcus epidermidis
	Streptococcus pyogenes
	Aspergillus species
	Candida species
Splenectomy	Encapsulated bacteria and fungi
Granulocyte and monocyte defects in movement, phagocytosis, or killing or decreased number of cells (neutropenia)	*S. aureus*
	S. pyogenes
	Haemophilus influenzae
	Gram-negative bacilli
	Escherichia coli
	Klebsiella species
	P. aeruginosa
	Nocardia species
	Aspergillus species
	Candida species
Individual components of complement system	*S. aureus*
	Streptococcus pneumoniae
	Pseudomonas species
	Proteus species
	Neisseria species
T cells	Cytomegalovirus
	Herpes simplex virus
	Herpes zoster virus
	Human herpesvirus 8
	Listeria monocytogenes
	Mycobacterium species
	Nocardia species
	Aspergillus species
	Candida species
	Cryptococcus neoformans

Continued

Table 12–9. Infections Associated with Defects in Immune Responses—cont'd

Defect	Pathogen
	Histoplasma capsulatum
	Pneumocystis jirovecii
	Strongyloides stercoralis
B cells	Enteroviruses
	S. aureus
	Streptococcus species
	H. influenzae
	Neisseria meningitidis
	E. coli
	Giardia lamblia
	P. carinii
Combined immunodeficiency	See pathogens listed for T cells and B cells

Immunosuppression

Immunosuppressive therapy is important for reducing excessive inflammatory or immune responses or for preventing the rejection of tissue transplants by T cells. Aspirin and nonsteroidal antiinflammatory drugs (NSAIDs) target the cyclooxygenases that generate inflammatory prostaglandins (e.g., PGD_2). Other **antiinflammatory treatments** target the production and action of TNF, IL-12, and IL-1. Corticosteroids prevent their production by macrophages and may be toxic to T cells. Soluble forms of the TNF receptor and antibody to TNF can be used to block the binding of TNF and prevent its action. **Immunosuppressive therapy for transplantation** generally inhibits the action or causes the lysis of T cells. Cyclosporin, tacrolimus (FK-506), and rapamycin prevent the activation of T cells (see Fig. 11-5). Anti-CD40 ligand and anti-IL-2 prevent activation of T cells, whereas anti-CD3 promotes complement lysis of T cells to suppress T-cell responses.

Hereditary Complement Deficiencies and Microbial Infection

Inherited **deficiencies of C1q, C1r, C1s, C4, and C2** components are associated with defects in activation of the classic complement pathway that lead to greater susceptibility to pyogenic (pus-producing) staphylococcal and streptococcal infections (Figure 12-16). These bacteria are

not controlled by γ/δ T cells. A **deficiency of C3** leads to a defect in activation of both the classic and the alternative pathways, which also results in a higher incidence of pyogenic infections. **Defects of the properdin factors** impair activation of the alternative pathway, which also results in an increased susceptibility to pyogenic infections. Finally, **deficiencies of C5 through C9** are associated with defective cell killing, which raises the susceptibility to disseminated infections by *Neisseria* spp.

Defects in Phagocyte Action

People with defective phagocytes are more susceptible to bacterial infections but not to viral or protozoal infections (Figure 12-17). The clinical relevance of oxygen-dependent killing is illustrated by **chronic granulomatous disease** in children who have diminished levels of cytochrome b and fail to form superoxide anions. Although phagocytosis is normal, these children have an impaired ability to oxidize NADPH and destroy bacteria through the oxidative pathway. In patients with **Chédiak-Higashi syndrome**, the neutrophil granules fuse when the cells are immature in the bone marrow. Thus neutrophils from these patients can phagocytose bacteria but have greatly diminished ability to kill them. **Asplenic individuals** are at risk for infection with encapsulated organisms because such people lack the filtration mechanism of spleen macrophages. Other deficiencies are shown in Figure 12-17.

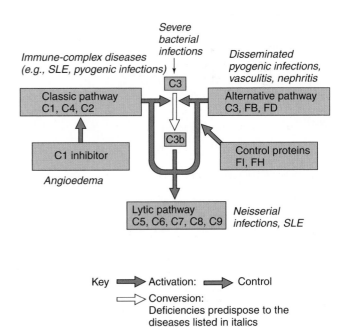

Figure 12–16. Consequences of deficiencies in the complement pathways. Factor B binds to C3b on cell surfaces, and the plasma serine protease D cleaves and activates B-C3b as part of the alternative pathway. Factors FI and FH limit the inappropriate activation of complement. FH binds to C3b and prevents activation and is a cofactor for FI. FI is a serine protease that cleaves C3b and C4b. SLE, systemic lupus erythematosus.

Figure 12—17. Consequences of phagocyte dysfunction. G6PD, glucose-6-phosphate dehydrogenase; Lad, leukocyte adhesion deficiency.

Deficiencies in Antigen-Specific Immune Responses

People deficient in **T-cell function** are susceptible to **opportunistic infections** by (1) viruses, especially enveloped and noncytolytic viruses and recurrences of viruses that establish latent infections, (2) intracellular bacteria, and (3) fungi. T-cell deficiencies can also prevent the maturation of B-cell antibody responses. T-cell deficiencies can arise from genetic disorders (e.g., X-linked immunodeficiency syndrome, Duncan disease, DiGeorge syndrome) (Table 12-10), infection (e.g., HIV and AIDS), cancer chemotherapy, or immunosuppressive therapy for tissue transplantation.

The immaturity of the immune system of **neonates** increases their susceptibility to infections resolved by TH1-associated responses, including infections by herpesviruses. Neonates are deficient in TH1 responses as a result of insufficient production of IFN-γ. Similarly the less-pronounced cell-mediated immune and inflammatory responses of **children** decrease the severity (in comparison with adults) of herpes (e.g., infectious mononucleosis, chickenpox) and hepatitis B infections but also increase the potential for the establishment of a chronic hepatitis B virus infection because of incomplete resolution. Pregnancy also induces immunosuppressive measures to prevent rejection of the fetus (a foreign tissue).

B-cell deficiencies may result in a complete lack of antibody production (hypogammaglobulinemia), inability to undergo class switching, or inability to produce specific subclasses of antibody. People deficient in antibody production are very susceptible to **bacterial infection**. IgA deficiency, which occurs in 1 of 700 Caucasians, results in a greater susceptibility to **respiratory infections**.

Table 12—10. Immunodeficiencies of Lymphocytes

Condition	T Cell No.	T-Cell Function	B Cell No.	Serum Antibodies	Incidence*
XLA, Bruton syndrome	✓	✓	↓↓	IgG, IgA, IgM↓↓	Rare
X-SCID	↓↓	↓	✓	↓	Rare
XLP, Duncan syndrome	✓	↓	✓	✓ or ↓	Rare
X-hyper IgM (CD40L mutation)	✓	↓	✓	IgG↓↓, IgA↓↓, IgM↑	Rare
Wiskott-Aldrich syndrome	✓	↓	✓	IgA↑, IgE↑, IgM↓	Rare
ADA deficiency (SCID)	↓↓	↓↓	↓	↓	Very rare
PNP deficiency (SCID)	↓	↓	✓	✓	Very rare
HLA deficiency	✓	↓	✓	Poor Ag response	Very rare
Ataxia telangiectasia	↓	↓	✓	IgE↓, IgA↓, IgG2↓	Uncommon
DiGeorge syndrome	↓↓	↓	✓	✓	Very rare
IgA deficiency	✓	✓	✓	IgA↓	Common

From Brostoff J, Male DK: Clinical Immunology: An Illustrated Outline, St Louis, Mosby, 1994.
ADA, adenosine deaminate; Ag, antigen; HLA, human leukocyte antigen; Ig, immunoglobulin; PNP, purine nucleoside phosphorylase; XLA, X-linked agammaglobulinemia; XLP, X-linked lymphoproliferative (syndrome); X-SCID, X-linked severe, combined immunodeficiency disease; ✓ = normal; ↑ = increased; ↓ = decreased or defective.
*Approximate incidence: Very rare = $<10^{-6}$; rare = 10^{-5} to 10^{-6}; common = 10^{-2} to 10^{-3}.

Questions

1. Describe the types of immune responses that would be generated to the following different types of vaccines. Consider the route of processing and presentation of the antigens and the cells and cytokines involved in generating each response.

   a. Tetanus toxoid: intramuscular injection of formalin-fixed, heat-inactivated tetanus toxin protein

   b. Inactivated polio vaccine: intramuscular injection of chemically inactivated poliovirus incapable of replication

   c. Live, attenuated measles vaccine: intramuscular injection of virus that replicates in cells and expresses antigen in cells and on cell surfaces

2. Reproduce (i.e., write out on a separate piece of paper) the following table and fill in the appropriate columns:

Immunodeficiency Disease	Immune Defect	Susceptibility to Specific Infections
Chédiak-Higashi syndrome		
Chronic granulomatous disease		
Complement C5 deficiency		
Complement C3 deficiency		
Complement C1 deficiency		
IgA deficiency		
X-linked agammaglobulinemia		
X-linked T-cell deficiency		
AIDS		
DiGeorge syndrome		
IgE deficiency		

Bibliography

Abbas AK, et al: Cellular and Molecular Immunology, 6th ed. Philadelphia, WB Saunders, 2007.

Alcami A, Koszinowski UH: Viral mechanisms of immune evasion. Trends Microbiol 8:410-418, 2000.

DeFranco AL, Locksley RM, Robertson M: Immunity: The Immune Response in Infectious and Inflammatory Disease. Sunderland, Mass, Sinauer Associates, 2007.

Janeway CA, et al: Immunobiology: The Immune System in Health and Disease, 6th ed. New York, Current Biology and Garland, 2004.

Kindt TJ, Goldsby RA, Osborne BA: Kuby Immunology, 6th ed. New York, WH Freeman, 2007.

Kumar V, Abbas AK, Fausto N: Robbins and Cotran Pathologic Basis of Disease, 7th ed. Philadelphia, Elsevier, 2005.

Male D: Immunology, 4th ed. London, Elsevier, 2004.

Mims C, et al: Medical Microbiology, 3rd ed. London, Elsevier, 2004.

Novak R: Crash Course Immunology. Philadelphia, Mosby, 2006.

Rosenthal KS: Are microbial symptoms "self-inflicted"?: The consequences of immunopathology. Infect Dis Clin Pract 13:306-310, 2005.

Rosenthal KS: Vaccines make good immune theater: Immunization as described in a three-act play. Infect Dis Clin Pract 14:35-45, 2006.

Rosenthal KS, Wilkinson JG: Flow cytometry and immunospeak. Infect Dis Clin Pract 15:183-191, 2007.

Sompayrac L: How the Immune System Works, 2nd ed. Malden, Mass, Blackwell Scientific, 2003.

Trends in Immunology: Issues contain understandable reviews on current topics in immunology.

Antimicrobial Vaccines

Immunity, whether generated in reaction to immunization or administered as therapy, can prevent or lessen the serious symptoms of disease by **blocking the spread** of a bacterium, bacterial toxin, virus, or other microbe to its target organ or by acting rapidly at the site of infection. The memory immune responses activated upon challenge of an immunized individual are faster and stronger than for an unimmunized individual. The immunization of a population, like personal immunity, stops the spread of the infectious agent by reducing the number of susceptible hosts (**herd immunity**). Immunization programs on national and international levels have achieved the following goals:

1. Protection of population groups from the symptoms of pertussis, diphtheria, tetanus, and rabies.
2. Control of the spread of measles, mumps, rubella, varicella-zoster virus, *Haemophilus influenzae* type B (Hib), and *Streptococcus pneumoniae*.
3. Elimination of wild-type poliomyelitis in the Western Hemisphere and smallpox worldwide.

In conjunction with immunization programs, measures can be taken to prevent disease by limiting the exposure of healthy people to infected people (**quarantine**) and by eliminating the source (e.g., water purification) or means of spread (e.g., mosquito eradication) of the infectious agent. Smallpox is an example of an infection that was controlled by such means. As of 1977, natural smallpox was eliminated through a successful World Health Organization (WHO) program that combined vaccination and quarantine.

Vaccine-preventable diseases still occur, however, where immunization programs (1) are unavailable or too expensive (developing countries) or (2) are neglected (e.g., the United States). An example is measles, which causes 2 million deaths annually worldwide for the first reason and outbreaks of which continue to occur in the United States for the second reason.

Types of Immunization

The injection of purified antibody or antibody-containing serum to provide rapid, temporary protection or treatment of a person is termed **passive immunization**. Newborns receive natural passive immunity from maternal immunoglobulin that crosses the placenta or is present in the mother's milk.

Active immunization occurs when an immune response is stimulated because of challenge with an immunogen, such as exposure to an infectious agent (**natural immunization**) or through exposure to microbes or their antigens in **vaccines**. On subsequent challenge with the virulent agent, a secondary immune response is activated that is faster and more effective at protecting the individual, or antibody is present to block the spread or function of the agent.

Passive Immunization

Passive immunization may be used as follows:

1. To prevent disease after a known exposure (e.g., needlestick injury with blood that is contaminated with hepatitis B virus)
2. To ameliorate the symptoms of an ongoing disease
3. To protect immunodeficient individuals
4. To block the action of bacterial toxins and prevent the diseases they cause (i.e., as therapy)

Immune serum globulin preparations derived from seropositive humans or animals (e.g., horses) are available as prophylaxis for several bacterial and viral diseases (Table 13-1). Human serum globulin is prepared from pooled plasma and contains the normal repertoire of antibodies for an adult. Special high-titer immune globulin preparations are available for hepatitis B virus (HBIg), varicella-zoster virus (VZIg), rabies (RIg), and tetanus (TIg). Human immunoglobulin is preferable to animal immunoglobulin

Table 13—1. Immune Globulins Available for Postexposure Prophylaxis*

Disease	Source
Hepatitis A	Human
Hepatitis B	Human
Measles	Human
Rabies	Human[†]
Chickenpox, varicella-zoster	Human[†]
Cytomegalovirus	Human
Tetanus	Human,[†] equine
Botulism	Equine
Diphtheria	Equine

*Immune globulins to other agents may also be available.
[†]Specific high-titer antibody is available and is the preferred therapy.

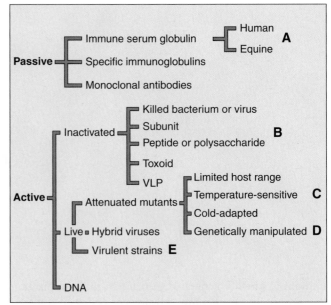

Figure 13—1. Types of immunizations. Antibodies (passive immunization) can be provided to block the action of an infectious agent, or an immune response can be elicited (active immunization) by natural infection or vaccination. The different forms of passive and active immunization are indicated. **A,** Equine antibodies can be used if human antibody is not available. **B,** Vaccine can consist of components purified from the infectious agent or can be developed through genetic engineering (VLP [virus-like protein]). **C,** Vaccine selected by passage in animals, embryonated eggs, or tissue culture cells. **D,** Deletion, insertion, reassortment, and other laboratory-derived mutants. **E,** Vaccine composed of a virus from a different species, which has a common antigen with the human virus.

because there is little risk of a hypersensitivity reaction (serum sickness).

Monoclonal antibody preparations are being developed for protection against various agents and diseases. In addition to infectious diseases, monoclonal antibodies are being used as therapy to block overzealous cytokine responses in inflammation and sepsis and for other therapies.

Active Immunization

The term *vaccine* is derived from vaccinia virus, a less virulent member of the poxvirus family that is used to immunize people against smallpox. Classical vaccines can be subdivided into two groups on the basis of whether they elicit an immune response on infection (**live vaccines** such as vaccinia) or not (**inactivated-subunit-killed vaccines**) (Figure 13-1). Deoxyribonucleic acid (**DNA**) **vaccines** represent a new means of immunization. In this approach, plasmid DNA is injected into muscle or skin, then taken up by dendritic, muscle, or macrophage cells, which express the gene for the immunogen as if for a natural infection. DNA vaccination stimulates T-cell immune responses, which can be boosted with antigen to elicit mature antibody responses.

Inactivated Vaccines

Inactivated vaccines utilize a large amount of antigen to produce a protective antibody response but without the risk of infection by the agent. Inactivated vaccines can be produced by chemical (e.g., formalin) or heat inactivation of bacteria, bacterial toxins, or viruses or by purification or synthesis of the components or subunits of the infectious agents.

These vaccines are usually administered with an **adjuvant**, which boosts their immunogenicity by enhancing uptake by or stimulating DCs and macrophages. Many adjuvants stimulate TLRs to activate these antigen-presenting cells. Most vaccines are precipitated onto alum to promote the slow release of antigen and uptake by DCs and macrophages. MF59 (squalene microfluidized in an oil and water emulsion) and monophosphoryl lipid A (MPL) are adjuvants used in some newer vaccines. Other adjuvants include emulsions, virus-like particles, liposomes (defined lipid complexes), bacterial cell wall components, molecular cages for antigen, and polymeric surfactants. Attenuated forms of cholera toxin and *Escherichia coli* lymphotoxin are potent adjuvants for secretory antibody (immunoglobulin [Ig] A) after intranasal or oral immunization.

Inactivated rather than live vaccines are used to confer protection against most bacteria and viruses that cannot be attenuated, may cause recurrent infection, or have oncogenic potential. Inactivated vaccines are generally safe, except in people who have allergic reactions to vaccine components. For example, many antiviral vaccines are produced in eggs and therefore cannot be administered to people who are allergic to eggs. The disadvantages of inactivated vaccines are listed below and compared to live vaccines in Table 13-2.

Table 13–2. Advantages and Disadvantages of Live versus Inactivated Vaccines

Property	Live	Inactivated
Route of administration	Natural* or injection	Injection
Dose of virus, cost	Low	High
Number of doses	Single†	Multiple
Need for adjuvant	No	Yes‡
Duration of immunity	Long-term	Short-term
Antibody response	IgG, IgA§	IgG
Cell-mediated immune response	Good	Poor
Heat lability in tropics	Yes‖	No
Interference¶	Occasional	None
Side effects	Occasional mild symptoms#	Occasional sore arm
Reversion to virulence	Rarely	None

From White DO, Fenner FJ: Medical Virology, 3rd ed. New York, Academic, 1986.
Ig, Immunoglobulin.
*Oral or respiratory, in certain cases.
†A single booster may be required (yellow fever, measles, rubella) after 6 to 10 years.
‡However, the commonly used alum is inefficient.
§IgA if delivered via the oral or respiratory route. Oral polio vaccine can prevent wild-type poliovirus from multiplying in the gut.
‖Magnesium chloride and other stabilizers and cold storage assist preservation.
¶Interference from other viruses or diseases.
#Especially rubella and measles.

1. Immunity is not usually lifelong.
2. Immunity may be only humoral and not cell-mediated (TH2).
3. The vaccine does not elicit a local IgA response.
4. Booster shots are required.
5. Larger doses must be used.

There are three major types of inactivated bacterial vaccines: **toxoid** (inactivated toxins), **inactivated (killed)** bacteria, and **capsule or protein subunits** of the bacteria. The bacterial vaccines currently available are listed in Table 13-3. Most antibacterial vaccines protect against the pathogenic action of toxins.

Inactivated viral vaccines are available for **polio, hepatitis A, influenza, and rabies**, among other viruses. The Salk polio vaccine (inactivated poliomyelitis vaccine, or **IPV**) is prepared through the formaldehyde inactivation of virions. In the past, a rabies vaccine was prepared by means of formalin inactivation of infected rabbit neurons or duck embryos. Now, however, it is prepared through the chemical inactivation of virions grown in human diploid tissue culture cells. Because of the slow course of rabies, the vaccine can be administered immediately after a person is exposed to the virus and still elicit a protective antibody response.

A **subunit vaccine** consists of the bacterial or viral components that elicit a protective immune response. Surface structures of bacteria and the viral attachment proteins (capsid or glycoproteins) elicit protective antibodies. T-cell epitopes may also be included in a subunit vaccine. The immunogenic component can be isolated from the bacterium, virus, or virally infected cells by biochemical means, or the vaccine can be prepared through genetic engineering by the expression of cloned viral genes in bacteria or eukaryotic cells. For example, the hepatitis B virus subunit vaccine was initially prepared from surface antigen obtained from human sera of chronic carriers of the virus. Today HBV vaccine is purified from yeast bearing the HBsAg gene. The antigen is purified, chemically treated, and absorbed onto alum to be used as a vaccine. The subunit proteins used in the HBV and the human papilloma virus vaccines form virus-like particles (**VLP**) which are more immunogenic than individual proteins.

The inactivated influenza vaccine consists of a mixture of strains of viruses grown in embryonated eggs and then inactivated or their protein subunits (hemagglutinin and neuraminidase). Tissue culture cell-derived and genetically engineered vaccines are in development. The vaccine is formulated annually to elicit protection from the virus strains predicted to threaten the population in the coming year.

Vaccines against *Haemophilus influenzae* B, *Neisseria meningitidis*, *Salmonella typhi*, and *Streptococcus pneumoniae* are prepared from capsular polysaccharides. Unfortunately polysaccharides are generally poor immunogens (T-independent antigens). The meningococcal vaccine contains the polysaccharides of four major serotypes (A, C, Y, and W-135). The pneumococcal vaccine contains polysaccharides from 23 serotypes. The immunogenicity of polysaccharides can be enhanced by chemical linkage to a protein carrier (conjugate vaccine) (e.g., diphtheria toxoid, *N. meningitidis* outer membrane protein, or *Corynebacterium diphtheriae* protein) (Figure 13-2). The *H. influenzae* B (Hib) polysaccharide—diphtheria toxoid carrier complex is approved for administration to infants and children. An *S. pneumoniae* "pneumococcal" conjugate vaccine has been developed in which polysaccharide from the seven most prevalent strains in the United States is attached to a nontoxic form of the diphtheria toxin. This vaccine is available for use in infants and young children. The other polysaccharide vaccines are less immunogenic and should be administered to individuals older than 2 years.

Live Vaccines

Live vaccines are prepared with organisms limited in their ability to cause disease (e.g., **avirulent** or **attenuated** organisms). Live vaccines are especially useful for protection

Table 13–3. Bacterial Vaccines*

Bacteria (Disease)	Vaccine Components	Who Should Receive Vaccinations
Corynebacterium diphtheriae (diphtheria)	Toxoid	Children and adults
Clostridium tetani (tetanus)	Toxoid	Children and adults
Bordetella pertussis (pertussis)	Killed cell or acellular	Children
Haemophilus influenzae B (Hib)	Capsule polysaccharide; capsule polysaccharide–protein conjugate	Children
Neisseria meningitidis A and C (meningococcal disease)	Capsule polysaccharide	People at high risk (e.g., those with asplenia), travelers to epidemic areas (e.g., military personnel), children
Streptococcus pneumoniae (pneumococcal disease; meningitis)	Capsule polysaccharides; capsule polysaccharide–protein conjugate	People at high risk (e.g., those with asplenia), children, the elderly
Vibrio cholerae (cholera)	Killed cell	Travelers at risk to exposure
Salmonella typhi (typhoid)	Killed cell; polysaccharide	Travelers at risk to exposure, household contacts, sewage workers
Bacillus anthracis (anthrax)	Killed cell	Handlers of imported fur, military personnel
Yersinia pestis (plague)	Killed cell	Veterinarians, animal handlers
Francisella tularensis (tularemia)	Live attenuated	Animal handlers in endemic areas
Coxiella burnetii (Q fever)	Inactivated	Sheep handlers, laboratory personnel working with *C. burnetii*
Mycobacterium tuberculosis (TB)	Live attenuated bacille Calmette-Guérin (*Mycobacterium bovis*)	Not recommended in United States

Listed in order of frequency of use.

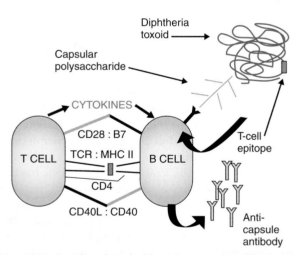

Figure 13–2. Capsular polysaccharide conjugate vaccines. Capsular polysaccharides are poor immunogens, do not elicit T-cell help, and only elicit IgM without memory. Capsule polysaccharide conjugated to a protein (e.g., diphtheria toxoid) binds to surface antipolysaccharide IgM on the B cell, the complex is internalized, processed and then a peptide is presented on MHC II to CD4 T cells. The T cells become activated, produce cytokines, and promote immunoglobulin class switching for the polysaccharide specific B cell. The B cell can become activated, make IgG, and memory cells will develop.

against infections caused by enveloped viruses, which require T-cell immune responses for resolution of the infection. Immunization with a live vaccine resembles the natural infection in that the immune response progresses through the natural innate, TH1, and then TH2 immune responses, and humoral, cellular, and memory immune responses are developed. Immunity is generally long lived and, depending on the route of administration, can mimic the normal immune response to the infecting agent. However, the following list includes three problems with live vaccines:

1. The vaccine virus may still be dangerous for immunosuppressed people or pregnant women, who do not have the immunologic resources to resolve even a weakened virus infection.
2. The vaccine may revert to a virulent viral form.
3. The viability of the vaccine must be maintained.

Live bacterial vaccines include the orally administered live, attenuated *S. typhi* strain (Ty2la) vaccine for typhoid; the Calmette-Guérin bacillus vaccine for tuberculosis, which consists of an attenuated strain of *Mycobacterium bovis;* and an attenuated tularemia vaccine. A combination of antibody and cell-mediated immune responses elicited by a live vaccine may be required against intracellularly growing bacteria. The Calmette-Guérin bacillus vaccine is not used in the United States because people vaccinated with it show a false-positive reaction to the purified protein derivative (PPD) test, which is the screening test used to control tuberculosis in the United States.

Live virus vaccines consist of less virulent mutants (**attenuated**) of the wild-type virus, viruses from other species that share antigenic determinants (vaccinia for smallpox, bovine or monkey rotavirus), or genetically engineered viruses lacking virulence properties (see Figure 13-1). Wild-type viruses are attenuated by growth in embryonated eggs or tissue culture cells at nonphysiologic temperatures (32° C to 34° C) and away from the selective pressures of the host immune response. These conditions **select** for or allow the growth of viral strains (mutants) that (1) are less virulent because they grow poorly at 37° C (**temperature-sensitive strains** [e.g., measles vaccine] and cold-adapted strains); (2) do not replicate well in any human cell (**host-range mutants**); (3) cannot escape immune control; or (4) can replicate at a benign site but do not disseminate, bind, or replicate in the target tissue characteristically affected by the disease (e.g., polio vaccine replicates in the gastrointestinal tract but does not reach or infect the brain). Table 13-4 lists examples of attenuated live virus vaccines currently in use.

The first vaccine—that for smallpox—was developed by Edward Jenner. The idea for the vaccine came to him when he noted that cowpox (vaccinia), a virulent virus from

Table 13—4. Viral Vaccines*

Virus	Vaccine Components	Who Should Receive Vaccinations
Polio	Inactivated (inactivated polio vaccine, Salk vaccine)	Children
	Attenuated (oral polio vaccine, Sabin vaccine)	Children
Measles	Attenuated	Children
Mumps	Attenuated	Children
Rubella	Attenuated	Children
Varicella-zoster	Attenuated	Children
Rotavirus	Human-bovine hybrids	Infants
Human papilloma virus (HPV)	Virus-like particle (VLP)	Girls aged 9-26
Influenza	Inactivated	Adults, especially medical personnel and the elderly
	Attenuated (nasal spray)	5-50 yr
Hepatitis B	Subunit (VLP)	Newborns, health care workers, high-risk groups (e.g., sexually promiscuous, intravenous drug users)
Hepatitis A	Inactivated Live (China)	Children, child-care workers, travelers to endemic areas, Native Americans and Alaskans
Adenovirus	Attenuated	Military personnel
Yellow fever	Attenuated	Travelers at risk to exposure, military personnel
Rabies	Inactivated	Anyone exposed to virus Preexposure: veterinarians, animal handlers
Smallpox	Live vaccinia virus	Protection from bioterrorism
Japanese encephalitis	Inactivated	Travelers at risk to exposure
Eastern and Western equine encephalitis, Russian spring-summer encephalitis	Inactivated	Military personnel

Listed in order of frequency of use.

another species that shares antigenic determinants with smallpox, caused benign infections in humans but conferred protective immunity against smallpox. In addition, a mixture of genetic reassortant human and bovine rotaviruses are the basis for the current vaccine administered to protect infants against human rotavirus.

Albert Sabin developed the first live **oral polio vaccine (OPV)** in the 1950s. The attenuated virus vaccine was obtained by multiple passage of the three types of poliovirus through monkey kidney tissue culture cells. At least 57 mutations accumulated in the polio type 1 vaccine strain. When this vaccine is administered orally, IgA is secreted in the gut and IgG in the serum, providing protection along the normal route of infection by the wild-type virus. This vaccine is inexpensive, easy to administer, and relatively stable. The vaccination program has been so successful that wild-type polio has been eliminated in the Western Hemisphere. Unfortunately, because of the risk of vaccine-virus-induced polio disease, the IPV rather than the OPV is used for routine well-baby immunizations (see Figure 13-2).

Live vaccines for measles, mumps, rubella (administered together as the MMR vaccine), **varicella-zoster**, and now **influenza** have been developed. Protection against these infections require a potent cellular immune response. To elicit a mature T-cell response, the vaccine must be administered after 1 year of age, when there will be no interference by maternal antibodies. A killed measles vaccine proved to be a failure because it conferred an incomplete immunity that induced more serious symptoms (atypical measles) on challenge with wild-type measles virus than the symptoms associated with the natural infection.

The initial live measles vaccine consisted of the Edmonston B strain, which was developed by Enders and colleagues. This virus underwent extensive passage at 35° C through primary human kidney cells, human amnion cells, and chicken embryo cells. The currently used Moraten (United States) and Schwarz (other countries) vaccine strains of measles were obtained by further passage of the Edmonston B strain in chick embryos at 32° C.

The mumps vaccine (Jeryl Lynn strain) and rubella vaccine (Wistar RA 27/3) viruses were also attenuated by extensive passage of the virus in cell culture. The varicella-zoster vaccine uses the Oka strain, an attenuated virus. The varicella-zoster vaccine is administered along with the MMR vaccine, or a stronger version is administered to adults to prevent zoster (shingles).

A new live influenza vaccine is administered nasally within a mist. Unlike the previous inactivated vaccine, T- and B-cell responses and mucosal immunity are elicited by this vaccine.

Future Directions for Vaccination

Molecular biology techniques are being used to develop new vaccines. New live vaccines can be created by genetic engineering mutations to inactivate or delete a virulence gene instead of through random attenuation of the virus by passage through tissue culture. Genes from infectious agents that cannot be properly attenuated can be inserted into safe viruses (e.g., vaccinia, canarypox) to form **hybrid virus vaccines** (see Figure 54-3). This approach holds the promise of allowing the development of a polyvalent vaccine to many agents in a single, safe, inexpensive, and relatively stable vector. On infection, the hybrid virus vaccine need not complete a replication cycle but simply promote the expression of the inserted gene to initiate an immune response to the antigens. The vaccinia and canarypox virus vector systems have been used in several experimental hybrid vaccines and are used to immunize forest animals against rabies. Other vectors that have been considered are attenuated retroviruses, adenovirus, and herpes simplex virus.

Genetically engineered **subunit vaccines** are being developed through cloning of genes that encode immunogenic proteins into bacterial and eukaryotic vectors. The greatest difficulties in the development of such vaccines are (1) identifying the appropriate subunit or peptide immunogen that can elicit protective antibody and, ideally, T-cell responses and (2) presenting the antigen in the correct conformation. Once identified, the gene can be isolated, cloned, and expressed in bacteria or yeast cells, and then large quantities of these proteins can be produced. Genes for protective immunogens, such as the surface antigen of hepatitis B (*in use*), the L protein of HPV 6, 11, 16, and 18 (*in use*), the envelope protein gp120 of the human immunodeficiency virus (HIV), the hemagglutinin of influenza, the G antigen of rabies, and the glycoprotein D of herpes simplex virus, have been cloned, and their proteins have been generated in bacteria or eukaryotic cells for use (or potential use) as subunit vaccines.

Peptide subunit vaccines consist of *specific epitopes* of microbial proteins that elicit neutralizing antibody or desired T-cell responses. To generate such a response, the peptide must contain sequences that bind to MHC I or MHC II (class I or class II major histocompatibility complex) proteins on dendritic cells for presentation and recognition by T cells to initiate an immune response. The immunogenicity of the peptide can be enhanced by its covalent attachment to a carrier protein (e.g., tetanus toxoid or keyhole limpet hemocyanin [KLH]) or an immunologic peptide that can specifically present the epitope to the appropriate immune response. Better vaccines are being developed as the mechanisms of antigen presentation and T-cell receptor—specific antigens are better understood.

Anti-idiotype antibodies are also being investigated as potential vaccines. Such antibodies recognize the variable region of a monoclonal antiviral antibody, which is like a cast of the viral epitope. The anti-idiotype antibody resembles the original viral epitope, as if it were molded in the cast. Immunization with an anti-idiotype antibody or the viral peptide would therefore elicit the production of similar antibodies.

Adjuvants in addition to alum are being developed to enhance the immunogenicity and direct the response of vaccines to a TH1 or TH2 type of response. These include activators of Toll-like receptors, such as the oligodeoxynucleotide CpG, derivatives of Lipid A from lipopolysaccharide, cytokines, liposomes, etc. Use of MF59 in a new influenza vaccine allows reduction in the amount of antigen required to elicit protective immunity.

DNA vaccines offer great potential for immunization against infectious agents that require T-cell responses but are not appropriate for use in live vaccines. For these vaccines, the gene for a protein that elicits protective responses is cloned into a plasmid that allows the protein to be expressed in eukaryotic cells. The naked DNA is injected into the muscle or skin of the vaccine recipient, where the DNA is taken up by cells, the gene is expressed, and the protein is produced, presented to, and activates T-cell responses. DNA vaccines usually require a boost with antigenic protein to produce antibody.

With the advent of new technology, it should be possible to develop vaccines against infectious agents such as *Streptococcus mutans* (to prevent tooth decay), the herpesviruses, HIV, and parasites such as *Plasmodium falciparum* (malaria) and *Leishmania*. In fact, it should be possible to produce a vaccine to almost any infectious agent once the appropriate protective immunogen is identified and its gene isolated.

Immunization Programs

An effective vaccine program can save millions of dollars in health care costs. Such a program not only protects each vaccinated person against infection and disease but also reduces the number of susceptible people in the population, thereby preventing the spread of the infectious agent within the population. Although immunization may be the best means of protecting people against infection, vaccines cannot be developed for all infectious agents. One reason is that it is very time consuming and costly to develop

---

Box 13–1. Properties of a Good Candidate for Vaccine Development

Organism causes significant illness.
    Organism exists as only one serotype.
    Antibody blocks infection or systemic spread.
    Organism does not have oncogenic potential.
    Vaccine is heat stable, so that it can be transported to
      endemic areas.

Box 13–2. Problems with Vaccine Use

Live vaccine can occasionally revert to virulent forms.
Interference by other organisms may prevent the infection produced by a live virus vaccine; for example, rubella prevents replication of poliovirus.
Vaccinating an immunocompromised person with a live vaccine can be life threatening. Side effects to vaccination can occur; these include hypersensitivity and allergic reactions to the antigen, to nonmicrobial material in the vaccine, and to contaminants (e.g., eggs).
Vaccine development and liability insurance for the manufacturer are very expensive with limited profit.
Microbes with many serotypes are difficult to control with vaccination.

---

vaccines. Box 13-1 lists the considerations that are weighed in the choice of a candidate for a vaccine program.

Natural smallpox was eliminated by means of an effective vaccine program because it was a good candidate for such a program; the virus existed in only one serotype, symptoms were always present in infected people, and the vaccine was relatively benign and stable. However, its elimination came about only as the result of a concerted, cooperative effort on the part of the WHO and local health agencies worldwide. Rhinovirus is an example of a poor candidate for vaccine development, because the viral disease is not serious and there are too many serotypes for vaccination to be successful. Practical aspects of and problems with vaccine development are listed in Box 13-2.

From the standpoint of the individual, the ideal vaccine should elicit dependable, lifelong immunity to infection without serious side effects. Factors that influence the success of an immunization program include not only the composition of the vaccine but also the timing, site, and conditions of its administration.

The recommended schedules of vaccinations for children are given in Figure 13-3. Tables of recommended schedules for vaccination of children, teens, adults, and for special cases are provided annually by the Advisory Committee on Immunization Practices (ACIP) of the Centers for Disease Control. **Booster immunizations** of inactivated vaccines and the live measles vaccine are required later in life. Women under the age of 26 years should receive the human papilloma vaccine, and college students should receive the meningococcal vaccine or a booster. Adults should be immunized with vaccines for *S. pneumoniae* (pneumococcus), influenza, rabies, hepatitis B virus, and other diseases, depending on their jobs, the type of traveling they do, and other risk factors that may make them particularly susceptible to specific infectious agents. Further discussion of each of the vaccines is presented with the disease they prevent.

Vaccine ▼ Age ▶	Birth	1 month	2 months	4 months	6 months	12 months	15 months	18 months	19-23 months	2-3 years	4-6 years
Hepatitis B	HepB	HepB				HepB					
Rotavirus			Rota	Rota	Rota						
Diphtheria, tetanus, pertussis			DTaP	DTaP	DTaP		DTaP				DTaP
Haemophilus influenzae type B			Hib	Hib	Hib	Hib					
Pneumococcal			PCV	PCV	PCV	PCV				PPV	
Inactivated poliovirus			IPV	IPV	IPV						IPV
Influenza					Influenza (yearly)						
Measles, mumps, rubella						MMR					MMR
Varicella						Varicella					Varicella
Hepatitis A						HepA (2 doses)				Hep A series	
Meningococcal										MSV4	

☐ Range of recommended ages   ☐ Certain high-risk groups

Figure 13—3. Recommended childhood immunization schedule from the Centers for Disease Control and Prevention. Vaccines are listed at the ages routinely recommended for their administration. Bars indicate the range of acceptable ages for vaccination. For example, hepatitis B vaccine should be administered to children at 11 to 12 years of age who have not been previously vaccinated; varicella-zoster virus vaccine should be administered to children who were not previously vaccinated and who lack a reliable history of chickenpox. Diphtheria and tetanus toxoids and acellular pertussis vaccines; tetanus and diphtheria toxoids, absorbed, for adult use. DTaP, diphtheria and tetanus; HepA, hepatitis A; HepB, hepatitis B; Hib, haemophilus influenzae type B; IPV, inactivated poliovirus; MMR, measles, mumps, and rubella; MSV4, meningococcal; PCV, pneumococcal conjugate; PPV, pneumococcal polysaccharide; Rota, rotavirus. (From the Centers for Disease Control and Prevention Advisory Committee on Immunization Practices: http://www.cdc.gov/nip/acip.)

Questions

1. Why is an inactivated rather than a live vaccine used for the following immunizations: rabies, influenza, tetanus, hepatitis B virus, *H. influenzae* B, diphtheria, polio, and pertussis?

2. Tetanus is treated with passive immunization and prevented by active immunization. Compare the nature and function of each of these therapies.

3. The inactivated polio vaccine is administered intramuscularly, whereas the live polio vaccine is administered as an oral vaccine. How do the course of the immune response and the immunoglobulins produced in response to each vaccine differ? What step in poliovirus infection is blocked in a person vaccinated by each vaccine?

4. Why have large-scale vaccine programs not been developed for rhinovirus, herpes simplex virus, and respiratory syncytial virus?

5. Describe the public or personal health benefits that justify the development of the following major vaccine programs: measles, mumps, rubella, polio, smallpox, tetanus, and pertussis.

Bibliography

Advisory Committee on Immunization Practices (ACIP): Statements available online at www.cdc.gov/nip/acip

Centers for Disease Control and Prevention (CDC): Immunization information page available online at www.cdc.gov

National Coalition for Adult Immunization online at www.nfid.org/ncai/

Plotkin SA, Orenstein WA: Vaccines, 4th ed. Philadelphia, WB Saunders, 2004.

Rosenthal KS: Vaccines make good immune theater: Immunization as described in a three-act play. Infect Dis Clin Pract 14:35-45, 2006.

Rosenthal KS, Zimmerman DH: Vaccines: All things considered. Clin Vaccine Immunol 13:821-829, 2006.

Vaccination information statements available online at www.immunize.org/vis

Vaccines: National Institute of Allergy and Infectious Diseases (NIAID) fact sheet available online at www.niaid.nih/gov/publications/vaccine.htm

World Health Organization: Diseases and vaccines fact sheet available online at www.who.int/vaccines-diseases/index.html

General Principles of Laboratory Diagnosis

Microscopic Principles and Applications

The true complexity of our surroundings was not appreciated until the first microbes were observed through the lens of a microscope. Indeed, the use of microscopy has helped define the relationships among a diversity of organisms, ranging from the smallest viruses consisting of a few proteins and minimal genetic information to multicellular parasites almost 10 meters long.

In general, microscopy is used in microbiology for two basic purposes: the initial detection of microbes and the preliminary or definitive identification of microbes. The microscopic examination of clinical specimens is used to detect bacterial cells, fungal elements, parasites (eggs, larvae, or adult forms), and viral inclusions present in infected cells. Characteristic morphologic properties can be used for the preliminary identification of most bacteria and are used for the definitive identification of many fungi and parasites. The microscopic detection of organisms stained with antibodies labeled with fluorescent dyes or other markers has proved to be very useful for the specific identification of many organisms. Five general microscopic methods are used (Box 14-1).

Microscopic Methods

Brightfield (Light) Microscopy

The basic components of light microscopes consist of a light source used to illuminate the specimen positioned on a stage, a condenser used to focus the light on the specimen, and two lens systems (**objective lens** and **ocular lens**) used to magnify the image of the specimen. In brightfield microscopy, the specimen is visualized by transillumination, with light passing up through the condenser to the specimen. The image is then magnified, first by the objective lens, then by the ocular lens. The total magnification of the image is the product of the magnifications of the objective and ocular lenses. Three different objective lenses are commonly used: low power (10-fold magnification), which can be used to scan a specimen; high dry (40-fold), which is used to look for large microbes such as parasites and filamentous fungi; and oil immersion (100-fold), which is used to observe bacteria, yeasts (single-cell stage of fungi), and the morphologic details of larger organisms and cells. Ocular lenses can further magnify the image (generally 10-fold to 15-fold).

The limitation of brightfield microscopy is the resolution of the image (i.e., the ability to distinguish that two objects are separate and not one). The **resolving power** of a microscope is determined by the wavelength of light used to illuminate the subject and the angle of light entering the objective lens (referred to as the **numerical aperture**). The resolving power is greatest when oil is placed between the objective lens (typically the 100× lens) and the specimen because oil reduces the dispersion of light. The best brightfield microscopes have a resolving power of approximately 0.2 μm, which allows most bacteria but not viruses to be visualized. Although most bacteria and larger microorganisms can be seen with brightfield microscopy, the **refractive indices** of the organisms and background are similar. Thus organisms must be stained with a dye so they can be observed, or an alternative microscopic method must be used.

Darkfield Microscopy

The same objective and ocular lenses used in brightfield microscopes are used in darkfield microscopes; however, a special **condenser** is used that prevents transmitted light from directly illuminating the specimen. Only oblique, scattered light reaches the specimen and passes into the lens systems, which causes the specimen to be brightly illuminated against a black background. The advantage of this method is that the resolving power of darkfield microscopy is significantly improved compared with that of brightfield microscopy (i.e., 0.02μm versus 0.2 μm), which makes it possible for extremely thin bacteria, such as *Treponema pallidum* (etiologic agent of syphilis) and *Leptospira* spp. (leptospirosis), to be detected. The disadvantage of this method is

---

Box 14–1. Microscopic Methods

Brightfield (light) microscopy
Darkfield microscopy
Phase-contrast microscopy
Fluorescent microscopy
Electron microscopy

---

that because light passes around rather than through organisms, their internal structure cannot be studied.

Phase-Contrast Microscopy

Phase-contrast microscopy enables the internal details of microbes to be examined. In this form of microscopy, as parallel beams of light are passed through objects of different densities, the wavelength of one beam moves out of "phase" relative to the other beam of light (i.e., the beam moving through the more dense material is retarded more than the other beam). Through the use of **annular rings** in the condenser and the objective lens, the differences in phase are amplified so that in-phase light appears brighter than out-of-phase light. This creates a three-dimensional image of the organism or specimen, which permits more detailed analysis of the internal structures.

Fluorescent Microscopy

Some compounds called **fluorochromes** can absorb short-wavelength ultraviolet or ultrablue light and emit energy at a higher visible wavelength. Although some microorganisms show natural fluorescence (**autofluorescence**), fluorescent microscopy typically involves staining organisms with fluorescent dyes and then examining them with a specially designed fluorescent microscope. The microscope uses a high-pressure mercury, halogen, or xenon vapor lamp that emits a shorter wavelength of light than that emitted by traditional brightfield microscopes. A series of filters are used to block the heat generated from the lamp, eliminate infrared light, and select the appropriate wavelength for exciting the fluorochrome. The light emitted from the fluorochrome is then magnified through traditional objective and ocular lenses. Organisms and specimens stained with fluorochromes appear brightly illuminated against a black background, although the colors vary depending on the fluorochrome selected. The contrast between the organism and background is great enough that the specimen can be screened rapidly under low magnification and then the material examined under higher magnification once fluorescence is detected.

Electron Microscopy

Unlike other forms of microscopy, **magnetic coils** (rather than lenses) are used in electron microscopes to direct a beam of electrons from a tungsten filament through a specimen and onto a screen. Because a much shorter wavelength of light is used, magnification and resolution are improved dramatically. Individual viral particles (as opposed to viral inclusion bodies) can be seen with electron microscopy. Samples are usually stained or coated with metal ions to create contrast. There are two types of electron microscopes: **transmission electron microscopes**, in which electrons such as light pass directly through the specimen, and **scanning electron microscopes**, in which electrons bounce off the surface of the specimen at an angle, and a three-dimensional picture is produced.

Examination Methods

Clinical specimens or suspensions of microorganisms can be placed on a glass slide and examined under the microscope (i.e., direct examination of a wet mount). Although large organisms and cellular material can be seen using this method, analysis of the internal detail is often difficult. Phase-contrast microscopy can overcome some of these problems; alternatively, the specimen or organism can be stained by a variety of methods (Table 14-1).

Direct Examination

Direct-examination methods are the simplest for preparing samples for microscopic examination. The sample can be suspended in water or saline (**wet mount**), mixed with alkali to dissolve background material (**potassium hydroxide [KOH] method**), or mixed with a combination of alkali and a contrasting dye (e.g., **lactophenol cotton blue, iodine**). The dyes nonspecifically stain the cellular material, increasing the contrast with the background, and permit examination of the detailed structures. A variation is the **India ink method**, in which the ink darkens the background rather than the cell. This method is used to detect capsules surrounding organisms, such as the yeast *Cryptococcus* (the dye is excluded by the capsule, creating a clear halo around the yeast cell), and is a rapid method for the preliminary detection and identification of this important fungus.

Differential Stains

A variety of differential stains are used to stain specific organisms or components of cellular material. The **Gram stain** is the best known and most widely used stain and forms the basis for the phenotypic classification of bacteria. Yeasts can also be stained with this method (yeasts are gram-positive). The **iron hematoxylin** and **trichrome** stains are invaluable for the identification of protozoan parasites, and the **Wright-Giemsa** stain is used to identify blood parasites and other selected organisms. Stains such as methenamine silver and toluidine blue O have largely been replaced by more sensitive or technically easier differential or fluorescent stains.

Table 14—1. Microscopic Preparations and Stains Used in the Clinical Microbiology Laboratory

Staining Method	Principle and Applications
Direct Examination	
Wet mount	Unstained preparation examined by brightfield, darkfield, or phase-contrast microscopy.
10% KOH	KOH used to dissolve proteinaceous material and facilitate detection of fungal elements that are not affected by strong alkali solution. Dyes such as lactophenol cotton blue can be added to increase contrast between fungal elements and background.
India ink	Modification of KOH procedure in which ink is added as contrast material. Dye primarily used to detect *Cryptococcus* spp. in cerebrospinal fluid and other body fluids. Polysaccharide capsule of *Cryptococcus* spp. excludes ink, creating halo around yeast cell.
Lugol iodine	Iodine is added to wet preparations of parasitology specimens to enhance contrast of internal structures. Facilitates differentiation of protozoa and host white blood cells.
Differential Stains	
Gram stain	Most commonly used stain in microbiology laboratory, forming basis for separating major groups of bacteria (e.g., gram-positive, gram-negative). After fixation of specimen to glass slide (by heating or alcohol treatment), specimen is exposed to crystal violet, and then iodine is added to form complex with primary dye. During decolorization with alcohol or acetone, complex is retained in gram-positive bacteria but lost in gram-negative organisms; counterstain safranin is retained by gram-negative organisms (hence their red color). Degree to which organism retains stain is function of organism, culture conditions, and staining skills of microscopist.
Iron hematoxylin stain	Used for detection and identification of fecal protozoa. Helminth eggs and larvae retain too much stain and are more easily identified with wet-mount preparation.
Methenamine silver	Generally performed in histology laboratories rather than in microbiology laboratories. Used primarily for detection of fungal elements in tissue, although other organisms, such as bacteria, can be detected. Silver staining requires skill, because nonspecific staining can render slides unable to be interpreted.
Toluidine blue O stain	Used primarily for detection of *Pneumocystis* organisms in respiratory specimens. Cysts stain reddish-blue to dark purple on light blue background. Background staining is removed by sulfation reagent. Yeast cells stain and are difficult to distinguish from *Pneumocystis* cells. Trophozoites do not stain. Many laboratories have replaced this stain with specific fluorescent stains.
Trichrome stain	Alternative to iron hematoxylin for staining protozoa. Protozoa have bluish-green to purple cytoplasms with red or purplish-red nuclei and inclusion bodies; specimen background is green.
Wright-Giemsa stain	Used to detect blood parasites, viral and chlamydial inclusion bodies, and *Borrelia*, *Toxoplasma*, *Pneumocystis*, and *Rickettsia* spp. Polychromatic stain that contains mixture of methylene blue, azure B, and eosin Y. Giemsa stain combines methylene blue and eosin. Eosin ions are negatively charged and stain basic components of cells orange to pink, whereas other dyes stain acidic cell structures various shades of blue to purple. Protozoan trophozoites have red nucleus and grayish-blue cytoplasm; intracellular yeasts and inclusion bodies typically stain blue; rickettsiae, chlamydiae, and *Pneumocystis* spp. stain purple.
Acid-Fast Stains	
Ziehl-Neelsen stain	Used to stain mycobacteria and other acid-fast organisms. Organisms are stained with basic carbol fuchsin and resist decolorization with acid-alkali solutions. Background is counterstained with methylene blue. Organisms appear red against light blue background. Uptake of carbol fuchsin requires heating specimen (hot acid-fast stain).
Kinyoun stain	Cold acid-fast stain (does not require heating). Same principle as Ziehl-Neelsen stain.
Auramine-rhodamine	Same principle as other acid-fast stains, except that fluorescent dyes (auramine and rhodamine) are used for primary stain, and potassium permanganate (strong oxidizing agent) is the counterstain and inactivates unbound fluorochrome dyes. Organisms fluoresce yellowish-green against black background.
Modified acid-fast stain	Weak decolorizing agent is used with any of three acid-fast stains listed. Whereas mycobacteria are strongly acid-fast, other organisms stain weaker (e.g., *Nocardia*, *Rhodococcus*, *Tsukamurella*, *Gordonia*, *Cryptosporidium*, *Isospora*, *Sarcocystis*, and *Cyclospora*). These organisms can be stained more efficiently by using weak decolorizing agent. Organisms that retain this stain are referred to as partially acid-fast.

Continued

Table 14–1. Microscopic Preparations and Stains Used in the Clinical Microbiology Laboratory—cont'd

Staining Method	Principle and Applications
Fluorescent Stains	
Acridine orange stain	Used for detection of bacteria and fungi in clinical specimens. Dye intercalates into nucleic acid (native and denatured). At neutral pH, bacteria, fungi, and cellular material stain reddish-orange. At acid pH (4.0), bacteria and fungi remain reddish-orange, but background material stains greenish-yellow.
Auramine-rhodamine stain	Same as acid-fast stains.
Calcofluor white stain	Used to detect fungal elements and *Pneumocystis* spp. Stain binds to cellulose and chitin in cell walls; microscopist can mix dye with KOH. (Many laboratories have replaced traditional KOH stain with this stain.)
Direct fluorescent antibody stain	Antibodies (monoclonal or polyclonal) are complexed with fluorescent molecules. Specific binding to an organism is detected by presence of microbial fluorescence. Technique has proved useful for detecting or identifying many organisms (e.g., *Streptococcus pyogenes*, *Bordetella*, *Francisella*, *Legionella*, *Chlamydia*, *Pneumocystis*, *Cryptosporidium*, *Giardia*, influenza virus, herpes simplex virus). Sensitivity and specificity of the test are determined by the number of organisms present in the test sample and quality of antibodies used in reagents.

KOH, potassium hydroxide.

Acid-Fast Stains

At least three different acid-fast stains are used, each exploiting the fact that some organisms retain a primary stain even when exposed to strong decolorizing agents such as mixtures of acids and alcohols. The **Ziehl-Neelsen** is the oldest method used but requires heating the specimen during the staining procedure. Many laboratories have replaced this method with either the cold acid-fast stain (**Kinyoun method**) or the fluorochrome stain (**auramine-rhodamine method**). The fluorochrome method is the stain of choice because a large area of the specimen can be examined rapidly by simply searching for fluorescing organisms against a black background. Some organisms are "partially acid-fast," retaining the primary stain only when they are decolorized with a weakly acidic solution. This property is characteristic of only a few organisms (see Table 14-1), making it quite valuable for their preliminary identification.

Fluorescent Stains

The auramine-rhodamine acid-fast stain is a specific example of a fluorescent stain. Numerous other fluorescent dyes have also been used to stain specimens. For example, the **acridine orange stain** can be used to stain bacteria and fungi, and **calcofluor white** stains the chitin in fungal cell walls. Although the acridine orange stain is rather limited in its applications, the calcofluor white stain has

replaced the potassium hydroxide stains. Another procedure is the examination of specimens with specific antibodies labeled with fluorescent dyes (**fluorescent antibody stains**). The presence of fluorescing organisms is a rapid method for both the detection and identification of the organism.

Questions

1. Explain the principles underlying brightfield, darkfield, phase-contrast, fluorescent, and electron microscopy. Give one example in which each method would be used.
2. List examples of direct microscopic examinations, differential stains, acid-fast stains, and fluorescent stains.

Bibliography

Chapin K: Principles of stains and media. In Murray P, et al (eds): Manual of Clinical Microbiology, 9th ed. Washington, DC, ASM Press, 2007.
Murray P, Shea Y: ASM Pocket Guide to Clinical Microbiology, 3rd ed. Washington, DC, ASM Press, 2004.
Wiedbrauk D: Microscopy. In Murray P, et al (eds): Manual of Clinical Microbiology, 9th ed. Washington, DC, ASM Press, 2007.
Zimbro M, Power D: Difco and BBL Manual: Manual of Microbiological Culture Media. Sparks, Md, Becton Dickinson, 2003.

15

In Vitro Culture: Principles and Applications

The foundation of microbiology was established in 1676 when Anton van Leeuwenhoek, using one of his early microscopes, observed bacteria in water. It was not until almost 200 years later that Pasteur was able to grow bacteria in the laboratory in a culture medium consisting of yeast extract, sugar, and ammonium salts. In 1881 Hesse used agar from his wife's kitchen to solidify the medium, which then permitted the growth of macroscopic colonies of bacteria. Over the years, microbiologists and cooks have returned to the kitchen to create hundreds of culture media that are now routinely used in all clinical microbiology laboratories. Although tests that rapidly detect microbial antigens and nucleic-acid-based molecular assays have replaced culture methods for the detection of many organisms, the ability to grow microbes in the laboratory remains an important procedure in all clinical labs. For many diseases, the ability to grow a specific organism from the site of infection is the definitive method to identify the cause of the infection.

The success of culture methods is defined by the biology of the organism, the site of the infection, the patient's immune response to the infection, and the quality of the culture media. The bacterium *Legionella* is an important respiratory pathogen; however, it was never grown in culture until it was recognized that recovery of the organism required using media supplemented with iron and L-cysteine. *Campylobacter*, an important enteric pathogen, was not recovered in stool specimens until highly selective media were incubated at 42° C in a microaerophilic atmosphere. *Chlamydia*, an important bacterium responsible for sexually transmitted diseases, is an obligate intracellular pathogen that must be grown in living cells. *Staphylococcus aureus*, the cause of staphylococcal toxic shock syndrome, produces disease by release of a toxin into the circulatory system. Culture of blood will almost always be negative, but culture of the site where the organism is growing will detect the organism. In many infections (e.g., gastroenteritis, pharyngitis,

urethritis) the organism responsible for the infection will be present with many other organisms that are part of the normal microbial population at the site of infection. Many media have been developed that suppress the normally present microbes and allow easier detection of clinically important organisms. The patient's innate and adaptive immunity may suppress the pathogen, so highly sensitive culture techniques are frequently required. Likewise, some infections are characterized by the presence of relatively few organisms (e.g., most septic patients have fewer than one organism per ml of blood), so the use of enrichment broths is frequently necessary. Finally, the quality of the media must be carefully monitored to demonstrate it will perform as designed.

Relatively few laboratories prepare their own media today. Most is produced by large commercial companies with expertise in media production. Although this has obvious advantages, it also means that most media are not "freshly produced." Although this is generally not a problem, it can impact on the recovery of some fastidious organisms (e.g., *Bordetella pertussis*). Thus laboratories that perform sophisticated testing frequently have the ability to make a limited amount of specialized media. Dehydrated formulations of most media are available so this can be accomplished with minimal difficulties. Please refer to the references in the Bibliography for additional information about the preparation and quality control of media.

Types of Culture Media

Culture media can be subdivided into four general categories: (1) enriched nonselective media, (2) selective media, (3) differential media, and (4) specialized media (Table 15-1). Some examples of these media are summarized below.

Table 15—1. Types of Culture Media

Type	Media (examples)	Purpose
Nonselective	Blood agar	Recovery of bacteria and fungi
	Chocolate agar	Recovery of bacteria, including *Haemophilus* and *Neisseria gonorrhoeae*
	Mueller-Hinton agar	Bacterial susceptibility test medium
	Thioglycolate broth	Enrichment broth for anaerobic bacteria
	Sabouraud dextrose agar	Recovery of fungi
Selective, differential	MacConkey agar	Selective for gram-negative bacteria; differential for lactose-fermenting species
	Mannitol salt agar	Selective for staphylococci; differential for *S. aureus*
	Xylose lysine deoxycholate agar	Selective, differential agar for *Salmonella* and *Shigella* in enteric cultures
	Lowenstein-Jensen medium	Selective for mycobacteria
	Middlebrook agar	Selective for mycobacteria
	CHROMagar	Selective, differential for yeast
	Inhibitory mold agar	Selective for molds
Specialized	Buffered charcoal yeast extract (BCYE) agar	Recovery of *Legionella* and *Nocardia*
	Cystine-tellurite agar	Recovery of *Corynebacterium diphtheriae*
	Lim broth	Recovery of *Streptococcus agalactiae*
	MacConkey sorbitol agar	Recovery of *Escherichia coli* O157
	Regan Lowe agar	Recovery of *Bordetella pertussis*
	Thiosulfate citrate bile salts sucrose (TCBS) agar	Recovery of *Vibrio* species

Enriched Nonselective Media

These media are designed to support the growth of most organisms without fastidious growth requirements. The following are some of the more commonly used media:

Blood agar. Many types of blood agar media are used in clinical laboratories. The media contain two primary components: (1) a basal medium (e.g., tryptic soy, brain heart infusion, *Brucella* base) and (2) blood (e.g., sheep, horse, and rabbit). Various other supplements can also be added to extend the range of organisms that can grow on the media.

Chocolate agar. This is a modified blood agar medium. When blood or hemoglobin is added to the heated basal media, it turns brown (hence the name). This medium supports the growth of most bacteria, including some that do not grow on blood agar (i.e., *Haemophilus*, some pathogenic *Neisseria* strains).

Mueller-Hinton agar. This is the recommended medium for routine susceptibility testing of bacteria.

It has a well-defined composition of beef and casein extracts, salts, divalent cations, and soluble starch that is necessary for reproducible test results.

Thioglycolate broth. This is one of a variety of enrichment broths used to recover low numbers of aerobic and anaerobic bacteria. Various formulations are used but most include casein digest, glucose, yeast extract, cysteine, and sodium thioglycolate. Supplementation with hemin and vitamin K will enhance the recovery of anaerobic bacteria.

Sabouraud dextrose agar. This is an enriched medium consisting of digests of casein and animal tissue supplemented with glucose; it is used for the isolation of fungi. A variety of formulations have been developed, but most mycologists use the formulation with a low concentration of glucose and neutral pH. By reducing the pH and adding antibiotics to inhibit bacteria, this medium can be made selective for fungi.

Selective Media and Differential Media

Selective media are designed for the recovery of specific organisms that may be present in a mixture of other organisms (e.g., an enteric pathogen in stool). The media are supplemented with inhibitors that suppress the growth of unwanted organisms. These media can be made differential by adding specific ingredients that allow the identification of an organism in a mixture (e.g., addition of lactose and a pH indicator to detect lactose-fermenting organisms). The following are some examples of selective and differential media:

MacConkey agar. This is a selective agar for gram-negative bacteria and differential for differentiation of lactose-fermenting and lactose-nonfermenting bacteria. The medium consists of digests of peptones, bile salts, lactose, neutral red, and crystal violet. The bile salts and crystal violet inhibit gram-positive bacteria. Bacteria that ferment lactose produce acid, which precipitates the bile salts and causes a red color in the neutral red indicator.

Mannitol salt agar. This is a selective medium used for the isolation of staphylococci. The medium consists of digests of casein and animal tissue, beef extract, mannitol, salts, and phenol red. Staphylococci can grow in the presence of a high salt concentration and *S. aureus* can ferment mannitol, producing yellow-colored colonies on this agar.

Xylose-lysine deoxycholate (XLD) agar. This is a selective agar used for the detection of *Salmonella* and *Shigella* in enteric cultures. This is an example of a very clever approach to detecting important bacteria in a complex mixture of insignificant bacteria. The medium consists of yeast extract with xylose, lysine, lactose, sucrose, sodium deoxycholate, sodium thiosulfate, ferric ammonium citrate, and phenol red. Sodium deoxycholate inhibits the growth of the majority of nonpathogenic bacteria. Those that do grow typically ferment lactose, sucrose, or xylose, producing yellow colonies. *Shigella* does not ferment these carbohydrates, so the colonies appear red. *Salmonella* ferments xylose but also decarboxylates lysine, producing the alkaline diamine product cadaverine. This neutralizes the acid fermentation products; thus the colonies appear red. Because most *Salmonella* produce hydrogen sulfide from sodium thiosulfate, the colonies will turn black in the presence of ferric ammonium citrate, thus differentiating *Salmonella* from *Shigella*.

Lowenstein-Jensen (LJ) medium. This medium, used for the isolation of mycobacteria, contains glycerol, potato flour, salts, and coagulated whole eggs (to solidify the medium). Malachite green is added to inhibit gram-positive bacteria.

Middlebrook agar. This agar medium is also used for the isolation of mycobacteria. It contains nutrients required for the growth of mycobacteria (i.e., salts, vitamins, oleic acid, albumin, catalase, glycerol, glucose) and malachite green for the inhibition of gram-positive bacteria. In contrast with LJ medium, it is solidified with agar.

CHROMagar. This is a selective, differential agar used for the isolation and identification of different species of the yeast *Candida*. The medium has chloramphenicol to inhibit bacteria and a mixture of proprietary chromogenic substrates. The different species of *Candida* have enzymes that can utilize one or more of the substrates, releasing the color compound and producing colored colonies. Thus *C. albicans* forms green colonies, *C. tropicalis* forms purple colonies, *C. krusei* forms pink colonies.

Inhibitory mold agar. This medium is an enriched, selective formulation that is used for the isolation of pathogenic fungi other than dermatophytes. Chloramphenicol is added to suppress the growth of contaminating bacteria.

Specialized Media

A large variety of specialized media have been created for the detection of specific organisms that may be fastidious or typically present in large mixtures of organisms. The more commonly used media are described in the specific organism chapters in this textbook.

Cell Culture

Some bacteria and all viruses are **strict intracellular microbes**; that is, they can only grow in living cells. In 1949, Enders described a technique for cultivating mammalian cells for the isolation of poliovirus. This technique has been expanded for the growth of most strict intracellular organisms. The cell cultures can either be cells that grow and divide on a surface (i.e., **cell monolayer**) or grow suspended in broth. Some cell cultures are well established and can be maintained indefinitely. These cultures are commonly commercially available. Other cell cultures must be prepared immediately before they are infected with the bacteria or viruses and cannot be maintained in the laboratory for more than a few cycles of division (**primary cell cultures**). Entry into cells is frequently regulated by the presence of specific receptors, so the differential ability to infect specific cell lines can be used to predict the identity of the bacteria or virus. Additional information about the use of cell cultures is described in the following chapters.

General Principles

The clinical presentation of most diseases (e.g., septicemia, pneumonia, gastroenteritis, intraabdominal infections) can be produced by a wide variety of organisms. Indeed, it is the exception where one specific organism is suspected (e.g., anthrax caused by *Bacillus anthracis*, histoplasmosis caused by *Histoplasma capsulatum*, influenza caused by influenza virus). Thus it is important for the diagnostic lab to select the appropriate media for the recovery of the most common organisms and to be able to select specialized media when the physician suspects a specific organism. In general, specimens collected from normally sterile sites (e.g., sterile fluids such as blood and spinal fluid, tissues) are inoculated onto enriched nonselective agars and broths (e.g., blood and chocolate agars, thioglycolate, or other enrichment broth). If the specimen is potentially contaminated with the patient's normal flora of organisms, selective and differential media is added (e.g., MacConkey agar). If a specific organism is suspected, then media to recover that organism is also added. Thus specimens can be inoculated onto a large variety of media. This is further complicated if media have to be selected for the recovery of bacteria, mycobacteria, and fungi. It is important that the number of cultures and other tests be carefully selected, particularly if only a limited quantity of specimen is available. If too many cultures, stains, antigen tests, and nucleic-acid-based tests are ordered, then the specimen may be diluted so much

that an inadequate quantity will be available for each of the ordered tests. For this reason, it is important for the microbiologist and clinician to work together to select the appropriate, most sensitive tests. In many cases, this will mean eliminating microscopic stains and antigen tests to maximize the amount of specimen that can be cultured.

Questions

1. Name three factors that affect the success of a culture.
2. Give three examples of enriched, nonselective media.
3. Give three examples of selective, differential media.

Bibliography

Atlas R: Handbook of Microbiologic Media, 3rd ed. New York, CRC, 2004.

Atlas R, Snyder J: Handbook of Media for Clinical Microbiology, 2nd ed. New York, CRC, 2006.

Difco & BBL Manual of Microbiological Culture Media. Sparks, Md, Becton Dickinson, 2003.

Murray P, et al: Manual of Clinical Microbiology, 9th ed. Washington, DC, ASM Press, 2007.

Murray P, Shea Y: ASM Pocket Guide to Clinical Microbiology, 3rd ed. Washington, DC, ASM Press, 2004.

Molecular Diagnosis

Like the evidence left at the scene of a crime, the DNA (deoxyribonucleic acid), RNA (ribonucleic acid), or proteins of an infectious agent in a clinical sample can be used to help identify the agent. In many cases the agent can be detected and identified in this way, even if it cannot be isolated or detected by immunologic means. New techniques and adaptations of older techniques are being developed for the analysis of infectious agents.

The advantages of molecular techniques are their sensitivity, specificity, and safety. From the standpoint of safety, these techniques do not require isolation of the infectious agent and can be performed on chemically fixed (inactivated) samples or extracts. Because of their sensitivity, very dilute samples of microbial DNA can be detected in a tissue, even if the agent is not replicating or producing other evidence of infection. These techniques can distinguish related strains on the basis of differences in their genotype (i.e., mutants). This is especially useful for distinguishing antiviral drug-resistant strains, which may differ by a single nucleotide.

Detection of Microbial Genetic Material

Electrophoretic Analysis of DNA and Restriction Fragment Length Polymorphism

The genome structure and genetic sequence are major distinguishing characteristics of the family, type, and strain of microorganism. Specific strains of microorganisms can be distinguished on the basis of their DNA or RNA or by the DNA fragments produced when the DNA is cleaved by specific restriction endonucleases (**restriction enzymes**). Restriction enzymes recognize specific DNA sequences that have a palindromic structure; an example follows:

$$\overset{\downarrow}{G}|A\ A\ T\ T\ C \quad \text{EcoR 1 recognition}$$
$$C\ T\ T\ A\ A|\underset{\uparrow}{G} \quad \text{sequence and cleavage}$$

The DNA sites recognized by different restriction endonucleases differ in their sequence, length, and frequency of occurrence. As a result, different restriction endonucleases cleave the DNA of a sample in different places, yielding fragments of different lengths. The cleavage of different DNA samples with one restriction endonuclease can also yield fragments of many different lengths. The differences in the length of the DNA fragments among the different strains of a specific organism produced on cleavage with one or more restriction endonucleases is termed **restriction fragment length polymorphism** (**RFLP**).

DNA or RNA fragments of different sizes or structures can be distinguished by their electrophoretic mobility in an agarose or polyacrylamide gel. Different forms of the same DNA sequence and different lengths of DNA move through the mazelike structure of an agarose gel at different speeds, allowing their separation. The DNA can be visualized by staining with ethidium bromide. Smaller fragments (fewer than 20,000 base pairs), such as those from bacterial plasmids or from viruses, can be separated and distinguished by normal electrophoretic methods. Larger fragments, such as those from whole bacteria, can be separated only by using a special electrophoretic technique called *pulsed-field gel electrophoresis*.

RFLP is useful, for example, for distinguishing different strains of herpes simplex virus (HSV). Comparison of the restriction endonuclease cleavage patterns of DNA from different isolates can identify a pattern of virus transmission from one person to another or distinguish HSV-1 from HSV-2. RFLP has also been used to show the spread of necrotizing fasciitis produced by a strain of *Streptococcus* from one patient to other patients, an emergency medical technician, and the emergency department and attending physicians (Figure 16-1).

Genetic Probes

DNA probes can be used like antibodies as sensitive and specific tools to detect, locate, and quantitate specific nucleic acid sequences in clinical specimens (Figure 16-2). Because of the specificity and sensitivity of DNA probe techniques,

Figure 16—1. Restriction fragment length polymorphism distinction of DNA from bacterial strains separated by pulsed-field gel electrophoresis. Lanes 1 to 3 show Sma 1 restriction endonuclease—digested DNA from bacteria from two family members with necrotizing fasciitis and from their physician (pharyngitis). Lanes 4 to 6 are from unrelated *Streptococcus pyogenes* strains. *(Courtesy of Dr. Joe DiPersio, Akron, Ohio.)*

Figure 16—2. DNA probe analysis of virus-infected cells. Such cells can be localized in histologically prepared tissue sections using DNA probes consisting of as few as nine nucleotides or bacterial plasmids containing the viral genome. A tagged DNA probe is added to the sample. In this case the DNA probe is labeled with biotin-modified thymidine, but radioactive agents can also be used. The sample is heated to denature the DNA and cooled to allow the probe to hybridize to the complementary sequence. Horseradish peroxidase—labeled avidin is added to bind to the biotin on the probe. The appropriate substrate is added to color the nuclei of virally infected cells. A, adenine; b, biotin; C, cytosine; G, guanine; T, thymine.

individual species or strains of an infectious agent can be detected, even if they are not growing or replicating.

DNA probes are chemically synthesized or obtained by cloning specific genomic fragments or an entire viral genome into bacterial vectors (plasmids, cosmids). DNA copies of RNA viruses are made with the retrovirus reverse transcriptase and then cloned into these vectors. After chemical or heat treatments melt (separate) the DNA strands in the sample, the DNA probe is added and allowed to **hybridize** (bind) with the identical or nearly identical sequence in the sample. The **stringency** (the requirement for an exact sequence match) of the interaction can be varied so that related sequences can be detected or different strains (mutants) can be distinguished. The DNA probes are labeled with radioactive or chemically modified nucleotides (e.g., biotinylated uridine) so that they can be detected and quantitated. The use of a biotin-labeled DNA probe allows the use of a fluorescent- or enzyme-labeled avidin or streptavidin (a protein that binds tightly to biotin) molecule to detect viral nucleic acids in a cell in a way similar to how indirect immunofluorescence or an enzyme immunoassay localizes an antigen.

The DNA probes can detect specific genetic sequences in fixed, permeabilized tissue biopsy specimens by **in situ hybridization**. The localization of cytomegalovirus- (Figure 16-3)

or papillomavirus-infected cells by in situ hybridization is preferable to an immunologic means of doing so and is the only commercially available means of localizing papillomavirus. There are now many commercially available viral probes and kits for detecting viruses.

Specific nucleic acid sequences in extracts from a clinical sample can be detected by applying a small volume of the extract to a nitrocellulose filter (**dot blot**) and then probing the filter with labeled, specific viral DNA. Alternatively, the electrophoretically separated restriction endonuclease cleavage pattern can be transferred onto a nitrocellulose filter (**Southern blot**—DNA:DNA probe hybridization), and then the specific sequence can be identified by hybridization with a specific genetic probe

Figure 16—3. In situ localization of cytomegalovirus (CMV) infection using a genetic probe. CMV infection of the renal tubules of a kidney is localized with a biotin-labeled, CMV-specific DNA probe and is visualized by means of the horseradish peroxidase—conjugated avidin conversion of substrate, in a manner similar to enzyme immunoassay. (*Courtesy of Donna Zabel, Akron, Ohio.*)

Figure 16—4. Polymerase chain reaction (PCR). This technique is a rapid means of amplifying a known sequence of DNA. A sample is mixed with a heat-stable DNA polymerase, excess deoxyribonucleotide triphosphates, and two DNA oligomers **(primers)**, which complement the ends of the target sequence to be amplified. The mixture is heated to denature the DNA, then cooled to allow binding of the primers to the target DNA and extension of the primers by the polymerase. The cycle is repeated 20 to 40 times. After the first cycle, only the sequence bracketed by the primers is amplified. In the **RT-PCR** technique, RNA can also be amplified after its conversion to DNA by reverse transcriptase. A and B, DNA oligomers used as primers; + and —, DNA strands. (*Modified from Blair GE, Blair Zajdel ME: Biochem Educ 20:87-90, 1992.*)

and by its characteristic electrophoretic mobility. Electrophoretically separated RNA (**Northern blot**—RNA: DNA probe hybridization) blotted onto a nitrocellulose filter can be detected in a similar manner.

The **polymerase chain reaction (PCR)** amplifies single copies of viral DNA millions of times over and is one of the newest techniques of genetic analysis (Figure 16-4). In this technique, a sample is incubated with two short DNA oligomers, termed **primers**, that are complementary to the ends of a known genetic sequence within the total DNA, a heat-stable DNA polymerase (Taq or other polymerase obtained from thermophilic bacteria), nucleotides, and buffers. The oligomers hybridize to the appropriate sequence of DNA and act as primers for the polymerase, which copies that segment of the DNA. The sample is then heated to denature the DNA (separating the strands of the double helix) and cooled to allow hybridization of the primers to the new DNA. Each copy of DNA becomes a new template. The process is repeated many (20 to 40) times to amplify the original DNA sequence in an exponential manner. A target sequence can be amplified 1,000,000-fold in a few hours using this method. This technique is especially useful for detecting latent and integrated virus sequences, such as in retroviruses, herpesviruses, papillomaviruses, and other DNA viruses.

The **RT-PCR** (reverse transcriptase polymerase chain reaction) technique is a variation of PCR, and it involves the use of the reverse transcriptase of retroviruses to convert viral RNA or messenger RNA to DNA before PCR amplification. In 1993, hantavirus sequences were used as primers for RT-PCR to identify the agent causing an outbreak of hemorrhagic pulmonary disease in the Four Corners area of New Mexico. It showed the infectious agent to be a hantavirus.

Real-time PCR can be used to quantitate the amount of DNA or RNA in a sample after it is converted to DNA by reverse transcriptase. Simply put, the more DNA in the sample, the faster new DNA is made in a PCR reaction, and the reaction kinetics are proportional to the amount of DNA. The production of double-stranded DNA is measured by the increase in fluorescence of a molecule bound to the amplified double-strand DNA molecule or by other means. This procedure is useful for quantitating the number of human immunodeficiency virus (HIV) genomes in a patient's blood to evaluate the course of the disease and antiviral drug efficacy.

Table 16–1. Molecular Techniques

Technique	Purpose	Clinical Examples
RFLP	Comparison of DNA	Molecular epidemiology, HSV-1 strains
DNA electrophoresis	Comparison of DNA	Viral strain differences (up to 20,000 bases)
Pulsed-field gel electrophoresis	Comparison of DNA (large pieces of DNA)	Streptococcal strain comparisons
In situ hybridization	Detection and localization of DNA sequences in tissue	Detection of nonreplicating DNA virus (e.g., cytomegalovirus, human papillomavirus)
Dot blot	Detection of DNA sequences in solution	Detection of viral DNA
Southern blot	Detection and characterization of DNA sequences by size	Identification of specific viral strains
Northern blot	Detection and characterization of RNA sequences by size	Identification of specific viral strains
PCR	Amplification of very dilute DNA samples	Detection of DNA viruses
RT-PCR	Amplification of very dilute RNA samples	Detection of RNA viruses
Real-time PCR	Quantification of very dilute DNA and RNA samples	Quantitation of HIV genome: virus load
Branched-chain DNA	Amplification of very dilute DNA or RNA samples	Quantitation of DNA and RNA viruses
Antibody capture solution hybridization DNA assay	Amplification of very dilute DNA or RNA samples	Quantitation of DNA and RNA viruses
SDS-PAGE	Separation of proteins by molecular weight	Molecular epidemiology of HSV

HSV, Herpes simplex virus; PCR, polymerase chain reaction; RFLP, restriction fragment length polymorphism; RT-PCR, reverse transcriptase polymerase chain reaction; SDS-PAGE, sodium dodecyl sulfate–polyacrylamide gel electrophoresis.

The **branched-chain DNA assay** is a hybridization technique that is an alternative to PCR and RT-PCR for detecting small amounts of specific RNA or DNA sequences. This technique is especially useful for quantitating plasma levels of HIV RNA (plasma viral load). In this case, plasma is incubated in a special tube lined with a short complementary DNA (cDNA) sequence to capture the viral RNA. Another cDNA sequence is added to bind to the sample, but this DNA is attached to an artificially branched chain of DNA. On development, each branch is capable of initiating a detectable signal. This amplifies the signal from the original sample. The **antibody capture solution hybridization assay** detects and quantitates RNA:DNA hybrids using an antibody specific for the complex in a technique similar to an ELISA (see Chapter 17).

Assay kits that use variations on the aforementioned techniques to detect, identify, and quantitate different microbes are commercially available.

Detection of Proteins

In some cases, viruses and other infectious agents can be detected on the basis of finding certain characteristic enzymes or specific proteins. For example, the detection of reverse transcriptase enzyme activity in serum or cell culture indicates the presence of a retrovirus. The pattern of proteins from a virus or another agent after sodium dodecyl sulfate–polyacrylamide gel electrophoresis (SDS-PAGE) can also be used to identify and distinguish different strains of viruses or bacteria. In the SDS-PAGE technique, SDS binds to the backbone of the protein to generate a uniform peptide structure and peptide length-to-charge ratio, such that the mobility of the protein in the gel is inversely related to the logarithm of its molecular weight. For example, the patterns of electrophoretically separated HSV proteins can be used to distinguish different types and strains of HSV-1 and HSV-2. Antibody can be used to identify specific proteins separated by SDS-PAGE using a Western blot technique (see Chapter 51). The molecular techniques used to identify infectious agents are summarized in Table 16-1.

Bibliography

DiPersio JR, et al: Spread of serious disease-producing M3 clones of group A *Streptococcus* among family members and health care workers. Clin Infect Dis 22:490-495, 1996.

Forbes BA, Sahm DF, Weissfeld AS: Bailey and Scott's Diagnostic Microbiology, 12th ed. St Louis, Mosby, 2007.

Fredericks DN, Relman DA: Application of polymerase chain reaction to the diagnosis of infectious diseases. Clin Infect Dis 29:475-486, 1999.

Murray PR, et al: Manual of Clinical Microbiology, 9th ed. Washington, DC, ASM Press, 2007.

Murray PR: ASM Pocket Guide to Clinical Microbiology, 3rd ed. Washington, DC, ASM Press, 2004.

Specter S, Hodinka RL, Young SA: Clinical Virology Manual, 3rd ed. Washington, DC, ASM Press, 2000.

Strauss JM, Strauss EG: Viruses and Human Disease, 2nd ed. San Diego, Academic, 2007.

Serologic Diagnosis

Immunologic techniques are used to detect, identify, and quantitate antigen in clinical samples, as well as to evaluate the antibody response to infection and a person's history of exposure to infectious agents. The specificity of the antibody-antigen interaction and the sensitivity of many of the immunologic techniques make them powerful laboratory tools (Table 17-1). *In most cases the same technique can be used to evaluate antigen and antibody.* Because many serologic assays are designed to give a positive or negative result, quantitation of the antibody strength is obtained as a titer. The **titer** of an antibody is defined as the lowest dilution of the sample that retains a detectable activity.

Antibodies

Antibodies can be used as sensitive and specific tools to detect, identify, and quantitate the antigens from a virus, bacterium, fungus, or parasite. Specific antibodies may be obtained from convalescent patients (e.g., antiviral antibodies) or prepared in animals. These antibodies are **polyclonal**; that is, they are heterogeneous antibody preparations that can recognize many epitopes on a single antigen. **Monoclonal** antibodies recognize individual epitopes on an antigen. Monoclonal antibodies for many antigens are commercially available, especially for lymphocyte cell surface antigens.

The development of monoclonal antibody technology revolutionized the science of immunology. For example, because of the specificity of these antibodies, lymphocyte subsets (e.g., CD4 and CD8 T cells) and lymphocyte cell surface antigens were identified. Monoclonal antibodies are the products of hybrid cells generated by the fusion and cloning of a spleen cell from an immunized mouse and a myeloma cell, which produces a hybridoma. The myeloma provides immortalization to the antibody-producing B cells of the spleen. *Each hybridoma clone is a factory for one antibody molecule, yielding a monoclonal antibody that recognizes only one epitope.* Monoclonal antibodies can

also be prepared and manipulated through genetic engineering and "humanized" for therapeutic usage.

The advantages of monoclonal antibodies are (1) that their specificity can be confined to a single epitope on an antigen and (2) that they can be prepared in "industrial-sized" tissue culture preparations. A major disadvantage of monoclonal antibodies is that they are often too specific, such that a monoclonal antibody specific for one epitope on a viral antigen of one strain may not be able to detect different strains of the same virus.

Methods of Detection

Antibody-antigen complexes can be detected directly, by precipitation techniques or by labeling the antibody with a radioactive, fluorescent, or enzyme probe; or they can be detected indirectly, through measurement of an antibody-directed reaction, such as complement fixation.

Precipitation and Immunodiffusion Techniques

Specific antigen-antibody complexes and cross-reactivity can be distinguished by immunoprecipitation techniques. Within a limited concentration range for both antigen and antibody, termed the **equivalence zone**, the antibody cross-links the antigen into a complex that is too large to stay in solution and therefore precipitates. This technique is based on the multivalent nature of antibody molecules (e.g., immunoglobulin [Ig] G has two antigen-binding domains). The antigen-antibody complexes are soluble at concentration ratios of antigen to antibody that are above and below the equivalence concentration.

Various immunodiffusion techniques make use of the equivalence concept to determine the identity of an antigen or the presence of antibody. **Single radial immunodiffusion** can be used to detect and quantify an antigen. In this technique, antigen is placed into a well and allowed to diffuse into antibody-containing agar. The higher the

Serologic Diagnosis

Immunologic techniques are used to detect, identify, and quantitate antigen in clinical samples, as well as to evaluate the antibody response to infection and a person's history of exposure to infectious agents. The specificity of the antibody-antigen interaction and the sensitivity of many of the immunologic techniques make them powerful laboratory tools (Table 17-1). *In most cases the same technique can be used to evaluate antigen and antibody.* Because many serologic assays are designed to give a positive or negative result, quantitation of the antibody strength is obtained as a titer. The **titer** of an antibody is defined as the lowest dilution of the sample that retains a detectable activity.

Antibodies

Antibodies can be used as sensitive and specific tools to detect, identify, and quantitate the antigens from a virus, bacterium, fungus, or parasite. Specific antibodies may be obtained from convalescent patients (e.g., antiviral antibodies) or prepared in animals. These antibodies are **polyclonal**; that is, they are heterogeneous antibody preparations that can recognize many epitopes on a single antigen. **Monoclonal** antibodies recognize individual epitopes on an antigen. Monoclonal antibodies for many antigens are commercially available, especially for lymphocyte cell surface antigens.

The development of monoclonal antibody technology revolutionized the science of immunology. For example, because of the specificity of these antibodies, lymphocyte subsets (e.g., CD4 and CD8 T cells) and lymphocyte cell surface antigens were identified. Monoclonal antibodies are the products of hybrid cells generated by the fusion and cloning of a spleen cell from an immunized mouse and a myeloma cell, which produces a hybridoma. The myeloma provides immortalization to the antibody-producing B cells of the spleen. *Each hybridoma clone is a factory for one antibody molecule, yielding a monoclonal antibody that recognizes only one epitope.* Monoclonal antibodies can

also be prepared and manipulated through genetic engineering and "humanized" for therapeutic usage.

The advantages of monoclonal antibodies are (1) that their specificity can be confined to a single epitope on an antigen and (2) that they can be prepared in "industrial-sized" tissue culture preparations. A major disadvantage of monoclonal antibodies is that they are often too specific, such that a monoclonal antibody specific for one epitope on a viral antigen of one strain may not be able to detect different strains of the same virus.

Methods of Detection

Antibody-antigen complexes can be detected directly, by precipitation techniques or by labeling the antibody with a radioactive, fluorescent, or enzyme probe; or they can be detected indirectly, through measurement of an antibody-directed reaction, such as complement fixation.

Precipitation and Immunodiffusion Techniques

Specific antigen-antibody complexes and cross-reactivity can be distinguished by immunoprecipitation techniques. Within a limited concentration range for both antigen and antibody, termed the **equivalence zone**, the antibody cross-links the antigen into a complex that is too large to stay in solution and therefore precipitates. This technique is based on the multivalent nature of antibody molecules (e.g., immunoglobulin [Ig] G has two antigen-binding domains). The antigen-antibody complexes are soluble at concentration ratios of antigen to antibody that are above and below the equivalence concentration.

Various immunodiffusion techniques make use of the equivalence concept to determine the identity of an antigen or the presence of antibody. **Single radial immunodiffusion** can be used to detect and quantify an antigen. In this technique, antigen is placed into a well and allowed to diffuse into antibody-containing agar. The higher the

Table 17–1. Selected Immunologic Techniques

Technique	Purpose	Clinical Examples
Ouchterlony immuno-double-diffusion	Detect and compare antigen and antibody	Fungal antigen and antibody
Immunofluorescence	Detection and localization of antigen	Viral antigen in biopsy (e.g., rabies, herpes simplex virus)
Enzyme immunoassay (EIA)	Same as immunofluorescence	Same as immunofluorescence
Immunofluorescence flow cytometry	Population analysis of antigen-positive cells	Immunophenotyping
Enzyme-linked immunosorbent assay (ELISA)	Quantitation of antigen or antibody	Viral antigen (rotavirus); viral antibody (anti-HIV)
Western blot	Detection of antigen-specific antibody	Confirmation of anti-HIV seropositivity
Radioimmunoassay (RIA)	Same as ELISA	Same as for ELISA
Complement fixation	Quantitate specific antibody titer	Fungal, viral antibody
Hemagglutination inhibition	Antiviral antibody titer; serotype of virus strain	Seroconversion to current influenza strain; identification of influenza
Latex agglutination	Quantitation and detection of antigen and antibody	Rheumatoid factor; fungal antigens; streptococcal antigens

HIV, Human immunodeficiency virus.

concentration of antigen, the farther it diffuses before it reaches equivalence with the antibody in the agar and precipitates as a ring around the well.

The **Ouchterlony immuno-double-diffusion** technique is used to determine the relatedness of different antigens, as shown in Figure 17-1. In this technique, solutions of antibody and antigen are placed in separate wells cut into agar, and the antigen and antibody are allowed to diffuse toward each other to establish concentration gradients of each substance. A visible precipitin line occurs where the concentrations of antigen and antibody reach equivalence. On the basis of the pattern of the precipitin lines, this technique can also be used to determine whether samples are identical, share some but not all epitopes (partial identity), or are distinct. This technique is used to detect antibody to fungal antigens (e.g., *Histoplasma* species, *Blastomyces* species, and coccidioidomycoses).

In other immunodiffusion techniques, the antigen may be separated by electrophoresis in agar and then reacted with antibody (immunoelectrophoresis); it may be pushed into agar that contains antibody by means of electrophoresis (rocket electrophoresis); or antigen and antibody may be placed in separate wells and allowed to move electrophoretically toward each other (countercurrent immunoelectrophoresis).

Immunoassays for Cell-Associated Antigen (Immunohistology)

Antigens on the cell surface or within the cell can be detected by **immunofluorescence** and **enzyme immunoassay (EIA)**.

In **direct immunofluorescence**, a fluorescent molecule is covalently attached to the antibody (e.g., fluorescein-isothiocyanate—labeled rabbit antiviral antibody). In **indirect immunofluorescence**, a second fluorescent antibody specific for the primary antibody (e.g., fluorescein-isothiocyanate—labeled goat anti—rabbit antibody) is used to detect the primary antiviral antibody and locate the antigen (Figures 17-2 and 17-3). In EIA, an enzyme such as horseradish peroxidase or alkaline phosphatase is conjugated to the antibody and converts a substrate into a chromophore to mark the antigen. Alternatively, an antibody modified by the attachment of a **biotin** (the vitamin) molecule can be localized by the very high affinity binding of avidin or streptavidin molecules. A fluorescent molecule or an enzyme attached to the avidin and streptavidin allows detection. These techniques are useful for the analysis of tissue biopsy specimens, blood cells, and tissue culture cells.

The **flow cytometer** can be used to analyze the immunofluorescence of cells in suspension and is especially useful for identifying and quantitating lymphocytes (immunophenotyping). A laser is used in the flow cytometer to excite the fluorescent antibody attached to the cell and to determine the size of the cell by means of light-scattering measurements. The cells flow past the laser at rates of more than 5000 cells per second, and analysis is performed electronically. The **fluorescence-activated cell sorter (FACS)** is a flow cytometer that can also isolate specific subpopulations of cells for tissue culture growth on the basis of their size and immunofluorescence.

The data obtained from a flow cytometer are usually presented in the form of a histogram, with the fluorescence intensity on the *x*-axis and the number of cells on the

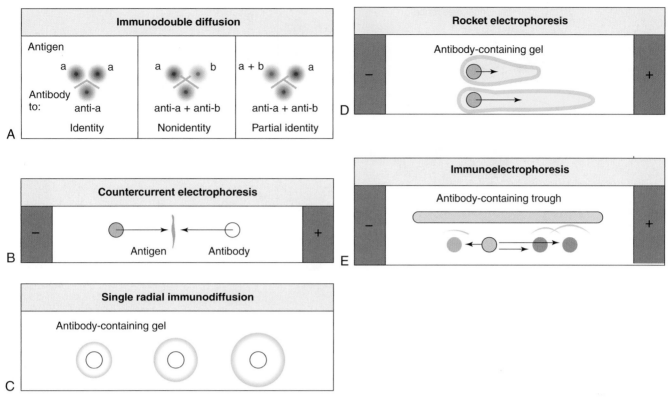

Figure 17–1. Analysis of antigens and antibodies by immunoprecipitation. The precipitation of protein occurs at the equivalence point, at which multivalent antibody forms large complexes with antigen. **A,** Ouchterlony immuno-double-diffusion. Antigen and antibody diffuse from wells, meet, and form a precipitin line. If identical antigens are placed in adjacent wells, the concentration of antigen between them is doubled, and precipitation does not occur in this region. If different antigens are used, two different precipitin lines are produced. If one sample shares antigen but is not identical, then a single spur results for the complete antigen. **B,** Countercurrent electrophoresis. This technique is similar to the Ouchterlony method, but antigen movement is facilitated by electrophoresis. **C,** Single radial immunodiffusion. This technique involves the diffusion of antigen into an antibody-containing gel. Precipitin rings indicate an immune reaction, and the area of the ring is proportional to the concentration of antigen. **D,** Rocket electrophoresis. Antigens are separated by electrophoresis into an agar gel that contains antibody. The length of the "rocket" indicates concentration of antigen. **E,** Immunoelectrophoresis. Antigen is placed in a well and separated by electrophoresis. Antibody is then placed in the trough, and precipitin lines form as antigen and antibody diffuse toward each other.

y-axis, or in the form of a dot plot, in which more than one parameter is compared for each cell. The flow cytometer can perform a differential analysis of white blood cells and compare CD4 and CD8 T-cell populations simultaneously (Figure 17-4). Flow cytometry is also useful for analyzing cell growth after the fluorescent labeling of deoxyribonucleic acid (DNA) and other fluorescent applications.

Immunoassays for Antibody and Soluble Antigen

The **enzyme-linked immunosorbent assay (ELISA)** uses antigen immobilized on a plastic surface, bead, or filter to capture and separate the specific antibody from other antibodies in a patient's serum (Figure 17-5). An antihuman antibody with a covalently linked enzyme (e.g., horseradish peroxidase, alkaline phosphatase, β-galactosidase) then detects the affixed patient antibody. It is quantitated spectrophotometrically according to the intensity of the color produced in response to the enzyme conversion of an appropriate substrate. The actual concentration of specific antibody can be determined by comparison with the reactivity of standard human antibody solutions. The many variations of ELISAs differ in the way in which they capture or detect antibody or antigen.

ELISAs can also be used to quantitate the soluble antigen in a patient's sample. In these assays, soluble antigen is captured and concentrated by an immobilized antibody and then detected with a different antibody labeled with the enzyme. An example of a commonly used ELISA is the home pregnancy test for the human chorionic gonadotropin hormone.

Western blot analysis is a variation of an ELISA. In this technique, viral proteins separated by electrophoresis

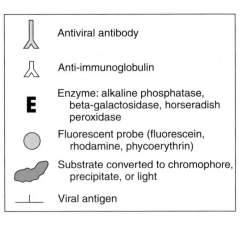

Figure 17—2. Immunofluorescence and enzyme immunoassays for antigen localization in cells. Antigen can be detected by *direct* assay with antiviral antibody modified covalently with a fluorescent or enzyme probe, or by *indirect* assay using antiviral antibody and chemically modified anti-immunoglobulin. The enzyme converts substrate to a precipitate, chromophore, or light.

according to their molecular weight or charge are transferred (blotted) onto a filter paper (e.g., nitrocellulose, nylon). When exposed to a patient's serum, the immobilized proteins capture virus-specific antibody and are visualized with an enzyme-conjugated antihuman antibody.

Figure 17—3. Immunofluorescence localization of herpes simplex virus (HSV)-infected nerve cells in a brain section from a patient with herpes encephalitis. *(From Emond RT, Rowland HAK: A Color Atlas of Infectious Diseases, 2nd ed. London, Wolfe, 1987.)*

This technique shows the proteins recognized by the patient serum. Western blot analysis is used to confirm ELISA results in patients suspected to be infected with the human immunodeficiency virus (HIV) (Figure 17-6; also see Figure 49-7).

In **radioimmunoassay (RIA)**, radiolabeled (e.g., with iodine-125) antibody or antigen is used to quantitate antigen-antibody complexes. RIA can be performed as a capture assay, as described previously for ELISA, or as a competition assay. In a competition assay, antibody in a patient's serum is quantitated according to its ability to compete with and replace a laboratory-prepared, radiolabeled antibody from antigen-antibody complexes. The antigen-antibody complexes are precipitated and separated from free antibody, and the radioactivity is measured for both fractions. The amount of the patient's antibody is then quantitated from standard curves prepared with use of known quantities of competing antibody. The radioallergosorbent assay is a variation of an RIA capture assay, in which radiolabeled anti-IgE is used to detect allergen-specific responses.

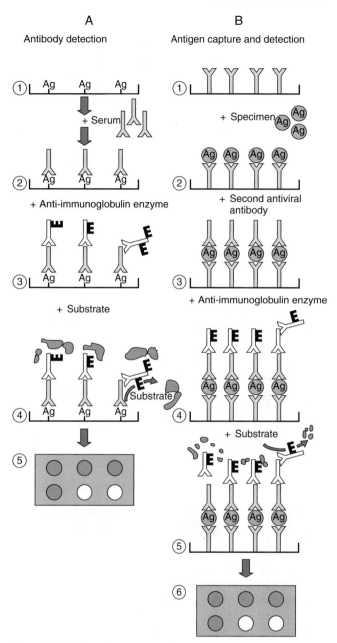

Figure 17—4. Flow cytometry. **A,** The flow cytometer evaluates individual cell parameters as the cells flow past a laser beam at rates of more than 5000 per second. Cell size and granularity are determined by light scattering (LS), and antigen expression is evaluated by immunofluorescence (F), using antibodies labeled with different fluorescent probes. Parts **B to D** depict T-cell analysis of a normal patient. **B,** Light-scatter analysis was used to define the lymphocytes (Ly), monocytes (Mo), and polymorphonuclear (neutrophil) leukocytes (PMN). *C,* The lymphocytes were analyzed for CD3 expression to identify T cells (presented in a histogram). **D,** CD4 and CD8 T cells were identified. Each dot represents one T cell. *(Data provided by Dr. Tom Alexander, Akron, Ohio.)*

Figure 17—5. Enzyme immunoassays for quantitation of antibody or antigen. **A,** Antibody detection. *1,* Viral antigen, obtained from infected cells, virions, or genetic engineering, is affixed to a surface. *2,* Patient serum is added and allowed to bind to the antigen. Unbound antibody is washed away. *3,* Enzyme-conjugated antihuman antibody is added, and unbound antibody is washed away. *4,* Substrate is added and converted *(5)* into chromophore, precipitate, or light. **B,** Antigen capture and detection. *1,* Antiviral antibody is affixed to a surface. *2,* A specimen that contains antigen is added, and unbound antigen is washed away. *3,* A second antiviral antibody is added to detect the captured antigen. *4,* Enzyme-conjugated anti-antibody is added, washed, and followed by substrate *(5),* which is converted *(6)* into chromophore, precipitate, or light.

Complement fixation is a standard but technically difficult serologic test (Box 17-1). In this test, the patient's serum sample is reacted with laboratory-derived antigen and extra complement. Antibody-antigen complexes bind, activate, and fix (use up) the complement. The residual complement is then assayed through the lysis of red blood cells coated with antibody. Antibodies measured by this system generally develop slightly later in an illness than those measured by other techniques.

Antibody inhibition assays make use of the specificity of an antibody to prevent infection (**neutralization**) or other activity (**hemagglutination inhibition**) to identify

Western blot

SDS-PAGE   NC
                paper

Figure 17–6. Western blot analysis. Proteins are separated by sodium dodecyl sulfate–polyacrylamide gel electrophoresis (SDS-PAGE), electroblotted onto nitrocellulose (NC) paper, and incubated with antigen-specific or patient's antisera (1°Ab) and then enzyme-conjugated antihuman serum (2°Ab). Enzyme conversion of substrate identifies the antigen.

Box 17–2. Viruses Diagnosed by Serology*

Epstein-Barr virus
Rubella virus
Hepatitis A, B, C, D, and E viruses
Human immunodeficiency virus
Human T-cell leukemia virus
Arboviruses (encephalitis viruses)

*Serologic testing is also used to determine a person's immune status with regard to other viruses

the strain of the infecting agent, usually a virus, or to quantitate antibody responses to a specific strain of virus. For example, hemagglutination inhibition is used to distinguish different strains of influenza A. These tests are discussed further in Chapter 49.

Latex agglutination is a rapid, technically simple assay for detecting antibody or soluble antigen. Virus-specific antibody causes latex particles coated with viral antigens to clump. Conversely, antibody-coated latex particles are used to detect soluble viral antigen. In passive hemagglutination, antigen-modified erythrocytes are used as indicators instead of latex particles.

Serology

The humoral immune response provides a history of a patient's infections. Serology can be used to identify the infecting agent, evaluate the course of an infection, or determine the nature of the infection—whether it is a primary infection or a reinfection, and whether it is acute or chronic. The antibody type and titer and the identity of the antigenic targets provide serologic data about an infection. Serologic

Box 17–1. Serologic Assays

Complement fixation
Hemagglutination inhibition*
Neutralization*
Immunofluorescence (direct and indirect)
Latex agglutination
In situ enzyme immunoassay (EIA)
Enzyme-linked immunosorbent assay (ELISA)
Radioimmunoassay (RIA)

*For detection of antibody or serotyping of virus

testing is used to identify viruses and other agents that are difficult to isolate and grow in the laboratory or that cause diseases that progress slowly (Box 17-2).

The relative antibody concentration is reported as a titer. A **titer** is the inverse of the greatest dilution, or lowest concentration (e.g., dilution of 1:64 = titer of 64), of a patient's serum that retains activity in one of the immunoassays just described. The amount of IgM, IgG, IgA, or IgE reactive with antigen can also be evaluated through the use of a labeled second antihuman antibody specific for the antibody isotype.

Serology is used to determine the time course of an infection. **Seroconversion** occurs when antibody is produced in response to a primary infection. *Specific IgM antibody, found during the first 2 to 3 weeks of a primary infection, is a good indicator of a recent primary infection.* Reinfection or recurrence later in life causes an **anamnestic** (secondary or booster) response. Antibody titers may remain high, however, in patients whose disease recurs frequently (e.g., herpesviruses). Seroconversion or reinfection is indicated by the finding *of at least a fourfold increase in the antibody titer between serum obtained during the acute phase of disease and that obtained at least 2 to 3 weeks later during the convalescent phase.* A twofold serial dilution will not distinguish between samples with 512 and 1023 units of antibody, both of which would give a reaction on a 512-fold dilution but not on a 1024-fold dilution, and both results would be reported as titers of 512. On the other hand, samples with 1020 and 1030 units are not significantly different but would be reported as titers of 512 and 1024, respectively.

Serology can also be used to determine the stage of a slower or chronic infection (e.g., hepatitis B or infectious mononucleosis caused by Epstein-Barr virus), based on the presence of antibody to specific microbial antigens. The first antibodies to be detected are those directed against antigens most available to the immune system (e.g., on the virion, on surfaces of infected cells, secreted). Later in the infection, when cells have been lysed by the infecting virus or the cellular immune response, antibodies directed against the intracellular proteins and enzymes are detected.

Questions

Describe the diagnostic procedure or procedures (molecular or immunologic) that would be appropriate for each of the following applications:

1. Determination of the apparent molecular weights of the HIV proteins

2. Detection of human papillomavirus 16 (a nonreplicating virus) in a Papanicolaou (Pap) smear

3. Detection of herpes simplex virus (a replicating virus) in a Pap smear

4. Presence of *Histoplasma* fungal antigens in a patient's serum

5. CD4 and CD8 T-cell concentrations in blood from a patient infected with HIV

6. The presence of antibody and the titer of anti-HIV antibody

7. Genetic differences between two herpes simplex viruses (DNA virus)

8. Genetic differences between two parainfluenza viruses (ribonucleic acid [RNA] virus)

9. Amount of rotavirus antigen in stool

10. Detection of group A streptococci and their distinction from other streptococci

Bibliography

Forbes BA, Sahm DF, Weissfeld AS: Bailey and Scott's Diagnostic Microbiology, 12th ed. St Louis, Mosby, 2007.
Murray PR: ASM Pocket Guide to Clinical Microbiology, 3rd ed. Washington, DC, American Society for Microbiology, 2004.
Murray PR et al: Manual of Clinical Microbiology, 9th ed. Washington, DC, ASM Press, 2007.
Rosenthal KS, Wilkinson MS: Flow cytometry and immunospeak. Infec Dis 15(3):183-191, 2007.
Specter S, Hodinka RL, Young SA: Clinical Virology Manual, 3rd ed. Washington, DC, ASM Press, 2000.
Strauss JM, Strauss EG: Viruses and Human Disease, 2nd ed. San Diego, Academic, 2007.

175

Bacteriology

Mechanisms of Bacterial Pathogenesis

To a bacterium, the human body is a collection of environmental niches that provide the warmth, moisture, and food necessary for growth. Bacteria have acquired genetic traits that enable them to enter (invade) the environment, remain in a niche (adhere or colonize), gain access to food sources (degradative enzymes), and escape clearance by host immune and nonimmune protective responses (e.g., **capsule**). Unfortunately, many of the mechanisms that bacteria use to maintain their niche and the byproducts of bacterial growth (e.g., acids, gas) cause damage and problems for the human host. Many of these genetic traits are **virulence factors**, which enhance the ability of bacteria to cause disease. Although many bacteria cause disease by directly destroying tissue, some release toxins, which are then disseminated by the blood to cause system-wide pathogenesis (Box 18-1). The surface structures of bacteria are powerful stimulators of host responses (acute phase: interleukin-1 [IL-1], interleukin-6 [IL-6], tumor necrosis factor [TNF]), which can be protective but are often the significant causes of the disease symptoms (e.g., sepsis). Production of disease results from the combination of damage caused by the bacteria and the consequences of the innate and immune responses to the infection (Box 18-2).

Not all bacteria or bacterial infections cause disease; however, some always cause disease. The human body is colonized with numerous microbes (**normal flora**), many of which serve important functions for their hosts. Normal flora bacteria aid in the digestion of food, produce vitamins (e.g., vitamin K), and can protect the host from colonization with pathogenic microbes. These endogenous bacteria normally reside in locations such as the gastrointestinal (GI) tract, mouth, skin, and upper respiratory tract, which are technically outside the body (Figure 18-1). Normal flora bacteria cause disease if they enter normally sterile sites of the body. **Virulent bacteria** have mechanisms that promote their growth in the host at the expense of the host's tissue or organ function. To grow and cause more serious disease, **opportunistic bacteria** take advantage of preexisting conditions such as immunosuppression

that enhance the susceptibility of the patient. For example, *Pseudomonas aeruginosa* infects burn victims and the lungs of patients with cystic fibrosis, and patients with the acquired immune deficiency syndrome (AIDS) are very susceptible to infection by intracellularly growing bacteria such as the mycobacteria.

Disease results from the damage or loss of tissue or organ function or the development of host inflammatory responses. The **signs and symptoms of a disease** are determined by the function of the affected tissue. **Systemic responses** are produced by toxins and the cytokines produced in response to the infection. The seriousness of the disease depends on the importance of the affected organ and the extent of the damage caused by the infection. Infections of the central nervous system are always serious. The **bacterial strain** and **inoculum size** are also major factors in determining whether disease occurs; however, the threshold for disease production is different for different bacteria (e.g., less than 200 *Shigella* are required for shigellosis but 10^8 *Vibrio cholerae* or *Campylobacter* organisms are required for GI tract infections). Host factors can also play a role. For example, although a million or more *Salmonella* organisms are necessary for gastroenteritis to become established in a healthy person, only a few thousand organisms are necessary in a person whose gastric pH is neutral. Congenital defects, immunodeficiency states (see Chapter 14), and other disease-related conditions might also increase a person's susceptibility to infection. The longer a bacterium remains in the body, the greater its numbers, its ability to spread, and its potential to cause tissue damage and disease.

Many of the virulence factors consist of complex structures or activities that are only expressed under special conditions. The components for these structures are often encoded together in a **pathogenicity island**. Pathogenicity islands are large chromosomal regions that contain sets of genes encoding numerous virulence factors. In many cases, a virulence process requiring coordinated expression of several genes is encoded in a pathogenicity island.

and *Staphylococcus epidermidis*, which are a part of the normal flora on skin, can enter the body through breaks in the skin and pose a major problem for people with indwelling catheters and intravenous lines.

The mouth, nose, respiratory tract, ears, eyes, urogenital tract, and anus are sites through which bacteria can enter the body. These natural openings in the skin and their associated body cavities are protected by natural defenses such as the mucus and ciliated epithelium that line the upper respiratory tract, the lysozyme and other antibacterial secretions in tears and mucus, and the acid and bile in the GI tract. However, many bacteria are unaffected or have the means to evade these defenses. For example, the outer membrane of the gram-negative bacteria makes these bacteria more resistant to lysozyme, acid, and bile. The enterobacteria are thus enabled to colonize the GI tract, where they serve the beneficial function of producing the vitamin K that the body needs. These endogenous bacteria are normally benign and restricted to the body cavities they colonize. However, these bacteria can enter normally sterile sites of the body, such as the peritoneum and the bloodstream, through a break in the normal barrier. An example of this is the patient whose colon tumor was diagnosed after detection of a septicemia (blood-borne infection) caused by enteric bacteria.

Colonization, Adhesion, and Invasion

As previously mentioned, the GI tract is naturally colonized by benign and potentially beneficial bacteria. In some cases, environmental conditions determine the bacteria that can or will colonize a site. For example, *Legionella* grows in the lungs but does not readily spread, because it cannot tolerate high temperatures (e.g., 35° C). Colonization of sites that are normally sterile implies the existence of a defect in a natural defense mechanism or a new portal of entry. Patients with cystic fibrosis have such defects because of the reduction in their ciliary mucoepithelial function and altered mucosal secretions; as a result, their lungs are colonized by *S. aureus* and *P. aeruginosa*.

Bacteria may use specific mechanisms to adhere to and colonize different body surfaces (Table 18-2). If the bacteria can adhere to epithelial or endothelial cell linings of the bladder, intestine, and blood vessels, they cannot be washed away, and this adherence allows them to colonize the tissue. For example, natural bladder function eliminates any bacteria not affixed to the bladder wall. *Escherichia coli* and other bacteria have **adhesins** that bind to specific receptors on the tissue surface and keep the organisms from being washed away. Many of these adhesin proteins are present at the tips of **fimbriae (pili)** and bind tightly to specific sugars on the target tissue. (This sugar-binding activity defines these proteins as lectins.) For example, most *E. coli* strains that cause pyelonephritis produce a fimbrial adhesin termed the *P fimbriae*. This adhesin can bind to

Table 18—2. Examples of Bacterial Adherence Mechanisms

Microbe	Adhesin	Receptor
Staphylococcus aureus	LTA	Unknown
Staphylococcus spp.	Slime	Unknown
Streptococcus, group A	LTA-M protein complex	Fibronectin
Streptococcus pneumoniae	Protein	*N*-acetylhexosamine-galactose
Escherichia coli	Type 1 fimbriae	D-Mannose
	Colonization factor antigen fimbriae	GM ganglioside 1
	P fimbriae	P blood group glycolipid
Neisseria gonorrhoeae	Fimbriae	GD_1 ganglioside
Treponema pallidum	P_1, P_2, P_3	Fibronectin
Chlamydia trachomatis	Cell surface lectin	*N*-acetylglucosamine
Mycoplasma pneumoniae	Protein P1	Sialic acid
Vibrio cholerae	Type 4 pili	Fucose and mannose

LTA, Lipoteichoic acid.

α-D-galactosyl-β-D-galactoside (Gal-Gal), which is part of the P blood group antigen structure on human erythrocytes and uroepithelial cells. *Neisseria gonorrhoeae* pili are also important virulence factors; they bind to oligosaccharide receptors on epithelial cells. *Yersinia* organisms, *Bordetella pertussis*, and *Mycoplasma pneumoniae* express adhesin proteins that are not on fimbriae. *Streptococcus pyogenes* uses **lipoteichoic acid** and the F protein (binds to fibronectin) to bind to epithelial cells.

A special bacterial adaptation that facilitates colonization, especially of surgical appliances such as artificial valves or indwelling catheters, is a **biofilm** produced by the bacteria. Bacteria in biofilms are bound within a sticky web of polysaccharide that binds the cells together and to the surface. Some bacteria, such as *Pseudomonas aeruginosa*, sense that sufficient bacteria are present to make a biofilm (quorum sensing) and create a bacterial community. Dental plaque is an example of a biofilm. The biofilm matrix can also protect the bacteria from host defenses and antibiotics.

Although bacteria do not have mechanisms that enable them to cross skin, several bacteria can cross mucosal membranes and other tissue barriers to enter normally sterile sites and more susceptible tissue. These invasive bacteria either destroy the barrier or penetrate into the cells of the barrier. *Shigella*, *Salmonella*, and *Yersinia* organisms are enteric bacteria that use fimbriae to bind to M (microfold) cells of the colon and then inject proteins into the M cell that stimulate the cell membrane to surround and take in the bacteria. These bacteria produce a type III secretion device that resembles a molecular syringe that injects pore-forming factors and effector molecules into the host cells. The effector proteins can facilitate uptake and invasion, promote the intracellular survival and replication of the bacteria, or the apoptotic death of the host cell. Enteropathogenic *E. coli* secretes proteins into the host cell that create a portable docking system for itself (see the animation at the Howard Hughes Institute website (http://www.hhmi.org/biointeractive/). *Salmonella* uses the device to promote its uptake into a vesicle that allows it to live intracellularly within the macrophage. *Shigella* uses a type III secretion device to enter cells; once inside cells, the organism causes cellular actin to polymerize and push the *Shigella* into an adjacent cell. *Listeria monocytogenes* causes the polymerization of actin at the rear of the cell to propel the bacteria into an adjacent cell, as if on the top of a battering ram.

Pathogenic Actions of Bacteria

Tissue Destruction

Byproducts of bacterial growth, especially fermentation, include acids, gas, and other substances that are toxic to tissue. In addition, *many bacteria release degradative enzymes* to break down tissue, thereby providing food for the growth of the organisms and promoting the spread of the bacteria. For example, *Clostridium perfringens* organisms are part of the normal flora of the GI tract but are also opportunistic pathogens that can establish infection in oxygen-depleted tissues and cause gas gangrene. These anaerobic bacteria produce enzymes (e.g., phospholipase C, collagenase, protease, and hyaluronidase), several toxins, and acid and gas from bacterial metabolism, which destroy the tissue. Staphylococci produce many different enzymes that modify the tissue environment. These enzymes include hyaluronidase, fibrinolysin, and lipases. Streptococci also produce enzymes, including streptolysins S and O, hyaluronidase, DNAases, and streptokinases; these enzymes facilitate the development of infection and spread into the tissue.

Toxins

Toxins are bacterial products that directly harm tissue or trigger destructive biologic activities. Toxin and toxin-like activities are degradative enzymes that cause lysis of cells or specific receptor-binding proteins that initiate toxic reactions in a specific target tissue. In addition, cell-wall components initiate a systemic response (e.g., fever) by promoting the inappropriate release of cytokines. In many cases, the toxin is completely responsible for causing the characteristic symptoms of the disease. For example, the **preformed toxin** present in food mediates the food poisoning caused by *S. aureus* and *Bacillus cereus* and the botulism caused by *Clostridium botulinum*. The symptoms caused by preformed toxin occur much sooner than for other forms of gastroenteritis because the effect is like eating a poison, and the bacteria do not need to grow for the symptoms to occur. Because a toxin can be spread systemically through the bloodstream, symptoms may arise at a site distant from the site of infection, such as occurs in tetanus, which is caused by *Clostridium tetani*.

Exotoxins

Exotoxins are proteins that can be produced by grampositive or gram-negative bacteria and include cytolytic enzymes and receptor-binding proteins that alter a function or kill the cell. In many cases, the toxin gene is encoded on a plasmid (tetanus toxin of *C. tetani*, LT and ST toxins of enterotoxigenic *E. coli*) or a lysogenic phage (*Corynebacterium diphtheriae* and *C. botulinum*).

Cytolytic toxins include membrane-disrupting enzymes such as the α-toxin (phospholipase C) produced by *C. perfringens*, which breaks down sphingomyelin and other membrane phospholipids. Hemolysins insert into and disrupt erythrocyte and other cell membranes. Pore forming toxins, including streptolysin O, can promote leakage of ions and water from the cell and disrupt cellular functions or cell lysis.

Many toxins are dimeric with A and B subunits (**A-B toxins**). The B portion of the A-B toxins binds to a specific cell surface receptor, and then the A subunit is transferred into the interior of the cell, where cell injury is induced. The tissues targeted by these toxins are very defined and limited (Figure 18-2 and Table 18-3). The biochemical targets of A-B toxins include ribosomes, transport mechanisms, and intracellular signaling (cyclic adenosine monophosphate [cAMP] production, G protein function), with effects ranging from diarrhea to loss of neuronal function to death. The functional properties of cytolytic and other exotoxins are discussed in greater detail in the chapters dealing with the specific diseases involved.

Superantigens are a special group of toxins (Figure 18-3). These molecules activate T cells by binding simultaneously to a T-cell receptor and a major histocompatibility complex class II (MHC II) molecule on an antigen-presenting cell without requiring antigen. *Superantigens activate large numbers of T cells to release large amounts of interleukins (cytokine storm)*, including IL-1, TNF, and IL-2, causing *life-threatening autoimmune-like responses*. This superantigen stimulation of T cells can also lead to death of the activated T cells, resulting in the loss of specific T-cell clones and the loss of their immune

A **Inhibition of protein synthesis**

B **Hyperactivation**

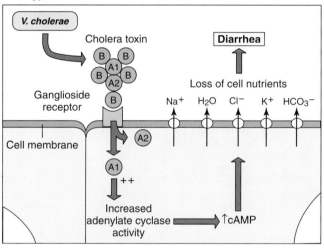

C **Effects on nerve–muscle transmission**

Figure 18–2. The mode of action of dimeric A-B exotoxins. The bacterial A-B toxins often consist of a two-chain molecule. The B chain promotes entry of the bacteria into cells, and the A chain has inhibitory activity against some vital function. ACH, acetylcholine; cAMP, cyclic adenosine monophosphate. *(Redrawn from Mims C, et al: Medical Microbiology. London, Mosby-Wolfe, 1993.)*

responses. Superantigens include the toxic shock syndrome toxin of *S. aureus*, staphylococcal enterotoxins, and the erythrogenic toxin A or C of *S. pyogenes*.

Endotoxin and Other Cell Wall Components

The presence of bacterial cell wall components acts as a signal of infection that provides a powerful multialarm warning to the body to activate the host's protective systems. The molecular patterns in these structures (**pathogen-associated molecular patterns [PAMPs]**) bind to Toll-like receptor (TLR) molecules and stimulate the production of cytokines. In some cases, the host response is excessive and may even be life threatening. On infection with gram-positive bacteria, **peptidoglycan** and its breakdown products, as well as **teichoic** and **lipoteichoic acids**, are released, and these stimulate endotoxin-like **pyrogenic** (fever) **acute-phase responses**. The **lipopolysaccharide** (LPS) produced by gram-negative bacteria is an even more powerful activator of acute-phase and inflammatory reactions and is termed **endotoxin**. The lipid A portion of

LPS is responsible for endotoxin activity. It is important to appreciate that endotoxin is not the same as exotoxin and that *only gram-negative bacteria make endotoxin.*

Gram-negative bacteria release endotoxin during infection. Endotoxin binds to specific receptors (CD14 and TLR4) on macrophages, B cells, and other cells and stimulates the production and release of **acute-phase cytokines** such as IL-1, TNF-α, IL-6, and prostaglandins (Figure 18-4). Endotoxin also stimulates the growth (mitogenic) of B cells.

At low concentrations, endotoxin stimulates the mounting of protective responses, such as fever, vasodilatation, and the activation of immune and inflammatory responses (Box 18-3). However, the endotoxin levels in the blood of patients with **gram-negative bacterial sepsis** (bacteria in the blood) can be very high, and the systemic response to these can be overpowering, resulting in shock and possibly death. High concentrations of endotoxin can also activate the alternative pathway of complement and production of anaphylotoxins (C3a, C5a), contributing to vasodilatation and capillary leakage. In combination with TNF and IL-1, this can lead to **hypotension** and **shock**. **Disseminated**

Table 18–3. Properties of A-B Type Bacterial Toxins

Toxin	Organism	Gene Location	Subunit Structure	Target Cell Receptor	Biologic Effects
Anthrax toxins	*Bacillus anthracis*	Plasmid	Three separate proteins (EF, LF, PA)	Tumor endothelial marker-8 (TEM-8); capillary morphogenesis protein 2 (CMG2)	EF + PA: increase in target cell cAMP level, localized edema; LF + PA: death of target cells and experimental animals
Bordetella adenylate cyclase toxin	*Bordetella* spp.	Chromosomal	A-B	Unknown, probably glycolipid	Increase in target cell cAMP level, modified cell function or cell death
Botulinum toxin	*Clostridium botulinum*	Phage	A-B	Polysialogangliosides plus synaptotagmin (co-receptors)	Decrease in peripheral presynaptic acetylcholine release, flaccid paralysis
Cholera toxin	*Vibrio cholerae*	Chromosomal	A-5B	Ganglioside (GM$_1$)	Activation of adenylate cyclase, increase in cAMP level, secretory diarrhea
Diphtheria toxin	*Corynebacterium diphtheriae*	Phage	A-B	Growth factor receptor precursor	Inhibition of protein synthesis, cell death
Heat-labile enterotoxins	*Escherichia coli*	Plasmid	Similar or identical to cholera toxin		
Pertussis toxin	*Bordetella pertussis*	Chromosomal	A-5B	Surface glycoproteins with terminal sialic acid residues	Block of signal transduction mediated by target G proteins
Pseudomonas exotoxin A	*Pseudomonas aeruginosa*	Chromosomal	A-B	α2-macroglobulin receptor (α2MR)	Similar or identical to diphtheria toxin
Shiga toxin	*Shigella dysenteriae*	Chromosomal	A-5B	Globotriasoyl ceramide (Gb3)	Inhibition of protein synthesis, cell death
Shiga-like toxins	*Shigella* spp., *E. coli*	Phage	Similar or identical to Shiga toxin		
Tetanus toxin	*Clostridium tetani*	Plasmid	A-B	Polysialogangliosides plus 15-kDa glycoprotein (co-receptors)	Decrease in neurotransmitter release from inhibitory neurons, spastic paralysis

Modified from Mandell G, Douglas G, Bennett J: Principles and Practice of Infectious Disease, 3rd ed. New York, Churchill Livingstone, 1990.
cAMP, cyclic adenosine monophosphate.

intravascular coagulation (DIC) can also result from the activation of blood coagulation pathways. The high fever, petechiae (skin lesions resulting from capillary leakage), and potential symptoms of shock (resulting from increased vascular permeability) associated with *Neisseria meningitidis* infection can be related to the large amounts of endotoxin released during infection.

Immunopathogenesis

In many cases, the symptoms of a bacterial infection are produced by excessive innate, immune, and inflammatory responses triggered by the infection. As described earlier, when limited and controlled, the acute-phase response to cell wall components is a protective antibacterial response. However, these responses also cause fever and malaise, and when systemic and out of control, the acute-phase response can cause life-threatening symptoms associated with sepsis and meningitis (see Figure 18-4). Activated neutrophils, macrophage, and complement can cause damage at the site of the infection. Activation of complement can also cause release of anaphylotoxins that initiate vascular permeability and capillary breakage. Cytokine storms generated by superantigens and endotoxin can cause shock and disruption of body function. Granuloma formation induced by CD4 T cells and macrophages for *Mycobacterium tuberculosis* can also lead to tissue destruction. Autoimmune responses can be triggered by bacterial proteins, such as the M protein of *S. pyogenes*, which antigenically mimics

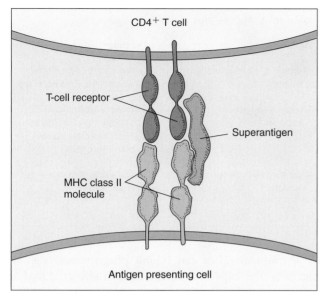

Figure 18—3. Superantigen binding to the external regions of the T-cell receptor and the major histocompatibility complex class II (MHC II) molecules.

heart tissue. The anti-M protein antibodies cross-react with and can initiate damage to the heart to cause rheumatic fever. Immune complexes deposited in the glomeruli of the kidney cause poststreptococcal glomerulonephritis. For *Chlamydia*, *Treponema* (syphilis), *Borrelia* (Lyme disease),

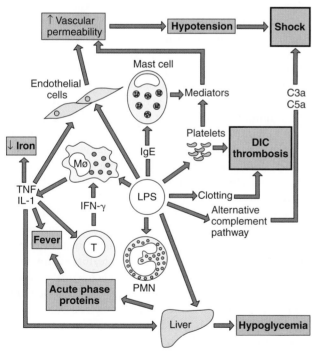

Figure 18—4. The many activities of lipopolysaccharide (LPS). This bacterial endotoxin activates almost every immune mechanism, as well as the clotting pathway, which together make LPS one of the most powerful immune stimuli known. DIC, disseminated intravascular coagulation; IFN-γ, interferon-γ; IgE, immunoglobulin E; IL-1, interleukin-1; PMN, polymorphonuclear (neutrophil) leukocytes; TNF, tumor necrosis factor. *(Redrawn from Mims C, et al: Medical Microbiology. London, Mosby-Wolfe, 1993.)*

Box 18—3. Endotoxin-Mediated Toxicity

Fever
Leukopenia followed by leukocytosis
Activation of complement
Thrombocytopenia
Disseminated intravascular coagulation
Decreased peripheral circulation and perfusion to major organs
Shock
Death

---

and other bacteria, the host immune response is the principal cause of disease symptoms in patients.

Mechanisms for Escaping Host Defenses

Bacteria are parasites, and evasion of host protective responses is a selective advantage. Logically, the longer a bacterial infection remains in a host, the more time the bacteria have to grow and also cause damage. Therefore bacteria that can evade or incapacitate the host defenses have a greater potential for causing disease. Bacteria evade recognition and killing by phagocytic cells, inactivate or evade the complement system and antibody, and even grow inside cells to hide from host responses (Box 18-4).

The capsule is one of the most important virulence factors (Box 18-5). These slime layers function by shielding the bacteria from immune and phagocytic responses. Capsules are typically made of polysaccharides, which are usually poor immunogens. The *S. pyogenes* capsule, for example, is made of hyaluronic acid, which mimics human connective tissue, thereby masking the bacteria and keeping them from being recognized by the immune system. The capsule also acts like a slimy football jersey, in that it is hard to grasp and tears away when grabbed by a phagocyte. The capsule also protects a bacterium from destruction within the phagolysosome of a macrophage or leukocyte. All of these properties can extend the time bacteria spend in blood (bacteremia) before being eliminated by host responses. Mutants of normally encapsulated bacteria that lose the ability to make a capsule also lose

---

Box 18—4. Microbial Defenses against Host Immunologic Clearance

Encapsulation
Antigenic mimicry
Antigenic masking
Antigenic shift
Production of antiimmunoglobulin proteases
Destruction of phagocyte
Inhibition of chemotaxis
Inhibition of phagocytosis
Inhibition of phagolysosome fusion
Resistance to lysosomal enzymes
Intracellular replication

Box 18—5. Examples of Encapsulated Microorganisms

Staphylococcus aureus
Streptococcus pneumoniae
Streptococcus pyogenes (group A)
Streptococcus agalactiae (group B)
Bacillus anthracis
Bacillus subtilis
Neisseria gonorrhoeae
Neisseria meningitidis
Haemophilus influenzae
Escherichia coli
Klebsiella pneumoniae
Salmonella spp.
Yersinia pestis
Campylobacter fetus
Pseudomonas aeruginosa
Bacteroides fragilis
Cryptococcus neoformans (yeast)

Table 18—4. Methods That Circumvent Phagocytic Killing

Method	Example
Inhibition of phagolysosome fusion	*Legionella* spp., *Mycobacterium tuberculosis*, *Chlamydia* spp.
Resistance to lysosomal enzymes	*Salmonella typhimurium*, *Coxiella* spp., *Ehrlichia* spp., *Mycobacterium leprae*, *Leishmania* spp.
Adaptation to cytoplasmic replication	*Listeria*, *Francisella*, and *Rickettsia* spp.

their virulence; examples of such bacteria are *Streptococcus pneumoniae* and *N. meningitidis*. A **biofilm**, which is made from capsular material, can prevent antibody and complement from getting to the bacteria.

Bacteria can evade antibody responses by **intracellular growth**, **antigenic variation**, or by **inactivation of antibody or complement**. Bacteria that grow intracellularly include mycobacteria, francisellae, brucellae, chlamydiae, and rickettsiae (Box 18-6). Unlike most bacteria, control of these infections requires TH1 T-helper cell immune responses, which activate macrophages to kill or create a wall (granuloma) around the infected cells (as for *Mycobacterium tuberculosis*). *Neisseria gonorrhoeae* can vary the structure of surface antigens to evade antibody responses and also produces a protease that degrades immunoglobulin A (IgA). By degrading the C5a component of complement, *Streptococcus pyogenes* can limit the chemotaxis of leukocytes to the site of infection.

Phagocytes (neutrophil, macrophage) are an important antibacterial defense, but many bacteria can circumvent phagocytic killing in various ways. They can produce enzymes capable of lysing phagocytic cells (e.g., the streptolysin produced by *S. pyogenes* or the α-toxin produced by

Box 18—6. Examples of Intracellular Pathogens

Mycobacterium spp.
Brucella spp.
Francisella spp.
Rickettsia spp.
Chlamydia spp.
Listeria monocytogenes
Salmonella Typhi
Shigella dysenteriae
Yersinia pestis
Legionella pneumophila

C. perfringens). They can inhibit phagocytosis (e.g., the effects of the **capsule** and the **M protein** produced by *S. pyogenes*) or block intracellular killing. Bacterial mechanisms for protection from intracellular killing include blocking phagolysosome fusion to prevent contact with its bactericidal contents (*Mycobacterium* species), capsule-mediated or enzymatic resistance to the bactericidal lysosomal enzymes or substances, and the ability to exit the phagosome into the host cytoplasm before being exposed to lysosomal enzymes (Table 18-4 and Figure 18-5). Production of catalase by staphylococci can break down the hydrogen peroxide produced by the myeloperoxidase system. Many of the bacteria that are internalized but survive phagocytosis can use the cell as a place to grow and hide from immune responses and as a means of being disseminated throughout the body.

Other important host defenses subverted by bacteria include the alternate pathway of complement and antibody. Bacteria evade complement action by masking themselves and by inhibiting activation of the cascade. The long O antigen of LPS prevents the complement from gaining access to the membrane and protects gram-negative bacteria from damage. *S. aureus* makes an immunoglobulin-G-binding protein, protein A, which masks the bacteria and thereby prevents antibody action.

S. aureus can also escape host defenses by walling off the site of infection. *S. aureus* can produce coagulase, an enzyme that promotes the conversion of fibrin to fibrinogen to produce a clotlike barrier; this feature distinguishes *S. aureus* from *S. epidermidis*. *M. tuberculosis* is able to survive in a host by promoting the development of a granuloma, within which viable bacteria may reside for the life of the infected person. The bacteria may resume growth if there is a decline in the immune status of the person.

Summary

The primary virulence factors of bacteria are the capsule, adhesins, invasins, degradative enzymes, toxins, and mechanisms for escaping elimination by host defenses.

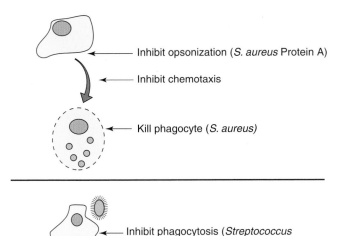

Inhibit opsonization (*S. aureus* Protein A)

Inhibit chemotaxis

Kill phagocyte (*S. aureus*)

Inhibit phagocytosis (*Streptococcus pneumoniae* capsule)

Phagocytosis

Inhibit lysosomal fusion (*M. tuberculosis*)

Escape lysosome and grow in cytoplasm

Resist antibacterial lysosomal action and multiply within cell   (*M. leprae, Salmonella* species, *S. aureus*)

Block activation by interferon-γ (Mycobacteria)

Interferon-γ

Figure 18–5. Bacterial mechanisms for escaping phagocytic clearance. Selected examples of bacteria that use the indicated antiphagocytic mechanisms are given.

Bacteria may only have one virulence mechanism. For example, *C. diphtheriae* has only one virulence mechanism, which is diphtheria toxin. Other bacteria express many virulence factors. *S. aureus* is an example of such a bacterium; it expresses adhesins, degradative enzymes, toxins, catalase, and coagulase, which are responsible for

producing a spectrum of diseases. In addition, different strains within a bacterial species may express different virulence mechanisms. For example, the symptoms and sequelae of gastroenteritis (diarrhea) caused by *E. coli* may include invasion and bloody stools, cholera-like watery stools, and even severe hemorrhagic disease, depending on the specific infecting strain.

Questions

1. Name three routes by which exogenous pathogens can infect a person. List five examples of organisms that use each route.

2. How are microbes able to resist immunologic clearance? Give at least one specific example of each mechanism.

3. What are the two general types of exotoxins? List examples of each type.

Reference to Student Consult Animation

Please visit **www.StudentConsult.com** to view an animation demonstrating the functions of *C. diphtheriae, B. anthracis, B. pertussis, P. aeruginosa, V. cholerae, E. coli* (enterotoxigenic), *C. botulinus, C. tetani,* and *C. difficile.*

Bibliography

Bisno AL, Brito MO, Collins CM: Molecular basis of group A streptococcal virulence. Lancet Infect Dis 3:191-200, 2003.

Bower S, Rosenthal KS: Bacterial cell walls: The armor, artillery and Achilles heel. Infect Dis Clin Pract 14:309-317, 2006.

Brodell LA, Rosenthal KS: Skin structure and function: The body's primary defense against infection. Infect Dis Clin Pract 16(2):113-117, 2008.

Cohen J, Powderly WC: Infectious Diseases, 2nd ed. London, Mosby, 2004.

Desvaux M, et al: Type III secretion: What's in a name? Trends Microbiol 14:157-160, 2006.

Finlay BB, Falkow S: Common themes in microbial pathogenicity revisited. Microbiol Mol Biol Rev 61:136-169, 1997.

Groisman EA, Ochman H: How *Salmonella* became a pathogen. Trends Microbiol 5:343-349, 1997.

Lee CA: Pathogenicity islands and the evolution of bacterial pathogens. Infect Agents Dis 5:1-7, 1996.

Mandell GL, Bennet JE, Dolin R, (eds): Principles and Practice of Infectious Diseases, 6th ed. Philadelphia, Churchill Livingstone, 2005.

McClane BA, et al: Microbial Pathogenesis: A Principles-Oriented Approach. Madison, CT, Fence Creek, 1999.

Papageorgiou AC, Acharya KR: Microbial superantigens: From structure to function. Trends Microbiol 8:369-375, 2000.

Reading N, Sperandio V: Quorum sensing: The many languages of bacteria. FEMS Microbiol Lett 254:1-11, 2006.

Rosenthal, KS: Are microbial symptoms "self-inflicted"?: The consequences of immunopathology. Infect Dis Clin Pract 13:306-310, 2005.

Laboratory Diagnosis of Bacterial Diseases

The laboratory diagnosis of bacterial diseases requires that the appropriate specimen is collected, delivered expeditiously to the laboratory in the appropriate transport system, and processed in a manner that will maximize detection of the most likely pathogens. Collection of the proper specimen and its rapid delivery to the clinical laboratory are primarily the responsibility of the patient's physician, whereas the clinical microbiologist selects the appropriate transport systems and detection method (i.e., microscopy, culture, antigen or antibody detection, and nucleic-acid-based tests). These responsibilities are not mutually exclusive. The microbiologist should be prepared to instruct the physician about what specimens should be collected if a particular diagnosis is suspected, and the physician must provide the microbiologist with information about the clinical diagnosis so the right tests are selected. This chapter is designed to provide an overview of specimen collection and transport, as well as the methods used in the microbiology laboratory for the detection and identification of bacteria. Because it is beyond the scope of this chapter to cover this subject exhaustively, the student is referred to the citations in the bibliography and the individual chapters that follow for more detailed information.

Specimen Collection, Transport, and Processing

Guidelines for the proper collection and transport of specimens are summarized in the following text and Table 19-1.

Blood

The culture of blood is one of the most important procedures performed in the clinical microbiology laboratory. The success of this test is directly related to the methods used to collect the blood sample. The most important factor that determines the success of a blood culture is the volume of blood processed. For example, 40% more cultures are positive for organisms if 20 ml rather than 10 ml of blood are cultured, because more than half of all septic patients have less than one organism per milliliter of blood. Approximately 20 ml of blood should be collected from an adult for each blood culture, and proportionally smaller volumes should be collected from children and neonates. Because many hospitalized patients are susceptible to infections with organisms colonizing their skin, careful disinfection of the patient's skin is important.

Bacteremia and **fungemia** are defined as the presence of bacteria and fungi, respectively, in the blood; these infections are referred to collectively as **septicemia**. Clinical studies have shown that septicemia can be continuous or intermittent. **Continuous septicemia** occurs primarily in patients with intravascular infections (e.g., endocarditis, septic thrombophlebitis, infections associated with intravascular catheters) or with overwhelming sepsis (e.g., septic shock). **Intermittent septicemia** occurs in patients with localized infections (e.g., lungs, urinary tract, soft tissues). The timing of blood collection is not important for patients with continuous septicemias, but it is important for patients with intermittent septicemia. In addition, because clinical signs of sepsis (e.g., fever, chills, and hypotension) are a response to the release of endotoxins or exotoxins from the organisms, these signs occur as long as 1 hour after the organisms entered the blood. Thus few to no organisms may be in the blood when the patient becomes febrile. For this reason, it is recommended that two to three blood samples should be collected at random times during a 24-hour period.

Most blood samples are inoculated directly into bottles filled with enriched nutrient broths. To ensure the maximal recovery of important organisms, two bottles of media should be inoculated for each culture (10 ml of blood per bottle). When these inoculated bottles are received in the laboratory, they are incubated at 37° C and inspected at regular intervals for evidence of microbial growth. In most laboratories, this is accomplished using automated blood culture instruments. When growth is detected, the broths

Table 19—1. Specimen Collection for Bacterial Pathogens

Specimen	Transport System	Specimen Volume	Other Considerations
Blood—routine bacterial culture	Blood culture bottle with nutrient media	Adults: 20 ml/culture Children: 5-10 ml/culture Neonates: 1-2 ml/culture	Skin should be disinfected with 70% alcohol followed by 2% iodine; 2-3 cultures collected every 24 hr unless patient is in septic shock or antibiotics will be started immediately; blood collections should be separated by 30-60 min; blood is divided equally into two bottles of nutrient media.
Blood—intracellular bacteria (e.g., *Brucella, Francisella, Neisseria* spp.)	Same as that for routine blood cultures; lysis-centrifugation system	Same as that for routine blood cultures	Considerations are same as those for routine blood cultures; release of intracellular bacteria may improve organism's recovery; *Neisseria* species are inhibited by some anticoagulants (sodium polyanetholsulfonate).
Blood—*Leptospira* spp.	Sterile heparinized tube	1-5 ml	Specimen is useful only during the first week of illness; afterward, urine should be cultured.
Cerebrospinal fluid	Sterile screw-capped tube	Bacteria culture: 1-5 ml Mycobacterial culture: as large a volume as possible	Specimen must be collected aseptically and delivered immediately to laboratory; it should not be exposed to heat or refrigeration.
Other normally sterile fluids (e.g., abdominal, chest, synovial, pericardial)	Small volume: sterile screw-capped tube; large volume: blood culture bottle with nutrient medium	As large a volume as possible	Specimens are collected with needle and syringe; swab is not used because quantity of collected specimen is inadequate; air should not be injected into culture bottle, because it will inhibit growth of anaerobes.
Catheter	Sterile screw-capped tube or specimen cup	N/A	The entry site should be disinfected with alcohol; catheter should be aseptically removed on receipt of specimen in laboratory; catheter is rolled across blood agar plate and then discarded.
Respiratory—throat	Swab immersed in transport medium	N/A	Area of inflammation is swabbed; exudate is collected if present; contact with saliva should be avoided, because it can inhibit recovery of group A streptococci.
Respiratory—epiglottis	Collection of blood for culture	Same as for blood culture	Swabbing the epiglottis can precipitate complete airway closure; blood cultures should be collected for specific diagnosis.
Respiratory—sinuses	Sterile anaerobic tube or vial	1-5 ml	Specimens must be collected with needle and syringe; culture of nasopharynx or oropharynx has no value; specimen should be cultured for aerobic and anaerobic bacteria.
Respiratory—lower airways	Sterile screw-capped bottle; anaerobic tube or vial only for specimens collected by avoiding upper tract flora	1-2 ml	Expectorated sputum: If possible, patient rinses mouth with water before collection of the specimen; patient should cough deeply and expectorate lower airway secretions directly into sterile cup; collector should avoid contamination with saliva. Bronchoscopy specimen: anesthetics can inhibit growth of bacteria, so specimens should be processed immediately; if "protected" bronchoscope is used, anaerobic cultures can be performed. Direct lung aspirate: specimens can be processed for aerobic and anaerobic bacteria.
Ear	Capped needleless syringe; sterile screw-capped tube	Whatever volume is collected	Specimen should be aspirated with needle and syringe; culture of external ear has no predictive value for otitis media.

Table 19–1. Specimen Collection for Bacterial Pathogens—cont'd

Specimen	Transport System	Specimen Volume	Other Considerations
Eye	Inoculate plates at bedside (seal and transport to laboratory immediately)	Whatever volume is collected	For infections on surface of eye, specimens are collected with swab or by corneal scrapings; for deep-seated infections, aspiration of aqueous or vitreous fluid is performed; all specimens should be inoculated onto appropriate media at collection; delays will result in significant loss of organisms.
Exudates (transudates, drainage, ulcers)	Swab immersed in transport medium; aspirate in sterile screw-capped tube	Bacteria: 1-5 ml Mycobacteria: 3-5 ml	Contamination with surface material should be avoided; specimens are generally unsuitable for anaerobic culture.
Wounds (abscess, pus)	Aspirate in sterile screw-capped tube or sterile anaerobic tube or vial	1-5 ml of pus	Specimens should be collected with sterile needle and syringe; curette is used to collect specimen at base of wound; swabbed specimens should be avoided.
Tissues	Sterile screw-capped tube; sterile anaerobic tube or vial	Representative sample from center and border of lesion	Specimen should be aseptically placed into appropriate sterile container; adequate quantity of specimen must be collected to recover small numbers of organisms.
Urine—midstream	Sterile urine container	Bacteria: 1 ml Mycobacteria: ≥10 ml	Contamination of specimen with bacteria from the urethra or vagina should be avoided; first portion of the voided specimen is discarded; organisms can grow rapidly in urine, so specimens must be transported immediately to laboratory, held in bacteriostatic preservative, or refrigerated.
Urine—catheterized	Sterile urine container	Bacteria: 1 ml Mycobacteria: ≥10 ml	Catheterization is not recommended for routine portion of cultures (risk of inducing infection); first collected specimen is contaminated with urethral bacteria, so it should be discarded (similar to midstream-voided specimen); specimen must be transported rapidly to laboratory.
Urine—suprapubic aspirate	Sterile anaerobic tube or vial	Bacteria: 1 ml Mycobacteria: ≥10 ml	This is an invasive specimen, so urethral bacteria are avoided; only valid method available for collecting specimens for anaerobic culture; also useful for collection of specimens from children or adults unable to void uncontaminated specimens.
Genitals	Specially designed swabs for *Neisseria gonorrhoeae* and *Chlamydia* probes	N/A	Area of inflammation or exudate should be sampled; endocervix (not vagina) and urethra should be cultured for optimal detection.
Feces (stool)	Sterile screw-capped container	N/A	Rapid transport to laboratory is necessary to prevent production of acid (bactericidal for some enteric pathogens) by normal fecal bacteria; unsuitable for anaerobic culture; because a large number of different media will be inoculated, swab should not be used for specimen collection.

are subcultured to isolate the organism for identification and antimicrobial susceptibility testing. Most clinically significant isolates are detected within the first 1 to 2 days of incubation; however, all cultures should be incubated for a minimum of 5 to 7 days. More prolonged incubation is generally unnecessary. Because few organisms are typically present in the blood of a septic patient, it is not

worthwhile to perform a Gram stain of blood for microscopic analysis.

Cerebrospinal Fluid

Bacterial meningitis is a serious disease associated with high morbidity and mortality if the etiologic diagnosis is delayed.

Because some common pathogens are labile (e.g., *Neisseria meningitidis*, *Streptococcus pneumoniae*), specimens of cerebrospinal fluid should be processed immediately after they are collected. Under no circumstance should the specimen be refrigerated or placed directly into an incubator. The patient's skin is disinfected before lumbar puncture, and the cerebrospinal fluid is collected into sterile screw-capped tubes. When the specimen is received in the microbiology laboratory, it is concentrated by centrifugation, and the sediment is used to inoculate bacteriologic media and prepare a Gram stain. The laboratory technologist should notify the physician immediately if organisms are observed microscopically or in culture.

Other Normally Sterile Fluids

A variety of other normally sterile fluids may be collected for bacteriologic culture, including abdominal (peritoneal), chest (pleural), synovial, and pericardial fluids. If a large volume of fluid can be collected by aspiration (e.g., abdominal or chest fluids), it should be inoculated into blood culture bottles containing nutrient media. A small portion should also be sent to the laboratory in a sterile tube so that appropriate stains (e.g., Gram, acid-fast) can be prepared. Many organisms are associated with infections at these sites, including polymicrobial mixtures of aerobic and anaerobic organisms. For this reason, biologic staining is useful for identifying the organisms responsible for the infection. Because relatively few organisms may be in the sample (as a result of the dilution of organisms or microbial elimination by the host immune response), it is important to culture as large a volume of fluid as possible. However, if only small quantities of fluid are collected, the specimen can be inoculated directly onto agar media and a tube of enriched broth media. Because anaerobes may also be present in the sample (particularly samples obtained from patients with intraabdominal or pulmonary infections), the specimen should not be exposed to oxygen.

Upper Respiratory Tract Specimens

Most bacterial infections of the pharynx are caused by group A *Streptococcus*. Other bacteria that may cause pharyngitis include *Corynebacterium diphtheriae*, *B. pertussis*, *Neisseria gonorrhoeae*, *Chlamydophila pneumoniae*, and *Mycoplasma pneumoniae*. However, special techniques are generally required to recover these organisms. Other potentially pathogenic bacteria, such as *Staphylococcus aureus*, *S. pneumoniae*, *Haemophilus influenzae*, Enterobacteriaceae, and *Pseudomonas aeruginosa*, may be present in the oropharynx but rarely cause pharyngitis.

A Dacron or calcium alginate swab should be used to collect pharyngeal specimens. The tonsillar areas, posterior pharynx, and any exudate or ulcerative area should be sampled. Contamination of the specimen with saliva should be avoided because bacteria in saliva can overgrow or inhibit the growth of group A streptococci. If a pseudomembrane is present (e.g., as with *C. diphtheriae* infections), a portion should be dislodged and submitted for culture. Group A streptococci and *C. diphtheriae* are very resistant to drying, so special precautions are not required for transport of the specimen to the laboratory. In contrast, specimens collected for the recovery of *B. pertussis* and *N. gonorrhoeae* should be inoculated onto culture media immediately after they are collected and before they are sent to the laboratory. Specimens obtained for the isolation of *C. pneumoniae* and *M. pneumoniae* should be transported in a special transport medium.

Group A streptococci can be detected directly in the clinical specimen through the use of immunoassays for the group-specific antigen. Although these tests are very specific and readily available, they are insensitive and cannot be used to reliably exclude the diagnosis of group A streptococcal pharyngitis. In other words, a negative assay must be confirmed by culture.

Other upper respiratory tract infections can involve the epiglottis and sinuses. Complete airway obstruction can be precipitated by attempts to culture the epiglottis (particularly in children); thus these cultures should never be performed. The specific diagnosis of a sinus infection requires (1) the direct aspiration of the sinus, (2) appropriate anaerobic transport of the specimen to the laboratory (using a system that avoids exposing anaerobes to oxygen and drying), and (3) prompt processing. Culture of the nasopharynx or oropharynx is not useful and should not be performed. *S. pneumoniae*, *H. influenzae*, *Moraxella catarrhalis*, *S. aureus*, and anaerobes are the most common pathogens that cause sinusitis.

Lower Respiratory Tract Specimens

A variety of techniques can be used to collect lower respiratory tract specimens; these include expectoration, induction with saline, bronchoscopy, and direct aspiration through the chest wall. Because upper airway bacteria may contaminate expectorated sputa, specimens should be inspected microscopically to assess the magnitude of oral contamination. Specimens containing many squamous epithelial cells and no predominant bacteria in association with neutrophils should not be processed for culture. The presence of squamous epithelial cells indicates that the specimen has been contaminated with saliva. Such contamination can be avoided by obtaining the specimen using specially designed bronchoscopes or direct lung aspiration. If an anaerobic lung infection is suspected, these invasive procedures must be used because contamination of the specimen with upper airway microbes would render the specimen worthless. Most lower respiratory tract pathogens grow rapidly (within 2 to 3 days); however, some slow-growing bacteria such as mycobacteria or nocardiae will require extended incubation.

Ear and Eye

Tympanocentesis (i.e., the aspiration of fluid from the middle ear) is required to make the specific diagnosis of a middle ear infection. This is unnecessary in most patients, however, because the most common pathogens that cause these infections (*S. pneumoniae, H. influenzae,* and *M. catarrhalis*) can be treated empirically. Outer ear infections are typically caused by *P. aeruginosa* ("swimmer's ear") or *S. aureus*. The proper specimen to be obtained for culture is a scraping of the involved area of the ear.

Collection of specimens for the diagnosis of ocular infections is difficult because the sample obtained is generally very small, and relatively few organisms may be present. Samples of the eye surface should be collected by a swab before topical anesthetics are applied, followed by corneal scrapings when necessary. Intraocular specimens are collected by directly aspirating the eye. The culture media should be inoculated when the specimens are collected and before they are sent to the laboratory. Although most common ocular pathogens grow rapidly (e.g., *S. aureus, S. pneumoniae, H. influenzae, P. aeruginosa, Bacillus cereus*), some may require prolonged incubation (e.g., coagulase-negative staphylococci) or the use of specialized culture media (*N. gonorrhoeae, Chlamydia trachomatis*).

Wounds, Abscesses, and Tissues

Open, draining wounds can often be contaminated with potentially pathogenic organisms unrelated to the specific infectious process. Therefore it is important to collect samples from deep in the wound after the surface has been cleaned. Whenever possible, a swab should be avoided, because it is difficult to obtain a representative sample without contamination by organisms colonizing the surface. Likewise, aspirates from a closed abscess should be collected from both the center and the wall of the abscess. Simply collecting pus from an abscess is generally nonproductive, because most organisms actively replicate at the base of the abscess rather than in the center. Drainage from soft-tissue infections can be collected by aspiration. If drainage material is not obtained, a small quantity of saline can be infused into the tissue and then withdrawn for culture. Saline containing a bactericidal preservative should not be used.

Tissues should be obtained from representative portions of the infectious process, with multiple samples collected whenever possible. The tissue specimen should be transported in a sterile screw-capped container, and sterile saline should be added to prevent drying if a small sample (e.g., biopsy specimen) is collected. A sample of tissue should also be submitted for histologic examination. Because collection of tissue specimens requires invasive procedures, every effort should be made to collect the proper specimen and ensure that it is cultured for all clinically significant organisms that may be responsible for the infection. This requires close communication between the physician and microbiologist.

Urine

Urine is one of the most frequently submitted specimens for culture. Because potentially pathogenic bacteria colonize the urethra, the first portion of urine collected by voiding or catheterization should be discarded. Urinary tract pathogens can also grow in urine, so there should be no delay in the transport of specimens to the laboratory. If the specimen cannot be cultured immediately, it should be refrigerated or placed into a bacteriostatic **urine preservative**. Once the specimen is received in the laboratory, 1 to 10 µl is inoculated onto each culture medium (generally one nonselective agar medium and one selective medium). This is done so that the number of organisms in the urine can be quantitated, which is useful for assessing the significance of an isolate, although small numbers of organisms in a patient with pyuria can be clinically significant. Numerous urine screening procedures (e.g., biochemical tests, microscopy stains) have been developed and are used widely; however, these procedures cannot be recommended, because they are invariably insensitive in detecting a clinically significant low-grade bacteriuria.

Genital Specimens

Despite the variety of bacteria associated with sexually transmitted diseases, most laboratories concentrate on detecting *N. gonorrhoeae* and *C. trachomatis*. Traditionally this was done by inoculating the specimen into a culture system selective for these organisms. This is a slow process, however, taking 2 or more days for a positive culture to be obtained and even more time for isolates to be identified definitively. Culture was also found to be insensitive, because the organisms are extremely labile and die rapidly during transit under less than optimal conditions. For these reasons, a variety of nonculture methods are now used. The most popular methods are nucleic acid amplification procedures (e.g., amplification of species-specific deoxyribonucleic acid [DNA] sequences by the polymerase chain reaction other methods) for both organisms. Detection of these amplified sequences with probes is both sensitive and specific. However, cross-contamination can occur if the test procedures are not controlled carefully. If urine is used for these tests, the first portion of voided urine and not the midstream portion (as is used for culture) should be tested.

The other major bacterium that causes sexually transmitted disease is *Treponema pallidum*, the etiologic agent of syphilis. This organism cannot be cultured in the clinical laboratory, so the diagnosis is made using microscopy or serology. Material from lesions must be examined using darkfield microscopy, because the organism is too thin to be detected using brightfield microscopy. In addition, the organism dies rapidly when exposed to air and drying conditions, so microscopic examination must be performed at the time the specimen is collected.

Fecal Specimens

A large variety of bacteria can cause gastrointestinal infections. For these bacteria to be recovered in culture, an adequate stool sample must be collected (generally not a problem in a patient with diarrhea), transported to the laboratory in a manner that ensures the viability of the infecting organism, and inoculated onto the appropriate selective media. Rectal swabs should not be submitted, because multiple selective media must be inoculated for the various possible pathogens to be recovered. The quantity of feces collected on a swab would be inadequate.

Stool specimens should be collected in a clean pan and then transferred into a tightly sealed waterproof container. The specimens should be transported promptly to the laboratory to prevent acidic changes in the stool (caused by bacterial metabolism), which are toxic for some organisms (e.g., *Shigella*). If a delay is anticipated, the feces should be mixed with a preservative such as phosphate buffer mixed with glycerol or Cary-Blair transport medium. In general, however, rapid transport of the specimen to the laboratory is always superior to the use of any transport medium.

It is important to notify the laboratory if a particular enteric pathogen is suspected, because this will help the laboratory select the appropriate specialized culture medium. For example, although *Vibrio* species can grow on the common media used for the culture of stool specimens, the use of media selective for *Vibrio* facilitates the rapid isolation and identification of this organism. In addition, some organisms are not isolated routinely by laboratory procedures. For example, enterotoxigenic *Escherichia coli* can grow on routine culture media but would not be readily distinguished from nonpathogenic *E. coli*. Likewise, other organisms would not be expected to be in a stool sample, because their disease is caused by toxin produced in the food and not by growth of the organism in the gastrointestinal tract (e.g., *S. aureus*, *Bacillus cereus*). The microbiologist should be able to select the appropriate test (e.g., culture, toxin assay) if the specific pathogen is indicated. *Clostridium difficile* is a significant cause of antibiotic-associated gastrointestinal disease. Although the organism can be cultured from stool specimens if the specimens are delivered promptly to the laboratory, the most specific way to diagnose the infection is by detecting in fecal extracts the *C. difficile* toxins responsible for the disease.

Because many bacteria, both pathogenic and nonpathogenic, are present in fecal specimens, it often takes at least 3 days for the enteric pathogen to be isolated and identified. For this reason, stool cultures are used to confirm the clinical diagnosis, and therapy, if indicated, should not be delayed pending the culture results.

Bacterial Detection and Identification

Detection of bacteria in clinical specimens is accomplished by 5 general procedures: (1) microscopy, (2) detection of bacterial antigens, (3) detection of specific bacterial nucleic acids, (4) culture, and (5) detection of an antibody response to the bacteria (serology). The specific techniques used for these procedures were presented in the preceding chapters and will not be repeated in this chapter. However, Table 19-2 summarizes the relative value of each procedure for the detection of organisms discussed in Chapters 21 to 46.

Although many organisms can be specifically identified by a variety of techniques, the most common procedure used in diagnostic laboratories is to identify an organism isolated in culture by biochemical tests. We believe most students using this textbook are not interested in the details of biochemical identification. Those who are interested should refer to textbooks such as *Bailey and Scott's Diagnostic Microbiology* and the *ASM Manual of Clinical Microbiology*. It is important for all students to appreciate that empiric antimicrobial therapy can be refined based on the preliminary identification of an organism using microscopic and macroscopic morphology and selected, rapid biochemical tests. Refer to Table 19-3 for specific examples.

Antimicrobial Susceptibility Tests

The results of in vitro antimicrobial susceptibility testing are valuable for selecting chemotherapeutic agents active against the infecting organism. Extensive work has been performed in an effort to standardize the testing methods and improve the clinical predictive value of the results. Despite these efforts, in vitro tests are simply a measurement of the effect of the antibiotic against the organism under specific conditions. The selection of an antibiotic and the patient's outcome are influenced by a variety of interrelated factors, including the pharmacokinetic properties of the antibiotic, drug toxicity, the clinical disease, and the patient's general medical status. Thus some organisms that are "susceptible" to an antibiotic will persist in an infection, and some organisms that are "resistant" to an antibiotic will be eliminated. For example, because oxygen is required for aminoglycosides to enter a bacterial cell, these antibiotics are ineffective in an anaerobic abscess. Likewise, very high concentrations of antibiotics can be achieved in urine, so "resistant" bacteria responsible for urinary tract infections can be eliminated by the high urine concentrations of some antibiotics.

Two general forms of antimicrobial susceptibility tests are performed in the clinical laboratory: **broth dilution tests** and **agar diffusion tests**. For broth dilution tests, serial dilutions of an antibiotic are prepared in a nutrient medium and then inoculated with a standardized concentration of the test bacterium. After overnight incubation, the lowest concentration of antibiotic that is able to inhibit the growth of the bacteria is referred to as the **minimum inhibitory concentration (MIC)**. For agar diffusion tests, a standardized concentration of bacteria is spread over the surface of an agar medium, and then paper disks or strips impregnated with antibiotics are placed on the agar surface. After overnight incubation, an area of inhibited growth is

Table 19–2. Detection Methods for Bacteria

Organism	Detection Methods				
	Microscopy	**Antigen Detection**	**Nucleic Acid–Based Tests**	**Culture**	**Antibody Detection**
Gram-Positive Cocci					
Staphylococcus aureus	A	B	C	A	D
Streptococcus pyogenes	B	A	A	A	B
Streptococcus agalactiae	B	B	B	A	D
Streptococcus pneumoniae	A	B	C	A	C
Enterococcus spp.	A	D	B	A	D
Gram-Positive Rods					
Bacillus anthracis	B	C	B	A	D
Bacillus cereus	B	D	D	B	D
Listeria monocytogenes	A	D	D	A	D
Erysipelothrix rhusiopathiae	A	D	D	A	D
Corynebacterium diphtheriae	B	D	C	A	D
Corynebacterium, other spp.	A	D	D	A	D
Tropheryma whippelii	B	D	A	D	D
Acid-Fast and Partially Acid-Fast Rods					
Nocardia spp.	A	D	D	A	D
Rhodococcus equi	A	D	D	A	D
Mycobacterium tuberculosis	A	B	B	A	C
Mycobacterium leprae	B	D	D	D	B
Mycobacterium, other spp.	A	D	B	A	D
Gram-Negative Cocci					
Neisseria gonorrhoeae	A	D	A	A	D
Neisseria meningitidis	A	B	D	A	D
Moraxella catarrhalis	A	D	D	A	D
Gram-Negative Rods					
Escherichia coli	A	B	C	A	D
Salmonella spp.	B	D	D	A	B
Shigella spp.	B	D	D	A	D
Yersinia pestis	B	C	B	A	C
Yersinia enterocolitica	B	D	D	A	B
Enterobacteriaceae, other genera	A	D	D	A	D
Vibrio cholerae	B	D	D	A	D

Continued

Table 19—2. Detection Methods for Bacteria—cont'd

Organism	Detection Methods				
	Microscopy	Antigen Detection	Nucleic Acid—Based Tests	Culture	Antibody Detection
Vibrio, other spp.	B	D	D	A	D
Aeromonas spp.	B	D	D	A	D
Campylobacter spp.	B	A	D	A	D
Helicobacter pylori	B	A	C	B	A
Pseudomonas aeruginosa	A	D	D	A	D
Burkholderia spp.	A	D	D	A	D
Acinetobacter spp.	A	D	D	A	D
Haemophilus influenzae	A	B	C	A	D
Haemophilus ducreyi	B	D	C	A	D
Bordetella pertussis	B	C	A	B	A
Brucella spp.	B	C	D	A	B
Francisella tularensis	B	C	D	A	B
Legionella spp.	B	A	B	A	B
Bartonella spp.	C	D	B	A	A
Anaerobes					
Clostridium perfringens	A	D	D	A	D
Clostridium tetani	B	D	D	A	D
Clostridium botulinum	B	A	D	B	D
Clostridium difficile	B	A	B	B	D
Anaerobic gram-positive cocci	A	D	D	A	D
Anaerobic gram-positive rods	A	D	D	A	D
Anaerobic gram-negative rods	A	D	D	A	D
Spiral-Shaped Bacteria					
Treponema pallidum	B	D	D	D	A
Borrelia burgdorferi	C	D	A	B	A
Borrelia, other spp.	A	D	D	B	D
Leptospira spp.	B	D	D	B	A
Mycoplasma *and Obligate Intracellular Bacteria*					
Mycoplasma pneumoniae	D	C	A	B	A
Rickettsia spp.	B	D	C	D	A
Orientia spp.	B	C	C	C	A
Ehrlichia spp.	B	C	C	C	A

Continued

Table 19–2. Detection Methods for Bacteria—cont'd

Organism	Detection Methods				
	Microscopy	Antigen Detection	Nucleic Acid–Based Tests	Culture	Antibody Detection
Anaplasma spp.	B	C	C	C	A
Coxiella burnetii	C	C	C	C	A
Chlamydia trachomatis	B	B	A	B	D
Chlamydophila pneumoniae	D	D	B	C	B
Chlamydophila psittaci	D	D	B	D	A

A: test generally useful for diagnosis; B: test useful under certain circumstances or for the diagnosis of specific forms of disease; C: test generally not used in diagnostic labs or used only in specialty reference labs; D: test generally not useful.

Table 19–3. Preliminary Identification of Bacteria Isolated in Culture

Organism	Properties
Staphylococcus aureus	Gram-positive cocci in clusters; large, β-hemolytic colonies; catalase-positive, coagulase-positive
Streptococcus pyogenes	Gram-positive cocci in long chains; small colonies with large zone of β hemolysis; catalase-negative, PYR-positive (ʟ-pyrrolidonyl arylamidase)
Streptococcus pneumoniae	Gram-positive cocci in pairs and short chains; small, α-hemolytic colonies; catalase-negative, soluble in bile
Enterococcus spp.	Gram-positive cocci in pairs and short chains; large, α- or nonhemolytic colonies; catalase-negative, PYR-positive
Listeria monocytogenes	Small, gram-positive rods; small, weakly β-hemolytic colonies; characteristic (tumbling) motility
Nocardia spp.	Weakly staining (Gram and modified acid-fast), thin, filamentous, branching rods; slow growth; fuzzy colonies (aerial hyphae)
Rhodococcus equi	Weakly staining (Gram and modified acid-fast); initially nonbranching rods, cocci in older cultures; slow growth; pink-red colonies
Mycobacterium tuberculosis	Strongly acid-fast rods; slow growth; nonpigmented colonies; identified using specific molecular probes
Enterobacteriaceae	Gram-negative rods with "bipolar" staining (more intense at ends); typically single cells; large colonies; growth on MacConkey agar (may/may not ferment lactose); oxidase-negative
Pseudomonas aeruginosa	Gram-negative rods with uniform staining; typically in pairs; large, spreading, fluorescent green colonies, usually β-hemolytic, fruity smell (grapelike); growth on MacConkey agar (nonfermenter); oxidase-positive
Stenotrophomonas maltophilia	Gram-negative rods with uniform staining; typically in pairs; lavender/green color on blood agar; growth on MacConkey agar (nonfermenter); oxidase-negative
Acinetobacter spp.	Large, gram-negative coccobacilli arranged as single cells or pairs; will retain crystal violet and may resemble fat, gram-positive cocci in pairs; growth on blood agar and MacConkey agar (may oxidize lactose and resemble weakly purple); oxidase-negative
Campylobacter spp.	Thin, curved, gram-negative rods arranged in pairs (S-shaped pairs); growth on highly selective media for *Campylobacter*; no growth on routine media (blood, chocolate, or MacConkey agars)
Haemophilus spp.	Small, gram-negative coccobacilli arranged as single cells; growth on chocolate agar but not blood or MacConkey agars; oxidase-positive
Brucella spp.	Very small, gram-negative coccobacilli arranged as single cells; slow-growing; no growth on MacConkey agar; biohazard

Continued

Table 19–3. Preliminary Identification of Bacteria Isolated in Culture—cont'd

Organism	Properties
Francisella spp.	Very small, gram-negative coccobacilli arranged as single cells; slow-growing, no growth on blood or MacConkey agars; biohazard
Legionella spp.	Weakly staining, thin, gram-negative rods; slow-growing; growth on specialized agar; no growth on blood, chocolate, or MacConkey agars
Clostridium perfringens	Large, rectangular rods with spores not observed; rapid growth of spreading colonies with "double zone" of hemolysis (large zone of α hemolysis with inner zone of β hemolysis); strict anaerobe
Bacteroides fragilis group	Weakly staining, pleomorphic (variable lengths), gram-negative rods; rapid growth stimulated by bile in media; strict anaerobe

observed surrounding the paper disks or strips. The size of the area of inhibition corresponds to the activity of the antibiotic—the more susceptible the organism is to the antibiotic, the larger the area of inhibited growth. By standardizing the test conditions for agar diffusion tests, the area of inhibition corresponds to the MIC value.

Broth dilution tests were originally performed in test tubes and were very labor intensive. Commercially prepared systems are now available; antibiotic dilutions are prepared in microtiter trays, and the inoculation of the trays and interpretation of the MICs are automated. The disadvantages of these systems are that the range of different antibiotics is determined by the manufacturer, and the number of dilutions of an individual antibiotic is limited. Thus results may not be available for newly introduced antibiotics. Diffusion tests are labor intensive, and the interpretation of the size of the area of inhibition can be subjective; however, the advantage of these tests is that virtually any antibiotic can be tested. The ability of both susceptibility testing methods to predict clinical response to an antibiotic is equivalent, so the selection of the tests is determined by practical considerations.

Question

1. What is the most important factor that influences the recovery of microorganisms in blood collected from patients with sepsis?
2. Which organisms are important causes of bacterial pharyngitis?
3. What criteria should be used to assess the quality of a lower respiratory tract specimen?
4. What methods are used to detect the three most common bacteria that cause sexually transmitted diseases?

Bibliography

Forbes B, et al: Bailey and Scott's Diagnostic Microbiology, 12th ed. St Louis, Mosby, 2007.

Mandell G, Bennett J, Dolin R: Principles and Practice of Infectious Diseases, 6th ed. New York, Churchill Livingstone, 2005.

Murray P, et al: Manual of Clinical Microbiology, 9th ed. Washington, DC, ASM Press, 2007.

Antibacterial Agents

This chapter provides an overview of the mechanisms of action and spectrum of the most commonly used antibacterial antibiotics, as well as a description of the common mechanisms of bacterial resistance. The terminology appropriate for this discussion is summarized in Box 20-1, and the basic mechanisms and sites of antibiotic activity are summarized in Table 20-1 and Figure 20-1, respectively.

The year 1935 was an important one for the chemotherapy of systemic bacterial infections. Although antiseptics had been applied topically to prevent the growth of microorganisms, the existing antiseptics were ineffective against systemic bacterial infections. In 1935, the dye prontosil was shown to protect mice against systemic streptococcal infection and to be curative in patients suffering from such infections. It was soon found that prontosil was cleaved in the body to release *p*-aminobenzene sulfonamide (sulfanilamide), which was shown to have antibacterial activity. This first "sulfa" drug ushered in a new era in medicine. Compounds produced by microorganisms (antibiotics) were eventually discovered to inhibit the growth of other microorganisms. For example, Alexander Fleming was the first to realize the mold *Penicillium* prevented the multiplication of staphylococci. A concentrate from a culture of this mold was prepared, and the remarkable antibacterial activity and lack of toxicity of the first antibiotic, penicillin, were demonstrated. Streptomycin and the tetracyclines were developed in the 1940s and 1950s, followed rapidly by the development of additional aminoglycosides, semisynthetic penicillins, cephalosporins, quinolones, and other antimicrobials. All these antibacterial agents greatly increased the range of infectious diseases that could be prevented or cured. Although the development of new antibacterial antibiotics has lagged in recent years, some new classes of agents have been introduced, including the ketolides (e.g., **telithromycin**), glycylcyclines (**tigecycline**), lipopeptides (**daptomycin**), streptogramins (**quinupristin-dalfopristin**), and oxazolidinones (**linezolid**).

Unfortunately, with the introduction of new chemotherapeutic agents, bacteria have shown a remarkable ability to develop resistance. Thus antibiotic therapy will not be the magical cure for all infections, as predicted; rather, it is only one weapon, albeit an important one, against infectious diseases. It is also important to recognize that because resistance to antibiotics is often not predictable, physicians must rely on their clinical experience for the initial selection of **empirical therapy**. Guidelines for the management of infections caused by specific organisms are discussed in the relevant chapters of this text.

Inhibition of Cell Wall Synthesis

The most common mechanism of antibiotic activity is interference with bacterial cell wall synthesis. Most of the cell-wall-active antibiotics are classified as β-lactam antibiotics (e.g., penicillins, cephalosporins, cephamycins, carbapenems, monobactams, β-lactamase inhibitors), so named because they share a common β-lactam ring structure. Other antibiotics that interfere with construction of the bacterial cell wall include vancomycin, daptomycin, bacitracin, and the following antimycobacterial agents: isoniazid, ethambutol, cycloserine, and ethionamide.

β-Lactam Antibiotics

The major structural component of most bacterial cell walls is the peptidoglycan layer. The basic structure is a chain of 10 to 65 disaccharide residues consisting of alternating molecules of *N*-acetylglucosamine and *N*-acetylmuramic acid. These chains are then cross-linked with peptide bridges that create a rigid mesh coating for the bacteria. The building of the chains and cross-links is catalyzed by specific enzymes (e.g., transpeptidases, transglycosylases, carboxypeptidases) that are members of a large family of **serine proteases**. These regulatory enzymes are also called **penicillin-binding proteins (PBPs)**, because they are the targets of β-lactam antibiotics. When growing bacteria are exposed to these antibiotics, the antibiotic binds to specific PBPs in the bacterial cell wall and inhibits assembly of the peptidoglycan chains. This in turn activates autolysins

Box 20–1. Terminology

Antibacterial spectrum:

Range of activity of an antimicrobial against bacteria. A **broad-spectrum** antibacterial drug can inhibit a variety of gram-positive and gram-negative bacteria, whereas a **narrow-spectrum** drug is active only against a limited variety of bacteria.

Bacteriostatic activity:

Level of antimicrobial activity that **inhibits** the growth of an organism. This is determined in vitro by testing a standardized concentration of organisms against a series of antimicrobial dilutions. The lowest concentration that inhibits the growth of the organism is referred to as the **minimum inhibitory concentration (MIC)**.

Bactericidal activity:

Level of antimicrobial activity that kills the test organism. This is determined in vitro by exposing a standardized concentration of organisms to a series of antimicrobial dilutions. The lowest concentration that kills 99.9% of the population is referred to as the **minimum bactericidal concentration (MBC)**.

Antibiotic combinations:

Combinations of antibiotics that may be used to (1) broaden the antibacterial spectrum for empirical therapy or the treatment of polymicrobial infections, (2) prevent the emergence of resistant organisms during therapy, and (3) achieve a synergistic killing effect.

Antibiotic synergism:

Combinations of two antibiotics that have enhanced bactericidal activity when tested together compared with the activity of each antibiotic.

Antibiotic antagonism:

Combination of antibiotics in which the activity of one antibiotic interferes with the activity of the other (e.g., the sum of the activity is less than the activity of the most active individual drug).

β-Lactamase:

An enzyme that hydrolyzes the β-lactam ring in the β-lactam class of antibiotics, thus inactivating the antibiotic. The enzymes specific for penicillins, cephalosporins, and carbapenems are the **penicillinases, cephalosporinases**, and **carbapenemases** (metallo-β-lactamases), respectively.

that degrade the cell wall, resulting in bacterial cell death. Thus the β-lactam antibiotics generally act as bactericidal agents.

Bacteria can become resistant to β-lactam antibiotics by three general mechanisms: (1) prevention of the interaction between the antibiotic and the target PBP, (2) modification of the binding of the antibiotic to the PBP, and (3) hydrolysis of the antibiotic by β-lactamases. The first mechanism of resistance is seen only in gram-negative bacteria (particularly *Pseudomonas* species), because they have an outer membrane that overlies the peptidoglycan layer. Penetration of β-lactam antibiotics into gram-negative rods requires transit through pores in the outer membrane. Changes in the proteins (**porins**) that form the walls of the pores can alter the size or charge of these channels and result in the exclusion of the antibiotic.

Resistance can also be acquired by modification of the β-lactam antibiotic binding to the PBP. This can be mediated by (1) an overproduction of PBP (a rare occurrence), (2) acquisition of a new PBP (e.g., methicillin resistance in *Staphylococcus aureus*), or (3) modification of an existing PBP through recombination (e.g., penicillin resistance in *Streptococcus pneumoniae*) or a point mutation (penicillin resistance in *Enterococcus faecium*).

Finally, bacteria can produce **β-lactamases** that inactivate the β-lactam antibiotics. Interestingly the β-lactamases are in the same family of serine proteases as the PBPs. More than 200 different β-lactamases have been described. Some are specific for penicillins (i.e., penicillinases), cephalosporins (i.e., cephalosporinases), or carbapenems (i.e., carbapenemases), whereas others have a broad range of activity, including some that are capable of inactivating most β-lactam antibiotics. An exhaustive discussion of β-lactamases is beyond the scope of this chapter; however, a brief discussion is germane for understanding the limitations of β-lactam antibiotics. By one classification scheme, β-lactamases have been separated into four classes (A to D). The most common class A β-lactamases are SHV-1 and TEM-1, penicillinases found in common gram-negative rods (e.g., *Escherichia, Klebsiella*), with minimal activity against cephalosporins. Unfortunately, simple point mutations in the genes encoding these enzymes have created β-lactamases with activity against all penicillins and cephalosporins. These β-lactamases are referred to as **extended-spectrum β-lactamases (ESBLs)** and are particularly troublesome because they are encoded on plasmids that can be transferred from organism to organism. The class B β-lactamases are zinc-dependent metalloenzymes that have a broad spectrum of activity against all β-lactam antibiotics, including the cephamycins and carbapenems. The **class C β-lactamases** are primarily cephalosporinases that are encoded on the bacterial chromosome. Expression of these enzymes is generally repressed, although this can be altered by exposure to certain "inducing" β-lactam antibiotics or by mutations in the genes controlling expression of the enzymes. Expression of this class of β-lactamases is particularly troublesome because they are active against the most potent expanded-spectrum cephalosporins. The class D β-lactamases are penicillinases found primarily in gram-negative rods.

Penicillins

Penicillin antibiotics (Table 20-2) are highly effective antibiotics with an extremely low toxicity. The basic compound is an organic acid with a β-lactam ring obtained from culture of the mold *Penicillium chrysogenum*. If the mold is grown by a fermentation process, large amounts of 6-aminopenicillanic acid (the β-lactam ring is fused with a thiazolidine ring) are produced. The biochemical

Table 20—1. Basic Mechanisms of Antibiotic Action

Antibiotic	Action
Disruption of Cell Wall	
Penicillins Cephalosporins Cephamycins Carbapenems Monobactams	Bind PBPs and enzymes responsible for peptidoglycan synthesis
β-lactam/β-lactamase inhibitor	Binds β-lactamases and prevents enzymatic inactivation of β-lactam
Vancomycin	Inhibits cross-linkage of peptidoglycan layers
Daptomycin	Causes depolarization of cytoplasmic membrane, resulting in disruption of ionic concentration gradients
Bacitracin	Inhibits bacterial cytoplasmic membrane and movement of peptidoglycan precursors
Polymyxins	Inhibit bacterial membranes
Isoniazid Ethionamide	Inhibit mycolic acid synthesis
Ethambutol	Inhibits arabinogalactan synthesis
Cycloserine	Inhibits cross-linkage of peptidoglycan layers
Inhibition of Protein Synthesis	
Aminoglycosides	Produce premature release of aberrant peptide chains from 30S ribosome
Tetracyclines	Prevent polypeptide elongation at 30S ribosome
Glycylcyclines	Bind to 30S ribosome and prevent initiation of protein synthesis
Oxazolidinone	Prevents initiation of protein synthesis at 50S ribosome
Macrolides Ketolides Clindamycin Streptogramins	Prevent polypeptide elongation at 50S ribosome
Inhibition of Nucleic Acid Synthesis	
Quinolones	Bind α subunit of DNA gyrase
Rifampin Rifabutin	Prevent transcription by binding DNA-dependent RNA polymerase
Metronidazole	Disrupts bacteria DNA (is cytotoxic compound)
Antimetabolite	
Sulfonamides	Inhibit dihydropteroate synthase and disrupt folic acid synthesis
Dapsone	Inhibits dihydropteroate synthase
Trimethoprim	Inhibits dihydrofolate reductase and disrupts folic acid synthesis

DNA, deoxyribonucleic acid; PBPs, penicillin-binding proteins; RNA, ribonucleic acid.

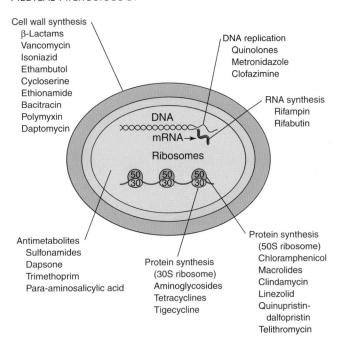

Cell wall synthesis
  β-Lactams
  Vancomycin
  Isoniazid
  Ethambutol
  Cycloserine
  Ethionamide
  Bacitracin
  Polymyxin
  Daptomycin

DNA replication
  Quinolones
  Metronidazole
  Clofazimine

RNA synthesis
  Rifampin
  Rifabutin

DNA
xxxxxxxxxxx
mRNA
Ribosomes

Antimetabolites
  Sulfonamides
  Dapsone
  Trimethoprim
  Para-aminosalicylic acid

Protein synthesis
(30S ribosome)
  Aminoglycosides
  Tetracyclines
  Tigecycline

Protein synthesis
(50S ribosome)
  Chloramphenicol
  Macrolides
  Clindamycin
  Linezolid
  Quinupristin-
    dalfopristin
  Telithromycin

Figure 20—1. Basic sites of antibiotic activity.

modification of this intermediate yields derivatives that have decreased acid lability and increased absorption in the gastrointestinal tract, resistance to destruction by penicillinase, or a broader spectrum of activity that includes gram-negative bacteria.

Penicillin G is incompletely absorbed because it is inactivated by gastric acid. Thus it is used mainly as an intravenous drug for the treatment of infections caused by the limited number of susceptible organisms. Penicillin V is more resistant to acid and is the preferred oral form for the treatment of susceptible bacteria. **Penicillinase-resistant penicillins** such as methicillin and oxacillin are used to treat infections caused by susceptible staphylococci. Ampicillin was the first **broad-spectrum penicillin**, although the spectrum of activity against gram-negative rods was limited primarily to *Escherichia*, *Proteus*, and *Haemophilus* species. Other penicillins (e.g., carbenicillin, ticarcillin, piperacillin) are effective against a broader range of gram-negative bacteria, including *Klebsiella*, *Enterobacter*, and *Pseudomonas* species.

Selected penicillins have been combined with **β-lactamase inhibitors**. The β-lactamase inhibitors (e.g., clavulanic acid, sulbactam, tazobactam) are relatively inactive by themselves; but when combined with certain penicillins (i.e., ampicillin, amoxicillin, ticarcillin, piperacillin), they are effective in treating some infections caused by β-lactamase-producing bacteria. The inhibitors irreversibly bind and inactivate susceptible bacterial β-lactamases (although not all are bound by these inhibitors), permitting the companion drug to disrupt bacterial cell wall synthesis.

Cephalosporins and Cephamycins

The cephalosporins (Table 20-3) are β-lactam antibiotics derived from 7-aminocephalosporanic acid (the β-lactam

Table 20—2. Penicillins

Antibiotics	Spectrum of Activity
Natural penicillins: benzylpenicillin (penicillin G), phenoxymethyl penicillin (penicillin V)	Active against all β-hemolytic streptococci and most other species; limited activity against staphylococci; active against meningococci and most gram-positive anaerobes; poor activity against aerobic and anaerobic gram-negative rods
Penicillinase-resistant penicillins: methicillin, nafcillin, oxacillin, cloxacillin, dicloxacillin	Similar to the natural penicillins, except enhanced activity against staphylococci
Broad-spectrum penicillins: aminopenicillins (ampicillin, amoxicillin); carboxypenicillins (carbenicillin, ticarcillin); ureidopenicillins (piperacillin)	Activity against gram-positive cocci equivalent to the natural penicillins; active against some gram-negative rods, with piperacillin the most active
β-Lactam with β-lactamase inhibitor (ampicillin-sulbactam, amoxicillin-clavulanate, ticarcillin-clavulanate, piperacillin-tazobactam)	Activity similar to natural β-lactams, plus improved activity against β-lactamase-producing staphylococci and selected gram-negative rods; not all β-lactamases are inhibited; piperacillin/tazobactam is the most active

Table 20—3. Selected Examples of Cephalosporins and Cephamycins

Antibiotics	Spectrum of Activity
Narrow spectrum (cephalexin, cephalothin, cefazolin, cephapirin, cephradine)	Activity equivalent to oxacillin against gram-positive bacteria; some gram-negative activity (e.g., *Escherichia coli*, *Klebsiella*, *Proteus mirabilis*)
Expanded-spectrum cephalosporins (cefaclor, cefuroxime)	Activity equivalent to oxacillin against gram-positive bacteria; improved gram-negative activity to include *Enterobacter*, *Citrobacter*, and additional *Proteus* species
Expanded-spectrum cephamycins (cefotetan, cefoxitin)	Activity similar to expanded-spectrum cephalosporins but less susceptible to β-lactamases
Broad spectrum (cefixime, cefotaxime, ceftriaxone, ceftazidime)	Activity equivalent to oxacillin against gram-positive bacteria; improved gram-negative activity to include *Pseudomonas*
Extended spectrum (cefepime, cefpirome)	Activity equivalent to oxacillin against gram-positive bacteria; marginally improved gram-negative activity

ring is fused with a dihydrothiazine ring) that was originally isolated from the mold *Cephalosporium*. The cephamycins are closely related to the cephalosporins, except that they contain oxygen in place of sulfur in the dihydrothiazine ring, rendering them more stable to β-lactamase hydrolysis. The cephalosporins and cephamycins have the same mechanism of action as the penicillins; however, they have a wider antibacterial spectrum, are resistant to many β-lactamases, and have improved pharmacokinetic properties (e.g., longer half-life).

Biochemical modifications in the basic antibiotic molecule resulted in the development of antibiotics with improved activity and pharmacokinetic properties. The cephalosporins have enhanced activity against gram-negative bacteria compared with the penicillins. This activity in turn varies among the different "generations" of cephalosporins. The activity of **narrow**-**spectrum** first-generation antibiotics is primarily restricted to *Escherichia coli, Klebsiella* species, *Proteus mirabilis*, and oxacillin-susceptible gram-positive cocci. Many of the **expanded-spectrum** second-generation antibiotics have additional activity against *Haemophilus influenzae, Enterobacter, Citrobacter*, and *Serratia* species and some anaerobes, such as *Bacteroides fragilis*. The **broad-spectrum** third-generation antibiotics and **extended-spectrum** fourth-generation antibiotics are active against most Enterobacteriaceae and *Pseudomonas aeruginosa*. Extended-spectrum antibiotics offer the advantage of increased stability to β-lactamases. Unfortunately, gram-negative bacteria have rapidly developed resistance to most cephalosporins and cephamycins (primarily as the result of β-lactamase production), which has significantly compromised the use of all these agents.

Other β-Lactam Antibiotics

Other classes of β-lactam antibiotics (Table 20-4) are the **carbapenems** (e.g., imipenem, meropenem, ertapenem) and **monobactams** (e.g., aztreonam). The carbapenems are important, widely prescribed broad-spectrum antibiotics

Table 20—4. Other β-Lactam Antibiotics

Antibiotics	Spectrum of Activity
Carbapenems (imipenem, meropenem, ertapenem)	Broad-spectrum antibiotics active against most aerobic and anaerobic gram-positive and gram-negative bacteria except oxacillin-resistant staphylococci, most *Enterococcus faecium*, and selected gram-negative rods (e.g., some *Burkholderia, Stenotrophomonas*, some *Pseudomonas*)
Monobactam (aztreonam)	Active against selected aerobic gram-negative rods but inactive against anaerobes or gram-positive cocci

that are active against virtually all groups of organisms, with only a few exceptions (e.g., resistance has been reported for all oxacillin-resistant staphylococci, selected Enterobacteriaceae and *Pseudomonas*, and other gram-negative rods). In contrast, the monobactams are narrow-spectrum antibiotics that are active only against aerobic, gram-negative bacteria. Anaerobic bacteria and gram-positive bacteria are resistant. The advantage of narrow-spectrum antibiotics is that they can be used to treat susceptible organisms without disruption of the patient's normal protective bacterial population. Despite this advantage, monobactams are not widely used.

Glycopeptides

Vancomycin, originally obtained from *Streptomyces orientalis*, is a complex glycopeptide that disrupts cell wall peptidoglycan synthesis in growing gram-positive bacteria. Vancomycin interacts with the D-alanine—D-alanine termini of the pentapeptide side chains, which interferes sterically with the formation of the bridges between the peptidoglycan chains. Vancomycin is used for the management of infections caused by oxacillin-resistant staphylococci and other gram-positive bacteria resistant to β-lactam antibiotics. Vancomycin is inactive against gram-negative bacteria because the molecule is too large to pass through the outer membrane pores and reach the peptidoglycan target site. In addition, some organisms are intrinsically resistant to vancomycin (e.g., *Leuconostoc, Lactobacillus, Pediococcus*, and *Erysipelothrix*) because the pentapeptide terminates in D-alanine—D-lactate, which does not bind vancomycin. Intrinsic resistance is also found in some species of enterococci that contain a D-alanine—D-serine terminus (i.e., *Enterococcus gallinarum, Enterococcus casseliflavus*). Finally, some species of enterococci (particularly *Enterococcus faecium* and *Enterococcus faecalis*) have acquired resistance to vancomycin. The genes for this resistance (primarily *van*A and *van*B), which also mediate changes in the pentapeptide terminus, can be carried on plasmids and have seriously compromised the usefulness of vancomycin for the treatment of enterococcal infections. More importantly, the gene for vancomycin resistance contained within a transposon on a multiresistance conjugative plasmid has been transferred in vivo from *E. faecalis* to a multiresistant *S. aureus*. The transposon then moved from the *E. faecalis* plasmid and recombined and integrated into the *S. aureus* multiresistance plasmid. This resulted in an *S. aureus* plasmid that encoded resistance to β-lactams, vancomycin, aminoglycosides, and other antibiotics—a plasmid that could be transferred to other staphylococci by conjugation. Obviously if this resistance becomes widespread, the medical implications are profound.

Lipopeptides

Daptomycin, a naturally occurring cyclic lipopeptide produced by *Streptomyces roseosporus*, binds irreversibly to the cytoplasmic membrane, resulting in membrane depolarization and disruption of the ionic gradients, ultimately leading to cell death. It has potent activity against gram-positive bacteria, but gram-negative bacteria are resistant to daptomycin because the drug cannot penetrate through the cell wall to the cytoplasmic membrane. Daptomycin has good activity against multidrug resistant staphylococci, streptococci, and enterococci (including vancomycin-resistant strains.

Polypeptides

Bacitracin, which was isolated from *Bacillus licheniformis*, is a mixture of polypeptides used in topically applied products (e.g., creams, ointments, sprays) for the treatment of skin infections caused by gram-positive bacteria (particularly those caused by *Staphylococcus* and group A *Streptococcus*). Gram-negative bacteria are resistant to this agent. Bacitracin inhibits cell wall synthesis by interfering with dephosphorylation and the recycling of the lipid carrier responsible for moving the peptidoglycan precursors through the cytoplasmic membrane to the cell wall. It may also damage the bacterial cytoplasmic membrane and inhibit ribonucleic acid (RNA) transcription. Resistance to the antibiotic is most likely caused by failure of the antibiotic to penetrate into the bacterial cell.

The **polymyxins** are a group of cyclic polypeptides derived from *Bacillus polymyxa*. These antibiotics insert into bacterial membranes like detergents by interacting with lipopolysaccharides and the phospholipids in the outer membrane, producing increased cell permeability and eventual cell death. **Polymyxins B** and **E** (**colistin**) are capable of causing serious nephrotoxicity. Thus their use has been limited chiefly to the external treatment of localized infections such as external otitis, eye infections, and skin infections caused by sensitive organisms, although colistin is used to treat some systemic infections caused by multidrug resistant gram-negative rods. Oral administration is used to sterilize the gut. These antibiotics are most active against gram-negative rods, because gram-positive bacteria do not have an outer membrane.

Isoniazid, Ethionamide, Ethambutol, and Cycloserine

Isoniazid, ethionamide, ethambutol, and cycloserine are cell-wall-active antibiotics used for the treatment of mycobacterial infections. **Isoniazid** (isonicotinic acid hydrazide [INH]) is bactericidal against actively replicating mycobacteria. Although the exact mechanism of action is unknown, the synthesis of mycolic acid is affected (the desaturation of the long-chain fatty acids and the elongation of fatty acids and hydroxy lipids are disrupted). **Ethionamide**, a derivative of INH, also blocks mycolic acid synthesis. **Ethambutol** interferes with the synthesis of arabinogalactan in the cell wall, and **cycloserine** inhibits two enzymes, D-alanine—D-alanine synthetase and alanine racemase,

which catalyze cell wall synthesis. Resistance to these four antibiotics results primarily from reduced drug uptake into the bacterial cell or alteration of the target sites.

Inhibition of Protein Synthesis

The primary action of the agents in the second largest class of antibiotics is the inhibition of protein synthesis (see Table 20-1).

Aminoglycosides

The aminoglycoside antibiotics (Table 20-5) consist of amino sugars linked through glycosidic bonds to an aminocyclitol ring. Streptomycin, neomycin, kanamycin, and tobramycin were originally isolated from *Streptomyces* species, and gentamicin and sisomicin were isolated from *Micromonospora* species. Amikacin and netilmicin are synthetic derivatives of kanamycin and sisomicin, respectively. These antibiotics exert their effect by passing through the bacterial outer membrane (in gram-negative bacteria), cell wall, and cytoplasmic membrane to the cytoplasm, where they inhibit bacterial protein synthesis by irreversibly binding to the 30S ribosomal proteins. This attachment to the ribosomes has two effects: production of aberrant proteins as the result of misreading of the messenger RNA (mRNA), and interruption of protein synthesis by causing the premature release of the ribosome from mRNA.

The aminoglycosides are bactericidal because of their ability to bind irreversibly to ribosomes and are commonly used to treat serious infections caused by many gram-negative rods (e.g., Enterobacteriaceae, *Pseudomonas*, *Acinetobacter*) and some gram-positive organisms. Penetration through the cytoplasmic membrane is an aerobic, energy-dependent process, so anaerobes are resistant to aminoglycosides, and susceptible organisms in an anaerobic environment (e.g., abscess) do not respond to treatment. Streptococci and enterococci are resistant to aminoglycosides because the aminoglycosides fail to penetrate through the cell wall of these bacteria. Treatment of these organisms requires co-administration of an aminoglycoside with an inhibitor of cell wall synthesis (e.g., penicillin, ampicillin, vancomycin) that facilitates uptake of the aminoglycoside.

The most commonly used antibiotics in this class are **amikacin**, **gentamicin**, and **tobramycin**. All three aminoglycosides are used to treat systemic infections caused by susceptible gram-negative bacteria. **Amikacin** has the best activity and is frequently reserved for treatment of infections caused by gram-negative bacteria that are resistant to gentamicin and tobramycin. **Streptomycin** is not readily available but has been used for the treatment of tuberculosis, tularemia, and gentamicin-resistant streptococcal or enterococcal infections (in combination with a penicillin).

Resistance to the antibacterial action of aminoglycosides can develop in one of four ways: (1) mutation of the

Table 20—5. Inhibitors of Protein Synthesis

Antibiotics	Spectrum of Activity
Aminoglycosides (streptomycin, kanamycin, gentamicin, tobramycin, amikacin)	Primarily used to treat infections with gram-negative rods; kanamycin with limited activity; tobramycin slightly more active than gentamicin against *Pseudomonas*; amikacin most active; streptomycin and gentamicin combined with cell-wall-active antibiotic to treat enterococcal infections; streptomycin active against mycobacteria and selected gram-negative rods
Aminocyclitol (spectinomycin)	Active against *Neisseria gonorrhoeae*
Tetracyclines (tetracycline, doxycycline, minocycline)	Broad-spectrum antibiotics active against gram-positive and some gram-negative bacteria (*Neisseria*, some Enterobacteriaceae), mycoplasmas, chlamydiae, and rickettsiae
Glycylcyclines (tigecycline)	Spectrum similar to tetracyclines but more active against gram-negative bacteria and rapidly growing mycobacteria
Oxazolidinone (linezolid)	Active against staphylococcus (including methicillin-resistant and vancomycin-intermediate strains), *Enterococcus*, *Streptococcus*, gram-positive rods, and *Clostridium* and anaerobic cocci; not active against gram-negative bacteria
Macrolides (erythromycin, azithromycin, clarithromycin)	Broad-spectrum antibiotics active against gram-positive and some gram-negative bacteria, *Neisseria*, *Legionella*, *Mycoplasma*, *Chlamydia*, *Chlamydophila*, *Treponema*, and *Rickettsia*; clarithromycin and azithromycin active against some mycobacteria
Ketolides (telithromycin)	Broad-spectrum antibiotic with activity similar to macrolides; active against some macrolide-resistant staphylococci and enterococci
Lincosamide (clindamycin)	Broad-spectrum activity against aerobic gram-positive cocci and anaerobes
Streptogramins (quinupristin-dalfopristin)	Primarily active against gram-positive bacteria; good activity against methicillin-susceptible and methicillin-resistant staphylococci, streptococci; vancomycin-susceptible and vancomycin-resistant *Enterococcus faecium* (no activity against *E. faecalis*); *Haemophilus*, *Moraxella*, and anaerobes (including *Bacteroides fragilis*); not active against Enterobacteriaceae or other gram-negative rods

ribosomal binding site, (2) decreased uptake of the antibiotic into the bacterial cell, (3) increased expulsion of the antibiotic from the cell, or (4) enzymatic modification of the antibiotic. The most common mechanism of resistance is enzymatic modification of aminoglycosides. This is accomplished by the action of phosphotransferases (APHs; seven described), adenyltransferases (ANTs; four described), and acetyltransferases (AACs; four described) on the amino and hydroxyl groups of the antibiotic. The differences in the antibacterial activity among the aminoglycosides are determined by their relative susceptibility to these enzymes. The other mechanisms by which bacteria develop resistance to aminoglycosides are relatively uncommon. Resistance caused by alteration of the bacterial ribosome requires systematic mutation of the multiple copies of the ribosomal genes that exist in the bacterial cell. Resistance caused by inhibited transport of the antibiotic into the bacterial cell is occasionally observed with *Pseudomonas* but is more commonly seen with anaerobic bacteria.

This mechanism produces low-level cross-resistance to all aminoglycosides. Active efflux of aminoglycosides occurs only in gram-negative bacteria and is rarely observed.

Tetracyclines

The tetracyclines (see Table 20-5) are broad-spectrum bacteriostatic antibiotics that inhibit protein synthesis in bacteria by binding reversibly to the 30S ribosomal subunits, thus blocking the binding of aminoacyl-transfer RNA (tRNA) to the 30S ribosome—mRNA complex. Tetracyclines (i.e., **tetracycline, doxycycline, minocycline**) are effective in the treatment of infections caused by *Chlamydia*, *Mycoplasma*, and *Rickettsia* species and other selected gram-positive and gram-negative bacteria. All tetracyclines have a similar spectrum of activity, with the primary difference among the antibiotics being in their pharmacokinetic properties (doxycycline and minocycline are easily absorbed and have a long half-life).

Resistance to the tetracyclines can stem from decreased penetration of the antibiotic into the bacterial cell, active efflux of the antibiotic out of the cell, alteration of the ribosomal target site, or enzymatic modification of the antibiotic. Mutations in the chromosomal gene encoding the outer membrane porin protein, OmpF, can lead to low-level resistance to the tetracyclines, as well as to other antibiotics (e.g., β-lactams, quinolones, chloramphenicol).

Researchers have identified a variety of genes that control the active efflux of the tetracyclines from the cell in different bacteria. This is the most common cause of resistance. Resistance to the tetracyclines can also result from the production of proteins similar to elongation factors that protect the 30S ribosome. When this happens, the antibiotic can still bind to the ribosome, but protein synthesis is not disrupted.

Glycylcyclines

Tigecycline, the first representative of this class of antibiotics, is a semisynthetic derivative of minocycline. It inhibits protein synthesis in the same manner as the tetracyclines. Tigecycline has a higher binding affinity for the ribosome and is less affected by efflux or enzymatic modification. It has a broad spectrum of activity against gram-positive, gram-negative, and anaerobic bacteria, although *Proteus, Morganella, Providencia,* and *Pseudomonas aeruginosa* are generally resistant.

Oxazolidinones

The oxazolidinones are a narrow-spectrum class of antibiotics, with **linezolid** being the agent currently used. Linezolid blocks initiation of protein synthesis by interfering with the formation of the initiation complex consisting of tRNA, mRNA, and the ribosome. The drug binds to the 50S ribosomal subunit, which distorts the binding site for tRNA, thus inhibiting formation of the 70S initiation complex. Because of this unique mechanism, cross-resistance with other protein inhibitors does not occur. Linezolid has activity against all staphylococci, streptococci, and enterococci (including those strains resistant to penicillins, vancomycin, and the aminoglycosides). Because the multidrug-resistant enterococci are difficult to treat, use of linezolid is generally reserved for these infections.

Chloramphenicol

Chloramphenicol has a broad antibacterial spectrum similar to that of tetracycline but is not commonly used in the United States. The reason for its limited use is that besides interfering with bacterial protein synthesis, it disrupts protein synthesis in human bone marrow cells and can produce blood dyscrasias such as aplastic anemia (one per 24,000 treated patients). Chloramphenicol exerts its bacteriostatic effect by binding reversibly to the peptidyl transferase component of the 50S ribosomal subunit, thus blocking peptide elongation. Resistance to chloramphenicol is observed in bacteria producing plasmid-encoded chloramphenicol acetyltransferase, which catalyzes the acetylation of the 3-hydroxy group of chloramphenicol. The product is incapable of binding to the 50S subunit. Less commonly, chromosomal mutations alter the outer membrane porin proteins, causing the gram-negative rods to be less permeable.

Macrolides

Erythromycin, derived from *Streptomyces erythreus*, is the model macrolide antibiotic (see Table 20-5). The basic structure of this class of antibiotics is a macrocyclic lactone ring bound to two sugars, desosamine and cladinose. Modification of the macrolide structure led to the development of **azithromycin** and **clarithromycin**. Macrolides exert their effect by their reversible binding to the 23S rRNA of the 50S ribosomal subunit, which blocks polypeptide elongation. Resistance to macrolides most commonly stems from the methylation of the 23S ribosomal RNA, preventing binding by the antibiotic. Other mechanisms of resistance include inactivation of the macrolides by enzymes (e.g., esterases, phosphorylases, glycosidase) or mutations in the 23S rRNA and ribosomal proteins. Macrolides are bacteriostatic antibiotics with a broad spectrum of activity. They have been used to treat pulmonary infections caused by *Mycoplasma, Legionella,* and *Chlamydia,* as well as to treat infections caused by *Campylobacter* species and gram-positive bacteria in patients allergic to penicillin. Most gram-negative bacteria are resistant to the macrolides. Azithromycin and clarithromycin have also been used to treat infections caused by mycobacteria (e.g., *Mycobacterium avium* complex).

Ketolides

Ketolides are semisynthetic derivatives of erythromycin, modified to increase stability in acid. **Telithromycin** is currently the only ketolide available for use in the United States. As with the macrolides, telithromycin binds to the 50S ribosomal subunity and blocks protein synthesis. Mutations in 23S rRNA or the ribosomal proteins can lead to resistance. Telithromycin has good activity against staphylococci (except strains that have constitutive resistance to erythromycin), *Streptococcus pneumoniae,* other respiratory pathogens (e.g., *Haemophilus influenzae, Moraxella catarrhalis*), gram-positive rods, and some anaerobes. It is not active against *Bacteroides fragilis* and most aerobic gram-negative rods (e.g., Enterobacteriaceae, *Pseudomonas, Acinetobacter, Stenotrophomonas*). Telithromycin also has good activity against intracellular pathogens (e.g., *Legionella, Mycoplasma, Chlamydia, Chlamydophila*), *Rickettsia, Bartonella, Coxiella, Francisella,* and *M. avium.*

reaction is positive (*S. pyogenes*) or negative (all other streptococci).

Antibody Detection

Patients with *S. pyogenes* disease produce antibodies to specific streptococcal enzymes. Although antibodies against the M protein are produced and are important for maintaining immunity, these type specific antibodies appear late in the clinical course of the disease and are not useful for diagnosis. In contrast, the measurement of antibodies against streptolysin O (**ASO test**) is useful for confirming rheumatic fever or acute glomerulonephritis resulting from a recent streptococcal pharyngeal infection. These antibodies appear 3 to 4 weeks after the initial exposure to the organism and then persist. An elevated ASO titer is not observed in patients with streptococcal pyoderma (as discussed above). The production of antibodies against other streptococcal enzymes, particularly DNase B, has been documented in patients with either streptococcal pyoderma or pharyngitis. The **anti-DNase B test** should be performed if streptococcal glomerulonephritis is suspected.

Treatment, Prevention, and Control

S. pyogenes is very sensitive to **penicillin**. An oral cephalosporin can be used in patients with a history of penicillin allergy. However, this therapy may be ineffective in patients with mixed infections that involve *Staphylococcus aureus*. Treatment in this case should include **oxacillin** or **vancomycin**. Resistance or poor clinical response has limited the usefulness of the tetracyclines and sulfonamides, and resistance to erythromycin and the newer macrolides (e.g., azithromycin, clarithromycin) is increasing in frequency. Drainage and aggressive surgical débridement must be promptly initiated in patients with serious soft-tissue infections.

Persistent oropharyngeal carriage of *S. pyogenes* can occur after a complete course of therapy. This state may stem from poor compliance with the prescribed course of therapy, reinfection with a new strain, or persistent carriage in a sequestered focus. Because penicillin resistance has not been observed in patients with oropharyngeal carriage, penicillin can be given for an additional course of treatment. If carriage persists, re-treatment is not indicated, because prolonged antibiotic therapy can disrupt the normal bacterial flora. Antibiotic therapy in patients with pharyngitis speeds the relief of symptoms and, if initiated within 10 days of the initial clinical disease, prevents rheumatic fever. Antibiotic therapy does not appear to influence the progression to acute glomerulonephritis.

Patients with a history of rheumatic fever require long-term **antibiotic prophylaxis** to prevent recurrence of the disease. Because damage to the heart valve predisposes these patients to endocarditis, they also require antibiotic prophylaxis before they undergo procedures that can induce transient bacteremias (e.g., dental procedures). Specific antibiotic therapy does not alter the course of acute glomerulonephritis, however, and prophylactic therapy is not indicated because recurrent disease is not observed in these patients.

Streptococcus agalactiae (Box 22-4)

S. agalactiae is the only species that carries the group B antigen. This organism was initially recognized as a cause of puerperal sepsis. Although this disease is now relatively

---

Box 22—4. Summary: *Streptococcus agalactiae* (group B)

Biology, Virulence, and Disease

Rapidly growing gram-positive cocci arranged in chains; group-specific carbohydrate (B antigen) and type-specific capsular carbohydrates (Ia, Ib, II-VIII)

Virulence determined primarily by ability to avoid phagocytosis (mediated by capsule)

Responsible for neonatal disease (early-onset and late-onset disease with meningitis, pneumonia, bacteremia), infections in pregnant women (endometritis, wound infections, urinary tract infections), and other adults (bacteremia, pneumonia, bone and joint infections, skin and soft-tissue infections)

Epidemiology

Asymptomatic colonization of the upper respiratory tract and genitourinary tract

Early-onset disease acquired by neonates from mother during pregnancy or at time of birth

Neonates are at higher risk for infection if (1) there is premature rupture of membranes, prolonged labor, preterm birth, or disseminated maternal group B streptococcal disease, and (2) mother is without type-specific antibodies and has low complement levels

Women with genital colonization are at risk for postpartum disease

Men and nonpregnant women with diabetes mellitus, cancer, or alcoholism are at increased risk for disease

No seasonal incidence

Diagnosis

Microscopy useful for meningitis (CSF), pneumonia (lower respiratory secretions), and wound infections (exudates)

Antigen tests are less sensitive than microscopy and should not be used

Culture most sensitive test; a selective broth (i.e., LIM) is needed to detect vaginal carriage

PCR-based assays to detect vaginal carriage in pregnant women are commercially available and as sensitive as culture

Isolates identified by catalase (negative), positive CAMP test and hippurate hydrolysis, and presence of group-specific carbohydrate (group B antigen)

Treatment, Prevention, and Control

Penicillin G is the drug of choice; a combination of penicillin and aminoglycoside is used in patients with serious infections; vancomycin is used for patients allergic to penicillin

For high-risk babies, penicillin is given at least 4 hours before delivery

Polyvalent conjugated vaccines to stimulate maternal antibodies are under development uncommon, *S. agalactiae* has become better known as an important cause of septicemia, pneumonia, and meningitis in newborn children, as well as a cause of serious disease in adults (see Box 22-3).

Physiology and Structure

Group B streptococci are gram-positive cocci (0.6 to 1.2 µm) that form short chains in clinical specimens and longer chains in culture, features that make them indistinguishable on Gram stain from *S. pyogenes*. They grow well on nutritionally enriched media, and in contrast with the colonies of *S. pyogenes*, the colonies of *S. agalactiae* are large with a narrow zone of β hemolysis (see Figure 22-2). Some strains (1% to 2%) are nonhemolytic, although their prevalence may be underestimated because nonhemolytic strains are not commonly screened for the group B antigen.

Strains of *S. agalactiae* can be characterized on the basis of three serologic markers: (1) the **group-specific cell wall polysaccharide B antigen** (Lancefield grouping antigen; composed of rhamnose, *N*-acetylglucosamine, and galactose), (2) nine **type-specific capsular polysaccharides** (Ia, Ib, and II to VIII), and (3) **surface proteins** (the most common is the **c antigen**). The type-specific polysaccharides are important epidemiologic markers, with serotypes Ia, III, and V most commonly associated with colonization and disease. Knowledge of the specific serotypes associated with disease and of shifting patterns of serotype prevalence is important for vaccine development.

Pathogenesis and Immunity

The most important virulence factor of *S. agalactiae* is the **polysaccharide capsule**, which interferes with phagocytosis until the patient develops type-specific antibodies. When antibodies develop against type-specific capsular antigens, they are protective, a factor that partly explains the predilection of this organism for neonates. In the absence of maternal antibodies, the neonate is at risk for disease. Additionally, genital colonization with group B streptococci has been associated with increased risk of premature delivery, and premature infants are at greater risk of disease. Functional classical and alternative complement pathways are required for killing group B streptococci, particularly types Ia, III, and V. As a result, there is a greater likelihood of systemic spread of the organism in colonized premature infants with physiologically **low complement levels** or for infants in whom the receptors for complement, or for the Fc fragment of IgG antibodies, are not exposed on neutrophils. It has also been found that the type-specific capsular polysaccharides of types Ia, Ib, and II streptococci have a terminal residue of sialic acid. **Sialic acid** can inhibit activation of the alternative complement pathway, thus interfering with the phagocytosis of these strains of group B streptococci.

Epidemiology

Group B streptococci colonize the lower gastrointestinal tract and the genitourinary tract. Transient vaginal carriage has been observed in 10% to 30% of pregnant women, although the incidence depends on the time during the gestation period when the sampling is done and the culture techniques used. A similar incidence has been observed in women who are not pregnant.

Approximately 60% of infants born to colonized mothers become colonized with their mothers' organisms. The likelihood of colonization at birth is higher if the mother is heavily colonized. Other risk factors for neonatal colonization are premature delivery, prolonged membrane rupture, and intrapartum fever. Disease in infants younger than 7 days of age is called **early-onset disease**; disease appearing between 1 week and 3 months of life is considered **late-onset disease**. The serotypes most commonly associated with early-onset disease are Ia (35% to 40%), III (30%), and V (15%). Serotype III is responsible for most late-onset disease. Serotypes Ia and V are the most common in **adult disease**.

Colonization with subsequent development of disease in the neonate can occur in utero, at birth, or during the first few months of life. *S. agalactiae* is the most common cause of septicemia and meningitis in newborns. The use of intrapartum antibiotic prophylaxis is responsible for a dramatic decline in neonatal disease—from approximately 8000 infections in 1993 to 1800 infections in 2002.

There are more group B streptococcal infections in adults (an estimated 17,000 invasive infections in 2002) than in neonates, but the overall incidence is higher in neonates. The risk of disease is greater in pregnant women than in men and nonpregnant women. Urinary tract infections, amnionitis, endometritis, and wound infections are the most common manifestations in pregnant women. Infections in men and nonpregnant women are primarily skin and soft-tissue infections, bacteremia, urosepsis (urinary tract infection with bacteremia), and pneumonia. Conditions that predispose to the development of disease in nonpregnant adults include diabetes mellitus, chronic liver or renal disease, cancer, and HIV infection.

Clinical Diseases

Early-Onset Neonatal Disease

Clinical symptoms of group B streptococcal disease acquired in utero or at birth develop during the first week of life. Early-onset disease, characterized by **bacteremia, pneumonia**, or **meningitis**, is indistinguishable from sepsis caused by other organisms. Because pulmonary involvement is observed in most infants, and meningeal involvement may be initially inapparent, examination of cerebrospinal fluid is required for all infected children. The mortality rate has decreased to less than 5% as a result of rapid diagnosis and better supportive care; however, 15% to 30% of infants who survive meningitis have neurologic sequelae, including blindness, deafness, and severe mental retardation.

Late-Onset Neonatal Disease (Clinical Case 22-2)

Late-onset disease is acquired from an exogenous source (e.g., mother, another infant) and develops between 1 week and 3 months of age. The predominant manifestation is **bacteremia with meningitis**, which resembles disease caused by other bacteria. Although the mortality rate is low (i.e., 3%), neurologic complications are common in children with meningitis (i.e., 25%-50%).

Infections in Pregnant Women

Postpartum endometritis, wound infection, and **urinary tract infections** occur in women during and immediately after pregnancy. Because childbearing women are generally in good health, the prognosis is excellent for those who receive appropriate therapy. Secondary complications of bacteremia, such as endocarditis, meningitis, and osteomyelitis, are rare.

Infections in Men and Nonpregnant Women

Compared with pregnant women who acquire group B streptococcal infection, men and nonpregnant women with group B streptococcal infections are generally older and have debilitating underlying conditions. The most common presentations are **bacteremia, pneumonia, bone and joint infections**, and **skin and soft-tissue infections**. Because these patients often have compromised immunity, mortality is higher in this population.

Laboratory Diagnosis

Antigen Detection

Tests for the direct detection of group B streptococci in urogenital specimens are available but are too insensitive to be used to screen mothers and predict which newborns are at increased risk for acquiring neonatal disease. Likewise, the antigen tests are too insensitive (<30%) to be used with CSF. A Gram stain of CSF has much better sensitivity and should be used.

Nucleic-Acid-Based Tests

A polymerase chain reaction (PCR)-based assay is approved by the Food and Drug Administration (FDA) for rectal/vaginal swabs from pregnant women. Because the test sensitivity and specificity approaches that of culture, this assay is a rapid alternative to standard culture for group B *Streptococcus*.

Culture

Group B streptococci readily grow on a nutritionally enriched medium, producing large colonies after 24 hours of incubation (see Figure 22-2). β Hemolysis may be difficult to detect or absent, posing a problem in the detection of the organism when other organisms are present in the culture (e.g., vaginal culture). Thus a selective broth medium with antibiotics added to suppress the growth of other organisms (e.g., LIM broth with colistin and nalidixic acid) is currently recommended by the CDC for the detection of group B streptococci in women between weeks 35 and 37 of pregnancy.

Identification

A preliminary identification of an isolate can be made by demonstration of a negative **catalase test,** positive Christie, Atkins, Munch-Petersen **(CAMP) test** (Figure 22-5), and **hydrolysis of hippurate**. Group B streptococci are identified definitively by the demonstration of the group-specific carbohydrate or the use of commercially prepared molecular probes.

Clinical Case 22-2. Group B Streptococcal Disease in a Neonate

The following is a description of late-onset group B streptococcal disease in a neonate (Hammersen, et al: Eur J Ped 126:189-197, 1977). An infant male weighing 3400 grams was delivered spontaneously at term. Physical examinations of the infant were normal during the first week of life; however, the child started feeding irregularly during the second week. On day 13, the baby was admitted to the hospital with generalized seizures. A small amount of cloudy CSF was collected by lumbar puncture and *Streptococcus agalactiae* serotype III was isolated in culture. Despite the prompt initiation of therapy, the baby developed hydrocephalus necessitating implantation of an atrioventricular shunt. The infant was discharged at age 3½ months with retardation of psychomotor development.

This patient illustrates neonatal meningitis caused by the most commonly implicated serotype of group B streptococci in late-onset disease and the complications associated with this infection.

Figure 22—5. CAMP reaction with group B streptococci. Group B streptococci produce a diffusible, heat-stable protein (CAMP factor) that enhances β hemolysis of *Staphylococcus aureus*. *S. aureus* (streaked from the top to the bottom of the agar plate) produces sphingomyelinase C, which can bind to erythrocyte membranes. When exposed to the group B CAMP factor, the cells undergo hemolysis (compare the two positive reactions of enhanced hemolysis to the left of the *S. aureus* streak, with the two negative reactions to the right). *(From Howard BJ: Clinical and Pathogenic Microbiology. St Louis, Mosby, 1987.)*

Treatment, Prevention, and Control

Group B streptococci are susceptible to **penicillin**, which is the drug of choice. However, the minimum inhibitory concentration (MIC) needed to inhibit the organism is approximately 10 times greater than that needed to inhibit *S. pyogenes*. In addition, tolerance to penicillin (the ability of the antibiotic to inhibit but not kill the organism) has been reported. For these reasons, a combination of penicillin and an aminoglycoside is frequently used in the management of serious infections. **Vancomycin** is an alternative therapy for patients allergic to penicillin. Antibiotic resistance to erythromycin and tetracycline has been observed.

In an effort to prevent neonatal disease, it is recommended that all pregnant women should be **screened for colonization** with group B streptococci at 35 to 37 weeks of gestation (refer to this CDC document for additional information: http://www.cdc.gov/mmwr/preview/mmwrhtml/rr5111a1.htm). **Chemoprophylaxis** should be used for all women who are either colonized or at high risk. A pregnant woman is considered to be at high risk to give birth to a baby with invasive group B disease if she has previously given birth to an infant with the disease or risk factors for the disease are present at birth. These risk factors are (1) intrapartum temperature of at least 38° C, (2) membrane rupture at least 18 hours before delivery, and (3) vaginal or rectal culture positive for organisms at 35 to 37 weeks of gestation. Intravenous penicillin G administered at least 4 hours before delivery is recommended; cefazolin or vancomycin is used for penicillin-allergic women. This approach ensures high protective antibiotic levels in the infant's circulatory system at the time of birth.

Because newborn disease is associated with decreased circulating antibodies in the mother, efforts have been directed at developing a polyvalent vaccine against serotypes Ia, Ib, II, III, and V. The capsular polysaccharides are poor immunogens; however, complexing them with tetanus toxoid has improved the immunogenicity of the vaccine. Trials with this polyvalent vaccine demonstrated that protective levels of antibodies are induced in animal models. However, commercial development of this vaccine for human use needs to be initiated.

Other β-Hemolytic Streptococci

Among the other β-hemolytic streptococci, groups C, F, and G are most commonly associated with human disease. Organisms of particular importance are the *Streptococcus anginosus* group (includes *S. anginosus*, *S. constellatus*, and *S. intermedius*) and *Streptococcus dysgalactiae*. β-Hemolytic members of the *S. anginosus* group can possess the group A, C, F, or G polysaccharide antigen (or not have any group specific antigen), and *S. dysgalactiae* can have either the group C or G antigen. It should be noted that an individual isolate possesses only one group antigen. Isolates of the *S. anginosus* group grow as small colonies (requiring 2 days of

Figure 22–6. Group C *Streptococcus*. **A**, *S. anginosus*, small-colony species. **B**, *S. dysgalactiae*, large-colony species.

incubation) with a narrow zone of β hemolysis (Figure 22-6A). These species are primarily associated with abscess formation and not pharyngitis, in contrast with the other group A *Streptococcus*, *S. pyogenes*. *S. dysgalactiae* produce large colonies with a large zone of β hemolysis on blood agar media (Figure 22-6B), a behavior similar to that of *S. pyogenes*. Like *S. pyogenes*, *S. dysgalactiae* causes pharyngitis, which is sometimes complicated by acute glomerulonephritis but never rheumatic fever.

Viridans Streptococci

The viridans group of streptococci is a heterogeneous collection of α-hemolytic and nonhemolytic streptococci. Their group name is derived from *viridis* (Latin for "green"), a reflection of the fact that many of these bacteria produce a green pigment on blood agar media (Figure 22-7). More than 30 species and subspecies have been identified, and most are classified into five subgroups. This classification scheme is clinically important because many of the species in the five subgroups are responsible for specific diseases (Table 22-2). Some members of the viridans streptococci (e.g., *S. anginosus* group) can have β-hemolytic strains with the group-specific cell

Figure 22–7. *Streptococcus mitis.* **A,** Gram stain from blood culture. **B,** α-Hemolytic colonies.

Table 22–2. Classification of Viridans Group of *Streptococcus*

Group	Representative Species	Diseases
Anginosus	*S. anginosus,* *S. constellatus,* *S. intermedius*	Abscesses in brain, oropharynx, or peritoneal cavity
Mitis	*S. mitis, S. pneumoniae, S. oralis*	Subacute endocarditis; sepsis in neutropenic patients; pneumonia; meningitis
Mutans	*S. mutans, S. sobrinus*	Dental caries; bacteremia
Salivarius	*S. salivarius*	Bacteremia; endocarditis
Bovis	*S. gallolyticus* subsp. *gallolyticus,* subsp. *pasteurianus*	Bacteremia associated with gastrointestinal cancer (subsp. *gallolyticus*); meningitis (subsp. *pasteurianus*)
Ungrouped	*S. suis*	Meningitis; bacteremia; streptococcal toxic shock syndrome

wall polysaccharides (thus contributing to the confusing taxonomy of this genus). Additionally, *S. pneumoniae* is a member of the *Streptococcus mitis* subgroup. Because *S. pneumoniae* is the most virulent member of the viridans group, it is discussed separately.

The viridans streptococci colonize the oropharynx, gastrointestinal tract, and genitourinary tract. They are rarely found on the skin surface, because the surface fatty acids are toxic to them. Like most other streptococci, viridans species are nutritionally fastidious, requiring complex media supplemented with blood products and frequently an incubation atmosphere augmented with 5% to 10% carbon dioxide.

In the past, most strains of viridans streptococci were highly susceptible to penicillin, with MICs of less than 0.1 μg/ml. However, moderately resistant (penicillin MIC of 0.2 to 2 μg/ml) and highly resistant (MIC >2 μg/ml) streptococci have become common in the *S. mitis* group, which includes *S. pneumoniae*. This issue is discussed in the next section. Infections with isolates that are moderately resistant can generally be treated with a combination of penicillin and an aminoglycoside. However, alternative antibiotics, such as a broad-spectrum cephalosporin or vancomycin, must be used to treat serious infections caused by penicillin-resistant strains.

Streptococcus pneumoniae (Box 22-5)

S. pneumoniae was isolated independently by Pasteur and Steinberg more than 100 years ago. Since that time, research with this organism has led to a greater understanding of molecular genetics, antibiotic resistance, and vaccine-related immunoprophylaxis. Unfortunately, pneumococcal disease is still a leading cause of morbidity and mortality.

Physiology and Structure

The pneumococcus is an **encapsulated** gram-positive coccus. The cells are 0.5 to 1.2 μm in diameter, oval or lancet-shaped, and arranged in pairs (**diplococci**) or short chains (Figure 22-8). Older cells decolorize readily and appear gram-negative. Colonial morphology varies. Colonies of encapsulated strains are generally large (1 to 3 mm in diameter on blood agar; smaller on chocolatized or heated blood agar), round, and mucoid; colonies of nonencapsulated strains are smaller and appear flat. All colonies undergo autolysis with aging—that is, the central portion of the colony dissolves, leaving a dimpled appearance. Colonies appear α-hemolytic on blood agar if incubated aerobically and may be β-hemolytic if grown anaerobically. The α-hemolytic appearance results from production of pneumolysin, an enzyme that degrades hemoglobin, producing a green product.

The organism has fastidious nutritional requirements and can grow only on enriched media supplemented with blood products. *S. pneumoniae* can ferment several carbohydrates, with lactic acid the primary metabolic byproduct. *S. pneumoniae* grows poorly in media with high glucose

Box 22—5. Summary: *Streptococcus pneumoniae*

Biology, Virulence, and Disease

Elongated or "lancet-shaped," gram-positive cocci arranged in pairs (diplococci) and short chains; teichoic acid rich in phosphocholine (C polysaccharide) and autolytic enzyme (amidase) in cell wall

Virulence determined by ability to colonize oropharynx (surface protein adhesions), spread into normally sterile tissues pneumolysin, IgA protease), stimulate local inflammatory response (teichoic acid, peptidoglycan fragments, pneumolysin), and evade phagocytic killing (polysaccharide capsule)

Responsible for pneumonia, sinusitis and otitis media, meningitis, and bacteremia

Epidemiology

Most infections are caused by endogenous spread from the colonized nasopharynx or oropharynx to distal site (e.g., lungs, sinuses, ears, blood, meninges); person-to-person spread through infectious droplets is rare

Colonization is highest in young children and their contacts

Individuals with antecedent viral respiratory tract disease or other conditions that interfere with bacterial clearance from respiratory tract are at increased risk for pulmonary disease

Children and the elderly are at greatest risk for meningitis

People with hematologic disorder (e.g., malignancy, sickle cell disease) or functional asplenia are at risk for fulminant sepsis

Although the organism is ubiquitous, disease is more common in cool months

Diagnosis

Microscopy is highly sensitive, as is culture, unless the patient has been treated with antibiotics

Antigen test for pneumococcal C polysaccharide is sensitive with CSF (meningitis) but not with urine (meningitis, pneumonia, other infections)

Nucleic-acid-based tests are not commonly used for diagnosis

Culture requires use of enriched-nutrient media (e.g., sheep blood agar); organism highly susceptible to many antibiotics, so culture can be negative in partially treated patients

Isolates identified by catalase (negative), susceptibility to optochin, and solubility in bile

Treatment, Prevention, and Control

Penicillin is the drug of choice for susceptible strains, although resistance is increasingly common

Fluoroquinolone or vancomycin combined with ceftriaxone is used for patients allergic to penicillin or for treatment of penicillin-resistant strains

Immunization with 7-valent conjugated vaccine is recommended for all children younger than 2 years of age; a 23-valent polysaccharide vaccine is recommended for adults at risk for disease

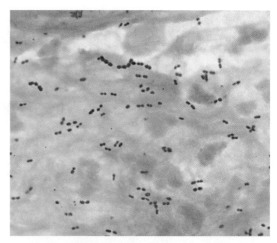

Figure 22—8. Gram stain of *Streptococcus pneumoniae*.

Virulent strains of *S. pneumoniae* are covered with a complex **polysaccharide capsule**. The capsular polysaccharides have been used for the serologic classification of strains; currently, 90 serotypes are recognized. Purified capsular polysaccharides from the most commonly isolated serotypes are used in a polyvalent vaccine.

The **peptidoglycan** layer of the cell wall of the pneumococcus is typical of gram-positive cocci. Attached to alternating subunits of *N*-acetylglucosamine and *N*-acetylmuramic acid are oligopeptide chains, which in turn are cross-linked by pentaglycine bridges. The other major component of the cell wall is teichoic acid. Two forms of **teichoic acid** exist in the pneumococcal cell wall, one exposed on the cell surface and a similar form covalently bound to the plasma membrane lipids. The exposed teichoic acid is linked to the peptidoglycan layer and extends through the overlying capsule. This species-specific structure, called the **C polysaccharide**, is unrelated to the group-specific carbohydrate observed by Lancefield in β-hemolytic streptococci. The C polysaccharide precipitates a serum globulin fraction (**C-reactive protein [CRP]**) in the presence of calcium. CRP is present in low concentrations in healthy people but in elevated concentrations in patients with acute inflammatory diseases (hence monitoring levels of CRP is used to predict inflammation). The lipid-bound teichoic acid in the bacterial cytoplasmic membrane is called the **F antigen** because it can cross-react with the Forssman surface antigens on mammalian cells. Both forms of teichoic acid are associated with phosphocholine residues. **Phosphocholine** is unique to the cell wall of *S. pneumoniae* and plays an important regulatory role in cell wall hydrolysis. Phosphocholine must be present for activity of the pneumococcal autolysin, **amidase**, during cell division.

Pathogenesis and Immunity

Although *S. pneumoniae* has been extensively studied, much remains to be learned about the pathogenesis of

concentrations because lactic acid rapidly reaches toxic levels in such preparations. Like all streptococci, the organism lacks catalase. Unless an exogenous source of catalase is provided (e.g., from blood), the accumulation of hydrogen peroxide inhibits the growth of *S. pneumoniae*, as observed on chocolatized blood agar.

pneumococcal disease. The disease manifestations are caused primarily by the host response to infection rather than the production of organism-specific toxic factors. However, an understanding of how *S. pneumoniae* colonizes the oropharynx, spreads into normally sterile tissues, stimulates a localized inflammatory response, and evades being killed by phagocytic cells is crucial.

Colonization and Migration

S. pneumoniae is a human pathogen that colonizes the oropharynx and then, in specific situations, is able to spread to the lungs, paranasal sinuses, or middle ear. It can also be transported in the blood to distal sites such as the brain. The initial colonization of the oropharynx is mediated by the binding of the bacteria to epithelial cells by means of **surface protein adhesins**. Subsequent migration of the organism to the lower respiratory tract can be prevented if the bacteria are enveloped in mucus and removed from the airways by the action of ciliated epithelial cells. The bacteria counteract this envelopment by producing **secretory IgA (sIgA) protease** and **pneumolysin**. Secretory IgA traps bacteria in mucin by attaching itself to the bacteria at the antigen-binding site and to mucin at the Fc region. The bacterial protease prevents this interaction. **Pneumolysin**, a cytotoxin similar to the streptolysin O in *S. pyogenes*, binds cholesterol in the host cell membrane and creates pores. This activity can destroy the ciliated epithelial cells and phagocytic cells.

Tissue Destruction

A characteristic of pneumococcal infections is the mobilization of inflammatory cells to the focus of infection. Pneumococcal teichoic acid, peptidoglycan fragments, and pneumolysin mediate the process. **Teichoic acid** and the **peptidoglycan fragments** activate the alternative complement pathway, producing C5a, which mediates the inflammatory process. This activity is augmented by the bacterial enzyme **amidase**, which enhances release of the cell wall components. **Pneumolysin** activates the classic complement pathway, resulting in the production of C3a and C5a. In turn, cytokines such as IL-1 and TNF-α are produced by the activated leukocytes, leading to the further migration of inflammatory cells to the site of infection, fever, tissue damage, and other signs characteristic of pneumococcal infection. The production of **hydrogen peroxide** by *S. pneumoniae* can also lead to tissue damage caused by reactive oxygen intermediates.

Finally, **phosphocholine** present in the bacterial cell wall can bind to receptors for platelet-activating factor that are expressed on the surface of endothelial cells, leukocytes, platelets, and tissue cells such as those in the lungs and meninges. By binding these receptors, the bacteria can enter the cells, where they are protected from opsonization and phagocytosis, and pass into sequestered areas, such as blood and the central nervous system. This activity facilitates the spread of disease.

Phagocytic Survival

S. pneumoniae survives phagocytosis because of the antiphagocytic protection afforded by its **capsule** and the pneumolysin-mediated suppression of the phagocytic cell oxidative burst, which is required for intracellular killing. The virulence of *S. pneumoniae* is a direct result of this capsule. Encapsulated (smooth) strains can cause disease in humans and experimental animals, whereas nonencapsulated (rough) strains are avirulent. Antibodies directed against the type-specific capsular polysaccharides protect against disease caused by immunologically related strains. The capsular polysaccharides are soluble and have been called **specific soluble substances**. Free polysaccharides can protect viable organisms from phagocytosis by binding with opsonic antibodies.

Epidemiology

S. pneumoniae is a common inhabitant of the throat and nasopharynx in healthy people, with colonization more common in children than in adults and more common in adults living in a household with children. Colonization initially occurs at approximately 6 months of age. Subsequently the child is transiently colonized with other serotypes of the organism. The duration of carriage decreases with each successive serotype carried, in part because of the development of serotype-specific immunity. Although new serotypes are acquired throughout the year, the incidence of carriage and associated disease is highest during the cool months. The strains of pneumococci that cause disease are the same as those associated with carriage.

Pneumococcal disease occurs when organisms colonizing the nasopharynx and oropharynx spread to the lungs (pneumonia), paranasal sinuses (sinusitis), ears (otitis media), or meninges (meningitis). Spread of *S. pneumoniae* in blood to other body sites can occur with all of these diseases.

Although the introduction of vaccines for pediatric and adult populations has reduced the incidence of disease caused by *S. pneumoniae*, the organism is still a common cause of bacterial pneumonia acquired outside the hospital, meningitis, otitis media and sinusitis, and bacteremia. Disease is most common in children and the elderly; both populations have low levels of protective antibodies directed against the pneumococcal capsular polysaccharides.

Pneumonia occurs when the endogenous oral organisms are aspirated into the lower airways. Although strains can spread on airborne droplets from one person to another in a closed population, epidemics are rare. Disease occurs when the natural defense mechanisms (e.g., epiglottal reflex, trapping of bacteria by the mucus-producing cells lining the bronchus, removal of organisms by the ciliated respiratory epithelium, and cough reflex) are circumvented, permitting organisms colonizing the oropharynx to gain access to the lungs. Pneumococcal disease is most commonly associated with an antecedent viral respiratory disease, such as influenza, or with other conditions that interfere with bacterial clearance, such as chronic pulmonary disease, alcoholism, congestive heart failure, diabetes mellitus, chronic renal disease, and splenic dysfunction or splenectomy.

Clinical Diseases

Pneumonia (Clinical Case 22-3)

Pneumococcal **pneumonia** develops when the bacteria multiply in the alveolar spaces. After aspiration, the bacteria grow rapidly in the nutrient-rich edema fluid. Erythrocytes, leaking from congested capillaries, accumulate in the alveoli, followed by the neutrophils, then the alveolar macrophages. Resolution occurs when specific anticapsular antibodies develop, facilitating phagocytosis of the organism and microbial killing.

The onset of the clinical manifestations of pneumococcal pneumonia is abrupt, consisting of a severe shaking chill and sustained fever of 39° C to 41° C. The patient often has symptoms of a viral respiratory tract infection 1 to 3 days before the onset. Most patients have a productive cough with blood-tinged sputum, and they commonly have chest pain (pleurisy). Because the disease is associated with aspiration, it is generally localized in the lower lobes of the lungs (hence the name **lobar pneumonia**; Figure 22-9). However, children and the elderly can have a more generalized bronchopneumonia. Patients usually recover rapidly after the initiation of appropriate antimicrobial therapy, with complete radiologic resolution in 2 to 3 weeks.

The overall mortality rate is 5%, although the likelihood of death is influenced by the serotype of the organism and the age and underlying disease of the patient. The mortality rate is considerably higher in patients with disease caused by *S. pneumoniae* type 3, as well as in elderly patients and patients with documented bacteremia. Patients with

Figure 22–9. Dense consolidation of left lower lobe in patient with pneumonia caused by *S. pneumoniae. (From Mandell G, Bennett J, Dolin R: Principles and Practice of Infectious Diseases, 6th ed. Philadelphia, Elsevier, 2005.)*

splenic dysfunction or splenectomy can also have severe pneumococcal disease as a result of decreased bacterial clearance from the blood and the defective production of early antibodies. In these patients, disease is associated with a fulminant course and high mortality rate.

Abscesses do not commonly form in patients with pneumococcal pneumonia, except in those infected with specific serotypes (e.g., serotype 3). Pleural effusions are seen in approximately 25% of patients with pneumococcal pneumonia, and empyema (purulent effusion) is a rare complication.

Sinusitis and Otitis Media

S. pneumoniae is a common cause of acute infections of the paranasal sinuses and ear. The disease is usually preceded by a viral infection of the upper respiratory tract, after which polymorphonuclear leukocytes (PMN) infiltrate and obstruct the sinuses and ear canal. Middle ear infection (**otitis media**) is primarily seen in young children, but bacterial **sinusitis** can occur in patients of all ages.

Meningitis

S. pneumoniae can spread into the central nervous system after bacteremia, infections of the ear or sinuses, or head trauma that causes a communication between the subarachnoid space and the nasopharynx. Although **pneumococcal meningitis** is relatively uncommon in neonates, *S. pneumoniae* is now a leading cause of disease in children and adults. Mortality and severe neurologic deficits are 4 to 20 times more common in patients with meningitis caused by *S. pneumoniae* than in those with meningitis resulting from other organisms.

Bacteremia

Bacteremia occurs in 25% to 30% of patients with pneumococcal pneumonia and in more than 80% of patients with

---

Clinical Case 22-3. Pneumonia Caused by *Streptococcus pneumoniae*

Costa, et al. (Am J Hematol 77:277-281, 2004) described a 68-year-old woman who was in good health until 3 days before hospitalization. She developed fever, chills, increased weakness, and a productive cough with pleuritic chest pain. On admission she was febrile, had an elevated pulse and respiration rate, and was in moderate respiratory distress. Initial laboratory values showed leucopenia, anemia, and acute renal failure. Chest radiograph demonstrated infiltrates in the right and left lower lobes, with pleural effusions. Therapy with a fluoroquinolone was initiated, and blood and respiratory cultures were positive for *S. pneumoniae*. Additional tests (serum and urine protein electrophoresis) revealed the patient had multiple myeloma. The patient's infection resolved with a 14-day course of antibiotics. This patient illustrates the typical picture of pneumococcal lobar pneumonia and the increased susceptibility to infection in patients with defects in their ability to clear encapsulated organisms.

meningitis. In contrast, bacteria are generally not present in the blood of patients with sinusitis or otitis media. Endocarditis can occur in patients with normal or previously damaged heart valves. Destruction of valve tissue is common.

Laboratory Diagnosis

Microscopy

Gram stain of sputum specimens is a rapid way to diagnose pneumococcal pneumonia and meningitis. The organisms characteristically appear as elongated pairs of gram-positive cocci (commonly referred to as "lancet-shaped diplococci") surrounded by an unstained capsule; however, they may also appear to be gram-negative, because they tend not to stain well (particularly in older cultures). In addition, their morphology may be distorted in a patient receiving antibiotic therapy. Gram stain consistent with *S. pneumoniae* can be confirmed with the **quellung** (German for "swelling") reaction. In this test, polyvalent anticapsular antibodies are mixed with the bacteria, and then the mixture is examined microscopically. A greater refractiveness around the bacteria is a positive reaction for *S. pneumoniae*.

Antigen Detection

Pneumococcal C polysaccharide is excreted in urine and can be detected using a commercially prepared immunoassay. Maximum sensitivity requires that the urine be concentrated by ultrafiltration before it is assayed. Sensitivity has been reported to be 70% in patients with bacteremic pneumococcal pneumonia; however, specificity can be low, particularly in pediatric patients. For this reason, the test is not recommended for pediatric patients. The test has a sensitivity approaching 100% for patients with pneumococcal meningitis if CSF is tested; however, the test has poor sensitivity and specificity if urine is tested in these patients.

Nucleic Acid-Based Tests

Nucleic acid probes and PCR assays have been developed for identification of *S. pneumoniae* isolates in culture but are not currently used for detection of bacteria in clinical specimens such as respiratory secretions or CSF.

Culture

Sputum specimens should be inoculated onto an enriched nutrient medium supplemented with blood. *S. pneumoniae* is recovered in the sputum cultures from only half of the patients who have pneumonia, because the organism has fastidious nutritional requirements and is rapidly overgrown by contaminating oral bacteria. Selective media have been used with some success to isolate the organism from sputum specimens, but it takes some technical skill to distinguish *S. pneumoniae* from the other α-hemolytic streptococci that are often present in the specimen.

For the organism responsible for sinusitis or otitis to be diagnosed definitively, an aspirate must be obtained from the sinus or middle ear. Specimens taken from the nasopharynx or outer ear should not be cultured. It is not difficult to isolate *S. pneumoniae* from specimens of cerebrospinal fluid if antibiotic therapy has not been initiated before the specimen is collected; however, as many as half of infected patients who have received even a single dose of antibiotics will have negative cultures.

Identification

Isolates of *S. pneumoniae* are lysed rapidly when the autolysins are activated after exposure to bile (**bile solubility test**). Thus the organism can be identified by placing a drop of bile on an isolated colony. Most colonies of *S. pneumoniae* are dissolved within a few minutes, whereas other α-hemolytic streptococci remain unchanged. *S. pneumoniae* can also be identified by its susceptibility to **optochin** (ethylhydrocupreine dihydrochloride). The isolate is streaked onto a blood agar plate, and a disk saturated with optochin is placed in the middle of the inoculum. A zone of inhibited bacterial growth is seen around the disk after overnight incubation. Additional biochemical, serologic, or molecular diagnostic tests can be performed for a definitive identification.

Treatment, Prevention, and Control

Before the advent of antibiotics, specific treatment of *S. pneumoniae* infection was guided by the passive infusion of type-specific capsular antibodies. These opsonizing antibodies enhanced phagocytosis and the killing of bacteria. However, this immunotherapy was discontinued once antimicrobial therapy became available.

Penicillin rapidly became the treatment of choice for pneumococcal disease. In 1977, researchers in South Africa reported isolates of *S. pneumoniae* resistant to multiple antibiotics, including penicillin. Until 1990, high-level resistance to penicillin (MIC of at least 2 μg/ml) was relatively uncommon, and only 5% of all strains of *S. pneumoniae* isolated in the United States were considered to be moderately resistant (MIC of 0.1 to 1.0 μg/ml). However, this situation has changed dramatically. Resistance to penicillin has now been observed for as many as a half of the strains isolated in the United States and in a higher number of those isolated in other countries. Greater resistance to penicillins is associated with a decreased affinity of the antibiotic for the penicillin-binding proteins present in the bacterial cell wall. Patients infected with resistant bacteria have an increased risk of an adverse outcome. Recently, resistance to macrolides (e.g., erythromycin), tetracyclines, and to a lesser extent cephalosporins (e.g., ceftriaxone) have also become commonplace. Thus for serious pneumococcal infections, treatment with a **fluoroquinolone** (e.g., levofloxacin) or **vancomycin combined with ceftriaxone** is recommended.

Efforts to prevent or control the disease have focused on the development of effective anticapsular vaccines. A 23-valent pneumococcal polysaccharide vaccine (with 23 different capsular polysaccharides) is recommended for children older than

2 years of age and adults. Polysaccharides are T-independent antigens, stimulating mature B lymphocytes but not T lymphocytes. Very young children respond poorly to T-independent antigens, so these polysaccharide vaccines are ineffective for this population. In contrast, conjugation of polysaccharides to proteins stimulates a T-helper cell response, resulting in a strong primary response among infants and effective booster response when reimmunized. This approach of using conjugated vaccines for pediatric immunizations has also been used for other neonatal pathogens such as *Haemophilus influenzae.* Immunization with the 7-valent conjugated pneumococcal vaccine is currently recommended for infants younger than 2 years of age. The effectiveness of these vaccines is determined by the prevalent serotypes of *S. pneumoniae* responsible for invasive disease in the population. Whereas these vaccines are generally effective in U.S. and European populations, they are less effective in developing countries, because the prevalent serotypes are not represented in the vaccines. Additionally, although the 23-valent vaccine is immunogenic in normal adults and immunity is long lived, the vaccine is less effective in some patients at high risk for pneumococcal disease, including: (1) patients with asplenia, sickle cell disease, hematologic malignancy, and HIV infection; (2) patients who have undergone renal transplant; and (3) the elderly.

Case Study and Questions

A 62-year-old man with a history of chronic obstructive pulmonary disease (COPD) came to the emergency department because of a fever of 40° C, chills, nausea, vomiting, and hypotension. The patient also produced tenacious, yellowish sputum that had increased in quantity over the preceding 3 days. His respiratory rate was 18 breaths/min, and his blood pressure was 94/52 mm Hg. Chest radiographic examination showed extensive infiltrates in the left lower lung that involved both the lower lobe and the lingula. Multiple blood cultures and culture of the sputum yielded *S. pneumoniae.* The isolate was susceptible to cefazolin, vancomycin, and erythromycin but resistant to penicillin.

1. What predisposing condition made this patient more susceptible to pneumonia and bacteremia caused by *S. pneumoniae?* What other populations of patients are susceptible to these infections? What other infections does this organism cause, and what populations are most susceptible?

2. What is the mechanism most likely responsible for this isolate's resistance to penicillin?

3. What infections are caused by *S. pyogenes, S. agalactiae, S. anginosus, S. dysgalactiae,* and viridans streptococci?

4. What are the major virulence factors of *S. pneumoniae, S. pyogenes,* and *S. agalactiae?*

5. *S. pyogenes* can cause streptococcal toxic shock syndrome. How does this disease differ from the disease produced by staphylococci?

6. What two nonsuppurative diseases can develop after localized *S. pyogenes* disease?

Bibliography

Barry AL: Antimicrobial resistance among clinical isolates of *Streptococcus pneumoniae* in North America. Am J Med 107:28S-33S, 1999.

Bisno AL, Stevens DL: Streptococcal infections of skin and soft tissues. N Engl J Med 334:240-245, 1996.

Cunningham M: Pathogenesis of group A streptococcal infections. Clin Microbiol Rev 13:470-511, 2000.

Hava D, LeMieux J, Camilli A: From nose to lung: The regulation behind *Streptococcus pneumoniae* virulence factors (review). Mol Microbiol 50:1103-1110, 2003.

Greene CM, et al: Preventability of invasive pneumococcal disease and assessment of current polysaccharide vaccine recommendations for adults: United States, 2001-2003. Clin Infect Dis 43:141-150, 2006.

Johnson D, et al: A comparison of group A streptococci from invasive and uncomplicated infections: Are virulent clones responsible for serious streptococcal infections? J Infect Dis 185:1586-1595, 2002.

Kaul R, et al: Population-based surveillance for group A streptococcal necrotizing fasciitis: Clinical features, prognostic indicators, and microbiologic analysis of seventy-seven cases. Am J Med 103:18-24, 1997.

Metlay J, et al: Impact of penicillin susceptibility on medical outcomes for adult patients with bacteremic pneumococcal pneumonia. Clin Infect Dis 30:520-528, 2000.

Schrag S, Schuchat A: Easing the burden: Characterizing the disease burden of neonatal group B streptococcal disease to motivate prevention. Clin Infect Dis 38:1209-1211, 2004.

Schuchat A: Epidemiology of group B streptococcal disease in the United States: Shifting paradigms. Clin Microbiol Rev 11:497-513, 1998.

Stevens DL: Streptococcal toxic shock syndrome: Spectrum of disease, pathogenesis, and new concepts in treatment. Emerging Infect Dis 1:69-78, 1995.

Enterococcus and Other Gram-Positive Cocci

The number of genera of catalase-negative, gram-positive cocci that are recognized as human pathogens continues to increase; however, *Streptococcus* (see Chapter 22) and *Enterococcus* (Box 23-1) are the genera most frequently isolated and most commonly responsible for human disease (Tables 23-1 and 23-2). The other genera are relatively uncommon and are discussed only briefly here.

Enterococcus (Box 23-2)

The enterococci ("enteric cocci") were previously classified as **group D streptococci** because they possess the **group D cell wall antigen**, a glycerol teichoic acid that is associated with the cytoplasmic membrane. In 1984, the enterococci were reclassified into the new genus *Enterococcus* and there are currently 38 species in this genus; however, relatively few species are important human pathogens. The most commonly isolated and clinically important species are *Enterococcus faecalis* and *Enterococcus faecium*. *Enterococcus gallinarum* and *Enterococcus casseliflavus* are also common colonizers of the human intestinal tract and are important because these species are inherently vancomycin-resistant.

Physiology and Structure

The enterococci are gram-positive cocci typically arranged in **pairs and short chains** (Figure 23-1). The microscopic morphology of these isolates frequently cannot be differentiated from that of *Streptococcus pneumoniae*. The cocci grow both aerobically and anaerobically and in a broad temperature range ($10°$ C to $45°$ C). Although the enterococci have complex nutritional needs (requiring B vitamins, nucleic acid bases, and a carbon source such as glucose), enriched sheep blood agar supports their growth. After 24 hours of incubation, the large colonies can appear non-hemolytic, α-hemolytic, or rarely β-hemolytic. The bacteria can grow in the presence of high concentrations of **NaCl** and **bile salts**. These basic properties can be used to distinguish enterococci from other catalase-negative, gram-positive cocci.

Pathogenesis and Immunity

Enterococci do not have a potent toxin or other well-defined virulence factors (Table 23-3). For this reason, these bacteria are typically considered to have a limited potential for causing disease, although life-threatening disease with antibiotic-resistant strains has become a serious problem in hospitalized patients.

These bacteria have **surface adhesin proteins** that allow them to bind to the cells lining the human intestine and vaginal host tissues, and they secrete proteins with **hemolytic activity** (cytolysin) and **proteolytic activity** (e.g., gelatinase, serine protease). The bacteria generally cannot avoid being engulfed and killed by phagocytic cells. Perhaps of greatest significance is that the enterococci either are **inherently resistant to many commonly used antibiotics** (e.g., oxacillin, cephalosporins) or have acquired resistance genes (e.g., to aminoglycosides, vancomycin).

Epidemiology

As their name implies, enterococci are enteric bacteria which are commonly recovered in feces collected from humans and from a variety of animals. *E. faecalis* is found in the large intestine in high concentrations (e.g., 10^7 organisms per gram of feces) and in the genitourinary tract. The distribution of *E. faecium* is similar to that of *E. faecalis*, but the organisms are found less frequently. Enterococci are not commonly isolated in the respiratory tract or on the skin surface, except in hospitalized patients who have been treated with broad-spectrum antibiotics. In these patients, use of the antibiotics allows the

Box 23—1. Important Enterococci

Organism	Historical Derivation
Enterococcus	*enteron*, "intestine"; *coccus*, "berry" (intestinal coccus)
E. faecalis	*faecalis*, relating to "feces"
E. faecium	*faecium*, "of feces"
E. gallinarum	*gallinarum*, "of hens" (original source was intestines of domestic fowl)
E. casseliflavus	*casseli*, "Kassel's"; *flavus*, "yellow" (Kassel's yellow)

Table 23—1. Frequency of Human Colonization and Disease Caused by Some Catalase-Negative, Gram-Positive Cocci

Genus	Human Colonization	Human Disease
Enterococcus	Common	Common
Streptococcus	Common	Common
Abiotrophia	Uncommon	Uncommon
Granulicatella	Uncommon	Uncommon
Leuconostoc	Uncommon	Uncommon
Aerococcus	Uncommon	Rare
Pediococcus	Uncommon	Rare
Lactococcus	Uncommon	Rare

Table 23—2. Catalase-Negative, Gram-Positive Cocci and Their Diseases

Organism	Diseases
Abiotrophia	Bacteremia, endocarditis (native and prosthetic valves), nosocomial brain abscesses and meningitis, eye infections
Aerococcus	Bacteremia, endocarditis, urinary tract infections
Enterococcus	Bacteremia, endocarditis, urinary tract infections, wound infections
Granulicatella	Bacteremia, endocarditis (native and prosthetic valves), eye infections
Lactococcus	Bacteremia in immunocompromised patients, endocarditis (native and prosthetic valves), urinary tract infections, osteomyelitis
Leuconostoc	Opportunistic infections including bacteremia, wound infections, central nervous system infections, and peritonitis
Pediococcus	Opportunistic infections including bacteremia in severely immunocompromised patients
Streptococcus	Refer to Chapter 22

Box 23—2. Summary: Enterococcus

Biology, Virulence, and Disease

Gram-positive cocci arranged in pairs and short chains (morphologically similar to *Streptococcus pneumoniae*)

Cell wall with group-specific antigen (group D glycerol teichoic acid)

Virulence mediated by ability to adhere to host surfaces, secrete cytolysins and proteases that cause localized tissue damage, and resist antibiotic treatment

Diseases include urinary tract infections, wound infections (particularly intraabdominal and usually polymicrobic), and bacteremia and endocarditis

Epidemiology

Colonizes the gastrointestinal tracts of humans and animals; spreads to other mucosal surfaces if broad spectrum antibiotics eliminate the normal bacterial population

Cell wall structure typical of gram-positive bacteria, which allows survival on environmental surfaces for prolonged periods

Most infections from patient's bacterial flora; some caused by patient-to-patient spread

Patients at increased risk include those hospitalized for prolonged periods and treated with broad-spectrum antibiotics (particularly cephalosporins, to which enterococci are naturally resistant)

Diagnosis

Grows readily on common, nonselective media. Differentiated from related organisms by simple tests (catalase negative, PYR positive, resistant to bile and optochin)

Treatment, Prevention, and Control

Therapy for serious infections requires combination of an aminoglycoside with a cell-wall-active antibiotic (penicillin, ampicillin, or vancomycin); newer agents include linezolid, quinupristin/dalfopristin, and selected fluoroquinolones

Antibiotic resistance to each of these drugs is becoming increasingly common, and infections with many isolates (particularly *E. faecium*) are not treatable with any antibiotics

Figure 23—1. Gram stain of blood culture with *Enterococcus faecalis*.

Table 23—3. Enterococcal Virulence Factors

Virulence Factor	Biologic Effect
Surface Adhesins	
Aggregation substance	Hairlike protein embedded in cytoplasmic membrane that facilitates plasmid exchange and binding to epithelial cells
Enterococcal surface protein	Collagen-binding adhesin present in *E. faecalis*
Carbohydrate adhesins	Present in individual bacterium in multiple types; mediate binding to host cells
Secreted Factors	
Cytolysin	Protein bacteriocin that inhibits growth of gram-positive bacteria (facilitates colonization); induces local tissue damage
Pheromone	Chemoattractant for neutrophils; may regulate inflammatory reaction
Gelatinase	Hydrolyzes gelatin, collagen, hemoglobin, and other small peptides
Antibiotic Resistance	
Multiple plasmid and chromosome genes	Resistant to aminoglycosides, β-lactams, and vancomycin

enterococci to spread from the intestinal tract to the other mucosal and skin surfaces. Thus patients who are treated with broad-spectrum antibiotics and who are typically quite ill are most likely to develop disease with the enterococci that are part of their normal microbial population.

The prevalence of the many other enterococcal species is unknown, although they are believed to colonize the intestines in small numbers. Two species that are commonly recovered in the human intestines are *E. gallinarum* and *E. casseliflavus*. These relatively avirulent species are important because, although they are rarely associated with human disease, they are inherently resistant to vancomycin and can be confused with the more important species, *E. faecalis* and *E. faecium*.

Clinical Diseases (Box 23-3; Clinical Case 23-1)

Despite the paucity of virulence factors, enterococci are important pathogens, particularly in hospitalized patients. Indeed, enterococci are one of the most common causes of infections acquired in the hospital (**nosocomial infection**). The urinary tract, peritoneum, and heart tissue are the sites involved most often. Enterococcal infections are particularly common in patients with urinary or intravascular catheters and in patients who have been hospitalized for prolonged periods and have received **broad-spectrum antibiotics**.

Box 23—3. Enterococcal Diseases: Clinical Summaries

Urinary tract infection: dysuria and pyuria most commonly in hospitalized patients with an indwelling urinary catheter and receiving broad-spectrum cephalosporin antibiotics
Peritonitis: abdominal swelling and tenderness after abdominal trauma or surgery; patients are typically acutely ill, febrile, and have positive blood cultures
Endocarditis: infection of the heart endothelium or valves; associated with persistent bacteremia; can present acutely or chronically

A particularly severe complication of enterococcal bacteremia is **endocarditis**, a disease with a high mortality rate. In contrast with bacteremia and urinary tract infections where enterococci are typically the only organism present, most abdominal and wound infections with enterococci are associated with other organisms (**polymicrobial infection**). Thus the importance of enterococci in these infections is less well defined.

Laboratory Diagnosis

Enterococci grow readily on nonselective media such as blood agar and chocolate agar. Despite the fact that enterococci may resemble *S. pneumoniae* on Gram-stained specimens, the organisms can be readily differentiated on the basis of simple biochemical reactions. For example, enterococci are resistant to optochin (*S. pneumoniae* is susceptible), do not dissolve when exposed to bile (*S. pneumoniae* is dissolved), and produce L-pyrrolidonyl arylamidase (the only *Streptococcus* that is PYR-positive is *Streptococcus pyogenes*). The **PYR test** is a commonly performed "5-minute spot test." Catalase-negative, PYR-positive cocci arranged

Clinical Case 23-1. Enterococcal Endocarditis

Zimmer, et al. (Clin Infect Dis 37:e29-e30, 2003) described the difficulties in treating a patient with enterococcal endocarditis. The patient was a 40-year-old man with hepatitis C, hypertension, and end-stage renal disease who developed fevers and chills during hemodialysis. In the two months before this episode, he was treated with ampicillin, levofloxacin, and gentamicin for group B streptococcal endocarditis. Cultures performed during the hemodialysis grew *Enterococcus faecalis* resistant to levofloxacin and gentamicin. Because the patient had an allergic reaction to ampicillin, he was treated with linezolid. Echocardiography showed vegetation on the mitral and tricuspid valves. Over a 3-week period, the patient's cardiac output deteriorated, so the patient was desensitized to ampicillin, and therapy was switched to ampicillin and streptomycin. After 25 days of hospitalization, the patient's damaged heart valves were replaced, and therapy was extended for an additional 6 weeks. Thus use of broad spectrum antibiotics predisposed this patient with previously damaged heart valves to endocarditis caused by *Enterococcus*, and treatment was complicated by resistance of the isolate to many commonly used antibiotics in pairs and short chains can be presumptively identified as enterococci. Phenotypic properties (e.g., pigment production, motility), biochemical tests, and nucleic acid sequencing are necessary to differentiate among *E. faecalis*, *E. faecium*, and the other *Enterococcus* species, but this topic is beyond the scope of this text.

Treatment, Prevention, and Control

Antimicrobial therapy for enterococcal infections is complicated, because most antibiotics are not bactericidal at clinically relevant concentrations. Therapy has traditionally consisted of the synergistic **combination of an aminoglycoside and a cell wall–active antibiotic** (e.g., ampicillin, vancomycin). However, resistance to aminoglycosides, ampicillin, penicillin, and vancomycin has become a major problem. Typically, more than 25% of enterococci are resistant to the aminoglycosides; virtually all isolates of *E. faecium* are resistant to ampicillin; and the majority of isolates of *E. faecium* are now resistant to vancomycin. The resistance in these strains to aminoglycosides and vancomycin is particularly troublesome, because it is mediated by plasmids and can be transferred to other bacteria.

Newer antibiotics have been developed specifically to treat enterococci resistant to ampicillin and vancomycin. They include linezolid, quinupristin/dalfopristin, and selected fluoroquinolones. Unfortunately, resistance to linezolid is steadily increasing, quinupristin/dalfopristin has no activity against *E. faecalis* (the most commonly isolated enterococcal species), and the fluoroquinolones have poor activity against vancomycin-resistant enterococci.

It is difficult to prevent and control enterococcal infections. Careful restriction of antibiotic therapy and the implementation of appropriate infection-control practices (e.g., isolation of infected patients, use of gowns and gloves by anyone in contact with patients) can reduce the risk of colonization with these bacteria, but the complete elimination of infections is unlikely.

Other Catalase-Negative, Gram-Positive Cocci

Other catalase-negative, gram-positive cocci associated with human disease are *Abiotrophia*, *Granulicatella*, *Leuconostoc*, *Lactococcus*, *Pediococcus*, *Aerococcus*, and other less commonly isolated genera. All are **opportunistic pathogens**.

Abiotrophia and *Granulicatella*, formerly called *nutritionally deficient streptococci*, are problematic, because they will initially grow in blood culture broths or in mixed cultures but do not grow when subcultured onto sheep blood agar media unless the media is supplemented with pyridoxal (vitamin B$_6$). *Leuconostoc* and *Pediococcus* can resemble streptococci but are **resistant to vancomycin**, a

trait that has not been seen in streptococci. *Lactococcus* can be misidentified as *Enterococcus*, and *Aerococcus* ("air coccus") is typically an airborne organism that can contaminate the patient's skin or the specimen while it is being collected or processed in the laboratory. It is difficult to identify most of these organisms precisely without using molecular tools such as gene sequencing, but having knowledge of their presence and clinical features is useful.

Case Study and Questions

A 72-year-old man was admitted to the hospital because of a fever that had risen as high as 40° C, myalgias, and respiratory complaints. The clinical diagnosis of influenza was confirmed by the laboratory isolation of influenza virus from respiratory secretions. This patient's hospitalization was complicated by the development of pneumonia caused by oxacillin-resistant *Staphylococcus aureus* that was treated with a 2-week course of vancomycin. Declining pulmonary function necessitated the use of a ventilator, which led to the development of a secondary infection with *Klebsiella pneumoniae*. Ceftazidime (a cephalosporin) and gentamicin were added to the patient's treatment. After 4 weeks of hospitalization, the patient became septic. *E. faecium* resistant to vancomycin, gentamicin, and ampicillin was cultured from three blood specimens.

1. What predisposing conditions made this patient more susceptible to infection with *E. faecium*?
2. What is the most likely source of this organism?
3. What factors contribute to the virulence of enterococci?

Bibliography

Bhavnani SM, et al: A nationwide, multicenter, case-control study comparing risk factors, treatment, and outcome for vancomycin-resistant and -susceptible enterococcal bacteremia. Diagn Microbiol Infect Dis 36:145-158, 2000.

Coburn PS, et al: *Enterococcus faecalis* senses target cells and in response expresses cytolysin. Science 306:2270-2272, 2004.

Elsner HA, et al: Virulence factors of *Enterococcus faecalis* and *Enterococcus faecium* blood culture isolates. Eur J Clin Infect Dis 19:39-42, 2000.

Facklam R, Elliott JA: Identification, classification, and clinical relevance of catalase-negative, gram-positive cocci, excluding the *streptococci* and *enterococci*. Clin Microbiol Rev 8:479-495, 1995.

Garbutt JM, et al: Association between resistance to vancomycin and death in cases of *Enterococcus faecium* bacteremia. Clin Infect Dis 30:466-472, 2000.

Gilmore MS, et al: *Enterococci*: Pathogenesis, Molecular Biology, and Antibiotic Resistance. Washington, DC, ASM Press, 2002.

Handwerger S, et al: Infection due to *Leuconostoc* species: Six cases and review. Rev Infect Dis 12:602-610, 1990.

Leclercq R, Courvalin P: Resistance to glycopeptides in *enterococci*. Clin Infect Dis 24:545-556, 1997.

Murray BE: Vancomycin-resistant *enterococci*. Am J Med 101:284-293, 1997.

Shay DK, et al: Epidemiology and mortality risk of vancomycin-resistant enterococcal bloodstream infections. J Infect Dis 172:993-1000, 1995.

Shepard BD, Gilmore, MS: Differential expression of virulence-related genes in *Enterococcus faecalis* in response to biological cues in serum and urine. Infect Immun 70:4344-4352, 2002.

Bacillus

The family Bacillaceae consists of a diverse collection of bacteria, including organisms that grow only aerobically or only anaerobically, organisms shaped as cocci or rods, and organisms that stain gram-positive or gram-negative. The one feature this diverse group of bacteria all share is the ability to form endospores (Figure 24-1). Despite the dozens of genera in this family, students need to know only two clinically important genera: **Bacillus** (the aerobic and facultative anaerobic spore formers; Box 24-1) and **Clostridium** (the strict, anaerobic spore formers; see Chapter 39).

Almost 200 species are in the genus *Bacillus*. Fortunately the species that are of medical interest are relatively limited. *Bacillus anthracis*, the organism responsible for anthrax, is the most important member of this genus. This species is considered one of the most feared agents of biologic warfare. Since the release of weaponized *B. anthracis* spores in the U.S. postal system in 2001, the potential danger associated with this organism has been re-emphasized. The other clinically important species in this genus is *Bacillus cereus*, an organism responsible for gastroenteritis, traumatic eye infections, catheter-associated sepsis, and rarely severe pneumonia.

Bacillus anthracis (Box 24-2)

Physiology and Structure

B. anthracis is a large (1×3 to $8~\mu m$) organism arranged as single or paired rods or as long, serpentine chains (Figure 24-2). Although spores are readily observed in 2- to 3-day-old cultures, they are not seen in clinical specimens.

Because of the unique medical importance of *B. anthracis*, it is important to understand the functional details of this organism's toxins. Virulent *B. anthracis* carries genes for three toxin protein components on a large plasmid, pXO1. The individual proteins, **protective antigen** (PA), **edema factor** (EF), and **lethal factor** (LF), are nontoxic individually but form important toxins when combined: Protective antigen plus edema factor forms **edema toxin**, and protective antigen plus lethal factor forms **lethal toxin**. *PA* is an **83-kDa protein** that binds to one of two receptors on host cell surfaces that are present on many cells and tissues (e.g., brain, heart, intestine, lung, skeletal muscle, pancreas, macrophages). After PA binds to its receptor, host proteases cleave PA, releasing a small fragment and retaining the 63-kDa fragment (PA_{63}) on the cell surface. The PA_{63} fragments self-associate on the cell surface, forming a ring-shaped complex of seven fragments (pore precursor or "prepore"). This heptameric complex can then bind up to three molecules of LF and/or EF. Both factors recognize the same binding site of PA_{63}, so the binding is competitive. Formation of the complex stimulates endocytosis and movement to an acidic compartment. In this environment, the heptameric complex forms a transmembrane pore and releases LF and EF into the cell cytosol. *LF* is **zinc-dependent protease** that is capable of cleaving mitogen-activated protein (MAP) kinase, leading to cell death by incompletely understood mechanisms. *EF* is a **calmodulin-dependent adenylate cyclase** that increases the intracellular cyclic adenosine monophosphate (cAMP) levels, resulting in edema. EF is related to the adenylate cyclases produced by *Bordetella pertussis* and *Pseudomonas aeruginosa*.

A second important virulence factor carried by *B. anthracis* is a prominent polypeptide **capsule** (consisting of poly-D-glutamic acid). The capsule is observed in clinical specimens but is not produced in vitro unless special growth conditions are used. Three genes (*cap*A, *cap*B, and *cap*C) are responsible for synthesis of this capsule and are carried on a second plasmid (pXO2). Only one type of capsule has been identified, presumably because it is composed of only glutamic acid.

Pathogenesis and Immunity

The major factors responsible for the virulence of *B. anthracis* are the capsule, edema toxin, and lethal toxin.

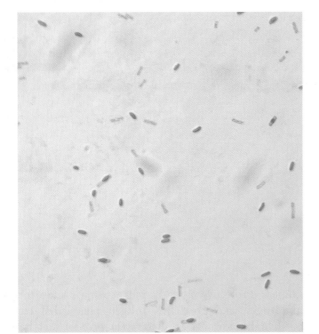

Figure 24—1. *Bacillus cereus*. Spores retain the malachite green dye in this special spore stain.

The capsule inhibits phagocytosis of replicating cells. The adenylate cyclase activity of edema toxin is responsible for the fluid accumulation observed in anthrax. The zinc metalloprotease activity of lethal toxin stimulates macrophages to release tumor necrosis factor-α (TNF-α), interleukin-1β (IL-1β), and other proinflammatory cytokines. This toxin also mediates lysis of macrophages in selected cell cultures. Of the major proteins of *B. anthracis*, PA is the most immunogenic (hence the name). Both LF and EF inhibit the host's innate immune system.

Epidemiology

Anthrax is primarily a disease of herbivores; humans are infected through exposure to contaminated animals or animal products. The disease is a serious problem in countries where animal vaccination is not practiced or is impractical (e.g., disease established in African wildlife). In contrast, natural infections with *B. anthracis* are rarely seen in the United States, with only five cases reported

Box 24—1. Important *Bacillus* Species

Organism	Historical Derivation
Bacillus	*bacillum*, "a small rod"
B. anthracis	*anthrax*, "charcoal," a carbuncle (refers to the black, necrotic wound associated with cutaneous anthrax)
B. cereus	*cereus*, "waxen, wax-colored" (refers to colonies with a typical dull or frosted-glass surface)

Box 24—2. Summary: *Bacillus anthracis*

Biology, Virulence, and Disease

Spore-forming, nonmotile, nonhemolytic gram-positive rods
Polypeptide capsule consisting of poly-D-glutamic acid observed in clinical specimens
Virulent strains also produce three exotoxins that combine to form edema toxin (combination of protective antigen and edema factor) and lethal toxin (protective antigen with lethal factor)
B. anthracis primarily infects herbivores, with humans as accidental hosts
Rarely isolated in developed countries but is prevalent in impoverished areas where vaccination of animals is not practiced
The greatest danger of anthrax in industrial countries is the use of *B. anthracis* as an agent of bioterrorism
Three forms of anthrax are recognized: cutaneous (most common in humans), gastrointestinal, and inhalation (bioterrorism)

Diagnosis

Organism is present in high concentrations in clinical specimens (microscopy typically positive) and grows readily in culture
Preliminary identification is based on microscopic (gram-positive, nonmotile rods) and colonial (nonhemolytic, adherent colonies) morphology. Confirmed by demonstrating capsule and either lysis with gamma phage, a positive DFA test for the specific cell wall polysaccharide, or positive nucleic acid amplification assay

Treatment, Prevention, and Control

Ciprofloxacin is the drug of choice for cutaneous anthrax; ciprofloxacin or doxycycline combined with additional antibiotics for inhalation anthrax
Vaccination of animal herds and people in endemic areas can control disease, but spores are difficult to eliminate from contaminated soils
Animal vaccination is effective, but human vaccines have limited usefulness
Alternative treatments interfering with the activity of anthrax toxins under investigation

Figure 24—2. *Bacillus anthracis* in the blood of a patient with inhalation anthrax.

between 1981 and 1999. This statistic may now be meaningless, with the deliberate contamination of the U.S. Postal Service with *B. anthracis* spores in 2001. The risk of exposing a large population to the dangerous pathogen has increased dramatically in this era of bioterrorism. A number of nations and independent terrorist groups have biologic warfare programs. Iraq, the former Soviet Union, and the Aum Shinrikyo terrorist group in Japan have experimented with using *B. anthracis* as a weapon. Indeed, much of what we know about anthrax acquired via the inhalation route was learned from the accidental release in 1979 of spores in Sverdlovsk in the former Soviet Union (at least 79 cases of anthrax with 68 deaths) and the terrorist contamination of employees of the U.S. Postal Service with letters containing *B. anthracis* (11 patients with inhalation anthrax and 11 patients with cutaneous anthrax).

Human *B. anthracis* disease (Box 24-3) is acquired by one of the following three routes: **inoculation, ingestion**, and **inhalation**. Approximately 95% of anthrax infections in humans result from the inoculation of *Bacillus* spores through exposed skin from either contaminated soil or infected animal products such as hides, goat hair, and wool.

Ingestion anthrax is very rare in humans, but ingestion is a common route of infection in herbivores. Because the organism can form resilient spores, contaminated soil or animal products can remain infectious for many years.

Inhalation anthrax was historically called **wool-sorters' disease** because most human infections resulted from the inhalation of *B. anthracis* spores during the processing of goat hair. This is currently an uncommon source for human infections; however, inhalation is the most likely route of infection with biologic weapons. The infectious dose of the organism is believed to be low, although this depends on the state of the spore preparation. Weaponized spores are treated in a way to minimize clumping so spores can reach the lower airways where alveolar macrophages can phagocytize the spores and initiate bacterial replication. Person-to-person transmission does not occur, because bacterial replication occurs in the mediastinal lymph nodes rather than the bronchopulmonary tree.

Clinical Diseases (Clinical Case 24-1)

Typically, **cutaneous anthrax** starts with the development of a painless papule at the site of inoculation that rapidly progresses to an ulcer surrounded by vesicles, then to a necrotic eschar (Figure 24-3). Systemic signs, painful lymphadenopathy, and massive edema may develop. The mortality rate in patients with untreated cutaneous anthrax is 20%.

Clinical symptoms of **gastrointestinal anthrax** are determined by the site of the infection. If organisms invade the upper intestinal tract, ulcers form in the mouth or esophagus, leading to regional lymphadenopathy, edema, and sepsis. If the organism invades the cecum or terminal ileum, the patient presents with nausea, vomiting, and malaise, which rapidly progress to systemic disease. The mortality associated with gastrointestinal anthrax is believed to approach 100%.

Unlike the other two forms of anthrax, **inhalation anthrax** can be associated with a prolonged latent period (2 months or more), during which the infected patient

---

Box 24-3. *Bacillus* Diseases: Clinical Summaries

Bacillus anthracis

Cutaneous anthrax: a painless papule progresses to ulceration with surrounding vesicles and then to eschar formation; painful lymphadenopathy, edema, and systemic signs may develop
Gastrointestinal anthrax: ulcers form at the site of invasion (e.g., mouth, esophagus, intestine) leading to regional lymphadenopathy, edema, and sepsis
Inhalation anthrax: initial nonspecific signs are followed by the rapid onset of sepsis with fever, edema, and lymphadenopathy (mediastinal lymph nodes); meningeal symptoms in half the patients, and most patients with inhalation anthrax will die unless treatment is initiated immediately

Bacillus cereus

Gastroenteritis: emetic form is characterized by a rapid onset of vomiting and abdominal pain and a short duration; diarrheal form is characterized by a longer onset and duration of diarrhea and abdominal cramps
Ocular infections: rapid, progressive destruction of the eye after traumatic introduction of the bacteria into the eye
Severe pulmonary disease: severe anthrax-like pulmonary disease in immunocompetent patients

---

Clinical Case 24-1. Inhalation Anthrax

Bush, et al. (N Engl J Med 345:1607-1610, 2001) reported the first case of inhalation anthrax in the 2001 bioterrorism attack in the United States. The patient was a 63-year-old man living in Florida who had a 4-day history of fever, myalgias, and malaise without localizing symptoms. His wife brought him to the regional hospital because he awoke from sleep with fever, emesis, and confusion. On physical examination, he had a temperature of 39° C, blood pressure of 150/80 mm Hg, pulse of 110, and respirations were 18. No respiratory distress was noted. Treatment was initiated for presumed bacterial meningitis. Basilar infiltrates and a widened mediastinum was noted on the initial chest radiograph. Gram stain of CSF revealed many neutrophils and large gram-positive rods. Anthrax was suspected, and penicillin treatment was initiated. Within 24 hours of admission, CSF and blood cultures were positive for *Bacillus anthracis*. During the first day of hospitalization, the patient had a grand mal seizure and was intubated. On the second hospital day, hypotension and azotemia developed, with subsequent renal failure. On the third hospital day, refractory hypotension developed, and the patient had a fatal cardiac arrest. This patient illustrates the rapidity with which patients with inhalation anthrax can deteriorate, despite a rapid diagnosis and appropriate antimicrobial therapy. Although the respiratory tract is the route of exposure, patients do not develop pneumonia; rather, the abnormal chest radiograph is caused by hemorrhagic mediastinitis.

Figure 24—3. Cutaneous anthrax demonstrating marked erythema, edema, and vesicle rupture. *(From Cohen J, Powderly WG: Infectious Diseases, 2nd ed. St Louis, Mosby, 2004.)*

remains asymptomatic. Spores can remain latent in the nasal passages or reach the lower airways, where alveolar macrophages ingest the inhaled spores and transport them to the mediastinal lymph nodes. The initial clinical symptoms of disease are nonspecific—fever, myalgias, nonproductive cough, and malaise. The second stage of disease is more dramatic, with a rapidly worsening course of fever, edema, massive enlargement of the mediastinal lymph nodes (this is responsible for the widened mediastinum observed on chest radiography; Figure 24-4), respiratory failure, and sepsis. Although the route of infection is by inhalation, pneumonia rarely develops. Meningeal symptoms are seen in half of patients with inhalation anthrax. Almost all cases progress to shock and death within 3 days of initial symptoms unless anthrax is suspected and treatment is initiated immediately. Serologic evidence indicates that a subclinical or asymptomatic form of inhalation anthrax does not exist. Virtually all patients who develop

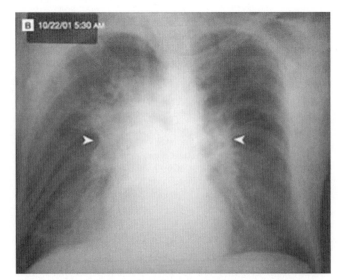

Figure 24—4. Inhalation anthrax demonstrating enlarged mediastinal lymph nodes.

disease progress to a fatal outcome unless there is immediate medical intervention.

Laboratory Diagnosis

Infections with *B. anthracis* are characterized by overwhelming numbers of organisms present in wounds, involved lymph nodes, and blood. Anthrax is one of the few bacterial diseases where organisms can be seen when peripheral blood is Gram stained (see Figure 24-2). Therefore the detection of organisms by microscopy and culture is not a problem. The diagnostic difficulty is distinguishing *B. anthracis* from other members of the taxonomically related *Bacillus cereus* group. A preliminary identification of *B. anthracis* is based on microscopic and colonial morphology. The organisms appear as long, thin, gram-positive rods arranged singly or in long chains. Spores are not observed in clinical specimens but only in cultures incubated in a low CO_2 atmosphere; they can be best seen with the use of a special spore stain (e.g., malachite green stain; see Figure 24-1). The **capsule** of *B. anthracis* is produced in vivo but is not typically observed in culture. The capsule can be observed with a contrasting stain such as India ink (the ink particles are excluded by the capsule so that the background but not the area around bacteria appears black), M'Fadyean methylene blue stain, or a direct fluorescent antibody (DFA) test developed against the capsular polypeptide. Colonies cultured on sheep blood agar are large, nonpigmented, and have a dry "ground glass" surface and irregular edges with projections along the lines, where the specimen was inoculated onto the agar plate (referred to as "Medusa head" morphology). The colonies are quite sticky and adherent to the agar, and if the edge is lifted with a bacteriologic loop, it will remain standing like a beaten egg white. Colonies are **not hemolytic** in contrast with *B. cereus*. *B. anthracis* will appear **nonmotile** in motility tests, such as the microscopic observation of individual rods in a suspended drop of culture medium. The definitive identification of nonmotile, nonhemolytic organisms resembling *B. anthracis* is made in a public health reference laboratory. This is accomplished by demonstrating capsule production (by microscopy or DFA) and either lysis of the bacteria with gamma phage or a positive DFA test for a specific *B. anthracis* cell wall polysaccharide. Additionally, nucleic acid amplification tests (e.g., polymerase chain reaction [PCR]) have been developed and are performed in reference laboratories. The PCR tests are also commercially available.

Treatment, Prevention, and Control

B. anthracis is susceptible to **penicillin**, doxycycline, and ciprofloxacin but resistant to sulfonamides and extended-spectrum cephalosporins. Because genes encoding resistance to penicillin and doxycycline have been transferred to *B. anthracis*, the current recommendation for treating a patient with suspected inhalation anthrax is use of the combination of either ciprofloxacin or doxycycline with one or two additional antibiotics (e.g., rifampin, vancomycin, penicillin, imipenem, clindamycin, clarithromycin.

The control of naturally acquired human disease requires the control of animal disease, which involves the **vaccination of animal herds** in endemic regions and the burning or burial of animals that die of anthrax. Complete eradication of anthrax is unlikely, because the spores of the organism can exist for many years in soil. Furthermore, complete eradication of anthrax infections is unlikely with the threat of bioterrorist-related infections a current reality.

Vaccination of animals is an effective control measure. Vaccination has also been used to protect (1) people who live in areas where the disease is endemic, (2) people who work with animal products imported from countries with endemic anthrax, and (3) military personnel. Although the current vaccine appears to be effective, work to develop a less toxic vaccine is underway. Alternative approaches to inactivating anthrax toxins have focused on protective antigen and its receptor target. Passive infusion of human monoclonal antibodies against *B. anthracis* protective antigen prevented death in an animal model of inhalation anthrax and was well tolerated in human volunteers. Synthetic peptide complexes that target the cell surface receptors for protective antigen have also been used to neutralize anthrax toxin in animal models. How these alternative approaches can be used to treat human disease remains to be demonstrated.

Bacillus cereus

Bacillus species other than *B. anthracis* are primarily opportunistic pathogens that have relatively low capacities for virulence. Although most of these species have been found to cause disease, *B. cereus* is clearly the most important pathogen, with gastroenteritis, ocular infections, and intravenous-catheter-related sepsis the diseases most commonly observed, and rare cases of severe pneumonia (Box 24-4).

Pathogenesis

Gastroenteritis caused by *B. cereus* is mediated by one of **two enterotoxins** (Table 24-1). The **heat-stable**, proteolysis-resistant enterotoxin causes the **emetic form** of the disease, and the **heat-labile** enterotoxin causes the **diarrheal form** of the disease. The heat-labile enterotoxin is similar to the enterotoxins produced by *Escherichia coli* and *Vibrio cholerae*; each stimulates the adenylate cyclase—cyclic adenosine monophosphate system in intestinal epithelial cells, leading to profuse watery diarrhea. The mechanism of action of the heat-stable enterotoxin is unknown.

Box 24—4. Summary: *Bacillus cereus*

Biology, Virulence, and Disease

Spore-forming, motile, gram-positive rods
Heat-stable and heat-labile enterotoxin
Tissue destruction mediated by cytotoxic enzymes, including cereolysin and phospholipase C
Ubiquitous in soils throughout the world
People at risk include those who consume food contaminated with the bacterium (e.g., rice, meat, vegetables, sauces), those with penetrating injuries (e.g., to eye), those who receive intravenous injections, and immunocompromised patients exposed to *B. cereus*
Capable of causing an anthrax-like disease in immunocompetent patients

Diagnosis

Isolation of the organism in implicated food product or nonfecal specimens (e.g., eye, wound)

Treatment, Prevention, and Control

Gastrointestinal infections are treated symptomatically
Ocular infectious or other invasive diseases require removal of foreign bodies and treatment with vancomycin, clindamycin, ciprofloxacin, or gentamicin
Gastrointestinal disease is prevented by proper preparation of food (e.g., foods should be consumed immediately after preparation or refrigerated)

The pathogenesis of *B. cereus* ocular infections is also incompletely defined. At least three toxins have been implicated; they are **necrotic toxin** (a heat-labile enterotoxin), **cereolysin** (a potent hemolysin named after the species), and **phospholipase C** (a potent lecithinase). It is likely that the rapid destruction of the eye that is characteristic of *B. cereus* infections results from the interaction of these toxins and other unidentified factors.

Bacillus species can colonize skin transiently and can be recovered as insignificant contaminants in blood cultures. In the presence of an intravascular foreign body, however, these organisms can be responsible for persistent bacteremia and signs of sepsis (i.e., fever, chills, hypotension, shock).

Table 24—1. *Bacillus cereus* Food Poisoning

	Emetic Form	Diarrheal Form
Implicated food	Rice	Meat, vegetables
Incubation period (hours)	< 6 (mean, 2)	> 6 (mean, 9)
Symptoms	Vomiting, nausea, abdominal cramps	Diarrhea, nausea, abdominal cramps
Duration (hours)	8-10 (mean, 9)	20-36 (mean, 24)
Enterotoxin	Heat stable	Heat labile

Epidemiology

B. cereus and other *Bacillus* species are ubiquitous organisms, present in virtually all environments. Virtually all infections originate from an environmental source (e.g., contaminated soil). Isolation of bacteria from clinical specimens in the absence of characteristic disease usually represents insignificant contamination.

Clinical Diseases

As mentioned previously, *B. cereus* is responsible for two forms of food poisoning: **vomiting disease (emetic form)** and **diarrheal disease (diarrheal form)**. In most patients, the emetic form of disease results from the consumption of contaminated **rice**. Most bacteria are killed during the initial cooking of the rice, but the heat-resistant spores survive. If the cooked rice is not refrigerated, the spores germinate, and the bacteria can multiply rapidly. The heat-stable enterotoxin that is released is not destroyed when the rice is reheated. The emetic form of disease is an intoxication, caused by ingestion of the enterotoxin and not the bacteria. Thus the incubation period after eating the contaminated rice is short (1 to 6 hours) and the duration of illness is also short (less than 24 hours). Symptoms consist of vomiting, nausea, and abdominal cramps. Fever and diarrhea are generally absent. Fulminant liver failure has also been associated with consumption of food contaminated with large amounts of emetic toxin, which impairs mitochondrial fatty acid metabolism. Fortunately this is a rare complication.

The diarrheal form of *B. cereus* food poisoning is a true infection, resulting from ingestion of the bacteria in contaminated meat, vegetables, or sauces. There is a longer incubation period, during which the organism multiplies in the patient's intestinal tract, followed by the release of the heat-labile enterotoxin. This enterotoxin is responsible for the diarrhea, nausea, and abdominal cramps that develop. This form of disease generally lasts 1 day or longer.

B. cereus **ocular infections** usually occur after traumatic penetrating injuries of the eye with a soil-contaminated object (Clinical Case 24-2). *Bacillus* panophthalmitis is a rapidly progressive disease that almost universally results in the complete loss of light perception within 48 hours of the injury. Disseminated infections with ocular manifestations can also develop in intravenous drug abusers.

Other infections with *B. cereus* and other *Bacillus* species are intravenous catheter and central nervous system shunt infections and endocarditis (most common in drug abusers), as well as pneumonitis, bacteremia, and meningitis in severely immunosuppressed patients. It has also been reported that ingestion of **tea** by immunocompromised patients is associated with an increased risk for invasive *B. cereus* disease.

One rare disease of *B. cereus* deserves special attention: **severe pneumonia mimicking anthrax in immunocompetent patients**. Four patients, all metal workers residing in

---

Clinical Case 24-2. *Bacillus cereus* Traumatic Endophthalmitis

Endophthalmitis caused by the traumatic introduction of *Bacillus cereus* into the eye is unfortunately not uncommon. This is a typical presentation. While working in a vegetable garden, a 44-year-old man suffered a traumatic eye injury when a piece of metal was deflected into his left eye, damaging the cornea and anterior and posterior lens capsule. Over the next 12 hours, he developed increasing pain and purulence in his eye. He underwent surgery to relieve the ocular pressure, drain the purulence, and introduce intravitreal antibiotics (vancomycin, ceftazidime) and dexamethasone. Culture of the aspirated fluid was positive for *Bacillus cereus*. Postoperatively, ciprofloxacin was added to his therapeutic regimen. Despite the prompt surgical and medical intervention and subsequent intravitreal antibiotic injections, the intraocular inflammation persisted, and enucleation was required. This patient illustrates the risks involved in penetrating eye injuries and the need to aggressively intervene if the eye is to be saved.

---

either Texas or Louisiana, have been described in the literature with this disease. What is most interesting is the strains contained the **B. anthracis pXO1 toxin genes** and all were **encapsulated**, although this was not the *B. anthracis* poly-γ-D-glutamic acid capsule. These strains demonstrate the potential danger and presumed ease of transferring *B. anthracis* virulence genes into the ubiquitous *B. cereus*.

Laboratory Diagnosis

Like *B. anthracis*, *B. cereus* and other species can be readily cultured from clinical specimens, except stool specimens collected from patients with the emetic form of food poisoning. For confirmation of the existence of foodborne disease, the implicated food (e.g., rice, meat, vegetables) should be cultured. Tests to detect the heat-stable or heat-labile enterotoxins are not commonly performed, so most cases of *B. cereus* gastroenteritis are diagnosed by epidemiologic criteria. *Bacillus* organisms grow rapidly and are readily detected with Gram stain and culture of specimens collected from infected eyes, intravenous culture sites, and other locations.

Treatment, Prevention, and Control

Because the course of *B. cereus* gastroenteritis is short and uncomplicated, symptomatic treatment is adequate. The treatment of other *Bacillus* infections is complicated by the fact that they have a rapid and progressive course and a high incidence of multiple-drug resistance (e.g., *B. cereus* carries genes for resistance to penicillins and cephalosporins). **Vancomycin, clindamycin, ciprofloxacin**, and **gentamicin** can be used to treat infections. Penicillins and cephalosporins are ineffective. Eye infections must be treated rapidly. Rapid consumption of foods after cooking and proper refrigeration of uneaten foods can prevent food poisoning.

Case Study and Questions

A 56-year-old female postal worker sought medical care for fever, diarrhea, and vomiting. She was offered symptomatic treatment and discharged from the community hospital emergency department. Five days later she returned to the hospital with complaints of chills, dry cough, and pleuritic chest pain. A chest radiograph showed a small right infiltrate and bilateral effusions but no evidence of a widened mediastinum. She was admitted to the hospital, and the next day her respiratory status and pleural effusions worsened. A computerized tomographic (CT) scan of her chest revealed enlarged mediastinal and cervical lymph nodes. Pleural fluid and blood was collected for culture and was positive within 10 hours for gram-positive rods in long chains.

1. The clinical impression is that this woman has inhalation anthrax. What tests should be performed to confirm the identification of the isolate?

2. What are the three primary virulence factors found in *B. anthracis*?

3. Describe the mechanisms of action of the toxins produced by *B. anthracis*.

4. Describe the two forms of *B. cereus* food poisoning. What toxin is responsible for each form? Why is the clinical presentation of these two diseases different?

5. *B. cereus* can cause eye infections. What are two risk factors for this disease?

Reference to Student Consult Animation

Please visit *www.StudentConsult.com* to view an animation demonstrating the functions of *B. anthracis* edema toxin with *B. anthracis* lethal toxin.

Bibliography

Avashia S, et al: Fatal pneumonia among metalworkers due to inhalation exposure to *Bacillus cereus* containing *Bacillus anthracis* toxin genes. Clin Infect Dis 44:414-416, 2006.

Baggett HC, et al: No evidence of a mild form of inhalational *Bacillus anthracis* infection during a bioterrorism-related inhalational anthrax outbreak in Washington, D.C., in 2001. Clin Infect Dis 41:991-997, 2005.

Basha S, et al: Polyvalent inhibitors of anthrax toxin that target host receptors. Proc Natl Acad Sci 103:13509-13513, 2006.

Bell CA, et al: Detection of *Bacillus anthracis* DNA by LightCycler PCR. J Clin Microbiol 40:2897-2902, 2002.

Collier RJ, Young JAT: Anthrax toxin. Annu Rev Cell Dev Biol 19:45-70, 2003.

Drobniewski FA: *Bacillus cereus* and related species. Clin Microbiol Rev 6:324-338, 1993.

Gaur AH, et al: *Bacillus cereus* bacteremia and meningitis in immunocompromised children. Clin Infect Dis 32:1456-1462, 2001.

Hoffmaster A, et al: Characterization of *Bacillus cereus* isolates associated with fatal pneumonias: Strains are closely related to *Bacillus anthracis* and harbor *B. anthracis* virulence genes. J Clin Microbiol 44:3352-3360, 2006.

Krantz BA, et al: A phenylalanine clamp catalyzes protein translocation through the anthrax toxin pore. Science 309:777-781, 2005.

Mahtab M, Leppla SH: The roles of anthrax toxin in pathogenesis. Curr Opin Microbiol 7:19-24, 2004.

Melnyk RA, et al: Structural determinants for the binding of anthrax lethal factor to oligomeric protective antigen. J Biol Chem 281:1630-1635, 2006.

Pickering AK, Merkel TJ: Macrophages release tumor necrosis factor alpha and interleukin-12 in response to intracellular *Bacillus anthracis* spores. Infect Immun 72:3069-3072, 2004.

Saleeby CM, et al: Association between tea ingestion and invasive *Bacillus cereus* infection among children with cancer. Clin Infect Dis 39:1536-1539, 2004.

Subramanian GM, et al: A Phase 1 study of PAmAb, a fully human monoclonal antibody against *Bacillus anthracis* protective antigen, in healthy volunteers. Clin Infect Dis 41:12-20, 2005.

Turnbull PC: Introduction: Anthrax history, disease and ecology. Curr Top Microbiol Immunol 271:1-19, 2002.

Listeria and *Erysipelothrix*

The aerobic, non-spore-forming, gram-positive rods are a heterogeneous group of bacteria. Some are well-known human pathogens (e.g., *Corynebacterium diphtheriae*, *Mycobacterium tuberculosis*), others are primarily animal pathogens that can cause human disease (e.g., *Erysipelothrix rhusiopathiae*, *Rhodococcus equi*), and others are opportunistic pathogens that typically infect hospitalized or immunocompromised patients (e.g., *Corynebacterium jeikeium*). Although the clinical presentation of the diseases can be characteristic, detection and identification of the organisms in the laboratory can be problematic. One technique that is useful for the preliminary identification of these bacteria involves their **microscopic morphology**. Gram-positive rods that are uniform in shape include *Listeria* and *Erysipelothrix* (Box 25-1), the subjects of this chapter. The coryneform rods (which include the genus *Corynebacterium*) comprise a large group of irregularly shaped rods (discussed in Chapter 26). The final group of rod-shaped bacteria is characterized by the presence of long-chain mycolic acids in their cell walls. This cell wall component makes it difficult to stain the bacteria with the Gram stain; thus the acid-fast stain was developed. Bacteria that are partially or completely acid-fast include *Nocardia*, *Rhodococcus*, and *Mycobacterium* (discussed in Chapters 27 and 28).

Listeria monocytogenes (Box 25-2)

The genus *Listeria* consists of six species, with ***Listeria monocytogenes*** and *Listeria ivanovii* the only recognized pathogens. *L. monocytogenes* is a significant human pathogen, and *L. ivanovii* is primarily an animal pathogen. *L. monocytogenes* is a short (0.4 to 0.5 × 0.5 to 2 μm), non-branching, gram-positive, facultatively anaerobic rod capable of growth at a broad temperature range (1° C to 45° C) and in a high concentration of salt. The **short rods** appear singly, in pairs, or in short chains (Figure 25-1) and can be mistaken for *Streptococcus pneumoniae* or *Enterococcus*. This is important because both *S. pneumoniae* and

L. monocytogenes can cause meningitis. The organisms are **motile** at room temperature but less so at 37° C, and they exhibit a characteristic end-over-end tumbling motion when a drop of broth is examined microscopically. *L. monocytogenes* exhibits **weak beta hemolysis** when grown on sheep blood agar plates. These differential characteristics (i.e., Gram-stain morphology, motility, β hemolysis) are useful for the preliminary identification of *Listeria*. Although the bacteria are widely distributed in nature, human disease is uncommon and is restricted primarily to several well-defined populations: neonates, the elderly, pregnant women, and patients with defective cellular immunity.

Pathogenesis and Immunity

L. monocytogenes is a **facultative intracellular pathogen**. Following ingestion in contaminated food, *L. monocytogenes* is able to survive exposure to proteolytic enzymes, stomach acid, and bile salts through the protective action of stress-response genes. The bacteria are then able to adhere to host cells via the interaction of proteins on the surface of the bacteria (i.e., internalin A, InlA) with glycoprotein receptors on the host cell surface (e.g., epithelial cadherin, E-cadherin). Other internalins (e.g., InlB) can recognize receptors on a wider range of host cells. Studies with animal models have shown that infection is initiated in the enterocytes or M cells in Peyer patches. After penetration into the cells, the acid pH of the phagolysosome that surrounds the bacteria activates a bacterial exotoxin (**listeriolysin O**) and two different **phospholipase C** enzymes, leading to release of the bacteria into the cell cytosol. The bacteria proceed to replicate and then move to the cell membrane. This movement is mediated by a bacterial protein, **ActA**, localized on the cell surface at one end of a bacterium, that coordinates **assembly of actin**. The distal ends of the actin tail remain fixed while assembly occurs adjacent to the end of the bacterium. Thus the bacterium is pushed to the cell membrane, where a protrusion

Box 25–1. *Listeria* and *Erysipelothrix*

Organism	Historical Derivation
Listeria	*Listeria*, named after the English surgeon Lord Lister
L. monocytogenes	*monocytum*, a "blood cell" or monocyte; *genero*, "produce" (monocyte-producing; membrane extracts stimulate monocyte production in rabbits, but this is not seen in human disease)
Erysipelothrix	*erythros*, "red"; *pella*, "skin"; *thrix*, "hair" (thin, hairlike organism that produces a red or inflammatory skin lesion)
E. rhusiopathiae	*rhusios*, "red"; *pathos*, "disease" (red disease)

Box 25–2. Summary: *Listeria*

Biology, Virulence, Disease

Gram-positive coccobacilli often arranged in pairs resembling enterococci
Facultative intracellular pathogen that can avoid antibody-mediated clearance
Virulent strains produce cell attachment factors (internalins), hemolysins (listeriolysin O, two phospholipase Cs), and a protein that mediates actin-directed intracellular motility (ActA)
Ability to grow at 4° C can lead to high concentrations of bacteria in contaminated foods

Epidemiology

Isolated in soil, water, and vegetation and from a variety of animals, including humans (low-level gastrointestinal carriage)
Disease associated with consumption of contaminated food products (e.g., soft cheese, milk, turkey, raw vegetables [esp. cabbage]) or transplacental spread from mother to neonate; sporadic cases and epidemics occur throughout the year but peak in warmer months
The young, elderly, and pregnant women, as well as patients with defects in cellular immunity, are at increased risk for disease

Diagnosis

Microscopy is insensitive; culture may require incubation for 2 to 3 days or enrichment at 4° C
Motile at room temperature, weakly β-hemolytic, and capable of growth at 4° C and in high-salt concentrations

Treatment, Prevention, and Control

The treatment of choice for severe disease is penicillin or ampicillin, alone or in combination with gentamicin
People at high risk should avoid eating raw or partially cooked foods of animal origin, soft cheese, and unwashed raw vegetables

Figure 25–1. Gram stain of *Listeria monocytogenes* in cerebrospinal fluid.

(filopod) is formed, pushing the bacterium into the adjacent cell. After the adjacent cell ingests the bacterium, the process of **phagolysosome lysis, bacterial replication**, and **directional movement** repeats. Entry into macrophages after passage through the intestinal lining carries the bacteria to the liver and spleen, leading to disseminated disease. The genes responsible for membrane lysis, intracellular replication, and directional movement are clustered together and regulated by a single gene, *prf*A or "positive regulatory factor" gene.

Humoral immunity is relatively unimportant for management of infections with *L. monocytogenes*. These bacteria can replicate in macrophages and move within cells, thus avoiding antibody-mediated clearance. For this reason, patients with defects in **cellular immunity** but not in humoral immunity are particularly susceptible to severe infections.

Epidemiology

L. monocytogenes is isolated from a variety of environmental sources and from the feces of mammals, birds, fish, insects, and other animals. The primary sources of this organism are believed to be soil and decaying vegetable matter. Fecal carriage is estimated to occur in 1% to 5% of healthy people. Because the organism is ubiquitous, exposure and transient colonization are likely to occur in most individuals. An estimated 2500 infections occur annually in the United States. However, many mild infections are not reported. Large outbreaks associated with **contaminated food products** have been documented. For example, 30 million pounds of contaminated meat were recalled in one outbreak in 1999, and 16 million pounds of processed turkey and chicken in a second multistate outbreak in 2000. Many people were exposed to the bacteria before the recall could be accomplished. The incidence of disease is also disproportionate in **high-risk**

populations, such as neonates, the elderly, pregnant women, and patients with severe defects in cell-mediated immunity (e.g., transplants, lymphomas, acquired immune deficiency syndrome [AIDS]).

Human listeriosis is a sporadic disease seen throughout the year, but the incidence peaks in the warmer months. Focal epidemics and sporadic cases of listeriosis have been associated with consumption of contaminated milk, soft cheese, undercooked meat and poultry (e.g., turkey franks, cold cuts), unwashed raw vegetables, and cabbage. Because *Listeria* can grow in a wide pH range and in cold temperatures, foods with small numbers of organisms can become grossly contaminated during prolonged refrigeration. Disease can occur if the food is uncooked or inadequately cooked (e.g., microwaved beef and turkey franks) before consumption. The mortality rate of symptomatic listeria infections (20% to 30%) is higher than that of almost all other foodborne diseases.

Clinical Diseases (Box 25-3)

Neonatal Disease

Two forms of neonatal disease have been described: (1) **early-onset disease**, acquired transplacentally in utero, and (2) **late-onset disease**, acquired at or soon after birth. Early-onset disease can result in abortion, stillbirth, or premature birth. **Granulomatosis infantiseptica** is a severe form of listeriosis characterized by the formation of disseminated abscesses and granulomas in multiple organs and a high mortality rate unless treated promptly.

Late-onset disease occurs 2 to 3 weeks after birth, in the form of meningitis or meningoencephalitis with septicemia. The clinical signs and symptoms are not unique; thus other causes of neonatal central nervous system disease, such as group B streptococcal disease, must be excluded.

Disease in Healthy Adults

Most listeria infections in healthy adults are asymptomatic or occur in the form of a mild influenza-like illness. Gastrointestinal symptoms develop in some patients. In contrast, illness in elderly patients and those with compromised cellular immunity is more severe.

Meningitis in Adults (Clinical Case 25-1)

Meningitis is the most common form of listeria infection in adults. Although the clinical signs and symptoms of meningitis caused by this organism are not specific, *Listeria* should always be suspected in patients with organ transplants or cancer and in pregnant women in whom meningitis develops. Disease is associated with high mortality (20% to 50%) and significant neurologic sequelae among the survivors.

Primary Bacteremia

Patients with bacteremia may have an unremarkable history of chills and fever (commonly observed in pregnant women) or a more acute presentation with high-grade fever and hypotension. Only severely immunocompromised patients and the infants of pregnant women with sepsis appear to be at risk of death.

Laboratory Diagnosis

Microscopy

Gram-stain preparations of cerebrospinal fluid (CSF) typically show no organisms, because the bacteria are generally present in concentrations below the limit of detection (e.g., 10^4 bacteria per mL CSF or less). This is

---

Box 25—3. *Listeria* and *Erysipelothrix*: Clinical Summaries

Listeria monocytogenes

Neonatal disease

Early-onset disease ("granulomatosis infantiseptica"): acquired transplacentally in utero and is characterized by disseminated abscesses and granulomas in multiple organs
Late-onset disease: acquired at or shortly after birth and presents as meningitis or meningoencephalitis with septicemia
Disease in healthy adults: typically an influenza-like illness with or without gastroenteritis
Disease in pregnant women or patients with cell-mediated immune defects: can present as a primary bacteremia or as disseminated disease with hypotension and meningitis

Erysipelothrix rhusiopathiae

Erysipeloid: a painful, pruritic inflammatory skin lesion with a raised violaceous edge and central clearing; a diffuse cutaneous infection can develop rarely with systemic manifestations
Septicemic disease: recovery of the bacteria in blood is typically associated with endocarditis (either the acute or the more commonly chronic form); rarely, abscess formation, meningitis, or osteomyelitis may develop

---

Clinical Case 25-1. *Listeria* meningitis in Immunocompromised Man

The following patient, described by Bowie, et al. (Ann Pharmacother 38:58-61, 2004), illustrates the clinical presentation of *Listeria* meningitis. A 73-year-old man with refractory rheumatoid arthritis was brought by his family to the local hospital because he had a decreased level of consciousness and a 3-day history of headache, nausea, and vomiting. His current medications were infliximab, methotrexate, and prednisone for his rheumatoid arthritis. On physical examination, the patient had a stiff neck, was febrile, had a pulse of 92 beat/min, and blood pressure of 179/72 mm Hg. Because meningitis was suspected, blood and cerebrospinal fluid were collected for culture. The Gram stain of the CSF was negative, but *Listeria* grew from both blood and CSF. The patient was treated with vancomycin, the infliximab was discontinued, and he made an uneventful recovery. Infliximab has been associated with a dose-dependent monocytopenia. Because monocytes are key effectors for clearance of *Listeria*, this immunocompromised patient was specifically at risk for infection with this organism. Failure to detect *Listeria* in CSF by Gram stain is typical of this disease.

in contrast with most other bacterial pathogens of the central nervous system, which are present in concentrations of 100-fold to 1000-fold higher. If the Gram stain shows organisms, they are intracellular and extracellular gram-positive coccobacilli. Care must be used to distinguish them from other bacteria such as *S. pneumoniae*, *Enterococcus*, and *Corynebacterium*.

Culture

Listeria grows on most conventional laboratory media, with small, round colonies observed on agar media after incubation for 1 to 2 days. It may be necessary to use selective media and **cold enrichment** (storage of the specimen in the refrigerator for a prolonged period) to detect listeriae in specimens contaminated with rapidly growing bacteria. Beta hemolysis on sheep blood agar media can serve to distinguish *Listeria* from morphologically similar bacteria; however, hemolysis is generally weak and may not be observed initially. Hemolysis is enhanced when the organisms are grown next to β-hemolytic *Staphylococcus aureus*. This enhanced hemolysis is referred to as a positive CAMP [Christie, Atkins, Munch-Petersen] test. The characteristic motility of the organism in a liquid medium or semisolid agar is also helpful for the preliminary identification of listeriae. All gram-positive rods isolated from blood and CSF should be identified to distinguish between *Corynebacterium* (presumably a contaminant) and *Listeria*.

Identification

Selected biochemical and serologic tests are used to identify the pathogen definitively. A total of 13 serotypes have been described, with 1/2a, 1/2b, and 4b responsible for most infections in neonates and adults. Serotyping is generally not useful in epidemiologic investigations because relatively few serotypes are isolated from humans with disease. Pulsed-field gel electrophoresis [PFGE] is used most commonly for epidemiologic investigations of suspected outbreaks. Strains of serotype. 1/2a are highly heterogeneous and can be easily subtyped; in contrast, serotype 4b is homogeneous and multiple typing methods are needed for optimal differentiation.

Treatment, Prevention, and Control

Because most antibiotics are only bacteriostatic with *L. monocytogenes*, the combination of **gentamicin with either penicillin or ampicillin** is the treatment of choice for serious infections. Listeriae are naturally resistant to cephalosporins and resistance to macrolides and tetracyclines has been observed, which can limit the utility of these drugs. Trimethoprim-sulfamethoxazole is bactericidal to *L. monocytogenes* and has been used successfully. Newer antibiotics such as linezolid, daptomycin, and tigecycline have good in vitro activity but have not been used to treat patients.

Because listeriae are ubiquitous and most infections are sporadic, prevention and control are difficult. People at high risk of infection should avoid eating raw or partially cooked foods of animal origin, soft cheeses, and unwashed raw vegetables. A vaccine is not available, and prophylactic antibiotic therapy for high-risk patients has not been evaluated.

Erysipelothrix rhusiopathiae (Box 25-4)

Physiology and Structure

The genus *Erysipelothrix* contains three species, of which *E. rhusiopathiae* is responsible for human disease. *E. rhusiopathiae* is a gram-positive, non-spore-forming rod that is distributed worldwide in wild and domestic animals. The rods are slender (0.2 to 0.5 × 0.8 to 2.5 μm) and sometimes pleomorphic, with a tendency to form filaments as long as 60 μm ("hairlike"). They decolorize readily and may appear gram-negative (Figure 25-2). The organisms are microaerophilic, preferring a reduced oxygen atmosphere and supplemented carbon dioxide (5% to 10%). Small, grayish, α-hemolytic colonies are observed after 2 to 3 days of incubation.

Box 25—4. Summary: *Erysipelothrix*

Biology, Virulence, and Disease

Slender, pleomorphic, gram-positive rods that form long (i.e., 60 μm) filaments
Production of neuraminidase is believed to be important for attachment and penetration into epithelial cells, and a polysaccharide-like capsule protects the bacteria from phagocytosis.
Disease in humans is most commonly a localized cutaneous infection or septicemia associated with endocarditis.

Epidemiology

Colonizes a variety of organisms, particularly swine and turkey
Found in soil rich in organic matter or groundwater contaminated with wastes from colonized animals
Uncommon pathogen in the United States
Occupational disease of butchers, meat processors, farmers, poultry workers, fish handlers, and veterinarians

Diagnosis

Long, filamentous, gram-positive rods seen on Gram stain of a biopsy collected at the advancing edge of the lesion
Grows well on blood and chocolate agars incubated in 5% to 10% CO_2

Treatment, Prevention, and Control

Penicillin is drug of choice; organism is susceptible to cephalosporins, fluoroquinolones, erythromycin, and clindamycin; variable susceptibility to aminoglycosides and sulfonamides; resistant to vancomycin
Workers should cover exposed skin when handling animals and animal products.
Swineherds should be vaccinated.

Figure 25–2. Gram stain of *Erysipelothrix rhusiopathiae* in culture. Note the variable lengths of the rods and the "gram-negative" appearance.

Clinical Case 25-2. *Erysipelothrix* Endocarditis

Endocarditis caused by *E. rhusiopathiae* is an uncommon but well recognized disease. The following case history reported by Artz, et al. (Eur J Clin Microbiol Infect Dis 20:587-588, 2001) is typical of this disease. A 46-year-old man who worked as a butcher and had a history of alcoholism was admitted to the hospital with an erythematous rash over his upper body and a complaint of arthralgias of both shoulders. Medical history revealed a 4-week history of night sweats and daily recurring chills, which the patient attributed to his drinking. Physical exam revealed hepatosplenomegaly, a systolic murmur detected on auscultation, and a calcified aortic valve with mild regurgitation but no vegetations on echocardiography. Five blood cultures were collected, and all were positive with *E. rhusiopathiae* after 2 days. The patient was transferred to surgery for valve replacement, and paravalvular abscesses were detected intraoperatively. After surgical repair, the patient was treated with clindamycin and penicillin and made a complete recovery. This case illustrates risk factors (i.e., butcher, alcoholism), a chronic course, and the value of surgery combined with treatment with effective antibiotics (i.e., penicillin, clindamycin).

Pathogenesis

Little is known about specific virulence factors in *Erysipelothrix*. Production of neuraminidase is believed to be important for attachment and penetration into epithelial cells, and a polysaccharide-like capsule protects the bacteria from phagocytosis.

Epidemiology

Erysipelothrix is a ubiquitous organism that is distributed worldwide. It can be recovered on the tonsils or in the digestive tracts of many wild and domestic animals, including mammals, birds, and fish. Colonization is particularly high in **swine** and **turkeys**. Soil rich in organic matter or groundwater contaminated with animal wastes can facilitate animal-to-animal spread. The bacteria are resistant to drying and can survive in soil for months to years. Additionally, *E. rhusiopathiae* is resistant to high concentrations of salt, pickling, and smoking. *Erysipelothrix* disease in humans is **zoonotic** (spread from animals to humans) and primarily occupational. Butchers, meat processors, farmers, poultry workers, fish handlers, and veterinarians are at greatest risk. Cutaneous infections typically develop after the organism is inoculated subcutaneously through an abrasion or puncture wound during the handling of contaminated animal products or soil. The incidence of human disease is unknown, because *Erysipelothrix* infection is not a reportable disease.

Clinical Diseases (see Box 25-3; Clinical Case 25-2)

Animal disease—particularly in swine—is widely recognized, but human disease is less common. Two primary forms of human infection with *E. rhusiopathiae* have been described: (1) a localized skin infection (**erysipeloid**) and (2) a **septicemic** form. Erysipeloid is an inflammatory skin lesion that develops at the site of trauma after 2 to 7 days of incubation. The lesion most commonly presents on the fingers or hands and appears violaceous with a raised edge. It slowly spreads peripherally as the discoloration in the central area fades. The painful lesion is pruritic, and the patient experiences a burning or throbbing sensation. Suppuration is uncommon, a feature distinguishing erysipeloid from streptococcal erysipelas. The resolution can be spontaneous but can be hastened with appropriate antibiotic therapy. A diffuse cutaneous infection can also develop. It is often associated with systemic manifestations, but blood culture results are typically negative for the organism.

The septicemic form of *Erysipelothrix* infections is uncommon, but when present it is frequently associated with endocarditis. *Erysipelothrix* endocarditis may have an acute onset but is usually subacute. Involvement of previously undamaged heart valves (particularly the aortic valve) is common. Other systemic complications (e.g., abscess formation, meningitis, osteomyelitis) are relatively uncommon.

Laboratory Diagnosis

The rods are located only in the deep tissue of the lesion. Thus full-thickness biopsy specimens or deep aspirates must be collected from the margin of the lesion. A Gram stain of the specimen is typically negative, although the presence of **thin, gram-positive rods** is useful. *E. rhusiopathiae* is not fastidious and grows on most conventional laboratory media incubated in the presence of 5% to 10% CO_2; however, growth is slow, and cultures must be incubated for 3 days or longer before considered negative. The absence of both motility and catalase production distinguishes this organism from *Listeria*. The organism is weakly fermentative and produces hydrogen sulfide on triple sugar iron agar.

Serology is not useful for diagnosis, because an antibody response is weak in human infections.

Treatment, Prevention, and Control

Erysipelothrix is susceptible to **penicillin**, which is the antibiotic of choice for both localized and systemic diseases. Cephalosporins, carbapenems, macrolides, fluoroquinolones, and clindamycin are also active in vitro, but the organism has variable susceptibility to sulfonamides and aminoglycosides and is resistant to vancomycin. Infections in people at a higher occupational risk are prevented by the use of gloves and other appropriate coverings on exposed skin. Vaccination is used to control disease in swine.

Case Study and Questions

A 35-year-old man was hospitalized because of headache, fever, and confusion. He had received a kidney transplant 7 months before, after which he had been given immunosuppressive drugs to prevent organ rejection. CSF was collected, which revealed a white blood cell count of 36 cells/mm^3 with 96% polymorphonuclear leukocytes, a glucose concentration of 40 mg/dL, and a protein concentration of 172 mg/dL. A Gram stain preparation of CSF was negative for organisms, but gram-positive coccobacilli grew in cultures of the blood and CSF.

1. What is the most likely cause of this patient's meningitis?

2. What are the potential sources of this organism?

3. What virulence factors are associated with this organism?

4. How would this disease be treated? Which antibiotics are effective in vitro? Which antibiotics are ineffective?

Bibliography

Gorby GL, Peacock JE Jr: *Erysipelothrix rhusiopathiae* endocarditis: Microbiologic, epidemiologic, and clinical features of an occupational disease. Rev Infect Dis 10:317-325, 1988.

Gray MJ, Freitag NE, Boor KJ: How the bacterial pathogen *Listeria monocytogenes* mediates the switch from environmental Dr. Jekyll to pathogenic Mr. Hyde. Infect Immun 74:2505-2512, 2006.

Hof H, Nichterlein T, Kretschmar M: Management of listeriosis. Clin Microbiol Rev 10:345-357, 1997.

Ireton K, Cossart P: Host-pathogen interactions during entry and actin-based movement of *Listeria monocytogenes*. Annu Rev Genet 31:113-138, 1997.

Liu D. Identification, subtyping and virulence determination of *Listeria monocytogenes*, an important foodborne pathogen. J Med Microbiol 55:645-659, 2006.

Lorber B: Listeriosis. Clin Infect Dis 24:1-11, 1997.

Olsen SJ, et al: Multistate outbreak of *Listeria monocytogenes* infection linked to delicatessen turkey meat. Clin Infect Dis 40:962-967, 2005.

Pamer EG: Immune responses to *Listeria monocytogenes*. Nature Rev Immunol 4:812-823, 2004.

Safdar A, Armstrong D: Listeriosis in patients at a comprehensive cancer center, 1955-1997. Clin Infect Dis 37:359-364, 2003.

Schlech W: Foodborne listeriosis. Clin Infect Dis 31:770-775, 2000.

Verbarg S, et al: *Erysipelothrix inopinata* sp. nov., isolated in the course of sterile filtration of vegetable peptone broth, and description of *Erysipelotrichaceae* fam. nov. Int J Syst Evol Microbiol 54:221-225, 2004.

Wing E, Gregory S: *Listeria monocytogenes*: Clinical and experimental update. J Infect Dis 185(Suppl 1):S18-S24, 2002.

Corynebacterium and Other Gram-Positive Rods

The aerobic gram-positive rods are a heterogeneous group of bacteria that have been loosely grouped on the basis of their cell morphology, staining properties, and guanine plus cytosine (G+C) content. The bacteria discussed in this chapter are broadly linked by their Gram stain morphology—they have an **irregular shape**. This group is commonly referred to as **coryneform** ("club-shaped") bacteria and includes *Corynebacterium* and related genera (Box 26-1).

The genus *Corynebacterium* is a large, heterogeneous collection of more than 100 species and subspecies that have a cell wall with arabinose, galactose, *meso*-diaminopimelic acid (*meso*-DAP), and (in most species) **short-chain mycolic acids** (22 to 36 carbon atoms). Although organisms with medium- and long-chain mycolic acids stain with acid-fast stains (refer to chapters 27 and 28), *Corynebacterium* organisms are not acid-fast. Gram stains of these bacteria reveal clumps and short chains of irregularly shaped (club-shaped) rods (Figure 26-1). **Metachromatic granules** (i.e., granules that stain a color different from the primary dye color) within the cells may be seen with special stains. Corynebacteria are aerobic or facultatively anaerobic, nonmotile, and catalase positive. Most (but not all) species ferment carbohydrates, producing lactic acid as a byproduct. Many species grow well on common laboratory media; however, some species require supplementation of media with lipids for good growth (**lipophilic** strains).

Corynebacteria are ubiquitous in plants and animals, and they normally colonize the skin, upper respiratory tract, gastrointestinal tract, and urogenital tract in humans. Although all species of corynebacteria can function as opportunistic pathogens, relatively few are associated with human disease (Table 26-1). The most famous of these is *Corynebacterium diphtheriae*, the etiologic agent of **diphtheria**.

A number of other genera of coryneform bacteria have been characterized. Four genera associated with human disease (*Arcanobacterium*, *Brevibacterium*, *Rothia*, *Tropheryma*) are discussed briefly at the end of this chapter.

Corynebacterium diphtheriae (Box 26-2)

Physiology and Structure

C. diphtheriae is an irregularly staining, pleomorphic rod (0.3 to 0.8 × 1.0 to 8.0 μm). Metachromatic granules have been observed in rods stained with methylene blue. After overnight incubation, large 1- to 3-mm colonies are observed on blood agar medium. More selective differential media can be used to recover this pathogen from specimens with other organisms present, such as pharyngeal specimens. This species is subdivided into four biotypes based on their colonial morphology and biochemical properties: *belfanti*, *gravis*, *intermedius*, and *mitis*. Most disease is caused by biotypes **gravis** and **mitis**, with biotypes *intermedius* and *belfanti* rarely associated with diphtheria.

Pathogenesis and Immunity

Diphtheria toxin is the major virulence factor of *C. diphtheriae*. This exotoxin is produced at the site of the infection and then disseminates through the blood to produce the systemic signs of diphtheria. The organism does not need to enter the blood to produce disease.

The *tox* gene that codes for the exotoxin is introduced into strains of *C. diphtheriae* by a lysogenic bacteriophage (**β-phage**). Two processing steps are necessary for the active gene product to be secreted: (1) proteolytic cleavage of the leader sequence from the toxin protein during secretion from the bacterial cell; and (2) cleavage of the toxin molecule into two polypeptides (A and B) that remain attached by a disulfide bond. This 58,300-Da protein is an example of the classic **A-B exotoxin**.

Box 26–1. Important Coryneform Bacteria

Organism	Historical Derivation
Corynebacterium	coryne, a "club"; Greek bakterion, a "small rod" (a small, club-shaped rod)
C. diphtheriae	diphthera, "leather" or "skin" (reference to the leathery membrane that forms initially on the pharynx)
C. jeikeium	jeikeium (species originally classified as group JK)
C. urealyticum	urea, urea; lyticum, lyse (capable of lysing urea; species rapidly hydrolyzes urea)
C. amycolatum	a, "without"; mycolatum, pertaining to mycolic acids (species does not have mycolic acids in the cell wall)
C. pseudotuberculosis	pseudo, "like"; tuberculosis (produces chronic, purulent infections [e.g., tuberculosis] in sheep and other warm-blooded animals)
C. ulcerans	ulcerans (can produce pharyngeal ulcers like C. diphtheriae)
Arcanobacterium	arcanus, "secretive"; Latin bacterium, "rod" (secretive bacterium; a slow-growing organism that can prove difficult to isolate)
Brevibacterium	brevis, "short"; Latin bacterium, "rod" (a short rod; this species appears as very small coccobacilli)
Rothia mucilaginosa	Named after Roth, the bacteriologist who originally studied this group of organisms; mucilaginosa, "slimy" (slimy or mucoid organisms)

Figure 26–1. Gram stain of *Corynebacterium* species in blood culture.

Table 26–1. *Corynebacterium* Species Associated with Human Disease

Organism	Diseases
C. diphtheriae	Diphtheria (respiratory, cutaneous); pharyngitis and endocarditis (nontoxigenic strains)
C. jeikeium (group JK)	Septicemia, endocarditis, wound infections, foreign body (catheter, shunt, prosthesis) infections
C. urealyticum	Urinary tract infections (including pyelonephritis and alkaline-encrusted cystitis), septicemia, endocarditis, wound infections
C. amycolatum	Wound infections, foreign body infections, septicemia, urinary tract infections, respiratory tract infections
C. pseudotuberculosis	Lymphadenitis, ulcerative lymphangitis, abscess formation
C. ulcerans	Respiratory diphtheria

Three functional regions exist on the toxin molecule, a **receptor-binding region** and a **translocation region** on the B subunit and a **catalytic region** on the A subunit. The receptor for the toxin is **heparin-binding epidermal growth factor**, which is present on the surface of many eukaryotic cells, particularly heart and nerve cells; its presence explains the cardiac and neurologic symptoms observed in patients with severe diphtheria. After the toxin becomes attached to the host cell, the translocation region is inserted into the endosomal membrane, facilitating the movement of the catalytic region into the cell cytosol. The A subunit then terminates host cell protein synthesis by inactivating **elongation factor 2 (EF-2)**, a factor required for the movement of nascent peptide chains on ribosomes. Because the turnover of EF-2 is very slow, and approximately only one molecule per ribosome is present in a cell, it has been estimated that one exotoxin molecule can inactivate the entire EF-2 content in a cell, completely terminating host cell protein synthesis. Toxin synthesis is regulated by a chromosomally encoded element, **diphtheria toxin repressor (DTxR)**. This protein, activated in the presence of high iron concentrations, can bind to the toxin gene operator and prevent toxin production.

Epidemiology

Diphtheria is a disease found worldwide, particularly in poor urban areas where there is crowding, and the protective level of vaccine-induced immunity is low. The largest outbreak in the latter part of the 20th century occurred in the former Soviet Union, where in 1994 almost 48,000 cases were documented, with 1746 deaths. *C. diphtheriae*

Box 26—2. Summary: *Corynebacterium diphtheriae*

Biology, Virulence, and Disease

Gram-positive pleomorphic rods
The major virulence factor is the diphtheria toxin,
    an A-B exotoxin; inhibits protein synthesis
Etiologic agent of diphtheria: respiratory and cutaneous forms

Epidemiology

Worldwide distribution maintained in asymptomatic carriers
    and infected patients
Humans are the only known reservoir, with carriage
    in oropharynx or on skin surface
Spread person to person by exposure to respiratory droplets or
    skin contact
Disease observed in unvaccinated people living in crowded urban
    areas and in children or adults with waning immunity
Diphtheria is very uncommon in the United States

Diagnosis

Microscopy is nonspecific; metachromatic granules observed
    in *C. diphtheriae* and other corynebacteria
Culture should be performed on nonselective (blood agar) and
    selective (cysteine-tellurite agar, Tinsdale medium,
    colistin-nalidixic agar) media
Presumptive identification of *C. diphtheriae* can be based on the
    presence of cysteinase and absence of pyrazinamidase;
    definitive identification by biochemical tests or species-specific
    gene sequencing
Demonstration of exotoxin is performed by polymerase chain
    reaction assay or Elek test

Treatment, Prevention, and Control

Infections treated with diphtheria antitoxin to neutralize
    exotoxin; penicillin or erythromycin to eliminate *C. diphtheriae*
    and terminate toxin production; and diphtheria toxoid
    immunization of convalescing patients to stimulate protective
    antibodies
Administration of diphtheria vaccine and booster shots
    to susceptible population

Box 26—3. *Corynebacterium diphtheriae*: Clinical Summaries

Respiratory diphtheria: sudden onset with exudative pharyngitis,
    sore throat, low-grade fever, and malaise; a thick
    pseudomembrane develops over the pharynx; in critically ill
    patients, cardiac and neurologic complications most significant
Cutaneous diphtheria: a papule can develop on the skin that
    progresses to a nonhealing ulcer; systemic signs can develop

Clinical Diseases

The clinical presentation of diphtheria is determined by (1) the site of infection, (2) the immune status of the patient, and (3) the virulence of the organism. Exposure to *C. diphtheriae* may result in asymptomatic colonization in fully immune people, mild respiratory disease in partially immune patients, or a fulminant, sometimes fatal disease in nonimmune patients (Box 26-3).

Respiratory Diphtheria (Clinical Case 26-1)

The symptoms of diphtheria involving the respiratory tract develop after a 2- to 4-day incubation period. Organisms multiply locally on epithelial cells in the pharynx or adjacent surfaces and initially cause localized damage as a result of exotoxin activity. The onset is sudden, with malaise, sore throat, **exudative pharyngitis**, and a low-grade fever. The exudate evolves into a thick **pseudomembrane** composed of bacteria, lymphocytes, plasma cells, fibrin, and dead cells that can cover the

---

Clinical Case 26-1. Respiratory Diphtheria

Lurie, et al. (J Am Med Assoc 291:937-938, 2004) reported the last patient with respiratory diphtheria seen in the United States. An unvaccinated 63-year-old man developed a sore throat while on a week-long trip in rural Haiti. Two days after he returned home to Pennsylvania, he visited a local hospital with complaints of a sore throat and difficulties in swallowing. He was treated with oral antibiotics but returned two days later with chills, sweating, difficulty swallowing and breathing, nausea, and vomiting. He had diminished breath sounds in the left lung, and radiographs confirmed pulmonary infiltrates, as well as enlargement of the epiglottis. Laryngoscopy revealed yellow exudates on the tonsils, posterior pharynx, and soft palate. He was admitted to the intensive care unit and treated with azithromycin, ceftriaxone, nafcillin, and steroids but over the next 4 days became hypotensive with a low-grade fever. Cultures were negative for *Corynebacterium diphtheriae*. By the eighth day of illness, a chest radiograph showed infiltrates in the right and left lung bases, and a white exudate consistent with *C. diphtheriae* pseudomembrane was observed over the supraglottic structures. Cultures at this time remained negative for *C. diphtheriae*, but PCR testing for the exotoxin gene was positive. Despite aggressive therapy, the patient continued to deteriorate, and on the 17th day of hospitalization developed cardiac complications and died. This patient illustrates the classic presentation of severe respiratory diphtheria in an unimmunized patient, as well as the difficulties that most labs would now have isolating the organism in culture.

---

is maintained in the population by **asymptomatic carriage** in the oropharynx or on the skin of immune people (after either exposure to *C. diphtheriae* or immunization). Respiratory droplets or skin contact transmit it from person to person. **Humans** are the **only known reservoir** for this organism.

Diphtheria has become uncommon in the United States as the result of an active immunization program, as shown by the fact that more than 200,000 cases were reported in 1921, but no cases have been reported since 2003. Diphtheria is primarily a pediatric disease, but the highest incidence has shifted toward older age groups in areas where there are active immunization programs for children. Skin infection with toxigenic *C. diphtheriae* (cutaneous diphtheria) also occurs, but it is not a reportable disease in the United States, so its incidence is unknown.

Figure 26—2. Pharynx of a 39-year-old woman with bacteriologically confirmed diphtheria. The photograph was taken 4 days after the onset of fever, malaise, and sore throat. Hemorrhage caused by removal of the membrane by swabbing appears as a dark area on the left. *(From Mandell G, Bennett J, Dolin R: Principles and Practice of Infectious Diseases, 6th ed. Churchill Livingstone, 2005.)*

tonsils, uvula, and palate and can extend up into the nasopharynx or down into the larynx (Figure 26-2). The pseudomembrane firmly adheres to the underlying tissue and is difficult to dislodge without making the tissue bleed (unique to diphtheria). As the patient recovers after the approximately 1-week course of the disease, the membrane dislodges and is expectorated. Systemic complications in patients with severe disease primarily involve the heart and nervous system. Evidence of **myocarditis** can be detected in the majority of patients with diphtheria, typically developing 1 to 2 weeks into the illness and at a time when the pharyngeal symptoms are improving. Symptoms can present acutely or gradually, progressing in severe disease to congestive heart failure, cardiac arrhythmias, and death. **Neurotoxicity** is proportional to the severity of the primary disease, which is influenced by the patient's immunity. The majority of patients with severe primary disease develop neuropathy, initially localized to the soft palate and pharynx, later involving oculomotor and ciliary paralysis, with progression to peripheral neuritis.

Cutaneous Diphtheria

Cutaneous diphtheria is acquired through skin contact with other infected persons. The organism colonizes the skin and gains entry into the subcutaneous tissue through breaks in the skin. A papule develops first and then evolves into a **chronic, nonhealing ulcer**, sometimes covered with a grayish membrane. *Staphylococcus aureus* or *Streptococcus pyogenes* is also frequently present in the wound.

Laboratory Diagnosis

The initial treatment of a patient with diphtheria is instituted on the basis of the clinical diagnosis, not laboratory

results, because definitive results are not available for at least a week.

Microscopy

The results of microscopic examination of clinical material are unreliable. Metachromatic granules in bacteria stained with methylene blue have been described, but this appearance is not specific to *C. diphtheriae*, and interpretation of the smear requires technical expertise.

Culture

Specimens for the recovery of *C. diphtheriae* should be collected from both the nasopharynx and the throat and should be inoculated onto a nonselective, enriched blood agar plate and a selective medium (e.g., cysteine-tellurite blood agar [CTBA], Tinsdale medium, colistin-nalidixic agar [CNA]). Tellurite inhibits the growth of most upper respiratory tract bacteria and gram-negative rods and is reduced by *C. diphtheriae*, producing characteristic gray to black color on agar containing tellurite. Degradation of cysteine by *C. diphtheriae* cysteinase activity produces a brown halo around the colonies. CTBA has a long shelf life (practical for cultures that are infrequently performed) but inhibits some strains of *C. diphtheriae*. Tinsdale medium is the best medium for recovering *C. diphtheriae* in clinical specimens, but it has a short shelf life and requires addition of horse serum (thus most labs do not use this medium). CNA is commonly used in the clinical lab, so this is a practical alternative medium. Regardless of the media that are used, all isolates resembling *C. diphtheriae* must be identified by biochemical testing and the presence of the diphtheria exotoxin confirmed.

Identification

The presumptive identification of *C. diphtheriae* can be based on the presence of cysteinase and absence of pyrazinamidase (two enzyme reactions that can be rapidly determined). More extensive biochemical tests or nucleic acid sequencing of species-specific genes is required for identification at the species level.

Toxigenicity Testing

All isolates of *C. diphtheriae* should be tested for the production of exotoxin. This has been done historically by an in vitro immunodiffusion assay (**Elek test**), a tissue culture neutralization assay using specific antitoxin. Currently a modification of the Elek test is what is done in most laboratories. An alternative method for detecting the exotoxin gene is a **PCR-based nucleic acid amplification method** developed by the Centers for Disease Control and Prevention (CDC). This test can detect the *tox* gene in clinical isolates and directly in clinical specimens (e.g., swabs from the diphtheritic membrane or biopsy material). Although this test is rapid and specific, strains with the *tox* gene not expressed (presumably because the **diphtheria toxin repressor** is expressed) can give a positive signal.

Nontoxigenic strains of *C. diphtheriae* should not be ignored, because these strains have been associated with significant disease, including septicemia, endocarditis, and septic arthritis, osteomyelitis, and abscess formation.

Treatment, Prevention, and Control

The most important aspect of the treatment for diphtheria is the early administration of **diphtheria antitoxin** to specifically neutralize the exotoxin before it is bound by the host cell. Once the cell internalizes the toxin, cell death is inevitable. Antibiotic therapy with **penicillin or erythromycin** is also used to eliminate *C. diphtheriae* and terminate toxin production. Bed rest, isolation to prevent secondary spread, and maintenance of an open airway in patients with respiratory diphtheria are all important. After the patient has recovered, **immunization** with toxoid is required because most patients fail to develop protective antibodies after a natural infection.

Symptomatic diphtheria can be prevented by actively immunizing people with diphtheria toxoid. The nontoxic immunogenic toxoid is prepared by formalin treatment of the toxin. Initially, children are given five injections of this preparation with pertussis and tetanus antigens (**DPT vaccine**) at ages 2 months, 4 months, 6 months, 15 to 18 months, and at 4 to 6 years. After that time, it is recommended that booster vaccinations with diphtheria toxoid combined with tetanus toxoid be given every 10 years. Serum antitoxin antibodies can be measured by a rabbit skin or Vero cell neutralization test.

People coming in close contact with patients who have documented diphtheria are at risk for acquiring the disease. Nasopharyngeal specimens for culture should be collected from all close contacts, and antimicrobial prophylaxis with penicillin or erythromycin started immediately. Any contact who has not completed the series of diphtheria immunizations or who has not received a booster dose within the previous 5 years should receive a booster dose of toxoid. People exposed to cutaneous diphtheria should be managed in the same manner as those exposed to respiratory diphtheria. If the respiratory or cutaneous infection is caused by a nontoxigenic strain, it is unnecessary to institute prophylaxis in contacts.

Other *Corynebacterium* Species

A large number of other *Corynebacterium* species have been found as part of the indigenous human flora and are capable of causing disease. The most common species are listed in Table 26-1 and summarized in Box 26-4.

Corynebacterium jeikeium (Figure 26-3) is a well-recognized opportunistic pathogen in immunocompromised patients, particularly those with hematologic disorders or intravascular catheters. Carriage of this organism is uncommon in healthy people, but the skin of as many as

---

Box 26—4. Summary: Other *Corynebacterium* Species

Biology, Virulence, and Disease

Gram-positive pleomorphic rods
Some clinically important species require lipids such as Tween 80 for good growth (e.g., *C. jeikeium*, *C. urealyticum*).
Diphtheria A-B exotoxin may be carried by *C. ulcerans* and *C. pseudotuberculosis*.
Urinary tract pathogens produce urease (e.g., *C. urealyticum*).
Many species able to adhere to foreign bodies (e.g., catheters, shunts, prosthetic devices)
Some species resistant to most antibiotics (e.g., *C. amycolatum*, *C. jeikeium*, *C. urealyticum*)
Diseases include septicemia, endocarditis, foreign body infections, wound infections, urinary tract infections, respiratory infections, including diphtheria.

Epidemiology

Most infections are endogenous (produced by species that are part of the host's normal bacterial population on the skin surface and mucosal membranes).

Diagnosis

Culture on nonselective media is reliable, although growth may be slow, and media may require supplementation with lipids.

Treatment, Prevention, and Control

Treatment with effective antibiotics to eliminate the organism
Removal of foreign body

40% of hospitalized patients can be colonized, regardless of their immune status. Predisposing conditions for disease include prolonged hospitalization, granulocytopenia, previous or concurrent antimicrobial therapy or chemotherapy, and the presence of an intravenous catheter. Most members of this species are very resistant to antibiotics,

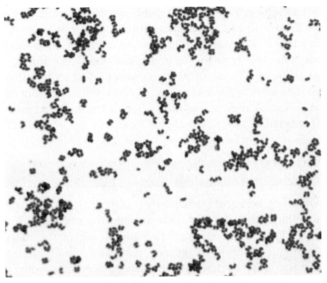

Figure 26—3. Gram stain of *Corynebacterium jeikeium* from a culture. Note the small, coccobacillary shape.

so antibiotic therapy during hospitalization may foster colonization of the skin. The organism then gains access through an intravenous catheter and establishes disease in the immunologically compromised patient.

Corynebacterium urealyticum is not a common isolate in healthy people; however, the species is an important pathogen of the urinary tract. As the name implies, *C. urealyticum*, which is a strong urease producer, can produce enough urease to make the urine alkaline, leading to the formation of **struvite calculi** or **renal stones**. Risk factors associated with *C. urealyticum* infections include immunosuppression, underlying genitourinary disorders, an antecedent urologic procedure, and previous antibiotic therapy. There are other urease-producing corynebacteria associated with urinary tract infections, but *C. urealyticum* is the most common.

C. amycolatum resides on the skin surface but not in the oropharynx. This species is the most commonly isolated species in clinical specimens, although its importance has been underappreciated because it is frequently misidentified as other corynebacteria species. This species, like *C. jeikeium* and *C. urealyticum*, is resistant to many antibiotics and is an important opportunistic pathogen, causing foreign-body infections, wound infections, and infections of the urinary tract and lower airways.

Corynebacterium pseudotuberculosis and *Corynebacterium ulcerans* are closely related to *C. diphtheriae* and can carry the diphtheria gene. Although *C. ulcerans* can cause a disease indistinguishable from diphtheria, human infections caused by *C. pseudotuberculosis* are rarely observed.

Numerous other *Corynebacterium* species have been associated with opportunistic infections. These bacteria are commonly present on the skin and mucosal surfaces, so their isolation in a clinical specimen may represent an important finding or may simply represent contamination of the specimen. Specific identification of these organisms beyond the genus level is probably not important.

Treatment of *Corynebacterium* infections can be problematic. *C. jeikeium*, *C. urealyticum*, and *C. amycolatum* are typically resistant to most antibiotics, so infected patients usually must be given vancomycin. The other species tend to be more susceptible to antibiotics, but in vitro testing may be required before a treatment regimen is selected.

Other Coryneform Genera

Other genera of irregularly shaped, gram-positive rods have been found to colonize humans and cause disease (Table 26-2). **Arcanobacterium** is one of the more common coryneform genera associated with human disease. This bacterium can cause pharyngitis with a "scarlet fever-like" rash that resembles streptococcal disease, as well as polymicrobic wound infections and

Table 26–2. Less Common Coryneform Gram-Positive Rods Associated with Human Disease

Organism	Diseases
Arcanobacterium	Pharyngitis, cellulitis, wound infections, abscess formation, septicemia, endocarditis
Brevibacterium	Septicemia, osteomyelitis, foreign body (catheter, shunt, prosthesis) infections
Rothia	Endocarditis, foreign body infections
Tropheryma	Whipple disease

(less commonly) systemic infections such as septicemia and endocarditis. Infections can be treated with penicillin or erythromycin.

Brevibacterium colonize the skin surface and, when grown in culture, produce a cheeselike odor. These bacteria have been blamed for malodorous feet in some colonized people. More important diseases attributed to *Brevibacterium* are septicemia, osteomyelitis, and foreign-body infections. The organisms grow readily in culture, appearing initially as small rods and developing coccoid forms in older cultures (which can complicate attempts to identify the organism). Treatment is complicated because many strains are resistant to β-lactam antibiotics, erythromycin, clindamycin, and ciprofloxacin. Use of vancomycin, tetracyclines, or gentamicin has proved effective.

Rothia mucilaginosa, the most important member of the genus, colonizes the oropharynx. Two properties are important: this species appears coccoid rather than rod-shaped, and the colonies are mucoid and sticky. This adherence property is expressed in vivo because the organisms can adhere to damaged heart valves and cause endocarditis. The activity of antibiotics against *R. mucilaginosa* is unpredictable, so in vitro susceptibility tests must be performed.

Tropheryma whippelii is the bacterium responsible for **Whipple disease**—a disorder characterized by arthralgia, diarrhea, abdominal pain, weight loss, lymphadenopathy, fever, and increased skin pigmentation. Historically the disease was diagnosed on the basis of the clinical presentation and the finding of periodic acid–Schiff positive inclusions in foamy macrophages that infiltrated the lamina propria of the small intestine. Although in vitro cultures of these specimens were uniformly negative, the bacterial etiology of this infection was confirmed through the use of molecular diagnostic techniques. The organism can grow slowly in tissue culture cells, but cell-free cultures have not been established. Laboratory confirmation of clinical disease is currently made using polymerase chain reaction (PCR) amplification of a species-specific sequence of bacterial DNA. Currently the recommended treatment is 2 weeks with parenteral penicillin and streptomycin, followed by oral trimethoprim-sulfamethoxazole for a year or more.

Case Study and Questions

A 78-year-old man with a history of hypertension was admitted to the hospital because of a severe headache of 4 hours' duration. Evidence of subarachnoid hemorrhage and hydrocephalus was found, and the patient required the placement of a left ventricular-atrial shunt. Fever developed 1 week after the operation. *C. jeikeium* was isolated from blood cultures and a subsequent culture of fluid collected from the shunt.

1. What risk factors are associated with infections with *C. jeikeium*?

2. What antibiotic therapy could be given for infections with this organism?

3. Name two other *Corynebacterium* species that are commonly resistant to multiple antibiotics. What diseases are associated with these organisms?

4. Explain the synthesis and mode of action of the diphtheria exotoxin.

Reference to Student Consult Animation

Please visit *www.StudentConsult.com* to view an animation demonstrating the function of diphtheria toxin.

Bibliography

Coyle MA, Lipsky BA: Coryneform bacteria in infectious diseases: Clinical and laboratory aspects. Clin Microbiol Rev 3:227-246, 1990.

Esteban J, et al: Microbiological characterization and clinical significance of *Corynebacterium amycolatum* strains. Eur J Clin Microbiol Infect Dis 18:518-521, 1999.

Fenollar F, et al: Whipple's disease. N Engl J Med 356:55-66, 2007.

Funke G, et al: Clinical microbiology of coryneform bacteria. Clin Microbiol Rev 10:125-159, 1997.

George MJ: Clinical significance and characterization of *Corynebacterium* species. Clin Microbiol Newsl 17:177-180, 1995.

Lipsky BA, et al: Infections caused by nondiphtheria corynebacteria. Rev Infect Dis 4:1220-1235, 1982.

McNeil M, Brown J: The medically important aerobic actinomycetes: Epidemiology and microbiology. Clin Microbiol Rev 7:357-417, 1994.

Pascual C, et al: Phylogenetic analysis of the genus *Corynebacterium* based on 16S rRNA gene sequences. Int J Syst Bacteriol 45:724-728, 1995.

Popovic T, et al: Molecular epidemiology of diphtheria in Russia, 1985-1994. J Infect Dis 174:1064-1072, 1996.

Soriano F, et al: Urinary tract infection caused by *Corynebacterium* group D2: Report of 82 cases and review. Rev Infect Dis 12:1019-1034, 1990.

Nocardia and Related Bacteria

The genera discussed in this chapter (Box 27-1) are aerobic gram-positive rods that stain **weakly acid-fast** (that is, resist decolorization with weak acid solutions) due to the medium-chain mycolic acids in their cell wall. Acid-fast bacteria with long-chain mycolic acids in their cell wall include the genus *Mycobacterium* and are discussed in the next chapter. The spectrum of the infections associated with the genera discussed here is extensive and includes insignificant colonization (many genera), pulmonary disease *(Nocardia, Rhodococcus)*, systemic infections *(Nocardia, Rhodococcus)*, mycetoma *(Nocardia)*, and opportunistic infections *(Nocardia, Rhodococcus, Gordonia, and Tsukamurella)* (Table 27-1).

Nocardia (Box 27-2)

Physiology and Structure

Nocardiae are strict aerobic rods that form branched filamentous form in tissues and culture. These filamentous forms resemble the hyphae formed by filamentous fungi (molds), and at one time *Nocardia* was thought to be a fungus. However, the organisms have a gram-positive cell wall and other cellular structures that are characteristic of bacteria. Most isolates stain poorly with the Gram stain and appear to be gram-negative with intracellular gram-positive beads (Figure 27-1). The reason for this staining property is that nocardiae have a cell-wall structure similar to that of mycobacteria (see Chapter 28), with 10-methyl stearic acid (**tuberculostearic acid**), *meso*-diaminopimelic acid (*meso*-DAP), arabinose, galactose, and mycolic acids present. The length of the mycolic acids in nocardiae (50 to 62 carbon atoms) is shorter than in mycobacteria (70 to 90 carbon atoms). This difference may explain why even though both genera stain acid-fast, *Nocardia* is described as "**weakly acid-fast**"; that is, a weak decolorizing solution of hydrochloric acid must be used to demonstrate the acid-fast property of nocardiae (Figure 27-2). This acid-fastness is

also a helpful characteristic for distinguishing *Nocardia* organisms from morphologically similar organisms such as *Actinomyces* (see Chapter 40). Most strains of *Nocardia* have trehalose linked to two molecules of mycolic acid (trehalose-6,6′-dimycolate; **cord factor**). Cord factor is an important virulence factor that facilitates intracellular survival (see Pathogenesis and Immunity Section).

Nocardia species are catalase-positive, use carbohydrates oxidatively, and can grow on most nonselective laboratory media used for the isolation of bacteria, mycobacteria, and fungi; however, their growth is slow, requiring 3 to 5 days of incubation before colonies may be observed on the culture plates. The appearance of colonies varies from dry to waxy and from white to orange (Figure 27-3). Aerial hyphae (hyphae that protrude upward from the surface of a colony) can be observed when the colonies are viewed with a dissecting microscope (Figure 27-4). The **presence of aerial hyphae and acid-fastness is unique** to *Nocardia* and can be used as a rapid test for the presumptive identification of the genus.

The taxonomic classification of this genus is—simply stated—a mess, with most of the organisms described in the literature now recognized as incorrectly identified. Historically, these organisms were classified by their ability to use carbohydrates and decompose a variety of substrates, as well as their antimicrobial susceptibility patterns. The true taxonomic relationships among the members of the genus were appreciated only recently through the use of gene sequencing and DNA-DNA hybridization. At the time the last edition of this textbook was published, 31 species of *Nocardia* were recognized. Four years later, 78 species have been named. Most likely by the time this edition is published, this number will be approaching 100 species. Fortunately, most infections are caused by a relatively few species, and identification of this group of organisms at the genus level, combined with in vitro susceptibility testing, is sufficient for the management of most patients.

Box 27—1. Weakly Acid-Fast Gram-Positive Rods

Organism	Historical Derivation
Nocardia	Named after the French veterinarian Edmond *Nocard*
Rhodococcus	*rhodo*, "rose" or "red-colored"; *coccus*, "berry" (red-colored coccus)
Gordonia	Named after the American microbiologist Ruth *Gordon*
Tsukamurella	Honoring the Japanese microbiologist, Michio *Tsukamura*, who first described the original isolate of this genus

Pathogenesis and Immunity

Nocardia causes **bronchopulmonary disease** in immuno-compromised patients, with a high predilection for hematogenous **spread to the central nervous system (CNS) or skin**. Patients at greatest risk for *Nocardia* infection are those with T-cell deficiencies produced by disease (e.g., leukemia, acquired immune deficiency syndrome [AIDS]) or by immunosuppressive therapy (e.g., corticosteroids for renal, cardiac, or bone marrow transplantation). Chronic localized pulmonary disease can occur in immunocompetent patients with bronchitis, emphysema, asthma, bronchiectasis, and alveolar proteinosis. **Cutaneous nocardiosis** can have four presentations: mycetoma, lymphocutaneous disease, superficial skin infection with abscess formation or cellulitis, and secondary cutaneous involvement following dissemination from a pulmonary site. *Nocardia brasiliensis* most commonly causes **primary cutaneous infections** in immunocompetent patients.

Bronchopulmonary disease develops after the initial colonization of the upper respiratory tract by inhalation and then aspiration of oral secretions into the lower airways. **Primary cutaneous nocardiosis** develops after traumatic introduction of organisms into subcutaneous tissues. Pulmonary and cutaneous diseases are characterized by necrosis and abscess formation similar to those caused by other pyogenic bacteria. Chronic infections with sinus tract formation can occur, particularly with primary cutaneous infections. Although "sulfur granules" (pigmented microcolonies of bacteria present in wound exudates) are observed with *Actinomyces* species, they are uncommon with nocardiae and seen only in cutaneous disease.

Although toxins and hemolysins have been described for nocardiae, the role these factors play in disease has not been defined. It would appear that the primary factor associated with virulence is the ability of pathogenic strains to **avoid phagocytic killing**. When phagocytes contact microbes, an oxidative burst occurs, with release of toxic oxygen metabolites (i.e., hydrogen peroxide, superoxide). Pathogenic strains of nocardiae are protected by their secretion of **catalase** and **superoxide dismutase**. Surface-associated superoxide dismutase also protects the bacteria. Nocardiae are also able to survive and **replicate in macrophages**. This is accomplished by (1) preventing fusion of the phagosome-lysosome (mediated by **cord factor**), (2) preventing acidification of the phagosome (by an undefined mechanism), and (3) avoiding acid phosphatase—mediated killing by metabolic utilization of the enzyme as a carbon source.

Epidemiology

Nocardia infections are **exogenous** (i.e., caused by organisms not part of the normal human flora). The ubiquitous presence of the organism in soil rich with organic matter and the increasing numbers of immunocompromised individuals living in communities have led to dramatic increases in disease caused by this organism. The increase is particularly noticeable in high-risk populations, such as ambulatory patients who are infected with human immunodeficiency virus (HIV) or who have received bone marrow or solid organ transplants.

Clinical Diseases (Box 27-3)

Bronchopulmonary disease (Clinical Case 27-1) caused by *Nocardia* species cannot be distinguished from infections

Table 27—1. Diseases of Selected Pathogenic Actinomycetes

Organism	Diseases	Frequency
Nocardia	Pulmonary diseases (bronchitis, pneumonia, lung abscesses); primary or secondary cutaneous infections (e.g., mycetoma, lymphocutaneous infections, cellulitis, subcutaneous abscesses); secondary CNS infections (e.g., meningitis, brain abscesses)	Common
Rhodococcus	Pulmonary diseases (pneumonia, lung abscesses); disseminated diseases (e.g., meningitis, pericarditis); opportunistic infections (e.g., wound infections, peritonitis, traumatic endophthalmitis)	Uncommon
Gordonia	Opportunistic infections	Rare
Tsukamurella	Opportunistic infections	Rare

Box 27–2. Summary: *Nocardia*

Biology, Virulence, and Disease

Gram-positive, partially acid-fast, filamentous rods; cell wall with mycolic acid

Strict aerobe capable of growth on most nonselective bacteria, fungal, and mycobacterial media; however, prolonged incubation (7 days or more) may be required

Virulence associated with ability to avoid intracellular killing

Catalase and superoxide dismutase: inactivate toxic oxygen metabolites (e.g., hydrogen peroxide, superoxide)

Cord factor: prevents intracellular killing in phagocytes by interfering with fusion of phagosomes with lysosomes

Primary disease most commonly bronchopulmonary (e.g., cavitary disease) or primary cutaneous infections (e.g., mycetoma, lymphocutaneous infection, cellulitis, subcutaneous abscesses)

Dissemination most commonly to central nervous system (e.g., brain abscesses) or skin

Epidemiology

Worldwide distribution in soil rich with organic matter

Exogenous infections acquired by inhalation (pulmonary) or traumatic introduction (cutaneous)

Opportunistic pathogen, causing disease most commonly in immunocompromised patients with T-cell deficiencies (transplant recipients, patients with malignancies, patients infected with the human immunodeficiency virus, patients receiving corticosteroids)

Diagnosis

Microscopy is sensitive and relatively specific when branching, partially acid-fast organisms are seen

Culture is slow, requiring incubation for up to 1 week; selective media (e.g., BCYE agar) may be required for isolating *Nocardia* in mixed cultures

Identification at the genus level can be made by the microscopic and macroscopic appearances (branching, weakly acid-fast rods forming colonies with aerial hyphae)

Identification at the species level requires genomic analysis for most isolates

Treatment, Prevention, and Control

Infections are treated with antibiotics and proper wound care

Trimethoprim-sulfamethoxazole is used for localized infections; combination of antibiotics such as amikacin with a carbapenem or broad-spectrum cephalosporin is used for severe, progressive disease; treatment for 6 weeks or more

Exposure cannot be avoided, because nocardiae are ubiquitous

Figure 27–1. Gram stain of *Nocardia* species in expectorated sputum. Note the delicate beaded filaments.

particularly if there is evidence of dissemination to the CNS or subcutaneous tissues. If a pulmonary or disseminated *Nocardia* infection is diagnosed in an individual with no underlying disease, then a comprehensive immunologic workup is indicated.

Cutaneous infections may be primary infections (e.g., mycetoma, lymphocutaneous infections, cellulitis, and subcutaneous abscesses) or the result of secondary spread of organisms from a primary pulmonary infection. **Mycetoma** is a painless, chronic infection primarily of the feet characterized by localized subcutaneous swelling, suppuration, and the formation of multiple sinus tracts. The underlying connective tissues, muscle, and bone can be involved, and draining sinus tracts usually open on the skin surface. A variety of organisms can cause mycetoma, although *N. brasiliensis* is the most common cause in North America, Central

Figure 27–2. Acid-fast stain of *Nocardia* species in expectorated sputum. In contrast with the mycobacteria, members of the genus *Nocardia* do not uniformly retain the stain ("partially acid-fast").

caused by other pyogenic organisms, although *Nocardia* infections tend to develop more slowly, and primary pulmonary disease caused by *Nocardia* occurs almost always in immunocompromised patients. Signs such as cough, dyspnea, and fever are usually present but are not diagnostic. Cavitation and spread into the pleura are common. Although the clinical picture is not specific for *Nocardia*, these organisms should be considered when immunocompromised patients experience pneumonia with cavitation,

Figure 27—3. Orange colonies of *Nocardia*.

America, and South America. **Lymphocutaneous infections** can manifest as cutaneous nodules and ulcerations along the lymphatics and regional lymph node involvement. These infections resemble cutaneous infections caused by some species of mycobacteria and by the fungus *Sporothrix schenckii*. *Nocardia* can also cause **chronic ulcerative lesions**, **subcutaneous abscesses**, and **cellulitis**; Figure 27-5).

As many as a third of all patients with *Nocardia* infections have dissemination to the brain, most commonly involving the formation of single or multiple **brain abscesses**. The disease can present initially as chronic meningitis.

Laboratory Diagnosis

Multiple sputum specimens should be collected from patients with pulmonary disease. Because nocardiae are usually

distributed throughout the tissue and abscess material, it is relatively easy to detect them by microscopy and to recover them in culture of specimens from patients with pulmonary, cutaneous, or CNS disease. The delicate hyphae of *Nocardia* in tissues cause them to resemble *Actinomyces* organisms; however, in contrast with *Actinomyces*, nocardiae are typically weakly acid-fast (see Figures 27-1 and 27-2).

The organisms grow on most laboratory media incubated in an atmosphere of 5% to 10% carbon dioxide, but the presence of these slow-growing organisms may be obscured by more rapidly growing commensal bacteria. If a specimen is potentially contaminated with other bacteria (e.g., oral bacteria in sputum), selective media should be inoculated. Success has been achieved with the medium used for the isolation of *Legionella* species (**buffered charcoal yeast extract [BCYE] agar**). Indeed, this medium can be used to recover both organisms from pulmonary specimens. *Nocardia* occasionally grows on media used for the

Figure 27—4. Aerial hyphae of *Nocardia*.

Figure 27—5. Cutaneous lesion caused by *Nocardia*. *(From Sorrell TC, et al: Nocardia species. In Mandell GL, Bennett JE, Dolin R (eds): Principles and Practice of Infectious Diseases, 6th ed. Philadelphia, Churchill Livingstone, 2005.)*

isolation of mycobacteria and fungi; however, this method is less reliable than the use of special bacterial media. It is important to notify the laboratory that nocardiosis is suspected, because most laboratories do not routinely use special culture media or incubate clinical specimens for more than 1 to 3 days. It takes more time (i.e., as long as a week) for *Nocardia* species to be detected in culture.

The preliminary identification of *Nocardia* is uncomplicated. Members of the genus can be classified initially on the basis of the presence of **filamentous**, **weakly acid-fast bacilli** and **aerial hyphae** on the colony surface. Definitive identification at the species level is more difficult. It is recognized that most species cannot be identified accurately by phenotypic (e.g., biochemical) tests, although many laboratories continue to use these tests. The accurate identification of most species requires molecular analysis of ribosomal ribonucleic acid (RNA) genes and "housekeeping" genes (e.g., heat-shock protein gene). Currently these tests are performed primarily in reference or research laboratories.

Treatment, Prevention, and Control

Nocardia infections are treated with the combination of antibiotics and appropriate surgical intervention. Trimethoprim-sulfamethoxazole is used most commonly to treat localized infections. In patients with severe, progressive disease, a combination of antibiotics is recommended, such as amikacin with a carbapenem (e.g., imipenem, meropenem) or broad-spectrum cephalosporin. In vitro susceptibility tests can be used to guide the selection of antibiotics. Because nocardiae can disseminate and produce significant disease, therapy should be extended for 6 weeks or more. Whereas the clinical response is favorable in patients with localized infections, the prognosis is poor for immunocompromised patients with disseminated disease.

Nocardiae are ubiquitous, so it is impossible to avoid exposure to them. However, bronchopulmonary disease caused by nocardiae is uncommon in immunocompetent persons,

and primary cutaneous infections can be prevented with proper wound care. If nocardiosis is considered in the differential diagnosis for immunocompromised patients with cavitary pulmonary disease and promptly treated, the complications associated with disseminated disease can be minimized.

Rhodococcus

The genus *Rhodococcus* consists of gram-positive, weakly acid-fast bacteria that initially appear rodlike and then revert to coccoid forms (Figure 27-6). Rudimentary branching may be present, but the delicate, branching filamentous forms commonly seen with nocardiae are not observed with rhodococci. Of the species currently recognized, ***Rhodococcus equi*** is the most important human pathogen. Originally, *R. equi* (formerly *Corynebacterium equi*) was considered a veterinary pathogen, particularly in herbivores, that occasionally caused occupational disease in farmers and veterinarians. However, this organism has become an increasingly more common **pathogen of immunocompromised patients** (e.g., patients infected with HIV, transplant recipients). Interestingly, most infected patients do not have a history of contact with grazing animals or of exposure to soil contaminated with herbivore manure. The rise in the incidence of human infection is most likely related to the increase in the number of patients with immunosuppressive diseases, particularly AIDS, and to the enhanced awareness of the organism. It is likely that many isolates were ignored previously or were misidentified as insignificant coryneform bacteria.

Like *Nocardia*, *R. equi* is a facultative, intracellular organism that survives in macrophages and causes granulomatous inflammation, which leads to **abscess formation**. Although numerous putative virulence factors have been identified, the precise pathophysiology of the infection is incompletely understood. A virulence-associated protein, *vap*A, has been implicated in disease in horses, but its role in human disease is less established. Individuals with depressed production of interferon-γ appear to be unable to clear bacteria from lung infections.

Immunocompromised patients most typically present with invasive pulmonary disease (e.g., pulmonary nodules, consolidation, lung abscesses), and evidence of dissemination in the blood to distal sites (lymph nodes, meninges, pericardium, and skin) is commonly observed. Rhodococci usually cause opportunistic infections in immunocompetent patients (e.g., posttraumatic cutaneous infections, peritonitis in patients undergoing long-term dialysis, traumatic endophthalmitis).

Rhodococci grow on nonselective media incubated aerobically, but the characteristic salmon-pink pigment may not be obvious for at least 4 days. Colonies are typically **mucoid**, although dry forms may also be seen. The organisms can be identified initially by their slow growth, macroscopic and

Figure 27–6. *Rhodococcus.* **A,** Gram stain after growth in nutrient broth for 4 hours. **B,** Gram stain after growth in nutrient broth for 18 hours. **C,** Acid-fast stain of organisms grown on mycobacterial Middlebrook agar for 2 days (note the paucity of red "acid-fast" cells). **D,** Gram stain of branching, filamentous forms.

microscopic morphology, and ability to weakly retain the **acid-fast** stain (particularly when grown on media for mycobacteria). Definitive identification at the species level is problematic because the organisms are relatively inert.

Rhodococcus infections have proved difficult to treat. Although in vitro tests and tests in animal models have identified specific combinations of drugs as effective, only limited success has been realized in the treatment of human infections, particularly in immunocompromised patients with low CD4 cell counts (50% mortality), compared with immunocompetent patients (20% mortality). The current recommendation for treating localized infections in immunocompetent patients is to use oral antibiotics (e.g., erythromycin, rifampin, and/or ciprofloxacin). Disseminated infections and infections in immunocompromised patients should be managed with combinations of intravenous antibiotics (e.g., vancomycin, imipenem, aminoglycosides, ciprofloxacin, rifampin, and/or erythromycin). Penicillins and cephalosporins should not be used, because resistance to these agents is common in rhodococci, and the effectiveness of any antibiotic must be confirmed by in vitro testing.

Gordonia and *Tsukamurella*

Gordonia (formerly *Gordona*) and *Tsukamurella* were previously classified with *Rhodococcus* because they are morphologically similar, contain mycolic acids, and are **partially acid-fast**. The organisms are present in soil and are rare opportunistic pathogens in humans. *Gordonia* has been associated with pulmonary and cutaneous infections, as well as nosocomial infections such as those resulting from contaminated intravascular catheters. *Tsukamurella* has been associated with catheter infections. The significance of isolating either organism in clinical specimens must be evaluated carefully.

Case Study and Questions

A 47-year-old renal transplant recipient who had been receiving prednisone and azathioprine for 2 years was admitted to the university medical center. Two weeks before, the patient had noticed the development of a dry, persistent cough. Five days before admission, the cough became productive, and pleuritic chest pain developed. On the day of admission, the patient was in mild respiratory arrest, and chest radiographs revealed a patchy right upper lobe infiltrate. Sputum specimens were initially sent for bacterial culture; results were reported as negative for organisms after 2 days of incubation. Antibiotic therapy with cephalothin was ineffective, so additional specimens were collected for the culture of bacteria, mycobacteria, *Legionella* species, and fungi. After 4 days of incubation, *Nocardia* was isolated on the media inoculated for mycobacteria, *Legionella* species, and fungi.

1. Why did the organism fail to grow initially? What can be done to correct this problem?

2. If this organism disseminates, what two target tissues are most likely to be involved?

3. What is the most common presentation of disease caused by *N. brasiliensis?*

4. What disease is caused by *Rhodococcus* in immunocompromised patients?

5. What microscopic property does *Rhodococcus* share with *Nocardia?* Which two other genera discussed in this chapter have the same property?

6. Which bacteria cause mycetoma? Which one is the most common cause in the United States?

Bibliography

Beaman B, Beaman L: *Nocardia* species: Host-parasite relationships. Clin Microbiol Rev 7:213-264, 1994.

Conville P, Witebsky F: *Nocardia* and other aerobic Actinomycetes. In Topley and Wilson's Microbiology and Microbial Infections, 10th ed. London, Hodder Arnold, 2005.

Conville P, Witebsky F: *Nocardia, Rhodococcus, Gordonia, Actinomadura, Streptomyces,* and other aerobic Actinomycetes. Manual of Clinical Microbiology, 9th ed. Washington DC, ASM Press, 2007.

Giguere S, et al: Role of the 85-kilobase plasmid and plasmid-encoded virulence-associated protein A in intracellular survival and virulence of *Rhodococcus equi.* Infect Immun 67:3548-3557, 1999.

Steingrube V, et al: Rapid identification of clinically significant species and taxa of aerobic Actinomycetes, including *Actinomadura, Gordona, Nocardia, Rhodococcus, Streptomyces,* and *Tsukamurella* isolates, by DNA amplification and restriction endonuclease analysis. J Clin Microbiol 35:817-822, 1997.

Weinstock D, Brown A: *Rhodococcus equi:* An emerging pathogen. Clin Infect Dis 34:1379-1385, 2002.

Mycobacterium

The genus *Mycobacterium* (Box 28-1) consists of nonmotile, non-spore-forming, aerobic rods that are 0.2 to 0.6 × 1 to 10 μm in size. The rods occasionally form branched filaments, but these can be readily disrupted. The cell wall is rich in lipids, making the surface hydrophobic and the mycobacteria resistant to many disinfectants and common laboratory stains. Once stained, the rods also cannot be decolorized with acid solutions; hence the name **acid-fast** bacteria. Because the mycobacterial cell wall is complex, and this group of organisms is fastidious, most mycobacteria grow slowly, dividing every 12 to 24 hours and requiring as long as 8 weeks before growth in detected in laboratory cultures.

Mycobacteria are a significant cause of morbidity and mortality, particularly in countries with limited medical resources. Currently, more than 130 species of mycobacteria have been described, many of which are associated with human disease (Table 28-1). Despite the abundance of mycobacterial species, the following few species or groups cause most human infections: *M. tuberculosis, M. leprae, M. avium* complex, *M. kansasii, M. fortuitum, M. chelonae,* and *M. abscessus.*

Physiology and Structure of Mycobacteria

Bacteria are classified in the genus *Mycobacterium* on the basis of (1) their acid-fastness, (2) the presence of **mycolic acids** containing 70 to 90 carbons, and (3) a high (61 to 71 mol%) guanine plus cytosine (G+C) content in their deoxyribonucleic acid (DNA). Although other species of bacteria can be acid-fast (i.e., *Nocardia, Rhodococcus, Tsukamurella, Gordonia*), they stain less intensely (are partially acid-fast), and their mycolic acids chains are shorter.

Mycobacteria possess a complex, **lipid-rich cell wall** (Figure 28-1). This cell wall is responsible for many of the characteristic properties of the bacteria (e.g., acid-fastness, slow growth, resistance to detergents, resistance to common antibacterial antibiotics, antigenicity, clumping).

The basic structure of the cell wall is typical of gram-positive bacteria: an inner plasma membrane overlaid with a thick peptidoglycan layer and no outer membrane. However, the mycobacterial cell wall structure is far more complex than that in other gram-positive bacteria. Anchored in the plasma membrane are proteins, phosphatidylinositol mannosides, and **lipoarabinomannan (LAM)**. LAM is functionally related to the O-antigenic lipopolysaccharides present in other bacteria. The peptidoglycan layer forms the foundation upon which are attached arabinogalactans, a branched polysaccharide consisting of D-arabinose and D-galactose. The terminal D-arabinose residue is esterified to high molecular weight, hydrophobic mycolic acids with attached glycolipid surface molecules. Additional lipids, glycolipids, and peptidoglycolipids are also present. The lipid components comprise 60% of the cell wall weight. Transport proteins and porins are interspersed throughout the cell wall layers, and these constitute 15% of the cell wall weight. The proteins are biologically important antigens, stimulating the patient's cellular immune response to infection. Extracted and partially purified preparations of these protein derivatives **(purified protein derivatives, or PPDs)** are used as skin test reagents to measure exposure to *M. tuberculosis*. Similar preparations from other mycobacteria have been used as species-specific skin test reagents.

Growth properties and colonial morphology are used for the preliminary classification of mycobacteria. As noted earlier, *M. tuberculosis* and closely related species in the *M. tuberculosis* complex are slow-growing bacteria. The colonies of these mycobacteria are either nonpigmented or a light tan color (Figure 28-2). The other mycobacteria, now referred to as "nontuberculous mycobacteria" or NTM, were classified originally by Runyon by their rate of growth and pigmentation (see Table 28-1). The pigmented mycobacteria produce intensely **yellow carotenoids** which may be stimulated by exposure to light (photochromogenic organisms; Figure 28-3) or produced in the absence of light (scotochromogenic organisms). The **Runyon classification**

Box 28–1. Important Mycobacteria

Organism	Historical Derivation
Mycobacterium	*myces*, a "fungus"; *bakterion*, a "small rod" (fungus-like rod)
M. abscessus	*abscessus*, of "abscess" (causes abscess formation)
M. avium	*avis*, of "birds" (causes tuberculosis-like illness in birds)
M. chelonae	*chelone*, a "tortoise"
M. fortuitum	*fortuitum*, "casual, accidental" (refers to fact this is an opportunistic pathogen)
M. haemophilum	*haema*, "blood"; *philos*, "loving" (blood-loving; refers to requirement for blood or hemin for in vitro growth)
M. intracellulare	*intra*, "within"; *cella*, "small room" (within cells; refers to the intracellular location of mycobacteria)
M. kansasii	*kansasii*, of "Kansas" (where the organism was originally isolated)
M. leprae	*lepra*, of "leprosy" (the cause of leprosy)
M. marinum	*marinum*, of the "sea" (bacterium associated with contaminated freshwater and salt waters)
M. tuberculosis	*tuberculum*, a "small swelling" or tubercle; *osis*, "characterized by" (characterized by tubercles; refers to the formation of tubercles in the lungs of infected patients)

Table 28–1. Classification of Selected Mycobacteria Pathogenic for Humans

Organism	Pathogenicity	Frequency in United States
***M. tuberculosis* Complex**		
M. tuberculosis	Strictly pathogenic	Common
M. leprae	Strictly pathogenic	Uncommon
M. africanum	Strictly pathogenic	Rare
M. bovis	Strictly pathogenic	Rare
M. bovis (BCG strain)	Sometimes pathogenic	Rare
Slow-Growing Nontuberculous Mycobacteria		
M. avium complex	Usually pathogenic	Common
M. kansasii	Usually pathogenic	Common
M. marinum	Usually pathogenic	Uncommon
M. simiae	Usually pathogenic	Uncommon
M. szulgai	Usually pathogenic	Uncommon
M. genavense	Usually pathogenic	Uncommon
M. haemophilum	Usually pathogenic	Uncommon
M. malmoense	Usually pathogenic	Uncommon
M. ulcerans	Usually pathogenic	Uncommon
M. scrofulaceum	Sometimes pathogenic	Uncommon
M. xenopi	Sometimes pathogenic	Uncommon
Rapidly Growing Nontuberculous Mycobacteria		
M. abscessus	Sometimes pathogenic	Common
M. chelonae	Sometimes pathogenic	Common
M. fortuitum	Sometimes pathogenic	Common
M. mucogenicum	Sometimes pathogenic	Uncommon

scheme consisted of four groups: slow-growing photochromogens (e.g., *M. kansasii, M. marinum*), slow-growing scotochromogens (e.g., *M. gordonae*—a commonly isolated nonpathogen), slow-growing nonpigmented mycobacteria (e.g., *M. avium, M. intracellulare*), and rapidly growing mycobacteria (e.g., *M. fortuitum, M. chelonae,* and *M. abscessus*). Currently used methods for the rapid detection and identification of mycobacteria have made this scheme less important. Nonetheless, a pigmented or a rapidly growing mycobacterium should never be mistaken for *M. tuberculosis*.

Mycobacterium tuberculosis (Box 28-2)

Pathogenesis and Immunity

M. tuberculosis is an intracellular pathogen that is able to establish lifelong infection. The complexity of the intracellular existence of this bacterium is still not completely understood but is slowly being unraveled. At the time of exposure, *M. tuberculosis* enters the respiratory airways and minute infectious particles penetrate to the alveoli, where they are phagocytized by alveolar macrophages. In contrast

Figure 28—1. Mycobacterial cell wall structure. The components include the *(A)* plasma membrane, *(B)* peptidoglycans, *(C)* arabinogalactan, *(D)* mannose-capped lipoarabinomannan, *(E)* plasma-associated and cell-wall—associated proteins, *(F)* mycolic acids, and *(G)* glycolipid surface molecules associated with the mycolic acids. *(P)*, phosphate molecule. *(Redrawn from Karakousis, et al: Cell Microbiol 6:105-116, 2004.)*

with most phagocytized bacteria, *M. tuberculosis* **prevents fusion of the phagosome with lysosomes** (by blocking the specific bridging molecule, early endosomal autoantigen 1 [EEA1]). At the same time, the phagosome is able to fuse with other intracellular vesicles, permitting access to nutrients and facilitating intravacuole replication. By inactivating the oxidants that are formed, phagocytized bacteria are also able to evade macrophage killing mediated by reactive nitrogen intermediates formed between nitric oxide and superoxide anions.

In response to infection with *M. tuberculosis*, macrophages secrete interleukin 12 (**IL-12**) and tumor necrosis factor alpha (**TNF-α**). These cytokines increase localized inflammation with the recruitment of T cells and natural killer (NK) cells into the area of the infected macrophages, inducing T-cell differentiation into TH1 cells (**T-helper cells**), with subsequent secretion of interferon gamma (**IFN-γ**). In the presence of IFN-γ, the infected macrophages are activated, leading to increased phagosome-lysosome fusion and intracellular killing. In addition, TNF-α stimulates production of nitric oxide and related reactive nitrogen intermediates, leading to enhanced intracellular killing. Patients with decreased production of IFN-γ or TNF-α, or who have defects in the receptors for these cytokines, are at increased risk for severe mycobacterial infections.

If a small antigenic burden is present at the time the macrophages are stimulated, the bacteria are destroyed with minimal tissue damage. If many bacteria are present, however, the

Figure 28—2. *Mycobacterium tuberculosis* colonies on Löwenstein-Jensen agar after 8 weeks of incubation. *(From Baron EJ, Peterson LR, Finegold SM: Bailey and Scott's Diagnostic Microbiology, 9th ed. St Louis, Mosby, 1994.)*

Figure 28—3. *Mycobacterium kansasii* colonies on Middlebrook agar 1 day after exposure to light.

Box 28–2. Summary: *Mycobacterium tuberculosis*

Biology, Virulence, and Disease

Weakly gram-positive, strongly acid-fast, aerobic rods
Lipid-rich cell wall, making the organism resistant to disinfectants, detergents, common antibacterial antibiotics, and traditional stains
Capable of intracellular growth in unactivated alveolar macrophages
Disease primarily from host response to infection
Primary infection is pulmonary
Dissemination to any body site occurs most commonly in immunocompromised patients

Epidemiology

Worldwide, a third of the world's population is infected with this organism
A total of 9 million new cases each year and 2 million deaths
Disease most common in Southeast Asia, sub-Saharan Africa, and Eastern Europe
Fewer than 14,000 new cases in United States in 2006
Populations at greatest risk for disease are immunocompromised patients (particularly those with HIV infection), drug or alcohol abusers, homeless persons, and individuals exposed to diseased patients
Humans are the only natural reservoir
Person-to-person spread by infectious aerosols

Diagnosis

Tuberculin skin test and IFN-γ release tests are sensitive markers for exposure to organism
Microscopy and culture are sensitive and specific
Direct detection by molecular probes is relatively insensitive, except for acid-fast smear-positive specimens
Identification most commonly made using species-specific molecular probes

Treatment, Prevention, and Control

Multiple-drug regimens and prolonged treatment are required to prevent development of drug-resistant strains
Isoniazid (INH), ethambutol, pyrazinamide, and rifampin for 2 months followed by 4 to 6 months of INH and rifampin or alternative combination drugs
Prophylaxis for exposure to tuberculosis can include INH for 6 to 9 months or rifampin for 4 months; pyrazinamide and ethambutol or levofloxacin are used for 6 to 12 months after exposure to drug-resistant *M. tuberculosis*
Immunoprophylaxis with bacille Calmette-Guerin (BCG) in endemic countries
Control of disease through active surveillance, prophylactic and therapeutic intervention, and careful case monitoring

cellular immune response results in tissue necrosis. Multiple host factors are involved in this process, including cytokine toxicity, local activation of the complement cascade, ischemia, and exposure to macrophage-derived hydrolytic enzymes and reactive oxygen intermediates. No known mycobacterial toxin or enzyme has been associated with tissue destruction.

The effectiveness of bacterial elimination is in part related to the size of the focus of infection. Alveolar macrophages, epithelioid cells, and **Langhans giant cells** (fused epithelioid

cells) with intracellular mycobacteria form the central core of a necrotic mass that is surrounded by a dense wall of CD4, CD8, and NK T cells and macrophages. This structure, a **granuloma**, prevents further spread of the bacteria. If the granuloma is small, then the intracellular bacteria are effectively killed. Large necrotic or caseous granulomas become encapsulated with fibrin that effectively protects the bacteria from macrophage killing. The bacteria can remain dormant in this stage or can be reactivated years later, when the patient's immunologic responsiveness wanes as the result of old age or immunosuppressive disease or therapy. This process is the reason why disease may not develop until late in life in patients exposed to *M. tuberculosis*.

Epidemiology

Although tuberculosis can be established in primates and laboratory animals such as guinea pigs, **humans are the only natural reservoir**. The disease is spread by close person-to-person contact through the inhalation of infectious aerosols. Large particles are trapped on mucosal surfaces and removed by the ciliary action of the respiratory tree. However, small particles containing one to three tubercle bacilli can reach the alveolar spaces and establish infection.

The World Health Organization (WHO) estimates that a third of the world's population is infected with *M. tuberculosis*. Currently there are almost 9 million new cases and 2 million deaths annually caused by *M. tuberculosis*. Regions with the highest incidence of disease are Southeast Asia, sub-Saharan Africa, and Eastern Europe. In the United States, the incidence of tuberculosis has decreased steadily since 1992 (Figure 28-4). In 2006, fewer than 14,000 cases were reported, with almost 60% of the infections in foreign-born persons. Other populations at increased risk for *M. tuberculosis* disease are homeless persons, drug and alcohol abusers, prisoners, and people infected with the human immunodeficiency virus (HIV). Because it is difficult to eradicate disease in these patients, spread of the infection to other populations, including health care workers, poses a significant public health problem. This is particularly true for drug-resistant *M. tuberculosis*, because patients who receive inadequate treatment may remain infectious for a long time.

Clinical Diseases (Clinical Case 28-1)

Although tuberculosis can involve any organ, most infections in immunocompetent patients are restricted to the lungs. The initial pulmonary focus is the middle or lower lung fields, where the tubercle bacilli can multiply freely. The patient's cellular immunity is activated, and mycobacterial replication ceases in most patients within 3 to 6 weeks after exposure to the organism. Approximately 5% of patients exposed to *M. tuberculosis* progress to having active disease within 2 years, and another 5% to 10% experience disease sometime later in life.

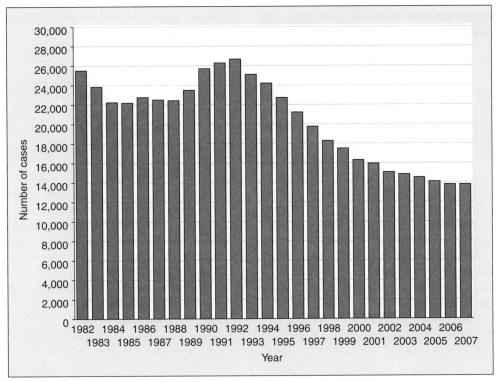

Figure 28—4. Incidence of *M. tuberculosis* infections in the United States, 1982-2007.

The likelihood that infection will progress to active disease is a function of both the infectious dose and the patient's immune competence. For example, active disease develops within 1 year of exposure in approximately 10% of patients who are infected with HIV and have a low CD4 T-cell count, compared with a 10% risk of disease during the lifetime of patients without HIV infection. In patients with HIV infection, disease usually appears before the onset of other opportunistic infections, is twice as likely to spread to extrapulmonary sites, and can progress rapidly to death.

The clinical signs and symptoms of tuberculosis reflect the site of infection, with primary disease usually restricted to the lower respiratory tract. The disease is insidious at onset. Patients typically have nonspecific complaints of malaise, weight loss, cough, and night sweats. Sputum may be scant or bloody and purulent. Sputum production with hemoptysis is associated with tissue destruction (e.g., **cavitary disease**). The clinical diagnosis is supported by (1) radiographic evidence of pulmonary disease (Figure 28-5), (2) positive skin test reactivity, and (3) the laboratory detection of mycobacteria, either with microscopy or in cultures. One or both upper lobes of the lungs are usually involved in patients with active disease that includes pneumonitis or abscess formation and cavitation.

Extrapulmonary tuberculosis can occur as the result of the hematogenous spread of the bacilli during the initial phase of multiplication. There may be no evidence of pulmonary disease in patients with **disseminated (miliary) tuberculosis**.

Clinical Case 28-1. Drug-resistant *Mycobacterium tuberculosis*

The risk of active tuberculosis is significantly increased in HIV-infected individuals. Unfortunately, this problem is complicated by the development of drug-resistant M. tuberculosis strains in this population. This was illustrated by the report by Gandhi, et al. (Lancet 368:1575-1580, 2006), who studied the prevalence of tuberculosis in South Africa from January 2005 to March 2006. They identified 475 patients with culture confirmed tuberculosis, of whom 39% had multidrug-resistant strains (MDR TB) and 6% had extensively drug-resistant strains (XDR TB). All patients with XDR TB were coinfected with HIV, and 98% of these patients died. The high prevalence of MDR TB and the evolution of XDR TB pose a serious challenge for tuberculosis treatment programs and emphasize the need for rapid diagnostic tests.

Figure 28—5. Pulmonary tuberculosis.

Mycobacterium leprae (Box 28-3)

Pathogenesis and Immunity

Leprosy (also called **Hansen disease**) is caused by *M. leprae*. Because the bacteria multiply very slowly, the incubation period is prolonged, with symptoms developing as long as 20 years after infection. As with *M. tuberculosis* infections, the clinical manifestations of leprosy depend on the patient's immune reaction to the bacteria. The clinical presentation of leprosy ranges from the tuberculoid form to the lepromatous form. Patients with **tuberculoid leprosy** (also called **paucibacillary Hansen disease**) have a strong cellular immune reaction, with many lymphocytes and granulomas present in the tissues and relatively few bacteria (Figure 28-6; Table 28-2). As in *M. tuberculosis* infections in immunocompetent patients, the bacteria induce cytokine production that mediate macrophage activation, phagocytosis, and bacillary clearance.

Patients with **lepromatous leprosy (multibacillary Hansen disease)**, however, have a strong antibody response but a specific defect in the cellular response to *M. leprae* antigens. Thus an abundance of bacteria is typically observed in dermal macrophages and the Schwann cells

---

Box 28–3. Summary: *Mycobacterium leprae*

Biology, Virulence, and Disease

Weakly gram-positive, strongly acid-fast rods
Lipid-rich cell wall
Unable to be cultured on artificial media
Disease primarily from host response to infection
Tuberculoid (paucibacillary) and lepromatous (multibacillary) forms of leprosy

Epidemiology

Fewer than 300,000 new cases were reported in 2005, with most cases in India, Nepal, and Brazil
Approximately 100 new cases reported in United States annually
Lepromatous form of disease, but not the tuberculoid form, is highly infectious
Person-to-person spread by direct contact or inhalation of infectious aerosols

Diagnosis

Microscopy is sensitive for the lepromatous form but not the tuberculoid form
Skin testing is required to confirm tuberculoid leprosy
Culture is not useful

Treatment, Prevention, and Control

Tuberculoid form is treated with rifampicin and dapsone for 6 months; clofazimine is added to this regimen for treatment of the lepromatous form, and therapy is extended to a minimum of 12 months
Disease is controlled through the prompt recognition and treatment of infected people

---

of the peripheral nerves. As would be expected, this is the most infectious form of leprosy.

Epidemiology

Leprosy was first described in 600 BC and was recognized in the ancient civilizations of China, Egypt, and India. The global **prevalence of leprosy has fallen dramatically** with the widespread use of effective therapy. More than 5 million cases were documented in 1985 and fewer than 300,000 cases 20 years later. Currently, 90% of the cases are in Brazil, Madagascar, Mozambique, Tanzania, and Nepal. In the United States, leprosy is uncommon, with approximately 100 cases reported annually. Most cases occur in California, Texas, and Hawaii and primarily in immigrants from Mexico, Asia, Africa, and the Pacific Islands. Interestingly, leprosy is endemic in **armadillos** found in Texas and Louisiana, producing a disease similar to the highly infectious lepromatous form of leprosy in humans. Thus these armadillos represent a potential endemic focus in this country.

Leprosy is spread by person-to-person contact. Although the most important route of infection is unknown, it is believed that *M. leprae* is spread either through the inhalation of infectious aerosols or through skin contact with respiratory secretions and wound exudates. Numerous *M. leprae* are found in the nasal secretions of patients with lepromatous leprosy.

***M. leprae* cannot grow in cell-free cultures**. Thus laboratory confirmation of leprosy requires histopathologic findings consistent with the clinical disease and either skin test reactivity to lepromin or observation of acid-fast bacteria in the lesions.

Clinical Diseases

Leprosy is a chronic infection that affects the skin and peripheral nerves. The spectrum of tissue involvement is influenced by the patient's immune status, as noted earlier (see Table 28-2). The tuberculoid form (Figure 28-7) is milder and is characterized by hypopigmented skin macules. The lepromatous form (Figure 28-8) is associated with disfiguring skin lesions, nodules, plaques, thickened dermis, and involvement of the nasal mucosa.

Mycobacterium avium Complex (Box 28-4)

The classification of mycobacteria in the *M. avium* complex has been defined recently by genomic-based studies. Two species, *M. avium* and *M. intracellulare*, and four subspecies are recognized currently (Table 28-3). Most reports in the literature refer to *M. avium* or *M. avium* complex as a cause of human disease. However, it appears that the strains responsible for avian disease (*M. avium* subsp. *avium*) are distinct from the strains responsible for most human disease (*M. avium* subsp. *hominissuis*). *M. avium* subsp. *silvaticum*

Figure 28—6. Acid-fast stains of skin biopsies from patients with (**A**) tuberculoid leprosy, (**B**) borderline tuberculoid leprosy, (**C**) borderline lepromatous leprosy, and (**D**) lepromatous leprosy. Note that there is a progressive increase in bacteria going from the tuberculoid form to the lepromatous form of the disease.

Table 28—2. Clinical and Immunologic Manifestations of Leprosy

Features	Tuberculoid Leprosy	Lepromatous Leprosy
Skin lesions	Few erythematous or hypopigmented plaques with flat centers and raised, demarcated borders; peripheral nerve damage with complete sensory loss; visible enlargement of nerves	Many erythematous macules, papules, or nodules; extensive tissue destruction (e.g., nasal cartilage, bones, ears); diffuse nerve involvement with patchy sensory loss; lack of nerve enlargement
Histopathology	Infiltration of lymphocytes around center of epithelial cells; presence of Langhans cells; few or no acid-fast rods observed	Predominantly "foamy" macrophages with few lymphocytes; lack of Langhans cells; numerous acid-fast rods in skin lesions and internal organs
Infectivity	Low	High
Immune response Delayed hypersensitivity	Reactivity to lepromin	Nonreactivity to lepromin
Immunoglobulin levels	Normal	Hypergammaglobulinemia
Erythema nodosum	Absent	Usually present

Figure 28—7. Tuberculoid leprosy. Early tuberculoid lesions are characterized by anesthetic macules with hypopigmentation. *(From Cohen J, Powderly WB: Infectious Diseases, 2nd ed. St Louis, Mosby, 2004.)*

has not been implicated in human disease, and a large body of literature has debated the role of *M. avium* subsp. *paratuberculosis*, the etiologic agent of chronic granulomatous enteritis (Johne disease) in ruminants, as a cause of chronic granulomatous enteritis in humans (Crohn disease). These taxonomic differences are important for understanding the epidemiology and pathogenesis of the *M. avium* complex strains responsible for human disease. However, for the purpose of this text, only the terms *M. avium* (*M. avium* subsp. *hominissuis*) and *M. avium* complex (*M. avium* and *M. intracellulare*) will be used.

Both species in the *M. avium* complex (*MAC*, a term commonly used today) produce disease in immunocompetent patients, whereas disease in HIV-infected patients is primarily caused by *M. avium*. Before the HIV epidemic,

Figure 28—8. Lepromatous leprosy. Diffuse infiltration of the skin by multiple nodules of varying size, each with many bacteria. *(From Cohen J, Powderly WB: Infectious Diseases, 2nd ed. St Louis, Mosby, 2004.)*

Box 28—4. Summary: *Mycobacterium avium* Complex

Biology, Virulence, and Disease

Weakly gram-positive, strongly acid-fast aerobic rods
Lipid-rich cell wall
Disease primarily from host response to infection
Disease includes: asymptomatic colonization, chronic localized pulmonary disease, solitary nodule, or disseminated disease, particularly in patients with AIDS

Epidemiology

Worldwide distribution, but disease is seen most commonly in countries where tuberculosis is less common
Acquired primarily through ingestion of contaminated water or food; inhalation of infectious aerosols is believed to play a minor role in transmission
Patients at greatest risk for disease are those who are immunocompromised (particularly patients with AIDS) and those with long-standing pulmonary disease

Diagnosis

Microscopy and culture are sensitive and specific

Treatment, Prevention, and Control

Infections treated for prolonged period with clarithromycin or azithromycin combined with ethambutol and rifabutin
Prophylaxis in patients with AIDS who have low CD4+ cell count consists of clarithromycin or azithromycin or rifabutin; has greatly reduced the incidence of disease

---

recovery of the organisms in clinical specimens typically represented transient colonization or, less commonly, chronic pulmonary disease. Pulmonary disease in immunocompetent patients presents in one of three forms. Most commonly, disease is seen in middle-age or older men with a history of smoking and **underlying pulmonary disease**. These patients typically have a slowly evolving cavitary disease that resembles tuberculosis on chest radiography.

Table 28—3. *Mycobacterium avium* Complex

Species	Disease
M. avium subsp. *avium*	Avian tuberculosis
M. avium subsp. *hominissuis*	Disease in humans and pigs; disseminated disease in HIV-infected patients; cervical lymphadenitis in children; chronic pulmonary disease in adolescents with cystic fibrosis and older adults with underlying pulmonary disease
M. avium subsp. *silvaticum*	Disease in wood pigeons
M. avium subsp. *paratuberculosis*	Chronic granulomatous enteric disease in ruminants (Johne disease) and possibly in humans (Crohn disease)
M. intracellulare	Pulmonary disease in immunocompetent patients

The second form of MAC infection is observed in elderly, female nonsmokers. These patients have lingular or middle lobe infiltrates with a patchy, nodular appearance on radiography and associated bronchiectasis (chronically dilated bronchi). This form of disease is indolent and has been associated with significant morbidity and mortality. It has been postulated that this disease is seen primarily in fastidious elderly women who chronically suppress their cough reflex, leading to nonspecific inflammatory changes in the lungs and predisposing them to superinfection with MAC. This specific disease has been called **Lady Windermere syndrome** after the principal character in the Oscar Wilde play. The third form of MAC disease is formation of a **solitary pulmonary nodule**. *M. avium* complex is the most common mycobacterial species that causes solitary pulmonary nodules.

A new spectrum of disease developed in **patients with AIDS**, making infection with *M. avium* complex the most common mycobacterial disease in these patients in the United States. *M. tuberculosis* infections are more common than *M. avium* infections in continents such as Africa and Asia, where tuberculosis is highly endemic. In contrast to disease in other groups of patients, MAC infection in patients with AIDS is typically disseminated, with virtually no organ spared (Clinical Case 28-2). The magnitude of these infections is remarkable; the tissues of some patients are literally filled with the mycobacteria (Figure 28-9), and there are hundreds to thousands of bacteria per milliliter of blood. Overwhelming disseminated infections with *M. avium* are

Figure 28–9. Tissue from a patient with AIDS who is infected with *Mycobacterium avium* complex photographed under low (**A**) and high (**B**) magnification.

Clinical Case 28-2. *Mycobacterium avium* Infection in an AIDS Patient

Woods and Goldsmith (Chest 95:1355-1357, 1989) described a patient with advanced AIDS who died of disseminated *M. avium* infection. The patient was a 27-year-old man who initially presented in October 1985 with a 2-week history of progressive dyspnea and a nonproductive cough. *Pneumocystis* was detected in a bronchoalveolar lavage, and serology confirmed the patient had an HIV infection. The patient was successfully treated with trimethoprim-sulfamethoxazole and discharged. The patient remained stable until May 1987, when he presented with persistent fever and dyspnea. Over the next week, he developed severe substernal chest pain and a pericardial friction rub. Echocardiogram revealed a small effusion. The patient left the hospital against medical advice but returned a week later with a persistent cough, fever, and pain in the chest and left arm. A diagnostic pericardiocentesis was performed and 220 mL of fluid was aspirated. Tuberculous pericarditis was suspected, and appropriate antimycobacterial therapy was initiated. However, over the next 3 weeks the patient developed progressive cardiac failure and died. *M. avium* was recovered from the pericardial fluid, as well as autopsy cultures of the pericardium, spleen, liver, adrenal glands, kidneys, small intestine, lymph nodes, and pituitary gland. Although *M. avium* pericarditis was unusual, extensive dissemination of the mycobacteria in patients with advanced AIDS was common before azithromycin prophylaxis became widely used.

particularly common in patients who are in the terminal stages of their immune disorder, when their CD4+ T lymphocyte counts fall below 10 cells/mm^3. Fortunately, with more effective antiretroviral therapy and the routine use of prophylactic antibiotics, *M. avium* disease infections in HIV-infected patients have become much less common. Although some patients with AIDS develop *M. avium* disease after pulmonary exposure (e.g., infectious aerosols of contaminated water), most infections are believed to develop after ingestion of the bacteria. Person-to-person transmission has not been demonstrated. After exposure to the mycobacteria, replication is initiated in localized lymph nodes and followed by systemic spread. The clinical manifestations of disease are not observed until the mass of replicating bacteria impairs normal organ function.

Other Slow-Growing Mycobacteria

Many other slow-growing mycobacteria can cause human disease, and new species continue to be reported as better diagnostic test methods are developed. The spectrum of diseases produced by these mycobacteria also continues to expand, in large part because diseases such as AIDS, malignancies, and organ transplantation with concomitant use of immunosuppressive drugs have created a population of patients who are highly susceptible to organisms with relatively low virulence potential. Some mycobacteria produce disease identical to pulmonary tuberculosis (e.g., *Mycobacterium bovis, M. kansasii*), other species commonly cause infections localized to lymphatic tissue (*Mycobacterium scrofulaceum*), and others that grow optimally at cool temperatures primarily produce cutaneous infections (*Mycobacterium ulcerans, Mycobacterium marinum, Mycobacterium haemophilum*). However, disseminated disease can be observed in patients with AIDS who are infected with these same species, as well as with relatively uncommon mycobacteria (e.g., *Mycobacterium genavense, Mycobacterium simiae*).

Most of these mycobacteria have been isolated in water and soil and occasionally from infected animals (e.g., *M. bovis* causes bovine tuberculosis). Often the isolation of these mycobacteria in clinical specimens simply represents transient colonization with organisms that the patient ingested. With the exception of *M. bovis* and other mycobacteria closely related to *M. tuberculosis*, person-to-person spread of these mycobacteria does not occur.

Rapidly Growing Mycobacteria

As discussed previously, nontuberculous mycobacteria can be subdivided into slow-growing species and rapidly growing species (growth in less than 7 days). This distinction is important because the rapidly growing species have a relatively low virulence potential, stain irregularly with traditional mycobacterial stains, and are more susceptible to "conventional" antibacterial antibiotics than to drugs used to treat other mycobacterial infections. The most common species associated with disease are *M. fortuitum, M. chelonae*, and *M. abscessus*.

The rapidly growing mycobacteria rarely cause disseminated infections. Rather, they are most commonly associated with disease occurring after bacteria are introduced into the deep subcutaneous tissues by **trauma or iatrogenic infections** (e.g., infections associated with an intravenous catheter, contaminated wound dressing, prosthetic device such as a heart valve, peritoneal dialysis, or bronchoscopy). Unfortunately the incidence of infections with these organisms is increasing as more invasive procedures are performed in hospitalized patients, and advanced medical care lengthens the life expectancy of immunocompromised patients. Opportunistic infections in immunocompetent patients are becoming commonplace (Clinical Case 28-3).

Laboratory Diagnosis

The various laboratory tests used in the diagnosis of infections caused by mycobacteria are listed in Box 28-5.

Immunodiagnosis

The traditional test to assess the patient's response to exposure to *M. tuberculosis* is the **tuberculin skin test**. Reactivity to an intradermal injection of mycobacterial antigens can differentiate between infected and noninfected people, with a positive PPD reaction usually developing 3 to 4 weeks after exposure to *M. tuberculosis*. The only evidence of infection with mycobacteria in most patients is a lifelong

Box 28—5. Laboratory Diagnosis of Mycobacterial Disease

Immunodiagnosis

Tuberculin skin test
IFN-γ release assays

Microscopy

Ziehl-Neelsen (hot acid-fast) stain
Kinyoun (cold acid-fast) stain
Truant fluorochrome acid-fast stain

Nucleic-Acid-Based Tests

Nucleic acid amplification (NAA) tests

Culture

Agar- or egg-based media
Broth-based media

Identification

Morphologic properties
Biochemical reactions
Analysis of cell wall lipids
Nucleic acid probes
Nucleic acid sequencing

positive skin test reaction and radiographic evidence of calcification of granulomas in the lungs or other organs.

The methods of antigen preparation have been changed many times since the tests were first developed. The currently recommended tuberculin antigen is a **purified protein derivative** (**PPD**) from the mycobacterial cell wall. In this test, a specific amount of the antigen (5 tuberculin units of PPD) is inoculated into the intradermal layer of the patient's skin. Skin test reactivity (defined by the diameter of the area of induration) is measured 48 hours later. Patients infected with *M. tuberculosis* may not show a response to the tuberculin skin test if they are anergic (nonreactive to antigens; particularly true of HIV-infected patients); thus control antigens should always be used with tuberculin tests. Additionally, individuals from countries where vaccination with attenuated *M. bovis* (bacille Calmette-Guérin [**BCG**]) is widespread (refer to the discussion headed **Immunoprophylaxis** later in this chapter) will have a positive skin test reaction.

In recent years, **in vitro IFN-γ release assays** have been introduced as a sensitive, more specific alternative to the PPD skin test. The tests use immunoassays to measure IFN-γ produced by sensitized T cells stimulated by *M. tuberculosis* antigens. If an individual was previously infected with *M. tuberculosis*, exposure of sensitized T cells present in whole blood to *M. tuberculosis*-specific antigens results in IFN-γ production. The initial assays that used PPD as the stimulating antigen have been replaced with second-generation assays that use more specific antigens (i.e, early secreted antigenic target 6 [**ESAT-6**], culture filtrate protein 10 [**CFP-10**]). Although the tests are sensitive and highly specific, the technical complexity of the assays currently limit their use. However, further modifications of these assays that show potential have been introduced, and the IFN-γ release assays are likely to be promising alternatives to the PPD skin test.

Reactivity to **lepromin**, which is prepared from inactivated *M. leprae*, is valuable for confirming the clinical diagnosis of tuberculoid leprosy. Papular induration develop 3 to 4 days after the intradermal injection of the antigen. This test is not useful for identifying patients with lepromatous leprosy, because such patients are anergic to the antigen.

Microscopy

The microscopic detection of acid-fast bacteria in clinical specimens is the most rapid way to confirm mycobacterial disease. The clinical specimen is stained with carbolfuchsin (**Ziehl-Neelsen** or **Kinyoun** methods) or fluorescent auramine-rhodamine dyes (Truant **fluorochrome** method), decolorized with an acid-alcohol solution, and then counterstained. The specimens are examined with a light microscope or, if fluorescent dyes are used, a fluorescent microscope (Figure 28-10). The Truant fluorochrome method is the most sensitive method, because the specimen can be scanned rapidly under low magnification for

Figure 28–10. Acid-fast stains of *Mycobacterium tuberculosis*. **A,** Stained with carbolfuchsin using the Kinyoun method. **B,** Stained with the fluorescent dyes auramine and rhodamine using the Truant fluorochrome method.

fluorescent areas, and then the presence of acid-fast bacteria can be confirmed with higher magnification.

In approximately half of all culture-positive specimens, acid-fast bacteria are detected by microscopy. The sensitivity of this test is high for (1) respiratory specimens (particularly from patients with radiographic evidence of cavitation) and (2) specimens for which many mycobacteria are isolated in culture. Thus a positive acid-fast stain reaction corresponds to higher infectivity. The specificity of the test is greater than 95% when it is performed carefully.

Nucleic-Acid-Based Tests

Although microscopy provides useful information regarding the presence of mycobacterial disease, it cannot identify the particular mycobacterial species involved. For this reason, techniques have been developed to detect specific mycobacterial nucleic acid sequences present in clinical specimens. Because only a few bacteria may be present, commercial companies have developed a variety of nucleic acid amplification techniques (e.g., polymerase chain reaction). The commercial assays currently used are specific for *M. tuberculosis* but are relatively insensitive. Additionally, the assays cannot be used to identify nontuberculous mycobacteria. Recently a gene encoding a secretory protein,

*Sec*A **gene**, has been demonstrated to be a useful target for directly identifying all species of mycobacteria in clinical specimens. The gene can be amplified by PCR and then the species-specific portion of the gene sequenced to determine the identity of the isolate. The test is highly sensitive and specific with acid-fast smear-positive specimens but is relatively insensitive in smear-negative specimens. With further refinements, however, these procedures will most likely prove to be useful diagnostic tools.

Culture

Mycobacteria that cause pulmonary disease, particularly in patients with evidence of cavitation, are abundant in the respiratory secretions (e.g., 10^8 bacilli per ml or more). Recovery of the organisms is virtually assured in patients from whom early morning respiratory specimens are collected for 3 consecutive days. However, it is more difficult to isolate *M. tuberculosis* and NTM species from other sites in patients with disseminated disease (e.g., genitourinary tract, tissues, cerebrospinal fluid). In such cases, additional specimens must be collected for cultures, and a large volume of fluid or tissue must be processed.

The in vitro growth of mycobacteria is complicated by the fact that most isolates grow slowly and can be obscured by the rapidly growing bacteria that normally colonize people. Thus specimens such as sputum are initially treated with a **decontaminating reagent** (e.g., 2% sodium hydroxide) to remove organisms that could confound results. Mycobacteria can tolerate brief alkali treatment, which kills the rapidly growing bacteria and permits the selective isolation of mycobacteria. Extended decontamination of the specimen kills mycobacteria, so the procedure is not performed when normally sterile specimens are being tested or when few mycobacteria are expected.

Formerly when specimens were inoculated onto egg-based (e.g., **Löwenstein-Jensen**) and agar-based (e.g., **Middlebrook**) media, it generally took a long time for *M. tuberculosis*, *M. avium* complex, and other important slow-growing mycobacteria to be detected. However, this time has been shortened through the use of specially formulated **broth cultures** that support the rapid growth of most mycobacteria. Thus the average time to grow mycobacteria has been decreased from 3 to 4 weeks to 10 to 14 days.

The ability of *M. tuberculosis* to grow rapidly in broth cultures has been used for performing rapid susceptibility tests. The technique, **MODS or microscopic observation drug susceptibility assay**, uses an inverted light microscope to examine 24-well plates inoculated with Middlebrook broth and decontaminated sputum. *M. tuberculosis* growth can generally be detected as tangles or cords of growth in the broth after a week of incubation. Incorporation of antimycobacterial drugs in the broth enables rapid, direct susceptibility testing with clinical specimens. This technique is widely available in laboratories servicing developing

countries where drug resistant strains of *M. tuberculosis* are widespread.

Some mycobacterial species (e.g., *M. marinum*, *M. haemophilum*, *M. malmoense*) require a lower **incubation temperature** than what is used for most cultures (30° C versus 37° C). Additionally, *M. haemophilum* requires supplementation of media with hemin or ferric ammonium citrate for growth. Because infections with these organisms characteristically involve the skin, most laboratories will culture superficial specimens (e.g., skin biopsies and lesions) at both 30° C and 37° C and on at least one medium supplemented with hemin.

Identification

Growth properties and colonial morphology can be used for the preliminary identification of the most common species of mycobacteria. The definitive identificazid of mycobacteria can made using a variety of techniques. Biochemical tests were the standard method for identifying mycobacteria, but because results are not available for at least 3 weeks or more, most laboratories do not rely on these tests. Mycobacterial species can also be identified through chromatographic analysis of their characteristic cell wall lipids. However, **species-specific molecular probes** are the most useful means of identifying commonly isolated mycobacteria (e.g., *M. tuberculosis*, *M. avium*, *M. kansasii*). Because many organisms are present after in vitro cultivation, it is not necessary to amplify the target genomic sequence. The commercially prepared probe identification systems currently used are rapid (test time, 2 hours), sensitive, and specific. Mycobacterial species for which probes are not available can be identified by amplifying species-specific gene sequences (e.g., hypervariable regions of the 16S rRNA gene or *Sec*A gene), followed by sequence analysis to identify the species. This method is rapid (1 to 2 days), is not limited by the availability of specific probes, and is likely to replace the alternative identification methods.

Treatment, Prevention, and Control

Treatment

The treatment and prophylaxis of mycobacterial infections, unlike those for most other bacterial infections, are complex and controversial. Slow-growing mycobacteria are resistant to most antibiotics used to treat other bacterial infections. In general, patients must take multiple antibiotics for an extended period (e.g., a minimum of 6 to 9 months), or antibiotic-resistant strains will develop. In 1990, the first outbreaks of **multidrug-resistant *M. tuberculosis*** (**MDR-TB**; resistant to at least isoniazid and rifampin) were observed in patients with AIDS and in homeless persons in New York City and Miami. Although these strains are relatively uncommon in the United States, they are dramatically increasing in prevalence in developing countries. Additionally, new strains of resistant *M. tuberculosis*, called **extensively drug-resistant (XDR) TB**, have emerged in every region of the world. These strains, defined as MDR-TB resistant to fluoroquinolones and at least one of the second line drugs (e.g., kanamycin, amikacin, capreomycin), are potentially untreatable.

The number of treatment regimens that have been developed for drug-susceptible and drug-resistant tuberculosis is too complex to comprehensively review here (refer to the CDC website, http://www.cdc.gov/tb/). Most treatment regimens begin with 2 months of isoniazid (INH), ethambutol, pyrazinamide, and rifampin, followed by 4 to 6 months of INH and rifampin or alternative combination drugs. Modifications to this treatment scheme are dictated by the drug susceptibility of the isolate and the patient population.

In the last decade, treatment of leprosy has successfully reduced the overall incidence of disease. The treatment regimens advanced by the WHO (http://WHO.int/lep) have distinguished between patients with the tuberculoid (paucibacillary) form and the lepromatous (multibacillary) form. The paucibacillary form should be treated with rifampicin and dapsone for a minimum of 6 months, whereas the multibacillary form should have clofazimine added to the regimen, and treatment should be extended to 12 months. It should be noted that many investigators believe much longer therapy is required for optimum management of patients. Single-drug treatment should not be used for either form.

M. avium complex and many other slow-growing mycobacteria are resistant to common antimycobacterial agents. One regimen currently recommended for MAC infections is clarithromycin or azithromycin, combined with ethambutol and rifampin. The American Thoracic Society has recommended that *M. kansasii* infections be treated with INH, rifampin, and ethambutol. The duration of treatment and final selection of drugs for these species and other slow-growing mycobacteria are determined by (1) the response to therapy and (2) interactions among these drugs and other drugs the patient is receiving (e.g., toxic and pharmacokinetic interactions of these drugs with protease inhibitors used to treat HIV infection). Refer to the publication by Griffith, et al. cited in the bibliography for additional information about treating NTM infections.

Unlike the slow-growing mycobacteria, the rapidly growing species are resistant to most commonly used antimycobacterial agents but are susceptible to antibiotics such as clarithromycin, imipenem, amikacin, cefoxitin, and the sulfonamides. The specific activity of these agents must be determined with in vitro tests. Because infections with these mycobacteria are generally confined to the skin or are associated with prosthetic devices, surgical debridement or removal of the prosthesis is also necessary.

Chemoprophylaxis

The American Thoracic Society and the Centers for Disease Control and Prevention have examined a number of prophylactic regimens for use in patients (HIV positive and HIV negative) exposed to *M. tuberculosis*. The regimens that have been recommended include daily or twice weekly INH for 6 to 9 months or daily rifampin for 4 months. Patients who have been exposed to drug-resistant *M. tuberculosis* should receive prophylaxis with pyrazinamide and either ethambutol or levofloxacin for 6 to 12 months. Because *M. avium* complex intracellulare infections are common in patients with AIDS, chemoprophylaxis is recommended for patients whose CD4+ T cell counts fall to less than 50 cells/μL. Prophylaxis with clarithromycin or azithromycin is recommended. Combinations of these drugs with rifabutin have been used, but they are generally more toxic and no more effective than the single agent. Chemoprophylaxis is unnecessary for patients with other mycobacterial infections.

Immunoprophylaxis

Vaccination with attenuated *M. bovis* BCG is commonly used in countries where tuberculosis is endemic and responsible for significant morbidity and mortality. This practice can lead to a significant reduction in the incidence of tuberculosis if BCG is administered to people when they are young (it is less effective in adults). Unfortunately, BCG immunization cannot be used in immunocompromised patients (e.g., those with HIV infection). Thus it is unlikely to be useful in countries with a high prevalence of HIV infections (e.g., Africa) or to control the spread of drug-resistant tuberculosis. An additional problem with BCG immunization is that positive skin test reactivity develops in all patients and may persist for a prolonged time. However, skin test reactivity is generally low, so a strongly reactive skin test (e.g., >20 mm of induration) is generally significant. The IFN-γ release assays are not affected by BCG immunization, so they can be used for screening this population. BCG immunization is not widely used in the United States or in other countries where the incidence of tuberculosis is low.

Control

Because a third of the world's population is infected with *M. tuberculosis*, the elimination of this disease is highly unlikely. Disease can be controlled, however, with a combination of active surveillance, prophylactic and therapeutic intervention, and careful case monitoring.

Case Study and Questions

A 35-year-old man with a history of intravenous drug use entered the local health clinic with complaints of a dry persistent cough, fever, malaise, and anorexia. Over the preceding 4 weeks, he had lost 15 pounds and experienced chills and sweats. A chest radiograph revealed patchy infiltrates throughout the lung fields. Because the patient had a nonproductive cough, sputum was induced and submitted for bacterial, fungal, and mycobacterial cultures, as well as examination for *Pneumocystis* organisms. Blood cultures and serologic tests for HIV infection were performed. The patient was found to be HIV positive. The results of all cultures were negative after 2 days of incubation; however, cultures were positive for *M. tuberculosis* after an additional week of incubation.

1. What is unique about the cell wall of mycobacteria, and what biologic effects can be attributed to the cell wall structure?

2. Why is *M. tuberculosis* more virulent in patients with HIV infection than in non-HIV-infected patients?

3. What is the definition of a positive skin test (PPD) result for *M. tuberculosis*?

4. What are the two clinical presentations of *M. leprae* infections? How do the diagnostic tests differ for these two presentations?

5. Why do mycobacterial infections have to be treated with multiple drugs for 6 months or more?

Bibliography

Appelberg R: Pathogenesis of *Mycobacterium avium* infection. Immunol Res 35:179-190, 2006.

Bottasso O, et al: The immuno-endocrine component in the pathogenesis of tuberculosis. Scan J Immunol 66:166-175, 2007.

Centers for Disease Control and Prevention: Guidelines for preventing opportunistic infections among HIV-infected persons—2002 recommendations of the U.S. Public Health Service and the Infectious Diseases Society of America. Morb Mortal Wkly Rep (MMWR) 51 (No. RR-8):1-53, 2002.

De Groote M, Huitt G: Infections due to rapidly growing mycobacteria. Clin Infect Dis 42:1756-1763, 2006.

Drobniewski F, et al: Antimicrobial susceptibility testing of *Mycobacterium tuberculosis*. Clin Microbiol Infect 13:1144-1156, 2007.

Flynn JL, Chan J: Immune evasion by *Mycobacterium tuberculosis*: Living with the enemy. Curr Opin Immunol 15:450-455, 2003.

Griffith D, et al: An official ATS/IDSA statement: Diagnosis, treatment, and prevention of nontuberculous mycobacterial diseases. Am J Respir Crit Care Med 175:367-416, 2007.

Jacobson K, et al: *Mycobacterium kansasii* infections in patients with cancer. Clin Infect Dis 30:965-969, 2000.

Karakousis PC, Bishai WR, Dorman SE. Microreview: *Mycobacterium tuberculosis* cell envelope lipids and the host immune response. Cell Microbiol 6:105-116, 2004.

Shah MK, et al: *Mycobacterium haemophilum* in immunocompromised patients. Clin Infect Dis 33:330-337, 2001.

Smith I: *Mycobacterium tuberculosis* pathogenesis and molecular determinants of virulence. Clin Microbiol Rev 16:463-496, 2003.

Turenne C, et al: *Mycobacterium avium* in the postgenomic era. Clin Microbiol Rev 20:205-229, 2007.

Ulrichs T, Kaufmann S: New insights into the function of granulomas in human tuberculosis. J Pathol 208:261-269, 2006.

Wells C, et al: HIV infection and multidrug-resistant tuberculosis—the perfect storm. J Infect Dis 196:S86-S107, 2007.

Yew W, Leung C: Update in tuberculosis 2006. Am J Respir Crit Care Med 175:541-546, 2007.

Neisseria and Related Bacteria

The three genera of medically important bacteria that are in the family Neisseriaceae are **Neisseria**, **Eikenella**, and **Kingella** (Box 29-1). Other genera in the family are rarely associated with human disease and will not be discussed in this chapter. The genus *Neisseria* consists of 10 species found in humans with two species, **Neisseria gonorrhoeae** and **Neisseria meningitidis**, strictly human pathogens. The remaining species are commonly present on mucosal surfaces of the oropharynx and nasopharynx and occasionally colonize the anogenital mucosal membranes. Although diseases caused by *N. gonorrhoeae* and *N. meningitidis* are well known, the other *Neisseria* species have limited virulence and generally produce disease only in compromised patients. **Eikenella corrodens** and **Kingella kingae** colonize the human oropharynx and are opportunistic pathogens.

Neisseria gonorrhoeae and *Neisseria meningitidis* (Boxes 29-2 and 29-3)

Infection with *N. gonorrhoeae* has been recognized for centuries. Despite effective antibiotic therapy, gonorrhea is still one of the most common sexually transmitted diseases in the United States. *N. gonorrhoeae* is always considered a pathogen. *N. meningitidis* is a paradox. This bacterium commonly colonizes the nasopharynx of healthy people. However, it is also the second most common cause of community-acquired meningitis in adults, can cause overwhelming and rapidly fatal sepsis, and can cause bronchopneumonia in patients with underlying pulmonary disease. The swift progression from good health to life-threatening disease can cause fear and panic in a community unlike the reaction to almost any other pathogen.

Physiology and Structure

Neisseria species are aerobic, **gram-negative** bacteria, typically coccoid shaped (0.6 to 1.0 μm in diameter) and arranged in pairs (**diplococci**) with adjacent sides flattened together (resembling coffee beans; Figure 29-1). The bacteria are not motile and do not form endospores. All species are oxidase positive, and most produce catalase—properties that combined with the Gram-stain morphology allow for a rapid, presumptive identification of a clinical isolate. Acid is produced by oxidation of carbohydrates (not by fermentation). *N. gonorrhoeae* strains produce acid by oxidizing glucose, and *N. meningitidis* strains oxidize both glucose and maltose. Other carbohydrates are not oxidized. This pattern of carbohydrate utilization is useful for differentiating these pathogenic strains from other *Neisseria* species.

Nonpathogenic species of *Neisseria* can grow on nutrient agar incubated at 35° C to 37° C. In contrast, *N. meningitidis* has variable growth on nutrient agar, and *N. gonorrhoeae* is a fastidious organism, **requiring complex media** for growth; it is adversely affected by exposure to dry conditions or fatty acids. All strains of *N. gonorrhoeae* require cystine and an energy source (e.g., glucose, pyruvate, and lactate) for growth, and many strains require supplementation of media with amino acids, purines, pyrimidines, and vitamins. Soluble starch is added to the media to neutralize the toxic effect of the fatty acids. Thus *N. gonorrhoeae* does not grow on blood agar but does grow on **chocolate agar** and other enriched supplemented media. The optimum growth temperature is **35° C to 37° C**, with poor survival of the organism at cooler temperatures. A humid atmosphere supplemented with **5% carbon dioxide (CO_2)** is either required or enhances growth of *N. gonorrhoeae*. Although the fastidious nature of this organism makes recovery from clinical specimens difficult, it is nevertheless easy for the organism to be transmitted sexually from person to person.

The structure of *N. gonorrhoeae* and *N. meningitidis* is typical of gram-negative bacteria, with the thin peptidoglycan layer sandwiched between the inner cytoplasmic membrane and the outer membrane. The major virulence factor for *N. meningitidis* is the polysaccharide capsule. Although the outer surface of *N. gonorrhoeae* is not covered with a true carbohydrate capsule, the cell surface of *N. gonorrhoeae* has a capsule-like negative charge. Antigenic differences in the

Box 29–1. Important Neisseriaceae

Organism	Historical Derivation
Neisseria	Named after the German physician Albert *Neisser*, who originally described the organism responsible for gonorrhea
N. gonorrhoeae	*gone*, "seed"; *rhoia*, a "flow" (a flow of seeds; reference to the disease gonorrhea)
N. meningitidis	*meningis*, the covering of the brain; *itis*, "inflammation" (inflammation of the meninges as in meningitis)
Eikenella	Named after M. *Eiken*, who first named the type species in this genus
E. corrodens	*corrodens*, "gnawing" or "eating" (reference to the observation that colonies of this species eat into the agar)
Kingella	Named after the American bacteriologist Elizabeth *King*

Box 29–2. Summary: *Neisseria gonorrhoeae*

Biology, Virulence, and Disease

Gram-negative diplococci with fastidious growth requirements
Growth best at 35° C to 37° C in a humid atmosphere supplemented with CO_2
Oxidase and catalase positive; acid produced from glucose oxidatively
Outer surface with multiple antigens: pili protein; Por proteins; Opa proteins; Rmp protein; protein receptors for transferrin, lactoferrin, and hemoglobin; lipooligosaccharide; immunoglobulin protease; β-lactamase
Refer to Table 29-1 for summary of virulence factors
Refer to Box 29-4 for summary of clinical diseases

Epidemiology

Humans are the only natural hosts
Carriage can be asymptomatic, particularly in women
Transmission is primarily by sexual contact
Almost 360,000 cases reported in United States in 2006 (true incidence of disease believed to be at least twice that)
Disease most common in blacks, people ages 15 to 24 years, residents of southeastern United States, people who have multiple sexual encounters
Higher risk of disseminated disease in patients with deficiencies in late components of complement

Diagnosis

Gram stain of urethral specimens is accurate for symptomatic males only
Culture is sensitive and specific but has been replaced with nucleic acid amplification assays in most laboratories

Treatment, Prevention, and Control

Ceftriaxone is currently the treatment of choice
Doxycycline or azithromycin should be added for infections complicated by *Chlamydia*
For neonates, prophylaxis with 1% silver nitrate; ophthalmia neonatorum is treated with ceftriaxone
Prevention consists of patient education, use of condoms or spermicides with nonoxynol-9 (only partially effective), and aggressive follow-up of sexual partners of infected patients
Effective vaccines are not available

polysaccharide capsule of *N. meningitidis* are the basis for serogrouping these bacteria. Thirteen serogroups are currently recognized (A, B, C, D, H, I, K, L, W-135, X, Y, Z, 29E), with most infections caused by serogroups A, B, C, Y, and W135.

Pathogenic and nonpathogenic strains of *Neisseria* have **pili** that extend from the cytoplasmic membrane through the outer membrane. Pili mediate a number of functions, including attachment to host cells, transfer of genetic material, and motility, and the presence of pili in *N. gonorrhoeae* and *N. meningitidis* appears to be important for pathogenesis. The pili are composed of repeating protein subunits (**pilins**), whose expression is controlled by the *pil* gene complex. Pili expression is associated with virulence, in part because the pili mediate attachment to nonciliated epithelial cells and provide resistance to killing by neutrophils. Pilin proteins have a conserved region at the amino terminal end and a highly variable region at the exposed carboxyl terminus. The carboxyl terminal portion of the pilin protein can be phosphorylated and glycosylated and is associated with a second protein, **PilC**, which contributes to its antigenic diversity. The lack of immunity to reinfection with *N. gonorrhoeae* results partially from the antigenic variation among the pilin proteins and partially from the phase variation in pilin expression; these factors complicate attempts to develop effective vaccines for gonorrhea.

Other prominent families of proteins are present in the outer membrane. The **porin proteins** are integral outer membrane proteins that form pores or channels for nutrients to pass into the cell and waste products to exit. *N. gonorrhoeae* and *N. meningitidis* have two porin genes, *porA* and *porB*. The gene products, **PorA and PorB proteins**, are both expressed in *N. meningitidis*, but the *porA* gene is silent in *N. gonorrhoeae*. Thus, not only is PorB the major outer membrane protein in *N. gonorrhoeae* (an estimated 60% of the gonococcal outer membrane proteins), but it must also be functionally active for *N. gonorrhoeae* to survive. PorB is expressed as two distinct classes of antigens, PIA and PIB, with many distinct serovars. The antigenic differences in the PorB protein are determined by differences in the exposed surface of the protein. Thus although the PorB protein is expressed in all gonococci, the large number of antigens

29

Summary: *Neisseria meningitidis*

Biology, Virulence, and Disease

Gram-negative diplococci with fastidious growth requirements

Grows best at 35° C to 37° C in a humid atmosphere

Oxidase and catalase positive; acid produced from glucose and maltose oxidatively

Outer surface antigens include polysaccharide capsule, pili, and lipooligosaccharide (LOS)

Capsule protects bacteria from antibody-mediated phagocytosis

Specific receptors for meningococcal pili allow colonization of nasopharynx

Bacteria can survive intracellular killing in the absence of humoral immunity

Endotoxin mediates most clinical manifestations

Refer to Box 29-4 for summary of clinical diseases

Epidemiology

Humans are the only natural hosts

Person-to-person spread occurs via aerosolization of respiratory tract secretions

Highest incidence of disease is in children younger than 5 years, institutionalized people, and patients with late complement deficiencies

Meningitis and meningococcemia most commonly caused by serogroups B, C, and Y; pneumonia most commonly caused by serogroups Y and W135; serogroups A and W135 associated with disease in underdeveloped countries

Disease occurs worldwide, most commonly in the dry, cold months of the year

Diagnosis

Gram stain of cerebrospinal fluid is sensitive and specific but is of limited value for blood specimens (too few organisms are generally present, except in overwhelming sepsis)

Culture is definitive, but organism is fastidious and dies rapidly when exposed to cold or dry conditions

Tests to detect meningococcal antigens are insensitive and nonspecific

Treatment, Prevention, and Control

Breast-fed infants have passive immunity (first 6 months)

Treatment is with penicillin (drug of choice)

Chemoprophylaxis for contact with persons with the disease is with rifampin, ciprofloxacin, or ceftriaxone

For immunoprophylaxis, vaccination is an adjunct to chemoprophylaxis; it is used only for serogroups A, C, Y, and W135; no effective vaccine is available for serogroup B

Figure 29—1. *Neisseria gonorrhoeae* in urethral exudate. Note the spatial arrangement of the pairs of cocci, with sides pressed together, which is characteristic of this genus.

Opa proteins (opacity proteins) are a family of membrane proteins that mediate intimate binding to epithelial and phagocytic cells and are important for cell-to-cell signaling. Multiple alleles of these proteins can be expressed by an individual isolate. *N. gonorrhoeae* expressing the Opa proteins appear opaque (versus transparent) when grown in culture. Expression of these proteins is **associated with clinical disease**. Opaque colonies are recovered most commonly in patients with localized disease (i.e., endocervicitis, urethritis, pharyngitis, proctitis), and transparent colonies are most commonly associated with pelvic inflammatory disease and disseminated infections.

The third group of proteins in the outer membrane is the highly conserved **Rmp proteins** (reduction-modifiable proteins). These proteins stimulate antibodies that **block serum bactericidal activity** against pathogenic neisseriae.

Iron is essential for the growth and metabolism of *N. gonorrhoeae* and *N. meningitidis*. These pathogenic neisseriae are able to complete with their human hosts for iron by **binding host cell transferrin** to specific bacterial surface receptors. The specificity of this binding for human transferrin is likely the reason these bacteria are strict human pathogens. The presence of this receptor is fundamentally different from most bacteria that synthesize siderophores to scavenge iron. The gonococci also have a variety of additional surface receptors for other host iron complexes, such as lactoferrin and hemoglobin.

Another major antigen in the cell wall is **lipooligosaccharide (LOS)**. This antigen is composed of lipid A and a core oligosaccharide but lacks the O-antigen polysaccharide found in lipopolysaccharide (LPS) in most gram-negative rods. The lipid A moiety possesses endotoxin activity. Both *N. gonorrhoeae* and *N. meningitidis* spontaneously **release outer membrane blebs** during rapid cell growth. These blebs contain LOS and surface proteins and may act

and antigenic variation of this protein makes it a **poor target for vaccine development**.

PorB is important for the virulence of *N. gonorrhoeae*. Purified PorB proteins can **interfere with degranulation of neutrophils** (i.e., phagolysosome fusion that would lead to killing of intracellular bacteria) and presumably protect the bacteria from the host's inflammatory response. Additionally, PorB with other adhesins **facilitates the bacterial invasion into epithelial cells**. Finally, expression of PIA PorB antigens makes the bacteria **resistant to complement-mediated serum killing**.

to both enhance endotoxin-mediated toxicity and protect replicating bacteria by binding protein-directed antibodies.

N. gonorrhoeae and *N. meningitidis* produce **immuno-globulin (Ig) A1 protease**, which cleaves the hinge region in IgA1. This action creates immunologically inactive Fc and Fab fragments. Some strains of *N. gonorrhoeae* also produce β-lactamases that can degrade penicillin.

Pathogenesis and Immunity (Table 29-1)

Gonococci attach to mucosal cells, penetrate into the cells and multiply, and then pass through the cells into the subepithelial space, where infection is established. Pili, PorB, and Opa proteins mediate attachment and penetration into host cells. The gonococcal LOS stimulates release of the proinflammatory cytokine, **tumor necrosis factor-α (TNF-α)**, which causes most of the symptoms associated with gonococcal disease.

IgG_3 is the predominant IgG antibody formed in response to gonococcal infection. Although the antibody response to PorB is minimal, serum antibodies to pilin,

Opa protein, and LOS are readily detected. Antibodies to LOS can activate complement, releasing complement component C5a, which has a chemotactic effect on neutrophils; however, IgG and secretory IgA1 antibodies directed against Rmp protein can block this bactericidal antibody response. Experiments with nasopharyngeal tissue organ cultures have shown that meningococci attach selectively to specific receptors for meningococcal pili on nonciliated columnar cells of the nasopharynx. Meningococci without pili are less able to bind to these cells.

Meningococcal disease occurs in the absence of specific antibodies directed against the polysaccharide capsule and other expressed bacterial antigens. Infants are initially afforded protection by the passive transfer of maternal antibodies. When the infant has reached age 6 months, however, this protective immunity has waned, a finding that is consistent with the observation that the incidence of disease is greatest in children younger than 2 years. Immunity can be stimulated by colonization with *N. meningitidis* or other bacteria with cross-reactive antigens (e.g., colonization with nonencapsulated *Neisseria* species; exposure to *Escherichia coli* K1 antigen, which cross-reacts with the group B capsular polysaccharide). Bactericidal activity also requires the existence of complement. Patients with **deficiencies in C5, C6, C7, or C8 of the complement system** are estimated to be at a 6000-fold greater risk for meningococcal disease. Although immunity is mediated primarily by the humoral immune response, lymphocyte responsiveness to meningococcal antigens is markedly depressed in patients with acute disease.

Like *N. gonorrhoeae*, meningococci are internalized into phagocytic vacuoles and are able to avoid intracellular death, replicate, and then migrate to the subepithelial spaces. The antiphagocytic properties of the polysaccharide capsule protect *N. meningitidis* from phagocytic destruction. The diffuse vascular damage associated with meningococcal infections (e.g., endothelial damage, inflammation of vessel walls, thrombosis, and disseminated intravascular coagulation) is largely attributed to the action of the **LOS endotoxin** present in the outer membrane.

Epidemiology

Gonorrhea occurs naturally only in humans; it has no other known reservoir. It is second only to chlamydia as the most commonly reported sexually transmitted disease in the United States. Infection rates are the same in males and females, are disproportionately higher in blacks than in Hispanic Americans and whites, and are highest in the southeastern United States. The peak incidence of the disease is in the age group 15 to 24 years. The incidence of disease decreased from 1978 to 1997; however, between 1998 and 2006, the incidence of gonorrhea has remained relatively constant. In 2006, almost 360,000 new infections were reported in the United States. However, even this large number is an underestimation of the true incidence

Table 29–1. Virulence Factors *in Neisseria gonorrhoeae*

Virulence Factor	Biologic Effect
Pilin	Protein that mediates initial attachment to nonciliated human cells (e.g., epithelium of vagina, fallopian tube, and buccal cavity); interferes with neutrophil killing
Por protein (protein I)	Porin protein: promotes intracellular survival by preventing phagolysosome fusion in neutrophils
Opa protein (protein II)	Opacity protein: mediates firm attachment to eukaryotic cells
Rmp protein (protein III)	Reduction-modifiable protein: protects other surface antigens (Por protein, LOS) from bactericidal antibodies
Transferrin-binding proteins	Mediate acquisition of iron for bacterial metabolism
Lactoferrin-binding proteins	Mediate acquisition of iron for bacterial metabolism
Hemoglobin-binding proteins	Mediate acquisition of iron for bacterial metabolism
LOS	Lipooligosaccharide: has endotoxin activity
IgA1 protease	Destroys immunoglobulin A1 (role in virulence is unknown)
β-Lactamase	Hydrolyzes the β-lactam ring in penicillin

of disease because the diagnosis and reporting of gonococcal infections are incomplete. Public health officials believe that at least half of the new infections are not reported.

N. gonorrhoeae is **transmitted primarily by sexual contact**. Women have a 50% risk of acquiring the infection as the result of a single exposure to an infected man, whereas men have a risk of approximately 20% as the result of a single exposure to an infected woman. The risk of infection rises as the person has more sexual encounters with infected partners.

The major reservoir for gonococci is the asymptomatically infected person. **Asymptomatic carriage is more common in women than in men**. As many as half of all infected women have mild or asymptomatic infections, whereas most men are initially symptomatic. The symptoms generally clear within a few weeks in people with untreated disease, and asymptomatic carriage may then become established. The site of infection also determines whether carriage occurs, with rectal and pharyngeal infections more commonly asymptomatic than genital infections.

Endemic meningococcal disease occurs worldwide, and epidemics are common in developing countries. Epidemic spread of disease results from the introduction of a new, virulent strain into an immunologically naïve population. Pandemics of disease have been uncommon in developed countries since World War II. Of the 13 serogroups, almost all infections are caused by serogroups A, B, C, Y, and W135. In Europe and the Americas, serogroups B, C, and Y predominate in meningitis or meningococcemia; serogroups A and W135 predominate in developing countries. Serogroups Y and W135 are most commonly associated with meningococcal pneumonia. *N. meningitidis* is **transmitted by respiratory droplets** among people in prolonged close contact, such as family members living in the same household and soldiers living together in military barracks. Classmates in schools and hospital employees are not considered close contacts and are not at significantly higher risk of acquiring the disease, unless they are in direct contact with the respiratory secretions of an infected person.

Humans are the only natural carriers for *N. meningitidis*. Studies of the asymptomatic carriage of *N. meningitidis* have shown that there is a tremendous variation in its prevalence, from less than 1% to almost 40%. The oral and nasopharyngeal carriage rates are highest for school-age children and young adults, are higher in lower socioeconomic populations (caused by person-to-person spread in crowded areas), and do not vary with the seasons, even though **disease is most common during the dry, cold months** of the year. Carriage is typically transient, with clearance occurring after specific antibodies develop. Endemic disease is most common in children younger than 5 years, particularly infants, and teenagers and young adults. People who are immunocompromised, the elderly, or those who live in closed populations (e.g., military barracks, prisons) are prone to infection during epidemics.

Neisseria gonorrhoeae

Clinical Diseases (Box 29-4)

Gonorrhea

Genital infection in men is primarily restricted to the **urethra**. A purulent urethral discharge (Figure 29-2) and dysuria develop after a 2- to 5-day incubation period. Approximately 95% of all infected men have acute symptoms. Although complications are rare, epididymitis, prostatitis, and periurethral abscesses may occur. The primary site of infection in women is the cervix, because the bacteria **infect the endocervical columnar epithelial cells**. The organism cannot infect the squamous epithelial cells that line the vagina of postpubescent women. Symptomatic patients commonly experience vaginal discharge, dysuria, and abdominal pain. Ascending genital infections, including salpingitis, tubo-ovarian abscesses, and pelvic inflammatory disease, are observed in 10% to 20% of women.

Gonococcemia (Clinical Case 29-1)

Disseminated infections with **septicemia and infection of skin and joints** occur in 1% to 3% of infected women and in a much lower percentage of infected men. The greater

---

Box 29—4. Neisseriaceae: Clinical Summaries

Neisseria gonorrhoeae

Gonorrhea: characterized by purulent discharge for involved site (e.g., urethra, cervix, epididymis, prostate, anus) after 2- to 5-day incubation period
Disseminated infections: spread of infection from genitourinary tract through blood to skin or joints; characterized by pustular rash with erythematous base and suppurative arthritis in involved joints
Ophthalmia neonatorum: purulent ocular infection acquired by neonate at birth

Neisseria meningitidis

Meningitis: purulent inflammation of meninges associated with headache, meningeal signs, and fever; high mortality rate unless promptly treated with effective antibiotics
Meningococcemia: disseminated infection characterized by thrombosis of small blood vessels and multiorgan involvement; small, petechial skin lesions coalesce into larger hemorrhagic lesions
Pneumonia: milder form of meningococcal disease characterized by bronchopneumonia in patients with underlying pulmonary disease

Eikenella corrodens

Human bite wounds: infection associated with traumatic (e.g., bite, fistfight injury) introduction of oral organisms into deep tissue
Subacute endocarditis: infection of endocardium characterized by gradual onset of low grade fevers, night sweats, and chills

Kingella kingae

Subacute endocarditis: as with *E. corrodens*

Figure 29–2. Purulent urethral discharge in man with urethritis. *(From Morse S, et al: Atlas of Sexually Transmitted Diseases and AIDS, 3rd ed. St Louis, Mosby, 2003.)*

Figure 29–3. Skin lesions of disseminated gonococcal infection. Classic large lesions with a necrotic, grayish central lesion on an erythematous base. *(From Morse S, et al: Atlas of Sexually Transmitted Diseases and AIDS, 3rd ed. St Louis, Mosby, 2003.)*

proportion of disseminated infections in women is caused by the numerous untreated asymptomatic infections in this population. The clinical manifestations of disseminated disease include fever; migratory arthralgias; suppurative arthritis in the wrists, knees, and ankles; and a pustular rash on an erythematous base (Figure 29-3) over the extremities but not on the head and trunk. *N. gonorrhoeae* is **a leading cause of purulent arthritis in adults.**

Other *N. gonorrhoeae* Syndromes

Other diseases associated with *N. gonorrhoeae* are perihepatitis (**Fitz-Hugh–Curtis syndrome**); purulent conjunctivitis (Figure 29-4), particularly in newborns infected during vaginal delivery (ophthalmia neonatorum); anorectal gonorrhea in homosexual men; and pharyngitis.

Clinical Case 29-1. Gonococcal Arthritis

Gonococcal arthritis is a common presentation of disseminated *Neisseria gonorrhoeae* infection. Fam, et al. (Can Med Assoc J 108:319-325, 1973) described six patients with this disease, including the following patient who has a typical presentation. A 17-year-old girl was admitted to the hospital with a 4-day history of fever, chills, malaise, sore throat, skin rash, and polyarthralgia. She reported being sexually active and a 5-week history of a profuse yellowish vaginal discharge, which was untreated. Upon presentation, she had erythematous maculopapular skin lesions over her forearm, thigh, and ankle, and her metacarpophalangeal joint, wrist, knee, ankle, and midtarsal joints were acutely inflamed. She had an elevated leukocyte count and sedimentation rate. Cultures of her cervix were positive for *N. gonorrhoeae*, but blood specimens, exudates for the skin lesions, and synovial fluid were all sterile. The diagnosis of disseminated gonorrhea with polyarthritis was made, and she was successfully treated with penicillin G for 2 weeks. This case illustrates the limitations of culture in disseminated infections and the value of a careful history.

Neisseria meningitidis

Clinical Diseases (see Box 29-4)

Meningitis

A total of 1245 cases of meningococcal disease (approximately 0.4 cases per 100,000 population) were reported in the United States in 2005. Most of these infections were meningitis. The disease usually begins abruptly with headache, meningeal signs, and fever. However, very young children may have only nonspecific signs such as fever and vomiting. Mortality approaches 100% in untreated patients but is less than 10% in patients in whom appropriate antibiotic therapy is instituted promptly. The incidence of neurologic sequelae is low, with hearing deficits and arthritis most commonly reported.

Figure 29–4. Gonococcal ophthalmia neonatorum. Lid edema, erythema, and marked purulent discharge are seen. A Gram-stained smear would reveal abundant organisms and inflammatory cells. *(From Morse S, et al: Atlas of Sexually Transmitted Diseases and AIDS, 3rd ed. St Louis, Mosby, 2003.)*

Gardner (N Engl J Med 355:1466-1473, 2006) described a previously healthy 18-year-old man who presented to a local emergency department with the acute onset of fever and headache. His temperature was elevated (40° C), he was tachycardic (pulse of 140 per minute), and hypotensive (blood pressure 70/40 mm Hg). Petechiae were noted over his chest. Although the result of a CSF culture was not reported, *Neisseria meningitidis* was recovered in the patient's blood cultures. Despite the prompt administration of antibiotics and other support measures, the patient's condition rapidly deteriorated, and he died 12 hours after arrival in the hospital. This patient illustrates the rapid progression of meningococcal disease, even in healthy young adults.

Meningococcemia (Clinical Case 29-2)

Septicemia (meningococcemia) with or without meningitis is a life-threatening disease. **Thrombosis of small blood vessels** and multiorgan involvement are the characteristic clinical features. Small, petechial skin lesions on the trunk and lower extremities are common and may coalesce to form larger hemorrhagic lesions (Figure 29-5). Overwhelming disseminated intravascular coagulation with shock, together with the bilateral destruction of the adrenal glands (**Waterhouse-Friderichsen syndrome**), may ensue. A milder, chronic septicemia has also been observed. Bacteremia can persist for days or weeks, and the only signs of infection are a low-grade fever, arthritis, and petechial skin lesions. The response to antibiotic therapy in patients with this form of the disease is generally excellent.

Other *N. meningitidis* Syndromes

Additional infections caused by *N. meningitidis* are pneumonia, arthritis, and urethritis. Meningococcal pneumonia is usually preceded by a respiratory tract infection. Symptoms include cough, chest pain, rales, fever, and chills. Evidence of pharyngitis is observed in most affected patients. The prognosis in patients with meningococcal pneumonia is good.

Laboratory Diagnosis

Microscopy

Gram stain is very sensitive (greater than 90%) and specific (98%) in detecting gonococcal infection in men with purulent urethritis (see Figure 29-1). However, its sensitivity in detecting infection in asymptomatic men is 60% or less. The test is also relatively insensitive in detecting gonococcal cervicitis in both symptomatic and asymptomatic women, although a positive result is considered reliable when an experienced microscopist sees gram-negative diplococci within polymorphonuclear leukocytes. Thus the Gram stain can be reliably used to diagnose infections in men with purulent urethritis and women with cervicitis, but all negative results in women and asymptomatic men must be confirmed by culture.

Gram stain is also useful for the early diagnosis of purulent arthritis but is insensitive and nonspecific for the detection of *N. gonorrhoeae* in patients with skin lesions, anorectal infections, or pharyngitis. Commensal *Neisseria* species in the oropharynx and morphologically similar bacteria in the gastrointestinal tract can be confused with *N. gonorrhoeae*.

N. meningitidis can be readily seen in the cerebrospinal fluid (CSF) of patients with meningitis (Figure 29-6), unless the patient has received prior antimicrobial therapy. Most patients with bacteremia caused by other organisms have so few organisms present in their blood that the Gram stain has no value. In contrast, patients with overwhelming meningococcal disease commonly have large numbers of organisms in their blood, which can be seen when the peripheral blood leukocytes are Gram stained.

Antigen Detection

Antigen testing for the detection of *N. gonorrhoeae* is less sensitive than culture or nucleic acid amplification tests

Figure 29—5. Skin lesions in a patient with meningococcemia. Note that the petechial lesions have coalesced and formed hemorrhagic bullae.

Figure 29—6. Gram stain of cerebrospinal fluid showing *Neisseria meningitidis*.

and is not recommended unless confirmatory tests are performed on negative specimens. Commercial tests to detect *N. meningitidis* capsular antigens in CSF, blood, and urine (where the antigens are excreted) were widely used in the past but have fallen into disfavor in recent years because the tests are less sensitive than Gram stains, and false-positive reactions, particularly with urine specimens, can occur.

Nucleic Acid-Based Tests

Nucleic acid amplification (NAA) assays specific for *N. gonorrhoeae* have been developed for the direct detection of bacteria in clinical specimens. Tests using these assays are sensitive, specific, and rapid (results are available in 4 hours). Combination NAA assays for both *N. gonorrhoeae* and *Chlamydia* organisms are available and have replaced culture in most labs. The primary problem with this approach is that it cannot be used to monitor antibiotic resistance of the identified pathogens.

Culture

N. gonorrhoeae can be readily isolated from genital specimens if care is taken in collecting and processing the specimens (Figure 29-7). Because other commensal organisms normally colonize mucosal surfaces, all genital, rectal, and pharyngeal specimens must be inoculated onto both **non-selective media** (e.g., chocolate blood agar) and **selective media** that suppress the growth of contaminating organisms (e.g., modified Thayer-Martin medium). A nonselective medium should be used because some gonococcal strains are inhibited by the vancomycin present in most selective media. The organisms are also inhibited by the fatty acids and trace metals present in the peptone hydrolysates and agar in other common laboratory media (e.g., blood agar, nutrient agar). The gonococci die rapidly if specimens are allowed to dry. Therefore drying and cold temperatures should be avoided by directly inoculating the specimen onto prewarmed media at the time of collection.

The endocervix must be properly exposed to ensure that an adequate specimen is collected. Although the endocervix is the most common site of infection in women, the rectal specimen may be the only one positive for gonococci in women who have asymptomatic infections, as well as in homosexual and bisexual men. Blood culture results are generally positive for gonococci only during the first week of the infection in patients with disseminated disease. In addition, special handling of blood specimens is required to ensure the adequate recovery of gonococci, because supplements present in the blood culture media can be toxic to *Neisseria*. Culture results of specimens from infected joints are positive for the organism if the specimens are collected at the time the arthritis develops, but skin specimen cultures are generally unrewarding.

N. meningitidis is generally present in large numbers in CSF, blood, and sputum. Although the organism is inhibited by toxic factors in media and by the anticoagulant in

NS, Not specific or sensitive.

Figure 29–7. Laboratory detection of *Neisseria gonorrhoeae*.

blood cultures, this appears to be less of a problem than with *N. gonorrhoeae*. Care should be used in processing CSF and blood specimens, because bacterial strains responsible for disseminated disease are more virulent and pose a safety risk for laboratory technologists.

Identification

Pathogenic *Neisseria* species are identified preliminarily on the basis of the isolation of oxidase-positive, gram-negative diplococci that grow on chocolate blood agar or on media that are selective for pathogenic *Neisseria* species. Definitive identification is guided by the pattern of oxidation of carbohydrates and other select tests.

Treatment, Prevention, and Control

Penicillin was historically the antibiotic of choice for treatment of gonorrhea; however, penicillin is not used today because the concentration of drug required to kill "susceptible" strains has steadily increased and frank resistance, because of β-lactamase production (plasmid-mediated) or chromosomally mediated changes in penicillin-binding proteins and in cell wall permeability, has become common. The chromosomally mediated penicillin resistance is also associated with resistance to tetracyclines, erythromycin, and aminoglycosides. Resistance to fluoroquinolones such as ciprofloxacin has also become prevalent in Asia, the Pacific Islands (including Hawaii), California, and in the male homosexual population in some U.S. cities.

Currently the Centers for Disease Control and Prevention (CDC) recommends that a fluoroquinolone not be used to treat gonorrhea infections acquired in areas where resistance is common. For these patients, **ceftriaxone** should be used as initial empiric therapy. If *Chlamydia trachomatis* infection has not been excluded, treatment should be combined with either a single dose of azithromycin or a 1-week course of doxycycline.

N. meningitidis remains susceptible to **penicillin**, although reports of strains with low-level resistance have been reported. For patients unable to receive penicillin, a broad-spectrum cephalosporin (e.g., ceftriaxone) or chloramphenicol can be used.

Although there is tremendous interest in developing a vaccine against **N. gonorrhoeae**, an **effective vaccine is not yet available**. Immunity to infection with *N. gonorrhoeae* is poorly understood. Antibodies can be detected to pili antigens, Por proteins, and LOS. However, multiple infections are common in sexually promiscuous people. This lack of protective immunity is explained in part by the antigenic diversity of gonococcal strains. The variable region at the carboxyl terminus of the pilin proteins is the immunodominant portion of the molecule. Antibodies developed against this region protect against reinfection with a homologous strain, but cross-protection against heterologous strains is incomplete. This antigenic diversity also explains the ineffectiveness of vaccines developed against pilin proteins.

Chemoprophylaxis is also ineffective, except in the protection of newborns against gonococcal eye infections (ophthalmia neonatorum), in which 1% silver nitrate, 1% tetracycline, or 0.5% erythromycin eye ointments are routinely used. Prophylactic use of penicillin to prevent genital disease is ineffective and may select for infection with a penicillin-resistant strain.

Major efforts to stem the epidemic of gonorrhea encompass education, aggressive detection, and follow-up screening of sexual contacts. It is important to realize that gonorrhea is not an insignificant disease. Chronic infections can lead to sterility, and asymptomatic infections perpetuate the reservoir of disease and lead to a higher incidence of disseminated infections.

Eradication of the pool of healthy carriers of *N. meningitidis* is unlikely. For this reason, efforts have been concentrated on the prophylactic treatment of people exposed to diseased patients and on the enhancement of immunity to the serogroups most commonly associated with disease.

Sulfonamides and penicillin are ineffective in eliminating the carrier state. Currently, rifampin, ciprofloxacin, or ceftriaxone are recommended for prophylaxis.

Vaccines directed against the group-specific capsular polysaccharides have been developed for antibody-mediated immunoprophylaxis. A **polyvalent polysaccharide-protein conjugate vaccine** effective against serogroups A, C, Y, and W135 was licensed in the United States in 2005. In 2007, the Advisory Committee on Immunization Practices (ACIP) recommended routine vaccination with one dose of this vaccine for all persons aged 11 to 18 years and other persons at increased risk for meningococcal disease. Unfortunately the group B polysaccharide is a weak immunogen and cannot induce a protective antibody response. Thus immunity to group B *N. meningitidis* must develop naturally after exposure to cross-reacting antigens. Vaccination with a suspension containing serogroup A can be used for control of an outbreak of disease, for travelers to hyperendemic areas, and for people at increased risk for disease (e.g., patients with complement deficiency).

Other *Neisseria* Species

Neisseria species such as *Neisseria sicca* and *Neisseria mucosa* are commensal organisms in the oropharynx. These organisms have been implicated in isolated cases of meningitis, osteomyelitis, endocarditis, bronchopulmonary infections, acute otitis media, and acute sinusitis. The true incidence of respiratory tract infections caused by these organisms is not known, because most specimens are contaminated with oral secretions. However, the observation of many gram-negative diplococci associated with inflammatory cells in a well-collected respiratory specimen would support the etiologic role of these organisms. Most isolates of *N. sicca* and *N. mucosa* are susceptible to penicillin, although low-level resistance caused by altered penicillin-binding protein (i.e., PBP2) has been observed.

Eikenella corrodens

In the early 1960s, a collection of small, fastidious, gram-negative rods were classified by workers at the CDC as members of the HB group (named after the patient infected with the original isolate). The organisms were subsequently subdivided into subgroup HB-1 (now known as *Eikenella corrodens*), subgroup HB-2 (*Aggregatibacter* [*Haemophilus*] *aphrophilus;* see Chapter 34), and subgroups HB-3 and HB-4 (*Aggregatibacter* [*Actinobacillus*] *actinomycetemcomitans;* see Chapter 34). In addition to being morphologically similar, these organisms colonize the human oropharynx; in the setting of preexisting heart disease, they can cause subacute bacterial endocarditis. In fact, the group of fastidious, gram-negative rods associated with subacute endocarditis is known by the now taxonomically incorrect acronym *HACEK* (*H. aphrophilus*, *A. actinomycetemcomitans*, *Cardiobacterium hominis*, *E. corrodens*, and *K. kingae*).

E. corrodens is a moderate-sized (0.2 × 2.0 μm), non-motile, non-spore-forming, facultatively anaerobic, gram-negative rod. The organism is named after Eiken, who characterized the bacterium and observed the ability of the organism to pit or "corrode" agar (from its ability to split polygalacturonic acid). *E. corrodens* is a normal inhabitant of the human upper respiratory tract, but because of its fastidious growth requirements, it is difficult to detect unless specific selective culture media are used. It is an opportunistic pathogen that causes infections in patients who are immunocompromised or have diseases or trauma of the oral cavity. *E. corrodens* is most commonly isolated in the settings of a human bite wound or fistfight injury. Other infections are endocarditis, sinusitis, meningitis, brain abscesses, pneumonia, and lung abscesses. Because most infections originate from the oropharynx, polymicrobial mixtures of aerobic and anaerobic bacteria are often present in cultures.

A slow-growing, fastidious organism, *E. corrodens* requires 5% to 10% carbon dioxide to grow. Small (0.5 to 1 mm) colonies are observed after 48 hours of incubation on blood or chocolate agar, but the organism grows poorly or not at all on selective media for gram-negative rods. Pitting in agar is a useful differential characteristic, but fewer than half of all isolates exhibit pitting. The organism also produces a characteristic bleachlike odor. Thus if a slow-growing, gram-negative rod is found to pit blood agar and produce a bleachlike order, a preliminary identification of the organism can be made. *E. corrodens* is susceptible to penicillin, ampicillin, extended-spectrum cephalosporins, tetracyclines, and fluoroquinolone but is resistant to oxacillin, first-generation cephalosporins, clindamycin, erythromycin, and the aminoglycosides. Thus *E. corrodens* is resistant to many antibiotics that are selected empirically to treat bite-wound infections.

Kingella kingae

Kingella species are small, gram-negative coccobacilli that morphologically resemble *Neisseria* species and reside in the human oropharynx. The bacteria are facultatively anaerobic, ferment carbohydrates, and have fastidious growth requirements. *K. kingae*, the most commonly isolated species, has been primarily responsible for septic arthritis in children and endocarditis in patients of all ages. Because

the organism grows slowly, it may take 3 or more days of incubation for the organism to be detected in clinical specimens. Most strains are susceptible to β-lactam antibiotics, including penicillin, tetracyclines, erythromycin, fluoroquinolones, and aminoglycosides.

Case Study and Questions

A 22-year-old female schoolteacher was brought to the emergency room after a 2-day history of headache and fever. On the day of admission, the patient had failed to come to school and could not be reached by telephone. When notified of this fact, the patient's mother went to her daughter's apartment, where she found her daughter in bed, confused and highly agitated. The patient was rushed to the local hospital, where she was comatose on arrival. Purpuric skin lesions were present on her trunk and arms. Analysis of her CSF revealed the presence of 380 cells/mm³ (93% polymorphonuclear leukocytes), a protein concentration of 220 mg/dL, and a glucose concentration of 32 mg/dL. Gram stain of CSF showed many gram-negative diplococci, and the same organisms were isolated from blood and CSF. The patient died despite prompt initiation of therapy with penicillin.

1. What is the most likely organism responsible for this fulminant disease? What is the most likely source of this organism?
2. Chemoprophylaxis should be administered to which people? What are the criteria for administering chemoprophylaxis?
3. What other diseases does this organism cause?
4. What virulence factors have been associated with other bacterial species in this genus?

Bibliography

Centers for Disease Control and Prevention: Revised recommendations of the Advisory Committee on Immunization Practices to vaccinate all persons aged 11-18 years with meningococcal conjugate vaccine. Morb Mortal Wkly Report 56:794-795, 2007.

Gardner P: Clinical practice: Prevention of meningococcal disease. N Engl J Med 355:1466-1473, 2006.

Glikman D, et al: Pneumonia and empyema caused by penicillin-resistant *Neisseria meningitidis*: A case report and literature review. Pediatrics 117:1061-1066, 2007.

Milonovich L: Meningococcemia: Epidemiology, pathophysiology, and management. J Pediatr Health Care 21:75-80, 2007.

Newman L, et al: Update on the management of gonorrhea in adults in the United States. Clin Infect Dis 44 (Suppl):S84-S101, 2007.

Stephens D: Conquering the meningococcus. FEMS Microbiol Rev 31:3-14, 2007.

Trotter C, Ramsay M: Vaccination against meningococcal disease in Europe: Review and recommendations for the use of conjugate vaccines. FEMS Microbiol Rev 31:101-107, 2007.

Whiley D, et al: Nucleic acid amplification testing for *Neisseria gonorrhoeae*: An ongoing challenge. J Mol Diagn 8:3-15, 2006.

Winstead JM, et al: Meningococcal pneumonia: Characterization and review of cases seen over the past 25 years. Clin Infect Dis 30:87-94, 2000.

Enterobacteriaceae

The family Enterobacteriaceae is the largest, most hetero-geneous collection of medically important **gram-negative rods**. More than 40 genera and hundreds of species and subspecies have been described. These genera have been classified based on biochemical properties, antigenic struc-ture, DNA-DNA hybridization, and 16S rRNA sequencing. Despite the complexity of this family, relatively few species are responsible for most human infections (Box 30-1).

Enterobacteriaceae are **ubiquitous** organisms, found worldwide in soil, water, and vegetation, and are part of the normal intestinal flora of most animals, including humans. These bacteria cause a variety of human diseases, including 30% to 35% of all bacteremias, more than 70% of urinary tract infections (UTIs), and many intestinal infections. Some organisms (e.g., *Salmonella* serotype Typhi, *Shigella* species, *Yersinia pestis*) are **always associated with human disease**, whereas others (e.g., *Escherichia coli*, *Klebsiella pneumoniae*, and *Proteus mirabilis*) are members of the normal commensal flora that can cause **opportunistic infections**. A third group of Enterobacteriaceae exists—those normally commensal organisms that become pathogenic when they acquire viru-lence factor genes on plasmids, bacteriophages, or pathoge-nicity islands (e.g., *E. coli* associated with gastroenteritis). Infections with the Enterobacteriaceae can originate from an animal reservoir (e.g., most *Salmonella* species, *Yersinia* species), from a human carrier (e.g., *Shigella* species, *Salmonella* serotype Typhi), or through the endogenous spread of organisms in a susceptible patient (e.g., *E. coli*) and can involve virtually all body sites (Figure 30-1).

Physiology and Structure

Members of the Enterobacteriaceae family are moderately sized (0.3 to 1.0 × 1.0 to 6.0 μm) gram-negative rods (Figure 30-2). They share a common antigen (**enterobac-terial common antigen**), are either motile with peritri-chous flagella (uniformly distributed over cell) or nonmotile and do not form spores. All members can grow rapidly, aerobically and anaerobically (**facultative anaerobes**), on a variety of nonselective (e.g., blood agar) and selective (e.g., MacConkey agar) media. The Enterobacteriaceae have simple nutritional requirements, **ferment glucose**, reduce nitrate, and are catalase positive and **oxidase negative**. The absence of cytochrome oxidase activity is an important characteristic because it can be measured rapidly with a simple test and is used to distin-guish the Enterobacteriaceae from many other fermentative and nonfermentative gram-negative rods. A few exceptions to these rules exist (e.g., *Plesiomonas shigelloides* is oxidase positive; *Klebsiella granulomatis* cannot be cultured on tra-ditional media).

Characteristics of the organisms' colonies on different media have been used to identify common members of the family Enterobacteriaceae. For example, the ability to **fer-ment lactose** (detected by color changes in lactose-containing media such as the commonly used MacConkey agar) has been used to differentiate lactose-fermenting strains (e.g., *Escherichia*, *Klebsiella*, *Enterobacter*, *Citrobacter*, and *Serratia* spp.; pink-purple colonies on MacConkey agar) from strains that do not ferment lactose or do so slowly (e.g., *Proteus*, *Salmonella*, *Shigella*, and *Yersinia* spp.; colorless colonies on MacConkey agar). **Resistance to bile salts** in some selective media has been used to sep-arate enteric pathogens (e.g., *Shigella*, *Salmonella*) from commensal organisms that are inhibited by bile salts (e.g., gram-positive and some gram-negative bacteria pres-ent in the gastrointestinal tract). Some Enterobacteriaceae have prominent **capsules** (e.g., most *Klebsiella*, some *Enterobacter* and *Escherichia* strains), whereas a loose fit-ting, diffusible slime layer surrounds other strains.

The heat-stable **lipopolysaccharide (LPS)** is the major cell wall antigen and consists of three components: the outermost somatic **O polysaccharide**, a **core polysaccharide** common to all Enterobacteriaceae (enterobacterial common antigen), and **lipid A** (Figure 30-3). The core polysaccharide is important for classifying an organism as a member of the Enterobacteriaceae; the O polysaccharide is important for

Box 30—1. Common Medically Important Enterobacteriaceae

Citrobacter freundii, Citrobacter koseri
Enterobacter aerogenes, Enterobacter cloacae
Escherichia coli
Klebsiella pneumoniae, Klebsiella oxytoca
Morganella morganii
Proteus mirabilis
Salmonella enterica
Serratia marcescens
Shigella sonnei, Shigella flexneri
Yersinia pestis, Yersinia enterocolitica, Yersinia pseudotuberculosis

Figure 30—2. Gram stain of *Salmonella* Typhi from a positive blood culture. Note the intense staining at the ends of the bacteria. This "bipolar staining" is characteristic of the Enterobacteriaceae.

the epidemiologic classification of strains within a species; and the lipid A component of LPS is responsible for endotoxin activity, an important virulence factor.

The epidemiologic (serologic) classification of the Enterobacteriaceae is based on three major groups of antigens: **somatic O polysaccharides, capsular K antigens** (type-specific polysaccharides), and the **flagellar H proteins.** Specific O antigens are present in each genus, although cross-reactions between closely related genera are common (e.g., *Salmonella* with *Citrobacter, Escherichia* with *Shigella*). The antigens are detected by agglutination with specific antibodies. The heat-labile K antigens are not commonly used for strain typing but are important because they may interfere with detection of the O antigens (i.e., a problem with some strains of *Salmonella*). Boiling of the organism to remove the heat-labile K antigen and expose the heat-stable O antigen circumvents this problem. The H antigens are heat-labile flagellin proteins. They may be absent from a cell, or they may undergo antigenic variation and be present in two phases.

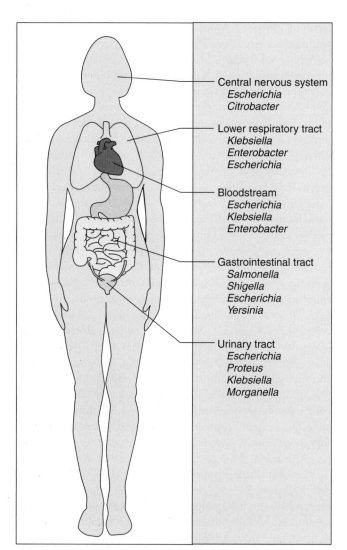

Figure 30—1. Sites of infections with common members of the Enterobacteriaceae listed in order of prevalence.

Central nervous system
Escherichia
Citrobacter

Lower respiratory tract
Klebsiella
Enterobacter
Escherichia

Bloodstream
Escherichia
Klebsiella
Enterobacter

Gastrointestinal tract
Salmonella
Shigella
Escherichia
Yersinia

Urinary tract
Escherichia
Proteus
Klebsiella
Morganella

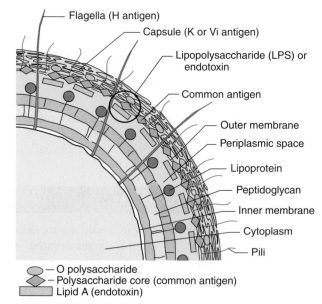

Flagella (H antigen)
Capsule (K or Vi antigen)
Lipopolysaccharide (LPS) or endotoxin
Common antigen
Outer membrane
Periplasmic space
Lipoprotein
Peptidoglycan
Inner membrane
Cytoplasm
Pili

— O polysaccharide
— Polysaccharide core (common antigen)
— Lipid A (endotoxin)

Figure 30—3. Antigenic structure of Enterobacteriaceae.

Most Enterobacteriaceae are motile, with the exception of the common isolates *Klebsiella*, *Shigella*, and *Yersinia*. The motile strains possess peritrichous **flagella**. Many Enterobacteriaceae also possess fimbriae (also referred to as *pili*), which have been subdivided into two general classes: chromosomally mediated common fimbriae and sex pili that are encoded on conjugative plasmids. The **common fimbriae** are important for the ability of bacteria to adhere to specific host cell receptors, whereas the **sex or conjugative pili** facilitate genetic transfer between bacteria.

Pathogenesis and Immunity

Numerous virulence factors have been identified in the members of the family Enterobacteriaceae. Some are common to all genera (Box 30-2), and others are unique to specific virulent strains.

Endotoxin

Endotoxin is a virulence factor shared among aerobic and some anaerobic gram-negative bacteria. The activity of this toxin depends on the **lipid A** component of LPS, which is released at cell lysis. Many of the systemic manifestations of gram-negative bacterial infections are initiated by endotoxin activation of complement, release of cytokines, leukocytosis, thrombocytopenia, disseminated intravascular coagulation, fever, decreased peripheral circulation, shock, and death.

Capsule

Encapsulated Enterobacteriaceae are protected from phagocytosis by the hydrophilic capsular antigens, which repel the hydrophobic phagocytic cell surface. These antigens interfere with the binding of antibodies to the bacteria and are poor immunogens or activators of complement. The protective role of the capsule is diminished, however, if the patient develops specific anticapsular antibodies.

Antigenic Phase Variation

The expression of capsular K and flagellar H antigens is under the genetic control of the organism. Each of these

Box 30–2. Common Virulence Factors Associated with Enterobacteriaceae

Endotoxin
Capsule
Antigenic phase variation
Type III secretion systems
Sequestration of growth factors
Resistance to serum killing
Antimicrobial resistance

antigens can be alternately expressed or not expressed (phase variation), a feature that protects the bacteria from antibody-mediated cell death.

Type III Secretion Systems

A variety of bacteria (e.g., *Yersinia*, *Salmonella*, *Shigella*, enteropathogenic *Escherichia*, *Pseudomonas*, and *Chlamydia*) have a common effector system for delivering their virulence factors into targeted eukaryotic cells. Think of the **type III secretion system** as a molecular syringe consisting of approximately 20 proteins that facilitate secretion of bacterial virulence factors when the bacteria come into contact with the host cells. Although the virulence factors and their effects differ among the various gram-negative rods, the general mechanism by which the virulence factors are introduced is the same. In the absence of the type III secretion system, the bacteria lose their virulence.

Sequestration of Growth Factors

Nutrients are provided to the organisms in enriched culture media, but the bacteria must become nutritional scavengers when growing in vivo. Iron is an important growth factor required by bacteria, but it is bound in **heme proteins** (e.g., hemoglobin, myoglobin) or in **iron-chelating proteins** (e.g., transferrin, lactoferrin). The bacteria counteract the binding by producing their own competitive **siderophores** or iron-chelating compounds (e.g., **enterobactin, aerobactin**). Iron can also be released from host cells by hemolysins produced by the bacteria.

Resistance to Serum Killing

Whereas many bacteria can be rapidly cleared from blood, virulent organisms capable of producing systemic infections are often resistant to serum killing. Although the bacterial capsule can protect the organism from serum killing, other factors prevent the binding of complement components to the bacteria and subsequent complement-mediated clearance.

Antimicrobial Resistance

As rapidly as new antibiotics are introduced, organisms can develop resistance to them. This resistance can be encoded on transferable plasmids and exchanged among species, genera, and even families of bacteria.

Escherichia coli (Box 30-3)

Escherichia coli is the most common and important member of the genus *Escherichia*. This organism is associated with a variety of diseases, including gastroenteritis and

Box 30—3. Summary: *Escherichia coli*

Biology, Virulence, and Disease

Gram-negative, facultative anaerobic rods
Fermenter; oxidase negative
Lipopolysaccharide consists of outer somatic O polysaccharide, core polysaccharide (common antigen), and lipid A (endotoxin)
Virulence—refer to Box 30-2; Table 30-1
At least five different pathogenic groups cause gastroenteritis (EPEC, ETEC, EHEC, EIEC, EAEC); most cause diseases in developing countries, although EHEC is an important cause of hemorrhagic colitis (HC) and hemolytic uremic syndrome (HUS) in the United States
Extraintestinal disease includes bacteremia, neonatal meningitis, urinary tract infections, and intraabdominal infections

Epidemiology

Most common aerobic, gram-negative rods in the gastrointestinal tract
Most infections are endogenous (patient's microbial flora), although strains causing gastroenteritis are generally acquired exogenously

Diagnosis

Organisms grow rapidly on most culture media
Enteric pathogens, with the exception of EHEC, are detected only in reference or research laboratories

Treatment, Prevention, and Control

Enteric pathogens are treated symptomatically unless disseminated disease occurs
Antibiotic therapy is guided by in vitro susceptibility tests
Appropriate infection-control practices are used to reduce the risk of nosocomial infections (e.g., restricting use of antibiotics, avoiding unnecessary use of urinary tract catheters)
Maintenance of high hygienic standards to reduce the risk of exposure to gastroenteritis strains
Proper cooking of beef products to reduce risk of EHEC infections

extraintestinal infections such as urinary tract infections (UTIs), meningitis, and sepsis. A multitude of strains are capable of causing disease, with some serotypes associated with greater virulence (e.g., *E. coli* O157 is the most common cause of hemorrhagic colitis).

Pathogenesis and Immunity

E. coli possesses a broad range of virulence factors (Table 30-1). In addition to the general factors possessed by all members of the family Enterobacteriaceae, *Escherichia* strains possess specialized virulence factors that can be placed into two general categories: adhesins and exotoxins. The function of these factors will be discussed in greater detail in the following sections.

Epidemiology

Large numbers of *E. coli* are present in the gastrointestinal tract. Although these organisms can be opportunistic pathogens when the intestines are perforated and the bacteria enter the peritoneal cavity, most *E. coli* that cause gastrointestinal and extraintestinal disease do so because they have acquired specific virulence factors encoded on plasmids, pathogenicity islands, or in bacteriophage DNA. The effectiveness of *E. coli* as a pathogen is illustrated by the fact the bacteria are (1) the most common gram-negative rods isolated from patients with sepsis (Figure 30-4), (2) responsible for causing more

than 80% of all community-acquired UTIs, as well as many hospital-acquired infections, and (3) a prominent cause of gastroenteritis in developing countries. Most infections (with the exception of neonatal meningitis and gastroenteritis) are endogenous; that is, the *E. coli* that are part of the patient's normal microbial flora are able to establish infection when the patient's defenses are compromised.

Table 30—1. Specialized Virulence Factors Associated with *Escherichia coli*

Bacteria	Adhesins	Exotoxins
ETEC	Colonization factor antigens (CFA/I, CFA/II, CFA/III)	Heat-labile toxin (LT-1); Heat-stable toxin (STa)
EPEC	Bundle-forming pili (Bfp); intimin	
EAEC	Aggregative adherence fimbriae (AAF/I, AAF/II, AAF/III)	Enteroaggregative heat-stable toxin (EAST); Plasmid encoded toxin (Pet)
EHEC	Bfp; intimin	Shiga toxins (Stx-1, Stx-2)
EIEC	Invasive plasmid antigen (Ipa)	Hemolysin (HlyA)
Uropathogens	P pili; Dr fimbriae	

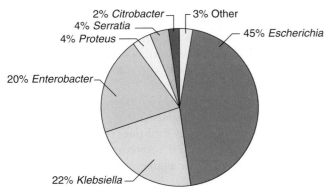

Figure 30—4. Incidence of Enterobacteriaceae associated with bacteremia. *(Data courtesy Barnes-Jewish Hospital, St. Louis, Missouri.)*

Clinical Diseases

Gastroenteritis

The strains of *E. coli* that cause gastroenteritis are subdivided into five major groups: enterotoxigenic (ETEC), enteropathogenic (EPEC), enteroaggregative (EAEC), enterohemorrhagic (EHEC), and enteroinvasive (EIEC) (Table 30-2). The first three groups primarily cause a secretory diarrhea involving the small intestine, and the last two groups primarily involve the large intestine.

ETEC

Disease caused by **enterotoxigenic *E. coli*** is seen most commonly in developing countries (an estimated 650 million cases per year), although almost 80,000 cases

are estimated to occur annually in travelers from the United States, and disease is endemic in Native American populations. Infections are observed most commonly in either young children in developing countries or travelers to these areas. The inoculum for disease is high, so infections are primarily **acquired through consumption of fecally contaminated food or water**. Person-to-person spread does not occur. **Secretory diarrhea** caused by ETEC develops after a 1- to 2-day incubation period and persists for an average of 3 to 5 days. The symptoms (watery diarrhea and abdominal cramps; nausea and vomiting are less commonly observed) are similar to those of cholera but are usually milder, particularly in adults. Neither histologic changes of the intestinal mucosa nor inflammation is observed.

ETEC produce two classes of enterotoxins: **heat-labile toxins** (LT-I, LT-II) and **heat-stable toxins** (STa and STb). Whereas LT-II is not associated with human disease, LT-I is functionally and structurally similar to cholera toxin (see Chapter 31) and is associated with human disease. This toxin consists of one A subunit and five identical B subunits. The B subunits bind to the same receptor as cholera toxin (GM_1 gangliosides), as well as other surface glycoproteins on epithelial cells in the small intestine.

After endocytosis, the A subunit of LT-I translocates across the membrane of the vacuole. The A subunit has adenosine diphosphate (ADP)-ribosyltransferase activity and interacts with a membrane protein (Gs) that regulates adenylate cyclase. The net effect of this interaction is an **increase in cyclic adenosine monophosphate (cAMP)** levels, with enhanced secretion of chloride and a decreased

Table 30—2. Gastroenteritis Caused by *Escherichia coli*

Organism	Site of Action	Disease	Pathogenesis
Enterotoxigenic *E. coli* (ETEC)	Small intestine	Traveler's diarrhea; infant diarrhea in developing countries; watery diarrhea, vomiting, cramps, nausea, low-grade fever	Plasmid-mediated, heat-stable and/or heat-labile enterotoxins that stimulate hypersecretion of fluids and electrolytes
Enteropathogenic *E. coli* (EPEC)	Small intestine	Infant diarrhea in underdeveloped countries; watery diarrhea and vomiting, nonbloody stools	Plasmid-mediated A/E histopathology with disruption of normal microvillus structure, resulting in malabsorption and diarrhea
Enteroaggregative *E. coli* (EAEC)	Small intestine	Infant diarrhea in underdeveloped countries; traveler's diarrhea; persistent watery diarrhea with vomiting, dehydration, and low-grade fever	Plasmid-mediated aggregative adherence of rods ("stacked bricks") with shortening of microvilli, mononuclear infiltration, and hemorrhage; decreased fluid absorption
Enterohemorrhagic *E. coli* (EHEC)	Large intestine	Initial watery diarrhea followed by grossly bloody diarrhea (hemorrhagic colitis) with abdominal cramps; little or no fever; may progress to hemolytic uremic syndrome (HUS)	Mediated by cytotoxic Shiga toxins (Stx-1, Stx-2), which disrupt protein synthesis; A/E lesions with destruction of intestinal microvilli, resulting in decreased absorption
Enteroinvasive *E. coli* (EIEC)	Large intestine	Disease in developing countries; fever, cramping, watery diarrhea; may progress to dysentery with scant, bloody stools	Plasmid-mediated invasion and destruction of epithelial cells lining colon

A/E, attachment/effacement.

absorption of sodium and chloride. These changes are manifested in a watery diarrhea. Exposure to the toxin also stimulates prostaglandin secretion and production of inflammatory cytokines, resulting in further fluid loss.

STa, but not STb, is associated with human disease. STa is a small, monomeric peptide that binds to the transmembrane guanylate cyclase receptor, leading to an **increase in cyclic guanosine monophosphate (cGMP)** and subsequent hypersecretion of fluids. Genes for LT-I and STa are present on a **transferable plasmid**, which can also carry the genes for **colonization factor adhesins (CFA/I, CFA/II, CFA/III)**. The colonization factors are fimbriae that recognize specific host glycoprotein receptors (define the host specificity). Both the toxin and colonization factors are required for disease to develop. Disease mediated by heat-stable toxin is indistinguishable from that mediated by heat-labile toxin.

EPEC

Enteropathogenic E. coli was the first *E. coli* associated with diarrheal disease and remains a **major cause of infant diarrhea in impoverished countries**. Disease is uncommon in developed countries, except in rare outbreaks in daycare nurseries, and is rare in older children and adults, presumably because they have developed protective immunity. In contrast with ETEC disease, **person-to-person spread** occurs with EPEC, so the infectious dose is likely to be low. Disease is characterized by **watery diarrhea** that may be severe and protracted. Fever and vomiting may also be present.

Infection is initiated by bacterial attachment to epithelial cells of the small intestine, with subsequent effacement (destruction) of the microvillus (**attachment/effacement [A/E] histopathology**). The initial aggregation of the bacteria leading to the formation of microcolonies on the epithelial cell surface is mediated by plasmid-encoded **bundle forming pili (BFP)**. The subsequent stages of attachment are regulated by genes encoded on the "**locus of enterocyte effacement (LEE)" pathogenicity island**. This island of more than 40 genes is responsible for attachment and destruction of the host cell surface. Following the loose attachment mediated by BFP, active secretion of proteins into the host epithelial cell occurs by the bacterial type III secretion system. One protein, **translocated intimin receptor (Tir)**, is inserted into the epithelial cell membrane and functions as a receptor for an outer membrane bacterial adhesin, **intimin**. Binding of intimin to Tir results in polymerization of actin and accumulation of cytoskeletal elements beneath the attached bacteria, loss of cell surface integrity, and cell death.

EAEC

Enteroaggregative E. coli strains have been implicated as a cause of persistent watery diarrhea with dehydration in infants in developing countries and in travelers to these countries. Outbreaks of gastroenteritis caused by EAEC

have also been reported in the United States, Europe, and Japan, and the organism is likely an important cause of childhood diarrhea in developed countries. This is one of the few bacteria associated with **chronic diarrhea and growth retardation** in children.

The bacteria are characterized by their autoagglutination in a "stacked-brick" arrangement. This process is mediated by **aggregative adherence fimbriae I (AAF1)**, adhesins that are similar to the BFP responsible for microcolony formation of EPEC. Other aggregative adherence fimbriae (AAF/II, AAF/III) have also been described. After EAEC adhere to the surface of the intestine, mucus secretion is stimulated, leading to the formation of a thick biofilm. This protects the aggregated bacteria from antibiotics and phagocytic cells. In addition, two groups of toxins are associated with EAEC: **enteroaggregative heat stable toxin (EAST)** and **plasmid encoded toxin (PET)**. EAST induces fluid secretion and is antigenically related to the heat-stable toxin of ETEC. PET also induces fluid secretion.

EHEC (Clinical Case 30-1)

Enterohemorrhagic E. coli are the most common strains producing disease in developed countries. It is estimated that these bacteria cause 73,000 infections and 60 deaths each year in the United States. EHEC disease is most common in the warm months, and the highest incidence is in children younger than 5 years. Most infections are attributed to the consumption of undercooked ground beef or other meat products, water, unpasteurized milk or fruit juices (e.g., cider made from apples contaminated with feces from cattle), uncooked vegetables such as spinach, and fruits. The **ingestion of fewer than 100 bacteria can produce disease**, and person-to-person spread occurs.

Disease caused by EHEC ranges from mild, uncomplicated diarrhea to **hemorrhagic colitis** with severe abdominal pain and bloody diarrhea. Initially, diarrhea with abdominal pain develops in patients after 3 to 4 days of incubation. Vomiting is observed in approximately half the patients, but a high fever is generally absent. Within 2 days

---

Clinical Case 30-1. Multistate Outbreak of EHEC Infections

In 2006, *Escherichia coli* O157 was responsible for a large, multistate outbreak of gastroenteritis. The outbreak was linked to contamination of spinach, with a total of 173 cases reported in 25 states, primarily over an 18-day period. The outbreak resulted in hospitalization of more than 50% of the patients with documented disease, a 16% rate of hemolytic uremic syndrome, and 1 death. Despite the wide distribution of the contaminated spinach, publication of the outbreak and the rapid determination that spinach was responsible promptly resulted in removal of spinach from grocery stores and termination of the outbreak. This outbreak illustrates how contamination of a food product, even with small numbers of organisms, can lead to a widespread outbreak with a particularly virulent organism such as strains of EHEC.

of onset, disease in 30% to 65% of patients progresses to a bloody diarrhea with severe abdominal pain. Complete resolution of symptoms typically occurs after 4 to 10 days in most untreated patients. **Hemolytic uremic syndrome (HUS)**, a disorder characterized by acute renal failure, thrombocytopenia, and microangiopathic hemolytic anemia, is a complication in 5% to 10% of infected children younger than 10 years. Resolution of symptoms occurs in uncomplicated disease after 4 to 10 days in most untreated patients; however, death can occur in 3% to 5% of patients with HUS, and severe sequelae (e.g., renal impairment, hypertension, CNS manifestations) can occur in as many as 30% of HUS patients.

The most common strain of EHEC is serotype O157:H7. This strain represents a clone that evolved from EPEC and expresses **attaching and effacing activity**. Additionally, these strains have acquired **Shiga toxin** (i.e., Stx-1, Stx-2, or both). Stx-1 is essentially identical to the Shiga toxin produced by *Shigella dysenteriae* (thus the source of the name); Stx-2 has 60% homology. Both toxins are acquired by lysogenic bacteriophages. Both have one A subunit and five B subunits, with the B subunits binding to a specific glycolipid on the host cell (globotriaosylceramide, GB_3). A high concentration of GB_3 receptors is found in the intestinal villus and renal endothelial cells. After the A subunit is internalized, it is cleaved into two molecules, and the A_1 fragment binds to 28S ribosomal ribonucleic acid (rRNA) and causes a cessation of protein synthesis. EHEC strains with both Shiga toxins and attaching and effacing activity are more pathogenic than strains only producing Shiga toxin.

HUS has been preferentially associated with the production of Stx-2, which has been shown to destroy glomerular endothelial cells. Damage to the endothelial cells leads to platelet activation and thrombin deposition, which in turn results in decreased glomerular filtration and acute renal failure. The Shiga toxins also stimulate expression of inflammatory cytokines (e.g., tumor necrosis factor [TNF]-γ, interleukin [IL]-6), which among other effects enhance expression of GB_3.

EIEC

Enteroinvasive *E. coli* strains are rare in the United States and uncommon in developing countries. Pathogenic strains are primarily associated with a few restricted O serotypes: O124, O143, and O164. The strains are closely related by phenotypic and pathogenic properties to *Shigella*. The bacteria are able to invade and destroy the colonic epithelium, producing a disease characterized initially by **watery diarrhea**. A minority of patients progress to the dysenteric form of disease, consisting of fever, abdominal cramps, and blood and leukocytes in stool specimens.

A series of genes on a plasmid mediate bacterial invasion (**pInv genes**) into the colonic epithelium. The bacteria then lyse the phagocytic vacuole and replicate in the cell cytoplasm. Movement within the cytoplasm and into adjacent epithelial cells is regulated by formation of actin tails (similar to that observed with *Listeria*). This process of epithelial cell destruction with inflammatory infiltration can progress to colonic ulceration.

Extraintestinal Infections

URINARY TRACT INFECTION

Most gram-negative rods that produce UTIs originate in the colon, contaminate the urethra, ascend into the bladder, and may migrate to the kidney or prostate. Although most strains of *E. coli* can produce UTIs, disease is more common with certain specific serogroups. These bacteria are particularly virulent because of their ability to produce **adhesins** (primarily P pili, AAF/I, AAF/III, and Dr), which bind to cells lining the bladder and upper urinary tract (preventing the elimination of the bacteria in voided urine), and **hemolysin HlyA**, which lyses erythrocytes and other cell types (leading to cytokine release and stimulation of an inflammatory response).

NEONATAL MENINGITIS

E. coli and group B streptococci cause the majority of CNS infections in infants younger than 1 month. Approximately 75% of the *E. coli* strains possess the **K1 capsular antigen**. This serogroup is also commonly present in the gastrointestinal tracts of pregnant women and newborn infants. However, the reason this serogroup has a predilection for causing disease in newborns is not understood.

SEPTICEMIA

Typically, septicemia caused by gram-negative rods such as *E. coli* originates from infections in the urinary or gastrointestinal tract (e.g., intestinal perforation leading to an intraabdominal infection). The mortality associated with *E. coli* septicemia is high for patients in whom immunity is compromised or the primary infection is in the abdomen or central nervous system (CNS).

Salmonella (Box 30-4)

The taxonomic classification of the genus *Salmonella* is problematic. DNA homology studies have revealed that most clinically significant isolates belong to the species *Salmonella enterica*. More than 2500 unique serotypes have been described for this single species; however, these serotypes are commonly listed as individual species (e.g., *Salmonella typhi*, *Salmonella choleraesuis*, *Salmonella typhimurium*, and *Salmonella enteritidis*). These designations are incorrect. For example, the correct nomenclature is "*Salmonella enterica*, serovar. Typhi." In an effort to prevent confusion and still retain the historical terms, individual serotypes are now commonly written with the serotype name capitalized and not in italics. For example, *Salmonella enterica*, serovar. Typhi is commonly designated as "*Salmonella* Typhi."

Box 30—4. Summary: *Salmonella*

Biology, Virulence, and Disease

Gram-negative, facultative anaerobic rods
Fermenter; oxidase negative
Lipopolysaccharide consists of outer somatic O polysaccharide, core polysaccharide (common antigen), and lipid A (endotoxin)
More than 2500 O serotypes
Virulence—refer to Box 30-2; tolerant of acids in phagocytic vesicles
Can survive in macrophages and spread from the intestine to other body sites
Diseases: enteritis (fever, nausea, vomiting, bloody or nonbloody diarrhea, abdominal cramps); enteric fever (typhoid fever, paratyphoid fever); bacteremia (most commonly seen with *Salmonella* Typhi, *Salmonella* Paratyphi, *Salmonella* Choleraesuis); asymptomatic colonization (primarily with *Salmonella* Typhi and *Salmonella* Paratyphi)

Epidemiology

Most infections are acquired by eating contaminated food products (poultry, eggs, and dairy products are the most common sources of infection)
Direct fecal-oral spread in children
Salmonella Typhi and *Salmonella* Paratyphi are strict human pathogens (no other reservoirs); these infections are passed person to person; asymptomatic long-term colonization occurs commonly
Individuals at risk for infection include those who eat improperly cooked poultry or eggs, patients with reduced gastric acid levels, and immunocompromised patients
Infections occur worldwide, particularly in the warm months of the year

Diagnosis

Isolation from stool specimens requires use of selective media

Treatment, Prevention, and Control

Antibiotic treatment not recommended for enteritis because may prolong duration of disease
Infections with *Salmonella* Typhi and *Salmonella* Paratyphi or disseminated infections with other organisms should be treated with an effective antibiotic (selected by in vitro susceptibility tests); fluoroquinolones (e.g., ciprofloxacin), chloramphenicol, trimethoprim-sulfamethoxazole, or a broad-spectrum cephalosporin may be used
Most infections can be controlled by proper preparation of poultry and eggs (completely cooked) and avoidance of contamination of other foods with uncooked poultry products
Carriers of *Salmonella* Typhi and *Salmonella* Paratyphi should be identified and treated
Vaccination against *Salmonella* Typhi can reduce the risk of disease for travelers into endemic areas

Pathogenesis and Immunity

After ingestion and passage through the stomach, salmonellae attach to the mucosa of the **small intestine** and invade into the **M (microfold) cells** located in Peyer patches, as well as into enterocytes. The bacteria remain in an endocytic vacuole, where they replicate. The bacteria can also be transported across the cytoplasm and released into the blood or lymphatic circulation. Regulation of the attachment, engulfment, and replication is controlled primarily by two large clusters of genes (**pathogenicity islands, PAI**) on the bacterial chromosome. **Pathogenicity island I (PAI I)** encodes salmonella-secreted invasion proteins (Ssps) and a type III secretion system that injects the proteins into the host cell. **Pathogenicity island II (PAI II)** contains genes that allow the bacteria to evade the host's immune response and a second type III secretion system for this function. With most infections, the inflammatory response confines the infection to the gastrointestinal tract, mediates the release of prostaglandins, and stimulates cAMP and active fluid secretion.

Epidemiology

Salmonella can colonize virtually all animals, including poultry, reptiles, livestock, rodents, domestic animals, birds, and humans. Animal-to-animal spread and the use of feeds contaminated with *Salmonella* maintain an **animal reservoir**. Serotypes such as *Salmonella* Typhi and *Salmonella* Paratyphi are highly **adapted to humans** and do not cause disease in nonhuman hosts. Other *Salmonella* serotypes (e.g., *Salmonella* Choleraesuis) are adapted to animals and can cause severe disease when they infect humans. Additionally, in contrast with other *Salmonella* serotypes, strains that are highly adapted to humans (i.e., *Salmonella* Typhi, *Salmonella* Paratyphi) can survive in the gall bladder and establish chronic carriage. Finally, many *Salmonella* strains have no host specificity and cause disease in both human and nonhuman hosts.

Most infections result from the **ingestion** of contaminated food products and from direct fecal-oral spread. The incidence of disease is greatest in children younger than 5 years and adults older than 60 years, who are commonly infected during the summer and autumn months when contaminated foods are consumed at outdoor social gatherings. The most common sources of human infections are **poultry, eggs, dairy products**, and foods prepared on contaminated work surfaces (e.g., cutting boards where uncooked poultry was prepared). Approximately 45,000 cases of nontyphoidal *Salmonella* infections were reported in the United States in 2005, although it has been estimated that more than 1.4 million infections and 600 deaths occur each year. *Salmonella* Typhi infections occur when food or water contaminated by infected food handlers is ingested. There is no animal reservoir. An average of 350 *Salmonella* Typhi infections are reported annually in the United States, most of which are acquired during foreign travel. In contrast, it is estimated that 21 million *Salmonella* Typhi infections and 200,000 deaths occur each year worldwide. The risk of disease is highest in children living in poverty in a developing country.

The infectious dose for *Salmonella* Typhi infections is low, so person-to-person spread is common. In contrast, a large inoculum (e.g., 10^6 to 10^8 bacteria) is required for symptomatic disease to develop with most other *Salmonella* serotypes. The organisms can multiply to this high density if contaminated food products are improperly stored (e.g., left at room temperature). The infectious dose is lower for people at high risk for disease because of age, immunosuppression or underlying disease (leukemia, lymphoma, sickle cell disease), or reduced gastric acidity.

Clinical Diseases

The following four forms of *Salmonella* infection exist: gastroenteritis, septicemia, enteric fever, and asymptomatic colonization.

Gastroenteritis

Gastroenteritis is the **most common form of salmonellosis** in the United States. Symptoms generally appear 6 to 48 hours after the consumption of contaminated food or water, with the initial presentation consisting of **nausea, vomiting, and nonbloody diarrhea**. Fever, abdominal cramps, myalgias, and headache are also common. Colonic involvement can be demonstrated in the acute form of the disease. Symptoms can persist from 2 days to 1 week before spontaneous resolution.

Septicemia

All *Salmonella* species can cause bacteremia, although infections with *Salmonella* Typhi, *Salmonella* Paratyphi, and *Salmonella* Choleraesuis more commonly lead to a bacteremic phase. The risk for *Salmonella* bacteremia is higher in pediatric and geriatric patients and in immunocompromised patients (HIV infections, sickle-cell disease, and congenital immunodeficiencies). The clinical presentation of *Salmonella* bacteremia is like that of other gram-negative bacteremias; however, localized suppurative infections (e.g., osteomyelitis, endocarditis, arthritis) can occur in as many as 10% of patients.

Clinical Case 30-2. *Salmonella* Typhi Infection

Scully, et al. (N Engl J Med 345:201-205, 2007) described a 25-year-old woman who was admitted into a Boston hospital with a history of persistent fever that did not respond to amoxicillin or acetaminophen or ibuprofen. She was a resident of the Philippines who had been traveling in the United States for the previous 11 days. On physical examination, she was febrile, had an enlarged liver, abdominal pain, and an abnormal urinalysis. Blood cultures were collected upon admission to the hospital and were positive the next day with *Salmonella* Typhi. Because the organism was susceptible to fluoroquinolones, this therapy was selected. Within 4 days, she had defervesced and was discharged to return home to the Philippines. Although typhoid fever can be a very serious, life-threatening illness, it can initially present with nonspecific symptoms, as was seen in this woman.

Enteric Fever (Clinical Case 30-2)

Salmonella Typhi produce a febrile illness called **typhoid fever**. A milder form of this disease, referred to as **paratyphoid fever**, is produced by *Salmonella* Paratyphi A, *Salmonella* Schottmuelleri (formerly *Salmonella* Paratyphi B), and *Salmonella* Hirschfeldii (formerly *Salmonella* Paratyphi C). Other *Salmonella* serotypes can rarely produce a similar syndrome. The bacteria responsible for enteric fever pass through the cells lining the intestines and are engulfed by macrophages. They replicate after being transported to the liver, spleen, and bone marrow. Ten to 14 days after ingestion of the bacteria, patients experience gradually increasing fever with nonspecific complaints of headache, myalgias, malaise, and anorexia. These symptoms persist for a week or longer and are followed by gastrointestinal symptoms. This cycle corresponds to an initial bacteremic phase that is followed by colonization of the gallbladder and then reinfection of the intestines. Enteric fever is a serious clinical disease and must be suspected in febrile patients who have recently traveled to developing countries where disease is endemic.

Asymptomatic Colonization

The strains of *Salmonella* responsible for causing typhoid and paratyphoid fevers are maintained by human colonization. **Chronic colonization** for more than 1 year after symptomatic disease develops in 1% to 5% of patients, the gallbladder being the reservoir in most patients. Chronic colonization with other species of *Salmonella* occurs in less than 1% of patients and does not represent an important source of human infection.

Shigella (Box 30-5)

The commonly used taxonomic classification of *Shigella* is simple, although technically incorrect. Four species consisting of more than 45 O antigen–based serogroups have been described: *S. dysenteriae, Shigella flexneri, Shigella boydii,* and *Shigella sonnei*. However, analysis of DNA has

Box 30–5. Summary: *Shigella*

Biology, Virulence, and Disease

Gram-negative, facultatively anaerobic rods
Fermenter; oxidase negative
Lipopolysaccharide consists of somatic O polysaccharide, core polysaccharide (common antigen), and lipid A (endotoxin)
Four species recognized: *S. sonnei* responsible for most infections in developed countries; *S. flexneri* for infections in developing countries; *S. dysenteriae* for the most severe infections; and *S. boydii* is not commonly isolated
Virulence—refer to Box 30-2; exotoxin (Shiga toxin) produced by *S. dysenteriae* disrupts protein synthesis and produces endothelial damage
Disease—most common form of disease is gastroenteritis (shigellosis), an initial watery diarrhea progressing within 1 to 2 days to abdominal cramps and tenesmus (with or without bloody stools); severe form of disease is caused by *S. dysenteriae* (bacterial dysentery); asymptomatic carriage develops in a small number of patients (reservoir for future infections)

Epidemiology

Humans are only reservoir for these bacteria
Disease spread person to person by fecal-oral route
Patients at highest risk for disease are young children in daycare centers, nurseries, and custodial institutions; siblings and parents of these children; male homosexuals
Relatively few organisms can produce disease (highly infectious)
Disease occurs worldwide with no seasonal incidence (consistent with person-to-person spread involving a low inoculum)

Diagnosis

Isolation from stool specimens requires use of selective media

Treatment, Prevention, and Control

Antibiotic therapy shortens the course of symptomatic disease and fecal shedding
Treatment should be guided by in vitro susceptibility tests
Empiric therapy can be initiated with a fluoroquinolone or trimethoprim-sulfamethoxazole
Appropriate infection control measures should be instituted to prevent spread of the organism, including handwashing and proper disposal of soiled linens

---

determined that these four species are actually biogroups within *E. coli*. Because it would be confusing to refer to these bacteria as *E. coli*, their historical names have been retained.

Pathogenesis and Immunity

Shigella cause disease by invading and replicating in cells lining the **colon**. Structural gene proteins mediate the adherence of the organisms to the cells, as well as their invasion, intracellular replication, and cell-to-cell spread. These genes are carried on a large virulence plasmid but are regulated by chromosomal genes. Thus the presence of the plasmid does not ensure functional gene activity.

Shigella species appear unable to attach to differentiated mucosal cells; rather, they first attach to and invade the M cells located in Peyer patches. The **type III secretion system** mediates secretion of four proteins (**IpaA, IpaB, IpaC, IpaD**) into epithelial cells and macrophages. These proteins induce membrane ruffling on the target cell, leading to engulfment of the bacteria. Shigellae lyse the phagocytic vacuole and replicate in the host cell cytoplasm (unlike *Salmonella*, which replicate in the vacuole). With the rearrangement of actin filaments in the host cells, the bacteria are propelled through the cytoplasm to adjacent cells, where **cell-to-cell passage** occurs. In this way, *Shigella* organisms are protected from immune-mediated clearance. Shigellae survive phagocytosis by inducing programmed cell death (**apoptosis**). This process also leads to the release of IL-1β, resulting in the attraction of polymorphonuclear leukocytes into the infected tissues. This in turn destabilizes the integrity of the intestinal wall and allows the bacteria to reach the deeper epithelial cells.

S. dysenteriae strains produce an exotoxin, **Shiga toxin**. Like Shiga toxin produced by EHEC, this toxin has one A subunit and five B subunits. The B subunits bind to a host cell glycolipid (GB_3) and facilitate transfer of the A subunit into the cell. The A subunit cleaves the 28S rRNA in the 60S ribosomal subunit, thereby preventing the binding of aminoacyl-transfer RNA and disrupting protein synthesis. The primary manifestation of toxin activity is damage to the intestinal epithelium; however, in a small subset of patients, the Shiga toxin can mediate damage to the glomerular endothelial cells, resulting in renal failure (HUS).

Epidemiology

Humans are the only reservoir for *Shigella*. It is estimated that almost 450,000 cases of *Shigella* infections occur each year in the United States. This figure pales in comparison with the estimated 150 million cases that occur annually worldwide. *S. sonnei* is responsible for almost 85% of the U.S. infections, while *S. flexneri* predominates in developing countries. Epidemics of *S. dysenteriae*, a particularly virulent species, occur in Africa and Central America, with case fatality rates of 5% to 15%.

Shigellosis is primarily a pediatric disease, with 60% of all infections in children younger than 10 years. Endemic disease in adults is common in male homosexuals and in household contacts of infected children. Epidemic outbreaks of disease occur in daycare centers, nurseries, and custodial institutions. Shigellosis is **transmitted person-to-person** by the fecal-oral route, primarily by people with contaminated hands, and less commonly in water or food. Because as few as 100 to 200 bacteria can establish disease, shigellosis spreads rapidly in communities where sanitary standards and the level of personal hygiene are low.

Clinical Diseases (Clinical Case 30-3)

Shigellosis is characterized by **abdominal cramps, diarrhea, fever, and bloody stools**. The clinical signs and symptoms of the disease appear 1 to 3 days after the bacteria are ingested. Shigella initially colonize the small intestine and begin to multiply within the first 12 hours. The first sign of infection (profuse, watery diarrhea without histologic evidence of mucosal invasion) is mediated by an enterotoxin. However, the cardinal feature of shigellosis is lower abdominal cramps and tenesmus (straining to defecate), with abundant pus and blood in the stool. It results from invasion of the colonic mucosa by the bacteria. Abundant neutrophils, erythrocytes, and mucus are found in the stool. Infection is generally self-limited, although antibiotic treatment is recommended to reduce the risk of secondary spread to family members and other contacts. Asymptomatic colonization of the organism in the colon develops in a small number of patients and represents a persistent reservoir for infection.

Clinical Case 30-3. Shigella Infections in Daycare Centers

In 2005, three states reported outbreaks of multidrug resistant Shigella infections in daycare centers. A total of 532 infections were reported in the Kansas City area with the median age of patients 6 years (MMWR 55:1068-1071, 2006). The predominant pathogen was a multidrug resistant stain of *Shigella sonnei*, with 89% of the isolates resistant to ampicillin and trimethoprim-sulfamethoxazole. Shigellosis spreads easily in daycare centers because of the increased risk of fecal contamination and the low infectious dose responsible for disease. Parents and teachers, as well as classmates, are at significant risk for disease.

Yersinia (Box 30-6)

The best-known human pathogens within the genus *Yersinia* are **Yersinia pestis, Yersinia enterocolitica**, and **Yersinia pseudotuberculosis**. *Y. pestis* is a highly virulent pathogen that causes the highly fatal systemic disease known as **plague**; *Y. enterocolitica* and *Y. pseudotuberculosis* are primarily enteric pathogens that are rarely cultured from blood.

Box 30—6. Summary: *Yersinia*

Biology, Virulence, and Disease

Gram-negative, facultatively anaerobic rods
Fermenter; oxidase negative
Lipopolysaccharide consists of somatic O polysaccharide, core polysaccharide (common antigen), and lipid A (endotoxin)
Y. pestis is covered with a protein capsule
Some species (e.g., *Y. enterocolitica*) can grow at cold temperatures (e.g., can grow to high numbers in contaminated, refrigerated food or blood products)
Virulence—refer to Box 30-2; capsule on *Y. pestis* is antiphagocytic; *Y. pestis* is resistant to serum killing; *Yersinia* with genes for adherence, cytotoxic activity, inhibition of phagocytic migration and engulfment, and inhibition of platelet aggregation
Disease—*Y. pestis* causes bubonic plague (most common) and pulmonary plague, both having a high mortality rate; other *Yersinia* species cause gastroenteritis (acute watery diarrhea or chronic diarrhea) and transfusion-related sepsis; enteric disease in children may manifest as enlarge mesenteric lymph nodes and mimic acute appendicitis

Epidemiology

Y. pestis is a zoonotic infection, with humans the accidental host; natural reservoirs include rats, squirrels, rabbits, and domestic animals
Disease is spread by flea bites or direct contact with infected tissues or person to person by inhalation of infectious aerosols from a patient with pulmonary disease
Other *Yersinia* infections are spread through exposure to contaminated food products or blood products *(Y. enterocolitica)*
Colonization with other *Yersinia* species can occur

Diagnosis

Organisms grow on most culture media; prolonged storage at 4° C can selectively enhance isolation

Treatment, Prevention, and Control

Y. pestis infections are treated with streptomycin; tetracyclines, chloramphenicol, or trimethoprim-sulfamethoxazole can be administered as alternative therapy
Enteric infections with other *Yersinia* species are usually self-limited. If antibiotic therapy is indicated, most organisms are susceptible to broad-spectrum cephalosporins, aminoglycosides, chloramphenicol, tetracyclines, and trimethoprim-sulfamethoxazole
Plague is controlled by reduction of the rodent population and vaccination of individuals at risk
Other *Yersinia* infections are controlled by the proper preparation of food products

Pathogenesis and Immunity

A common characteristic of the pathogenic *Yersinia* species is their ability to **resist phagocytic killing**. The type III secretion system mediates this property. On contact with phagocytic cells, the bacteria secrete proteins into the phagocyte that dephosphorylate several proteins required for phagocytosis (*Yop*H gene product), induce cytotoxicity by disrupting actin filaments (*Yop*E gene product), and initiate apoptosis in macrophages (*Yop*J/P gene product). The type III secretion system also suppresses cytokine production, in turn diminishing the inflammatory immune response to infection.

Y. pestis has two plasmids that encode virulence genes: (1) fraction 1 (F1) gene, which codes for an antiphagocytic **protein capsule**, and (2) **plasminogen activator (Pla) protease** gene, which degrades complement components C3b and C5a, preventing opsonization and phagocytic migration, respectively. The Pla gene also degrades fibrin clots, permitting *Y. pestis* to spread rapidly. Other virulence factors specifically associated with *Y. pestis* are serum resistance and the ability of the organism to absorb organic iron as a result of a siderophore-independent mechanism.

Epidemiology

All *Yersinia* infections are **zoonotic**, with humans the accidental hosts. There are two forms of *Y. pestis* infection: **urban plague**, for which rats are the natural reservoirs, and **sylvatic plague**, which causes infections in squirrels, rabbits, field rats, and domestic cats. Pigs, rodents, livestock, and rabbits are the natural reservoirs for *Y. enterocolitica*, whereas rodents, wild animals, and game birds are the natural reservoirs for *Y. pseudotuberculosis*.

Plague caused by *Y. pestis* was one of the most devastating diseases in history. Epidemics of the plague were recorded in the Old Testament. The first of three major pandemics (urban plague) started in Egypt in 541 AD and spread throughout North Africa, Europe, central and southern Asia, and Arabia. By the time this pandemic ended in the mid-700s, a major proportion of the population in these countries had died from the plague. The second pandemic, which started in the 1320s, resulted (over a 5-year period) in more than 25 million deaths in Europe alone (30% to 40% of the population). The third pandemic began in China in the 1860s and spread to Africa, Europe, and the Americas. Epidemic and sporadic cases of the disease continue to this day. In the last decade, an average of 10 cases annually were reported in the United States, with **disease (sylvatic plague) primarily in the western United States.**

Urban plague is maintained in rat populations and is spread among **rats**, or between rats and humans by infected **fleas**. Fleas become infected during a blood meal from a bacteremic rat. After the bacteria replicate in the flea gut, the organisms can be transferred to another rodent or to humans. Urban plague has been eliminated from most communities by the effective control of rats and better hygiene. In contrast, **sylvatic plague** is difficult or impossible to eliminate because the **mammalian reservoirs** and **flea vectors** are widespread. *Y. pestis* produces a fatal infection in the animal reservoir. Thus cyclic patterns of human disease occur as the opportunity for contact with the reservoir population increases or decreases. Infections can also be acquired through the ingestion of contaminated animals or the handling of contaminated animal tissues. Although the organism is highly infectious, human-to-human spread is uncommon unless the patient has pulmonary involvement.

Y. enterocolitica is a common cause of enterocolitis in Scandinavian and other European countries and in the colder areas of North America. In the United States, approximately one culture-confirmed infection occurs per 100,000 persons each year, with 90% of the infections being associated with consumption of contaminated meat, milk, or water. Most studies show that infections are more common during the cold months. Virulence with this organism is associated with specific serogroups. The most common serogroups found in Europe, Africa, Japan, and Canada are O3 and O9. Serogroup O8 has been identified in the United States. *Y. pseudotuberculosis* is a relatively uncommon cause of human disease.

Clinical Diseases (Clinical Case 30-4)

The two clinical manifestations of *Y. pestis* infection are bubonic plague and pneumonic plague. **Bubonic plague** is characterized by an incubation period of no more than 7 days after a person has been bitten by an infected flea. Patients have a high fever and a painful **bubo** (inflammatory swelling of the lymph nodes) in the groin or axilla. Bacteremia develops rapidly if patients are not treated, and as many as 75% die. The incubation period

---

Clinical Case 30-4. Human Plague in the United States

In 2006, a total of 13 human plague cases were reported in the United States—7 in New Mexico, 3 in Colorado, 2 in California, and 1 in Texas (Morb Mortal Wkly Rev [MMWR] 55:940-943, 2006). The following is a description of a 30-year-old man with a classical presentation of bubonic plague. On July 9, the man presented to his local hospital with a 3-day history of fever, nausea, vomiting, and right inguinal lymphadenopathy. He was discharged without treatment. Three days later he returned to the hospital and was admitted with sepsis and bilateral pulmonary infiltrates. He was placed on respiratory isolation and treated with gentamicin, to which he responded. Cultures of his blood and enlarged lymph node were positive for *Yersinia pestis*. The bacteria were also recovered in fleas collected near the patient's home. Typically the reservoirs for sylvatic plague are small mammals, and the vectors are fleas. When the mammals die off, the fleas will seek human hosts. In this example, a total of 5 human cases of plague were reported in the county over a 1-year period.

(2 to 3 days) is shorter in patients with **pneumonic plague**. Initially these patients experience fever and malaise, and pulmonary signs develop within 1 day. The patients are highly infectious; person-to-person spread occurs by aerosols. The mortality rate in untreated patients with pneumonic plague exceeds 90%.

Approximately two-thirds of all *Y. enterocolitica* infections are **enterocolitis**, as the name implies. The gastroenteritis is typically associated with ingestion of contaminated food products or water. After an incubation period of 1 to 10 days (average, 4 to 6 days), the patient experiences disease characterized by diarrhea, fever, and abdominal pain that last for as long as 1 to 2 weeks. A chronic form of the disease can also develop and persist for months. Disease involves the terminal ileum and, if the mesenteric lymph nodes become enlarged, can mimic acute appendicitis. *Y. enterocolitica* infection is most common in children, with **pseudoappendicitis** posing a particular problem in this age group. *Y. pseudotuberculosis* can also produce an enteric disease with the same clinical features. Other manifestations seen in adults are septicemia, arthritis, intraabdominal abscess, hepatitis, and osteomyelitis.

In 1987, *Y. enterocolitica* was first reported to cause **blood transfusion—related bacteremia** and endotoxic shock. Because *Yersinia* organisms **can grow at 4° C**, this organism can multiply to high concentrations in nutritionally rich blood products that are stored in a refrigerator.

Other Enterobacteriaceae

Klebsiella

Members of the genus *Klebsiella* have a prominent capsule that is responsible for the mucoid appearance of isolated colonies and the enhanced virulence of the organisms in vivo. The most commonly isolated members of this genus are ***Klebsiella pneumoniae*** and ***Klebsiella oxytoca***, which can cause community- or hospital-acquired primary **lobar pneumonia**. Pneumonia caused by *Klebsiella* species frequently involves the necrotic destruction of alveolar spaces, formation of cavities, and the production of blood-tinged sputum. These bacteria also cause wound, soft tissue, and urinary tract infections.

The organism formerly called *Donovania granulomatis* and then *Calymmatobacterium granulomatis* has been reclassified as ***Klebsiella granulomatis***. *K. granulomatis* is the etiologic agent of **granuloma inguinale**, a granulomatous disease affecting the genitalia and inguinal area (Figures 30-5 and 30-6). Unfortunately, this disease is commonly called **donovanosis** in reference to the historical origin of the genus name. Granuloma inguinale is a rare disease in the United States but is endemic in parts of Papua New Guinea, the Caribbean, South America, India, southern Africa, Vietnam, and Australia. It can be transmitted after repeated exposure through sexual intercourse

Figure 30—5. Penile ulcer caused by *K. granulomatis*. This can mimic the chancre of syphilis. *(From Morse SA, et al: Atlas of Sexually Transmitted Diseases, 3rd ed. St Louis, Mosby, 2003.)*

or nonsexual trauma to the genitalia. After a prolonged incubation of weeks to months, subcutaneous nodules appear on the genitalia or in the inguinal area. The nodules subsequently break down, revealing one or more painless granulomatous lesions that can extend and coalesce.

Two other *Klebsiella* species of clinical importance are ***Klebsiella rhinoscleromatis***, cause of a granulomatous disease of the nose, and ***Klebsiella ozaenae***, cause of chronic atrophic rhinitis. Both diseases are relatively uncommon in the United States.

Proteus

Infections of the urinary tract with ***Proteus mirabilis*** are the most common diseases produced by this genus. *P. mirabilis* produces large quantities of urease, which splits urea into carbon dioxide and ammonia. This process raises the

Figure 30—6. Light microscopy of impression smear of granulation tissue from genital lesion of patient infected with *K. granulomatis*. Note the numerous bacteria in the cytoplasmic vacuole of the mononuclear cell; modified Giemsa stain. *(From Morse SA, et al: Atlas of Sexually Transmitted Diseases, 3rd ed. St Louis, Mosby, 2003.)*

urine pH, precipitating magnesium and calcium in the form of struvite and apatite crystals, respectively, and results in the formation of **renal (kidney) stones**. The increased alkalinity of the urine is also toxic to the uro-epithelium. *Proteus* also produces as many as six different types of fimbriae, some of which are important for adher-ence to the uroepithelium.

Enterobacter, Citrobacter, Morganella, Serratia

Primary infections caused by *Enterobacter, Citrobacter, Morganella*, and *Serratia* are rare in immunocompetent patients. They are more common causes of hospital-acquired infections in neonates and immunocompromised patients. For example, **Citrobacter koseri** has been recognized to have a predilection for causing meningitis and brain abscesses in neonates. Antibiotic therapy for these genera can be ineffective because the organisms are frequently resistant to multiple antibiotics. Resistance is a particularly serious problem with *Enterobacter* species.

Laboratory Diagnosis

Culture

Members of the family Enterobacteriaceae grow readily on culture media. Specimens of normally sterile material, such as spinal fluid and tissue collected at surgery, can be inoculated onto nonselective blood agar media. Selective media (e.g., MacConkey agar, eosin–methylene blue [EMB] agar) are used for the culture of specimens normally contaminated with other organisms (e.g., sputum, feces). Use of these selective differential agars enables the separa-tion of lactose-fermenting Enterobacteriaceae from nonfer-menting strains, thereby providing information that can be used to guide empirical antimicrobial therapy.

Diagnosis of *E. coli* strains responsible for gastroenteritis is most commonly performed by reference laboratories. The exception is detection of EHEC. Two approaches have been used: culture and toxin detection. In contrast with most *E. coli*, many strains of EHEC do not ferment sorbitol. Thus, **sorbitol-containing MacConkey agar** (S-MAC) has been used to screen stool specimens for sorbitol-negative (colorless), gram-negative bacteria that are then confirmed by serogrouping and biochemical tests to be *E. coli* O157, the most common serotype of EHEC. The limitation to this approach is that some strains of O157 and many other EHEC serotypes ferment sorbitol and would be missed by this screening approach. The preferred method to detect EHEC is to culture stool specimens on nonselective MacConkey agar and then assay isolated colonies for toxin production by commercially available immunoassays. Unfortunately, this is a slow and labor-intensive procedure.

Highly selective or organism-specific media are useful for the recovery of organisms such as *Salmonella* and *Shigella* in stool specimens, where an abundance of normal flora can obscure the presence of these important pathogens.

It is difficult to recover *Y. enterocolitica*, because this organism grows slowly at traditional incubation tempera-tures and prefers cooler temperatures, at which it is more active metabolically. Clinical laboratories have exploited this property, however, by mixing the fecal specimen with saline and then storing the specimen at 4° C for 2 weeks or more before subculturing it to agar media. This **cold enrichment** permits the growth of *Yersinia* but inhi-bits or kills other organisms in the specimen. Although use of the cold enrichment method does not aid in the initial management of a patient with *Yersinia* gastroenteritis, it has helped elucidate the role of this organism in chronic intestinal disease.

Biochemical Identification

There are many diverse species in the family Enterobacteriaceae. The citations listed in the bibliography at the end of this chapter provide additional information about their biochemical identification. Biochemical test systems have become increasingly sophisticated, and the most common members of the family can be identified accurately in less than 24 hours with one of the many com-mercially available identification systems. Sequencing of species-specific genes is used to identify the less common species.

Serologic Classification

Serologic testing is very useful for determining the clinical significance of an isolate (e.g., serotyping specific pathogenic strains, such as *E. coli* O157 or *Y. enterocolitica* O8) and for classifying isolates for epidemiologic purposes. The usefulness of this procedure is limited, however, by cross-reactions with antigenically related Enterobacteriaceae and with organisms from other bacterial families.

Treatment, Prevention, and Control

Antibiotic therapy for infections with Enterobacteriaceae must be guided by in vitro susceptibility test results and clinical experience. Whereas some organisms such as *E. coli* and *P. mirabilis* are susceptible to many antibiotics, others can be highly resistant. Furthermore, susceptible organisms exposed to subtherapeutic concentrations of antibiotics in a hospital setting can rapidly develop resistance. In general, **antibiotic resistance** is more common in hospital-acquired infections than in commu-nity-acquired infections. Antibiotic therapy is not recom-mended for some infections. For example, symptomatic relief but not antibiotic treatment is usually recommended

ENTEROBACTERIACEAE

30

for patients with enterohemorrhagic *E. coli* and *Salmonella* gastroenteritis because antibiotics can prolong the fecal carriage of these organisms or increase the risk of secondary complications (e.g., HUS with EHEC infections in children). Treatment of *Salmonella* Typhi infections or other systemic *Salmonella* infections is indicated; however, increasing resistance to antibiotics such as the fluoroquinolones has complicated therapy.

It is difficult to prevent infections with Enterobacteriaceae, because these organisms are a major part of the endogenous microbial population. However, some risk factors for the infections should be avoided. These include the unrestricted use of antibiotics that can select for resistant bacteria; the performance of procedures that traumatize mucosal barriers without prophylactic antibiotic coverage; and the use of urinary catheters. Unfortunately, many of these factors are present in patients at greatest risk for infection (e.g., immunocompromised patients confined to the hospital for extended periods).

Exogenous infection with Enterobacteriaceae is theoretically easier to control. For example, the source of infections with organisms such as *Salmonella* is well defined. However, these bacteria are ubiquitous in poultry and eggs. Unless care is taken in the preparation and refrigeration of such foods, little can be done to control these infections. *Shigella* organisms are predominantly transmitted in young children, but it is difficult to interrupt the fecal-hand-mouth transmission responsible for spreading the infection in this population. Outbreaks of these infections can be effectively prevented and controlled only through education, and the introduction of appropriate infection-control procedures (e.g., handwashing, and proper disposal of soiled diapers and linens) in the settings where these infections typically occur.

A vaccine for *Y. pestis* is no longer available, although this is likely to change in light of the concern that this organism can be used by bioterrorists. Two vaccines for *Salmonella* Typhi are available—an oral, live, attenuated vaccine and a Vi capsular polysaccharide vaccine. Both vaccines protect 50% to 80% of the recipients, are administered in multiple doses, and require booster immunization because immunity is short-lived. Refer to the CDC website (www.cdc.gov) for current recommendations.

Reference to Student Consult Animation

Please visit ***www.StudentConsult.com*** to view an animation demonstrating the functions of *E.coli* heat-labile enterotoxin, *E.coli* shiga toxin, *Shigella dysenteriae* shiga toxin, and *Shigella* shiga toxin with *E.coli* shiga toxin.

Case Study and Questions

A 25-year-old, previously healthy woman came to the emergency room for the evaluation of bloody diarrhea and diffuse abdominal pain of 24 hours' duration. She complained of nausea and had vomited twice. She reported no history of inflammatory bowel disease, previous diarrhea, or contact with other people with diarrhea. The symptoms began 24 hours after she had eaten an undercooked hamburger at a local fast food restaurant. Rectal examination revealed watery stool with gross blood. Sigmoidoscopy showed diffuse mucosal erythema and petechiae with a modest exudation but no ulceration or pseudomembranes.

1. Name four genera of Enterobacteriaceae that can cause gastrointestinal disease. Name the two genera that can cause hemorrhagic colitis.
2. What virulence factor mediates this disease?
3. Name the five groups of *Escherichia coli* that can cause gastroenteritis. What is characteristic of each group of organisms?
4. What are the four forms of *Salmonella* infection?
5. Differentiate between disease caused by *Salmonella* Typhi and that caused by *Shigella sonnei*.
6. Describe the epidemiology of the two forms of disease caused by *Yersinia pestis*.

Bibliography

Abbott S: *Klebsiella, Enterobacter, Citrobacter, Serratia, Plesiomonas,* and other Enterobacteriaceae. In Murray PR, et al (eds): Manual of Clinical Microbiology, 9th ed. Washington, DC, ASM Press, 2007.

Ackers ML, et al: Laboratory-based surveillance of *Salmonella* serotype Typhi infections in the United States: Antimicrobial resistance on the rise. J Am Med Assoc 283:2668-2673, 2000.

Farmer JJ, et al: Enterobacteriaceae: Introduction and identification. In Murray PR, et al (eds): Manual of Clinical Microbiology, 9th ed. Washington, DC, ASM Press, 2007.

Nataro J, et al: *Escherichia, Shigella,* and *Salmonella.* In Murray PR, et al (eds): Manual of Clinical Microbiology, 9th ed. Washington, DC, ASM Press, 2007.

Qadri F, et al: Enterotoxigenic *Escherichia coli* in developing countries: Epidemiology, microbiology, clinical features, treatment, and prevention. Clin Microbiol Rev 18:465-483, 2005.

Wanger A: *Yersinia.* In Murray PR, et al (eds): Manual of Clinical Microbiology, 9th ed. Washington, DC, ASM Press, 2007.

Wong CS, et al: The risk of the hemolytic-uremic syndrome after antibiotic treatment of *Escherichia coli* O157:H7 infections. N Engl J Med 342:1930-1936, 2000.

Zaharik ML, et al: Delivery of dangerous goods: Type III secretion in enteric pathogens. Int J Med Microbiol 291:593-603, 2002.

315

Vibrio and Aeromonas

The second major group of **gram-negative, facultatively anaerobic, fermentative rods** are the genera *Vibrio* and *Aeromonas*. These organisms were at one time classified together in the family Vibrionaceae and were separated from the Enterobacteriaceae on the basis of a **positive oxidase reaction** and the presence of **polar flagella**. These organisms were also classified together because they are primarily found in water and are able to cause gastrointestinal disease. However, molecular biology techniques have established that these genera are only distantly related and belong in separate families: *Vibrio* and *Aeromonas* are now classified in the families Vibrionaceae and Aeromonadaceae, respectively (Box 31-1). Despite this taxonomic reorganization, it is appropriate to consider these bacteria together because their epidemiology and range of diseases are similar.

Vibrio

The genus *Vibrio* has undergone numerous changes in recent years, with a number of less common species described or reclassified. Currently the genus is composed of 76 species of **curved rods**. A number of species are associated with human disease, but three species are particularly important human pathogens (Table 31-1): ***Vibrio cholerae*** (Box 31-2), ***Vibrio parahaemolyticus*** (Box 31-3), and ***Vibrio vulnificus*** (Box 31-4).

Physiology and Structure

Vibrio species can grow on a variety of simple media within a broad temperature range (from $14°$ C to $40°$ C). All species of **Vibrio require salt** for growth. *V. cholerae* can grow on most media without added salt, but most other species (halophilic species) require the addition of NaCl. Vibrios tolerate a wide range of pH (e.g., pH of 6.5 to 9.0) but are **susceptible to stomach acids**. If gastric acid production is reduced or neutralized, patients are more susceptible to *Vibrio* infections.

Most vibrios have **polar flagella** (important for motility), as well as various pili that are important for virulence. For example, epidemic strains of *V. cholerae*, the etiologic agent of cholera, have the **toxin co-regulated pilus** (see the next section). The cell wall structure of vibrios is also important. All strains possess **lipopolysaccharides** consisting of lipid A (endotoxin), core polysaccharide, and an O polysaccharide side chain. The O polysaccharide is used to subdivide *Vibrio* species into **serogroups**: there are 140 serogroups of *V. cholerae* (O1-O140), 7 O serogroups of *V. vulnificus*, and 13 O serogroups of *V. parahaemolyticus*. The interest in this classification scheme is more than academic—***V. cholerae* O1 and O139** produce **cholera toxin** and are associated with epidemics of cholera. Other strains of *V. cholerae* generally do not produce cholera toxin and do not cause epidemic disease. *V. cholerae* serogroup O1 is further subdivided into serotypes and biotypes. Three **serotypes** are recognized: **Inaba, Ogawa,** and **Hikojima.** Strains can shift between serotype Inaba and serotype Ogawa, with Hikojima a transitional state in which both Inaba and Ogawa antigens are expressed. Two **biotypes** of *V. cholerae* O1 are recognized: **Classical** and **El Tor.** These biotypes are subdivided by differences in phenotypic and morphologic properties. Seven worldwide pandemics of *V. cholerae* infections have been documented. *V. cholerae* strains responsible for the sixth worldwide pandemic of cholera were the Classical biotype, whereas most strains responsible for the current seventh pandemic are the El Tor biotype.

V. vulnificus and non-O1 *V. cholerae* produce acidic **polysaccharide capsules** that are important for disseminated infections. *V. cholerae* O1 does not produce a capsule, so infections with this organism do not spread beyond the confines of the intestine.

V. cholerae and *V. parahaemolyticus* possess two circular chromosomes, each of which contain essential genes for these bacteria. It is not known if other *Vibrio* species have a similar genomic structure. Plasmids, including those encoding antimicrobial resistance, are also commonly found in *Vibrio* species.

Box 31—1. Important *Vibrio* and *Aeromonas* Species

Organism	Historical Derivation
Vibrio	*vibrio*, "move rapidly" or "vibrate" (rapid movement caused by polar flagella)
V. cholerae	*cholera*, "cholera" or an intestinal disease
V. parahaemolyticus	*para*, "by the side of"; *haema*, "blood"; *lyticus*, "dissolving" (dissolving blood; Kanagawa-toxin-positive strains are hemolytic)
V. vulnificus	*vulnificus*, "inflicting wounds" (associated with prominent wound infections)
Aeromonas	*aero*, "gas" or "air"; *monas*, "unit" or "monad" (gas-producing bacteria)
A. caviae	*cavia*, "guinea pig" (first isolated in guinea pigs)
A. hydrophila	*hydro*, "water"; *phila*, "loving" (water loving)
A. veronii	*veron*, named after the bacteriologist *Veron*

Pathogenesis and Immunity (Table 31-2)

The **bacteriophage CTXΦ** encodes the genes for the two subunits of **cholera toxin** (*ctx*A and *ctx*B). This bacteriophage binds to the **toxin co-regulated pilus** (*tcp*) and moves into the bacterial cell, where it becomes integrated into the *V. cholerae* genome. The lysogenic bacteriophage chromosomal locus also contains other virulence factors: the *ace* gene for **accessory cholera enterotoxin**, *zot* gene for the **zonula occludens toxin**, and the *cep* gene for **chemotaxis proteins**. Multiple copies of these genes are found in *V. cholerae* O1 and O139, and their expression is coordinated by regulatory genes.

The cholera toxin is a **complex A-B toxin** that is structurally and functionally similar to the heat-labile enterotoxin of *Escherichia coli*. A ring of five identical B subunits of cholera toxin binds to the ganglioside GM_1 receptors on the intestinal epithelial cells. The active portion of the A subunit is internalized and interacts with G proteins that control adenylate cyclase, leading to the catabolic conversion of adenosine triphosphate (ATP) to cyclic adenosine

Table 31—1. *Vibrio* Species Commonly Associated with Human Disease

Species	Source of Infection	Clinical Disease
V. cholerae	Water, food	Gastroenteritis, bacteremia
V. parahaemolyticus	Shellfish, seawater	Gastroenteritis, wound infection, bacteremia
V. vulnificus	Shellfish, seawater	Bacteremia, wound infection

Box 31—2. Summary: *Vibrio cholerae*

Biology, Virulence, and Disease

Curved, gram-negative rods
Fermentative, facultatively anaerobic; require salt for growth
Strains subdivided into 140 serogroups (O cell-wall antigens)
V. cholerae serogroup O1 is further subdivided into serotypes (Inaba, Ogawa, Hikojima) and biotypes (Classical, El Tor)
Disease mediated by cholera toxin (complex A-B toxin) and toxin co-regulated pilus
Infection can range from asymptomatic colonization or mild diarrhea to severe, rapidly fatal diarrhea

Epidemiology

Serotype O1 is responsible for major pandemics (worldwide epidemics) with significant mortality in developing countries; O139 can cause similar diseases
Organism found in estuarine and marine environments worldwide (including along the coast of the United States); associated with chitinous shellfish
Organism can multiply freely in water
Bacterial levels in contaminated waters increase during the warm months
Spread by consumption of contaminated food or water
Direct person-to-person spread is rare because the infectious dose is high; the infectious dose is high because most organisms are killed by stomach acids

Diagnosis

Microscopic examination of stool generally nonproductive because the organism is diluted in the large volume of watery diarrhea
Culture should be performed early in course of disease with fresh stool specimens maintained in a neutral to alkaline pH

Treatment, Prevention, and Control

Fluid and electrolyte replacement are crucial
Antibiotics (e.g., azithromycin) reduce the bacterial burden and exotoxin production, as well as duration of diarrhea
Improved hygiene is critical for control
Combination inactivated whole cell and cholera toxin B subunit vaccines provide limited protection and herd immunity

monophosphate (cAMP). This results in a hypersecretion of water and electrolytes. Severely infected patients can lose as much as 1 liter of fluid per hour during the height of the disease. Such a tremendous loss of fluid would normally flush the organisms out of the gastrointestinal tract; however, *V. cholerae* are able to **adhere to the mucosal cell layer** by means of (1) the **toxin co-regulated pili** encoded by the *tcp* gene complex and (2) **chemotaxis proteins** encoded by the *cep* genes. Thus the toxin co-regulated pilus is important both as a receptor for the cholera toxin carrying phage and for adherence to the mucosa lining the intestines. Nonadherent strains are unable to establish infection.

In the absence of cholera toxin, *V. cholerae* O1 can still produce significant diarrhea through the action of the **zonula occludens toxin** and **accessory cholera enterotoxin**. As the name implies, the zonula occludens toxin loosens

Box 31–3. Summary: *Vibrio parahaemolyticus*

Biology, Virulence, and Disease

Curved, gram-negative rods
Fermentative, facultatively anaerobic; require salt for growth
Production of thermostable direct hemolysin (TDH; Kanagawa hemolysin) associated with pathogenic strains
Most symptomatic infections are self-limited diarrhea

Epidemiology

Organism found in estuarine and marine environments worldwide
Associated with consumption of contaminated raw shellfish
Most common cause of bacterial gastroenteritis in Japan and Southeast Asia
Most common cause of seafood-associated gastroenteritis in United States

Diagnosis

Culture should be performed as with *V. cholerae*

Treatment, Prevention, and Control

Self-limited disease, although antibiotics can shorten length of symptoms and fluid loss
Disease prevented by proper cooking of shellfish
No vaccines are available

Box 31–4. Summary: *Vibrio vulnificus*

Biology, Virulence, and Disease

Curved, gram-negative rods
Fermentative, facultatively anaerobic; require salt for growth
Virulence associated with presence of polysaccharide capsule and hydrolytic enzymes
High mortality associated with primary septicemia and wound infections, particularly in patients with underlying hepatic disease

Epidemiology

Infection associated with exposure of a wound to contaminated salt water or ingestion of improperly prepared shellfish

Diagnosis

Culture wounds and blood

Treatment, Prevention, and Control

Life-threatening illnesses that must be promptly treated with antibiotics
Minocycline combined with a fluoroquinolone or cefotaxime is the treatment of choice
No vaccine is available

the tight junctions (zonula occludens) of the small intestine mucosa, leading to increased intestinal permeability, and the enterotoxin produces increased fluid secretion.

Unlike other non-O1 serotypes, *V. cholerae* O139 possesses the same virulence complex as that of the O1 strains. Thus the ability of the O139 strains to adhere to the intestinal mucosa and produce cholera toxin is the reason these strains can produce a watery diarrhea similar to cholera.

The means by which other *Vibrio* species cause disease is less clearly understood, although a variety of potential

virulence factors have been identified. Most virulent strains of *V. parahaemolyticus* produce a thermostable direct hemolysin (TDH; also called **Kanagawa hemolysin**). TDH is an enterotoxin that induces chloride ion secretion in epithelial cells by increasing intracellular calcium. An important method for classifying virulent strains of *V. parahaemolyticus* is detection of this hemolysin, which produces β-hemolytic colonies on agar media with human blood but not sheep blood. These virulent strains are referred to as **Kanagawa positive. Capsule** production in

Table 31–2. Virulence Factors of *Vibrio* Species

Species	Virulence Factor	Biologic Effect
V. cholerae	Cholera toxin	Hypersecretion of electrolytes and water
	Toxin co-regulated pilus	Binding site for CTXΦ; mediates adherence to intestinal mucosal cells
	Chemotaxis protein	Adhesin factor
	Accessory cholera enterotoxin	Increases intestinal fluid secretion
	Zonula occludens toxin	Increases intestinal permeability
	Neuraminidase	Modifies cell surface to increase GM_1 binding sites for cholera toxin
V. parahaemolyticus	Kanagawa hemolysin	Enterotoxin that induces chloride ion secretion (watery diarrhea)
V. vulnificus	Polysaccharide capsule	Antiphagocytic
	Cytolysins, proteases, collagenase	Mediates tissue destruction

V. vulnificus is important for the ability of this organism to produce severe, disseminated infections.

Epidemiology

Vibrio species, including *V. cholerae*, grow naturally in **estuarine and marine environments** worldwide. All *Vibrio* species are able to survive and replicate in contaminated waters with increased salinity. Pathogenic vibrios can also flourish in waters with chitinous **shellfish** (e.g., oysters, clams, mussels)—hence the association between *Vibrio* infections and the consumption of shellfish. Asymptomatically infected humans can also be an important reservoir for this organism in areas where *V. cholerae* disease is endemic.

Seven major pandemics of cholera have occurred since 1816, resulting in thousands of deaths and major socioeconomic changes. Sporadic disease and epidemics occurred before this time, but worldwide spread of the disease became possible only with intercontinental travel resulting from increased commerce and wars.

The seventh pandemic, which is caused by *V. cholerae* **O1 biotype El Tor**, began in Asia in 1961 and spread to Africa, Europe, and Oceania in the 1970s and 1980s. In 1991, the pandemic strain spread to Peru and subsequently caused disease in most countries in South and Central America, as well as in the United States and Canada. A second epidemic strain emerged in 1992 in India and rapidly spread across Asia. This strain, *V. cholerae* **O139 Bengal**, produces the cholera toxin and shares other traits with *V. cholerae* O1. This is the first non-O1 strain capable of causing epidemic disease and produced disease in adults who were previously infected with the O1 strain (showing that no protective immunity is conferred).

Cholera is spread by **contaminated water and food**, rather than direct person-to-person spread, because a high inoculum (e.g., more than 10^8 organisms) is required to establish infection in a person with normal gastric acidity. In a person with achlorhydria or hypochlorhydria, the infectious dose can be as low as 10^3 to 10^5 organisms. Cholera is usually seen in communities with **poor sanitation**. Indeed, one outcome from the cholera pandemics was recognition of the role of contaminated water in the spread of disease and the need to improve community sanitation systems so that the disease could be controlled.

Infections caused by *V. parahaemolyticus*, *V. vulnificus*, and other pathogenic vibrios result from the consumption of improperly cooked seafood, particularly oysters, or exposure to contaminated seawater. *V. parahaemolyticus* is the most common cause of bacterial gastroenteritis in Japan and Southeast Asia and is the most common *Vibrio* species responsible for gastroenteritis in the United States. *V. vulnificus* is not frequently isolated but is responsible for severe wound infections and a high incidence of fatal outcomes. *V. vulnificus* is the most common cause of vibrio septicemia. Gastroenteritis caused by vibrios occurs

throughout the year, because oysters are typically contaminated with abundant organisms year-round. In contrast, septicemia and wound infections with *Vibrio* occur during the warm months, when the organisms in seawater can multiply to high numbers.

Clinical Diseases (Box 31-5)

Vibrio cholerae (Clinical Case 31-1)

The majority of individuals exposed to toxigenic *V. cholerae* **O1** have asymptomatic infections or self-limited diarrhea; however, some individuals develop severe, rapidly fatal diarrhea. The clinical manifestations of cholera begin an average of 2 to 3 days after ingestion of the bacteria, with the abrupt onset of watery diarrhea and vomiting. As more fluid is lost, the feces-streaked stool specimens become colorless and odorless, free of protein, and speckled with mucus (**"rice-water" stools**). The resulting severe fluid and electrolyte loss can lead to dehydration, painful muscle cramps, metabolic acidosis (bicarbonate loss), and hypokalemia and hypovolemic shock (potassium loss), with cardiac arrhythmia and renal failure. The mortality rate is 60% in untreated patients but less than 1% in patients who are promptly treated with replacement of lost fluids and electrolytes. Disease caused by *V. cholerae* **O139** can be as severe as disease caused by *V. cholerae* O1. Other serotypes of *V. cholerae* (commonly called *V. cholerae* **non-O1**) do not produce cholera toxin and are usually responsible for mild watery diarrhea. These strains can also cause extraintestinal infections such as septicemia, particularly in patients with liver disease or hematologic malignancies.

Vibrio parahaemolyticus (Clinical Case 31-2)

The severity of gastroenteritis caused by *V. parahaemolyticus* can range from a self-limited diarrhea to a mild, cholera-like illness. In general, the disease develops after a 5- to 72-hour

---

Box 31–5. Clinical Summaries

Vibrio cholerae

Cholera: begins with an abrupt onset of watery diarrhea and vomiting and can progress to severe dehydration, metabolic acidosis and hypokalemia, and hypovolemic shock

Gastroenteritis: milder forms of diarrheal disease can occur in toxin-negative strains of *V. cholerae* O1 and in non-O1 serotypes

Vibrio parahaemolyticus

Gastroenteritis: generally self-limited with an explosive onset of watery diarrhea and nausea, vomiting, abdominal cramps, headache, and low-grade fever

Wound infection: associated with exposure to contaminated water

Vibrio vulnificus

Wound infection: severe, potentially fatal infections characterized by erythema, pain, bullae formation, tissue necrosis, and septicemia incubation period (mean, 24 hours), with explosive, **watery diarrhea**. No grossly evident blood or mucus is found in stool specimens except in severe cases. Headache, abdominal cramps, nausea, vomiting, and low-grade fever may persist for 72 hours or more. The patient usually experiences an uneventful recovery. Wound infections with this organism can occur in people exposed to contaminated seawater.

Vibrio vulnificus (Clinical Case 31-3)

V. vulnificus is a particularly virulent species of *Vibrio* responsible for more than 90% of the vibrio-related deaths in the United States. The most common presentations are

primary septicemia after consumption of contaminated raw oysters or rapidly progressive **wound infection** after exposure to contaminated seawater. Patients with primary septicemia present with a sudden onset of fever and chills, vomiting, diarrhea, and abdominal pain. Secondary skin lesions with tissue necrosis are often present. The mortality in patients with *V. vulnificus* septicemia can be as high as 50%. The wound infections are characterized by initial swelling, erythema, and pain at the wound site, followed by the development of vesicles or bullae and eventual tissue necrosis, together with systemic signs of fever and chills. Mortality associated with wound infections ranges from 20% to 30%. *V. vulnificus* infections are most severe in patients with hepatic disease, hematopoietic disease, or chronic renal failure and in those receiving immunosuppressive drugs.

Laboratory Diagnosis

Microscopy

Vibrio species are small (0.5 to 1.5 $\times$ 3 μm), curved, gram-negative rods. The organisms cannot be differentiated from other enteric organisms, so the direct **microscopic examination of stool specimens is not recommended**. Examination of Gram-stained wound specimens may be useful and support clinical and epidemiologic evidence of a vibrio infection.

Culture

Vibrio organisms **survive poorly in an acidic or dry environment**. Specimens must be collected early in the disease and inoculated promptly onto culture media. If culture will be delayed, the specimen should be mixed in a Cary-Blair transport medium and refrigerated. Vibrios have low survival rates in buffered glycerol-saline, the transport medium used for most enteric pathogens.

Vibrios grow on most media used in clinical laboratories for stool and wound cultures, including blood agar and

MacConkey agar. Special selective agar for vibrios (e.g., thiosulfate citrate bile salts sucrose [**TCBS**] agar), as well as an enrichment broth (e.g., **alkaline peptone broth;** pH. 8.6), can also be used to recover vibrios in specimens with a mixture of organisms (e.g., stools). Isolates are identified with selective biochemical tests and serotyped using polyvalent antisera. In tests performed to identify halophilic vibrios, the media for biochemical testing must be supplemented with 1% sodium chloride.

Treatment, Prevention, and Control

Patients with cholera must be promptly treated with **fluid and electrolyte replacement** before the resultant massive fluid loss leads to hypovolemic shock. Antibiotic therapy, although of secondary value, can reduce toxin production and more rapidly eliminate the organism. **Azithromycin** is the drug of choice for children and adults. Resistance to ciprofloxacin, furazolidone, and trimethoprim-sulfamethoxazole (drugs previously recommended) now limit their effectiveness.

V. parahaemolyticus gastroenteritis is usually a self-limited disease, although antibiotic therapy can be used in addition to fluid and electrolyte therapy in patients with severe infections. *V. vulnificus* wound infections and septicemia must be promptly treated with antibiotic therapy. The combination of minocycline and a fluoroquinolone or cefotaxime appears to be the most effective treatment.

People infected with *V. cholerae* can shed bacteria for the first few days of acute illness and represent important sources of new infections. Although long-term carriage of *V. cholerae* does not occur, vibrios are free living in estuarine and marine reservoirs. **Only improvements in sanitation can lead to effective control of the disease.** This involves adequate sewage management, the use of purification systems to eliminate contamination of the water supply, and the implementation of appropriate steps to prevent contamination of food.

A variety of **cholera vaccines** have been developed, none providing long-term protection. Field trials with an oral vaccine consisting of inactivated whole cell *V. cholerae* combined with B subunits demonstrated protection for 62% of the vaccine recipients at 1 year. It was also noted that the incidence of cholera was reduced in the entire population (i.e., **herd immunity**) if a significant proportion of the population was vaccinated. Unfortunately, multiple doses are required for immunity, and protection fades 2 to 3 years after immunization. Other vaccines, including a live, attenuated vaccine, are in development. There is no vaccine for the O139 strains. Tetracycline prophylaxis has also been used to reduce the risk of infection in people traveling to areas where the disease is endemic but has not prevented the spread of cholera. Because the infectious dose of *V. cholerae* is high, antibiotic prophylaxis is generally unnecessary in people who use appropriate hygiene.

Aeromonas

Aeromonas is a **gram-negative, facultatively anaerobic fermentative rod** that morphologically resembles members of the family Enterobacteriaceae. As with *Vibrio*, extensive reorganization of the taxonomy of these bacteria has occurred. Twenty-one species of *Aeromonas* have been described, many of which are associated with human disease. The most important pathogens are **Aeromonas hydrophila**, **Aeromonas caviae**, and **Aeromonas veronii** biovar *sobria*. The organisms are ubiquitous in fresh and brackish water.

Aeromonas species cause three forms of disease: (1) **diarrheal disease** in otherwise healthy people, (2) **wound infections**, and (3) **opportunistic systemic disease** in immunocompromised patients (particularly those with hepatobiliary disease or an underlying malignancy). Intestinal disease can present as acute watery diarrhea, dysenteric diarrhea characterized by severe abdominal pain and blood and leukocytes in the stools, or a chronic illness with intermittent diarrhea. Gastrointestinal carriage has been observed in individuals, with the highest carriage in the warm months. Thus the significance of isolating *Aeromonas* in enteric specimens must be determined by the clinical presentation of the patient. Gastroenteritis typically occurs after the ingestion of contaminated water or food (e.g., fresh produce, meats, dairy products), whereas wound infections most commonly result from a traumatic injury associated with exposure to contaminated water. One unusual form of *Aeromonas* wound infections is associated with the use of medicinal leeches whose gut is colonized with *A. veronii* biovar *sobria* (Clinical Case 31-4).

Although numerous potential virulence factors (e.g., endotoxin, hemolysins, heat-labile and heat-stable

---

Clinical Case 31-4. Medicinal Leeches and *Aeromonas* Wound Infections

Medicinal leeches (*Hiruda medicinalis*) are commonly used in plastic surgery to stimulate blood flow in surgical skin grafts. Leeches remove stagnant blood and stimulate oozing of blood into the skin graft for up to 48 hours after removal of the leech. This bleeding is mediated by an inhibitor of thrombin, hirudin (source of the genus name), that is present in the saliva of leeches. *Aeromonas* is present in the leech gut and produces proteolytic enzymes used by the leech to digest blood. One complication of using leeches is wound infections with *Aeromonas*, as illustrated by the patient described by Snower D, et al. (J Clin Microbiol 27:1421-1422, 1989). A 62-year-old woman had basal cell epitheliomas removed from her forehead, with the surgical site covered with skin grafts. Medicinal leeches were used to relieve swelling at the graft site. The leeches were removed from a leech tank and applied to the wound for 1 hour on four separate occasions. Eleven days after the initial surgery, the graft appeared infected and was removed. Culture of this graft, as well as leeches and water from the leech tank, were positive for *Aeromonas*. The patient was treated with parenteral antibiotics, and regrafting without the use of leeches was successful.

enterotoxins) have been identified for *Aeromonas*, their precise role in disease is unknown.

Acute diarrheal disease is self-limited, and only supportive care is indicated in affected patients. Antimicrobial therapy is necessary in patients with chronic diarrheal disease, wound infections or systemic disease. *Aeromonas* species are resistant to penicillins, most cephalosporins, and erythromycin. **Ciprofloxacin** is consistently active against *Aeromonas* strains isolated in the United States and Europe; however, resistance has been reported in strains recovered in Asia. Thus the long-term effectiveness of fluoroquinolones remains to be seen. Gentamicin, amikacin, and trimethoprim-sulfamethoxazole are also active against most aeromonads.

Case Study and Questions

A 57-year-old man was hospitalized in New York with a 2-day history of severe, watery diarrhea. The illness had begun 1 day after his return from Ecuador. The patient was dehydrated and suffering from an electrolyte imbalance (acidosis, hypokalemia). The patient made an uneventful recovery after fluid and electrolyte replacement was instituted to compensate for the losses resulting from the watery diarrhea. Stool cultures were positive for *V. cholerae*.

1. What are the characteristic clinical symptoms of cholera?

2. What is the most important virulence factor in this disease? What other virulence factors have been described? What are the modes of their action?

3. How did this patient acquire this infection? How does this situation differ from the acquisition of infections caused by *V. parahaemolyticus* or *V. vulnificus*?

4. How can cholera be controlled in areas where infection is endemic?

Reference to Student Consult Animation

Please visit *www.StudentConsult.com* to view an animation demonstrating the functions of cholera toxin and cholera toxin with *E.coli* heat-labile enterotoxin.

Bibliography

Albert MJ, Nair GB: *Vibrio cholerae* O139—10 years on. Rev Med Microbiol 16:135-143, 2005.

Ali M, et al: Herd immunity conferred by killed oral cholera vaccines in Bangladesh: A reanalysis. Lancet 366:44-48, 2005.

Klose KE: Regulation of virulence in *Vibrio cholerae*. Int J Med Microbiol 291:81-88, 2001.

Ko W-C, Chuang Y-C: *Aeromonas* bacteremia: Review of 59 episodes. Clin Infect Dis 20:1298-1304, 1995.

Lacey SW: Cholera: Calamitous past, ominous future. Clin Infect Dis 20:1409-1419, 1995.

McLaughlin JB, et al: Outbreak of *Vibrio parahaemolyticus* gastroenteritis associated with Alaskan oysters. N Engl J Med 353:1463-1470, 2005.

Oliver JD: Wound infections caused by *Vibrio vulnificus* and other marine bacteria. Epidemiol Infect 133:383-391, 2005.

Saha D, et al: Single-dose azithromycin for the treatment of cholera in adults. N Engl J Med 354:2452-2462, 2006.

Snower DP, et al: *Aeromonas hydrophila* infection associated with the use of medicinal leeches. J Clin Microbiol 27:1421-1422, 1989.

Yeung PSM, Boor KJ: Epidemiology, pathogenesis, and prevention of foodborne *Vibrio parahaemolyticus*. Foodborne Pathog Dis 1:74-88, 2004.

Campylobacter and *Helicobacter*

The classification of *Campylobacter* and *Helicobacter* (Box 32-1) has undergone many changes since the bacteria were first discovered. However, molecular biology techniques (e.g., sequence analysis of 16S rRNA genes), characterization of cell wall proteins and lipids, serologic characterization, and analysis of biochemical properties have been used to resolve much of the taxonomic confusion. These genera belong to the same rRNA superfamily, which consists of spiral, gram-negative rods with (1) a low DNA guanosine-plus-cytosine base ratio, (2) an inability to ferment or oxidize carbohydrates, and (3) microaerophilic growth requirements (i.e., growth only in the presence of a reduced oxygen level).

Campylobacter (Box 32-2)

The genus *Campylobacter* consists of small (0.2 to 0.5 μm wide × 0.5 to 5.0 μm long), **comma-shaped, gram-negative rods** (Figure 32-1) that are motile by means of a polar flagellum. Most species are **microaerobic**, requiring an atmosphere with decreased oxygen and increased hydrogen and carbon dioxide levels for aerobic growth. A total of 25 species and 11 subspecies are now recognized, many of which are associated with human disease, but only four species are significant human pathogens (Table 32-1).

The primary diseases caused by campylobacters are gastroenteritis and septicemia. *Campylobacter jejuni* is the most common cause of bacterial gastroenteritis in the United States, and *Campylobacter coli* is responsible for 2% to 5% of the cases of *Campylobacter* gastroenteritis. The latter is a more common cause of gastroenteritis in developing countries.

Campylobacter upsaliensis is most likely an important cause of gastroenteritis in humans; however, the true incidence of disease caused by this organism is underestimated by conventional culture methods (*C. upsaliensis* is inhibited by the antibiotics used in isolation media for other campylobacters). A variety of other species are rare causes of gastroenteritis or systemic infections. Unlike other species,

Campylobacter fetus is most commonly responsible for causing systemic infections such as bacteremia, septic thrombophlebitis, arthritis, septic abortion, and meningitis.

Physiology and Structure

Campylobacters have a typical gram-negative cell wall structure. The major antigen of the genus is the lipopolysaccharide of the outer membrane. In addition, the different somatic O polysaccharide antigens and the heat-labile capsular and flagellar antigens have been used for the epidemiologic classification of clinical isolates.

Recognition of the role of campylobacters in gastrointestinal disease was delayed because the organisms grow best in an atmosphere of reduced oxygen (5% to 7%, **microaerophilic**) and increased carbon dioxide (5% to 10%). In addition, **C. jejuni grows better at 42° C** than at 37° C. These properties have been exploited for the selective isolation of pathogenic campylobacters in stool specimens. The **small size** of the organisms (0.2 to 0.5 μm in diameter) has also been used to recover the bacteria by filtration of stool specimens. Campylobacters pass through 0.45-μm filters, whereas other bacteria are retained. Although this property led to the initial discovery of campylobacters (stools were filtered looking for viruses), filtration of stool specimens is a cumbersome procedure and is not used routinely in clinical laboratories.

Pathogenesis and Immunity

Efforts to define the role of specific virulence factors in *Campylobacter* disease have been thwarted by a lack of an animal model to study the disease. *C. jejuni* is the best studied species. Although adhesins, cytotoxic enzymes, and enterotoxins have been detected in this species, their specific role in disease remains poorly defined. It is clear that the risk of disease is influenced by the infectious dose. The organisms are killed when exposed to gastric acids, so conditions that decrease or neutralize gastric-acid secretion

Box 32—1. Important *Campylobacter* and *Helicobacter* Species

Organism	Historical Derivation
Campylobacter	*kampylos*, "curved"; *bacter*, "rod" (a curved rod)
C. jejuni	*jejuni*, of the jejunum
C. coli	*coli*, of the colon
C. fetus	*fetus*, refers to the initial observation that these bacteria caused fetal infections
C. upsaliensis	*upsaliensis*, original isolates recovered from the feces of dogs at an animal clinic in *Uppsala, Sweden*
Helicobacter	*helix*, "spiral"; *bacter*, "rod" (a spiral rod)
H. pylori	*pylorus*, lower part of the stomach
H. cinaedi	*cinaedi*, of a "homosexual" (the organism was first isolated from homosexuals with gastroenteritis)
H. fennelliae	*fennelliae*, named after C. *Fennell*, who first isolated the organism

Box 32—2. Summary: *Campylobacter*

Biology, Virulence, and Disease

Thin, curved, gram-negative rods
Factors that regulate adhesion, motility, and invasion into intestinal mucosa are poorly defined
Guillain-Barré syndrome believed to be an autoimmune disease caused by antigenic cross-reactivity between oligosaccharides in bacterial capsule and glycosphingolipids on surface of neural tissues
Most common disease is acute enteritis with diarrhea, malaise, fever, and abdominal pain
Most infections are self-limited but can persist for a week or more
C. fetus is associated with septicemia and is disseminated to multiple organs

Epidemiology

Zoonotic infection; improperly prepared poultry is a common source of human infections
Infections acquired by ingestion of contaminated food, unpasteurized milk, or contaminated water
Person-to-person spread is unusual
Dose required to establish disease is high, unless the gastric acids are neutralized or absent
Worldwide distribution with enteric infections seen throughout the year

Diagnosis

Detection of thin, "S-shaped," gram-negative rods in stool specimens is insensitive but specific
Culture requires use of specialized media incubated with reduced oxygen, increased carbon dioxide, and (for thermophilic species) elevated temperatures; requires incubation for 2 or more days
Detection of *Campylobacter* antigens in stool specimens is moderately sensitive and very specific compared with culture

Treatment, Prevention, and Control

For gastroenteritis, infection is self-limited and is managed by fluid and electrolyte replacement
Severe gastroenteritis and septicemia are treated with erythromycin or azithromycin
Gastroenteritis is prevented by proper preparation of food and consumption of pasteurized milk; preventing contamination of water supplies also controls infection

favor disease. The patient's immune status also affects the severity of disease. People living in a population of high endemic disease develop measurable levels of specific serum and secretory antibodies and have less severe disease. Patients with hypogammaglobulinemia have prolonged, severe disease with *C. jejuni*.

C. jejuni gastrointestinal disease characteristically produces **histologic damage to the mucosal surfaces of the jejunum** (as implied by the name of the species), ileum, and colon. The mucosal surface appears ulcerated, edematous, and bloody, with crypt abscesses in the epithelial glands and infiltration of the lamina propria with neutrophils, mononuclear cells, and eosinophils. This inflammatory process is consistent with invasion of the organisms into the intestinal tissue. However, the precise roles of cytopathic toxins, enterotoxins, and endotoxic activity that have been detected in *C. jejuni* isolates have not been defined. For example, strains lacking enterotoxin activity are still fully virulent.

C. jejuni and *C. upsaliensis* have been associated with **Guillain-Barré syndrome**, an autoimmune disorder of the peripheral nervous system characterized by development of symmetrical weakness over several days and recovery requiring months or longer. Although this is an uncommon complication of *Campylobacter* disease (approximately one in 1000 diagnosed infections), the syndrome has been associated with specific serotypes (primarily *C. jejuni* serotype O:19). It is believed that the pathogenesis of this disease is related to **antigenic cross-reactivity** between the surface lipopolysaccharides of some strains

of *Campylobacter* and peripheral nerve gangliosides. Thus antibodies directed against specific strains of *Campylobacter* can damage neural tissue in the peripheral nervous system. Another immune-related late complication of campylobacter infections is **reactive arthritis**, a condition characterized by painful joint swellings that may last for weeks to a year.

Whereas *C. jejuni* and *C. coli* rarely cause bacteremia (1.5 cases per 1000 intestinal infections), *C. fetus* has a propensity to spread from the gastrointestinal tract to the blood and distal foci. This spread is particularly common in debilitated and immunocompromised patients, such as

Figure 32–1. Mixed culture of bacteria from a fecal specimen. *Campylobacter jejuni* is the thin, curved, gram-negative bacteria (arrow).

those with liver disease, diabetes mellitus, chronic alcoholism, or malignancies. In vitro studies have shown that *C. fetus* is resistant to complement- and antibody-mediated serum killing, whereas *C. jejuni* and most other *Campylobacter* species are killed rapidly. *C. fetus* is covered with a heat-stable, capsule-like protein (**S protein**) that prevents complement-mediated killing in serum (inhibition of C3b binding to the bacteria). *C. fetus* loses its virulence if this protein layer is removed.

Table 32–1. Common *Campylobacter* Species Associated with Human Disease

Species	Common Reservoir Hosts	Human Disease
C. jejuni	Poultry, cattle, sheep	Gastroenteritis, extraintestinal infections, Guillain-Barré syndrome, reactive arthritis
C. coli	Pigs, poultry, sheep, birds	Gastroenteritis, extraintestinal infections
C. fetus	Cattle, sheep	Vascular infections (e.g., septicemia, septic thrombophlebitis, endocarditis), meningoencephalitis, gastroenteritis
C. upsaliensis	Dogs, cats	Gastroenteritis, extraintestinal infections

Epidemiology

Campylobacter infections are **zoonotic**, with a variety of animals serving as reservoirs (see Table 32-1). Humans acquire the infections with *C. jejuni* and *C. coli* after consumption of contaminated food, milk, or water; **contaminated poultry** are responsible for more than half of the *Campylobacter* infections in developed countries. In contrast, *C. upsaliensis* infections are acquired primarily after contact with domestic dogs (either healthy carriers or pets with diarrheal disease). Food products that neutralize gastric acids (e.g., milk) effectively reduce the infectious dose. Fecal-oral transmission from person to person may also occur, but it is **uncommon for the disease to be transmitted by food handlers**.

The actual incidence of *Campylobacter* infections is unknown because disease is not reported to public health officials. Epidemiologic surveys indicate that the incidence of disease has decreased in the last decade, most likely due to improved food handling techniques; however, it is estimated that between 1.4 and 2 million infections occur annually in the United States, and these infections are more common than *Salmonella* and *Shigella* infections combined. The number of *Campylobacter* infections may be even higher, because *C. upsaliensis* is believed to be responsible for approximately 10% of the *Campylobacter* infections, and this species would not be isolated by commonly used techniques. Disease occurs throughout the year, but epidemics are most common in the spring and fall months. The peak incidence of disease is in **infants and young children**, with a second peak of disease in 20- to 40-year-old adults. The incidence of disease is higher in developing countries, with symptomatic disease in infants and young children and asymptomatic carriage frequently observed in adults.

C. fetus infections are relatively uncommon, with fewer than 250 cases reported annually. Unlike *C. jejuni*, *C. fetus* primarily infects immunocompromised elderly people.

Clinical Diseases (Clinical Case 32-1)

Gastrointestinal infections with *C. jejuni*, *C. coli*, and *C. upsaliensis* present most commonly as **acute enteritis** with diarrhea, fever, and abdominal pain. Affected patients can have 10 or more bowel movements per day during the peak of disease, and stools may be bloody on gross examination. The disease is generally self-limited, although symptoms may last for a week or longer. The range of clinical manifestations includes colitis, **abdominal pain mimicking acute appendicitis**, and bacteremia. Chronic enteric infections may develop in immunocompromised patients (e.g., patients with AIDS) and be difficult to treat. A variety of extraintestinal infections are reported but are relatively uncommon. **Guillain-Barré syndrome** and **reactive arthritis** are well-recognized complications of Campylobacter infections. *C. fetus* differs from other *Campylobacter* species in that this species is primarily responsible for **intravascular**

(e.g., septicemia, endocarditis, septic thrombophlebitis) and **extraintestinal** (e.g., meningoencephalitis, abscesses) **infections.** Most *C. fetus* infections are in elderly or immunocompromised patients.

Laboratory Diagnosis

Microscopy

Campylobacters are thin and are not easily seen when specimens are Gram stained. Despite the low sensitivity of a Gram stain, observation of the characteristic **thin, "S-shaped" organisms** in a stool specimen (see Figure 32-1) is very specific.

Antigen Detection

A commercial immunoassay for detection of *C. jejuni* and *C. coli* is available. When compared with culture, the test has a sensitivity of 80% to 90% and a specificity of >95%. Some strains of *C. upsaliensis* are also reactive in this test.

Culture

C. jejuni, *C. coli*, and *C. upsaliensis* went unrecognized for many years because their isolation requires growth in a **microaerophilic atmosphere** (i.e., 5% to 7% oxygen, 5% to 10% carbon dioxide, and the balance nitrogen), at an **elevated incubation temperature** (i.e., 42° C), and on selective agar media. The appropriate atmosphere for growing campylobacters can be produced by a disposable commercial gas-generator system that is added to an incubation jar with the inoculated culture media. The selective media must contain blood or charcoal to remove toxic oxygen radicals, and antibiotics are added to inhibit the growth of contaminating organisms. Unfortunately the antibiotics used in most campylobacter media may inhibit some species (e.g., *C. upsaliensis*). Campylobacters are **slow-growing** organisms, usually requiring incubation for 48 to 72 hours or longer. *C. fetus* is not thermophilic and cannot grow at 42° C; however, its isolation still requires a microaerophilic atmosphere.

Identification

A presumptive identification of isolates is based on growth under selective conditions, typical microscopic morphology, and positive oxidase and catalase tests.

Antibody Detection

Serologic testing for IgM and IgG is useful for epidemiologic surveys but is not used for diagnosis in an individual patient.

Treatment, Prevention, and Control

Campylobacter gastroenteritis is typically a self-limited infection managed by the replacement of lost fluids and electrolytes. Antibiotic therapy may be used in patients with severe infections or septicemia. Campylobacters are susceptible to a variety of antibiotics, including macrolides (i.e., erythromycin, azithromycin, and clarithromycin), tetracyclines, aminoglycosides, chloramphenicol, fluoroquinolones, clindamycin, amoxicillin/clavulanic acid, and imipenem. Most isolates are resistant to penicillins, cephalosporins, and sulfonamide antibiotics. **Erythromycin or azithromycin** are the antibiotics of choice for the treatment of enteritis, with tetracycline or fluoroquinolones used as secondary antibiotics. Resistance to fluoroquinolones has increased, so these drugs may be less effective. Amoxicillin/clavulanic acid can be used in place of tetracycline, which is contraindicated in young children. Systemic infections are treated with an aminoglycoside, chloramphenicol, or imipenem.

Exposure to enteric campylobacters is prevented by the proper preparation of food (particularly poultry), avoidance of unpasteurized dairy products, and the implementation of safeguards to prevent the contamination of water supplies. It is unlikely that *Campylobacter* carriage in animal reservoirs such as chickens and turkeys will be eliminated, so the risk of infections from these sources remains.

Helicobacter (Box 32-3)

In 1983, **spiral, gram-negative rods** resembling campylobacters were found in patients with type B gastritis (chronic inflammation of the stomach antrum [pyloric end]). The organisms were originally classified as *Campylobacter* but were subsequently reclassified as a new genus, *Helicobacter*. The bacteria *Helicobacter pylori* (a **gastric helicobacter**) have now been associated with **gastritis, peptic ulcers, gastric adenocarcinoma**, and **gastric mucosa—associated**

Box 32–3. Summary: *Helicobacter pylori*

Biology, Virulence, and Disease

Curved, gram-negative rods
Urease production at very high levels is typical of gastric
  helicobacters (e.g., *H. pylori*) and uncommon in intestinal
  helicobacters (important diagnostic test for *H. pylori*)
Multiple factors contribute to gastric colonization, inflammation,
  alteration of gastric acid production and tissue destruction
H. pylori is an important cause of acute and chronic gastritis,
  peptic ulcers, gastric adenocarcinoma, and MALT lymphoma

Epidemiology

Infections are common, particularly in people in a low
  socioeconomic class or in developing nations
Humans are the primary reservoir
Person-to-person spread is important (typically fecal-oral)
Ubiquitous and worldwide with no seasonal incidence of disease

Diagnosis

Microscopy: histologic examination of biopsy specimens is
  sensitive and specific
Urease test relatively sensitive and highly specific; urea breath
  test is a noninvasive test
H. pylori antigen test is sensitive and specific; performed with
  stool specimens
Culture requires incubation in microaerophilic conditions; growth
  is slow; relatively insensitive unless multiple biopsies are
  cultured
Serology useful for demonstrating exposure to *H. pylori*

Treatment, Prevention, and Control

Multiple regimens have been evaluated for treatment of *H. pylori*
  infections. Combined therapy with a proton pump inhibitor
  (e.g., omeprazole), a macrolide (e.g., clarithromycin), and a
  beta-lactam (e.g., amoxicillin) for 2 weeks has had a high
  success rate
Prophylactic treatment of colonized individuals has not been
  useful and potentially has adverse effects, such as
  predisposing patients to adenocarcinomas of the lower
  esophagus
Human vaccines are not currently available

Table 32–2. *Helicobacter* Species Associated with Human Disease*

Species	Common Reservoir Hosts	Human Disease
H. pylori	Humans, primates, pigs	Gastritis, peptic ulcers, gastric adenocarcinoma, MALT B-cell lymphomas
H. cinaedi	Humans, hamster	Gastroenteritis, septicemia, proctocolitis
H. fennelliae	Humans	Gastroenteritis, septicemia, proctocolitis

fatty acids, and the presence of polar flagella. Currently, 30 species have been characterized, but this taxonomy is changing rapidly. Helicobacters have a bacillary or **spiral shape** in young cultures (0.5 to 1.0 μm wide × 2 to 4 μm long) but can assume coccoid forms in older cultures (Figure 32-2).

All gastric helicobacters, including *H. pylori*, are highly **motile** (corkscrew motility) via polar flagella and produce an abundance of **urease**. These properties are believed to be important for survival in gastric acids and rapid movement through the viscous mucus layer towards a neutral pH environment. Most helicobacters are catalase- and oxidase-positive and do not ferment or oxidize carbohydrates, although they can metabolize amino acids by fermentative pathways. Lipopolysaccharide (LPS), consisting of lipid A, core oligosaccharide, and an O side chain, is present in the outer membrane. *H. pylori* lipid A has low endotoxin activity compared with other gram-negative bacteria, and the O side chain is antigenically similar to the Lewis blood group antigens, which may protect the bacteria from immune clearance.

lymphoid tissue (MALT) B-cell lymphomas (Table 32-2). The intestinal tract of humans is colonized by other helicobacter species (i.e., **enterohepatic helicobacters**), including *Helicobacter cinaedi* and *Helicobacter fennelliae*, which have been isolated from homosexual men with proctitis, proctocolitis, or enteritis. Helicobacters are also isolated from the stomachs and intestines of many other mammals (e.g., monkeys, dogs, cats, cheetahs, ferrets, mice, rats). Most of the discussion in this chapter will be restricted to the gastric helicobacter, *H. pylori*.

Physiology and Structure

Helicobacter species are characterized according to sequence analysis of their 16S rRNA genes, their cellular

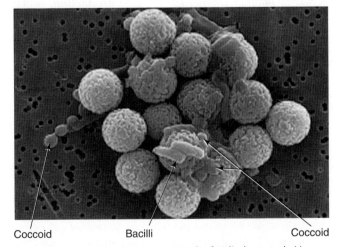

Coccoid   Bacilli   Coccoid

Figure 32–2. Scanning electron micrograph of *Helicobacter pylori* in a 7-day culture. Bacillary and coccoid forms (*arrows*) are bound to paramagnetic beads used in immunomagnetic separation. (*Courtesy Dr. L. Engstrand, Uppsala, Sweden.*)

Growth of *H. pylori* and other helicobacters requires a complex medium supplemented with blood, serum, charcoal, starch, or egg yolk; microaerophilic conditions (decreased oxygen and increased carbon dioxide); and a temperature range between 30° C and 37° C. Because helicobacters are relatively difficult to isolate in culture and identify by biochemical testing, most diseases caused by *H. pylori* are confirmed by nonculture techniques (see below).

Pathogenesis and Immunity

H. pylori is a remarkable bacterium in its ability to establish lifelong colonization in the stomach of untreated humans. Most research into the virulence factors in helicobacters has focused on *H. pylori*. Multiple factors contribute to the gastric colonization, inflammation, alteration of gastric acid production, and tissue destruction that are characteristic of *H. pylori* disease. Initial colonization is facilitated by (1) blockage of acid production by a bacterial acid-inhibitory protein and (2) neutralization of gastric acids by the ammonia produced by bacterial urease activity. The actively motile helicobacters can then pass through the gastric mucus and adhere to the gastric epithelial cells by multiple surface-adhesion proteins. Surface proteins can also bind host proteins and help the bacteria evade immune detection. Localized tissue damage is mediated by urease byproducts, **mucinase, phospholipases**, and the activity of the **vacuolating cytotoxin A (VacA)**, a protein that after endocytosis by epithelial cells, damages the cells by producing vacuoles. Another important virulence factor of *H. pylori* is the **cytotoxin-associated gene (cagA)** that resides on a pathogenicity island containing approximately 30 genes. These genes encode a structure (type IV secretion system) that acts like a syringe to inject the CagA protein into the host epithelial cells, which interferes with the normal cytoskeletal structure of the epithelial cells. The *cag* PAI (*phosphoribosylanthranilate isomerase*) genes also induce **interleukin-8 (IL-8) production**, which attracts neutrophils. Release of proteases and reactive oxygen molecules by the neutrophils is believed to contribute to gastritis and gastric ulcers.

Epidemiology

An enormous amount of information about the prevalence of *H. pylori* has been collected since 1984, when the organism was first isolated in culture. The highest incidence of carriage is found in developing countries, where 70% to 90% of the population is colonized, most before the age of 10 years. The prevalence of *H. pylori* in industrial countries such as the United States is less than 40% and is decreasing due to improved hygiene and active treatment of colonized individuals. These studies have also demonstrated that 70% to 100% of patients with gastritis, gastric ulcers, or duodenal ulcers are infected with *H. pylori*. **Humans are the primary reservoir for H. pylori**, and colonization is believed to persist for life unless the host is specifically treated. Transmission is most likely via the **fecal-oral route**.

An interesting observation about *H. pylori* colonization has been made. This organism is clearly associated with diseases such as gastritis, gastric ulcers, gastric adenocarcinoma, and gastric MALT lymphomas. It is anticipated that treatment of colonized or infected individuals will lead to a reduction of these diseases. However, colonization with *H. pylori* appears to offer protection from gastroesophageal reflux disease and adenocarcinomas of the lower esophagus and gastric cardia. Thus it may be unwise to eliminate *H. pylori* in patients without symptomatic disease. Certainly the complex relationship between *H. pylori* and its host remains to be defined.

Clinical Diseases (Clinical Case 32-2)

Helicobacter species are subdivided into gastric helicobacters (e.g., *H. pylori*) and enterohepatic helicobacters (e.g., *H. cinaedi*, *H. fennelliae*). Disease caused by helicobacters is directly related to their site of colonization. For example, *H. pylori* is associated with gastritis, whereas the enterohepatic species cause gastroenteritis.

Colonization with *H. pylori* invariably leads to histological evidence of **gastritis** (that is, infiltration of neutrophils and mononuclear cells into the gastric mucosa). The acute phase of gastritis is characterized by a feeling of fullness, nausea, vomiting, and hypochlorhydria (decreased acid production in the stomach). This can evolve into chronic gastritis, with disease confined to the gastric antrum (where few acid-secreting parietal cells are present) in individuals with normal acid secretion, or involve the entire stomach (pangastritis) if acid secretion is suppressed. Approximately 10% to 15% of patients with chronic gastritis will progress to develop peptic ulcers. The ulcers develop at the sites of intense inflammation, commonly involving the junction between the corpus and antrum (**gastric ulcer**) or the proximal duodenum (**duodenal ulcer**). *H. pylori* is responsible

---

Clinical Case 32-2. The Discovery of *Helicobacter pylori*

In 1984, Australian physicians Marshall and Warren reported a discovery that completely changed the approach to treatment of gastritis and peptic ulcer disease, as well as set the foundation for understanding the cause of gastric adenocarcinomas and MALT lymphomas (Lancet 1:1311-1315, 1984). In an analysis of gastric biopsy specimens from 100 consecutive patients presenting for gastroscopy, they demonstrated curved, gram-negative rods resembling *Campylobacter* in 58 patients. The bacteria were observed in most patients with active gastritis, gastric ulcers, and duodenal ulcers. Although similar organisms were observed associated with gastric tissues 45 years before, this report stimulated resurgence in investigations of the role of this "new" organism in gastric diseases. Despite the skepticism that greeted their initial report, the significance of their work with *Campylobacter* was recognized when Marshall and Warren received the 2005 Nobel Prize in Medicine.

for 85% of gastric ulcers and 95% of duodenal ulcers. Recognition of the role of *H. pylori* has dramatically changed the treatment and prognosis of peptic ulcer disease.

Chronic gastritis eventually leads to replacement of the normal gastric mucosa with fibrosis and proliferation of intestinal-type epithelium. This process increases the patient's risk for **gastric cancer** by almost 100-fold. This risk is influenced by the strain of *H. pylori* and the host's response (*cag*A-positive strains and high levels of IL-1 production are associated with a higher risk for cancer).

Infection with *H. pylori* is also associated with infiltration of lymphoid tissue into the gastric mucosa. In a small number of patients, a monoclonal population of B cells may develop and evolve into a **MALT lymphoma**.

H. cinaedi and *H. fennelliae* can cause **gastroenteritis** and **bacteremia**, most commonly in immunocompromised patients (e.g., homosexual men with HIV infections). Another species of uncertain taxonomy, currently termed "*Helicobacter* species flexispira taxon 8," causes bacteremia with cellulitis in immunocompromised patients.

Laboratory Diagnosis

Microscopy

H. pylori is detected by histologic examination of gastric biopsy specimens. Although the organism can be seen in specimens stained with hematoxylin-eosin or Gram stain, the Warthin-Starry silver stain is the most sensitive. When an adequate quantity of the specimen is collected and examined by an experienced microscopist, the test sensitivity and specificity approaches 100% and is considered the diagnostic gold standard. Because this is an invasive test, alternative test procedures are preferred for routine diagnosis.

Antigen Detection

Biopsy specimens can also be tested for the presence of bacterial urease activity. The abundance of urease produced by *H. pylori* permits detection of the alkaline byproduct in less than 2 hours. The sensitivity of the direct test with biopsy specimens varies from 75% to 95%; however, the specificity approaches 100%, so a positive reaction is compelling evidence of an active infection. As with microscopy, the limitation of this method is the requirement for a biopsy specimen. Noninvasive urease testing of human breath following consumption of an isotopically labeled urea solution has excellent sensitivity and specificity. Unfortunately, this assay is relatively expensive because of the cost of the detection instruments.

A number of polyclonal and monoclonal immunoassays for *H. pylori* antigens excreted in stool have been developed and demonstrated to have sensitivities and specificities exceeding 95%. These tests are easy to perform, inexpensive, and able to be used on stool specimens rather than biopsies. Although enterohepatic helicobacters are uncommon in most patients, the reactivity of these immunoassays with other helicobacter species must still be determined.

Nucleic-Acid-Based Tests

At the present time, nucleic-acid-based amplification tests for *H. pylori* and enterohepatic helicobacters are restricted to research labs and not in clinical use.

Culture

H. pylori adheres to gastric mucosa and is not recovered in stool or blood specimens. The bacteria can be isolated in culture if the specimen is inoculated onto enriched medium supplemented with blood, hemin, or charcoal and incubated in a microaerophilic atmosphere for up to 2 weeks. However, diagnosis of *H. pylori* infections is most commonly by noninvasive methods (e.g., immunoassay), with culture reserved for antibiotic susceptibility tests.

Identification

Presumptive identification of isolates is based on their growth characteristics under selective conditions, typical microscopic morphologic findings, and detection of oxidase, catalase, and urease activity.

Antibody Detection

Serology is an important screening test for the diagnosis of *H. pylori*, with a variety of commercial tests available. Although IgM antibodies disappear rapidly, IgA and IgG antibodies can persist for months to years. Because the **antibody titers persist** for many years, the test cannot be used to discriminate between past and current infection. Furthermore, the titer of antibodies measured does not correlate with the severity of the disease or the response to therapy. However, the tests are useful for documenting exposure to the bacteria, either for epidemiologic studies or for the initial evaluation of a symptomatic patient.

Treatment, Prevention, and Control

Numerous antibiotic regimens have been evaluated for treating *H. pylori* infections. Use of a single antibiotic or an antibiotic combined with bismuth is ineffective. The greatest success in curing gastritis or peptic ulcer disease has been accomplished with the combination of a **proton pump inhibitor** (e.g., omeprazole), a **macrolide** (e.g., clarithromycin), and a **beta-lactam** (e.g., amoxicillin), with administration for 7 to 10 days initially. Treatment failure is most commonly associated with clarithromycin resistance. Routine susceptibility testing should be performed if the patient does not respond to therapy. Metronidazole can also be used in combination therapy, but resistance is commonplace.

Infection with *H. pylori* stimulates a strong TH1-cell-mediated inflammatory response. Use of *H. pylori* antigens in experimental vaccines that stimulate TH1 cells leads to enhanced inflammation. In contrast, use of antigens in combination with mucosal adjuvants that induce a TH2 cell response is protective in an animal model and can eradicate existing infections. The effectiveness of these vaccines in humans remains to be demonstrated.

Case Study and Questions

A mother and her 4-year-old son came to the local emergency room with a 1-day history of diarrhea and abdominal cramping. Both patients had low-grade fevers, and blood was grossly evident in the child's stool specimen. The symptoms had developed 18 hours after the patients had consumed a dinner consisting of mixed green salad, chicken, corn, bread, and apple pie. Culture of blood samples was negative for organisms, but *C. jejuni* was isolated from stool specimens of both the mother and the child.

1. Which food that they consumed is most likely responsible for these infections? What measures should be used to prevent these infections?

2. Name three *Campylobacter* species that have been associated with gastroenteritis. Name the species of *Campylobacter* that is most commonly associated with septicemia.

3. What diseases have been associated with *H. pylori*? *H. cinaedi*? *H. fennelliae*?

4. *H. pylori* has multiple virulence factors. Which factors are responsible for interfering with gastric acid secretion? For adhering to the gastric epithelium? For disrupting the gastric mucosa? For interfering with phagocytic killing?

Bibliography

Algood H, Cover T: *Helicobacter pylori* persistence: An overview of interactions between *H. pylori* and host immune defenses. Clin Microbiol Rev 19:597-613, 2006.

Farinha P, Gascoyne R: *Helicobacter pylori* and MALT lymphoma. Gastroenterology 128:1579-1605, 2005.

Friedman L: *Helicobacter pylori* and nonulcer dyspepsia [editorial]. N Engl J Med 339:1928-1930, 1998.

Kabir S: The current status of *Helicobacter pylori* vaccines: A review. Helicobacter 12:89-102, 2007.

Kusters JG, van Vliet A, Kuipers EJ: Pathogenesis of *Helicobacter pylori* infection. Clin Microbiol Rev 19:449-490, 2006.

Lastovica A: Emerging *Campylobacter* spp.: The tip of the iceberg. Clin Microbiol Newslett 28:49-55, 2006.

Marshall B: *Helicobacter pylori*: 20 years on. Clin Med 2:147-152, 2002.

Nachamkin I, et al: *Campylobacter* species and Guillain-Barré syndrome. Clin Microbiol Rev 11:555-567, 1998.

Passaro D, Chosy EJ, Parsonnet J: *Helicobacter pylori*: Consensus and controversy. Clin Infect Dis 35:298-304, 2002.

Samuel MC, et al: Epidemiology of sporadic *Campylobacter* infection in the United States and declining trend in incidence, FoodNet 1996-1999. Clin Infect Dis 38:S165-S174, 2004.

Solnick J: Clinical significance of *Helicobacter* species other than *Helicobacter pylori*. Clin Infect Dis 36:348-354, 2003.

Pseudomonas and Related Bacteria

Pseudomonas and related nonfermentative rods are a mixture of opportunistic pathogens of plants, animals, and humans. To complicate our understanding of these organisms, their taxonomic classification has undergone numerous changes in recent years. Despite the many genera, most clinically significant isolates are members of five genera: *Pseudomonas*, *Burkholderia*, *Stenotrophomonas*, *Acinetobacter*, and *Moraxella* (Box 33-1). These organisms will be the focus of this chapter.

Pseudomonas (Box 33-2)

The genus *Pseudomonas* originally consisted of a large, heterogeneous collection of nonfermentative bacteria that were grouped together because of their morphologic similarity. They were referred to as *pseudomonads* because they are commonly arranged in pairs of cells that resemble a single cell (Figure 33-1). In 1992, this genus was subdivided into a number of new genera (including *Burkholderia* and *Stenotrophomonas*); however, there are still almost 200 species in *Pseudomonas*. **P. aeruginosa** is the most important species and the one discussed here.

Members of the genus are **ubiquitous**, found in soil, decaying organic matter, vegetation, and water. Unfortunately, they are also found throughout the hospital environment in moist reservoirs such as food, cut flowers, sinks, toilets, floor mops, respiratory therapy and dialysis equipment, and even in disinfectant solutions. It is uncommon for carriage to persist in humans as part of the normal microbial flora, except in hospitalized patients and ambulatory, immunocompromised hosts.

The broad environmental distribution of *Pseudomonas* is made possible by their simple growth requirements and nutritional versatility. They are capable of using many organic compounds as sources of carbon and nitrogen, and some strains can even grow in distilled water by using trace nutrients. These organisms also possess many structural factors, enzymes, and toxins that enhance their

virulence and render them resistant to most commonly used antibiotics. Indeed, it is surprising that they are not more common pathogens, considering their ubiquitous presence, ability to grow in virtually any environment, virulence properties, and resistance to many antibiotics. Fortunately, *Pseudomonas* infections are **primarily opportunistic** (i.e., restricted to patients receiving broad-spectrum antibiotics that suppress the normal intestinal bacterial population or patients with compromised host defenses).

Physiology and Structure

Pseudomonas species are usually motile, straight or slightly curved, gram-negative rods (0.5 to 1.0 × 1.5 to 5.0 µm) typically **arranged in pairs** (see Figure 33-1). The organisms utilize carbohydrates through **aerobic respiration** (refer to Chapter 2), with oxygen the terminal electron acceptor. Although described as obligate aerobes, they can grow anaerobically using nitrate or arginine as an alternate electron acceptor. The presence of cytochrome **oxidase** (detected in a rapid 5-minute test) in *Pseudomonas* species is used to differentiate them from the Enterobacteriaceae. Some strains appear **mucoid** because of the abundance of a polysaccharide capsule (Figure 33-2); these strains are particularly common in patients with cystic fibrosis. Some species produce **diffusible pigments** (e.g., pyocyanin [blue], pyoverdin [yellow-green], and pyorubin [reddish-brown]) that give them a characteristic appearance in culture.

Pathogenesis and Immunity

P. aeruginosa has many virulence factors, including structural components, toxins, and enzymes. Additionally, the delivery system used by *Pseudomonas*, the type III secretion system, is particularly effective in injecting toxins into the host cell. Despite the diversity of virulence factors, most experts believe that multiple factors must work together for *P. aeruginosa* to cause disease.

Box 33—1. Important Nonfermentative Gram-Negative Rods

Organism	Historical Derivation
Acinetobacter	*akinetos*, "unable to move"; *bactrum*, "rod" (nonmotile rods)
A. baumannii	*baumannii*, named after the microbiologist *Baumann*
A. lwoffii	*lwoffii*, named after the microbiologist *Lwoff*
Burkholderia	*Burkholderia*, named after the microbiologist *Burkholder*
B. cepacia	*cepacia*, like an "onion" (original strains isolated from rotten onions)
B. mallei	*mallei*, from "malleus," Latin name of the equine disease glanders
B. pseudomallei	*pseudes*, "false"; *mallei* (refers to the fact this species closely resembles *B. mallei*)
Moraxella	*Moraxella*, named after the Swiss ophthalmologist *Morax*, who first recognized the species
M. catarrhalis	*catarrhus*, "downflowing" or catarrh (refers to inflammation of the respiratory tract mucous membranes)
Pseudomonas	*pseudes*, "false"; *monas*, a "unit" (refers to Gram stain appearance of pairs of organisms that resemble a single cell)
P. aeruginosa	*aeruginosa*, full of "copper rust" or green (refers to green pigmentation resulting from blue and yellow pigments produced by this species)
Stenotrophomonas	*Stenos*, "narrow"; *trophos*, "one who feeds"; *monas*, "unit" (refers to observation that these are narrow bacteria that require few substrates for growth)
S. maltophilia	*malt*, malt (sprouted grain); *philia*, "friend" (friend of malt)

Box 33—2. Summary: *Pseudomonas aeruginosa*

Biology, Virulence, and Disease

Small, gram-negative rods typically arranged in pairs
Obligate aerobe; glucose oxidizer; simple nutritional needs
Mucoid polysaccharide capsule
Multiple virulence factors, including adhesins (e.g., flagella, pili, LPS, alginate capsule), secreted toxins and enzymes (e.g., exotoxin A, pyocyanin, pyoverdin, elastases, proteases, phospholipase C, exoenzymes S and T), and antimicrobial resistance
Diseases include infections of the respiratory tract, urinary tract, skin and soft tissues, ears and eyes, as well as bacteremia and endocarditis

Epidemiology

Ubiquitous in nature and moist environmental hospital sites (e.g., flowers, sinks, toilets, mechanical ventilation and dialysis equipment)
No seasonal incidence of disease
Can transiently colonize the respiratory and gastrointestinal tracts of hospitalized patients, particularly those treated with broad-spectrum antibiotics, exposed to respiratory therapy equipment, or hospitalized for extended periods

Diagnosis

Grows rapidly on common laboratory media
Identified by colonial characteristics (e.g., beta hemolysis, green pigment, grapelike odor) and simple biochemical tests (e.g., positive oxidase reaction; oxidative utilization of carbohydrates)

Treatment, Prevention, and Control

Combined use of effective antibiotics (e.g., aminoglycoside and β-lactam antibiotics) frequently required; monotherapy is generally ineffective and can select for resistant strains
Hospital infection-control efforts should concentrate on preventing contamination of sterile medical equipment and nosocomial transmission; unnecessary use of broad-spectrum antibiotics can select for resistant organisms

Figure 33—1. Gram stain of *Pseudomonas aeruginosa* with cells arranged singly and in pairs.

Figure 33–2. Gram stain of *Pseudomonas aeruginosa* surrounded by mucoid capsular material in cystic fibrosis patient.

Adhesins

Adherence to host cells is critical for establishing infection. At least four structural components on the surface of *P. aeruginosa* facilitate this adherence: (1) flagella, (2) pili, (3) lipopolysaccharide (LPS), and (4) alginate. Flagella and pili also mediate motility in *P. aeruginosa*, and the lipid-A component of LPS is responsible for endotoxin activity. Alginate is a mucoid exopolysaccharide that forms a prominent **capsule** on the bacterial surface and protects the organism from phagocytosis and the activity of antibiotics. The production of this mucoid polysaccharide is under complex regulation. The genes controlling production of the alginate polysaccharide can be activated in patients such as those with cystic fibrosis or other chronic respiratory diseases, who are predisposed to long-term colonization with these mucoid strains of *P. aeruginosa*.

Secreted Toxins and Enzymes

Exotoxin A (ETA) is believed to be one of the most important virulence factors produced by pathogenic strains of *P. aeruginosa*. This toxin **disrupts protein synthesis** by blocking peptide chain elongation in eukaryotic cells, much like the diphtheria toxin produced by *Corynebacterium diphtheriae*. However, the toxins produced by these two organisms are structurally and immunologically different, and exotoxin A is less potent than diphtheria toxin. Exotoxin A most likely contributes to the dermatonecrosis that occurs in burn wounds, corneal damage in ocular infections, and tissue damage in chronic pulmonary infections. The toxin is also immunosuppressive.

A blue pigment, **pyocyanin**, produced by *P. aeruginosa* catalyzes the production of superoxide and hydrogen peroxide, toxic forms of oxygen. This pigment also stimulates interleukin-8 (IL-8) release, leading to enhanced attraction of neutrophils.

A yellow-green pigment, **pyoverdin**, is a siderophore that binds iron for use in metabolism. This pigment also

regulates secretion of other virulence factors, including exotoxin A.

Two enzymes, LasA (**serine protease**) and LasB (**zinc metalloprotease**), act synergistically to degrade elastin, resulting in damage to elastin-containing tissues and producing the lung parenchymal damage and hemorrhagic lesions (**ecthyma gangrenosum**) associated with disseminated *P. aeruginosa* infections. These enzymes can also degrade complement components and inhibit neutrophil chemotaxis and function, leading to further spread and tissue damage in acute infections. Chronic *Pseudomonas* infections are characterized by the formation of antibodies to LasA and LasB, with the deposition of immune complexes in the infected tissues.

Like the elastases, **alkaline protease** contributes to tissue destruction and spread of *P. aeruginosa*. It also interferes with the host immune response.

Phospholipase C is a heat-labile hemolysin that breaks down lipids and lecithin, facilitating tissue destruction. The exact role of this enzyme in respiratory and urinary tract infections (UTIs) is unclear, although an important association between hemolysin production and disease has been recognized.

Exoenzymes S and **T** are extracellular toxins produced by *P. aeruginosa*. They possess adenosine diphosphate (ADP)-ribosyltransferase activity, the function of which is unclear. However, when the type III secretion system introduces the proteins into their target eukaryotic cells, epithelial cell damage occurs, facilitating bacterial spread, tissue invasion, and necrosis. This cytotoxicity is mediated by actin rearrangement.

Antibiotic Resistance

P. aeruginosa is inherently **resistant to many antibiotics** and can mutate to even more resistant strains during therapy. Although numerous resistance mechanisms have been identified, the **mutation of porin proteins** constitutes the major mechanism of resistance. Penetration of antibiotics into the pseudomonad cell is primarily through pores in the outer membrane. If the proteins forming the walls of these pores are altered to restrict flow into the cell, resistance to many classes of antibiotics can develop simultaneously. *P. aeruginosa* also produces a number of different β-lactamases that can inactivate many β-lactam antibiotics (e.g., penicillins, cephalosporins, and carbapenems).

Epidemiology

Pseudomonas is an opportunistic pathogen present in a variety of environments. The ability to isolate this organism from moist surfaces may be limited only by the efforts to look for the organism. *Pseudomonas* has minimal nutritional requirements, tolerates a wide range of temperatures (4° C to 42° C), and is resistant to many antibiotics and disinfectants. Indeed, the recovery of *Pseudomonas* from an environmental source (e.g., hospital sink or floor) means very little unless there is epidemiologic evidence that the contaminated site is a reservoir for infection.

Furthermore, isolation of *Pseudomonas* from a hospitalized patient is worrisome but does not normally justify therapeutic intervention unless there is evidence of disease. The recovery of *Pseudomonas* from a clinical specimen, particularly species other than *P. aeruginosa*, may represent simple transient colonization of the patient or environmental contamination of the specimen during collection or laboratory processing.

Clinical Diseases

Pulmonary Infections

P. aeruginosa infections of the lower respiratory tract can range in severity from **asymptomatic colonization** or benign **tracheobronchitis** to severe **necrotizing bronchopneumonia**. Colonization is seen in patients with cystic fibrosis, other chronic lung diseases, or neutropenia. Infections in patients with cystic fibrosis have been associated with exacerbation of the underlying disease and invasive pulmonary disease. Mucoid strains are commonly isolated from specimens from such patients and are difficult to eradicate because the bacteria are frequently resistant to many antibiotics.

Conditions that predispose immunocompromised patients to infections with *Pseudomonas* include: (1) previous therapy with broad-spectrum antibiotics that eliminate the normal, protective bacterial population, and (2) use of mechanical ventilation equipment, which may introduce the organism into the lower airways. Invasive disease in this population is characterized by a diffuse, typically bilateral bronchopneumonia with microabscess formation and tissue necrosis. The mortality rate is as high as 70%.

Primary Skin and Soft Tissue Infections

P. aeruginosa can cause a variety of primary skin infections. The most recognized are infections of **burn wounds** (Figure 33-3). Colonization of a burn wound, followed by localized

Figure 33—4. *Pseudomonas* folliculitis. *(From Cohen J, Powderly WB: Infectious Diseases, 2nd ed. St Louis, Mosby, 2004.)*

vascular damage, tissue necrosis, and ultimately bacteremia, is common in patients with severe burns. The moist surface of the burn and inability of neutrophils to penetrate into the wounds predispose patients to such infections. Wound management with topical antibiotic creams has had only limited success in controlling these infections.

Folliculitis (Figure 33-4; Clinical Case 33-1) is another common infection caused by *Pseudomonas*; it results from immersion in contaminated water (e.g., hot tubs, whirlpools, swimming pools). Secondary infections with *Pseudomonas* also occur in people who have acne or who depilate their legs. Finally, *P. aeruginosa* can cause fingernail infections in people whose hands are frequently exposed to water or who frequent "nail salons."

P. aeruginosa is also the most common cause of **osteochondritis** (inflammation of bone and cartilage) of the foot after a penetrating injury (e.g., associated with stepping on a nail).

Figure 33—3. *Pseudomonas* infection of burn wound. *(From Cohen J, Powderly WB: Infectious Diseases, 2nd ed. St Louis, Mosby, 2004.)*

Clinical Case 33-1. *Pseudomonas* folliculitis

Ratnam, et al. (J Clin Microbiol 23:655-659, 1986) described an outbreak of folliculitis caused by *P. aeruginosa* in guests of a Canadian hotel. A number of guests complained of a skin rash, which began as pruritic erythematous papules and progressed to erythematous pustules distributed in the axilla and over the abdomen and buttocks. For most patients, the rash resolved spontaneously over a 5-day period. The local health department investigated the outbreak and determined the source was a whirlpool contaminated with a high concentration of *P. aeruginosa*. The outbreak was terminated when the whirlpool was drained, cleaned, and superchlorinated. Skin infections such as this are common in individuals with extensive exposure to contaminated water.

Urinary Tract Infections

Infection of the urinary tract is seen primarily in patients with long-term **indwelling urinary catheters**. Typically, such patients are treated with multiple courses of antibiotics, which tend to select for the more resistant strains of bacteria, such as *Pseudomonas*.

Ear Infections

External otitis is frequently caused by *P. aeruginosa*, with swimming an important risk factor (**"swimmer's ear"**). This localized infection can be managed with topical antibiotics and drying agents. **Malignant external otitis** is a virulent form of disease seen primarily in persons with diabetes and elderly patients. It can invade the underlying tissues, damage the cranial nerves and bones, and be life threatening. Aggressive, antimicrobial, and surgical intervention is required for patients with the latter disease. *P. aeruginosa* is also associated with **chronic otitis media**.

Eye Infections

Infections of the eye occur after initial trauma to the cornea (e.g., abrasion from a contact lens, scratch on the eye surface) and then exposure to *P. aeruginosa* in contaminated water. **Corneal ulcers** develop and can progress to eye-threatening disease unless prompt treatment is instituted.

Bacteremia and Endocarditis

Bacteremia caused by *P. aeruginosa* is clinically indistinguishable from that caused by other gram-negative bacteria. However, the mortality rate in affected patients is higher with *P. aeruginosa* bacteremia because of (1) the predilection of the organism for immunocompromised patients and (2) the inherent virulence of *Pseudomonas*. Bacteremia occurs most often in patients with neutropenia, diabetes mellitus, extensive burns, and hematologic malignancies. Most bacteremias originate from infections of the lower respiratory tract, urinary tract, and skin and soft tissue (particularly burn wound infections). Although seen in a minority of bacteremic patients, characteristic skin lesions (**ecthyma gangrenosum**) may develop. The lesions manifest as erythematous vesicles that become hemorrhagic, necrotic, and ulcerated. Microscopic examination of the lesion shows abundant organisms, vascular destruction (which explains the hemorrhagic nature of the lesions), and an absence of neutrophils, as would be expected in neutropenic patients.

Pseudomonas **endocarditis** is uncommon, primarily seen in intravenous-drug abusers. These patients acquire the infection from the use of drug paraphernalia contaminated with the waterborne organisms. The tricuspid valve is often involved, and the infection is associated with a chronic course but with a more favorable prognosis than that in patients who have infections of the aortic or mitral valve.

Other Infections

P. aeruginosa is also the cause of a variety of other infections, including those localized in the gastrointestinal tract, central nervous system, and musculoskeletal system. The underlying conditions required for most infections are (1) the presence of the organism in a moist reservoir and (2) the compromised host defenses (e.g., cutaneous trauma, elimination of normal microbial flora as a result of antibiotic usage, neutropenia).

Laboratory Diagnosis

Microscopy

Observation of thin, gram-negative rods arranged singly and in pairs is suggestive of *Pseudomonas* but not pathognomonic; *Burkholderia*, *Stenotrophomonas*, and other pseudomonads have a similar morphology. However, observation of these bacteria in the appropriate clinical setting can guide empiric therapy.

Culture

Because *Pseudomonas* has simple nutritional requirements, the bacteria are readily recovered on common isolation media such as blood agar and MacConkey agar. They do require aerobic incubation (unless nitrate is available), so their growth in broth is generally confined to the broth-air interface where the oxygen concentration is the highest.

Identification

The colonial morphology (e.g., colony size, hemolytic activity, pigmentation, odor; Figure 33-5) and the results of selected rapid biochemical tests (e.g., positive **oxidase** reaction) are sufficient for the preliminary identification of these isolates. For example, *P. aeruginosa* grows rapidly and has flat colonies with a spreading border, **β-hemolysis**, a **green pigmentation** caused by the production of the blue (pyocyanin) and yellow-green (pyoverdin) pigments, and a characteristic sweet, **grapelike odor**. Although definitive identification of *P. aeruginosa* is relatively easy, an extensive battery of physiologic tests may be required to identify other species.

Figure 33—5. Colonial morphology of *Pseudomonas aeruginosa*; note the green pigmentation that results from the production of two water-soluble dyes: blue pyocyanin and yellow fluorescein.

Treatment, Prevention, and Control

The antimicrobial therapy for *Pseudomonas* infections is frustrating, because (1) the bacteria are typically resistant to most antibiotics and (2) the infected patient with compromised host defenses cannot augment the antibiotic activity. Even susceptible organisms can become resistant during therapy by inducing the formation of antibiotic-inactivating enzymes (e.g., β-lactamases), mutation of the genes coding the outer membrane pore proteins (so antibiotics cannot penetrate into the cell), or through the transfer of plasmid-mediated resistance from a resistant organism to a susceptible one. A **combination of active antibiotics** is generally required for therapy to be successful in patients with serious infections.

Attempts to eliminate *Pseudomonas* from the hospital environment are practically useless, given the ubiquitous presence of the organism in water supplies. Effective infection-control practices should concentrate on **preventing the contamination of sterile equipment**, such as mechanical ventilation equipment and dialysis machines, and the cross-contamination of patients by medical personnel. The inappropriate use of broad-spectrum antibiotics should also be avoided because such use can suppress the normal microbial flora and permit the overgrowth of resistant strains of *Pseudomonas*.

Burkholderia

In 1992, seven species formerly classified as *Pseudomonas* were reclassified as members of the new genus *Burkholderia*. It was subsequently appreciated that the most common species, *B. cepacia*, was actually a complex of nine species. Because most labs cannot identify the individual species, the collection is commonly referred to as *B. cepacia* complex. **B. cepacia complex**, **Burkholderia gladioli**, and **Burkholderia pseudomallei** are important human pathogens in this genus (Box 33-3); other species (e.g., *Burkholderia mallei*) are less commonly associated with human disease.

Like *P. aeruginosa*, *Burkholderia* species can colonize a variety of moist environmental surfaces and are **opportunistic pathogens** (Clinical Case 33-2). Patients particularly susceptible to pulmonary infections with *B. cepacia* complex and *B. gladioli* are those with cystic fibrosis or chronic granulomatous disease (a primary immunodeficiency in which white blood cells have defective intracellular microbicidal activity). Colonization of the respiratory tract of cystic fibrosis patients with *B. cepacia* complex has such a poor prognosis that this is a contraindication for lung transplantation. *B. cepacia* complex is also responsible for urinary tract infections in catheterized patients, septicemia (particularly in patients with contaminated intravascular catheters), and other opportunistic infections. With the exception of pulmonary infections, *B. cepacia* complex has a relatively low level of virulence, and infections with the organism do not commonly result in death.

Box 33—3. Clinical Summaries

Pseudomonas aeruginosa

Pulmonary infections: range from mild irritation of the bronchi (tracheobronchitis) to necrosis of the lung parenchyma (necrotizing bronchopneumonia)

Primary skin infections: opportunistic infections of existing wounds (e.g., burns) to localized infections of hair follicles (e.g., associated with immersion in contaminated waters such as hot tubs)

Urinary tract infections: opportunistic infections in patients with indwelling urinary catheters and exposure to broad-spectrum antibiotics (selects for these antibiotic-resistant bacteria)

Ear infections: can range from mild irritation of external ear ("swimmer's ear") to invasive destruction of cranial bones adjacent to the infected ear

Eye infections: opportunistic infections of exposed, mildly damaged corneas

Bacteremia: dissemination of bacteria from primary infection (e.g., pulmonary) to other organs and tissues; can be characterized by necrotic skin lesions (ecthyma gangrenosum)

***Burkholderia cepacia* Complex**

Pulmonary infections: range from colonization to bronchopneumonia primarily in patients with cystic fibrosis or chronic granulomatous disease

Opportunistic infections: urinary tract infections in catheterized patients; bacteria in immunocompromised patients with contaminated intravascular catheters

Burkholderia pseudomallei

Pulmonary infections: can range from asymptomatic colonization to abscess formation

Stenotrophomonas maltophilia

Opportunistic infections: a variety of infections (most commonly bacteremia and pneumonia) in immunocompromised patients previously exposed to broad-spectrum antimicrobial therapy

***Acinetobacter* Species**

Pulmonary infections: opportunistic pathogen in patients receiving respiratory therapy

Wound infections: nosocomial infections in soldiers with traumatic wounds

***Moraxella* Species**

Pulmonary infections: tracheobronchitis or bronchopneumonia in patients with chronic pulmonary diseases (most commonly caused by *M. catarrhalis*)

B. pseudomallei is a saprophyte found in soil, water, and vegetation. It is endemic in Southeast Asia, India, Africa, and Australia. Infections are acquired by either inhalation or less commonly by percutaneous inoculation. Most persons exposed to *B. pseudomallei* remain asymptomatic; however, alcoholics, diabetics, and individuals with chronic renal or lung disease are susceptible to opportunistic infections caused by this organism. Infections are called

melioidosis (*melis*, "distemper"; *eidos*, "resemblance"; *osis*, "condition": disease resembling equine distemper or glanders caused by *B. mallei*). Exposure by the percutaneous route presents as a localized, suppurative **cutaneous infection** accompanied by regional lymphadenitis, fever, and malaise. This form of disease can resolve without incident or can progress rapidly to overwhelming sepsis. **Pulmonary disease** that develops after respiratory exposure may range in severity from a mild bronchitis to necrotizing pneumonia. Cavitation progressing to overwhelming sepsis and death can develop if appropriate antimicrobial therapy is not instituted. *B. pseudomallei* has been used in biologic weapons programs, so work with this organism is restricted to appropriately licensed laboratories, and the recovery from a patient justifies intervention by the public health department. Isolation of *B. pseudomallei* for diagnostic purposes should be approached carefully because the organism is highly infectious.

Burkholderia species are susceptible to **trimethoprim-sulfamethoxazole**, which distinguishes them from *P. aeruginosa*. Although the organisms appear to be susceptible in vitro to piperacillin, broad-spectrum cephalosporins, and ciprofloxacin, the clinical response is generally poor.

Stenotrophomonas maltophilia

S. maltophilia was originally classified in the genus *Pseudomonas*, moved to the genus *Xanthomonas*, and then transferred to the genus *Stenotrophomonas*. Despite the confusion created by these taxonomic changes, the clinical importance of this opportunistic pathogen is well known. It is responsible for infections in debilitated patients with impaired host-defense mechanisms. Also, because *S. maltophilia* is resistant to most commonly used β-lactam and aminoglycoside antibiotics, patients receiving long-term antibiotic therapy with these drugs are particularly at risk for acquiring infections.

The most common nosocomial infections caused by *S. maltophilia* are bacteremia and pneumonia, with both associated with a high incidence of complications and death (Clinical Case 33-3). Hospital infections with this organism have been traced to contaminated intravenous catheters, disinfectant solutions, mechanical ventilation equipment, and ice machines.

Antimicrobial therapy is complicated, because the organism is resistant to many commonly used drugs. In contrast with most gram-negative rods, *Stenotrophomonas* is **resistant to carbapenems** (e.g., imipenem, meropenem, ertapenem). **Trimethoprim-sulfamethoxazole** is the agent most active against the organism; in vitro activity is also seen with doxycycline and ceftazidime.

Acinetobacter

Acinetobacters are strictly aerobic, oxidase-negative, plump, gram-negative coccobacilli (Figure 33-6). They are **ubiquitous** saprophytes, recovered in nature and in the hospital and able to survive on both moist surfaces, such as mechanical ventilation equipment, and on dry surfaces, such as human skin (the latter feature is unusual for gram-negative rods). These bacteria are also part of the normal oropharyngeal flora of a small number of healthy people and can proliferate to large numbers during hospitalization. The genus *Acinetobacter* is subdivided into two groups:

Figure 33–6. Gram stain of *Acinetobacter baumannii* (*black arrow*) and *Pseudomonas aeruginosa* (*red arrow*). Note *Acinetobacter* are more coccobacillary in shape and appear gram-positive.

Figure 33–7. Gram stain of *Moraxella catarrhalis* (*black arrow*). Note the cells resemble gram-negative diplococci (similar to *Neisseria*).

glucose-oxidizing species (**A. baumannii** is the most common) and glucose nonoxidizing species (**A. lwoffii** and **A. haemolyticus** are the most common). Most human infections are caused by *A. baumannii*.

Acinetobacters are **opportunistic pathogens** (see Box 33-3) that cause infections in the respiratory tract, urinary tract, and wounds; they also cause septicemia. Patients at risk for *Acinetobacter* infections are those receiving broad-spectrum antibiotics, recovering from surgery, or on respiratory ventilation. Nosocomial wound infections in hospitalized soldiers has also been a significant problem. Treatment of *Acinetobacter* infections is difficult because these organisms, particularly *A. baumannii*, are often **resistant to antibiotics**, including the carbapenems. Specific therapy must be guided by in vitro susceptibility tests.

Moraxella

Like other genera discussed in this chapter, the genus *Moraxella* was reorganized on the basis of nucleic acid analysis. Although the species classified in this genus continue to change, *M. catarrhalis* is the most important pathogen. **M. catarrhalis** is a strictly aerobic, oxidase-positive, gram-negative diplococci (Figure 33-7). This organism is a common cause of bronchitis and bronchopneumonia (in elderly patients with chronic pulmonary disease), sinusitis, and otitis (see Box 33-3). The latter two infections occur most commonly in previously healthy people. Most isolates produce β-lactamases and are **resistant to penicillins**; however, these bacteria are uniformly susceptible to most other antibiotics, including cephalosporins, erythromycin, tetracycline, trimethoprim-sulfamethoxazole, and the combination of penicillins with a β-lactamase inhibitor (e.g., clavulanic acid). Two other species of *Moraxella* colonize humans and are recovered with some frequency: *Moraxella osloensis* and

Moraxella nonliquefaciens. Both species are found on the skin surface and mucosal membranes of the mouth and genitourinary tract. These species are rare causes of opportunistic infections.

Case Study and Questions

A 63-year-old man has been hospitalized for 21 days for the management of newly diagnosed leukemia. Three days after the patient entered the hospital, a urinary tract infection with *Escherichia coli* developed. He was treated for 14 days with broad-spectrum antibiotics. On day 21 of his hospital stay, the patient experienced fever and shaking chills. Within 24 hours he became hypotensive, and ecthymic skin lesions appeared. Despite aggressive therapy with antibiotics, the patient died. Multiple blood cultures were positive for *P. aeruginosa*.

1. What factors put this man at increased risk for infection with *P. aeruginosa*?

2. What virulence factors possessed by the organism make it a particularly serious pathogen? What are the biologic effects of these factors?

3. What three mechanisms are responsible for the antibiotic resistance found in *P. aeruginosa*?

4. What diseases are caused by *B. cepacia* complex? *S. maltophilia*? *A. baumannii*? *M. catarrhalis*? What antibiotics can be used to treat these infections?

Reference to Student Consult Animation

Please visit **www.StudentConsult.com** to view an animation demonstrating the function of *Pseudomonas* exotoxin A.

Clinical Case 33-2. Granulomatous Disease Caused by *Burkholderia*.

McLean-Tooke, et al. (BMC Clin Pathol 7:1-5, 2007) described a 21-year-old man with granulomatous lymphadenitis. The man presented with a history of weight loss, fevers, hepatosplenomegaly, and cervical lymphadenopathy. During the preceding 3 years, he had presented on two occasions with enlarged lymph nodes that were biopsied, and histological examination revealed granulomatous lymphadenitis. A clinical diagnosis of sarcoidosis was made, and the man was discharged on 20 mg prednisolone. Over the next 24 months, the patient remained clinically well; however, he developed pancytopenia, and granulomas were observed on a bone marrow biopsy. During this hospitalization, the patient developed a cough. Chest radiograph revealed consolidation in the base of the lungs. A lung biopsy and bronchoalveolar lavage was submitted for culture, and *Burkholderia cepacia* was isolated from both specimens. A subsequent immunologic evaluation of the patient confirmed that he had genetic disease: chronic granulomatous disease (CGD). This case illustrates the susceptibility of CGD patients to infections with *Burkholderia*.

Clinical Case 33-3. Disseminated *Stenotrophomonas* Infections in a Neutropenic Patient.

Wan-Yee, et al. (Ann Acad Med Singapore 35:897-900, 2006) described an 8-year-old Chinese girl with acute myeloid leukemia and a complex history of recurrent fungal and bacterial infections during treatment of her leukemia. Infections included pulmonary aspergillosis and septicemia with *Klebsiella*, *Enterobacter*, *Staphylococcus*, *Streptococcus*, and *Bacillus*. While receiving treatment with meropenem (a carbapenem antibiotic) and amikacin (an aminoglycoside), and during a period of severe neutropenia, she became bacteremic with *Stenotrophomonas maltophilia* that was sensitive to trimethoprim-sulfamethoxazole (TMP-SMX). Over the next few days, she developed painful, erythematous, nodular skin lesions. *S. maltophilia* was isolated from a biopsy of one of the lesions. Treatment with intravenous TMP-SMX led to gradual resolution of the skin lesions. This case illustrates the predilection for *Stenotrophomonas* to cause disease in immunocompromised patients receiving a carbapenem antibiotic. Characteristically, *Stenotrophomonas* is one of the few gram-negative bacteria that are resistant to carbapenems and susceptible to TMP-SMX.

melioidosis (*melis*, "distemper"; *eidos*, "resemblance"; *osis*, "condition": disease resembling equine distemper or glanders caused by *B. mallei*). Exposure by the percutaneous route presents as a localized, suppurative **cutaneous infection** accompanied by regional lymphadenitis, fever, and malaise. This form of disease can resolve without incident or can progress rapidly to overwhelming sepsis. **Pulmonary disease** that develops after respiratory exposure may range in severity from a mild bronchitis to necrotizing pneumonia. Cavitation progressing to overwhelming sepsis and death can develop if appropriate antimicrobial therapy is not instituted. *B. pseudomallei* has been used in biologic weapons programs, so work with this organism is restricted to appropriately licensed laboratories, and the recovery from a patient justifies intervention by the public health department. Isolation of *B. pseudomallei* for diagnostic purposes should be approached carefully because the organism is highly infectious.

Burkholderia species are susceptible to **trimethoprim-sulfamethoxazole**, which distinguishes them from *P. aeruginosa*. Although the organisms appear to be susceptible in vitro to piperacillin, broad-spectrum cephalosporins, and ciprofloxacin, the clinical response is generally poor.

Stenotrophomonas maltophilia

S. maltophilia was originally classified in the genus *Pseudomonas*, moved to the genus *Xanthomonas*, and then transferred to the genus *Stenotrophomonas*. Despite the confusion created by these taxonomic changes, the clinical importance of this opportunistic pathogen is well known. It is responsible for infections in debilitated

patients with impaired host-defense mechanisms. Also, because *S. maltophilia* is resistant to most commonly used β-lactam and aminoglycoside antibiotics, patients receiving long-term antibiotic therapy with these drugs are particularly at risk for acquiring infections.

The most common nosocomial infections caused by *S. maltophilia* are bacteremia and pneumonia, with both associated with a high incidence of complications and death (Clinical Case 33-3). Hospital infections with this organism have been traced to contaminated intravenous catheters, disinfectant solutions, mechanical ventilation equipment, and ice machines.

Antimicrobial therapy is complicated, because the organism is resistant to many commonly used drugs. In contrast with most gram-negative rods, *Stenotrophomonas* is **resistant to carbapenems** (e.g., imipenem, meropenem, ertapenem). **Trimethoprim-sulfamethoxazole** is the agent most active against the organism; in vitro activity is also seen with doxycycline and ceftazidime.

Acinetobacter

Acinetobacters are strictly aerobic, oxidase-negative, plump, gram-negative coccobacilli (Figure 33-6). They are **ubiquitous** saprophytes, recovered in nature and in the hospital and able to survive on both moist surfaces, such as mechanical ventilation equipment, and on dry surfaces, such as human skin (the latter feature is unusual for gram-negative rods). These bacteria are also part of the normal oropharyngeal flora of a small number of healthy people and can proliferate to large numbers during hospitalization. The genus *Acinetobacter* is subdivided into two groups:

Bibliography

Forster D, Dashner F: *Acinetobacter* species as nosocomial pathogens. Eur J Clin Microbiol Infect Dis 17:73-77, 1998.

Govan J, Deretic V: Microbial pathogenesis in cystic fibrosis: Mucoid *Pseudomonas aeruginosa* and *Burkholderia cepacia*. Microbiol Rev 60:539-574, 1996.

Kipnis E, et al: Targeting mechanisms of *Pseudomonas aeruginosa* pathogenesis. Med Mal Infect 36:78-91, 2006.

Mahenthiralingam E, et al: The multifarious, multireplicon *Burkholderia cepacia* complex. Nat Rev Microbiol 3:144-156, 2005.

Mahenthiralingam E, Vandamme P: Taxonomy and pathogenesis of the *Burkholderia cepacia* complex. Chron Respir Dis 2:209-217, 2005.

McGregor K, et al: *Moraxella catarrhalis*: Clinical significance, antimicrobial susceptibility and BRO beta-lactamases. Eur J Clin Microbiol Infect Dis 17:219-234, 1998.

Peacock S: Melioidosis. Curr Opin Infect Dis 19:421-428, 2006.

Sadikot R, et al: Pathogen-host interactions in *Pseudomonas aeruginosa* pneumonia. Am J Respir Crit Care Med 171:1209-1223, 2005.

Senol E: *Stenotrophomonas maltophilia*: The significance and role as a nosocomial pathogen. J Hosp Infect 57:1-7, 2004.

Yahr T, Wolfgang M: Transcriptional regulation of the *Pseudomonas aeruginosa* type III secretion system. Mol Microbiol 62:631-640, 2006.

Yates S, et al: Stealth and mimicry by deadly bacterial toxins. Trends Biochem Sci 31:123-133, 2006.

Haemophilus and Related Bacteria

The four most important genera in the family Pasteurellaceae are **Haemophilus**, **Actinobacillus**, **Aggregatibacter**, and **Pasteurella** (Box 34-1); they are responsible for a broad spectrum of diseases (Box 34-2). The members of this family are small (0.2 to 0.3 × 1.0 to 2.0 µm), gram-negative, facultative anaerobic rods. Most have fastidious growth needs, requiring enriched media for isolation. Members of the genus *Haemophilus* are the most commonly isolated and significant human pathogens and will be the main focus of this chapter (Table 34-1).

Haemophilus (Box 34-3)

Haemophilae are small, sometimes pleomorphic, gram-negative rods present on the mucous membranes of humans (Figure 34-1). **Haemophilus influenzae** is the species most commonly associated with disease, with infections most often reported in pediatric patients before the introduction of the *H. influenzae* type b (HIB) vaccine. **Haemophilus aegyptius** is an important cause of acute, purulent conjunctivitis. **Haemophilus ducreyi** is well recognized as the etiologic agent of the sexually transmitted disease **soft chancre**, or **chancroid**. The other members of the genus are commonly isolated in clinical specimens (e.g., *Haemophilus parainfluenzae* is the most common species in the mouth) but are rarely pathogenic, being responsible primarily for opportunistic infections.

Physiology and Structure

The growth of most species of *Haemophilus* requires supplementation of media with one or both of the following growth-stimulating factors: (1) **hemin** (also called **X factor** for unknown factor), and (2) **nicotinamide adenine dinucleotide** (NAD; also called **V factor** for "vitamin"). Although both factors are present in blood-enriched media, sheep blood agar must be gently heated to destroy the inhibitors of V factor. For this reason, heated blood ("chocolate") agar is used for the in vitro isolation of *Haemophilus*.

The cell wall structure of *Haemophilus* is typical of other gram-negative rods. Lipopolysaccharide with endotoxin activity is present in the cell wall, and strain-specific and species-specific proteins are found in the outer membrane. Analysis of these strain-specific proteins is valuable in epidemiologic investigations. The surface of many but not all strains of *H. influenzae* is covered with a **polysaccharide capsule**, and six antigenic **serotypes** (**a** through **f**) have been identified. Before the introduction of the HIB vaccine, *H. influenzae* serotype b was responsible for more than 95% of all invasive *Haemophilus* infections. After the introduction of the vaccine, most disease caused by this serotype disappeared, and more than half of all invasive disease is now caused by nonencapsulated (nontypeable) strains.

In addition to the serologic differentiation of *H. influenzae*, the species is subdivided into eight **biotypes** (I through VIII), as determined by three biochemical reactions: indole production, urease activity, and ornithine decarboxylase activity. The separation of these biotypes is useful for epidemiologic purposes.

Pathogenesis and Immunity

Haemophilus species, particularly *H. parainfluenzae* and nonencapsulated *H. influenzae*, colonize the upper respiratory tract in virtually all people within the first few months of life. These organisms can spread locally and cause disease in the ears (otitis media), sinuses (sinusitis), and lower respiratory tract (bronchitis, pneumonia). Disseminated disease, however, is relatively uncommon. In contrast, encapsulated *H. influenzae* (particularly serotype b [biotype I]) is uncommon in the upper respiratory tract or is present in only very small numbers but is a common cause of **disease in unvaccinated children** (i.e., meningitis, epiglottitis [obstructive laryngitis], cellulitis). Pili and nonpilus adhesins mediate colonization of the oropharynx with *H. influenzae*. Cell wall components of the bacteria (e.g., lipopolysaccharide and a low-molecular-weight glycopeptide) impair ciliary function, leading to damage of the

Box 34–1. Important Pasteurellaceae

Organism	Historical Derivation
Haemophilus	*haemo*, "blood"; *hilos*, "lover" ("blood lover"; requires blood for growth on agar media)
H. influenzae	Originally thought to be the cause of *influenza*
H. aegyptius	*aegyptius*, "Egyptian" (observed by R. Koch in 1883 in exudates from Egyptians with conjunctivitis)
H. ducreyi	Named after the bacteriologist *Ducrey*, who first isolated this organism)
Actinobacillus	*actinis*, "ray"; *bacillus*, "small staff" or "rod" ("ray bacillus"; refers to the growth of filamentous forms [rays])
Aggregatibacter	*aggregare*, to "come together"; *bacter*, bacterial "rod"; rod-shaped bacteria that aggregate or clump together
A. actinomycetemcomitans	*comitans*, "accompanying" ("accompanying actinomycetes"; isolates are frequently associated with *Actinomyces*)
A. aphrophilus	*aphros*, "foam"; *philos*, "loving" ("foam-loving")
Pasteurella	Named after Louis *Pasteur*
P. multocida	*multus*, "many"; *cidus*, "to kill" ("many-killing"; pathogenic for many species of animals)
P. canis	*canis*, "dog" (isolated from the mouths of dogs)

Box 34–2. Pasteurellaceae: Clinical Summaries

Haemophilus influenzae

Meningitis: primarily a disease of unimmunized children; characterized by fever, severe headache, and systemic signs
Epiglottitis: primarily a disease of unimmunized children; characterized by initial pharyngitis, fever, and difficulty breathing, and progressing to cellulitis and swelling of the supraglottic tissues, with obstruction of the airways possible
Pneumonia: inflammation and consolidation of the lungs observed primarily in the elderly with underlying chronic pulmonary disease; typically caused by nontypeable strains

Haemophilus aegyptius

Conjunctivitis: an acute, purulent conjunctivitis ("pink eye")

Haemophilus ducreyi

Chancroid: sexually transmitted disease characterized by a tender papule with an erythematous base, progressing to painful ulceration with associated lymphadenopathy

Aggregatibacter actinomycetemcomitans

Endocarditis: responsible for subacute form of endocarditis in patients with underlying damage to the heart valve

Aggregatibacter aphrophilus

Endocarditis: as with *A. actinomycetemcomitans*

Pasteurella multocida

Bite wound: most common manifestation is infected cat- or dog-bite wound; particularly common with cat bites, because the wounds are deep and difficult to disinfect

Table 34–1. *Haemophilus* Species Associated with Human Disease

Species	Primary Diseases	Frequency
H. influenzae	Pneumonia, sinusitis, otitis, meningitis, epiglottitis, cellulitis, bacteremia	Common
H. aegyptius	Conjunctivitis	Uncommon
H. ducreyi	Chancroid	Uncommon (in United States)
H. parainfluenzae	Bacteremia, endocarditis, opportunistic infections	Rare
H. haemolyticus	Opportunistic infections	Rare
H. parahaemolyticus	Opportunistic infections	Rare

respiratory epithelium. The bacteria can then be translocated across both epithelial and endothelial cells and can enter the blood. In the absence of specific opsonic antibodies directed against the polysaccharide capsule, high-grade bacteremia can develop, with dissemination to the meninges or other distal foci.

The major virulence factor in *H. influenzae* type b is the antiphagocytic polysaccharide capsule, which contains ribose, ribitol, and phosphate (commonly referred to as **polyribitol phosphate [PRP]**). Antibodies directed against the capsule greatly stimulate bacterial phagocytosis and

Box 34—3. Summary: *Haemophilus*

Biology, Virulence, and Disease

Small, pleomorphic, gram-negative rods or coccobacilli
Facultative anaerobes, fermentative
Most species require X and/or V factor for growth
H. influenzae subdivided serologically (types a to f) and
   biochemically (biotypes I to VIII)
H. influenzae type b is clinically most virulent (with PRP,
   [polyribitol phosphate] in capsule)
Haemophilus adhere to host cells via pili and nonpilus structures
Refer to Table 34-1 for a summary of diseases

Epidemiology

Haemophilus species commonly colonized in humans although
   encapsulated *Haemophilus* species, particularly *H. influenzae*
   type b, are uncommon members of normal flora
Disease caused by *H. influenzae* type b was primarily a pediatric
   problem; eliminated in immunized populations
H. ducreyi disease is uncommon in the United States
With the exception of *H. ducreyi*, which is spread by sexual
   contact, most *Haemophilus* infections are caused by the
   patient's oropharyngeal flora (endogenous infections)
Patients at greatest risk for disease are those with inadequate
   levels of protective antibodies, those with
   depleted complement, and those who have undergone
   splenectomy

Diagnosis

Microscopy is a sensitive test for detecting *H. influenzae* in
   cerebrospinal fluid (CSF), synovial fluid, and lower respiratory
   specimens but not from other sites
Culture is performed using chocolate agar
Antigen tests are specific for *H. influenzae* type b; therefore,
   these tests are nonreactive for infections caused by other
   organisms

Treatment, Prevention, and Control

Haemophilus infections are treated with broad-spectrum
   cephalosporins, azithromycin, or fluoroquinolones; many
   strains are resistant to ampicillin
Active immunization with conjugated PRP vaccines prevents most
   H. influenzae type b infections

Figure 34—1. Gram stains of *Haemophilus influenzae*. **A,** Small coccobacilli forms seen in sputum from patient with pneumonia. **B,** Thin, pleomorphic forms seen in 1-year-old, unvaccinated child in Africa with overwhelming meningitis.

complement-mediated bactericidal activity. These antibodies develop as a result of natural infection, vaccination with purified PRP, or the passive transfer of maternal antibodies. The severity of systemic disease is inversely related to the rate of clearance of bacteria from the blood. The risk of meningitis and epiglottitis is significantly greater in patients with no anti-PRP antibodies, those with depletion of complement, and those who have undergone splenectomy. The lipopolysaccharide **lipid A** component induces meningeal inflammation in an animal model and may be responsible for initiating this response in humans. Immunoglobulin **IgA1 proteases** are produced by *H. influenzae* (both encapsulated and nonencapsulated strains) and may facilitate colonization of the organisms on mucosal surfaces by interfering with humoral immunity.

Epidemiology

Haemophilus species are present in almost all individuals, primarily colonizing the mucosal membranes of the respiratory tract. *H. parainfluenzae* is the predominant *Haemophilus* species in the mouth. Nonencapsulated strains of *H. influenzae* are also commonly found in the upper respiratory tract; however, encapsulated strains are detectable only in small numbers and only when highly selective culture methods are used. Before the introduction of the *H. influenzae* vaccine, although *H. influenzae* type b was the most common serotype that caused systemic disease, it was rarely isolated in healthy children (a fact that emphasizes the virulence of this bacterium).

The epidemiology of *Haemophilus* disease has changed dramatically. Before the introduction of **conjugated *H. influenzae* type b vaccines**, an estimated 20,000 cases of invasive *H. influenzae* type b disease occurred annually in children younger than age 5 in the United States. The first polysaccharide vaccines for *H. influenzae* type b were not protective for children younger than 18 months (the population at greatest risk for disease) because there is a natural delay in the maturation of the immune response to polysaccharide antigens. Vaccines containing purified PRP antigens conjugated to protein carriers (i.e., diphtheria toxoid, tetanus toxoid, meningococcal outer membrane protein), however, were found to elicit a protective antibody response in infants 2 months and older. Since the introduction of the conjugated vaccine in December 1987, systemic disease in children younger than 5 years has been virtually eliminated in the United States, with only 15 cases reported in 2006. Most of the *H. influenzae* type b infections now occur in children who are not immune (because of incomplete vaccination or a poor response to the vaccine) and in elderly adults with waning immunity. In addition, invasive *H. influenzae* disease caused by other serotypes of encapsulated bacteria and by nonencapsulated strains has now become proportionally more common than that resulting from serotype b. It should be noted that the successful elimination of *H. influenzae* type b disease in the United States has not been seen in many developing countries where vaccination programs have been difficult to implement. Thus *H. influenzae* type b remains the most significant pediatric pathogen in many countries of the world. It is estimated that 3 million cases of serious disease and up to 700,000 fatalities occur in children each year worldwide. The epidemiology of disease caused by nonencapsulated *H. influenzae* and other *Haemophilus* species is distinct. Ear and sinus infections caused by these organisms are primarily pediatric diseases but can occur in adults. Pulmonary disease most commonly affects elderly people, particularly those with a history of underlying obstructive pulmonary disease or conditions predisposing to aspiration (e.g., alcoholism, altered mental state).

H. ducreyi is an important cause of genital ulcers (chancroid) in Africa and Asia but is less common in Europe and North America. The incidence of disease in the United States is cyclic. A peak incidence of more than 5000 cases was reported in 1988, which decreased to 33 cases in 2006. Despite this favorable trend, the Centers for Disease Control and Prevention have documented that the disease is significantly underreported, making the true incidence unknown.

Clinical Diseases (Table 34-1)

The clinical syndromes seen in patients with *H. influenzae* infections are represented in Figure 34-2. The diseases caused by all *Haemophilus* species are described in the following sections.

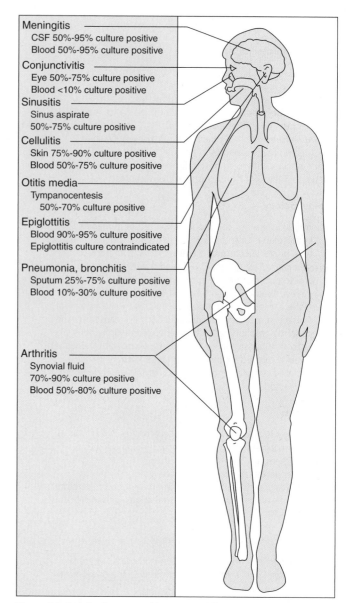

Meningitis
  CSF 50%-95% culture positive
  Blood 50%-95% culture positive
Conjunctivitis
  Eye 50%-75% culture positive
  Blood <10% culture positive
Sinusitis
  Sinus aspirate
  50%-75% culture positive
Cellulitis
  Skin 75%-90% culture positive
  Blood 50%-75% culture positive
Otitis media
  Tympanocentesis
    50%-70% culture positive
Epiglottitis
  Blood 90%-95% culture positive
  Epiglottitis culture contraindicated
Pneumonia, bronchitis
  Sputum 25%-75% culture positive
  Blood 10%-30% culture positive
Arthritis
  Synovial fluid
  70%-90% culture positive
  Blood 50%-80% culture positive

Figure 34—2. Infections caused by *Haemophilus influenzae*. With the advent of the conjugated vaccine, most infections in adults involve areas contiguous with the oropharynx (i.e., lower respiratory tract, sinuses, and ears). Serious systemic infections (e.g., meningitis, epiglottitis) can occur in nonimmune patients. CSF, cerebrospinal fluid.

Meningitis

H. influenzae type b was the most common cause of pediatric meningitis, but this situation changed rapidly when the conjugated vaccines became widely used. Disease in nonimmune patients results from the bacteremic spread of the organisms from the nasopharynx and cannot be differentiated clinically from other causes of bacterial meningitis. The initial presentation is a 1- to 3-day history of mild upper respiratory disease, after which the typical signs and symptoms of meningitis appear. Mortality is less than 10% in patients who receive prompt therapy, and carefully designed studies have documented a low incidence of serious neurologic sequelae (in contrast with the 50%

incidence of severe residual damage in nonimmune children seen in initial studies). Person-to-person spread in a nonimmune population is well documented, so appropriate epidemiologic precautions must be used.

Epiglottitis

Epiglottitis, characterized by cellulitis and the swelling of the supraglottic tissues, represents a life-threatening emergency. Although epiglottitis is a pediatric disease, the peak incidence of this disease during the prevaccine era occurred in children 2 to 4 years of age; in contrast, the peak incidence of meningitis was seen in children 3 to 18 months of age. Children with epiglottitis have pharyngitis, fever, and difficulty breathing, which can progress rapidly to obstruction of the airway and death. Since the introduction of the vaccine, the incidence of this disease has also decreased dramatically in children and remains relatively rare in adults.

Cellulitis

Like meningitis and epiglottitis, *H. influenzae* cellulitis is a pediatric disease that has largely been eliminated by vaccination. When it is observed, patients have fever and cellulitis characterized by the development of reddish-blue patches on the cheeks or periorbital areas. The diagnosis is strongly suggested by the typical clinical presentation, cellulitis proximal to the oral mucosa, and lack of documented vaccination in the child.

Arthritis

Before the advent of conjugated vaccines, the most common form of arthritis in children younger than 2 years was an infection of a single, large joint secondary to the bacteremic spread of *H. influenzae* type b. Disease does occur in older children and adults, but it is very uncommon and generally affects immunocompromised patients and patients with previously damaged joints.

Otitis, Sinusitis, and Lower Respiratory Tract Disease (Clinical Case 34-1)

Nonencapsulated strains of *H. influenzae* (primarily biotypes II and III) are opportunistic pathogens that can cause infections of the upper and lower airways. Most studies have shown that *H. influenzae* and *Streptococcus pneumoniae* are the two most common causes of acute and chronic otitis and sinusitis. Primary pneumonia is uncommon in children and adults who have normal pulmonary function. These organisms commonly colonize patients who have chronic pulmonary disease (including cystic fibrosis) and frequently are associated with exacerbation of bronchitis and frank pneumonia.

Conjunctivitis

H. aegyptius, also called the **Koch-Weeks bacillus**, causes an acute, purulent conjunctivitis. This contagious organism is associated with epidemics, particularly during the warm months of the year.

Chancroid

Chancroid is a sexually transmitted disease that is most commonly diagnosed in men, presumably because women can have asymptomatic or inapparent disease. Approximately 5 to 7 days after exposure, a tender papule with an erythematous base develops on the genitalia or perianal area. Within 2 days the lesion ulcerates and becomes **painful**, and inguinal **lymphadenopathy** is commonly present. Other causes of genital ulcers, such as syphilis and herpes simplex disease, must be excluded to confirm the diagnose chancroid.

Other Infections

Other species of *Haemophilus* can cause opportunistic infections, such as otitis media, conjunctivitis, sinusitis, endocarditis, meningitis, and dental abscesses.

Laboratory Diagnosis

Specimen Collection and Transport

Because most *Haemophilus* infections in vaccinated individuals originate from the oropharynx and are restricted to the upper and lower respiratory tract, contamination of the specimen with oral secretions should be avoided. Direct needle aspiration should be used for the microbiologic diagnosis of sinusitis or otitis, and sputum produced from the lower airways is used for the diagnosis of pneumonia. Culture of blood for patients with pneumonia may be useful but would be predictably negative in patients with upper respiratory infections. Both blood and cerebrospinal fluid (CSF) should be collected from nonimmune children with the diagnosis of meningitis. Because there are approximately 10^7 bacteria per mL of CSF in patients with untreated meningitis, 1 to 2 mL of fluid is generally adequate for microscopy, culture, and antigen-detection tests. Microscopy and culture are less sensitive if the patient has been exposed to antibiotics before the CSF is collected. Blood cultures should also be collected for the diagnosis of epiglottitis, cellulitis, and arthritis. Specimens should not be collected from the posterior pharynx in patients with suspected epiglottitis because the procedure may stimulate coughing and obstruct the airway. Specimens for the detection of *H. ducreyi* should be collected with a moistened

---

Clinical Case 34-1. Pneumonia Caused by *Haemophilus influenzae*

Holmes and Kozinn (J Clin Microbiol 18:730-732, 1983) described a 61-year-old woman with pneumonia caused by *H. influenzae* serotype d. The patient had a long history of smoking, chronic obstructive lung disease, diabetes mellitus, and congestive heart failure. She presented with a left upper lobe pneumonia, producing purulent sputum with many gram-negative bacteria. Both sputum and blood cultures were positive for *H. influenzae* serotype d. The organism was susceptible to ampicillin, to which the patient responded. This case illustrates the susceptibility of patients with chronic underlying pulmonary disease to infections with nonserotype b strains of *H. influenzae*.

swab from the base or margin of the ulcer. Culture of pus collected by aspiration from an enlarged lymph node can be performed but is generally less sensitive than culture of the ulcer. The laboratory should be notified that *H. ducreyi* is suspected, because special culture techniques must be used for recovery of the organism.

Microscopy

If microscopy is performed carefully, the detection of *Haemophilus* species in clinical specimens is both sensitive and specific. Gram-negative rods ranging in shape from coccobacilli to long, pleomorphic filaments can be detected in more than 80% of CSF specimens from patients with untreated *Haemophilus* meningitis (see Figure 34-1). The microscopic examination of Gram-stained specimens is also useful for the rapid diagnosis of the organism in arthritis and lower respiratory tract disease.

Antigen Detection

The immunologic detection of *H. influenzae* antigen, specifically the PRP capsular antigen, is a rapid and sensitive way to diagnose *H. influenzae* type b disease. PRP can be detected with the particle agglutination test, which can detect less than 1ng/ml of PRP in a clinical specimen. In this test, antibody-coated latex particles are mixed with the clinical specimen; agglutination occurs if PRP is present. Antigen can be detected in CSF and urine (in which the antigen is eliminated intact). However, this test has limited use because it can detect only *H. influenzae* type b, which is now uncommon in the United States and other countries with an established vaccine program. Other capsular serotypes and nonencapsulated strains do not give a positive reaction.

Culture

It is relatively easy to isolate *H. influenzae* from clinical specimens inoculated onto media supplemented with the appropriate growth factors. Chocolate agar or Levinthal agar is used in most laboratories. However, if chocolate agar is overheated during preparation, V factor is destroyed, and *Haemophilus* species requiring this growth factor (e.g., *H. influenzae*, *H. aegyptius*, *H. parainfluenzae*) will not grow. The bacteria appear as 1- to 2-mm, smooth, opaque colonies after 24 hours of incubation. They can also be detected growing around colonies of *Staphylococcus aureus* on unheated blood agar (**satellite phenomenon**; Figure 34-3). The staphylococci provide the requisite growth factors by lysing the erythrocytes in the medium and releasing intracellular heme (X factor) and excreting NAD (V factor). The colonies of *H. influenzae* in these cultures are much smaller than they are on chocolate agar, because the V factor inhibitors present in blood are not inactivated.

The growth of *Haemophilus* in blood cultures is generally delayed, because most commercially prepared blood culture broths are not supplemented with optimum concentrations of X and V factors and inhibitors of V factor. Furthermore, the growth factors are released only when the blood cells

Figure 34—3. Satellite phenomenon. *Staphylococcus aureus* excretes nicotinamide adenine dinucleotide (NAD, or V factor) into the medium, providing a growth factor required for *H. influenzae* (small colonies surrounding *S. aureus* colonies).

lyse. Isolates of *H. influenzae* often grow better in anaerobically incubated blood cultures because under these conditions, the organisms do not require X factor for growth.

H. aegyptius and *H. ducreyi* are fastidious and require specialized growth conditions. *H. aegyptius* grows best on chocolate agar supplemented with 1% IsoVitaleX (mixture of chemically defined supplements), with growth detected after incubation in a carbon dioxide atmosphere for 2 to 4 days. Culture for *H. ducreyi* is relatively insensitive (less than 85% of cultures yield organisms under optimal conditions) but reportedly is best on gonococcal (GC) agar supplemented with 1% to 2% hemoglobin, 5% fetal bovine serum, IsoViteleX enrichment, and vancomycin (3 μg/ml). Cultures should be incubated at 33° C in 5% to 10% carbon dioxide for 7 days or more. Because the media and incubation conditions are not used for other bacterial cultures, success in recovering *H. ducreyi* requires that the microbiologist look specifically for this organism.

Identification

A presumptive identification of *H. influenzae* can be made by the Gram stain morphology and demonstration of a requirement for both X and V factors. Further subgrouping of *H. influenzae* can be done with biotyping, electrophoretic characterization of the membrane protein antigens, and analysis of the strain-specific nucleic acid sequences. Biochemical tests or nucleic acid analysis is used to identify other species in this genus.

Treatment, Prevention, and Control

Patients with systemic *H. influenzae* infections require prompt antimicrobial therapy, because the mortality rate in patients with untreated meningitis or epiglottitis approaches 100%. Serious infections are treated with **broad-spectrum cephalosporins**. Less severe infections such as sinusitis and otitis can be treated with ampicillin (if susceptible, approximately 30% of strains are resistant), an active cephalosporin, azithromycin, or a fluoroquinolone. Most isolates of *H. ducreyi* are susceptible to **erythromycin**, the drug recommended for treatment.

The primary approach to preventing *H. influenzae* type b disease is through active immunization with purified capsular PRP. As discussed previously, the use of conjugated vaccines has been remarkably successful in reducing the incidence of *H. influenzae* type b disease and colonization. Currently, it is recommended that children receive three doses of vaccine against *H. influenzae* type b disease before the age of 6 months, followed by booster doses.

Antibiotic chemoprophylaxis is used to eliminate the carriage of *H. influenzae* type b in children at high risk for disease (e.g., children younger than 2 years in a family or daycare center where systemic disease is documented). Rifampin prophylaxis has been used in these settings.

Actinobacillus

Actinobacillus species are small, facultatively anaerobic, gram-negative rods that grow slowly (generally requiring 2 to 3 days of incubation). *Actinobacillus actinomycetemcomitans* was the most important human pathogen in this genus; however, in 2006 this species and *Haemophilus aphrophilus* were transferred into a new genus, *Aggregatibacter*. The remaining members of the genus *Actinobacillus* colonize the oropharynx of humans and animals and are rare causes of periodontitis, endocarditis, bite wound infections, and opportunistic infections (Table 34-2).

Aggregatibacter (Clinical Case 34-2)

Two members of this genus are important human pathogens: **A. actinomycetemcomitans** and **A. aphrophilus** (Table 34-3). Both species colonize the human mouth and can spread from the mouth into the blood and then stick to a previously damaged heart valve or artificial valve, leading to the development of endocarditis. **Endocarditis** caused by these bacteria is particularly difficult to diagnose, because clinical signs and symptoms develop slowly (subacute endocarditis), and the

Clinical Case 34-2. Endocarditis Caused by *Aggregatibacter actinomycetemcomitans*

Steitz, et al. (Clin Infect Dis 27:224-225, 1998) described a 54-year-old woman who was admitted to their hospital with a history of fever, night sweats, and fatigue. Physical examination revealed a tricuspid systolic murmur and splenomegaly, and echocardiography revealed a vegetation on the tricuspid valve. Cultures of blood collected on admission were positive after 5 days of incubation for *Aggregatibacter (Actinobacillus) actinomycetemcomitans*. Her clinical history was incomplete, because it is not known how chronic her course was, but this case illustrates the slow growth of the organism in routine culture.

bacteria grow slowly in blood cultures. Both species form adherent colonies that can be observed on the glass surface of the blood culture bottles and on agar media. The treatment of choice for endocarditis caused by these organisms is a cephalosporin such as ceftriaxone.

Pasteurella (Clinical Case 34-3)

Pasteurella are small, facultatively anaerobic, fermentative coccobacilli (Figure 34-4) commonly found as commensals in the oropharynx of healthy animals. Most human infections result from animal contact (e.g., animal bites, scratches, shared food). **Pasteurella multocida** (the most common isolate) and **Pasteurella canis** are human pathogens; the other *Pasteurella* species are rarely associated with human infections (Table 34-4). The following three general forms of disease are reported: (1) localized **cellulitis** and **lymphadenitis** that occur after an animal bite or scratch (*P. multocida* from contact with cats or dogs; *P. canis* from dogs); (2) an exacerbation of chronic **respiratory disease** in patients with underlying pulmonary dysfunction (presumably related to colonization of the patient's oropharynx followed by the aspiration of oral secretions); and (3) a **systemic infection in immunocompromised patients**, particularly those with underlying hepatic disease.

P. multocida grows well on blood and chocolate agars but poorly on MacConkey agar and other media typically selective for gram-negative rods. After overnight incubation on blood agar, large, buttery colonies with a

Table 34-2. *Actinobacillus* Species Associated with Human Disease

Species	Primary Diseases	Frequency
A. equuli	Bite-wound infections	Rare
A. hominis	Opportunistic infections (bacteremia, pneumonia)	Rare
A. lignieresii	Bite-wound infections	Rare
A. ureae	Opportunistic infections (bacteremia, meningitis, pneumonia)	Rare

Table 34-3. *Aggregatibacter* Species Associated with Human Disease

Species	Primary Diseases	Frequency
A. actinomycetemcomitans	Periodontitis, endocarditis, bite-wound infections	Common
A. aphrophilus	Endocarditis, opportunistic infections	Uncommon

Clinical Case 34-3. Fatal *Pasteurella multocida* Infection

Chang, et al. (Scan J Infect Dis 39:167-192, 2007) described a fatal case of *P. multocida* bacteremia and necrotizing fasciitis. The 58-year-old man had a history of chronic renal insufficiency, gouty arthritis, and Cushing syndrome treated with steroids. Upon admission to the hospital, his left hand was erythematous, warm, and tender with reddish to purplish macules over the surface. Over a 2-day period, bullae developed and extended rapidly to the left arm, left calf, and right foot, and the patient began to exhibit systemic signs of shock and gastrointestinal bleeding. Blood cultures collected at the time of admission were positive for *P. multocida*. Despite aggressive antibiotic and surgical treatment, the lesions progressed rapidly, and the patient eventually expired. A careful history at the time of admission revealed that the patient allowed his pet dog to lick his open wounds. It is likely that this was the source of the bacteria, and the steroid treatments allowed the organism to invade the wound and rapidly spread in the tissues.

Figure 34—4. *Pasteurella multocida* in respiratory specimen from patient with pneumonia.

Table 34—4. *Pasteurella* Species Associated with Human Disease

Species	Primary Disease	Frequency
P. multocida	Bite-wound infections, chronic pulmonary disease, bacteremia, meningitis	Common
P. canis	Bite-wound infections	Uncommon
P. bettyae	Opportunistic infections (abscesses, bite-wound infections, urogenital infections, bacteremia)	Rare
P. dagmatis	Bite-wound infections	Rare
P. stomatis	Bite-wound infections	Rare

characteristic musty odor caused by the production of indole are present. *P. multocida* is susceptible to a variety of antibiotics. **Penicillin** is the antibiotic of choice, and expanded spectrum cephalosporins, macrolides, tetracyclines, or fluoroquinolones are acceptable alternatives. Semisynthetic penicillins (e.g., oxacillin), first-generation cephalosporins, and aminoglycosides have poor activity.

Case Study and Questions

A 78-year-old man confined to a nursing home awoke with a severe headache and stiff neck. Because he had a high fever and signs of meningitis, the nursing home staff took him to a local emergency department. The CSF specimen was cloudy. Analysis revealed 400 white blood cells per mm^3 (95% polymorphonuclear neutrophils), a protein concentration of 75 mg/dL, and a glucose concentration of 20 mg/dL. Small, gram-negative rods were seen on Gram stain of the CSF, and cultures of CSF and blood were positive for *Haemophilus influenzae*.

1. Discuss the epidemiology of *H. influenzae* meningitis, and compare it with the epidemiology of meningitis caused by *Streptococcus pneumoniae* and by *Neisseria meningitidis*.

2. Compare the biology of the *H. influenzae* strain that is likely to be the cause of this patient's disease with that of the strains that historically caused pediatric diseases (prior to vaccination).

3. What other diseases does this organism cause? What other *Haemophilus* species cause disease, and what are the diseases?

4. Why is chocolate agar needed for the isolation of *Haemophilus* organisms?

5. What diseases are caused by *Aggregatibacter actinomycetemcomitans*? What is the source of this organism?

6. What diseases are caused by *Pasteurella multocida*? What is the source of this organism?

Bibliography

Chen HI, Hulten K, Clarridge JE: Taxonomic subgroups of *Pasteurella multocida* correlate with clinical presentation. J Clin Microbiol 40:3438-3441, 2002.

Dworkin M, Park L, Borchardt S: The changing epidemiology of invasive *Haemophilus influenzae* disease, especially in persons >65 years old. Clin Infect Dis 44:810-816, 2007.

Holst E, et al: Characterization and distribution of *Pasteurella* species recovered from infected humans. J Clin Microbiol 30:2984-2987, 1992.

Norskov-Lauritsen N, Kilian M: Reclassification of *Actinobacillus actinomycetemcomitans*, *Haemophilus aphrophilus*, *Haemophilus paraphrophilus* and *Haemophilus segnis* as *Aggregatibacter actinomycetemcomitans*, *Aggregatibacter aphrophilus*, and *Aggregatibacter segnis*, and emended description of *Aggregatibacter aphrophilus* to include V factor-dependent and V factor-independent isolates. Int J Syst Evol Microbiol 56:2135-2146, 2006.

Peltola H: Worldwide *Haemophilus influenzae* type b disease at the beginning of the 21st century: Global analysis of the disease burden 25 years after the use of the polysaccharide vaccine and a decade after the advent of conjugates. Clin Microbiol Rev 13:302-317, 2000.

Talan D, et al: Bacteriologic analysis of infected dog and cat bites. N Engl J Med 340:85-92, 1999.

Trees D, Morse S: Chancroid and *Haemophilus ducreyi*: An update. Clin Microbiol Rev 8:357-375, 1995.

Tristram S, Jacobs M, Appelbaum P: Antimicrobial resistance in *Haemophilus influenzae*. Clin Microbiol Rev 20:368-389, 2007.

Tsang R, et al: Characterization of invasive *Haemophilus influenzae* disease in Manitoba, Canada, 2000-2006: Invasive disease due to non-Type B strains. Clin Infect Dis 44:1611-1614, 2007.

Bordetella

Bordetella is an extremely **small** (0.2 to 0.5 × 1 μm), **strictly aerobic, gram-negative coccobacillus**. Eight species are currently recognized, with four species responsible for human disease (Box 35-1): *Bordetella pertussis* (Box 35-2), the agent responsible for pertussis or whooping cough; *Bordetella parapertussis*, responsible for a milder form of pertussis; *Bordetella bronchiseptica*, responsible for respiratory disease in dogs, swine, laboratory animals, and occasionally respiratory disease in humans; and *Bordetella holmesii*, an uncommon cause of sepsis.

Bordetella pertussis

Physiology and Structure

Bordetella species are differentiated on the basis of their growth characteristics, biochemical reactivity, and antigenic properties. Despite phenotypic differences, genetic studies have shown that the four species pathogenic for humans are closely related or identical species, differing only in the expression of virulence genes. At this time, however, the species have not been reclassified and should be considered as distinct.

Bordetella species have simple nutritional requirements, but some species are highly **susceptible to toxic substances and metabolites** in common laboratory media. These species (particularly *B. pertussis*) require media supplemented with charcoal, starch, blood, or albumin to absorb these toxic substances. The more fastidious species also grow slowly in culture. The organisms are nonmotile and oxidize amino acids, but they do not ferment carbohydrates.

Pathogenesis and Immunity

Infection with *B. pertussis* and the development of whooping cough require exposure to the organism, bacterial attachment to the ciliated epithelial cells of the respiratory tract, proliferation of the bacteria, and production of localized tissue damage and systemic toxicity. Attachment of the organisms to ciliated epithelial cells is mediated by protein adhesions (Table 35-1). **Pertactin** and **filamentous hemagglutinin** contain an Arg-Gly-Asp sequence (RGD motif) that promotes binding to sulfated glycoprotein integrins on the membranes of ciliated respiratory cells. These adhesins also bind to CR3, a glycoprotein receptor on the surface of macrophages. This interaction initiates the phagocytosis of the bacteria without initiating an oxidative burst, which is important in the intracellular survival and replication of the bacteria. This also protects *B. pertussis* from humoral antibodies. Similar proteins are also found in *B. parapertussis* and *B. bronchiseptica*. **Pertussis toxin** is a classic A-B toxin consisting of a toxic subunit (S1) and five binding subunits (S2 to S5; two S4 subunits are present in each toxin molecule). The S2 subunit binds to lactosylceramide, a glycolipid present on ciliated respiratory cells. The S3 subunit binds to receptors on phagocytic cells, leading to an increase in CR3 on the cell surface, which facilitates attachment mediated by the pertactin and filamentous hemagglutinin and subsequent bacterial phagocytosis. Another adhesin, **fimbria**, has been identified in *B. pertussis* and demonstrated to mediate the binding to cultured mammalian cells. The role of fimbriae in the attachment to ciliated cells in vivo is unknown; however, fimbriae and the other *B. pertussis* adhesins stimulate humoral immunity in vivo and are incorporated into acellular vaccines.

B. pertussis produces several toxins that mediate the localized and systemic manifestations of disease. The S1 portion of **pertussis toxin** has adenosine diphosphate (ADP)–ribosylating activity for the membrane surface G proteins (guanine nucleotide–binding regulatory proteins). These proteins regulate adenylate cyclase activity. Pertussis toxin inactivates $G_{i\alpha}$, the inhibitory protein that controls adenylate cyclase activity. The uncontrolled expression of the enzyme leads to an increase in cyclic adenosine monophosphate (cAMP) levels and a subsequent increase in respiratory secretions and mucus production characteristic of the paroxysmal stage of pertussis.

Box 35–1. *Bordetella* Species Associated with Human Disease

Organism	Historical Derivation
Bordetella	Named after Jules *Bordet*, who first isolated the organism responsible for pertussis
B. pertussis	*per*, very or "severe"; *tussis*, "cough" (a severe cough)
B. parapertussis	*para*, "resembling" (resembling pertussis)
B. bronchiseptica	*bronchus*, the trachea; *septicus*, septic (an infected bronchus)
B. holmesii	Named after the microbiologist Barry *Holmes*

Adenylate cyclase/hemolysin is a bifunctional toxin that is activated in the target mammalian cell by intracellular calmodulin and catalyzes the conversion of endogenous adenosine triphosphate (ATP) to cAMP in eukaryotic cells (as pertussis toxin does). Adenylate cyclase toxin also inhibits leukocyte chemotaxis, phagocytosis, and killing. This toxin may be important for the initial protection of the bacteria during the early stages of disease.

Dermonecrotic toxin is a heat-labile toxin that at low doses causes vasoconstriction of peripheral blood vessels in mice; this is accompanied by localized ischemia, the movement of leukocytes to extravascular spaces, and hemorrhage. At high doses this toxin causes fatal reactions in mice. The toxin probably is responsible for the localized tissue destruction in human infections, although further research is necessary to confirm this theory.

Tracheal cytotoxin is a low-molecular-weight cell wall peptidoglycan monomer that has a specific affinity for ciliated epithelial cells. At low concentrations, it causes ciliostasis (inhibition of cilia movement), and at the higher concentrations produced later in the infection, it causes extrusion of ciliated cells. Tracheal cytotoxin specifically interferes with deoxyribonucleic acid (DNA) synthesis, thereby impairing the regeneration of damaged cells. This process disrupts the normal clearance mechanisms in the respiratory tree and leads to the characteristic cough associated with pertussis. The toxin also stimulates the release of the cytokine interleukin-1 (IL-1), which leads to fever.

B. pertussis produces two distinct **lipopolysaccharides**, one with lipid A and the other with lipid X. Both lipopolysaccharide molecules can activate the alternate complement pathway and stimulate cytokine release. Their role in the disease process is unknown.

Epidemiology

B. pertussis is a **human disease** with no other recognized animal or environmental reservoir. Although the incidence of pertussis, with its associated morbidity and mortality,

Box 35–2. Summary: *Bordetella pertussis*

Biology, Virulence, and Disease

Very small, gram-negative coccobacilli
Nonfermentative but can oxidize amino acids as an energy source
Strict aerobe
Growth in vitro requires prolonged incubation in media supplemented with charcoal, starch, blood, or albumin
Many virulence factors responsible for adherence to eukaryotic cells and production of localized tissue destruction (see Table 35-1)
Pertussis characterized by three stages: catarrhal, paroxysmal, and convalescent
Most severe disease is in nonvaccinated individuals

Epidemiology

Human reservoir host
Worldwide distribution
Children younger than 1 year at greatest risk for infection, but disease is now most common in older children and adults
Nonvaccinated individuals at greatest risk for disease
Disease spread person to person by infectious aerosols

Diagnosis

Microscopy is insensitive and nonspecific
Culture is specific but insensitive
Nucleic acid amplification tests are the most sensitive and specific tests
Detection of IgG or IgA can be used as a confirmatory test

Treatment, Prevention, and Control

Treatment with macrolide (i.e., erythromycin, azithromycin, clarithromycin) is effective in eradicating organisms and reducing length of infectious stage
Erythromycin has been used for prophylaxis, but the effectiveness is unknown
Vaccines containing inactivated pertussis toxin, filamentous hemagglutinin, and pertactin are highly effective
Pediatric vaccine administered in five doses (at ages 2 months, 4 months, 6 months, and 15 to 18 months, and between ages 4 and 6 years); adult vaccine administered at 11 to 12 years and again between 19 and 65 years

was reduced considerably after the introduction of vaccines in 1949, the disease is still endemic worldwide, with an estimated 20 to 40 million infections and 200,000 to 400,000 deaths each year, primarily in unvaccinated children. The incidence of reported disease in the United States has **risen dramatically in recent years**, with more than 25,000 reported cases in 2005 (Figure 35-1); however, this is certainly an underestimation of the true incidence of disease. It has been projected that more than 3 million new cases of pertussis occur each year in the United States. Historically, pertussis was considered a pediatric disease, but now the majority of infections are found in **adolescents and adults** (Figure 35-2). A satisfactory explanation does not exist for the increase in disease and shift to older populations in recent years; however, the recognition of milder forms of disease in older children and adults and improved diagnostic tests certainly have contributed to the increase in reported disease.

Table 35–1. Virulence Factors Associated with *Bordetella pertussis*

Virulence Factor	Biologic Effect
Adhesins	
Filamentous hemagglutinin	Required for binding to sulfated glycoproteins on membranes of ciliated cells in trachea; highly immunogenic
Pertactin	As with filamentous hemagglutinin
Pertussis toxin	S2 subunit binds to glycolipid on surface of ciliated respiratory cells; S3 subunit binds to ganglioside on surface of phagocytic cells
Fimbriae	Bind to mammalian cells; role in disease is unknown but stimulates humoral immunity
Toxins	
Pertussis toxin	S1 subunit inactivates $G_{1\alpha}$, the membrane surface protein that controls adenylate cyclase activity; uncontrolled expression leads to increased cAMP levels; toxin inhibits phagocytic killing and monocyte migration
Adenylate cyclase/hemolysin toxin	Increases intracellular level of adenylate cyclase; inhibits phagocytic killing and monocyte migration
Dermonecrotic toxin	Causes dose-dependent skin lesions or fatal reactions in experimental animal model; role in disease is unknown
Tracheal cytotoxin	A peptidoglycan fragment that kills ciliated respiratory cells and stimulates the release of interleukin-1 (fever)
Lipopolysaccharide	Two distinct lipopolysaccharide molecules with either lipid A or lipid X; activates alternate complement pathway and stimulates cytokine release; role in disease is unknown

cAMP, cyclic adenosine monophosphate.

Clinical Diseases (Box 35-3; Clinical Case 35-1)

Infection is initiated when infectious aerosols are inhaled, and the bacteria become attached to and proliferate on ciliated epithelial cells. After a 7- to 10-day incubation period, the classical presentation of pertussis proceeds through three stages (Figure 35-3). The first stage, the **catarrhal stage**, resembles a common cold, with serous rhinorrhea, sneezing, malaise, anorexia, and low-grade fever. Because the peak number of bacteria is produced during this stage, and the cause of the disease is not yet recognized,

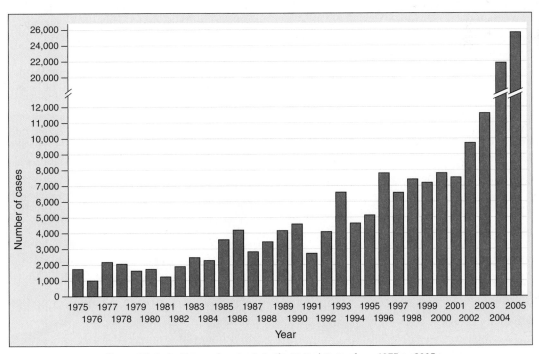

Figure 35–1. Incidence of pertussis in the United States from 1975 to 2005.

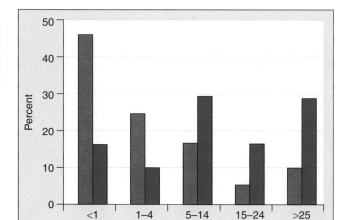

Figure 35—2. Age distribution for pertussis infections reported in 1988 *(red bars)* and 2005 *(blue bars)*.

patients in the catarrhal stage pose the highest risk to their contacts. After 1 to 2 weeks, the **paroxysmal stage** begins. During this time, ciliated epithelial cells are extruded from the respiratory tract, and the clearance of mucus is impaired. This stage is characterized by the **classic whooping cough paroxysms** (i.e., a series of repetitive coughs followed by an inspiratory whoop). Mucus production in the respiratory tract is common and is partially responsible for causing airway restriction. The paroxysms are frequently terminated with vomiting and exhaustion. A marked lymphocytosis is also prominent during this stage. Affected patients may experience as many as 40 to 50 paroxysms daily during the height of the illness. After 2 to 4 weeks, the disease enters the **convalescent stage**; at this time, the paroxysms diminish in number and severity, but secondary complications can occur. It is now appreciated that this classic presentation of pertussis may not be seen in patients with partial immunity. Such patients may have a history of a chronic persistent cough without

Box 35—3. *Bordetella* Species: Clinical Summaries

Bordetella pertussis

After a 7- to 10-day incubation period, disease is characterized by the **catarrhal stage** (resembles the common cold), progressing to the **paroxysmal stage** (repetitive coughs followed by inspiratory whoops), then the **convalescence stage** (diminishing paroxysms and secondary complications)

Bordetella parapertussis

Produces a milder form of pertussis

Bordetella bronchiseptica

Primarily a respiratory disease of animals but can cause bronchopneumonia in humans

Bordetella holmesii

Uncommon cause of sepsis

whooping or vomiting. Because this presentation is not distinctive, appropriate diagnostic tests should be performed for *Bordetella*, as well as other bacterial respiratory pathogens (e.g., *Mycoplasma pneumoniae*, *Chlamydophila pneumoniae*, *Legionella pneumophila*).

Laboratory Diagnosis

Specimen Collection and Transport

B. pertussis organisms are extremely sensitive to drying and do not survive unless care is taken during the collection and transport of the specimen to the laboratory. The optimal diagnostic specimen is a nasopharyngeal aspirate. Calcium alginate or Dacron fiber swabs must be used, because cotton swabs contain fatty acids that are toxic to *B. pertussis*. Oropharyngeal swabs should not be used, because sufficient numbers of ciliated epithelial cells are not collected. The specimen should be inoculated onto freshly prepared isolation media (e.g., Regan-Lowe agar) at the patient's bedside. If this is not possible, the specimen should be placed in a suitable transport medium (e.g., Regan-Lowe transport medium) and promptly delivered to the lab.

Microscopy

A direct fluorescent antibody procedure using either monoclonal or polyclonal antibodies can be used to examine

	Incubation	Catarrhal	Paroxysmal	Convalescent
Duration	7-10 days	1-2 weeks	2-4 weeks	3-4 weeks (or longer)
Symptoms	None	Rhinorrhea, malaise, fever, sneezing, anorexia	Repetitive cough with whoops, vomiting, leukocytosis	Diminished paroxysmal cough, development of secondary complications (pneumonia, seizures, encephalopathy)
Bacterial culture				

Figure 35—3. Clinical presentation of *Bordetella pertussis* disease.

specimens. In this method, the aspirated specimen is smeared onto a microscopic slide, air-dried and heat fixed, and then stained with fluorescein-labeled antibodies directed against *B. pertussis*. Antibodies against *B. parapertussis* should also be used to detect mild forms of pertussis caused by this organism. The direct fluorescent antibody test results are positive in about half of the patients with pertussis, but false-positive results can occur as a result of cross-reactions with other bacteria. Because of the sensitivity and specificity problems with this test, PCR and/or culture should also be performed.

Nucleic-Acid-Based Tests

Nucleic acid amplification methods such as polymerase chain reaction (PCR) are the most sensitive diagnostic test available for pertussis. These methods have replaced microscopy and culture in most laboratories that offer laboratory testing. Currently no FDA-approved test is commercially available, so many laboratories have developed their own molecular assay targeting a variety of genes. For this reason, the performance characteristics of the assays (e.g., sensitivity, specificity) are not well defined but appear to be superior to microscopy and culture.

Culture

At the present time, culture is generally offered by laboratories unable to perform nucleic-acid-based assays or in conjunction with these assays. The sensitivity of culture is affected by patient factors (i.e., stage of illness, use of antibiotics), the quality of the specimen, transport conditions, and culture methods. The traditional use of **Bordet-Gengou** medium has been replaced by **Regan-Lowe charcoal medium** supplemented with glycerol, peptones, and horse blood. The media should be incubated in air at 35° C and in a humidified chamber. **Prolonged incubation** (e.g., 7 to 12 days) is necessary. Because the quality of the media dramatically affects the success of culture, laboratories that infrequently culture specimens for *Bordetella* should arrange for the state public health department to process these specimens. Despite use of optimized culture conditions, fewer than half the infected patients have positive cultures.

Identification

B. pertussis organisms are identified by their characteristic microscopic and colonial morphology on selective media and their reactivity with a specific antiserum (either in an agglutination reaction or with the reagents used in the direct fluorescent antibody test). Phenotypic reactions (e.g., biochemical testing) can be used to differentiate the *Bordetella* species.

Antibody Detection

It is difficult to interpret the results of serologic tests, because microscopy and culture techniques are relatively insensitive standards by which these test have been evaluated. Enzyme-linked immunosorbent assay (ELISA) tests have been developed to detect IgA, IgM, and IgG antibodies against pertussis toxin, filamentous hemagglutinin, pertactin, and fimbriae. Antibodies directed against pertussis toxin are specific for *B. pertussis;* however, antibodies to the other antigens may occur with infections caused by other *Bordetella* species and other bacteria.

Treatment, Prevention, and Control

The **treatment for pertussis is primarily supportive**, with nursing supervision during the paroxysmal and convalescent stages of the illness. Antibiotics can ameliorate the clinical course, but convalescence depends primarily on the rapidity and degree to which the layer of ciliated epithelial cells regenerates. **Macrolides** (i.e., erythromycin, azithromycin, clarithromycin) are effective in eradicating the organisms and can reduce the duration of infectivity; however, this effect has limited value because the illness is usually unrecognized during the peak of contagiousness. Strains resistant to erythromycin have been reported but are not widespread. Trimethoprim-sulfamethoxazole or fluoroquinolones can be used in patients unable to tolerate macrolides. The use of pertussis immunoglobulins may reduce the severity of disease in children, but clinical trials have not been performed.

In U.S. practice, whole-cell, inactivated vaccines for pertussis have been associated with unacceptable levels of complications and have been replaced with acellular vaccines. Two **acellular vaccines** (one for children, one for adults) administered in combination with vaccines for tetanus and diphtheria are currently approved in the United States. Both vaccines contain inactivated pertussis toxin, filamentous hemagglutinin, and pertactin. The pediatric vaccine is administered to children at the ages of 2 months, 4 months, 6 months, and 15 to 18 months, with the fifth dose given between the ages of 4 and 6 years. The current recommendations for the adult vaccine is to administer it at 11 or 12 years of age and then again between the ages of 19 and 65. Studies to measure humoral and cellular immunity to the pertussis antigens demonstrated detectable immunity in >90% of adolescent vaccine recipients more than 5 years after vaccination.

Because pertussis is highly contagious in a susceptible population, and unrecognized infections in family members of a symptomatic patient can maintain disease in a community, erythromycin has been used for prophylaxis in select instances.

Other *Bordetella* Species

B. parapertussis is responsible for causing 10% to 20% of the cases of mild pertussis occurring annually in the United States. *B. bronchiseptica* causes respiratory disease primarily in animals but has been associated with human respiratory tract colonization and bronchopulmonary disease. Investigators at the Centers for Disease Controls in Atlanta reported that *B. holmesii* is primarily associated with septicemia.

Case Study and Questions

A 5-year-old girl was brought to the local public health clinic because of a severe, intractable cough. During the previous 10 days, she had a persistent cold that had worsened. The cough developed the previous day and was so severe that vomiting frequently followed it. The child appeared exhausted from the coughing episodes. A blood cell count showed a marked leukocytosis with a predominance of lymphocytes. The examining physician suspected that the child had pertussis.

1. What laboratory tests can be performed to confirm the physician's clinical diagnosis? What specimens should be collected, and how should they be submitted to the laboratory?

2. What virulence factors are produced by *B. pertussis*, and what are their biologic effects? What is the natural progression and prognosis for this disease? How can it be prevented?

Reference to Student Consult Animation

Please visit *www.StudentConsult.com* to view an animation demonstrating the function of pertussis toxin.

Bibliography

Carbonetti N, et al: Pertussis toxin plays an early role in respiratory tract colonization by *Bordetella pertussis*. Infect Immun 71:6358-6366, 2003.

Cassiday P, et al: Polymorphism in *Bordetella pertussis* pertactin and pertussis toxin virulence factors in the United States, 1935-1999. J Infect Dis 182:1402-1408, 2000.

Cherry J: Immunity to pertussis. Clin Infect Dis 44:1278-1279, 2007.

Cherry J, Robbins J: Pertussis in adults: Epidemiology, signs, symptoms, and implications for vaccination. Clin Infect Dis 28(Suppl 2), 1999.

Edelman K, et al: Immunity to pertussis 5 years after booster immunization during adolescence. Clin Infect Dis 44:1271-1277, 2007.

Kirimanjeswara G, Mann P, Harvill E: Role of antibodies in immunity to *Bordetella infections*. Infect Immun 71:1719-1724, 2003.

Mattoo S, Cherry J: Molecular pathogenesis, epidemiology, and clinical manifestations of respiratory infections due to *Bordetella pertussis* and other *Bordetella* subspecies. Clin Microbiol Rev 18:326-382, 2005.

Preziosi M, Halloran M: Effects of pertussis vaccination on disease: Vaccine efficacy in reducing clinical severity. Clin Infect Dis 37:772-779, 2003.

Tilley P, et al: Detection of *Bordetella pertussis* in a clinical laboratory by culture, polymerase chain reaction, and direct fluorescent antibody staining: Accuracy and cost. Diagn Microbiol Infect Dis 37:17-23, 2000.

Ward J, et al: *Bordetella pertussis* infections in vaccinated and unvaccinated adolescents and adults, as assessed in a national prospective randomized acellular pertussis vaccine trial (APERT). Clin Infect Dis 43:151-157, 2006.

Weyant R, et al: *Bordetella holmesii* sp. nov., a new gram-negative species associated with septicemia. J Clin Microbiol 33:1-7, 1995.

Francisella and *Brucella*

Francisella and *Brucella* are important **zoonotic pathogens** that occasionally cause human disease (Box 36-1). These organisms have also gained notoriety as potential agents of bioterrorism. Although the organisms have some common properties (e.g., **very small coccobacilli**, fastidious and slow growth requirements, always pathogenic in humans), they are taxonomically unrelated. In the phylogenetic tree of bacterial life, the α-proteobacteria occupy one limb and the γ-proteobacteria another. **Brucella** is a member of the α-proteobacteria group (with organisms such as *Rickettsia, Ehrlichia, Bartonella,* and other genera), and **Francisella** is a member of the γ-proteobacteria group (with many genera, including *Legionella, Pasteurella,* and *Pseudomonas*).

Francisella tularensis (Box 36-2)

The genus *Francisella* consists of two species, *Francisella tularensis* and *Francisella philomiragia*. *F. tularensis* is the causative agent of **tularemia** (also called **glandular fever, rabbit fever, tick fever,** and **deer fly fever**) in animals and humans. *F. tularensis* is subdivided into four subspecies that are subdivided based on their biochemical properties. **Subspecies *tularensis* (type A)** and **subspecies *holarctica* (type B)** are the most important, while *F. tularensis* subsp. *mediasiatica* and subsp. *novicida* are rarely associated with human disease. *F. philomiragia* is also an uncommon opportunistic pathogen that is associated with exposure to salt water. It has a particular predilection for patients with immunologic deficiencies (i.e., chronic granulomatous disease, myeloproliferative diseases). Because this pathogen is rarely isolated, it will not be discussed further in this chapter.

Physiology and Structure

F. tularensis is a **very small** (0.2 × 0.2 to 0.7 μm), faintly staining, gram-negative coccobacillus (Figure 36-1). The organism is nonmotile, has a thin lipid capsule, and has fastidious growth requirements (i.e., most strains **require cysteine** for growth). It is **strictly aerobic** and requires 3 or more days before growth is detected in culture.

Pathogenesis and Immunity

F. tularensis is an **intracellular pathogen** that can survive for prolonged periods in macrophages of the reticuloendothelial system, because the organism inhibits phagosome-lysosome fusion. Pathogenic strains possess an antiphagocytic, **polysaccharide-rich capsule**, and loss of the capsule is associated with decreased virulence. The capsule protects the bacteria from complement-mediated killing during the bacteremia phase of disease. Like most gram-negative rods, this organism has endotoxin, but it is considerably less active than the endotoxin found in other gram-negative rods (e.g., *Escherichia coli*).

A strong, innate immune response with production of interferon-γ and tumor necrosis factor (TNF) are important for controlling bacterial replication in macrophages in the early phase of infection. Specific T-cell immunity is required for activation of macrophages for intracellular killing in the late stages of disease. B-cell mediated immunity is less important for elimination of this facultative intracellular pathogen.

Epidemiology

F. tularensis subsp. *tularensis* (type A) is restricted to North America, but subsp. *holarctica* (type B) is endemic throughout the Northern Hemisphere. Type A strains are further subdivided into **type A-west** that predominate in the arid region from the Rocky Mountains to the Sierra Nevada Mountains, and **type A-east** that occur in the central southeast states of Arkansas, Missouri, and Oklahoma and along the Atlantic Coast. **Type B** strains cluster along major waterways such as the upper Mississippi River and in areas with high rainfall such as the Pacific Northwest. The distribution of these strains is important because the epidemiologic features of the individual diseases is distinct,

Box 36—1. Important *Brucella* and *Francisella* Species

Organism	Historical Derivation
Brucella	Named after Sir David *Bruce*, who first recognized the organism as a cause of "undulant fever"
B. abortus	*abortus*, abortion or miscarriage (this organism is responsible for abortion in infected animals)
B. melitensis	*melitensis*, pertaining to the Island of Malta (*Melita*), where the first outbreak was recognized by Bruce
B. suis	*suis*, of the "pig" (a swine pathogen)
B. canis	*canis*, of the "dog" (a dog pathogen)
Francisella	Named after the American microbiologist Edward *Francis*, who first described tularemia
F. tularensis subsp. *tularensis* (type A)	*tularensis*, pertaining to *Tulare* County, California, where the disease was first described
F. tularensis subsp. *holarctica* (type B)	*holos*, "whole"; *arctos*, "northern regions" (reference to distribution in the arctic or northern regions)
F. tularensis subsp. *mediasiatica*	*media*, "middle"; *asiatica*, "Asian" (pertaining to middle Asia)
F. tularensis subsp. *novicida*	*novus*, "new"; *cida*, to "cut" (a "new killer")
F. philomiragia	*philos*, "loving"; *miragia*, "mirage" (loving of mirages, reference to presence in water)

and the course of clinical disease significantly different. The geographic distribution of type A-west, type A-east, and type B strains is defined by the distribution of the natural reservoirs and vectors of *F. tularensis*. More than 200 species of mammals, as well as birds and blood-sucking arthropods, are infected naturally with *F. tularensis*. Type A infections are most commonly associated with exposure to **lagomorphs** (rabbits, hares) and **cats**; type B infections are associated with **rodents** and cats, but not lagomorphs. Infections caused by **biting arthropods** (e.g., hard shell ticks [*Ixodes, Dermacentor, Amblyomma* spp.], deer flies) are more common with type A than with type B strains. The spread to type A-east strains from the central southeast states to the Atlantic Coast states occurred when infected rabbits were imported from the central states to East Coast hunting clubs in the 1920s and 1930s. Type A-east infections are more commonly associated with disseminated disease and a high mortality rate when compared with disease caused by type A-west strains; the course of disease caused by type B stains is intermediate.

Box 36—2. Summary: *Francisella tularensis*

Biology, Virulence, and Disease

Very small, gram-negative coccobacilli (0.2 × 0.2 to 0.7 μm)
Strict aerobe; nonfermenter
Requires specialized media and prolonged incubation for growth in culture
Antiphagocytic capsule
Intracellular pathogen resistant to killing in serum and by phagocytes
Clinical symptoms and prognosis determined by route of infection: ulceroglandular, oculoglandular, glandular, typhoidal, oropharyngeal, gastrointestinal, pneumonic (see Box 36-3)

Epidemiology

Wild mammals, domestic animals, birds, fish, and blood-sucking arthropods are reservoirs; rabbits, cats, hard ticks, and biting flies are most commonly associated with human disease; humans are accidental hosts
Worldwide distribution; most common in United States in Oklahoma, Missouri, and Arkansas
Approximately 100 cases seen in United States, although the actual number may be much higher
The infectious dose is small when exposure is by arthropod, through skin, or by inhalation; large numbers of organisms must be ingested for infection by this route

Diagnosis

Microscopy is insensitive
Culture on cysteine-supplemented media (e.g., chocolate agar, BCYE agar) is sensitive and specific if prolonged incubation is used
Serology can be used to confirm the clinical diagnosis; fourfold increase in titer or single titer >1:160; high titers can persist for months to years; cross-reactive with *Brucella*

Treatment, Prevention, and Control

Gentamicin is the antibiotic of choice; fluoroquinolones (e.g., ciprofloxacin) and doxycycline have good activity; penicillins and some cephalosporins are ineffective
Disease prevented by avoiding reservoirs and vectors of infection; clothing and gloves are protective
Live attenuated vaccine available but rarely used in human disease

Figure 36—1. Gram stain of *Francisella tularensis* isolated in culture; note that the extremely small coccobacilli look like fine sand.

The reported incidence of disease is low. In 2006, almost 100 cases were reported in the United States; however, the actual number of infections is likely to be much higher, because tularemia is frequently unsuspected and is difficult to confirm by laboratory tests. Most of the infections occur during summer (when exposure to infected ticks is greatest) and winter (when hunters are exposed to infected rabbits) months. The incidence of disease increases dramatically when a relatively warm winter is followed by a wet summer, causing the tick population to proliferate. People at greatest risk for infection are hunters, laboratory personnel, and those exposed to ticks and other biting arthropods. In areas where the organism is endemic, it is said that if a rabbit is moving so slowly that it can be shot by a hunter or caught by a pet, the rabbit could be infected.

Clinical Diseases (Box 36-3; Clinical Case 36-1)

Disease caused by *F. tularensis* is subdivided into several forms, based on the clinical presentation: **ulceroglandular** (cutaneous ulcer and swollen lymph node), **oculoglandular** (eye involvement and swollen cervical lymph nodes), glandular (primarily swollen lymph nodes with no other localized symptoms), **typhoidal** (systemic signs of sepsis), **pneumonic** (pulmonary symptoms), and **oropharyngeal** and **gastrointestinal** disease after ingestion of *F. tularensis*. Variations of these presentations are also common (e.g., pneumonic tularemia typically has systemic signs of sepsis).

Ulceroglandular tularemia is the most common manifestation. The skin lesion, which starts as a painful papule, develops at the site of the tick bite or direct inoculation of the organism into the skin (e.g., a laboratory accident).

Box 36—3. *Brucella* and *Francisella*: Clinical Summaries

Brucella

Brucellosis: initial nonspecific symptoms of malaise, chills, sweats, fatigue, myalgias, weight loss, arthralgias, and fever; can be intermittent (undulant fever); can progress to systemic involvement (gastrointestinal tract, bones or joints, respiratory tract, other organs)
Brucella melitensis: severe, acute disease with complications common
Brucella abortus: mild disease with suppurative complications
Brucella suis: chronic, suppurative, destructive disease
Brucella canis: mild disease with suppurative complications

Francisella

Ulceroglandular tularemia: painful papule develops at site of inoculation and progresses to ulceration; localized lymphadenopathy
Oculoglandular tularemia: following inoculation into the eye (e.g., rubbing eye with a contaminated finger), painful conjunctivitis develops, with regional lymphadenopathy
Pneumonic tularemia: pneumonitis with signs of sepsis develops rapidly after exposure to contaminated aerosols; high mortality unless promptly diagnosed and treated

---

Clinical Case 36-1. Cat-Associated Tularemia

Capellan and Fong (Clin Infect Dis 16:472-475, 1993) described a 63-year-old man who developed ulceroglandular tularemia complicated by pneumonia after a cat bite. He initially presented with pain and localized swelling of his thumb 5 days after the bite. Oral penicillins were prescribed, but the patient's condition worsened, with increased local pain, swelling, and erythema at the wound site and systemic signs (fever, malaise, vomiting). Incision of the wound was performed, but no abscess was found; culture of the wound was positive for a light growth of coagulase-negative staphylococci. Intravenous penicillins were prescribed, but the patient continued to deteriorate, with the development of tender axillary lymphadenopathy and pulmonary symptoms. Chest radiograph revealed pneumonic infiltrates in the right middle and lower lobes of the lung. The patient's therapy was changed to clindamycin and gentamicin, which was followed by defervescence and improvement of his clinical status. After 3 days of incubation, tiny colonies of faintly staining gram-negative coccobacilli were observed on the original wound culture. The organism was referred to a national reference lab, where it was identified as *F. tularensis*. A more complete history revealed the patient's cat lived outdoors and fed on wild rodents. This case illustrates the difficulty in making the diagnosis of tularemia and the lack of responsiveness to penicillins.

The papule then ulcerates and has a necrotic center and raised border. Localized lymphadenopathy and bacteremia are also typically present (although bacteremia may be difficult to document).

Oculoglandular tularemia (Figure 36-2) is a specialized form of the disease and results from direct contamination of the eye. The organism can be introduced into the eyes, for example, by contaminated fingers or through exposure to water or aerosols. Affected patients have a painful conjunctivitis and regional lymphadenopathy.

Pneumonic tularemia (Figure 36-3) results from inhalation of infectious aerosols and is associated with high morbidity and mortality unless the organism is recovered rapidly in blood cultures (it is generally difficult to detect in respiratory cultures). There is also concern that *F. tularensis* could be used as a biologic weapon. As such, creation of an infectious aerosol would be the most likely method of dispersal.

Figure 36—2. Patient with oculoglandular tularemia.

Figure 36—3. Chest radiograph of patient with pulmonary tularemia.

Laboratory Diagnosis

Specimen Collection

The collection and processing of specimens for the isolation of *F. tularensis* are hazardous for both the physician and the laboratory worker. The organism, by virtue of its small size, can penetrate through unbroken skin and mucous membranes during collection of the sample, or it can be inhaled if aerosols are produced (a particular concern during processing of specimens in the laboratory). Although tularemia is rare, laboratory-acquired infections are disproportionately common. Gloves should be worn during collection of the specimen (e.g., aspiration of an ulcer or lymph node), and all laboratory work (both initial processing and identification tests) should be performed in a biohazard hood.

Microscopy

Detection of *F. tularensis* in Gram-stained aspirates from infected nodes or ulcers is almost always **unsuccessful**, because the organism is extremely small and stains faintly (see Figure 36-1). A more sensitive and specific approach is direct staining of the clinical specimen with fluorescein-labeled antibodies directed against the organism. Antibody reagents against types A and B are available from the Centers for Disease Control and Prevention (CDC) and state public health facilities but are not available in most clinical laboratories.

Nucleic-Acid-Based Tests

Polymerase chain reaction (PCR)-based assays are under development but are not widely available at this time. This may change rapidly with the increased interest in the development of diagnostic tests for this organism in the event of a bioterrorist attack.

Culture

It has been stated that *F. tularensis* cannot be reliably recovered on common laboratory media because the organism requires sulfhydryl-containing substances (e.g., **cysteine**) for growth. However, *F. tularensis* can grow on **chocolate agar** or **buffered charcoal yeast extract** (**BCYE**) agar, media supplemented with cysteine that are used in most laboratories. Thus it is usually not necessary for a laboratory to use specialized media such as cysteine blood agar or glucose cysteine agar. However, if infection with *F. tularensis* is suspected, the laboratory should be notified, because *F. tularensis* grows slowly and may be overlooked if the cultures are not incubated for a prolonged period. Additionally, because this organism is highly infectious, special care is required for microbiologic testing. Blood cultures are generally negative for the organism unless the cultures are incubated for a week or longer. Cultures of respiratory specimens will be positive if appropriate selective media are used to suppress the more rapidly growing bacteria from the upper respiratory tract. *F. tularensis* also grows on the selective media used for *Legionella* (e.g., BCYE agar). Aspirates of lymph nodes or draining sinuses are usually positive if the cultures are incubated for 3 days or longer.

Identification

Preliminary identification of *F. tularensis* is based on the slow growth of very small gram-negative coccobacilli. Growth on chocolate agar but not blood agar (blood agar is not supplemented with cysteine) is also helpful. The identification is confirmed by demonstrating the reactivity of the bacteria with specific antiserum (i.e., agglutination of the organism with antibodies against *Francisella*). Further biochemical testing is not helpful and can be hazardous.

Antibody Detection

Tularemia is diagnosed in most patients by the finding of a fourfold or greater increase in the titer of antibodies during the illness or a single titer of 1:160 or greater. However, antibodies (including IgG, IgM, and IgA) can persist for many years, making it difficult to differentiate between past and current disease. Reagents that are currently available react with subspecies *tularensis* and *holarctica* but not the other subspecies or *F. philomiragia*. Antibodies directed against *Brucella* can cross-react with *Francisella*. Therefore the diagnosis of tularemia should not be based solely on serologic tests.

Treatment, Prevention, and Control

Streptomycin was the traditional antibiotic of choice for the treatment of all forms of tularemia; however, this antibiotic is not readily available and is associated with a high level of toxicity. **Gentamicin** is now considered the antibiotic of choice. The **fluoroquinolones** (e.g., ciprofloxacin) have good bactericidal activity in vitro and in a mouse animal model. Doxycycline is also bactericidal in the mouse model. *F. tularensis* strains produce β-lactamase, which renders penicillins and cephalosporins ineffective. The mortality rate is less than

1% if patients are treated promptly but is much higher in untreated patients, particularly those infected with type A-east strains.

To prevent infection, people should avoid the reservoirs and vectors of infection (e.g., rabbits, ticks, biting insects), but this is often difficult. At a minimum, people should not handle ill-appearing rabbits and should wear gloves when skinning and eviscerating animals. Because the organism is present in the arthropod's feces and not saliva, the tick must feed for a prolonged time before the infection is transmitted. Prompt removal of the tick can therefore prevent infection. Wearing protective clothing and using insect repellents reduce the risk of exposure. Persons who have a high risk of exposure (e.g., exposure to an infectious aerosol) should be treated with prophylactic antibiotics. Live attenuated vaccines are not completely effective in preventing disease but can lessen the severity of the disease. These are recommended for people at a significantly increased risk of exposure to the organism. Inactivated vaccines do not elicit protective cellular immunity.

Brucella (Box 36-4)

Molecular studies of the genus *Brucella* demonstrate a close relationship among the strains and are consistent with a single genus; however, the genus has historically been subdivided into a number of species. Currently, there are six species of *Brucella*, with four species associated with human disease: **Brucella abortus, Brucella melitensis, Brucella suis,** and **Brucella canis** (see Box 36-1). The diseases caused by members of this genus are characterized by a number of names, based on the original microbiologists who isolated and described the organisms (e.g., Sir David Bruce [**brucellosis**], Bernhard Bang [**Bang's disease**]), clinical presentation (**undulant fever**), and the sites of recognized outbreaks (e.g., Malta fever, Mediterranean remittent fever, rock fever of Gibraltar, county fever of Constantinople, fever of Crete). However, the most commonly used term is **brucellosis**, which will be used in this chapter.

Physiology and Structure

Brucellae are small (0.5×0.6 to 1.5 µm), nonmotile, non-encapsulated, gram-negative coccobacilli. The organism grows slowly in culture (taking a week or more) and generally requires complex growth media; is strictly aerobic, with some strains requiring supplemental carbon dioxide for growth; and does not ferment carbohydrates.

Colonies can assume both smooth (translucent, homogeneous) and rough (opaque, granular, or sticky) forms, as determined by the O antigen of the cell wall lipopolysaccharide (LPS). Antisera to one form (e.g., smooth) do not cross-react with the other form (e.g., rough). *Brucella* species can be further characterized by the relative proportion of antigenic epitopes, referred to as **A antigens** and **M antigens** that reside on the O polysaccharide chain of the smooth LPS.

Box 36—4. Summary: *Brucella*

Biology, Virulence, and Disease

Very small, gram-negative coccobacilli (0.5×0.6 to 1.5 µm)
Strict aerobe; nonfermenter
Requires complex media and prolonged incubation for in vitro growth
Intracellular pathogen that is resistant to killing in serum and by phagocytes
Smooth colonies associated with virulence
Refer to Box 36-3 for diseases

Epidemiology

Animal reservoirs are goats and sheep (*Brucella melitensis*); cattle and American bison (*Brucella abortus*); swine, reindeer, and caribou (*Brucella suis*); and dogs, foxes, and coyotes (*Brucella canis*)
Infects animal tissues rich in erythritol (e.g., breast, uterus, placenta, epididymis)
Worldwide distribution, particularly in Latin America, Africa, the Mediterranean basin, Middle East, and Western Asia
Vaccination of herds has controlled disease in the United States
Most disease in the United States is reported in California and Texas in travelers from Mexico
Individuals at greatest risk for disease are people who consume unpasteurized dairy products, people in direct contact with infected animals, and laboratory workers

Diagnosis

Microscopy is insensitive
Culture (blood, bone marrow, infected tissue if localized infection) is sensitive and specific if prolonged incubation is used (minimum of 3 days to 2 weeks)
Serology can be used to confirm the clinical diagnosis; fourfold increase in titer or single titer >1:160; high titers can persist for months to years; cross-reactive with other bacteria

Treatment, Prevention, and Control

Recommended treatment is doxycycline combined with rifampin for a minimum of 6 weeks for nonpregnant adults; trimethoprim-sulfamethoxazole for pregnant women and for children younger than 8 years
Human disease is controlled by eradication of the disease in the animal reservoir through vaccination and serologic monitoring of the animals for evidence of disease; pasteurization of dairy products; and use of proper safety techniques in clinical laboratories working with this organism

Pathogenesis and Immunity

Brucella does not produce a detectable exotoxin, and the endotoxin is less toxic than that produced by other gram-negative rods. Reversion of smooth strains to the rough morphology is associated with greatly reduced virulence, so the O chain of the smooth LPS is an important marker for virulence. *Brucella* is also an **intracellular parasite** of the **reticuloendothelial system**. After initial exposure, the organisms are phagocytosed by macrophages and monocytes. Brucellae survive and replicate in phagocytic cells by inhibiting phagolysosome fusion, preventing release of toxic enzymes from intracellular granules, suppressing production of TNF-α, and inactivating hydrogen peroxide and superoxide by production of catalase and superoxide dismutase. Phagocytosed bacteria are carried to the spleen, liver, bone marrow, lymph nodes, and kidneys. The bacteria secrete proteins that induce granuloma formation in these organs and destructive changes in these and other tissues occur in patients with advanced disease.

Epidemiology

Brucella infections have a **worldwide distribution**, with endemic disease most common in Latin America, Africa, the Mediterranean basin, the Middle East, and Western Asia. More than 500,000 documented cases are reported annually worldwide. In contrast, the incidence of disease in the United States is much lower (121 reported infections in 2006). The highest number of U.S. cases are reported in **California** and **Texas**, and most of these infections occur in residents from Mexico or visitors to that country. Laboratory personnel are also at significant risk for infection through direct contact or inhalation of the organism. Disease in cattle, swine, sheep, and goats in the United States has been effectively eliminated through the destruction of infected animals and the vaccination of domestic animals; thus infections in veterinarians, slaughterhouse workers, and farmers are much less common than before 1980.

Brucellosis in humans can be acquired by direct contact with the organism (e.g., a laboratory exposure), ingestion (e.g., consumption of contaminated food products), or inhalation. Of particular concern is the potential use of *Brucella* as a biologic weapon, in which exposure would most likely be by inhalation.

Brucella causes mild or asymptomatic disease in the natural host: *B. abortus* infects cattle and American bison; *B. melitensis*, goats and sheep; *B. suis*, swine, reindeer, and caribou; and *B. canis*, dogs, foxes, and coyotes. The organism has a predilection for infecting organs rich in **erythritol**, a sugar metabolized by many *Brucella* strains in preference to glucose. Animal (but not human) tissues, including breast, uterus, placenta, and epididymis, are rich in erythritol. The organisms thus localize in these tissues in nonhuman reservoirs and can cause sterility, abortions, or asymptomatic lifelong carriage. Brucellae are shed in high numbers in milk, urine, and birth products. Human disease in the United States is most commonly caused by **B. melitensis** and results primarily from consumption of contaminated unpasteurized milk and other **dairy products**.

Clinical Diseases (See Box 36-3; Clinical Case 36-2)

The disease spectrum of brucellosis depends on the infecting organism. *B. abortus* and *B. canis* tend to produce mild

---

Clinical Case 36-2. Brucellosis

Lee and Fung (Hong Kong Med J 11:403-406, 2005) described a 34-year-old woman who developed brucellosis caused by *Brucella melitensis*. The woman presented with recurrent headaches, fever, and malaise that developed after she had handled goat placenta in China. Blood cultures were positive for *B. melitensis* after extended incubation. She was treated for 6 weeks with doxycycline and rifampicin and had a successful response. The case was a classic description of exposure to contaminated tissues high in erythritol, a presentation of recurrent fevers and headaches, and response to the combination of doxycycline and rifampicin.

---

disease with rare suppurative complications. In contrast, *B. suis* causes the formation of destructive lesions and has a prolonged course. *B. melitensis* also causes severe disease with a high incidence of serious complications, because the organisms can multiply to high concentrations in phagocytic cells.

Acute disease develops in approximately half of the patients infected with *Brucella*, with symptoms typically first appearing 1 to 3 weeks after exposure. Initial symptoms are nonspecific and consist of malaise, chills, sweats, fatigue, weakness, myalgias, weight loss, arthralgias, and nonproductive cough. Almost all patients have fever, and this can be intermittent in untreated patients, hence the name **undulant fever**. Patients with advanced disease can have gastrointestinal tract symptoms (70% of patients), osteolytic lesions or joint effusions (20% to 60%), respiratory tract symptoms (25%), and less commonly, cutaneous, neurologic, or cardiovascular manifestations. Chronic infections can also develop in inadequately treated patients, with symptoms developing within 3 to 6 months after discontinuing antibiotic therapy. Relapses are associated with a persistent focus on infections (e.g., in bone, spleen, liver) and not with the development of antibiotic resistance.

Laboratory Diagnosis

Specimen Collection

Several blood samples should be collected for culture and serologic testing. Bone marrow cultures and cultures of infected tissues may also be useful. To ensure safe handling of the specimen, the laboratory should be notified if brucellosis is suspected.

Microscopy

Brucella organisms are readily stained using conventional techniques, but their intracellular location and small size make them difficult to detect in clinical specimens. Currently, specific immunofluorescent antibody tests are not available.

Culture

Brucella organisms grow slowly during primary isolation. The organisms can grow on most enriched blood agars and occasionally on MacConkey agar; however, incubation for 3 or more days may be required. **Blood cultures should be incubated for 2 weeks** before they are considered negative. More extended incubation of blood cultures is now unnecessary with the use of automated culture systems.

Identification

Preliminary identification of *Brucella* is based on the isolate's microscopic and colonial morphology, positive oxidase and urease reactions, and reactivity with antibodies directed against *B. abortus* and *B. melitensis*. *B. melitensis*, *B. abortus*, and *B. suis* will react with antisera prepared against *B. abortus* or *B. melitensis* (illustrating the close relationship among these species). In contrast, *B. canis* is not reactive with either antisera. Identification at the genus level can also be accomplished by sequencing the 16S ribosomal ribonucleic acid (rRNA) gene. Because brucellosis is uncommon in the United States, most laboratories refer the organism to a state public health laboratory for definitive identification.

Antibody Detection

Subclinical brucellosis and many cases of acute and chronic diseases are identified by a specific antibody response in the infected patient. Antibodies are detected in virtually all patients. Immunoglobulin M (IgM) response is initially observed, after which both IgG and IgA antibodies are produced. Antibodies can persist for many months or years; thus a significant increase in the antibody titer is required to provide definitive serologic evidence of current disease. A **presumptive diagnosis** can be made if there is a fourfold increase in the titer or a single titer is greater than or equal to 1:160. High antibody titers (1:160 or more) are noted in 5% to 10% of the population living in endemic areas; thus serologic tests should be used to confirm the clinical diagnosis of brucellosis and not to form the basis of the diagnosis. The antigen used in the *Brucella* serum agglutination test (SAT) is from *B. abortus*. Antibodies directed against *B. melitensis* or *B. suis* cross-react with this antigen; however, there is no cross-reactivity with *B. canis*. The specific *B. canis* antigen must be used to diagnose infections with this organism. Antibodies directed against other genera of bacteria (e.g., some strains of *Escherichia*, *Salmonella*, *Vibrio*, *Yersinia*, *Stenotrophomonas*, and *Francisella*) are also reported to cross-react with the *B. abortus* antigen.

Treatment, Prevention, and Control

Tetracyclines, with **doxycycline** the preferred agent, are generally active against most strains of *Brucella*; however, because this is a bacteriostatic drug, relapse is common after an initially successful response. The World Health Organization currently recommends the combination of **doxycycline with rifampin**. Because the tetracyclines are toxic to young children and fetuses, doxycycline should be replaced with trimethoprim-sulfamethoxazole for pregnant women and for children younger than 8 years.

Treatment must be continued for 6 weeks or longer for it to be successful. Fluoroquinolones, macrolides, penicillins, and cephalosporins are either ineffective or have unpredictable activity. Relapse of disease is caused by inadequate therapy and not the development of antibiotic resistance.

Control of human brucellosis is accomplished through control of the disease in livestock, as demonstrated in the United States. This requires systematic identification (by serologic testing) and elimination of infected herds and **animal vaccination** (currently with the rough strain of *B. abortus* strain RB51). The avoidance of unpasteurized dairy products, the observance of appropriate safety procedures in the clinical laboratory, and the wearing of protective clothing by abattoir workers are further ways to prevent brucellosis. The live attenuated *B. abortus* and *B. melitensis* vaccines have been used successfully to prevent infection in animal herds. Vaccines have not been developed against *B. suis* or *B. canis*, and the existing vaccines cannot be used in humans because they produce symptomatic disease. The lack of an effective human vaccine is of concern, because *Brucella* (as well as *Francisella*) could be used as an agent of bioterrorism.

Case Study and Questions

A 27-year-old man was mowing his field when he ran over two young rabbits. When he stopped his mower, he realized that two other rabbits were dead in the unmowed part of the lawn. He removed all the rabbits and buried them. Three days later, he developed a fever, muscle aches, and a dry, nonproductive cough. Over the next 12 hours, he got progressively sicker and was transported by his wife to the area hospital. Results of a chest x-ray showed infiltrates in both lung fields. Blood cultures and respiratory secretions were collected, and antibiotics were initiated. Blood cultures became positive with small gram-negative rods after 3 days of incubation, and the same organism grew from the respiratory specimen that was inoculated onto BCYE agar.

1. What test should be performed to confirm the tentative diagnosis of *Francisella tularensis*?

2. This infection was presumably acquired by inhalation of aerosolized contaminated blood. What are the most common sources of *F. tularensis* infections and the most common routes of exposure?

3. What are the different clinical manifestations of *F. tularensis*?

Bibliography

Boschiroli M, et al: Brucellosis: A worldwide zoonosis. Curr Opin Microbiol 4:58-64, 2001.

Dennis D, et al: Tularemia as a biological weapon: Medical and public health management. J Am Med Assoc 285:2763-2773, 2001.

Farlow J, et al: *Francisella tularensis* in the United States. Emerg Infect Dis 12:1835-1841, 2005.

Feldman K, et al: Outbreak of primary pneumonic tularemia on Martha's Vineyard. N Engl J Med 345:1601-1606, 2001.

Pappas G, et al: Brucellosis. N Engl J Med 352:2325-2336, 2005.

Staples J, et al: Epidemiologic and molecular analysis of human tularemia, United States, 1964-2004. Emerg Infect Dis 12:1113-1118, 2006.

Legionella

In the summer of 1976, public attention was focused on an outbreak of severe pneumonia that caused many deaths in American Legion members attending a convention in Philadelphia. After months of intensive investigations, a previously unknown gram-negative rod was isolated. Subsequent studies found this organism, named *Legionella pneumophila*, to be the cause of multiple epidemics and sporadic infections. The organism was not previously recognized, because it stains poorly with conventional dyes and does not grow on common laboratory media. Despite the initial problems with the isolation of *Legionella* organisms, it is now known to be a ubiquitous aquatic saprophyte.

Legionellaceae

Taxonomic studies have shown that the family Legionellaceae consists of one genus, *Legionella*, with 50 species. Approximately half of these species have been implicated in human disease, with the others found in environmental sources. *L. pneumophila* is the cause of 90% of all infections; serotypes 1 and 6 are most commonly isolated (Figure 37-1).

Physiology and Structure

Members of the genus *Legionella* are **slender, pleomorphic, gram-negative rods** measuring 0.3 to 0.9 × 2 μm (Box 37-1). The organisms characteristically appear as short coccobacilli when observed in tissue but are very pleomorphic (up to 20 μm long) on artificial media (Figure 7-2). Legionellae in clinical specimens do not stain with common reagents but can be seen in tissues stained with Dieterle silver stain. One species, *Legionella micdadei*, can also be stained with weak acid-fast stains, but the organism loses this property when grown in vitro.

Legionellae are obligate aerobes and nutritionally fastidious. They require media supplemented with L-cysteine and iron for primary isolation. Growth of these bacteria on supplemented media but not on conventional blood agar media has been used as the basis for the preliminary identification of clinical isolates. The bacteria have developed multiple methods to acquire iron from their host cells or in vitro media, and loss of this ability is associated with loss of virulence. The organisms are nonfermentative and derive energy from the metabolism of amino acids.

Pathogenesis and Immunity

Respiratory tract disease caused by *Legionella* species develops in susceptible people who inhale infectious aerosols. Legionellae are facultative **intracellular parasites** that multiply in free-living amoebae in nature and in alveolar macrophages, monocytes, and alveolar epithelial cells in infected hosts. This ability to infect and replicate in macrophages is critical for pathogenesis. The replicative cycle is initiated by binding complement to an outer membrane porin protein and depositing complement component C3b on the bacterial surface. The bacteria bind to the CR3 complement receptors on mononuclear phagocytes, after which the organisms penetrate the cell through endocytosis. The bacteria are not killed in the cells by exposure to toxic superoxide, hydrogen peroxide, and hydroxyl radicals, because **phagolysosome fusion is inhibited**. Chemokines and cytokines released by the infected macrophages stimulate a severe inflammatory response, characteristic of infections with *Legionella*. The organisms proliferate in their intracellular vacuole and produce proteolytic enzymes, phosphatase, lipase, and nuclease that eventually kill the host cell when the vacuole is lysed. Immunity to disease is primarily cell mediated, with humoral immunity playing a minor role. The bacteria are not killed until sensitized helper T cells (TH1 cells) activate the parasitized macrophages. Production of interferon-γ (IFN-γ) is critical for elimination of *Legionella* organisms.

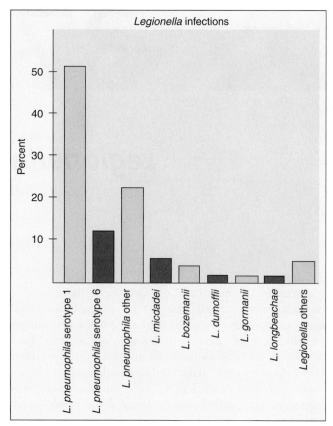

Figure 37–1. *Legionella* species associated with human disease.

Figure 37–2. Gram stain of *Legionella pneumophila* grown on buffered charcoal yeast extract agar. Note the pleomorphic forms characteristic of *Legionella*. *(Courtesy Dr. Janet Stout; Pittsburgh, Pennsylvania.)*

Epidemiology

Sporadic and epidemic legionellosis has a **worldwide distribution**. The bacteria are commonly present in natural bodies of water such as lakes and streams, as well as in air conditioning cooling towers and condensers and in water systems (e.g., showers, hot tubs). Human infections are most commonly associated with **exposure to contaminated aerosols** (e.g., air conditioning cooling towers,

---

Box 37–1. Summary: *Legionella*

Biology, Virulence, and Disease

Slender, pleomorphic, nonfermentative, gram-negative rods
Stains poorly with common reagents
Nutritionally fastidious with requirement for L-cysteine and enhanced growth with iron salts
Capable of replication in alveolar macrophages (and amoebae in nature)
Prevents phagolysosome fusion
Responsible for legionnaires disease and Pontiac fever

Epidemiology

Capable of sporadic, epidemic, and nosocomial infections
Commonly found in natural bodies of water, cooling towers, condensers, and water systems (including hospital systems)
Estimated to be between 10,000 and 20,000 cases of infection in United States annually
Patients at high risk for symptomatic disease include patients with compromised pulmonary function and patients with decreased cellular immunity (particularly transplant patients)

Diagnosis

Microscopy is insensitive
Antigen tests are sensitive for *L. pneumophila* serogroup 1 but have poor sensitivity for other serogroups and species
Culture on buffered charcoal yeast extract (BCYE) agar is the diagnostic test of choice
Seroconversion must be demonstrated; this can take as long as 6 months to develop; positive serology may persist for months
Nucleic acid amplification assays are as sensitive and specific as culture

Treatment, Control, and Prevention

Newer macrolides (e.g., azithromycin, clarithromycin) or fluoroquinolones (e.g., ciprofloxacin, levofloxacin) are the treatment of choice
Decrease environmental exposure to reduce risk of disease
For environmental sources associated with disease, treat with hyperchlorination, superheating, or copper-silver ionization

whirlpool spas, shower heads, or water misters). The organisms can survive in moist environments for a long time, at relatively high temperatures, and in the presence of disinfectants such as chlorine. One reason for their survival is that the bacteria can parasitize amoebae in the water and replicate in this protected environment (similar to their replication in human macrophages). The bacteria also survive in biofilms that develop in the pipes of water systems.

The incidence of infections caused by *Legionella* species is unknown because disease is difficult to document. The number of reported cases has steadily risen since the year 2000, with 2834 cases reported in 2006. However, the Centers for Disease Control and Prevention (CDC) estimate that between 10,000 and 20,000 cases of legionnaires disease occur each year in the United States. Serologic studies have also shown that a significant proportion of the population has acquired immunity to this group of organisms. It is reasonable to conclude that contact with the organism and acquisition of immunity after an asymptomatic infection are common.

Although sporadic outbreaks of the disease occur throughout the year, most epidemics of the infection occur in late summer and autumn, presumably because the organism proliferates in water reservoirs during the warm months. More than 80% of the documented infections in the United States are in individuals 40 years of age or older, presumably because they are more likely to have decreased cellular immunity and compromised pulmonary function. Almost 25% of reported cases are acquired in hospitals because of the predominance of high-risk patients. Person-to-person spread or an animal reservoir has not been demonstrated.

Clinical Diseases

Asymptomatic *Legionella* infections are believed to be relatively common. Symptomatic infections primarily affect the lungs and present in one of two forms (Table 37-1): (1) an influenza-like illness (referred to as **Pontiac fever**) and (2) a severe form of pneumonia (i.e., **legionnaires disease**).

Pontiac Fever

L. pneumophila was responsible for causing a self-limited, febrile illness in people working at the Pontiac, Michigan, Public Health Department in 1968. Fever, chills, myalgia, malaise, and headache, without clinical evidence of pneumonia, are characteristic of the disease. The symptoms developed over 12 hours, persisted for 2 to 5 days, and then resolved spontaneously without antibiotic treatment and with minimal morbidity and no deaths. Other outbreaks of Pontiac fever, with and without *Legionella* pneumonia, have been reported. The precise pathogenesis of this syndrome is unknown, although it is believed that the pathology of this disease is caused by a hypersensitivity reaction to bacterial toxin (e.g., endotoxin).

Table 37–1. Comparison of Diseases Caused by *Legionella*

	Legionnaires Disease	Pontiac Fever
Epidemiology		
Presentation	Epidemic, sporadic	Epidemic
Attack rate (%)	<5	>90
Person-to-person spread	No	No
Underlying pulmonary disease	Yes	No
Time of onset	Epidemic disease in late summer or autumn; endemic disease throughout year	Throughout year
Clinical Manifestations		
Incubation period (days)	2-10	1-2
Pneumonia	Yes	No
Course	Requires antibiotic therapy	Self-limited
Mortality (%)	15-20; higher if diagnosis is delayed	<1

Legionnaires Disease (Clinical Case 37-1)

Legionnaires disease (legionellosis) is characteristically more severe than Pontiac fever and if untreated, promptly causes considerable morbidity, often leading to death in 15% of previously healthy individuals and up to 75% in

Clinical Case 37-1. Outbreak of Legionnaires Disease

Kirrage, et al. (Respir Med, 101:1639, 2007) described an outbreak of legionnaires disease (LD) that occurred in Hereford, England. On Oct 24, 2007, the public health agency was notified that an elderly man had died of LD. Three days later, the agency was notified that an elderly woman had also died of LD. As part of an active surveillance investigation, two additional patients with positive *Legionella* urine antigen tests were identified in a local hospital. Further investigations revealed 28 epidemiologically linked patients, with the onset of disease from October 8 to November 20. All patients had positive urine antigen tests, four had high antibody titers, and two were culture positive. The implicated source of the outbreak was a cooling tower that had recently been restarted after a period of inactivity. After the tower was closed and recleaned, the epidemic was terminated. This outbreak illustrates the difficulty of recognizing the problem when the individuals infected may present to different hospitals. This is particularly a problem when the source is located in a hotel or vacation place.

immunocompromised patients. After an incubation period of 2 to 10 days, systemic signs of an acute illness appear abruptly (e.g., fever and chills, a dry, nonproductive cough, headache). Multiorgan disease involving the gastrointestinal tract, central nervous system, liver, and kidneys is common. The primary manifestation is pneumonia with multilobar consolidation, evident on x-ray, and inflammation and microabscesses in lung tissue observed on histopathologic studies. Pulmonary function steadily deteriorates in susceptible patients with untreated disease. The clinical presentation of pneumonia caused by *Legionella* is not unique, so laboratory tests are required to confirm the diagnosis.

Laboratory Diagnosis

Since *Legionella* was first isolated, the laboratory diagnosis of infections caused by this organism has undergone a significant transition. Initial testing depended on microscopy, culture, and serology. Although culture remains the gold standard for diagnosis, microscopy and serology have been replaced by immunoassays for the detection of *Legionella*-specific antigens in urine and nucleic acid amplification assays.

Microscopy

Legionellae in clinical specimens **stain poorly** with Gram stain and the small, intracellular bacteria are rarely recognized. The organism will stain with nonspecific methods, such as Dieterle silver stain, but this stain is used with tissue specimens and not sputum. The most sensitive way of detecting legionellae microscopically in clinical specimens is to use the **direct fluorescent antibody (DFA)** test, in which fluorescein-labeled monoclonal or polyclonal antibodies directed against *Legionella* species are used. Tests using monoclonal reagents are specific; however, false-positive reactions are common with the polyclonal reagents. Unfortunately the sensitivity of the DFA test is low (reported to range from 25% to 75%), because (1) the antibody preparations are serotype- or species-specific and (2) many organisms must be present for detection. The latter problem is a result of the relatively small size and predominantly intracellular location of the bacteria. Because of the problems with the DFA test, antigen detection tests are now used in most laboratories.

Urinary Antigen Tests

Immunoassays are used to detect soluble ***Legionella* serogroup 1–specific lipopolysaccharide antigens** excreted in the urine of infected patients. The sensitivity of these assays for *L. pneumophila* serogroup 1 is relatively high (range, 60% to 90%), particularly with concentrated urines, but the assays cannot be used to detect other serogroups or *Legionella* species. This is an important distinction because *L. pneumophila* serogroup 1 is responsible for 80% to 90% of community-acquired infections but is responsible for fewer

than 50% of hospital-acquired infections. Antigens persist in the urine of treated patients, with almost 50% of patients remaining positive at 1 month and 25% at 2 months. Persistence is particularly common with immunosuppressed patients, in whom antigens can persist for up to 1 year.

Nucleic Acid Amplification Assays

Nucleic acid amplification (NAA) assays are highly specific and have a sensitivity equivalent to culture for the detection of *Legionella* species in respiratory secretions (i.e., bronchial alveolar lavage [BAL] fluid). Although these assays are not widely available, it is anticipated that they will be the diagnostic method of choice in the future. The presence of inhibitors in respiratory secretions may cause false-negative reactions, so all specimens should still be cultured. Additionally, culture has been demonstrated to be more sensitive than NAA assays for tissue specimens.

Culture

Although legionellae were difficult to grow initially, commercially available media now make culture easy (test sensitivity 80% to >90%). As mentioned above, legionellae require L-cysteine and iron salts (supplied in hemoglobin or ferric pyrophosphate) for primary isolation. The medium most commonly used for the isolation of legionellae is **buffered charcoal yeast extract (BCYE) agar**, although other supplemented media have been used. Antibiotics can be added to suppress the growth of rapidly growing, contaminating bacteria. Legionellae grow in air or 3% to 5% carbon dioxide at 35° C after 3 to 5 days. The small (1 to 3 mm) colonies have a characteristic ground-glass appearance.

Identification

It is easy to identify an isolate as *Legionella* from the findings of typical morphology and specific growth requirements. Legionellae appear as weakly staining, pleomorphic, thin, gram-negative rods. Their growth on BCYE agar but not on media without L-cysteine is presumptive evidence that the organism is *Legionella*. Specific staining with fluorescein-labeled antibodies can confirm the identity of the organisms. In contrast to the identification of the genus, species classification is problematic and generally relegated to reference laboratories. Although biochemical tests and the ability of rods to fluoresce under long-wave ultraviolet light are useful for differentiating species, the species can be identified definitively only through analysis of the major branched-chain fatty acids in the cell wall and sequencing species-specific gene targets.

Antibody Detection

Legionellosis caused by *L. pneumophila* serogroup 1 is commonly diagnosed with the use of enzyme immunoassays (EIA) or indirect fluorescent antibody (IFA) tests to measure a serologic response to infection. A fourfold or greater increase in the antibody titer (to a level of 1:128 or greater) is considered diagnostic. However, these tests are relatively insensitive and nonspecific, particularly when polyclonal reagents are used. The response may be delayed. Although a significant increase in the titer can be detected in 25% to 40% of patients in the first week of disease, up to 6 months may be required before seroconversion is demonstrated for the remaining patients. Because high titers can persist for prolonged periods, a single, high-antibody ctiter cannot be used to define active disease.

Treatment, Prevention, and Control

In vitro susceptibility tests are not performed with legionellae, because the organisms grow poorly on the media commonly used for these tests. Additionally, some antibiotics that appear active in vitro are ineffective in treating infections. One explanation is that these antibiotics cannot penetrate the macrophages where the legionellae survive and multiply. Accumulated clinical experience indicates that **macrolides** (e.g., azithromycin, clarithromycin) or **fluoroquinolones** (e.g., ciprofloxacin, levofloxacin) should be used to treat *Legionella* infections. Newer macrolide antibiotics have replaced erythromycin. β-Lactam antibiotics are ineffective because most isolates produce β-lactamases, and these antibiotics do not penetrate macrophages. Specific therapy for Pontiac fever is generally unnecessary, because it is a self-limited hypersensitivity disease.

Prevention of legionellosis requires identification of the environmental source of the organism and reduction of the microbial burden. Hyperchlorination of the water supply and the maintenance of elevated water temperatures have proved moderately successful. However, elimination of *Legionella* organisms from a water supply is often difficult or impossible to achieve. Because the organism has a low potential for causing disease, reducing the number of organisms in the water supply is often an adequate control measure. Hospitals with patients at high risk for disease should monitor their water supply on a regular basis for the presence of *Legionella* and their hospital population for disease. If hyperchlorination or superheating of the water does not eliminate disease (complete elimination of the organisms in the water supply is probably not possible), continuous copper-silver ionization of the water supply may be necessary.

Case Study and Questions

A 73-year-old man was admitted to the hospital because of breathing difficulties, chest pain, chills, and fever of several days' duration. He had been well until 1 week before admission, when he noted the onset of a persistent headache and a productive cough. The patient smoked two packs of cigarettes a day for more than 50 years and drank a six-pack of beer daily; he also had a history of bronchitis. Physical examination results revealed an elderly man in severe respiratory distress with a temperature of 39° C, pulse of 120 beats/minute, respiratory rate of 36 breaths/minute, and blood pressure of 145/95 mm Hg. Chest radiograph revealed an infiltrate in the middle and lower lobes of the right lung. The white blood cell count was 14,000 cells/mm³ (80% polymorphonuclear neutrophils). Gram stain of the sputum showed neutrophils but no bacteria, and routine bacterial cultures of sputum and blood were negative for organisms. Infection with *Legionella pneumophila* was suspected.

1. What laboratory tests can be used to confirm this diagnosis? Why were the routine culture and Gram-stained specimen negative for *Legionella* organisms?
2. How are *Legionella* species able to survive phagocytosis by the alveolar macrophages?
3. What environmental factors are implicated in the spread of *Legionella* infections? How can this risk be eliminated or minimized?

Bibliography

Edelstein P: Antimicrobial chemotherapy for Legionnaires disease: Time for a change. Ann Intern Med 129:328-330, 1998.
Edelstein P: Urine antigen tests positive for Pontiac fever: Implications for diagnosis and pathogenesis. Clin Infect Dis 44:229-231, 2007.
Fields BS, Benson RF, Besser RE: Legionella and legionnaires disease: 25 years of investigation. Clin Microbiol Rev 15:506-526, 2002.
Greenberg D, et al: Problem pathogens: Paediatric legionellosis — implications for improved diagnosis. Lancet 6:529-535, 2006.
Hayden RT, et al: Direct detection of Legionella species from bronchoalveolar lavage and open lung biopsy specimens: Comparison of LightCycler PCR, in situ hybridization, direct fluorescence antigen detection, and culture. J Clin Microbiol 39:2618-2626, 2001.
Helbig JH, et al: Clinical utility of urinary antigen detection for diagnosis of community-acquired, travel-associated, and nosocomial legionnaires disease. J Clin Microbiol 41:837-840, 2003.
Kim MJ, et al: Characterization of a lipoprotein common to Legionella species as a urinary broad-spectrum antigen for diagnosis of legionnaires disease. J Clin Microbiol 41:2974-2979, 2003.
Modol J, et al: Hospital-acquired legionnaires disease in a university hospital: Impact of the copper-silver ionization system. Clin Infect Dis 44:263-265, 2007.
Sopena N, et al: Factors related to persistence of Legionella urinary antigen excretion in patients with legionnaires disease. Eur J Clin Microbiol Infect Dis 21:845-848, 2002.
Stout J, Yu V: Legionellosis. N Engl J Med 337:681-687, 1997.

Miscellaneous Gram-Negative Rods

Miscellaneous clinically important gram-negative rods not discussed in the preceding chapters are the subject of this chapter (Box 38-1).

Bartonella

As with many groups of bacteria studied in recent years, analysis of the 16S ribosomal ribonucleic acid (rRNA) gene has led to the reorganization of the genus *Bartonella*. Currently, 19 species are included in the genus, with three species most commonly associated with human disease: ***B. bacilliformis***, ***B. henselae***, and ***B. quintana*** (Box 38-2). Members of the genus are short (0.3 to 0.5 × 1.0 to 1.7 μm), gram-negative, aerobic rods with fastidious growth requirements. Although the organisms can grow on enriched blood agar, prolonged incubation (1 to 6 weeks) in a humid (37° C) atmosphere supplemented with carbon dioxide is required for their initial recovery.

Members of the genus *Bartonella* are found in a variety of animal reservoirs and are typically present without evidence of disease. The spread of most *Bartonella* species from colonized animals to humans is either by direct contact or by **insect vectors** (e.g., *B. bacilliformis*, **sand flies**; *B. quintana*, **lice**; *B. henselae*, **fleas**). Most infections with *Bartonella* are characterized by **recurrent fevers** and/or **angioproliferative lesions** (blood-filled cysts).

B. bacilliformis, the original member of the genus, is responsible for Carrión disease, an **acute febrile illness** consisting of severe **anemia (Oroya fever)** followed by a chronic **cutaneous** form (**verruga peruana**). The disease is restricted to the Andes mountain region of Peru, Ecuador, and Colombia, the endemic area of the sand fly vector *Phlebotomus*. After the bite of an infected sand fly, the bacteria enter the blood, multiply, and penetrate into erythrocytes. This process increases the fragility of the infected cells and facilitates their clearance by the reticuloendothelial system, leading to acute anemia. Myalgia, arthralgia, and headache are also common. This stage of illness ends with the development of humoral immunity. In the chronic stage of Carrión disease, 1- to 2-cm cutaneous nodules, often engorged with blood (angioproliferative), appear over the course of 1 to 2 months and may persist for months to years. The link between verruga peruana skin lesions and Oroya fever was demonstrated by a nineteenth-century Peruvian medical student, Daniel Alcides Carrión, who infected himself with aspirates from the skin lesions and died of Oroya fever in 1885. This act of scientific recklessness immortalized him.

Bartonella quintana was originally described as the causative organism of **trench fever** (also called **"5-day" fever**; see Box 38-2), a disease prevalent during World War I. Infection can vary from asymptomatic to a severe, debilitating illness. Typically patients have severe headache, fever, weakness, and pain in the long bones (particularly the tibia). The fever can recur at 5-day intervals, hence the name of the disease. Although trench fever does not cause death, the illness can be very severe. No animal reservoir for this disease has been identified. Rather, exposure to contaminated feces of the **human body louse** spreads disease from person to person.

B. quintana is also associated with a spectrum of diseases in immunocompromised patients, particularly patients infected with the human immunodeficiency virus (HIV). Infection manifests as **recurrent fevers with bacteremia** (Clinical Case 38-1) and **bacillary angiomatosis**. Bacteremia is characterized by an insidious onset of malaise, body aches, fatigue, weight loss, headaches, and recurrent fevers. This can lead to endocarditis or, more commonly, vascular proliferative diseases of the skin (bacillary angiomatosis; Figure 38-1), subcutaneous tissues, or bone. The vascular lesions appear as multiple blood-filled nodules (resembling verruga peruana). As with trench fever, the vector of these diseases appears to be the human body louse, and disease is primarily restricted to the homeless population, in whom personal hygiene is substandard.

B. henselae is also responsible for bacillary angiomatosis; however, it primarily involves the skin, lymph nodes, liver

Box 38—1. Miscellaneous Medically Important Gram-Negative Rods

Organism	Historical Derivation
Bartonella	Bartonella, named after Barton, who originally described B. bacilliformis
B. bacilliformis	bacillus, "rod"; forma, "shape" (rod-shaped)
B. henselae	hensel, named after D.M. Hensel, who worked with this organism
B. quintana	quintana, "fifth" (refers to 5-day fever)
Cardiobacterium hominis	cardia, "heart"; bakterion, "small rod"; hominis, of "man" (refers to the predilection of this bacterium to cause endocarditis in humans)
Capnocytophaga	capno, "smoke"; cytophaga, "eater" (literally, eater of smoke; refers to the requirement for carbon dioxide for growth)
Streptobacillus moniliformis	streptos, "twisted" or "curved"; bacillus, "rod"; monile, "necklace"; forma, "shape" (twisted, necklace-shaped bacillus; refers to the pleomorphic morphology of the bacteria)

Box 38—2. Clinical Summaries

Bartonella bacilliformis

Carrión disease: the disease is characterized by acute febrile illness consisting of severe anemia (**Oroya fever**) followed by chronic, cutaneous, blood-filled nodules (**verruga peruana**)

Bartonella quintana

Trench fever: disease is characterized by severe headache, fever, weakness, and pain in the long bones; the fever recurs at 5-day intervals
Bacillary angiomatosis: vascular proliferative disease in immunocompromised patients; involves the skin, subcutaneous tissues, and bones
Subacute endocarditis: mild but progressive infection of the endocardium

Bartonella henselae

Bacillary angiomatosis: same as above, except primarily involving the skin, lymph nodes, or liver and spleen
Subacute endocarditis: same as above
Cat-scratch disease: chronic regional lymphadenopathy associated with cat scratch

Cardiobacterium hominis

Subacute endocarditis: same as above

***Capnocytophaga* species**

Opportunistic infections: variety of infections, including periodontitis, bacteremia, and endocarditis (from dysgonic fermenter 1 [DF-1] species); dog- or cat-bite wounds (from DF-2 species)

Streptobacillus moniliformis

Rat-bite fever: irregular fever, headache, chills, myalgia, and arthralgia associated with rodent bite; pharyngitis and vomiting is associated with exposure to bacteria in food or water

(**peliosis hepatis**), or spleen (**splenic peliosis**). The reasons for this differential tissue affinity are not known. Also like *B. quintana*, *B. henselae* can cause subacute endocarditis. The reservoirs for *B. henselae* are cats and their fleas. The bacterium is carried asymptomatically in the feline oropharynx and can cause transient bacteremia, particularly in young or feral cats. *B. henselae* is responsible for another disease acquired after exposure to cats (e.g., scratches, bites, contact with the contaminated feces of cat fleas): **cat-scratch disease.** Typically, cat-scratch disease is a benign infection in children, characterized by **chronic regional adenopathy** of the lymph nodes draining the site of contact. Although bacteria can be seen in the lymph node tissues, culture is virtually always negative. A definitive diagnosis is based on the characteristic presentation and serologic evidence of a recent infection. Cultures are not useful, because relatively few organisms are present in the tissues as a result of the vigorous cellular immune reaction in immunocompetent patients. In contrast, *B. henselae* can be isolated from blood collected from immunocompromised patients with chronic bacteremia if the cultures are incubated for 3 weeks or more (Figure 38-2).

Clinical Case 38-1. Fever and Bacteremia Caused by *Bartonella*

Slater, et al. (N Engl J Med 3323:1587-93, 1990) described the first *Bartonella henselae* infection in an HIV-infected patient. A 31-year-old man with advanced HIV infection presented with high fevers, chills, sweats, and weight loss. Blood cultures were negative after 2 days of incubation. Despite an initial response to oral antibiotic therapy, the fevers returned after 2 weeks. The patient was pancytopenic and had elevated liver enzyme levels. Hepatomegaly was the only abnormality detected by computed tomography. All diagnostic tests were negative until after more than 2 weeks of incubation, when gram-negative rods were recovered in the blood cultures. Subsequent studies characterized this as a newly discovered organism and named it *B. henselae*. The patient was treated with parenteral erythromycin and, despite recurrent fevers, subsequently became culture negative. This patient illustrates the susceptibility of HIV patients to this organism and the insidious onset and prolonged course of the disease.

Figure 38–1. Skin lesions of bacillary angiomatosis caused by *Bartonella henselae*. (*From Cohen J, Powderly WG: Infectious Diseases, 2nd ed. St Louis, Mosby, 2004.*)

Treatment of *B. bacilliformis* infections is with oral chloramphenicol, doxycycline, or rifampin. Oral erythromycin or doxycycline is most commonly used for treatment of other *Bartonella* infections. Although the value of treating cat-scratch disease is controversial, azithromycin is the drug of choice if treatment is prescribed. Penicillinase-resistant penicillins, first-generation cephalosporins, and clindamycin do not appear active in vitro against *Bartonella*. The incidence of *Bartonella* infections in HIV-infected patients has declined in recent years because these patients are treated routinely with azithromycin or clarithromycin for prevention of *Mycobacterium avium* infections.

Figure 38–2. *B. henselae* growing on blood agar plates; note the two typical colonial morphologies. (*From Cohen J, Powderly WG: Infectious Diseases, 2nd ed. St Louis, Mosby, 2004.*)

Cardiobacterium

Cardiobacterium hominis is named for the predilection of this bacterium to cause endocarditis in humans. These bacteria are nonmotile, facultatively anaerobic, and characteristically small (1 × 1 to 2 µm) pleomorphic, gram-negative or gram-variable rods. The bacteria are fermentative, oxidase positive, and catalase negative. *C. hominis* is present in the upper respiratory tract of almost 70% of healthy people.

Although uncommon, **endocarditis** is the primary human disease caused by *C. hominis* (Clinical Case 38-2). Many infections are likely to be unreported or undiagnosed because of the low virulence of this organism and its slow growth in vitro. Most patients with *C. hominis* endocarditis have **preexisting heart disease** and either have a history of oral disease or have undergone dental procedures before the clinical symptoms develop. The organisms are able to enter the blood from the oropharynx, adhere to the damaged heart tissue, and then slowly multiply. The course of disease is insidious and subacute; patients typically have symptoms (e.g., fatigue, malaise, and low-grade fever) for months before seeking medical care. Complications are rare, and complete recovery after appropriate antibiotic therapy is common.

The isolation of *C. hominis* from blood cultures confirms the diagnosis of endocarditis. The organism grows slowly in culture, requiring 1 week or more for growth to be detected. *C. hominis* appears in broth cultures as discrete clumps that can be easily overlooked. The organism requires enhanced carbon dioxide and humidity levels to grow on agar media, with pinpoint (1 mm) colonies seen on blood or chocolate agar plates after 2 days of incubation. The organism does not grow on MacConkey agar or other selective media commonly used for gram-negative rods. *C. hominis* can be readily identified from its growth

Clinical Case 38-2. *Cardiobacterium* Endocarditis

Hoover, et al. (Ann Intern Med 142(3):229-230, 2005) described the first patient infected with *Cardiobacterium valvarum* (a newly described species in the genus *Cardiobacterium*). The patient was a 46-year-old man who over the course of 1 month developed anorexia and fatigue. The symptoms developed 2 weeks after a dental extraction. His physical examination was notable for fatigue, lower extremity edema, and a new heart murmur. Bilateral pleural effusions were revealed on chest radiography. All blood cultures collected over a 24-hour period were positive for a pleomorphic gram-negative rod that was subsequently identified as *C. valvarum*. Management of the patient involved replacement of the aortic valve with a prosthetic valve and 4 weeks of treatment with ceftriaxone. Follow-up visits with the patient documented complete recovery. This case illustrates the subacute presentation and generally successful outcome for patients with *Cardiobacterium* endocarditis. What is unique is that the patient did not have a history of previous heart disease, although it is likely to have been present.

properties, microscopic morphology, and reactivity in biochemical tests.

C. hominis is susceptible to many antibiotics, and most infections are treated successfully with **penicillin or ampicillin** for 2 to 6 weeks (although penicillin-resistant strains have been reported). *C. hominis* endocarditis in people with preexisting heart disease is prevented by the maintenance of good oral hygiene and the use of antibiotic prophylaxis at the time of dental procedures. Long-acting penicillin is effective prophylaxis, but erythromycin should not be used, because *C. hominis* is commonly resistant to it.

Capnocytophaga and Dysgonomonas

Members of the genus *Capnocytophaga* are filamentous, gram-negative rods capable of aerobic and anaerobic growth in the presence of carbon dioxide. The genus is subdivided into two groups: (1) dysgonic fermenter 1 (DF-1), with five species; and (2) dysgonic fermenter 2 (DF-2), with two species. DF-1 strains colonize the human oropharynx and are associated with periodontitis, septicemia (particularly in patients who have undergone splenectomy or have compromised hepatic function [cirrhosis]), and rarely endocarditis. DF-2 strains colonize the oral cavities of cats and dogs and are associated with bite wounds. A third group of three species was transferred from this genus to a new genus, *Dysgonomonas*. These bacteria are associated with gastroenteritis in immunocompromised patients.

Capnocytophaga initially grows slowly in culture, requiring 2 or more days before colonies are observed on blood agar plates. The bacterial cells are long and thin with tapered ends ("fusiform" shaped). Because some strains of *Capnocytophaga* produce beta-lactamases, treatment with the combination of a β-lactam/β-lactamase inhibitor such as **amoxicillin-clavulanate** is recommended. Resistance of some strains to fluoroquinolones is reported, and most strains are resistant to the aminoglycosides.

Streptobacillus

Streptobacillus moniliformis, the causative agent of **rat-bite fever**, is a long, thin (0.1 to 0.5 × 1 to 5 μm), gram-negative rod that tends to stain poorly and to be more pleomorphic in older cultures. Granules, bulbous swellings resembling a string of beads, and extremely long filaments may be seen (Figure 38-3).

Streptobacillus is found in the nasopharynx of rats and other small rodents, as well as transiently in animals that feed on rodents (e.g., dogs, cats). Human infections result from rodent bites (**rat-bite fever**; Clinical Case 38-3) or much less commonly from consumption of contaminated food or water (**Haverhill fever**). Most cases of rat-bite fever

Figure 38—3. Gram stain of *Streptobacillus moniliformis*; note the pleomorphic forms and bulbous swellings.

in the United States are in children with pet rats, laboratory workers, and pet shop employees. After a 2- to 10-day incubation period, the onset of rat-bite fever is abrupt, characterized by irregular fever, headache, chills, muscle pain, and migratory pain in multiple joints (polyarthralgias). A maculopapular or petechial rash develops a few days later, with involvement extending to the hands and feet. This hemorrhagic rash in a patient with a recent history of a rat bite and migratory polyarthralgias is diagnostic. In the absence of effective antibiotics, rat-bite fever is associated with a 10% mortality rate. Despite effective treatment, some patients have persistent polyarthralgias, fatigue, and a slowly resolving rash. *S. moniliformis* is susceptible to many antibiotics, including **penicillin** (not active against cell-wall-defective forms) and **tetracycline**.

Laboratory confirmation of *Streptobacillus* infections is difficult. Blood and joint fluid should be collected, and the laboratory should be notified that *S. moniliformis* is

Clinical Case 38-3. Rat-Bite Fever

Irvine (Clin Microbiol Newsl 28:15-17, 2006) described a 60-year-old man who developed rat-bite fever. The patient was admitted to the hospital complaining of fever, confusion, headaches, and pustular lesions on both hands. The diagnosis of sepsis was made, and blood cultures, CSF, and the purulent material from the lesions were collected. Lymphocytes were the predominant cells in the CSF, and no bacteria were seen on Gram stain, consistent with aseptic meningitis. A Gram stain of purulent material revealed pleomorphic gram-negative rods. After 3 days of incubation, the bacteria grew from both the blood and wound cultures. Growth in the blood culture broths appeared as clumps of organisms resembling "bread crumbs." The organism was subsequently identified as *Streptobacillus moniliformis*. The patient was treated with penicillin, and within 24 hours, his fever resolved and sensorium cleared. A more complete social history revealed the patient had a pet snake and maintained mice to feed the snake. Although he did not remember recent bites from the mice, exposure of open cuts on his hands to the rodents is sufficient for an infection to develop.

suspected, because growth of the organism requires use of enriched media supplemented with 15% blood, 20% horse or calf serum, or 5% ascitic fluid. *S. moniliformis* grows slowly, taking at least 3 days to be isolated. When grown in broth, it has the appearance of "puffballs"; small, round colonies are seen on agar, as are cell-wall-defective forms, with their typical fried-egg appearance. It is difficult to identify the organisms, because they are relatively inactive, although acid is produced from glucose and other selected carbohydrates. The most reliable method for identifying isolates is sequencing the 16S rRNA gene.

Case Study and Questions

A previously healthy 12-year-old girl developed a slowly enlarging, swollen axillary lymph node. One week before the onset of disease, she had suffered a scratch while playing with a kitten. Her physician suspected the diagnosis of cat-scratch disease.

1. What is the most sensitive diagnostic test for confirming this diagnosis?

2. What infections are caused by *Bartonella quintana* and *Bartonella henselae*? How does the epidemiology of these infections differ?

3. What infection is caused by *Cardiobacterium*? *Streptobacillus*?

Bibliography

Agan BK, Dolan MJ: Laboratory diagnosis of *Bartonella* infections. Clin Lab Med 22:937-962, 2002.

Anderson B, Neuman M: *Bartonella* spp. as emerging human pathogens. Clin Microbiol Rev 10:203-219, 1997.

Elliott S: Rat bite fever and *Streptobacillus moniliformis*. Clin Microbiol Rev 20:13-22, 2007.

Koehler J, et al: Molecular epidemiology of *Bartonella* infections in patients with bacillary angiomatosis-peliosis. N Engl J Med 337:1876-1883, 1997.

Koehler J, et al: Prevalence of *Bartonella* infection among human immunodeficiency virus-infected patients with fever. Clin Infect Dis 37:550-666, 2003.

La Scola B, Raoult D: Culture of *Bartonella quintana* and *Bartonella henselae* from human samples: A 5-year experience (1993 to 1998). J Clin Microbiol 37:1899-1905, 1999.

Malani A, et al: *Cardiobacterium hominis* endocarditis: Two cases and a review of the literature. Eur J Clin Microbiol Infect Dis 25:587-595, 2006.

Maurin M, Raoult D: *Bartonella (Rochalimaea) quintana* infections. Clin Microbiol Rev 9:273-292, 1996.

Metzkor-Cotter E, et al: Long-term serological analysis and clinical follow-up of patients with cat scratch disease. Clin Infect Dis 37:1149-1154, 2003.

Resto-Ruiz S, Burgess A, Anderson B: The role of the host immune response in pathogenesis of *Bartonella henselae*. DNA Cell Biol 22:431-440, 2003.

Spach D, et al: *Bartonella (Rochalimaea)* species as a cause of apparent "culture-negative" endocarditis. Clin Infect Dis 20:1044-1047, 1995.

Zeaiter Z, et al: Phylogenetic classification of *Bartonella* species by comparing groEL sequences. Int J Syst Evol Microbiol 52:165-171, 2002.

Clostridium

Historically, the collection of all anaerobic, gram-positive rods capable of forming endospores was placed in the genus *Clostridium*. This genus was defined by four properties: (1) presence of endospores, (2) strict anaerobic metabolism, (3) inability to reduce sulfate to sulfite, and (4) gram-positive cell wall structure. Even with this broad classification scheme, some clinically significant members of the genus can be misclassified. Spores are only rarely demonstrated in some species (*Clostridium perfringens*, *Clostridium ramosum*), some species are aerotolerant and can grow on agar media exposed to air (e.g., *Clostridium tertium*, *Clostridium histolyticum*), and some clostridia consistently stain gram-negative (e.g., *Clostridium ramosum*, *Clostridium clostridioforme*). The traditional method for classifying an isolate in the genus *Clostridium* was based on a combination of diagnostic tests, including the demonstration of spores, optimal growth in anaerobic conditions, a complex pattern of biochemical reactivity, and detection of characteristic volatile fatty acids by gas chromatography. With these methods, 191 species have been defined, although most of the clinically important isolates fall within a few species (Table 39-1). It should not be surprising that the use of gene-sequencing techniques has led to the reorganization of this heterogeneous collection of organisms into a number of groups that should appropriately represent new genera. However, most clinically significant *Clostridium* species cluster in homology group I and will remain in the genus *Clostridium*.

The organisms are **ubiquitous** in soil, water, and sewage and are part of the normal microbial flora in the gastrointestinal tracts of animals and humans. Most clostridia are harmless saprophytes, but some are well-recognized human pathogens with a clearly documented history of causing diseases such as **tetanus** (*C. tetani*), **botulism** (*Clostridium botulinum*, *Clostridium baratii*, *Clostridium butyricum*), myonecrosis or **gas gangrene** (*C. perfringens*, *Clostridium novyi*, *Clostridium septicum*, *C. histolyticum*), and **diarrhea** and **colitis** (*C. perfringens*, *Clostridium difficile*). The majority of infections seen today are skin and soft-tissue infections, food poisoning, and antibiotic-associated diarrhea and colitis. The remarkable capacity of clostridia to cause diseases is attributed to their (1) ability to survive adverse environmental conditions through spore formation; (2) rapid growth in a nutritionally enriched, oxygen-deprived environment, and (3) production of numerous histolytic toxins, enterotoxins, and neurotoxins. The most common or important human pathogens in the genus are discussed in this chapter (Box 39-1).

Clostridium perfringens (Box 39-2)

Physiology and Structure

C. perfringens can be associated with simple colonization or can cause life-threatening disease. *C. perfringens* is a large (0.6 to 2.4 × 1.3 to 19.0 μm), rectangular, gram-positive rod (Figure 39-1), with **spores rarely observed** either in vivo or after in vitro cultivation. This organism is one of the few nonmotile clostridia, but **rapidly spreading growth** on laboratory media (resembling the growth of motile organisms) is characteristic (Figure 39-2). The organism grows rapidly in tissues and in culture, is hemolytic, and is metabolically active, features that make possible its identification in the laboratory. The production of one or more "major lethal" toxins by *C. perfringens* (alpha, beta, epsilon, and iota toxins) is used to subdivide isolates into five types (A through E).

Pathogenesis and Immunity

C. perfringens can cause a spectrum of diseases, from a self-limited gastroenteritis to an overwhelming destruction of tissue (e.g., clostridial myonecrosis) associated with a very high mortality, even in patients who receive early medical intervention. This pathogenic potential is attributed primarily to at least 12 toxins and enzymes produced by this organism. **Alpha toxin**, the most important toxin and the one produced by all five types of *C. perfringens*, is a

Table 39–1. Pathogenic Clostridia and Their Associated Human Diseases*

Species	Human Disease	Frequency
C. difficile	Antibiotic-associated diarrhea, pseudomembranous colitis	Common
C. perfringens	Soft-tissue infections (e.g., cellulitis, suppurative myositis, myonecrosis, gas gangrene), food poisoning, enteritis necroticans, septicemia	Common
C. septicum	Gas gangrene, septicemia	Uncommon
C. botulinum	Botulism	Uncommon
C. tetani	Tetanus	Uncommon
C. tertium	Opportunistic infections	Uncommon
C. baratii	Botulism	Rare
C. butyricum	Botulism	Rare
C. clostridioforme	Opportunistic infections	Rare
C. histolyticum	Gas gangrene	Rare
C. innocuum	Opportunistic infections	Rare
C. novyi	Gas gangrene	Rare
C. sordellii	Gas gangrene, septic shock syndrome	Rare
C. sporogenes	Opportunistic infections	Rare

*Other clostridial species have been associated with human disease but primarily as opportunistic pathogens. Additionally, some species (e.g., C. clostridioforme, C. innocuum, C. ramosum) are commonly isolated but are rarely associated with disease.

Box 39–1. Important Clostridia

Organism	Historical Derivation
Clostridium	closter, a "spindle"
C. botulinum	botulus, "sausage" (the first major outbreak was associated with insufficiently smoked sausage)
C. difficile	difficile, "difficult" (difficult to isolate and grow; refers to the extreme oxygen sensitivity of this organism)
C. perfringens	perfringens, "breaking through" (associated with highly invasive tissue necrosis)
C. septicum	septicum, "putrefactive" (associated with sepsis and a high mortality)
C. sordellii	sordellii, named after the bacteriologist Sordelli, who first described the organism
C. tertium	tertium, "third" (historically, the third most commonly isolated anaerobe from war wounds
C. tetani	tetani, related to "tension" (disease caused by this organism characterized by muscle spasms)

from vegetative cells to spores and is released with the formed spores when the cells undergo the terminal stages of spore formation (**sporulation**). The alkaline conditions in the small intestine stimulate sporulation. The released enterotoxin binds to receptors on the brush border membrane of the small intestine epithelium in the ileum (primarily) and jejunum but not duodenum. Insertion of the toxin into the cell membrane leads to altered membrane permeability and loss of fluids and ions. The enterotoxin also acts as a superantigen simulating T lymphocyte activity. Antibodies to enterotoxin, indicating previous exposure, are commonly found in adults but are not protective.

Epidemiology

Type A *C. perfringens* commonly inhabits the intestinal tract of humans and animals and is widely distributed in nature, particularly in **soil and water contaminated with feces** (see Box 39-2). Spores are formed under adverse environmental conditions and can survive for prolonged periods. Strains of types B through E do not survive in soil but rather colonize the intestinal tracts of animals and occasionally humans. **Type A *C. perfringens*** is responsible for most human infections, including soft-tissue infections, food poisoning, and primary septicemia. Type C *C. perfringens* is responsible for one other important infection in humans—**enteritis necroticans**.

lecithinase (phospholipase C) that lyses erythrocytes, platelets, leukocytes, and endothelial cells. This toxin mediates massive hemolysis, increased vascular permeability and bleeding (augmented by destruction of platelets), tissue destruction (as found in myonecrosis), hepatic toxicity, and myocardial dysfunction (bradycardia, hypotension). The largest quantities of alpha toxin are produced by *C. perfringens* type A. Beta toxin is responsible for intestinal stasis, loss of mucosa with formation of the necrotic lesions, and progression to necrotizing enteritis (**enteritis necroticans, pig-bel**). **Epsilon toxin**, a protoxin, is activated by trypsin and increases the vascular permeability of the gastrointestinal wall. **Iota toxin**, the fourth major lethal toxin, is produced by type E *C. perfringens*. This toxin has necrotic activity and increases vascular permeability.

The *C. perfringens* **enterotoxin** is produced primarily by type A strains. The heat-labile toxin is susceptible to pronase. Exposure to trypsin enhances toxin activity threefold. The enterotoxin is produced during the phase transition

Box 39-2. Summary: *Clostridium perfringens*

Biology, Virulence, and Disease

Organisms multiply rapidly in culture and in patients
Produces many toxins and enzymes that lyse blood cells and destroy tissues, leading to diseases such as overwhelming sepsis, massive hemolysis, and myonecrosis
Produces a heat-sensitive enterotoxin that binds to receptors on the epithelium of the small intestine, leading to loss of fluids and ions (watery diarrhea)

Epidemiology

Ubiquitous; present in soil, water, and intestinal tract of humans and animals
Type A strains are responsible for most human infections
Soft tissue infections typically associated with bacterial contamination of wounds or localized trauma
Food poisoning associated with contaminated meat products held at temperatures below 60° C, which allow the organisms to grow to large numbers

Diagnosis

Reliably seen in Gram-stained tissue specimens (large, gram-positive rods)
Grows rapidly in culture

Treatment, Prevention, and Control

Rapid treatment is essential for serious infections
Severe infections require surgical débridement and high-dose penicillin therapy
Symptomatic treatment for food poisoning
Proper wound care and judicious use of prophylactic antibiotics will prevent most infections

Clinical Diseases (Box 39-3)

Soft-Tissue Infections

Soft-tissue infections caused by *C. perfringens* are subdivided into (1) cellulitis, (2) fasciitis or suppurative myositis, and (3) myonecrosis or gas gangrene. Clostridial species

Figure 39–1. Gram stain of *Clostridium perfringens* in a wound specimen. Note the rectangular shape of the rods, the presence of many decolorized rods appearing gram-negative, and the absence of blood cells.

Figure 39–2. Growth of *Clostridium perfringens* on sheep blood agar. Note the flat, spreading colonies and the hemolytic activity of the organism. A presumptive identification of *C. perfringens* can be made by detection of a zone of complete hemolysis (caused by the theta toxin) and a wider zone of partial hemolysis (caused by the alpha toxin), combined with the characteristic microscopic morphology.

can colonize wounds and skin with no clinical consequences. Indeed, most strains of *C. perfringens* and other clostridial species isolated in wound cultures are insignificant. However, these organisms can also initiate **cellulitis** (Figure 39-3) with gas formation in the soft tissue. This process can progress to **suppurative myositis** characterized by an accumulation of pus in the muscle planes, but muscle necrosis and systemic symptoms are absent.

Clostridial myonecrosis is a life-threatening disease that illustrates the full virulence potential of histotoxic clostridia. The onset of disease, characterized by intense pain, generally develops within a week after clostridia are introduced into tissue by trauma or surgery. The onset is followed rapidly by extensive muscle necrosis, shock, renal failure, and death, often within 2 days of initial onset. Macroscopic examination of muscle reveals devitalized necrotic tissue. Gas found in the tissue is caused by the metabolic activity of the rapidly dividing bacteria (hence the name **gas gangrene**). Microscopic examination reveals abundant rectangular, gram-positive rods in the absence of inflammatory cells (resulting from lysis by clostridial toxins). The clostridial toxins characteristically cause extensive hemolysis and bleeding. Clostridial myonecrosis is most commonly caused by *C. perfringens*, although other species (e.g., *C. septicum*, *C. histolyticum*, and *C. novyi*) can also produce this disease.

Food Poisoning (Clinical Case 39-1)

Clostridial food poisoning, a relatively common but underappreciated intoxication, is characterized by (1) a short incubation period (8 to 24 hours), (2) a clinical presentation that includes abdominal cramps and watery diarrhea but no fever, nausea, or vomiting, and (3) a clinical course lasting 24 to 48 hours. Disease results from the ingestion of meat products (e.g., beef, chicken, turkey) contaminated with large numbers (10^8 to 10^9 organisms) of

Box 39—3. Clostridial Diseases: Clinical Summaries

Clostridium perfringens

Soft-Tissue Infections

Cellulitis: localized edema and erythema with gas formation in the soft tissue; generally nonpainful

Suppurative myositis: accumulation of pus (suppuration) in the muscle planes without muscle necrosis or systemic symptoms

Myonecrosis: painful, rapid destruction of muscle tissue; systemic spread with high mortality

Gastroenteritis

Food poisoning: rapid onset of abdominal cramps and watery diarrhea with no fever, nausea, or vomiting; short duration and self-limited

Necrotizing enteritis: acute, necrotizing destruction of jejunum with abdominal pain, vomiting, bloody diarrhea, and peritonitis

Clostridium tetani

Generalized tetanus: generalized musculature spasms and involvement of the autonomic nervous system in severe disease (e.g., cardiac arrhythmias, fluctuations in blood pressure, profound sweating, dehydration)

Localized tetanus: musculature spasms restricted to localized area of primary infection

Neonatal tetanus: neonatal infection primarily involving the umbilical stump; very high mortality

Clostridium botulinum

Foodborne botulism: initial presentation of blurred vision, dry mouth, constipation, and abdominal pain; progresses to bilateral descending weakness of the peripheral muscles with flaccid paralysis

Infant botulism: initially nonspecific symptoms (e.g., constipation, weak cry, failure to thrive) that progress to flaccid paralysis and respiratory arrest

Wound botulism: clinical presentation same as with foodborne disease, although the incubation period is longer and fewer gastrointestinal symptoms

Inhalation botulism: inhalation exposure to botulinum toxin would be expected to have a rapid onset of symptoms (flaccid paralysis, pulmonary failure) and high mortality

Clostridium difficile

Antibiotic-associated diarrhea: acute diarrhea generally developing 5 to 10 days after initiation of antibiotic treatment (particularly clindamycin, penicillins, cephalosporins, fluoroquinolones); may be brief and self-limited or more protracted

Pseudomembranous colitis: most severe form of *C. difficile* disease with profuse diarrhea, abdominal cramping, and fever; whitish plaques (pseudomembranes) over intact colonic tissue seen on colonoscopy

enterotoxin-containing type A *C. perfringens*. Holding contaminated foods at temperatures below 60° C (46° C is optimal) allows spores that survived the cooking process to germinate and multiply to high numbers. Rapid refrigeration of food after preparation prevents this bacterial

Figure 39—3. Clostridial cellulitis. Clostridia can be introduced into tissue during surgery or by a traumatic injury. This patient suffered a compound fracture of the tibia. Five days after the injury, the skin became discolored, and bullae and necrosis developed. A serosanguineous exudate and subcutaneous gas were present, but there was no evidence of muscle necrosis. The patient had an uneventful recovery. *(From Lambert H, Farrar W (eds): Infectious Diseases Illustrated. London, Gower, 1982.)*

growth. Alternatively, reheating of the food to 74° C can destroy the heat-labile enterotoxin.

Necrotizing Enteritis

Necrotizing enteritis (also called **enteritis necroticans** or **pig-bel**) is a rare, acute necrotizing process in the jejunum characterized by acute abdominal pain, vomiting, bloody

Clinical Case 39-1. *Clostridium perfringens* Gastroenteritis

The Centers for Disease Control and Prevention reported an outbreak of *C. perfringens* gastroenteritis associated with corned beef served at St. Patrick's Day celebrations (Morb Mortal Wkly Rep 43:137, 1994). On March 18, 1993, the Cleveland City Health Department received telephone calls from 15 persons who became ill after eating corned beef purchased from one delicatessen. After the outbreak was publicized, 156 persons contacted the Health Department with a similar history. In addition to a history of diarrhea, 88% complained of abdominal cramps and 13% vomiting, which developed an average of 12 hours after eating the implicated meat. An investigation revealed the delicatessen had purchased 1400 pounds of raw, salt-cured meat, and beginning on March 12, portions of the corned beef were boiled for 3 hours, allowed to cool at room temperature, and then refrigerated. On March 16 and 17, the meat was removed from the refrigerator, heated to 48.8° C, and served. Cultures of the meat yielded >10^5 colonies of *C. perfringens* per gram. The Health Department recommended that if the meat could not be served immediately after cooking, it should have been rapidly cooled in ice and refrigerated. Before it was served, it should have been warmed to at least 74° C to destroy the heat-sensitive enterotoxin.

diarrhea, ulceration of the small intestine, and perforation of the intestinal wall, leading to peritonitis and shock. The mortality in patients with this infection approaches 50%. Beta toxin produced by *C. perfringens* type C is responsible for this disease. Necrotizing enteritis is most common in Papua New Guinea, with sporadic cases reported from other countries. It is associated with eating undercooked, contaminated pork with sweet potatoes, which contain a heat-resistant trypsin inhibitor. This inhibitor protects the beta toxin from inactivation by trypsin. Other risk factors for the disease are exposure to large numbers of organisms and malnutrition (with loss of the proteolytic activity that inactivates the toxin).

Septicemia

The isolation of *C. perfringens* or other clostridial species in blood cultures can be alarming. However, more than half of the isolates are clinically insignificant, representing a transient bacteremia or more likely contamination of the culture with clostridia colonizing the skin. The significance of an isolate must be viewed in light of other clinical findings. When *C. perfringens* is isolated in the blood from patients with significant infections (e.g., myonecrosis, necrotizing enteritis), the organism is typically associated with massive hemolysis.

Laboratory Diagnosis

The laboratory performs only a confirmatory role in the diagnosis of clostridial soft-tissue diseases, because therapy must be initiated immediately. The microscopic detection of gram-positive rods in clinical specimens, usually in the absence of leukocytes, can be a very useful finding, because these organisms have a characteristic morphology. It is also relatively simple to culture these anaerobes. *C. perfringens* can be detected on simple media after incubation for 1 day or less. Under appropriate conditions, *C. perfringens* divides every 8 to 10 minutes, so growth on agar media or in blood culture broths can be detected after incubation for only a few hours. The role of *C. perfringens* in food poisoning is documented by recovery of more than 10^5 organisms per gram of food or more than 10^6 bacteria per gram of feces collected within 1 day of the onset of disease. Immunoassays have also been developed for detection of the enterotoxin in fecal specimens, although culture or immunoassays are not commonly used in clinical labs for this diagnosis.

Treatment, Prevention, and Control

C. perfringens soft-tissue infections, such as suppurative myositis and myonecrosis, must be treated aggressively with **surgical débridement** and **high-dose penicillin therapy**. Hyperbaric oxygen treatment has been used to manage these infections; however, the results are inconclusive. Treatment with antiserum against alpha toxin also has not been successful and is no longer available. Despite all

therapeutic efforts, the prognosis in patients with these diseases is poor, with reported mortality ranging from 40% to almost 100%. Less serious, localized soft-tissue infections can be successfully treated with penicillin.

Antibiotic therapy for clostridial food poisoning is unnecessary, because this is a self-limiting disease (i.e., the diarrhea washes the bacteria out of the intestines, and the normal intestinal flora reestablishes itself).

Prevention and control of *C. perfringens* infections are difficult because the organisms are ubiquitous. Disease requires introduction of the organism into devitalized tissues and maintenance of an anaerobic environment favorable for bacterial growth. Thus proper wound care and the judicious use of prophylactic antibiotics can do much to prevent most infections.

Clostridium tetani (Box 39-4)

Physiology and Structure

C. tetani is a large (0.5 to 2 × 2 to 18 μm), motile, spore-forming rod. The organism produces round, terminal spores that give it the appearance of a drumstick.

Box 39—4. Summary: *Clostridium tetani*

Biology, Virulence, and Disease

Organism extremely oxygen-sensitive, which makes detection by culture difficult
The primary virulence factor is tetanospasmin, a heat-labile neurotoxin that blocks release of neurotransmitters (i.e., gamma-aminobutyric acid, glycine) for inhibitory synapses
Disease is characterized by muscle spasms and involvement of the autonomic nervous system

Epidemiology

Ubiquitous; spores are found in most soils and can colonize gastrointestinal tract of humans and animals
Exposure to spores is common, but disease is uncommon, except in developing countries where there is poor access to vaccine and medical care
Risk is greatest for people with inadequate vaccine-induced immunity
Disease does not induce immunity

Diagnosis

Diagnosis is based on clinical presentation and not laboratory tests
Microscopy and culture are insensitive, and neither tetanus toxin nor antibodies are typically detected

Treatment, Prevention, and Control

Treatment requires débridement, antibiotic therapy (metronidazole), passive immunization with antitoxin globulin, and vaccination with tetanus toxoid
Prevention through use of vaccination, consisting of three doses of tetanus toxoid followed by booster doses every 10 years

Unlike *C. perfringens*, *C. tetani* is difficult to grow. The organism is extremely sensitive to oxygen toxicity, and when growth is detected on agar media, it typically appears as a film over the surface of the agar rather than discrete colonies. The bacteria are proteolytic but unable to ferment carbohydrates.

Pathogenesis and Immunity

Although the vegetative cells of *C. tetani* die rapidly when exposed to oxygen, spore formation allows the organism to survive in the most adverse conditions. Of greater significance is the fact that *C. tetani* produces two toxins, an oxygen-labile hemolysin (**tetanolysin**) and a plasmid-encoded, heat-labile neurotoxin (**tetanospasmin**). The plasmid carrying the gene for tetanospasmin is nonconjugative, so a nontoxic *C. tetani* strain cannot be converted to a toxigenic strain. Tetanolysin is serologically related to streptolysin O and *C. perfringens* and *Listeria monocytogenes* hemolysins. The clinical significance of this enzyme is unknown, however, because it is inhibited by oxygen and serum cholesterol.

Tetanospasmin is produced during the stationary phase of growth, is released when the cell is lysed, and is responsible for the clinical manifestations of tetanus. Tetanospasmin (an **A-B toxin**) is synthesized as a single, 150,000-Da peptide that is cleaved into a light (A-chain) subunit and a heavy (B-chain) subunit by an endogenous protease when the cell releases the neurotoxin. A disulfide bond and noncovalent forces hold the two chains together. The carbohydrate-binding domain of the heavy (100,000-Da) chain, carboxyl-terminal portion, binds to specific sialic acid receptors (e.g., polysialogangliosides) and adjacent glycoproteins on the surface of motor neurons. The intact toxin molecules are internalized in endosomal vesicles and transported in the neuron axon to motor neuron soma located in the spinal cord. In this location, the endosome becomes acidified, which results in a conformational change in the N-terminus domain of the heavy chain, which is followed by its insertion into the endosome membrane and passage of the toxin light chain into the cytosol of the cell. The light chain is a **zinc endopeptidase** that cleaves core proteins involved in the trafficking and release of neurotransmitters. Specifically, tetanospasmin **inactivates proteins that regulate release of the inhibitory neurotransmitters** glycine and gamma-aminobutyric acid (GABA). This leads to unregulated excitatory synaptic activity in the motor neurons, resulting in **spastic paralysis**. The toxin binding is irreversible, so recovery depends on whether new axonal terminals form.

Epidemiology

C. tetani is **ubiquitous**. It is found in fertile soil and transiently colonizes the gastrointestinal tracts of many animals, including humans. The vegetative forms of *C. tetani* are extremely susceptible to oxygen toxicity, but the organisms sporulate readily and can survive in nature for a long time. Disease is relatively rare in the United States because of the high incidence of vaccine-induced immunity. Fewer than 40 cases are reported annually, and the disease occurs primarily in elderly patients with waning immunity. However, tetanus is still responsible for many deaths in developing countries where vaccination is unavailable or medical practices are lax. It is estimated that more than 1 million cases occur worldwide, with a mortality rate ranging from 30% to 50%. At least half the deaths occur in neonates.

Clinical Diseases (see Box 39-3; Clinical Case 39-2)

The incubation period for tetanus varies from a few days to weeks. The duration of the incubation period is directly related to the distance of the primary wound infection from the central nervous system.

Generalized tetanus is the most common form. Involvement of the masseter muscles (trismus or lockjaw) is the presenting sign in most patients. The characteristic sardonic smile that results from the sustained contraction of the facial muscles is known as **risus sardonicus** (Figure 39-4). Other early signs are drooling, sweating, irritability, and persistent back spasms (**opisthotonos**) (Figure 39-5). The autonomic nervous system is involved in patients with more severe disease; the signs and symptoms include cardiac arrhythmias, fluctuations in blood pressure, profound sweating, and dehydration.

Another form of *C. tetani* disease is **localized tetanus**, in which the disease remains confined to the musculature at the site of primary infection. A variant is **cephalic tetanus**, in which the primary site of infection is the head. In contrast to the prognosis for patients with localized tetanus, the prognosis for patients with cephalic tetanus is very poor.

Neonatal tetanus (tetanus neonatorum) is typically associated with an initial infection of the umbilical stump

---

Clinical Case 39-2. Tetanus

The following is a typical history of a patient with tetanus (Morb Mortal Wkly Rep 51:613-615, 2002). An 86-year-old man saw a physician for care of a splinter wound in his right hand acquired 3 days earlier while gardening. He was not treated with either a tetanus toxoid vaccine or tetanus immune globulin (TIG). Seven days later, he developed pharyngitis, and after an additional 3 days he presented to the local hospital with difficulty talking, swallowing, and breathing and with chest pain and disorientation. He was admitted to the hospital with the diagnosis of stroke. On his fourth hospital day, he had developed neck rigidity and respiratory failure requiring tracheostomy and mechanical ventilation. He was transferred to the medical intensive care unit, where the clinical diagnosis of tetanus was made. Despite treatment with tetanus toxoid and immune globulin, the patient died 1 month after admission to the hospital. This case illustrates that *C. tetani* is ubiquitous in soil, can contaminate relatively minor wounds, and can initiate unrelenting progression of neurologic disease in untreated patients.

Figure 39–4. Facial spasm and risus sardonicus in a patient with tetanus. *(From Cohen J, Powderly WG: Infectious Diseases, 2nd ed. St Louis, Mosby, 2004.)*

that progresses to become generalized. The mortality in infants exceeds 90%, and developmental defects are present in survivors. This is almost exclusively a disease in developing countries.

Laboratory Diagnosis

The diagnosis of tetanus, as with that of most other clostridial diseases, is made on the basis of the clinical presentation. The microscopic detection of *C. tetani* or recovery in culture is useful but frequently unsuccessful. Culture results are positive in only approximately 30% of patients with tetanus, because disease can be caused by relatively few organisms, and the slow-growing bacteria are killed rapidly when exposed to air. Neither tetanus toxin nor antibodies to the toxin are detectable in the patient, because the toxin is rapidly bound to motor neurons and

internalized. If the organism is recovered in culture, production of toxin by the isolate can be confirmed with the tetanus antitoxin neutralization test in mice (a procedure performed only in public health reference laboratories).

Treatment, Prevention, and Control

The mortality associated with tetanus has steadily decreased during the past century, resulting in large part from the decreased incidence of tetanus in the United States. The highest mortality is in newborns and in patients in whom the incubation period is shorter than 1 week.

Treatment of tetanus requires **débridement** of the primary wound (which may appear innocuous), use of **metronidazole, passive immunization** with human tetanus immunoglobulin, and **vaccination** with tetanus toxoid. Wound care and metronidazole therapy eliminate the vegetative bacteria that produce toxin, and the antitoxin antibodies work by binding free tetanospasmin molecules. Metronidazole and penicillin have equivalent activity against *C. tetani*; however, penicillin, like tetanospasmin, inhibits GABA activity and hence should not be used. Toxin bound to nerve endings is protected from antibodies. Thus the toxic effects must be controlled symptomatically until the normal regulation of synaptic transmission is restored. Vaccination with a series of three doses of tetanus toxoid, followed by booster doses every 10 years, is highly effective in preventing tetanus.

Clostridium botulinum (Box 39-5)

Physiology and Structure

C. botulinum, the etiologic agent of botulism, is a heterogeneous group of large (0.6 to 1.4 × 3.0 to 20.2 μm),

Figure 39–5. A child with tetanus and opisthotonos resulting from persistent spasms of the back muscles. *(From Emond RT, Rowland HAK, Welsby P: Colour Atlas of Infectious Diseases, 3rd ed. London, Wolfe, 1995.)*

fastidious, spore-forming, anaerobic rods. These bacteria are subdivided into four groups, based on phenotypic and genetic properties, and certainly represent four separate species that have been historically classified within a single species. Seven antigenically distinct botulinum toxins (A to G) have been described; human disease is associated with types A, B, E, and F. Other species of clostridia produce botulinum toxins, including *C. butyricum* (type E toxin), *C. baratii* (type F toxin), and *Clostridium argentinense* (type G toxin). Human disease has only rarely been associated with *C. butyricum* and *C. baratii* and not definitively demonstrated with *C. argentinense*.

Pathogenesis and Immunity

Like tetanus toxin, *C. botulinum* toxin is a 150,000-Da progenitor protein (A-B toxin) consisting of a small subunit (light or A chain) with **zinc-endopeptidase** activity and a large, nontoxic subunit (heavy or B chain). In contrast with the tetanus neurotoxin, the *C. botulinum* toxin is complexed with nontoxic proteins that protect the neurotoxin during passage through the digestive tract (this is unnecessary for tetanus neurotoxin). The carboxyl-terminal portion of the botulinum heavy chain binds specific sialic acid receptors and glycoproteins (different from those targeted by tetanospasmin) on the surface of motor neurons and stimulates endocytosis of the toxin molecule. Also in contrast with tetanospasmin, the botulinum neurotoxin remains at the neuromuscular junction. Acidification of the endosome stimulates N-terminal, heavy-chain-mediated release of the light chain. The botulinum endopeptidase then **inactivates the proteins that regulate release of acetylcholine**, blocking neurotransmission at peripheral cholinergic synapses. Because acetylcholine is required for excitation of muscle, the resulting clinical presentation of botulism is a **flaccid paralysis**. As with tetanus, recovery of function after botulism requires regeneration of the nerve endings.

Epidemiology

C. botulinum is commonly isolated in soil and water samples throughout the world. In the United States, type A strains are found mainly in neutral or alkaline soil west of the Mississippi River; type B strains are found primarily in the eastern part of the country in rich, organic soil; and type E strains are found only in wet soil. Although *C. botulinum* is commonly found in soil, disease is uncommon in the United States.

Four forms of botulism have been identified: (1) classic or foodborne botulism, (2) infant botulism, (3) wound botulism, and (4) inhalation botulism. In the United States, fewer than 30 cases of **foodborne botulism** are seen annually; most are associated with the consumption of home-canned foods (types A and B toxins) and occasionally with the consumption of preserved fish (type E toxin). The food may not appear spoiled, but even a small taste can cause full-blown clinical disease. **Infant botulism** is more common (although fewer than 100 cases are reported annually) and has been associated with the consumption of foods (honey, infant milk powder) contaminated with botulinum spores and ingestion of spore-contaminated soil and dust (now the most common source of infant exposure). The incidence of **wound botulism** is unknown, but the disease is very rare. **Inhalation botulism** is a major concern in this era of bioterrorism. Botulinum toxin has been concentrated for purposes of aerosolization as a biologic weapon. When administered in this manner, inhalation disease has a rapid onset and potentially high mortality.

Clinical Diseases (Box 39-3)

Foodborne Botulism (Clinical Case 39-3)

Patients with foodborne botulism typically become weak and dizzy 1 to 3 days after consuming the contaminated

Clinical Case 39-3. Foodborne Botulism with Commercial Carrot Juice

The Centers for Disease Control and Prevention reported an outbreak of foodborne botulism associated with contaminated carrot juice (Morb Mortal Wkly Rep 55:1098, 2006). On September 8, 2006, three patients went to a hospital in Washington County, Georgia, with cranial nerve palsies and progressive descending flaccid paralysis resulting in respiratory failure. The patients had shared meals on the previous day. Because botulism was suspected, the patients were treated with botulinum antitoxin. The patients had no progression of their neurologic symptoms, but they remained hospitalized and on ventilators. An investigation determined that the patients had consumed contaminated carrot juice produced by a commercial vendor. Botulinum toxin type A was detected in the serum and stool of all three patients and in leftover carrot juice. An additional patient in Florida was also hospitalized with respiratory failure and descending paralysis after drinking carrot juice sold in Florida. Because carrot juice has a low acid content (pH 6.0), *C. botulinum* spores can germinate and produce toxin if contaminated juice is left at room temperature.

Clinical Case 39-4. Infant Botulism

In January 2003, four children with infant botulism were reported by the Centers for Disease Control and Prevention (Morb Mortal Wkly Rep 52:24, 2003). The following is the description of one of the children. A 10-week-old infant with a history of constipation in the first month of life was admitted to a hospital after having difficulty in sucking and swallowing for 2 days. The infant was irritable and had loss of facial expression, generalized muscle weakness, and constipation. Mechanical ventilation was required for 10 days because of respiratory failure. A diagnosis of infant botulism was established 29 days after onset of symptoms by detection of *C. botulinum* producing toxin type B in stool enrichment cultures. The patient was treated with Botulism Immune Globulin Intravenous (BIG-IV) and discharged fully recovered after 20 days. In contrast with foodborne botulism, diagnosis of infant botulism can be made by detecting the organism in the baby's stools.

food. The initial signs include blurred vision with fixed, dilated pupils, dry mouth (indicative of the anticholinergic effects of the toxin), constipation, and abdominal pain. Fever is absent. Bilateral descending weakness of the peripheral muscles develops in patients with progressive disease (flaccid paralysis), and death is most commonly attributed to respiratory paralysis. Patients maintain a clear sensorium throughout the disease. Despite aggressive management of the patient's condition, the disease may continue to progress, because the neurotoxin is irreversibly bound and inhibits the release of excitatory neurotransmitters for a prolonged period. Complete recovery in patients often requires many months to years, or until the affected nerve endings regrow. Mortality in patients with foodborne botulism, which once approached 70%, has been reduced to 5% to 10% through the use of better supportive care, particularly in the management of respiratory complications.

Infant Botulism (Clinical Case 39-4)

Infant botulism was first recognized in 1976 and is now the most common form of botulism in the United States. In contrast with foodborne botulism, this disease is caused by neurotoxin produced in vivo by *C. botulinum* colonizing the gastrointestinal tracts of infants. Although adults are exposed to the organism in their diet, *C. botulinum* cannot survive and proliferate in their intestines. In the absence of competitive bowel microbes, however, the organism can become established in the gastrointestinal tracts of infants. The disease typically affects infants younger than 1 year (most between 1 and 6 months), and the symptoms are initially nonspecific (e.g., constipation, weak cry, or "failure to thrive"). Progressive disease with flaccid paralysis and respiratory arrest can develop; however, mortality in documented cases of infant botulism is very low

(1% to 2%). Some infant deaths attributed to other conditions (e.g., sudden infant death syndrome) may actually be caused by botulism.

Wound Botulism

As the name implies, wound botulism develops from toxin production by *C. botulinum* in contaminated wounds. Although the symptoms of disease are identical to those of foodborne disease, the incubation period is generally longer (4 days or more), and the gastrointestinal tract symptoms are less prominent.

Laboratory Diagnosis

The clinical diagnosis of foodborne botulism is confirmed if toxin activity is demonstrated in the implicated food or in the patient's serum, feces, or gastric fluid. Infant botulism is confirmed if toxin is detected in the infant's feces or serum or the organism cultured from feces. Wound botulism is confirmed if toxin is detected in the patient's serum or wound or the organism cultured from the wound. Toxin activity is most likely to be found early in the disease. No single test for foodborne botulism has sensitivity greater than 60%; in contrast, toxin is detected in the serum of more than 90% of infants with botulism.

Isolation of *C. botulinum* from specimens contaminated with other organisms can be improved by heating the specimen for 10 minutes at 80° C to kill all nonclostridial cells. Culture of the heated specimen on nutritionally enriched anaerobic media allows the heat-resistant *C. botulinum* spores to germinate. Demonstration of toxin production (typically performed at public health laboratories) must be done with a mouse bioassay. This procedure consists of the preparation of two aliquots of the isolate, mixing of one aliquot with antitoxin, and intraperitoneal inoculation of each aliquot into mice. If the antitoxin treatment protects the mice, toxin activity is confirmed. Samples of the implicated food, stool specimen, and patient's serum should also be tested for toxin activity.

Treatment, Prevention, and Control

Patients with botulism require the following treatment measures: (1) adequate **ventilatory support**; (2) elimination of the organism from the gastrointestinal tract through the judicious use of gastric lavage and **metronidazole or penicillin** therapy; and (3) the use of **trivalent botulinum antitoxin** versus toxins A, B, and E to bind toxin circulating in the bloodstream. Ventilatory support is extremely important in reducing mortality. Protective levels of antibodies do not develop after disease, so patients are susceptible to multiple infections.

Disease is prevented by destroying the spores in food (virtually impossible for practical reasons), preventing spore germination (by maintaining the food in an acid pH or storage at 4° C or colder), or destroying the preformed toxin (all botulinum toxins are inactivated by heating at 60° C to 100° C for 10 minutes). Infant botulism has been associated with the consumption of honey contaminated with *C. botulinum* spores, so children younger than 1 year should not eat honey.

Clostridium difficile (Box 39-6)

Until the mid-1970s the clinical importance of *C. difficile* was not appreciated. This organism was infrequently isolated in fecal cultures, and its role in human disease was unknown. Systematic studies now clearly show, however, that toxin-producing *C. difficile* is responsible for antibiotic-associated gastrointestinal diseases ranging from a relatively benign, self-limited diarrhea to severe, life-threatening pseudomembranous colitis (Figures 39-6 and 39-7).

C. difficile produces two toxins, an **enterotoxin (toxin A)** and a **cytotoxin (toxin B)**. The enterotoxin is chemotactic for neutrophils, stimulating the infiltration of polymorphonuclear neutrophils into the ileum with release of cytokines. Toxin A also produces a cytopathic effect, resulting in disruption of the tight cell—cell junction, increased permeability of the intestinal wall, and subsequent diarrhea. The cytotoxin causes actin to depolymerize, with the resultant destruction of the cellular cytoskeleton both in vivo and in vitro. Although both toxins appear to interact synergistically in the pathogenesis of disease, enterotoxin A—negative isolates can still produce disease. Additionally, production of one or both toxins does not appear to be sufficient alone for disease (e.g., carriage of *C. difficile* and high levels of toxins are common in young children, but disease is rare). Bacterial "surface-layer proteins" (SLPs) are important for the binding of *C. difficile* to the intestinal epithelium, leading to localized production of toxins and subsequent tissue damage.

C. difficile is part of the normal intestinal flora in a small number of healthy people and hospitalized patients. The disease develops in people taking antibiotics, because the drugs alter the normal enteric flora, either permitting the overgrowth of these relatively resistant organisms or making the patient more susceptible to the exogenous acquisition of *C. difficile*. The disease occurs if the organisms proliferate in the colon and produce their toxins.

In 2003, disease caused by a highly virulent stain of *C. difficile* was reported in communities and hospitals in Canada, the United States, and Europe. This strain is responsible for more severe disease, a high mortality rate, increased risk of relapse, and more complications. The increased virulence of this strain is the result of a mutation in the gene that regulates production of the enterotoxin and cytotoxin. Because the regulatory gene is nonfunctional, there is a 16- to 23-fold **increase in toxin production**. This new strain of *C. difficile* also produces another toxin, binary toxin, that is a useful marker for this strain but has unknown clinical significance. Unlike most isolates of *C. difficile*, this strain is resistant to fluoroquinolone

Box 39—6. Summary: *Clostridium difficile*

Biology, Virulence, and Disease

Most strains produce two toxins: an enterotoxin that attracts neutrophils and stimulates their release of cytokines, and a cytotoxin that increases permeability of the intestinal wall, producing subsequent diarrhea

Spore formation allows the organism to persist in the hospital environment and resist decontamination efforts

Resistance to antibiotics such as clindamycin, cephalosporins, and fluoroquinolones allows *C. difficile* to overgrow the normal intestinal bacteria and produce disease in patients exposed to these antibiotics

Epidemiology

Colonizes the intestines of a small proportion of healthy individuals (<5%)

Exposure to antibiotics is associated with overgrowth of *C. difficile* and subsequent disease (endogenous infection)

Spores can be detected in hospital rooms of infected patients (particularly around beds and in the bathrooms); these can be an exogenous source of infection

A highly virulent stain of *C. difficile* currently causes disease in communities and hospitals in Canada, the United States, and Europe

Diagnosis

C. difficile disease is confirmed by detecting the cytotoxin or enterotoxin in the patient's feces

Treatment, Prevention, and Control

The implicated antibiotic should be discontinued

Treatment with metronidazole or vancomycin should be used in severe disease

Relapse is common because antibiotics do not kill spores; a second course of therapy with the same antibiotic is usually successful, although multiple courses may be necessary

The hospital room should be carefully cleaned after the infected patient is discharged

Figure 39—6. Antibiotic-associated colitis: gross section of the lumen of the colon. Note the white plaques of fibrin, mucus, and inflammatory cells overlying the normal red intestinal mucosa.

antibiotics. Because fluoroquinolones are widely used in the community and hospitals, it is believed that this practice has selected for this virulent strain.

The diagnosis of *C. difficile* infection is confirmed by demonstration of the enterotoxin or cytotoxin in a stool specimen from a patient with compatible clinical symptoms. Isolation of the organism in stool culture documents colonization but not disease. The enterotoxin and cytotoxin can be detected with a number of commercial immunoassays. These assays vary in sensitivity and specificity, so care must be used in selecting the appropriate test, and a negative test result does not exclude the diagnosis.

The cytotoxin can also be detected by an in vivo cytotoxicity assay using tissue culture cells and specific neutralizing antibodies for the cytotoxin; however, this assay is technically cumbersome and requires 1 to 2 days before results are available. Most laboratories have replaced the cytotoxicity assay with immunoassay methods.

Discontinuation of the implicated antibiotic (e.g., ampicillin, clindamycin, fluoroquinolones) is generally sufficient to alleviate mild disease. However, specific therapy with **metronidazole** or **vancomycin** is necessary for the management of severe diarrhea or colitis. Relapses may occur in as many as 20% to 30% of patients after the completion of therapy, because only the vegetative forms of *C. difficile* are killed by the antibiotics; the spores are resistant. A second course of treatment with the same antibiotic is frequently successful, although multiple relapses are well documented in some patients. It is difficult to prevent the disease, because the organism commonly exists in hospitals, particularly in areas adjacent to infected patients (e.g., beds, bathrooms). The spores of *C. difficile* are difficult to eliminate unless thorough housekeeping measures are used. Thus the organism can contaminate an environment for many months and can be a major source of nosocomial outbreaks of *C. difficile* disease.

Other Clostridial Species

Many other clostridia have been associated with clinically significant disease. Their virulence is a result of their ability to survive exposure to oxygen by forming spores and producing many diverse toxins and enzymes. ***C. septicum*** (Figures 39-8 and 39-9) is a particularly important pathogen because it is a cause of nontraumatic myonecrosis and often exists in patients with occult colon cancer, acute

Figure 39—7. Antibiotic-associated colitis caused by *Clostridium difficile*. A histologic section of colon shows an intense inflammatory response, with the characteristic "plaque" (*black arrow*) overlying the intact intestinal mucosa (*white arrow*). (Hematoxylin and eosin stain.) (*From Lambert HP, Farrar WE (eds): Infectious Diseases Illustrated. London, Gower, 1982.*)

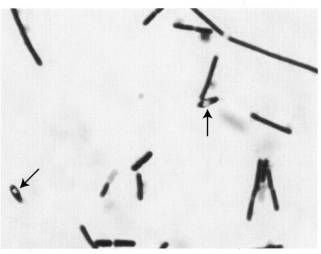

Figure 39—8. *Clostridium septicum*: note the spores (*arrows*) within the rods.

Figure 39—9. *Clostridium septicum.* Note how the growth "swarms" across the surface of the blood agar plate (*arrow*). This rapid spreading growth is also characteristic of rapid progression of disease in an infected patient.

leukemia, or diabetes. If the integrity of the bowel mucosa is compromised and the patient's body is less able to mount an effective response to the organism, *C. septicum* can spread into tissue and rapidly proliferate, producing gas and tissue destruction (Figure 39-10). Most patients have a fulminant course, dying within 1 to 2 days after initial presentation. *C. sordellii* is implicated in fatal toxic shock syndrome associated with natural childbirth or medically induced abortions (Clinical Case 39-5). *C. tertium* is another important clostridia that is commonly isolated in soil samples. It has primarily been associated with traumatic wound infections (e.g., war wounds, a fall producing a soil-contaminated wound). This organism can pose a diagnostic challenge because it can grow on aerobically incubated agar media. The correct identification can be made once spores are observed and it is zdetermined that the organism grows better anaerobically.

Figure 39—10. Radiograph of the leg of a patient with myonecrosis caused by *C. septicum.* Note the gas (*arrows*) in the tissue.

Case Study and Questions

A 61-year-old woman with left-sided face pain came to the emergency department of a local hospital. She was unable to open her mouth because of facial muscle spasms and had been unable to eat for 4 days because of severe pain in her jaw. Her attending physician had noted trismus and risus sardonicus. The patient reported that 1 week before presentation, she had incurred a puncture wound to her toe while walking in her garden. She had cleaned the wound and removed small pieces of wood from it, but she had not sought medical attention. Although she had received tetanus immunizations as a child, she had not had a booster vaccination since she was 15 years old. The presumptive diagnosis of tetanus was made.

1. How should this diagnosis be confirmed?
2. What is the recommended procedure for treating this patient? Should management wait until the laboratory results are available? What is the long-term prognosis for this patient?
3. Compare the mode of action of the toxins produced by *C. tetani* and *C. botulinum.*
4. What virulence factors are produced by *C. perfringens*?
5. *C. perfringens* causes what diseases?
6. *C. difficile* causes what diseases? Why is it difficult to manage infections caused by this organism?

Reference to Student Consult Animation

Please visit *www.StudentConsult.com* to view an animation demonstrating the functions of *Clostridium difficile* enterotoxin and cytotoxin, *Clostridium botulinum* toxin, and *Clostridium tetani* toxin.

Bibliography

Boone J, Carman R: *Clostridium perfringens*: Food poisoning and antibiotic-associated diarrhea. Clin Microbiol Newsl 19:65-67, 1997.

Bryant A, et al: Clostridial gas gangrene, I and II. J Infect Dis 182:799-807, 808-815, 2000.

Calabi E, et al: Binding of *Clostridium difficile* surface layer proteins to gastrointestinal tissues. Infect Immun 70:5770-5778, 2002.

Fischer M, et al: Fatal toxic shock syndrome associated with *Clostridium sordellii* after medical abortion. N Engl J Med 353:2352-2360, 2005.

Gergen P, et al: A population-based serologic survey of immunity to tetanus in the United States. N Engl J Med 332:761-766, 1995.

Kelly C, LaMont JT: *Clostridium difficile* infection. Annu Rev Med 49:375-390, 1998.

Kuijper EJ, Coignard B, Tull P: Emergence of *Clostridium difficile*-associated disease in North America and Europe. Clin Microbiol Infect 12(6):2-18, 2006.

Lalli G, et al: The journey of tetanus and botulinum neurotoxins in neurons. Trends Microbiol 11:431-437, 2003.

Lindstrom M, Korkeala H: Laboratory diagnostics of botulism. Clin Microbiol Rev 19:298-314, 2006.

Midura T: Update: Infant botulism. Clin Microbiol Rev 9:119-125, 1996.

Shapiro R, Hatheway C, Swerdlow D: Botulism in the United States: A clinical and epidemiologic review. Ann Intern Med 129:221-228, 1998.

Stevens DL, Bryant AE: The role of clostridial toxins in the pathogenesis of gas gangrene. Clin Infect Dis 35(Suppl 1):S93-S100, 2002.

Voth DE, Ballard JD: *Clostridium difficile* toxins: Mechanism of action and role in disease. Clin Microbiol Rev 18:247-263, 2005.

Wilkins TD, Lyerly DM: *Clostridium difficile* testing: After 20 years, still challenging. J Clin Microbiol 41:531-534, 2003.

Anaerobic, Non-Spore-Forming, Gram-Positive Bacteria

The anaerobic gram-positive cocci and non-spore-forming rods are a heterogeneous group of bacteria that characteristically colonize the skin and mucosal surfaces. These organisms are opportunistic pathogens, typically responsible for endogenous infections and usually recovered in mixtures of aerobic and anaerobic bacteria. Additionally, most of these anaerobes have fastidious nutritional requirements and grow slowly on laboratory media. Thus the isolation and identification of individual strains are difficult and often time consuming. Fortunately, the appropriate management and treatment of most infections with these organisms can be based on the knowledge that a mixture of aerobic and anaerobic organisms is present in the clinical specimen and does not require the isolation and identification of the individual organisms.

Anaerobic Gram-Positive Cocci (Box 40-1)

At one time, all clinically significant anaerobic cocci were included in the genus *Peptostreptococcus*. Unfortunately, it was recognized that these organisms were organized in a single genus based primarily on their Gram stain morphology and inability to grow aerobically. More sophisticated methods have since been used to reclassify many of these species into six genera. The most common isolates are listed in Table 40-1. Although some anaerobic cocci are more virulent than others, and some are associated with specific diseases, biochemical separation of the different genera is generally unnecessary, and knowledge that an anaerobic coccus is associated with an infection is typically sufficient.

The anaerobic gram-positive cocci normally colonize the oral cavity, gastrointestinal tract, genitourinary tract, and skin. They produce infections when they spread from these sites to normally sterile sites. For example, bacteria colonizing the upper airways can cause sinusitis and pleuropulmonary infections; bacteria in the intestines can cause intraabdominal infections; bacteria in the genitourinary tract can cause endometritis, pelvic abscesses, and salpingitis; bacteria on the skin can cause cellulitis and soft-tissue infections; and bacteria that invade the blood can produce infections in bones and solid organs (Figure 40-1).

Laboratory confirmation of infections with anaerobic cocci is complicated by the following three factors: (1) care must be taken to prevent contamination of the clinical specimen with the anaerobic cocci that normally colonize the skin and mucosal surface; (2) the collected specimen must be transported in an oxygen-free container to prevent loss of the organisms; and (3) specimens should be cultured on nutritionally enriched media for a prolonged period (i.e., 5 to 7 days). Additionally, some species of staphylococci and streptococci grow initially in an anaerobic atmosphere only and may be mistaken for anaerobic cocci. However, these organisms eventually grow well in air supplemented with 10% carbon dioxide (CO_2), so they cannot be classified as anaerobes.

Anaerobic cocci are usually susceptible to **penicillin** and **carbapenems** (e.g., imipenem, meropenem). They have intermediate susceptibility to broad-spectrum cephalosporins, clindamycin, erythromycin, and the tetracyclines, and are resistant to the aminoglycosides (as are all anaerobes). Specific therapy is generally indicated in monomicrobic infections; however, because most infections with these organisms are polymicrobic, broad-spectrum therapy against aerobic and anaerobic bacteria is usually selected.

Anaerobic, Non-spore-forming, Gram-Positive Rods (see Box 40-1)

The non-spore-forming, gram-positive rods are a diverse collection of facultatively anaerobic or strictly anaerobic bacteria that colonize the skin and mucosal surfaces (Table 40-2). *Actinomyces*, *Mobiluncus*, *Lactobacillus*, and

Box 40–1. Important Anaerobic Gram-Positive Bacteria

Organism	Historical Derivation
Anaerobic Cocci	
Anaerococcus	*an*, "without"; *aer* "air"; *coccus*, "berry" or coccus (anaerobic coccus)
Finegoldia	Named after the American microbiologist S. *Finegold*
Micromonas	*micro*, "tiny"; *monas*, "cell" (tiny cell)
Peptostreptococcus	*pepto*, "cook" or "digest" (the digesting streptococcus)
Schleiferella	Named after the German microbiologist K.H. *Schleifer*
Anaerobic Rods	
Actinomyces	*aktinos*, "ray"; *mykes*, "fungus" (ray fungus, referring to the radial arrangement of filaments in granules)
Bifidobacterium	*bifidus*, "cleft"; *bakterion*, "small rod" (a small clefted or bifurcated rod)
Eubacterium	*eu*, "good" or "beneficial" (a beneficial rod; that is, a rod normally present)
Lactobacillus	*lacto*, "milk" (milk bacillus; organism originally recovered in milk; also, lactic acid is the primary metabolic product of fermentation)
Mobiluncus	*mobilis*, "capable of movement" or being active; *uncus*, "hook" (motile, curved rod)
Propionibacterium	*propionicum*, propionic acid (propionic acid is the primary metabolic product of fermentation)

Propionibacterium are well recognized opportunistic pathogens, whereas other genera such as *Bifidobacterium* and *Eubacterium* can be isolated in clinical specimens but rarely cause human disease.

Actinomyces

Physiology and Structure

Actinomyces organisms are facultatively anaerobic or strictly anaerobic, gram-positive rods. They are not acid-fast

Table 40–1. New Classification of Selected Anaerobic Cocci Formerly in the Genus *Peptostreptococcus*

Former Classification	New Classification
P. anaerobius	Unchanged
P. asaccharolyticus	*Peptoniphilus asaccharolyticus*
P. magnus	*Finegoldia magna*
P. micros	Unchanged
P. parvulus	*Atopobium parvulum*
P. prevotii	*Anaerococcus prevotii*

(in contrast to the morphologically similar *Nocardia* species), they grow slowly in culture, and they tend to produce **chronic, slowly developing infections**. They typically develop delicate filamentous forms or hyphae (resembling fungi) in clinical specimens or when isolated in culture

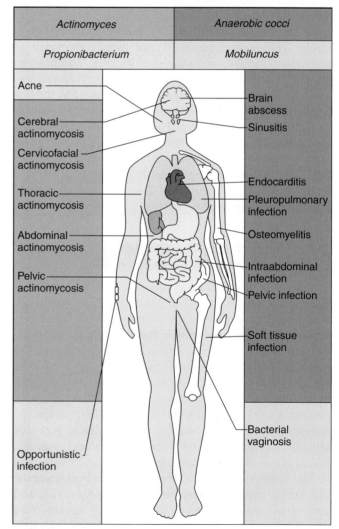

Figure 40–1. Diseases associated with anaerobic cocci, *Actinomyces*, *Propionibacterium*, and *Mobiluncus*, which are all anaerobic, non-spore-forming, gram-positive rods.

Table 40–2. Anaerobic, Non-spore-Forming, Gram-Positive Rods

Organism	Human Disease
Actinomyces spp.	Localized oral infections, actinomycosis (cervicofacial, thoracic, abdominal, pelvic, central nervous system)
Propionibacterium spp.	Acne, lacrimal canaliculitis, opportunistic infections
Mobiluncus spp.	Bacterial vaginosis, opportunistic infections
Lactobacillus spp.	Endocarditis, opportunistic infections
Eubacterium spp.	Opportunistic infections
Bifidobacterium spp.	Opportunistic infections

Figure 40–3. Sulfur granule collected from the sinus tract in a patient with actinomycosis. Delicate filamentous rods *(arrow)* are seen at the periphery of the crushed granule.

(Figure 40-2). However, these organisms are true bacteria in that they lack mitochondria and a nuclear membrane, reproduce by fission, and are inhibited by penicillin but not antifungal antibiotics. Numerous species have been described: *Actinomyces israelii*, *Actinomyces naeslundii*, *Actinomyces radingae*, and *Actinomyces turicensis* are responsible for most human infections

Pathogenesis and Immunity

Actinomyces organisms colonize the upper respiratory, gastrointestinal, and female genital tracts. These bacteria are not normally present on the skin surface. The organisms have a low virulence potential and cause disease only when the normal mucosal barriers are disrupted by trauma, surgery, or infection.

Classic disease caused by *Actinomyces* is termed **actinomycosis** (in keeping with the original idea that these organisms were fungi or "mycoses"). Actinomycosis is characterized by the development of chronic granulomatous lesions that become suppurative and form abscesses connected by sinus

tracts. Macroscopic colonies of organisms resembling grains of sand can frequently be seen in the abscesses and sinus tracts. These colonies, called **sulfur granules** because they appear yellow or orange, are masses of filamentous organisms bound together by calcium phosphate (Figure 40-3). The areas of suppuration are surrounded by fibrosing granulation tissue, which gives the surface overlying the involved tissues a hard or woody consistency. Actinomycosis is now relatively uncommon. Currently, most infections involving *Actinomyces* are polymicrobic, oral infections, such as endodontic infections, odontogenic abscesses, and dental-implant–associated infections.

Epidemiology

Infections caused by *Actinomyces* are **endogenous**, with no evidence of person-to-person spread or disease originating from an external source such as soil or water. Cervicofacial infections are seen in patients who have poor oral hygiene or have undergone an invasive dental procedure or oral trauma. In these patients, the *Actinomyces* that are present in the mouth invade into the diseased tissue and initiate the infectious process.

Patients with thoracic infections generally have a history of aspiration, with the disease becoming established in the lungs and then spreading to adjoining tissues. Abdominal infections most commonly occur in patients who have undergone gastrointestinal surgery or have suffered trauma to the bowel. Pelvic infection can be a secondary manifestation of abdominal actinomycosis or may be a primary infection in a woman with an intrauterine device (Figure 40-4). Central nervous system infections usually represent hematogenous spread from another infected tissue, such as the lungs.

Clinical Diseases (Clinical Case 40-1)

Most *Actinomyces* infections are the **cervicofacial** type (Figure 40-5). The disease may occur as an acute, pyogenic

Figure 40–2. Macroscopic colony *(left)* and Gram stain *(right)* of Actinomyces.

Figure 40—4. *Actinomyces* species can colonize the surface of foreign bodies, such as this intrauterine device, leading to the development of pelvic actinomycosis. *(From Smith E: In Lambert H, Farrar W (eds): Infectious Diseases Illustrated. London, Gower, 1982.)*

Clinical Case 40-1. Pelvic Actinomycosis

Quercia, et al. (Med Mal Infect 36:393-395, 2006) described a classic presentation of pelvic actinomycosis associated with an intrauterine contraceptive device (IUD). The patient is a 41-year-old woman who presented with a 5-month history of abdominal and pelvic pain, weight loss, malaise, and a yellow vaginal discharge. Since 1994 she had used an IUD, which was removed in June 2004. Her symptoms began soon after removal of the IUD. A CT-scan revealed a large pelvic mass involving the fallopian tubes, as well as numerous hepatic abscesses. A surgical biopsy was performed and *Actinomyces* was recovered in culture. She underwent surgical débridement and received oral therapy with a penicillin antibiotic for 1 year. The medical team thought the woman's pelvis was infected with *Actinomyces* at the time the IUD was removed. This episode illustrates the chronic nature of actinomycosis and the need for surgical drainage and long-term antibiotic therapy.

infection or as a slowly evolving, relatively painless process. The finding of tissue swelling with fibrosis and scarring, as well as draining sinus tracts along the angle of the jaw and neck, should alert the physician to the possibility of actinomycosis. Symptoms of **thoracic actinomycosis** are nonspecific. Abscesses may form in the lung tissue early in the disease and then spread into adjoining tissues as the disease progresses. **Abdominal actinomycosis** can spread throughout the abdomen, potentially involving virtually every organ system. **Pelvic actinomycosis** can occur as a relatively benign form of vaginitis or more commonly there can be extensive tissue destruction, including the development of tubo-ovarian abscesses or ureteral obstruction. The most common manifestation of **central nervous system actinomycosis** is a solitary brain abscess, but meningitis, subdural empyema, and epidural abscess are also seen.

Laboratory Diagnosis

Laboratory confirmation of actinomycosis is often difficult. Care must be used during collection of clinical specimens that they not become contaminated with *Actinomyces* that are part of the normal bacterial population on mucosal surfaces. The significance of *Actinomyces* isolated from contaminated specimens cannot be determined. Because the organisms are concentrated in sulfur granules and are sparse in involved tissues, a large amount of tissue or pus should be collected. If sulfur granules are detected in a sinus tract or in tissue, the granule should be crushed between two glass slides, stained, and examined microscopically. Thin, gram-positive, branching rods can be seen along the periphery of the granules.

    Actinomyces are fastidious and grow slowly under anaerobic conditions; it can take 2 weeks or more for the organisms to be isolated. Colonies appear white and have a domed surface that can become irregular after incubation for a week or more, resembling the top of a molar (Figure 40-6). The individual species of *Actinomyces* can be

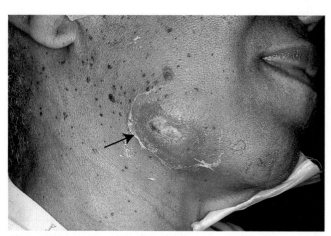

Figure 40—5. This patient is suffering from cervicofacial actinomycosis. Note the draining sinus tract.

Figure 40—6. Molar tooth appearance of *Actinomyces israelii* after incubation for 1 week. This colonial morphology serves as a reminder that the bacteria are normally found in the mouth.

differentiated by biochemical tests; however, this process can be time consuming. Generally, it is necessary to determine only that the isolate is a member of the genus *Actinomyces*.

Recovery of *Actinomyces* in blood cultures should be evaluated carefully. Most isolates represent transient, insignificant bacteremia from the oropharynx or gastrointestinal tract. If the isolate is clinically significant, evidence of tissue pathology should be obtained.

Treatment, Prevention, and Control

Treatment for actinomycosis involves the combination of drainage of a localized abscess or **surgical débridement** of the involved tissues and the prolonged administration of antibiotics. *Actinomyces* are uniformly susceptible to **penicillin** (considered the antibiotic of choice), carbapenems, macrolides, and clindamycin. Most species are resistant to metronidazole, and the tetracyclines have variable activity. An undrained focus should be suspected in patients with infections that do not appear to respond to prolonged therapy (e.g., 4 to 12 months). The clinical response is generally good, even in patients who have suffered extensive tissue destruction. Maintenance of good oral hygiene and the use of appropriate antibiotic prophylaxis when the mouth or gastrointestinal tract is penetrated can lower the risk of these infections.

Propionibacterium

Propionibacteria are small, gram-positive rods often arranged in short chains or clumps (Figure 40-7). They are commonly found on the skin (in contrast with the *Actinomyces*), conjunctiva, external ear, and in the oropharynx and female genital tract. The organisms are anaerobic or aerotolerant, nonmotile, catalase positive, and capable of fermenting carbohydrates, producing propionic acid as their major byproduct (hence the name). The two most commonly isolated species are *Propionibacterium acnes* and *Propionibacterium propionicum*.

Figure 40—7. Gram stain of *Propionibacterium* in a blood culture.

Clinical Case 40-2. Shunt Infected with *Propionibacterium*

Chu, et al. (Neurosurgery 49:717-720, 2001) reported three patients with central nervous system (CNS) infections with *Propionibacterium acnes*. The following patient illustrates the problems with this organism. A 38-year-old woman with congenital hydrocephalus presented with a 1-week history of decreased level of consciousness, headaches, and emesis. She had undergone numerous ventriculoperitoneal shunt placements in the past, with the last one placed 5 years before this presentation. The patient was afebrile and had no meningeal signs, but she was somnolent and arousable only to deep stimuli. CSF collected from the shunt contained no erythrocytes but had 55 WBCs; protein levels were high and glucose slightly low. Pleomorphic, gram-positive rods were observed on Gram stain, and *P. acnes* grew in the anaerobic culture of the CSF. After 1 week of therapy with high-dose penicillin, the CSF remained positive by Gram stain and culture. The patient was taken to surgery, where all foreign material was removed, and the patient was treated with penicillin for an additional 10 weeks. This patient illustrates the chronic, relatively asymptomatic nature of this disease, the need to remove the shunt and other foreign bodies, and the need to treat for a prolonged period of time.

P. acnes is responsible for two types of infections: (1) **acne vulgaris** (as the name implies) in teenagers and young adults and (2) **opportunistic infections** (Clinical Case 40-2) in patients with prosthetic devices (e.g., artificial heart valves or joints) or intravascular lines (e.g., catheters, cerebrospinal fluid shunts). Propionibacteria are also commonly isolated in blood cultures, but this finding usually represents contamination with bacteria on the skin at the phlebotomy site.

The central role of *P. acnes* in acne is to stimulate an inflammatory response. Production of a low-molecular-weight peptide by bacteria residing in sebaceous follicles attracts leukocytes. The bacteria are phagocytized and, after release of bacterial hydrolytic enzymes (lipases, proteases, neuraminidase, and hyaluronidase), stimulate a localized inflammatory response. *P. propionicum* is associated with endodontic abscesses and lacrimal canaliculitis (inflammation of the tear duct).

Propionibacteria can grow on most common media, although it may take 2 to 5 days for growth to appear. Care must be taken to avoid contamination of the specimen with the organisms normally found on the skin. The significance of the recovery of an isolate must also be interpreted in light of the clinical presentation (e.g., a catheter or other foreign body can serve as a focus for these opportunistic pathogens).

Acne is unrelated to the effectiveness of skin cleansing, because the lesion develops within the sebaceous follicles. For this reason, acne is managed primarily through the topical application of benzoyl peroxide and antibiotics. Antibiotics such as erythromycin and clindamycin have proved effective for treatment.

Figure 40—8. Gram stain of *Mobiluncus*. The cells are curved and have pointed ends.

Mobiluncus

Members of the genus *Mobiluncus* are obligate anaerobic, gram-variable or gram-negative, curved rods with tapered ends. Despite their appearance in Gram-stained specimens (Figure 40-8), they are classified as gram-positive rods because they (1) have a gram-positive cell wall, (2) lack endotoxin, and (3) are susceptible to vancomycin, clindamycin, erythromycin, and ampicillin but resistant to colistin. The organisms are fastidious, growing slowly even on enriched media supplemented with rabbit or horse serum.

Of the two species of *Mobiluncus*, **M. curtisii** is rarely found in the vaginas of healthy women but is abundant in women with **bacterial vaginosis** (vaginitis). Their microscopic appearance is a useful marker for this disease, but the precise role of these organisms in the pathogenesis of bacterial vaginosis is unclear.

Lactobacillus

Lactobacillus species are facultatively anaerobic or strictly anaerobic rods. They are found as part of the normal flora of the mouth, stomach, intestines, and genitourinary tract. The organisms are most commonly isolated in urine specimens and blood cultures. Because lactobacilli are the most common organism in the urethra, their recovery in urine cultures usually is a result of contamination of the specimen, even when large numbers of the organisms are present. The reason lactobacilli rarely cause infections of the urinary tract is their inability to grow in urine. Invasion into blood occurs in one of the following three settings: (1) **transient bacteremia** from a genitourinary source (e.g., after childbirth or a gynecologic procedure), (2) **endocarditis** (Clinical Case 40-3), and (3) **opportunistic septicemia** in an immunocompromised patient. Strains of lactobacilli are used as probiotics and have occasionally been associated with human infections.

Treatment of endocarditis and opportunistic infections is difficult because lactobacilli are resistant to vancomycin (an antibiotic commonly active against gram-positive bacteria) and are inhibited but not killed by other antibiotics. A combination of **penicillin with an aminoglycoside** is required for bactericidal activity.

Bifidobacterium and Eubacterium

Bifidobacterium and *Eubacterium* species are commonly found in the oropharynx, large intestine, and vagina. These bacteria can be isolated in clinical specimens but have a very low virulence potential and usually represent clinically insignificant contaminants. Confirmation of their etiologic role in an infection requires their repeated isolation in large numbers from multiple specimens and the absence of other pathogenic organisms.

Case Study and Questions

A 41-year-old man entered the university hospital for the treatment of a chronically draining wound in his jaw. The patient had undergone extraction of many teeth 3 months before admission and had poor oral hygiene and fetid breath at the time of admission. Multiple pustular nodules were observed overlying the carious teeth, and some nodules had ruptured. The drainage material consisted of serosanguineous fluid containing small, hard granules.

1. The diagnosis of actinomycosis is considered. How would you collect and transport specimens for confirmation of this diagnosis? What diagnostic tests can be performed?

2. Describe the epidemiology of actinomycosis. What is the risk factor for this patient?

3. What diseases does *Propionibacterium* cause? What is the most common source of this organism?

Bibliography

Brook I, Frazier EH: Infections caused by *Propionibacterium* species. Rev Infect Dis 3:819-822, 1991.

Cannon JP, et al: Pathogenic relevance of *Lactobacillus*: A retrospective review of over 200 cases. Eur J Clin Microbiol Infect Dis 24:31-40, 2005.

Hofstad T: Current taxonomy of medically important nonsporing anaerobes. Rev Infect Dis 12(Suppl):122-126, 1990.

Hollick G: Isolation and identification of aerobic actinomycetes. Clin Microbiol Newsl 17:25-29, 1995.

Murdoch D: Gram-positive anaerobic cocci. Clin Microbiol Rev 11:81-120, 1998.

Pulverer G, Schutt-Gerowitt H, Schaal KP: Human cervicofacial actinomycoses: Microbiological data for 1997 cases. Clin Infect Dis 37:490-497, 2003.

Smego RA: Actinomycosis of the central nervous system. Rev Infect Dis 9:855-865, 1987.

Stackebrandt E, Rainey F, Ward-Rainey N: Proposal for a new hierarchic classification system, *Actinobacteria classis* nov. Int J Syst Bacteriol 47:479-491, 1997.

Tiveljung A, Forsum U, Monstein HJ: Classification of the genus *Mobiluncus* based on comparative partial 16S rRNA gene analysis. Int J Syst Bacteriol 46:332-336, 1996.

Mycoplasma and *Ureaplasma*

The class of organisms Mollicutes is subdivided into five families with almost 200 species. Sixteen species of the family Mycoplasmataceae colonize humans, and five species are associated with human disease. The most important species is *Mycoplasma pneumoniae* (also called **Eaton agent** after the investigator who originally isolated it). *M. pneumoniae* causes respiratory tract diseases such as tracheobronchitis and pneumonia (Box 43-1). Other commonly isolated pathogens include *Mycoplasma genitalium*, *Mycoplasma hominis*, and *Ureaplasma urealyticum* (Table 43-1).

Physiology and Structure

Mycoplasma and *Ureaplasma* organisms are the **smallest free-living bacteria**. They are unique among bacteria because they **do not have a cell wall**, and their cell membrane contains **sterols**. In contrast, other cell-wall-deficient bacteria (called **L forms**) do not have sterols in their cell membrane and can form cell walls under the appropriate growth conditions. The absence of the cell wall renders the mycoplasmas resistant to penicillins, cephalosporins, vancomycin, and other antibiotics that interfere with synthesis of the cell wall.

The mycoplasmas form pleomorphic shapes varying from 0.2 to 0.3 μm coccoid forms to rods 0.1 to 0.2 μm in width and 1 to 2 μm long. Many can pass through the 0.45-μm filters used to remove bacteria from solutions, which was why the mycoplasmas were originally thought to be viruses. However, the organisms divide by binary fission (typical of all bacteria), grow on artificial cell-free media, and contain both ribonucleic acid (RNA) and deoxyribonucleic acid (DNA). Mycoplasmas are facultatively anaerobic (except *M. pneumoniae*, which is a **strict aerobe**) and require exogenous sterols supplied by animal serum added to the growth medium. The mycoplasmas **grow slowly**, with a generation time of 1 to 16 hours, and most form small colonies that are difficult to detect without extended incubation.

Because the Mycoplasmataceae do not have a cell wall, the major antigenic determinants are membrane glycolipids and proteins. These antigens cross-react with human tissues and other bacteria.

Pathogenesis and Immunity

M. pneumoniae is an extracellular pathogen that adheres to the respiratory epithelium by means of a specialized attachment structure that forms at one end of the cell. The structure consists of a complex of adhesions proteins, with the **P1 adhesin** the most important. The adhesions interact specifically with sialated glycoprotein receptors at the base of cilia on the epithelial cell surface (and on the surface of erythrocytes). Ciliostasis then occurs, after which first the cilia, then the ciliated epithelial cells, are destroyed. The loss of these cells interferes with the normal clearance of the upper airways and permits the lower respiratory tract to become contaminated with microbes and mechanically irritated. This process is responsible for the persistent cough present in patients with symptomatic disease. *M. pneumoniae* functions as a superantigen, stimulating inflammatory cells to migrate to the site of infection and release cytokines, initially tumor necrosis factor-α (TNF-α) and interleukin-1 (IL-1) and later, IL-6. This process contributes to both the clearance of the bacteria and the observed disease.

Epidemiology

M. pneumoniae is a strict human pathogen. Respiratory disease (e.g., tracheobronchitis, pneumonia) caused by *M. pneumoniae* occurs worldwide throughout the year, with no consistent increase in seasonal activity. However, because disease caused by other infectious agents (e.g., *Streptococcus pneumoniae*, viruses) is more common during the cold months, *M. pneumoniae* disease is proportionally more

Box 43–1. Summary of *Mycoplasma pneumoniae*

Biology, Virulence, and Disease

The smallest free-living bacterium; able to pass through 0.45-μm pore filters
Absence of cell wall and a cell membrane containing sterols are unique among bacteria
Slow rate of growth (generation time, 6 hours); strict aerobe
P1 adhesin protein binds to base of cilia on epithelial cells, leading to eventual loss of ciliated epithelial cells
Stimulates migration of inflammatory cells and release of cytokines
Strict human pathogen
Refer to Table 43-1 for disease

Epidemiology

Worldwide disease with no seasonal incidence (in contrast to disease caused by most respiratory pathogens)
Primarily infects children between ages 5 and 15 years, but all populations susceptible to disease
Transmitted by inhalation of aerosolized droplet

Diagnosis

Refer to Table 43-2

Treatment, Prevention, and Control

Drug of choice is erythromycin, doxycycline, or newer fluoroquinolones
Immunity to reinfection is not lifelong, and vaccines have proved ineffective

common during the summer and fall. Epidemic disease occurs every 4 to 8 years. Disease is most common in school-age children and young adults (ages 5 to 15 years), although all age groups are susceptible.

It has been estimated that 2 million cases of *M. pneumoniae* pneumonia and 100,000 pneumonia-related hospitalizations occur annually in the United States. However, *M. pneumoniae* disease is not a reportable disease, and reliable diagnostic tests are not widely available, so the true incidence is not known.

M. pneumoniae colonizes the nose, throat, trachea, and lower airways of infected individuals and is spread via large respiratory droplets during coughing episodes. Infection usually spreads among classmates, family members, or other close contacts. The attack rate is higher in children than in adults (overall average, approximately 60%), presumably because most adults are partially immune from previous exposure. The incubation period and time of infectivity are prolonged; thus disease can persist for months. Infants, particularly females, are colonized with *M. hominis*, *M. genitalium*, and *Ureaplasma* species, with *Ureaplasma* organisms being isolated most often. Although carriage of these mycoplasmas usually does not persist, a small proportion of prepubertal children remains colonized. The incidence of genital mycoplasmas rises after puberty, corresponding to sexual activity. Approximately 15% of sexually active men and women are colonized with *M. hominis*, and 45% to 75% are colonized with *Ureaplasma*. The incidence of carriage in adults who are sexually inactive is no greater than that in prepubertal children. *M. pneumoniae* is not part of the normal mucosal flora of humans; however, prolonged carriage can occur following symptomatic disease.

Clinical Diseases (Clinical Case 43-1)

Exposure to *M. pneumoniae* typically results in **asymptomatic carriage**. The most common clinical presentation of *M. pneumoniae* infection is **tracheobronchitis**. Low-grade fever, malaise, headache, and a dry, nonproductive cough develop 2 to 3 weeks after exposure. Acute **pharyngitis** may also be present. Symptoms gradually worsen over the next few days and can persist for 2 weeks or longer. The bronchial passages primarily become infiltrated with lymphocytes and plasma cells. Pneumonia (referred to as primary **atypical pneumonia** or walking pneumonia) can also develop, with a patchy bronchopneumonia seen on chest radiographs that is typically more impressive than the physical findings. Myalgias and gastrointestinal tract symptoms are uncommon. Secondary complications include neurologic abnormalities (e.g., meningoencephalitis, paralysis, and myelitis), pericarditis, hemolytic anemia, arthritis, and mucocutaneous lesions.

Table 43–1. Clinically Important Mycoplasmataceae

Organism	Site	Human Disease
Mycoplasma pneumoniae	Respiratory tract	Tracheobronchitis, pharyngitis, pneumonia, secondary complications (neurologic, pericarditis, hemolytic anemia, arthritis, mucocutaneous lesions)
Mycoplasma genitalium	Genitourinary tract	Nongonococcal urethritis (NGU), pelvic inflammatory disease
Mycoplasma hominis	Respiratory tract, genitourinary tract	Pyelonephritis, postpartum fever, systemic infections in immunocompromised patients
Ureaplasma urealyticum	Respiratory tract, genitourinary tract	NGU, pyelonephritis, spontaneous abortion, premature birth

Clinical Case 43-1. Fatal *Mycoplasma pneumoniae* Pneumonia in a Young Adult

Caxboeck, et al. (Wien Klin Wochenschr 119:379-384, 2007) described an unusual case of fatal *M. pneumoniae* pneumonia in a previously healthy 18-year-old woman. Prior to admission to the hospital, she had seen her physician with respiratory complaints, and a chest radiograph was consistent with pneumonia. A fluoroquinolone antibiotic was prescribed, but she failed to respond. Upon admission to the hospital, she had a temperature of 40° C and a productive cough. Her antibiotic was changed to a macrolide and cephalosporin; however, she continued to deteriorate, with progression of the pulmonary infiltrates, development of bilateral pleural effusions, and evidence of liver failure. Despite aggressive antibiotic therapy and respiratory support, her disease progressed to hemorrhagic pneumonia with multiorgan failure, and she died on hospital day 35. Diagnosis of *M. pneumoniae* infection was based on positive serology and the lack of other respiratory pathogens by microscopy, culture, and antigen testing. Although diagnosis by culture or PCR would be more convincing, the case illustrates the susceptibility of adults to mycoplasma infections and the uncommon but well-recognized occurrence of serious complications in susceptible patients. It should also be noted that this patient most likely had an undiagnosed immune defect that increased her susceptibility to this pathogen.

Because the genitourinary tract is colonized with other *Mycoplasma* species and *Ureaplasma*, it is difficult to determine the role of these organisms in disease in individual patients. However, it is generally accepted that *M. genitalium* can cause nongonococcal urethritis (NGU) and pelvic inflammatory disease; *U. urealyticum* can cause NGU, pyelonephritis, and spontaneous abortion or premature birth; and *M. hominis* can cause pyelonephritis, postpartum fevers, and systemic infections in immunocompromised patients. The evidence implicating the organisms in these diseases is based on (1) recovery of the bacteria from specimens from infected patients, (2) a serologic response to the organism, (3) clinical improvement after treatment with specific antibiotics, (4) demonstration of disease in animal models, or (5) a combination of these findings.

Laboratory Diagnosis

The diagnostic tests for *M. pneumoniae* infections are summarized in Table 43-2.

Microscopy

Microscopy is of no diagnostic value. Mycoplasmas stain poorly because they have no cell wall.

Antigen Detection

Although antigen tests have been developed for the rapid diagnosis of *M. pneumoniae*, the tests have poor sensitivity and specificity and are not recommended.

Nucleic-Acid-Based Tests

PCR amplification tests of species-specific targets have been developed for all pathogenic *Mycoplasma* and *Ureaplasma* species. The tests have excellent sensitivity, but the specificity is not well defined; that is, these assays may cross-react with avirulent species that colonize humans. In addition, commercial PCR assays are not available at this time, so testing is primarily restricted to research and reference laboratories.

Culture

Unlike other mycoplasmas, *M. pneumoniae* is a strict aerobe. These mycoplasmas can be isolated from throat

Table 43–2. Diagnostic Tests for *Mycoplasma pneumoniae* Infections

Test	Assessment
Microscopy	Test is not useful, because organisms do not have a cell wall and do not stain with conventional reagents
Culture	Test is slow (2 to 6 weeks before positive diagnosis) and insensitive; it is not available in most laboratories
Molecular diagnosis	PCR-based amplification assays with excellent sensitivity; specificity is not well defined; expected to be the diagnostic test of choice when assays become more widely available
Serology: Complement fixation	Antibody titers vs. glycolipid antigens peak in 4 weeks and persist for 6-12 months; poor sensitivity and specificity
Enzyme immunoassays	Multiple assays available with varying sensitivity and specificity; assays directed vs. P1 adhesin protein may be most specific
Cold agglutinin	Sensitivity and specificity poor, with cross-reactions with other respiratory pathogens (e.g., Epstein-Barr virus, cytomegalovirus, adenovirus); test commonly used but not recommended

PCR, polymerase chain reaction.

washings, bronchial washings, or expectorated sputum. Washings are more reliable than sputum specimens, because most infected patients have a dry, nonproductive cough and do not produce sputum. The specimen should be inoculated into special media supplemented with serum (provides sterols), yeast extract (for nucleic acid precursors), glucose, a pH indicator, and penicillin (to inhibit other bacteria). The organisms grow slowly in culture, with a generation time of 6 hours.

Although a positive culture result is definitive evidence of disease, it is relatively **insensitive**. In one well-designed study, 36% of the isolates were detected within 2 weeks, whereas detection of the remaining isolates required prolonged incubation (as long as 6 weeks). In another study, only 64% of cultures from patients with serologic evidence of an acute *Mycoplasma* infection had positive results. Growth of the organisms in culture is indicated by the metabolism of glucose with a corresponding pH change.

Colonies of *M. pneumoniae* are small and have a homogeneous granular appearance ("mulberry shaped"), unlike the fried-egg morphology of other mycoplasmas. Identification of isolates can be confirmed by inhibition of their growth with specific antisera. However, because this organism is difficult to grow, and results are typically not available for many weeks, most laboratories do not perform cultures.

M. hominis is a facultative anaerobe that grows within 1 to 4 days and metabolizes arginine but not glucose. The colonies have a typical, large fried-egg appearance. Inhibition of their growth with specific antisera is used to differentiate them from other genital mycoplasmas. *Ureaplasma* requires urea for growth but is inhibited by the higher alkalinity resulting from the metabolism of urea. Thus the growth medium must be supplemented with urea and be highly buffered. Even if these steps are taken, ureaplasmas die rapidly after initial isolation.

Antibody Detection

Antibody-specific tests are available only for *M. pneumoniae*. Detection of antibodies directed against *M. pneumoniae* by complement fixation is the traditional serologic reference standard. However, the test has poor sensitivity, and antibodies directed against the target glycolipid antigen are also elicited by other *Mycoplasma* species and by host tissues. A number of enzyme immunoassays for the detection of immunoglobulin M (IgM) and IgG antibodies are available. In general, the tests are more sensitive than complement fixation tests and culture. The disadvantage with these tests is that sera have to be collected early in the course of disease and again after 3 to 4 weeks to demonstrate a rise in antibody levels.

Historically, it was also possible to measure nonspecific reactions to the outer membrane glycolipids of *M. pneumoniae*. The most useful of these reactions is the production of **cold agglutinins** (e.g., IgM antibodies that bind the I antigen on the surface of human erythrocytes at 4° C).

This test is insensitive and nonspecific, so it should not performed.

Treatment, Prevention, and Control

Erythromycin, tetracyclines (particularly doxycycline), and fluoroquinolones are equally effective in treating *M. pneumoniae* infections, although the tetracyclines and fluoroquinolones are reserved for use in adults. Tetracyclines have the advantage of also being active against most other mycoplasmas and chlamydia, a common cause of nongonococcal urethritis. Erythromycin is used to treat *Ureaplasma* infections because these organisms are resistant to tetracycline. Unlike the other mycoplasmas, *M. hominis* is resistant to erythromycin and occasionally to the tetracyclines. Clindamycin has been used to treat infections caused by these resistant strains.

The prevention of *Mycoplasma* disease is problematic. *M. pneumoniae* infections are spread by close contact; thus the isolation of infected people could theoretically reduce the risk of infection. Isolation is impractical, however, because patients are typically infectious for a prolonged period, even while receiving appropriate antibiotics. Inactivated vaccines and attenuated live vaccines have also proved disappointing. The protective immunity conferred by infection has been low. Infections with *M. hominis*, *M. genitalium*, and *Ureaplasma* are transmitted by sexual contact. Therefore these diseases can be prevented by avoidance of sexual activity or the use of proper barrier precautions.

Case Study and Questions

Increased lethargy, headache, cough, a low-grade fever, and chills and sweats at night developed in a 21-year-old university student. When she was seen at the student health center, she had a nonproductive cough and shortness of breath on exertion. Her pulse rate was 95 beats/min, and her respiratory rate was 28 breaths/min. Her pharynx was erythematous; scattered rhonchi and rales but no consolidation were noted on auscultation. Results of a chest radiograph showed patchy infiltrates. A Gram stain of sputum revealed many white blood cells but no organisms. The antibody titer for a *Mycoplasma* complement fixation test performed on a specimen collected at admission was 1:8; the titer for a specimen collected a week later was 1:32. The patient was treated with erythromycin, to which her disease responded slowly during the next 2 weeks.

1. If cultures were performed, what would be the best specimen? When would the results be available? What are the sensitivity and specificity of culture in a patient infected with *M. pneumoniae*?

2. How do *Mycoplasma* species differ from other bacteria?

3. Describe the epidemiology of *M. pneumoniae* infections. What aspects of this case are characteristic of such infections?

4. What other mycoplasmas cause human disease? What diseases do they cause?

Bibliography

Blasi F, et al: *Chlamydia pneumoniae* and *Mycoplasma pneumoniae*. Semin Respir Crit Care Med 26:617-624, 2005.

Loens K, et al: Molecular diagnosis of *Mycoplasma pneumoniae* respiratory tract infections. J Clin Microbiol 41:4915-4923, 2003.

Templeton KE, et al: Comparison and evaluation of real-time PCR, real-time nucleic acid sequence-based amplification, conventional PCR, and serology for diagnosis of *Mycoplasma pneumoniae*. J Clin Microbiol 41:4366-4371, 2003.

Waites K, Katz B, Schelonka R: Mycoplasmas and ureaplasmas as neonatal pathogens. Clin Microbiol Rev 18:757-789, 2005.

Waites K, Talkington D: *Mycoplasma pneumoniae* and its role as a human pathogen. Clin Microbiol Rev 17:697-728, 2004.

Waites K, Talkington D: New developments in human diseases due to mycoplasmas. In Blanchard A, Browning G (eds): Mycoplasmas: Pathogenesis, Molecular Biology, and Emerging Strategies for Control. Norwich, United Kingdom, Horizon Scientific, 2005, pp 289-354.

Rickettsia and Orientia

Rickettsia (named after Howard Ricketts), *Ehrlichia* (named after Paul Ehrlich), and *Coxiella* (named after Harold Cox) were historically classified in a single family, Rickettsiaceae, based on the observation that they were obligate, intracellular, aerobic, gram-negative rods. Analysis of their deoxyribonucleic acid (DNA) sequences revealed that this classification was invalid. Furthermore, it was observed that *Rickettsia* should be subdivided into two genera (*Rickettsia* and *Orientia*) and *Ehrlichia* into two genera (*Ehrlichia* and *Anaplasma*). *Rickettsia* and *Orientia* are discussed in this chapter, and the other two genera of intracellular organisms are discussed in Chapter 45.

The organisms of the family Rickettsiaceae are small (0.3 × 1 to 2 μm), structurally similar to gram-negative rods, although they stain poorly with the Gram stain, and grow only in the cytoplasm of eukaryotic cells. The pathogenic species of *Rickettsia* and *Orientia* (Box 44-1) are maintained in animal and arthropod reservoirs and are transmitted by arthropod vectors (e.g., ticks, mites, lice, fleas). Humans are accidental hosts. *Rickettsia* species are subdivided into the **spotted fever group** and the **typhus group**. At least 17 species of *Rickettsia* in the spotted fever group have been associated with human disease. ***Rickettsia rickettsii*** (Rocky Mountain spotted fever) and ***Rickettsia akari*** (rickettsialpox) will be discussed in this chapter. For a comprehensive review of other members of the spotted fever group distributed throughout the world, please refer to the review by Parola, et al. Two species of *Rickettsia* are members of the typhus group: ***R. prowazekii*** and ***R. typhi***. A single species is in the genus *Orientia*: ***O. tsutsugamushi***.

Rickettsiae are maintained in reservoir hosts, primarily rodents and their arthropod vectors (e.g., ticks, mites, fleas) (Figure 44-1). **Transovarian transmission** also maintains the bacteria in the arthropods, so they serve as both vector and host. The exception to this is *Rickettsia prowazekii*, for which humans are the primary host, and the arthropod vector is the human body louse. The bacteria kill the louse, so transovarian transmission is not important. The distribution of rickettsial diseases is determined by the distribution of the arthropod host/vector. Most infections with tick vectors (e.g., spotted fevers) have a restricted geographic distribution, whereas rickettsial infections with other vectors such as lice *(R. prowazekii)*, fleas *(Rickettsia typhi)*, and mites *(Rickettsia akari, Orientia tsutsugamushi)* have worldwide distribution (Table 44-1).

Physiology and Structure

The cell wall structures of *Rickettsia* are typical of gram-negative rods, with a peptidoglycan layer and lipopolysaccharide (LPS). However, the peptidoglycan layer is minimal (stains poorly with the Gram stain), and the LPS has only weak endotoxin activity. *Orientia* lacks both the peptidoglycan layer and LPS. The organisms are seen best with Giemsa or Gimenez stains (Figure 44-2). The bacteria do not have flagella, and *Rickettsia* is surrounded by a loosely adherent slime layer. *Rickettsia* and *Orientia* are strict intracellular parasites found free in the cytoplasm of infected cells.

The bacteria enter eukaryotic cells by attaching to host cell surface receptors and stimulating phagocytosis. After engulfment, *Rickettsia* and *Orientia* must degrade the phagosome membrane by producing a phospholipase and be released into the cytoplasm, or the organism will not survive. Multiplication in the host cell by binary fission is slow (generation time, 9 to 12 hours). *Orientia* and the spotted fever group of *Rickettsia* grow in the cytoplasm and nucleus of infected cells and are continually released from cells through long, cytoplasmic projections. In contrast, the typhus group accumulates in the cell cytoplasm until the cell membranes lyse, signaling cell death and bacterial release. It is believed that the fundamental difference is caused by intracellular motility—the spotted fever group is able to polymerize host cell actin, whereas the typhus group lacks the required gene. Once these bacteria are released from the host cell, they are unstable and die quickly.

The genomes of *R. prowazekii* have been sequenced, providing information about the parasitic nature of these bacteria.

Box 44–1. Important *Rickettsia* and *Orientia*

Organism	Historical Derivation
Rickettsia rickettsii	Named after Howard *Ricketts*, who implicated the wood tick as the vector of Rocky Mountain spotted fever
R. akari	*akari*, "mite"; the vector of rickettsialpox
R. prowazekii	Named after Stanislav von *Prowazek*, an early investigator of typhus who was a victim of this disease
R. typhi	*typhi*, "typhus" or "fever"
Orientia tsutsugamushi	*Orientia*, "Orient"; *tsutsugamushi*, "mite disease," the popular name of this disease in the Orient

Table 44–1. Distribution of *Rickettsia* and *Orientia* Species

Organism	Human Disease	Distribution
R. rickettsii	Rocky Mountain spotted fever	Western hemisphere (United States, Canada, Mexico, Panama, Costa Rica, Brazil, Colombia, Argentina)
R. akari	Rickettsialpox	United States, Ukraine, Croatia, Korea
R. prowazekii	Epidemic typhus	Worldwide
	Recrudescent typhus	Worldwide
	Sporadic typhus	United States
R. typhi	Endemic (murine) typhus	Worldwide
O. tsutsugamushi	Scrub typhus	Japan, eastern Asia, northern Australia, west and southwest Pacific

The bacteria depend on their host cell for many functions: carbohydrate metabolism, lipid biosynthesis, nucleotide synthesis, and amino acid synthesis. The bacteria are able to produce adenosine triphosphate (ATP) by means of the tricarboxylic acid cycle, or they can act as energy parasites, using the host cell ATP as long as it is available. *R. prowazekii* has a parasitic enzyme (ATP/ADP translocase) that facilitates transfer of ATP from the host cell to the bacteria.

Rickettsia rickettsii (Box 44-2)

Pathogenesis and Immunity

The most common rickettsiae causing human disease in the United States is *R. rickettsii*, the agent responsible for

Disease	Organism	Vector	Reservoir
Rocky Mountain spotted fever	*R. rickettsii*	Tick-borne	Ticks, wild rodents
Rickettsialpox	*R. akari*	Mite-borne	Mites, wild rodents
Scrub typhus	*O. tsutsugamushi*		Mites (chiggers), wild rodents
Epidemic typhus	*R. prowazekii*	Louse-borne	Humans, squirrel fleas, flying squirrels
Murine endemic typhus	*R. typhi*	Flea-borne	Wild rodents

Figure 44–1. Epidemiology of common *Rickettsia* and *Orientia* infections.

Rocky Mountain spotted fever. There is no evidence that *R. rickettsii* produces toxins or that the host's immune response is responsible for the pathologic manifestations of Rocky Mountain spotted fever. Outer membrane protein A (**OmpA**), expressed on the surface of *R. rickettsii*, is responsible for the ability of the bacteria to adhere to endothelial cells. After the bacteria penetrate into the cell, they are released from the phagosome, freely multiply in both the cytoplasm and nucleus, and move from cell to adjacent cell. The primary clinical manifestations appear to result from the replication of bacteria in endothelial cells, with subsequent damage to the cells and leakage of

Figure 44–2. Gimenez stain of tissue culture cells infected with spotted fever group *Rickettsia*. (*From Cohen J, Powderly WG: Infectious Diseases, 2nd ed. St Louis, Mosby, 2004.*)

Box 44-2. Summary: *Rickettsia rickettsii*

Biology, Virulence, and Disease

Small, intracellular bacteria
Stain poorly with Gram stain; best with Giemsa or Gimenez
 stains
Replication occurs in cytoplasm and nucleus of endothelial cells,
 with resulting vasculitis
Intracellular growth protects the bacteria from immune clearance
Rocky Mountain spotted fever characterized by high fever, severe
 headache, myalgias, and rash; complications common in
 untreated patients or where diagnosis is delayed

Epidemiology

R. rickettsii is most common rickettsial pathogen in United States
Hard ticks (e.g., dog tick, wood tick) are the primary reservoirs
 and vectors
Transmission requires prolonged contact
Distribution in Western hemisphere; in United States, infection is
 most common in south-Atlantic region
Disease is most common April through September

Diagnosis

Serology (e.g., microimmunofluorescence test) is used most
 commonly for diagnosis

Treatment, Prevention, and Control

Doxycycline is the drug of choice
People should avoid tick-infested areas, wear protective clothing,
 and use effective insecticides
People should remove attached ticks immediately
No vaccine is currently available

---

the blood vessels. Hypovolemia and hypoproteinemia caused by the loss of plasma into tissues can lead to reduced perfusion of various organs and organ failure. The host immune response to infection is based on cytokine-mediated intracellular killing and clearance by cytotoxic CD8 lymphocytes. Antibody response to rickettsial outer membrane proteins may also be important.

Epidemiology

In 2006, almost 2300 cases of Rocky Mountain spotted fever were reported in the United States, the highest incidence ever recorded (Figure 44-3). Over 90% of the infections occurred from **April to September**, corresponding to the period of greatest tick activity, with the majority of infections reported in the south-Atlantic region of the United States. The distribution of disease mimics the distribution of the principal reservoir and vector for *R. rickettsii*, **hard ticks** in the family Ixodidae. The two hard ticks most commonly associated with disease in the United States are the **dog tick (Dermacentor variabilis)** in the southeastern states and the West Coast and the **wood tick (Dermacentor andersoni)** in the Rocky Mountain states and southwestern Canada. Other tick vectors have been identified in Central and South America. To become infected, a person must be exposed to the tick for a lengthy period (e.g., 6 hours or more). The dormant avirulent rickettsiae are activated by the warm blood meal, then must be released from the tick salivary glands to penetrate into the blood of the human host.

Clinical Diseases (Clinical Case 44-1)

Clinically symptomatic diseases develop 7 days (range, 2 to 14 days) after the tick bite (Table 44-2). The patient may not

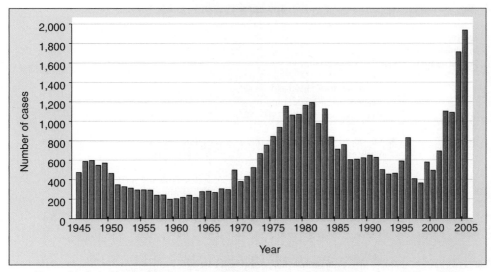

Figure 44–3. Incidence of Rocky Mountain spotted fever in the United States from 1945 to 2005.

Clinical Case 44-1. Rocky Mountain Spotted Fever

Oster and associates (N Engl J Med 297:859-863, 1977) described a series of patients who acquired Rocky Mountain spotted fever after working with *R. rickettsii* in the laboratory. One patient, a 21-year-old veterinary technician, presented to a clinic with complaints of myalgia and a nonproductive cough. He was treated with penicillin and discharged. Over the next few days, he developed chills and a headache. When he returned to the hospital, he had a temperature of 40° C and a macular rash on his extremities and trunk. Intramuscular tetracycline was started, but he remained febrile, and the rash evolved to petechiae on his trunk, extremities, and soles of his feet. Bilateral pleural effusions developed, and IV tetracycline was begun. Over the next 2 weeks, the effusions resolved, and the patient made a slow but uneventful recovery. Although this patient was not working directly with *R. rickettsii*, he had visited a lab that was processing the bacterium. This patient illustrates the characteristic presentation of Rocky Mountain spotted fever: headache, fever, myalgias, and a macular rash that can evolve into a petechial or "spotted" rash.

recall the painless tick bite. The onset of disease is heralded by a high fever and headache that may be associated with malaise, myalgias, nausea, vomiting, abdominal pain, and diarrhea. A macular rash develops in 90% of patients after 3 days, initially on the wrists, arms, and ankles, and then spreads to the trunk. The palms and soles can also be involved. The rash can evolve to the "spotted" or petechial form, which is a harbinger of more severe disease. Complications of Rocky Mountain spotted fever include neurologic manifestations, pulmonary and renal failure, and cardiac abnormalities. A delay in diagnosis, either because the clinical presentation is not characteristic or the physician does not recognize the disease, is associated with a worse prognosis. The fatality rate in untreated disease is 10% to 25%.

Laboratory Diagnosis

Microscopy

Although rickettsiae stain poorly with Gram stain, they can be stained with Giemsa or Gimenez stains. Specific fluorescein-labeled antibodies can also be used to stain the intracellular bacteria in biopsy tissue specimens. This direct detection of rickettsial antigens is a rapid, specific method for confirming the clinical diagnosis of Rocky Mountain spotted fever but is primarily available only through reference labs.

Nucleic-Acid-Based Tests

PCR assays and gene sequencing are now used in many reference laboratories for the diagnosis of rickettsial diseases. A variety of gene targets is used, including gene sequences for outer membrane proteins (OmpA, OmpB), 17-kDa lipoprotein, and citrate synthase. Unfortunately, conventional PCR assays are relatively insensitive when blood samples are used.

Culture

Although isolation of rickettsiae in tissue culture systems or embryonated eggs is relatively easy, only reference labs with extensive experience with rickettsiae routinely perform these cultures. If culture is attempted, buffy coat preparations of blood or skin biopsy specimens should be processed.

Antibody Detection

Although the **Weil-Felix test** (which involves the differential agglutination of cross-reacting *Proteus* antigens) has been used historically for the diagnosis of rickettsial infections, it is no longer recommended, because it is insensitive and nonspecific. Unfortunately, this test is frequently used in laboratories with limited resources. The serology test

Table 44—2. Clinical Course of Human Diseases Caused by *Rickettsia* and *Orientia* Species

Disease	Average Incubation Period (days)	Clinical Presentation	Rash	Eschar	Mortality without Treatment (%)
Rocky Mountain spotted fever	7	Abrupt onset; fever, headache, malaise, myalgias, nausea, vomiting, abdominal pain	>90%; macular; centripetal spread	No	10-25
Rickettsialpox	9-14	Abrupt onset; fever, headache, chills, myalgias, photophobia	100%; papulovesicular; generalized	Yes	Low
Epidemic typhus	8	Abrupt onset; fever, headache, chills, myalgias, arthralgia	20%-80%; macular; centrifugal spread	No	20
Endemic typhus	7-14	Gradual onset; fever, headache, myalgias, cough	50%; maculopapular rash on trunk	No	Low
Scrub typhus	10-12	Abrupt onset; fever, headache, myalgias	<50%; maculopapular rash; centrifugal spread	No	1-15

that is considered the reference method is the microimmunofluorescence (MIF) test. The test detects antibodies directed against outer membrane proteins (species-specific) and the LPS antigen. Because the LPS antigen is shared among rickettsial species, the Western blot immunoassay must be performed to define the individual species. The sensitivity and specificity of MIF is high, with diagnostic levels of antibodies generally detected in the second week of illness. Commercially prepared enzyme immunoassays are also available but generally have a lower sensitivity and specificity when compared with MIF.

Treatment, Prevention, and Control

The drug of choice for treating all rickettsial infections is **doxycycline**. Although the tetracyclines are generally contraindicated for pregnant women and young children, this antibiotic is recommended for all patients with suspected rickettsial disease, because it is the most effective antibiotic, and inadequately treated disease is associated with a high morbidity and mortality. Fluoroquinolones (e.g., ciprofloxacin) have good in vitro activity, but clinical experience is inadequate to recommend this for primary therapy. Chloramphenicol also has activity in vitro against rickettsiae, but its use for treatment of infections is associated with a higher incidence of relapse. The prompt diagnosis and institution of appropriate therapy usually result in a satisfactory prognosis; unfortunately, this scenario may not occur if key clinical signs (e.g., rash) develop late or not at all. In addition, the serologic findings often are not available until 2 or more weeks after the onset of disease, also delaying the start of treatment. Therefore, it is recommended that empiric therapy with doxycycline be started as soon as the diagnosis is considered.

There is no vaccine for Rocky Mountain spotted fever. Thus avoidance of tick-infested areas, the use of protective clothing and insect repellents, and the prompt removal of attached ticks are the best preventive measures. It is virtually impossible to eliminate the tick reservoir, because the ticks can survive for as long as 4 years without feeding.

Rickettsia akari

R. akari, the agent responsible for causing **rickettsialpox**, is one of the few rickettsiae in the spotted fever group that has a **cosmopolitan** distribution and is transmitted by infected **mites**. Culture-confirmed disease has been reported from the Ukraine, Croatia, Korea, and the United States, primarily in the New York City area. A cluster of cases was documented in New York City following the release of *Bacillus anthracis* in 2001, when biopsies of eschars from city residents were demonstrated to contain *R. akari* and not *B. anthracis* (Clinical Case 44-2). Based on this experience, it is likely that rickettsialpox is underdiagnosed in endemic areas.

Clinical Case 44-2. Rickettsialpox in New York City

Koss, et al. (Arch Dermatol 139:1545-1552, 2003) described 18 patients with rickettsialpox who were diagnosed at Columbia Presbyterian Medical Center in New York City in a 20-month period after the anthrax bioterrorism attack in the fall of 2001. The patients presented to the hospital because they had a necrotic eschar and were thought to have cutaneous anthrax. The patients also had fever, headache, and a papulovesicular rash. Many patients also complained of myalgias, sore throat, arthralgias, and gastrointestinal symptoms. Immunohistochemical staining of eschar and skin biopsies confirmed the diagnosis of rickettsialpox and not cutaneous anthrax. These patients illustrate the diagnostic difficulties of recognizing uncommon diseases, even when the clinical presentation is characteristic.

Infections with *R. akari* are maintained in the rodent population through the bite of mouse ectoparasites (e.g., mites) and in mites by transovarian transmission. Humans become accidental hosts when bitten by infected mites.

Clinical infection with *R. akari* is biphasic. First, a papule develops at the site where the mite has bitten the host. The papule appears approximately 1 week after the bite and quickly progresses to ulceration and then **eschar formation**. During this period, the rickettsiae spread systemically. After an incubation period of 7 to 24 days (average, 9 to 14 days), the second phase of the disease develops abruptly, with high **fever**, severe headache, chills, sweats, myalgias, and photophobia. A generalized papulovesicular **rash** forms within 2 to 3 days. A poxlike progression of the rash is then seen, in which vesicles form and then crust over. Presence of the rash distinguishes this disease from anthrax and, in a patient with a high fever and eschar, should raise the clinical diagnosis of rickettsialpox. Despite the appearance of the disseminated rash, rickettsialpox is usually mild and uncomplicated, and complete healing is seen within 2 to 3 weeks without treatment. Specific therapy with doxycycline speeds the process.

Rickettsia prowazekii (Box 44-3)

Epidemiology

R. prowazekii, one of two members of the typhus group of rickettsiae, is the etiologic agent of **epidemic** or **louse-borne typhus**. *Humans are the principal reservoir* of this disease, and the vector is the **human body louse**, *Pediculus humanus*. Epidemic typhus occurs among people living in crowded, unsanitary conditions that favor the spread of body lice—conditions such as those that arise during wars, famines, and natural disasters. Lice die from their infection within 2 to 3 weeks, preventing the transovarian transmission of *R. prowazekii*. The disease is present in Central and South America, Africa, and less commonly in the United States.

Box 44–3. Summary: *Rickettsia prowazekii*

Biology, Virulence, and Disease

Small, intracellular bacteria
Stain poorly with Gram stain; best with Giemsa or Gimenez stains
Replicate in cytoplasm of endothelial cells, with resulting vasculitis
Intracellular growth protects the bacteria from immune clearance
Epidemic typhus (louse-borne typhus) characterized by high fever, severe headache, and myalgias
Recrudescent typhus (Brill-Zinsser disease) is a milder form of the disease

Epidemiology

Humans are the primary reservoir, with person-to-person transmission by louse vector
It is believed that sporadic disease is spread from squirrels to humans via squirrel fleas
Recrudescent disease can develop years after initial infection
People at greatest risk are those living in crowded, unsanitary conditions
Disease is worldwide, with most infections in Central and South America and Africa
Sporadic disease is seen in the eastern United States

Diagnosis

The MIF test is the test of choice

Treatment, Prevention, and Control

Doxycycline is the drug of choice
Controlled through improvements in living conditions and reduction of the lice population through use of insecticides
Inactivated vaccine is available for high-risk populations

The incidence of the disease in the United States is unknown, because it is not a disease reportable to public health departments. Sporadic disease in the United States is primarily restricted to rural areas of the eastern states. In this area **flying squirrels**, as well as squirrel fleas and lice, are infected with *R. prowazekii*. Squirrel lice do not feed on humans, but the fleas are less discriminating and may be responsible for transmitting the *Rickettsia* from squirrels to humans. Epidemiologic and serologic evidence supports this hypothesis, but such transmission has not been documented.

Recrudescent disease with *R. prowazekii* (**Brill-Zinsser disease**) can occur in people years after their initial infection. Such people in the United States are primarily Eastern European immigrants who were exposed to epidemic typhus during World War II.

Clinical Diseases

In one study of epidemic typhus in Africa, clinical disease was found to develop an average of 8 days after exposure

(range, 2 to 30 days). Most of the patients initially had nonspecific symptoms; then within 1 to 3 days, high **fever**, severe **headache**, and **myalgias**. Other symptoms can include pneumonia, arthralgia, and neurological involvement (stupor, confusion, and coma). A petechial or macular rash develops in 20% to 80% of patients, but this may be obscured in darkly pigmented individuals. The mortality rate in the absence of treatment is 20% to 30% but may be much higher in populations with poor general health and nutrition and lacking proper supportive medical care. In patients with uncomplicated disease, the body temperature returns to normal within 2 weeks, but complete convalescence may take 3 months or longer. The rickettsiae may remain dormant for years and then reactivate to cause recrudescent epidemic typhus or Brill-Zinsser disease. At the time symptoms develop, bacteremia occurs, and the patient is potentially infectious for lice. The course of this form of disease is generally milder, and a rash is frequently absent, making diagnosis more difficult.

Laboratory Diagnosis

The MIF test is the diagnostic method of choice for documenting disease with *R. prowazekii*.

Treatment, Prevention, and Control

The tetracyclines are highly effective in the treatment of epidemic typhus; however, antibiotic treatment must be combined with effective louse-control measures for the management of an epidemic. A formaldehyde-inactivated typhus vaccine is available, and its use is recommended in high-risk populations.

Rickettsia typhi

Epidemiology

Endemic or **murine typhus** is caused by *R. typhi*. Disease is distributed worldwide, primarily in warm, humid areas. In the United States, 50 to 100 cases are reported annually, with most cases in the Gulf states (especially Texas) and southern California. Endemic disease continues to be reported in people living in the temperate and subtropical coastal areas of Africa, Asia, Australia, Europe, and South America. **Rodents** are the primary reservoir, and the **rat flea** (*Xenopsylla cheopis*) is the principal vector. However, the **cat flea** (*Ctenocephalides felis*), which infests cats, opossums, raccoons, and skunks, is considered an important vector for disease in the United States. Most cases occur during the warm months.

Clinical Disease

The incubation period for *R. typhi* disease is 7 to 14 days. The symptoms appear abruptly, with fever, severe headache, chills, myalgias, and nausea most common. A rash develops in approximately half of infected patients, most commonly late in the illness. It is typically restricted to the chest and abdomen. The course of disease is generally uncomplicated, lasting less than 3 weeks even in untreated patients.

Laboratory Diagnosis

An *R. typhi*—specific indirect fluorescent assay (IFA) test is used to confirm the diagnosis of murine typhus. Significant titers are usually detectable within 1 to 2 weeks of the onset of disease.

Treatment, Prevention, and Control

The **tetracyclines** are effective in the treatment of murine typhus, and patients respond promptly to these agents. It is difficult to control or prevent endemic typhus, because the reservoir and vector are widely distributed. Any such efforts should be directed at controlling the rodent reservoir. An effective vaccine is not available.

Orientia tsutsugamushi

O. tsutsugamushi, formerly classified with the *Rickettsia*, is the etiologic agent for **scrub typhus**, a disease transmitted to humans by **mites** (chiggers, red mites). The reservoir is the mite population, in which the bacteria are transmitted by transovarian means. Infection is also present in the **rodent** population, which can serve as a reservoir for mite infections. Because mites feed only once during their life span, rodents are not believed to be an important reservoir for human disease. Scrub typhus is present in people living in eastern Asia, Australia, and Japan and other western Pacific islands. It can also be imported into the United States.

O. tsutsugamushi disease develops suddenly after a 6- to 18-day incubation period (average, 10 to 12 days), with severe **headache, fever**, and **myalgias**. A macular to papular rash develops on the trunk in less than half of patients and spreads centrifugally to the extremities. Generalized lymphadenopathy, splenomegaly, central nervous system complications, and heart failure can occur. Fever in untreated patients disappears after 2 to 3 weeks, whereas fever in patients who receive appropriate treatment with **doxycycline** respond promptly. No vaccine is available, so the disease is prevented by avoidance of exposure to mites (i.e., the wearing of protective clothing, the use of insect repellents).

Case Study and Questions

A 24-year-old man living in North Carolina came to the local emergency department because of fever, arthralgias, myalgias, and malaise. He was well until 4 days before admission, when he developed a fever reaching 40° C, chills, severe headache, and muscle aches. Physical examination revealed a critically ill man with a temperature of 39.7° C, pulse of 110 beats/min, respiratory rate of 28 breaths/min, blood pressure of 100/60 mm Hg, and a rash over his extremities, including his palms and soles. The patient recalled having had numerous tick bites 10 days before the onset of symptoms. Rocky Mountain spotted fever was considered in the diagnosis, and serologic tests for *Rickettsia* species confirmed this diagnosis.

1. What antibiotics can be used to treat this infection? Which antibiotics should not be used?

2. Which rickettsiae are associated with the following vectors: ticks, lice, mites, fleas?

3. Why is use of the Gram stain inappropriate for the diagnosis of rickettsial infections?

Bibliography

Archibald L, Sexton D: Long-term sequelae of Rocky Mountain spotted fever. Clin Infect Dis 20:1122-1125, 1995.

Dumler JS, Walker D: Rocky Mountain spotted fever—changing ecology and persisting virulence. N Engl J Med 353:551-553, 2005.

Koss T, et al: Increased detection of rickettsialpox in a New York City hospital following the anthrax outbreak of 2001. Arch Dermatol 139:1545-1552, 2003.

Paddock C, et al: Isolation of *Rickettsia akari* from eschars of patients with rickettsialpox. Am J Trop Med Hyg 75:732-738, 2006.

Parola P, Paddock C, Raoult D: Tick-borne rickettsioses around the world: Emerging diseases challenging old concepts. Clin Microbiol Rev 18:719-756, 2005.

Raoult D, Dumler JS: *Rickettsia* and *Orientia*. In Borriello SP, Murray P, Funke G (eds): Topley and Wilson's Microbiology and Microbial Infections, 10th ed. London Holder-Arnold 2005, pp 2026-2047.

Richards A: Rickettsial vaccines: The old and the new. Expert Rev Vaccines 3:541-555, 2004.

Rolain J, et al: In vitro susceptibilities of 27 rickettsiae to 13 antimicrobials. Antimicrob Agents Chemother 42:1537-1541, 1998.

Spach D, et al: Tick-borne diseases in the United States. N Engl J Med 329:936-947, 1993.

Walker D, Bouyer D: *Rickettsia* and *Orientia*. In Murray P, Baron E, Jorgensen J, et al (eds): Manual of Clinical Microbiology, 9th ed. Washington, DC, ASM Press, pp 1036-1045.

Ehrlichia, Anaplasma, and Coxiella

All tick-borne bacteria in the family Anaplasmataceae are grouped into two genera: *Ehrlichia* and *Anaplasma* (Box 45-1). They are **obligate intracellular** bacteria that **survive in cytoplasmic vacuoles** of mammalian **hematopoietic cells**. *Coxiella* is an intracellular pathogen that was once thought to be closely related to *Rickettsia* and *Ehrlichia*. Although it is now recognized that *Coxiella* is not a member of the families Rickettsiaceae or Anaplasmataceae, it will also be discussed in this chapter.

Ehrlichia and *Anaplasma* (Box 45-2)

Physiology and Structure

The genera *Ehrlichia* and *Anaplasma* consist of intracellular bacteria that parasitize granulocytes, monocytes, erythrocytes, and platelets. In contrast with *Rickettsia* and *Orientia*, *Ehrlichia* and *Anaplasma* remain in the phagocytic vacuole after entry into the host cell. Fusion with lysosomes is prevented because expression of appropriate receptors on the phagocytic vacuole surface is interrupted. Thus the bacteria can multiple by binary fission in the phagosome without exposure to the hydrolytic lysosome enzymes. Two morphologic forms of the bacteria exist: small (0.2 to 0.4 μm) **elementary bodies** and larger (0.8 to 1.5 μm) **reticulate bodies**. A few days after the cell is infected, the replicating elementary bodies assemble into membrane-enclosed masses called **morulae** (Figure 45-1). Progressive infection leads to lysis of the infected cell, release of bacteria, and subsequent infection of new cells. Detection of morulae when the cells are stained with **Giemsa** or **Wright stains** is a rapid, specific diagnostic test; however, relatively few infected cells may be seen, so a negative test is not helpful. Analysis of the genome revealed that these bacteria lack the genes for cell-wall peptidoglycan synthesis, as well as genes for the glycolytic pathway.

The cell wall structure of *Ehrlichia* and *Anaplasma* is similar to that of gram-negative bacteria; however, the bacteria lack genes for synthesis of peptidoglycan or lipopolysaccharide (LPS). Additionally, many of the genes of the glycolytic pathway are also absent. A number of protein antigens are shared among species in these genera, as well as with species of other genera. For this reason, cross-reactive antibodies are commonly observed in serologic assays.

Pathogenesis and Immunity

The intracellular location of the organisms protects them from the host's antibody response. However, bacterial stimulation of proinflammatory cytokine production is believed to play an important role in activating macrophages that act either directly on infected cells or on antibody-opsonized bacteria during their extracellular phase.

Epidemiology (Table 45-1)

The first human infection in the United States with these organisms was reported in 1986. *Ehrlichia canis* was initially believed to be responsible for the newly named disease, **human monocytic ehrlichiosis;** however, a new species, *Ehrlichia chaffeensis*, was recognized as the etiologic agent. Between 1987 and 2005, more than 1500 cases were reported. The prevalence of this disease is underestimated because serologic studies have shown that antibodies to *E. chaffeensis* are at least as common as antibodies to *Rickettsia rickettsii*, which has a similar geographic distribution. Disease in the United States is found predominantly in the southeastern, mid-Atlantic, midwestern, and south-central states (e.g., Arkansas, Georgia, Maryland, Missouri, North and South Carolina, Oklahoma, and Texas). This area corresponds to the geographic distribution of *Amblyomma americanum* (Lone Star tick), the primary vector responsible for transmitting the organism, and of white-tailed deer, an important reservoir for *E. chaffeensis*. Other animals that can serve as hosts include domestic dogs, foxes, coyotes, and wolves.

Box 45—1. *Ehrlichia*, *Anaplasma*, and *Coxiella*

Organism	Historical Derivation
Ehrlichia	Named after the German microbiologist Paul *Ehrlich*
E. chaffeensis	First isolated in an Army reservist at Fort *Chaffee*, Ark.
E. ewingii	Named after the American microbiologist William *Ewing*
Anaplasma	*an*, "without"; *plasma*, anything "formed" (a thing without form, referring to the intracytoplasmic inclusions)
A. phagocytophilum	*phago*, to "eat"; *kytos*, a "vessel" or "enclosure"; *philein*, to "love" (found in phagocytes)
Coxiella burnetii	Named after Harold *Cox* and F.M. *Burnet*, who isolated the bacterium from ticks in Montana and patients in Australia, respectively

Box 45—2. Summary of *Ehrlichia* and *Anaplasma*

Biology, Virulence, Disease

Small, intracellular bacteria that stain poorly with Gram stain; best with Giemsa or Gimenez stains
Replicates in phagosome of infected cells
Intracellular growth protects bacteria from immune clearance
Able to prevent fusion of phagosome with lysosome of monocytes or granulocytes
Initiates inflammatory response that contributes to pathology
Diseases are human monocytic ehrlichiosis and human anaplasmosis (formerly called *human granulocytic ehrlichiosis*)

Epidemiology

Depending on the species of *Ehrlichia*, important reservoirs are white-tailed deer, white-footed mouse, chipmunks, voles, and canines
Ticks are important vectors, but transovarian transmission in inefficient
Disease in United States is most common in the southeastern, mid-Atlantic, midwestern, and south-central states
People at greatest risk are those exposed to ticks in the endemic areas
Disease is most common from April to October

Diagnosis

Microscopy of limited value
Serology and DNA probe tests are methods of choice

Treatment, Prevention, and Control

Doxycycline is drug of choice; rifampin is an acceptable alternative
Prevention involves avoidance of tick-infested areas, use of protective clothing and insect repellents, and prompt removal of embedded ticks
Vaccines are not available

Figure 45—1. Multiple morulae of *Ehrlichia canis* in DH82 tissue culture cells. *(From Cohen J, Powderly WG: Infectious Diseases, 2nd ed. St Louis, Mosby, 2004.)*

Granulocytic ehrlichiosis is caused by two bacteria: *Ehrlichia ewingii* and *Anaplasma phagocytophilum*. *E. ewingii* has a geographic distribution similar to *E. chaffeensis* because they share the same tick vector *(Amblyomma americanum)*. The frequency with which it is associated with human disease is unknown because serologic response to this organism cross-reacts with antibodies against *E. chaffeensis*. Disease caused by *A. phagocytophilum* is found primarily in the northern and central midwestern states and northeast and central Atlantic states. The reservoirs are small mammals (e.g., white-footed mouse, chipmunks, voles), and the vectors are *Ixodes* ticks. More than 90% of all disease caused by *Ehrlichia* and *Anaplasma* in the United States occurs between mid-April and late October.

Transovarian transmission of *Ehrlichia* and *Anaplasma* in ticks does not occur (in contrast with *Rickettsia* and *Orientia*), so these bacteria must be maintained in reservoir vertebrate hosts. Ticks become infected when an immature stage (e.g., larva, nymph) ingests blood from a naturally infected host and then transmits the bacteria to another mammalian host (e.g., human) during the next blood meal. Humans are accidental hosts, and thus transmission terminates at this stage.

Clinical Diseases

Human Monocytic Ehrlichiosis

Human monocytic ehrlichiosis is caused by *E. chaffeensis*, following infection of blood monocytes and mononuclear phagocytes in tissues and organs. Approximately 1 to 3 weeks after a tick bite, patients develop a flulike illness with high fever, headache, malaise, and myalgias. A late-onset rash develops in 30% to 40% of patients (more common in children than in adults). Leukopenia, thrombocytopenia, and elevated serum transaminases develop in the majority of patients and can range from mild to severe. Although mortality is low (2% to 3%), more than half the infected patients require hospitalization and experience a prolonged recovery period. The pathology of this infection

Table 45–1. Epidemiology of *Ehrlichia* and *Anaplasma*

	E. chaffeensis	*E. ewingii*	*A. phagocytophilum*
Geographic distribution	North America	North America	North and South America, Europe, Asia
Reservoir host	Deer, dogs, and other *Canis*	Dogs	Small rodents, deer, sheep
Vector (ticks)	*Amblyomma americanum*	*Amblyomma americanum*	*Ixodes species*
Host with clinical symptoms	Humans, dogs	Dogs, humans	Ruminants, horses, dogs, humans
Infected host cell	Monocytes, macrophages	Neutrophils	Neutrophils, eosinophils, basophils

is disproportionate to the number of infected cells or microbial burden present in tissue. It is believed that *E. chaffeensis* disturbs mononuclear phagocytic function and the regulation of the inflammatory response. Thus the immune response both eliminates the pathogen and produces much of the tissue damage.

Canine Granulocytic Ehrlichiosis

E. ewingii primarily causes disease in canines, with humans the accidental hosts. Because there is serologic cross-reactivity between *E. ewingii* and *E. chaffeensis*, the incidence of infections with this organism is likely to be underestimated. The clinical presentation is similar to that of *E. chaffeensis*, with fever, headaches, and myalgias. Leukopenia, thrombocytopenia, and elevated serum transaminases are also seen.

Human Anaplasmosis (Clinical Case 45-1)

Human anaplasmosis, formerly called *human granulocytic ehrlichiosis*, is caused by *A. phagocytophilum*. Granulocytes (i.e., neutrophils, eosinophils, basophils) are primarily infected. The disease presents 5 to 11 days after exposure as a flulike illness with a high fever, headache, malaise, and myalgias; a skin rash is observed in less than 10% of

---

Clinical Case 45-1. Clinical Human Anaplasmosis

Heller, et al. (N Engl J Med 352:1358-1364, 2005) described a 73-year-old man who presented to their hospital with fever, weakness, and leg myalgias. Six days before his admission, he had traveled to South Carolina, and 3 days later he developed intense leg pains, a high fever, and generalized weakness. Upon admission he was febrile, tachycardic, and hypertensive; the liver and spleen could not be palpated, and no cutaneous rash was noted. Cultures for bacteria, fungi, and viruses were negative. A peripheral blood smear showed rare intracytoplasmic inclusion in the granulocytes, suggestive of morulae. PCR analysis of blood samples collected on the second and third hospital days were positive for *A. phagocytophilum* DNA, confirming the diagnosis of anaplasmosis. The patient was treated successfully with a 14-day course of doxycycline, although residual muscle weakness and residual pain persisted. Serum collected during the convalescent period was positive for *Anaplasma*. It is noteworthy that the patient did not remember a tick bite during his South Carolina trip, consistent with the observation that the early tick stages, larva and nymphs, are most commonly associated with human disease.

---

the patients. Leukopenia, thrombocytopenia, and serum transaminase elevation are observed in most patients. More than half the infected patients require hospitalization, and severe complications are common. Despite the potential severity of this disease, mortality is less than 1%. As with *E. chaffeensis* infections, the pathology of this disease appears related to macrophage activation.

Laboratory Diagnosis

Microscopy is of limited value for diagnosing infections. *Ehrlichia* and *Anaplasma* stain poorly with the Gram stain. Giemsa-stained preparations of peripheral blood should be performed, because detection of intracellular organisms (**morulae**) is diagnostic; however, morulae are detected in less than 10% of patients with monocytic ehrlichiosis and in 20% to 80% of patients with granulocytic ehrlichiosis and anaplasmosis. Likewise, although *Ehrlichia* have been cultured in vitro in established cell lines, this procedure is not performed in most clinical laboratories. The most common methods for confirming the clinical diagnosis of ehrlichiosis are deoxyribonucleic acid (DNA) amplification tests and serology. Species-specific DNA amplification tests are available in some reference laboratories and can provide a sensitive, specific diagnostic test for acute disease. An increase in the antibody titer is typically observed 3 to 6 weeks after the initial presentation, so these tests are primarily confirmatory. *E. chaffeensis* and *E. ewingii* are closely related and cannot be differentiated by serology. The specificity of the serology tests is compromised by cross-reactions with organisms responsible for Rocky Mountain spotted fever, Q fever, Lyme disease, brucellosis, and Epstein-Barr virus infections.

Treatment, Prevention, and Control

Patients with suspected ehrlichiosis should be treated with **doxycycline**. Therapy should not be delayed to wait for laboratory confirmation of the disease. Rifampin has been used to treat patients who are unable to tolerate doxycycline. Both doxycycline and rifampin are bactericidal in vitro. The fluoroquinolones are bacteriostatic in vitro, and resistance has been detected in some *Ehrlichia* species, so use of these drugs is contraindicated. Penicillins, cephalosporins, chloramphenicol, aminoglycosides, and macrolides are ineffective. Infection is prevented by avoidance of tick-infested areas, wearing of protective clothing, and use of insect repellents. Embedded ticks should be removed promptly. Vaccines are not available.

Coxiella burnetii (Box 45-3)

Coxiella burnetii was originally classified with *Rickettsia* because the gram-negative bacteria stain weakly with the Gram stain, **grow intracellularly** in eukaryotic cells, and are associated with arthropods (e.g., **ticks**). However, it is

---

Box 45–3. Summary of *Coxiella*

Biology, Virulence, Disease

Small, intracellular bacteria that stain poorly with Gram stain; best with Giemsa or Gimenez stains
Replicate in phagolysosome of infected cells
Capable of phase transition with phase I (infectious) and phase II lipopolysaccharide antigens
Intracellular growth protects the bacteria from immune clearance
Able to replicate in acidic environment of fused phagosomes and lysosomes
Phase I forms are protected from antibody interaction with bacterial surface proteins
Extracellular form extremely stable; can survive in nature for a prolonged period
Most infections are asymptomatic; most common acute presentation is nonspecific influenza-like syndrome; <5% develop significant acute disease (pneumonia, hepatitis, pericarditis, fever)
Chronic diseases include endocarditis, hepatitis, pulmonary disease, and infection of pregnant women

Epidemiology

Many reservoirs, including mammals, birds, and ticks
Most human infections associated with contact with infected cattle, sheep, goats, dogs, and cats
Most disease acquired through inhalation; possible disease from consumption of contaminated milk; ticks are not an important vector for human disease
Worldwide distribution
No seasonal incidence

Diagnosis

Detection of antibody response to phase I and phase II antigens is test of choice

Treatment, Prevention, and Control

Tetracyclines are the drugs of choice for acute infections; rifampin or hydroxychloroquine combined with doxycycline is used to treat chronic infections
Phase I antigen vaccines are protective and safe if administered in a single dose before the animal or human has been exposed to *Coxiella*; not available in the United States for animals or humans

---

now recognized that these bacteria are not related to *Rickettsia* but rather to *Legionella*. The disease caused by *C. burnetii* is **Q (query) fever**.

Physiology and Structure

Two structural forms of *C. burnetii* are recognized: **small cell variants (SCV)** that are extremely resistant to environmental stress (e.g., heat, desiccation, chemical agents), and **large cell variants (LCV)** that multiply in the host **monocytes** or **macrophages**. Upon exposure to *C. burnetii* in the environment, the SCV are phagocytosed, rearranged into the LCV, and fusion of the phagosome and lysosome follows. In the acidic environment of the phagolysosome, the LCV replicate. At some point in the replication cycle, LCV reorganize into SCV, which are released from the infected cell and can pass into the environment and remain infectious for months to years.

Pathogenesis and Immunity

An important characteristic of *Coxiella* infections is the ability to undergo **antigenic variation** in expression of the cell wall LPS antigen. The highly infectious form of the bacteria possesses LPS with a complex carbohydrate (**phase I antigen**) that blocks antibody interaction with surface proteins. After cultivation of the bacterium, the phase I antigen gene undergoes a deletion mutation, producing the **phase II antigen**. This antigenic change exposes the surface proteins to antibodies. Antibody response to these antigens in disease is a useful marker for acute and chronic diseases. Acute disease is characterized by antibodies against the exposed phase II antigen, whereas high antibody titers against the phase I and II antigens are detected in patients with chronic infections. Clearance of *C. burnetii* requires both specific antibody production and T-cell dependent immunity. Thus immunocompromised patients are more susceptible to persistent infections.

Epidemiology (See Table 45-1)

C. burnetii is extremely stable in harsh environmental conditions and *can survive in soil and milk for months to years*. The range of hosts for *C. burnetii* is wide, with infections being found in mammals, birds, and numerous genera of ticks. Farm animals such as sheep, cattle, and goats and recently infected cats, dogs, and rabbits are the primary reservoirs for human disease. Ticks are an important vector for disease in animals but not in humans. The bacteria can reach high concentrations in the placenta of infected livestock. Dried placentas left on the ground after parturition and feces, urine, and tick feces can contaminate soil, which in turn can serve as a focus for infection if these bacteria become airborne and are inhaled. Human infections occur after the inhalation of airborne particles from a **contaminated environmental source** or, less commonly, following ingestion of contaminated **unpasteurized milk** or other dairy products.

Q fever has a worldwide distribution. Relatively few cases are reported annually in the United States (from 21 in 2000 to 169 in 2006); however, this figure is certainly an underestimation of the actual prevalence of the disease. Infection is common in livestock in the United States, but symptomatic disease in livestock is rare. Human exposure, particularly for ranchers, veterinarians, and food handlers, is frequent, and experimental studies have shown that the infectious dose of *C. burnetii* is small. Thus most human infections are asymptomatic or mild. This finding is confirmed by serologic studies, which have shown that more than half of all patients with detectable antibodies do not have a history of disease. Infections also go undiagnosed because diagnostic tests for *C. burnetii* are often not considered in patients.

Clinical Diseases (Clinical Case 45-2)

The majority of individuals exposed to *C. burnetii* have an **asymptomatic infection**, and most symptomatic infections are mild, presenting with nonspecific **flulike symptoms**. Less than 5% of acutely infected individuals develop symptoms severe enough to require hospitalization, with **pneumonia, hepatitis**, or isolated **fevers** the most common presentations. Histologically, diffuse granulomas are typically seen in the involved organs. Chronic Q fever can develop months to years after the initial exposure and occurs almost exclusively in patients with predisposing conditions such as underlying valvular heart disease or immunosuppression. **Subacute endocarditis** is the most common presentation and can be difficult to diagnose because of the lack of specific signs and symptoms.

Clinical Case 45-2. *Coxiella burnetii* Endocarditis

Karakousis, et al. (J Clin Microbiol 44:2283-2287, 2006) described a 31-year-old man from West Virginia who developed chronic endocarditis caused by *C. burnetii*. At the time the patient was admitted to the hospital, he described an 11-month history of fevers, night sweats, paroxysmal coughing, fatigue, and weight loss. He had received various antibiotic treatments for bronchitis, with no relief. His past medical history was significant for congenital heart disease, with placement of a shunt as an infant. He lived on a farm and participated in birthing his calves. His cardiac exam upon admission revealed a murmur; no hepatosplenomegaly or peripheral stigmata of endocarditis were noted, but his liver enzymes were elevated. All bacterial and fungal blood cultures were negative; however, serology for *Coxiella* phase I and phase II antibodies were markedly elevated. Treatment with doxycycline and rifampin was initiated, and the patient rapidly defervesced. Although prolonged treatment was recommended, the patient was noncompliant, and he rapidly became symptomatic every time he discontinued one or both antibiotics. He also refused to take hydroxychloroquine because of his concerns about retinal toxicity. This patient typifies the risk for patients with underlying heart disease and the difficulties in treating this infection.

However, chronic Q fever is a serious illness with a mortality rate that approaches 65% in untreated patients.

Laboratory Diagnosis

At present, Q fever can be diagnosed by culture (not commonly performed), serology, or the polymerase chain reaction (PCR). Currently, **serology** is the most commonly used diagnostic test. As previously mentioned, *C. burnetii* undergoes phase variation characterized by the development of phase I and II antigens. The phase I antigens are only weakly antigenic. A variety of methods is used to measure antibody production: the microagglutination tests, indirect immunofluorescent-antibody (IFA) test, and enzyme-linked immunosorbent assay (ELISA). IFA is the test of choice, although ELISA is used in many laboratories and appears to be as sensitive. Cross-reactions occur with *Bartonella* (which can cause a similar disease), so all serologic tests should include an assay for both organisms. In acute Q fever, immunoglobulin (Ig)M and IgG antibodies are developed primarily against **phase II antigens**. A diagnosis of chronic Q fever is confirmed by the demonstration of antibodies against both **phase I and II antigens**, with the titers to the phase I antigen typically higher. Nucleic acid amplification techniques such as PCR have been developed in reference laboratories and are generally not available for routine diagnosis. Additionally, although the tests are sensitive when tissue samples are examined, the sensitivity is poor with serum. PCR-based tests are not required for the diagnosis of chronic *C. burnetii* infections, because these patients characteristically have high levels of antibodies present.

Treatment, Prevention, and Control

In vitro susceptibility tests have not proved useful for predicting clinical efficacy. For this reason, treatment of acute and chronic *C. burnetii* infections is guided by clinical experience. Currently, it is recommended that acute infections be treated with a tetracycline (e.g., **doxycycline**). Chronic disease should be treated for a prolonged period with a bactericidal combination of drugs, doxycycline, and the alkalinizing agent hydroxychloroquine. Doxycycline and rifampin or doxycycline combined with a fluoroquinolone can also be used, although the treatment interval must be increased to at least 3 years. Macrolides, aminoglycosides, and beta-lactam antibiotics are not effective.

Inactivated whole-cell vaccines and partially purified antigen vaccines for Q fever have been developed, and the vaccines prepared from phase I organisms have been shown to provide the best protection. Vaccination of animal herds appears efficacious, unless the animals have been previously infected naturally. Vaccination does not eradicate *Coxiella* in infected animals or decrease asymptomatic shedding. Likewise, vaccination of humans with phase I vaccines is protective if the vaccinees are uninfected. Vaccination of previously infected individuals is contraindicated because immune stimulation can lead to an increase in adverse reactions. For this reason, a single-dose vaccine with no booster immunizations is recommended. Commercial vaccines for humans or livestock are not available at this time in the United States.

Case Study and Questions

A 46-year-old man went to his physician with a 2-month history of weight loss (15 lbs), night sweats, and a low-grade fever. Results of a chest examination revealed a new heart murmur. The physician suspected his patient had subacute endocarditis, and three sets of blood cultures were collected. After 1 week of incubation, the cultures remained negative.

1. What diagnostic test(s) should be performed to determine if this patient has endocarditis caused by *Coxiella burnetii*?

2. If this diagnosis is confirmed, how did the patient most likely acquire his infection?

3. How should this infection be treated?

Bibliography

Cutler S, et al: Review: Q fever. J Infect 54:313-318, 2007.

Dumler JS: Laboratory diagnosis of human rickettsial and ehrlichial infections. Clin Microbiol Newsl 18:57-61, 1996.

Dumler J, et al: Human granulocytic anaplasmosis and *Anaplasma phagocytophilum*. Emerg Infect Dis 11:1828-1834, 2005.

Raoult D, et al: Natural history and pathophysiology of Q fever. Lancet Infect Dis 5:219-226, 2005.

Paddock C, Childs J: *Ehrlichia chaffeensis*: A prototypical emerging pathogen. Clin Microbiol Rev 16:37-64, 2003.

Parker N, et al: Q fever. Lancet 367:679-688, 2006.

Schutze GE: Ehrlichiosis. Pediatr Infect Dis J 25:71-72, 2006.

Chlamydia and Chlamydophila

The family Chlamydiaceae consists of two clinically important genera, *Chlamydia* and *Chlamydophila*, with three species responsible for human disease: ***Chlamydia trachomatis***, ***Chlamydophila psittaci***, and ***Chlamydophila pneumoniae*** (Box 46-1). Other species have been placed into the two genera, but they are uncommon human pathogens and are not discussed in this chapter.

The Chlamydiaceae are **obligate intracellular parasites** that were once considered viruses because they are small enough to pass through 0.45 μm filters. However, the organisms have the following properties of bacteria: They (1) possess inner and outer membranes similar to those of gram-negative bacteria; (2) contain both deoxyribonucleic acid (DNA) and ribonucleic acid (RNA); (3) possess prokaryotic ribosomes; (4) synthesize their own proteins, nucleic acids, and lipids; and (5) are susceptible to numerous antibacterial antibiotics.

Unlike other bacteria, the Chlamydiaceae have a unique developmental cycle, forming metabolically inactive infectious forms (**elementary bodies [EBs]**) and metabolically active, noninfectious forms (**reticulate bodies [RBs]**). Properties that differentiate the three important human pathogens in this family are summarized in Table 46-1.

Family Chlamydiaceae

Physiology and Structure

Much like a spore, elementary bodies are resistant to many harsh environmental factors. Although these bacteria lack the rigid peptidoglycan layer found in most other bacteria, their central dense core is surrounded by a cytoplasmic membrane and a double-layer outer membrane. The cell wall contains a lipopolysaccharide (**LPS**) that is common to all members of the family. The LPS has only **weak endotoxin activity**. The **major outer membrane protein (MOMP)** in the cell wall is an important structural component of the outer membrane and is unique for each species. Variable regions in the gene encoding this

protein are found in *C. trachomatis* and are responsible for 18 serologic variants (called **serovars**). Similar variable regions are found in *C. psittaci* MOMP; in contrast, the *C. pneumoniae* MOMP is homogeneous, and only a single serovar has been described. A second, highly conserved outer membrane protein, **OMP 2**, is shared by all members of the family Chlamydiaceae. This cysteine-rich protein is responsible for the extensive disulfide cross-links that provide the stability in the elementary bodies.

The elementary bodies cannot replicate but are infectious; that is, they can bind to receptors on host cells and stimulate uptake by the infected cell. In this intracellular location, the elementary bodies convert into reticulate bodies, the metabolically active, replicating chlamydial form. Because the extensive cross-linked proteins are absent in reticulate bodies, this form is osmotically fragile; however, they are protected by their intracellular location.

The Chlamydiaceae replicate by means of a unique growth cycle that occurs within susceptible host cells (Figure 46-1). The cycle is initiated when the small (300 to 400 nm), infectious elementary bodies become attached to the microvilli of susceptible cells, followed by active penetration into the host cell. After they are internalized, the bacteria remain within cytoplasmic phagosomes, where the replicative cycle proceeds. If the outer membrane of the elementary body is intact, fusion of cellular lysosomes with the EB-containing phagosome is inhibited, thus preventing intracellular killing. If the outer membrane is damaged or the bacteria are inactivated by heat or coated with antibodies, phagolysosomal fusion occurs with subsequent bacterial killing. Within 6 to 8 hours after entering the cell, the elementary bodies reorganize into the larger (800 to 1000 nm), metabolically active reticulate bodies. The Chlamydiaceae are **energy parasites**, because they use host cell adenosine triphosphate for their energy requirements. Some strains may also depend on the host to provide specific amino acids. The reticulate bodies replicate by binary fission, similar to other bacteria, and histologic stains can readily detect the phagosome with accumulated reticulate bodies, called an **inclusion**. Approximately 18 to 24 hours

Box 46—1. Important Chlamydiaceae

Organism	Historical Derivation
Chlamydia	*chlamydis*, a "cloak"
C. trachomatis	*trachomatis*, of "trachoma" or "rough" (the disease trachoma is characterized by rough granulations on the conjunctival surfaces that lead to chronic inflammation and blindness)
Chlamydophila	*chlamydis*, a "cloak"; *phila*, "dear" (dear to the cloak; related to *Chlamydia*)
C. pneumoniae	*pneumoniae*, related to pneumonia
C. psittaci	*psittacus*, a "parrot" (disease associated with birds)

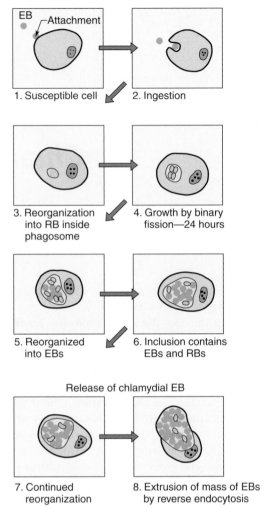

Figure 46—1. The growth cycle of *Chlamydia trachomatis*. *(Redrawn from Batteiger B, Jones R: Infect Dis Clin North Am 1:55-81, 1987.)*

after infection, the reticulate bodies begin reorganizing into the smaller elementary bodies, and between 48 and 72 hours, the cell ruptures and then releases the infectious bacteria.

Chlamydia trachomatis (Box 46-2)

C. trachomatis has a limited host range, with infections restricted to humans (Box 46-3). The species responsible for human disease are subdivided into two **biovars**: **trachoma** and **LGV (lymphogranuloma venereum)**. The biovars have been further divided into **serovars** on the basis of antigenic differences in the major outer membrane protein (MOMP). Specific serovars are associated with specific diseases (Table 46-2).

Table 46—1. Differentiation of Chlamydiaceae That Cause Human Disease

Property	*Chlamydia trachomatis*	*Chlamydophila pneumoniae*	*Chlamydophila psittaci*
Host range	Primarily human pathogen	Primarily human pathogen	Primarily animal pathogen; occasionally infects humans
Biovars	LGV and trachoma	TWAR	Many
Diseases	LGV; ocular trachoma, oculogenital disease, infant pneumonia	Bronchitis, pneumonia, sinusitis, pharyngitis, coronary artery disease (?)	Pneumonia (psittacosis)
Elementary body morphology	Round, narrow periplasmic space	Pear-shaped, large periplasmic space	Round, narrow periplasmic space
Inclusion body morphology	Single, round inclusion per cell	Multiple uniform inclusions per cell	Multiple, variably sized inclusions per cell
Plasmid DNA	Yes	No	Yes
Iodine-staining glycogen in inclusions	Yes	No	No
Susceptibility to sulfonamides	Yes	No	No

DNA, deoxyribonucleic acid; LGV, lymphogranuloma venereum

Box 46–2. Summary: *Chlamydia trachomatis*

Biology, Virulence, and Disease

Small, gram-negative rods with no peptidoglycan layer in cell wall
Strict intracellular parasite of humans
Two distinct forms: infectious elementary bodies and noninfectious reticulate bodies
Lipopolysaccharide antigen shared by *Chlamydia* and *Chlamydophila* species
Major outer membrane proteins are species specific
Two biovars associated with human disease: trachoma and lymphogranuloma venereum (LGV)
Infects nonciliated columnar, cuboidal, and transitional epithelial cells
Prevents fusion of phagosome with cellular lysosomes
Pathologic effects of trachoma caused by repeated infections
Diseases—refer to Box 46-3

Epidemiology

Most common sexually transmitted bacteria in United States
Ocular trachoma primarily in North and sub-Sahara Africa, the Middle East, southern Asia, South America
LGV highly prevalent in Africa, Asia, and South America

Diagnosis

Culture is highly specific but is relatively insensitive
Antigen tests (DFA, ELISA) are relatively insensitive
Molecular amplification tests are the most sensitive and specific tests currently available

Treatment, Prevention, and Control

Treat LGV with doxycycline or erythromycin
Treat ocular or genital infections with azithromycin or doxycycline
Treat newborn conjunctivitis or pneumonia with erythromycin
Safe sex practices and prompt treatment of patient and sexual partners help control infections

DFA, direct fluorescent antibody; ELISA, enzyme-linked immunosorbent assay.

Box 46–3. Chlamydiaceae: Clinical Summaries

Chlamydia trachomatis

Trachoma: chronic, inflammatory, granulomatous process of eye surface, leading to corneal ulceration, scarring, pannus formation, and blindness
Adult inclusion conjunctivitis: acute process with mucopurulent discharge, dermatitis, corneal infiltrates, and corneal vascularization in chronic disease
Neonatal conjunctivitis: acute process characterized by a mucopurulent discharge
Infant pneumonia: after a 2- to 3-week incubation period, the infant develops rhinitis, followed by bronchitis with a characteristic dry cough
Urogenital infections: acute process involving the genitourinary tract, with characteristic mucopurulent discharge; asymptomatic infections common in women
Lymphogranuloma venereum: a painless ulcer develops at the site of infection that spontaneously heals; followed by inflammation and swelling of lymph nodes draining the area, then progression to systemic symptoms

Chlamydophila pneumoniae

Respiratory infections: can range from asymptomatic or mild disease to severe, atypical pneumonia requiring hospitalization
Atherosclerosis: *C. pneumoniae* has been associated with inflammatory plaques in blood vessels; the etiologic role in this disease is controversial

Chlamydophila psittaci

Respiratory infections: can range from asymptomatic colonization to severe bronchopneumonia with localized infiltration of inflammatory cells, necrosis, and hemorrhage

Pathogenesis and Immunity

The range of cells that *C. trachomatis* can infect is limited. Receptors for EBs are primarily restricted to nonciliated columnar, cuboidal, and transitional epithelial cells, which are found on the mucous membranes of the urethra, endocervix, endometrium, fallopian tubes, anorectum, respiratory tract, and conjunctivae. The LGV serovars are more invasive than the other serovars, because they replicate in mononuclear phagocytes. The clinical manifestations of chlamydial infections are caused by (1) the direct destruction of cells during replication and (2) the proinflammatory cytokine response they stimulate.

Chlamydiae gain access through minute abrasions or lacerations. In LGV, the lesions form in the lymph nodes, draining the site of primary infection (Figure 46-2). Granuloma formation is characteristic. The lesions may become necrotic, attract polymorphonuclear leukocytes, and cause the inflammatory process to spread to surrounding tissues. Subsequent rupture of the lymph node leads to formation of abscesses or sinus tracts. Infection with non-LGV serovars of *C. trachomatis* stimulates a severe inflammatory response consisting of neutrophils, lymphocytes, and plasma cells.

Infection does not confer long-lasting immunity. Rather, reinfection characteristically induces a vigorous inflammatory response with subsequent tissue damage. This response produces vision loss in patients with chronic ocular infections and scarring with sterility and sexual dysfunction in patients with genital infections.

Table 46–2. Clinical Spectrum of *Chlamydia trachomatis* Infections

Serovars	Disease
A, B, Ba, C	Trachoma
D-K	Urogenital tract disease
L1, L2, L2a, L2b, L3	Lymphogranuloma venereum

Figure 46–2. Patient with lymphogranuloma venereum causing unilateral vulvar lymphedema and inguinal buboes. *(From Cohen J, Powderly W: Infectious Diseases, 2nd ed. St Louis, Mosby, 2004.)*

Epidemiology

C. trachomatis is found worldwide and causes trachoma (chronic keratoconjunctivitis), oculogenital disease, pneumonia, and LGV. Trachoma is endemic in North and sub-Sahara Africa, the Middle East, southern Asia, and South America. The World Health Organization estimates 6 million people are blind due to trachoma, and more than 150 million are in need of treatment. Trachoma is the **leading cause of preventable blindness**. Infections occur predominantly in children, who are the chief reservoir of *C. trachomatis* in endemic areas. The incidence of infection is lower in older children and adolescents; however, the incidence of blindness continues to rise through adulthood as the disease progresses. Trachoma is transmitted eye-to-eye by droplet, hands, contaminated clothing, and eye-seeking flies, which transmit ocular discharges from the eyes of infected children to the eyes of uninfected children. Because a high percentage of children in endemic areas harbor *C. trachomatis* in their respiratory and gastrointestinal tracts, the pathogen may also be transmitted by respiratory droplet or through fecal contamination. Trachoma generally is endemic in communities where the living conditions are crowded, sanitation is poor, and the personal hygiene of the people is poor—all risk factors that promote the transmission of infections.

Most cases of *C. trachomatis* **adult inclusion conjunctivitis** occur in people who are 18 to 30 years of age, and genital infection probably precedes eye involvement. Autoinoculation and oral-genital contact are believed to be the routes of transmission. A third form of *C. trachomatis* eye infections is **newborn inclusion conjunctivitis**, an infection acquired during passage of the infant through an infected birth canal. *C. trachomatis* conjunctivitis develops in approximately 25% of infants whose mothers have active genital infections.

Pulmonary infection with *C. trachomatis* also occurs in newborns. A diffuse **interstitial pneumonia** develops in 10% to 20% of infants exposed to the pathogen at birth.

C. trachomatis is thought to be the most common **sexually transmitted bacterial disease** in the United States. In 2006, 1 million infections were reported in the United States. However, this figure is believed to be an underestimate, because most infected patients either do not seek medical treatment or are treated without a specific diagnosis. It is estimated that 2.8 million Americans are infected each year, and as many as 50 million new infections occur annually worldwide. Most genital tract infections are caused by serotypes D through K.

LGV is a chronic sexually transmitted disease caused by *C. trachomatis* serotypes L1, L2, L2a, L2b, and L3. It occurs sporadically in the United States and other industrialized countries but is highly prevalent in Africa, Asia, and South America. Acute LGV is seen more frequently in men, primarily because symptomatic infection is less common in women.

Clinical Diseases

Trachoma

Trachoma is a **chronic disease** caused by serovars A, B, Ba, and C. Initially, patients have a **follicular conjunctivitis** with diffuse inflammation that involves the entire conjunctiva. The conjunctivae become scarred as the disease progresses, causing the patient's eyelids to turn inward. The turned-in eyelashes abrade the cornea, eventually resulting in corneal ulceration, scarring, pannus formation (invasion of vessels into the cornea), and loss of vision. It is common for trachoma to recur after apparent healing, most likely a result of subclinical infections that have been documented in children in endemic areas and in immigrants to the United States who acquired trachoma during childhood in their native countries.

Adult Inclusion Conjunctivitis

An acute follicular conjunctivitis caused by the *C. trachomatis* strains associated with genital infections (serovars A, B, Ba, D to K) has been documented in sexually active adults. The infection is characterized by mucopurulent discharge, keratitis, corneal infiltrates, and occasionally some corneal vascularization. Corneal scarring has been observed in patients with chronic infection.

Neonatal Conjunctivitis

Eye infections can also develop in **infants exposed to *C. trachomatis* at birth**. After an incubation of 5 to 12 days, the infant's eyelids swell, hyperemia occurs, and copious purulent discharge appears. Untreated infections may run a course as long as 12 months, during which time conjunctival scarring and corneal vascularization occur. Infants who are untreated or are treated with topical therapy only are at risk for *C. trachomatis* pneumonia.

Infant Pneumonia (Clinical Case 46-1)

The incubation period for infant pneumonia is variable, but the onset generally occurs 2 to 3 weeks after birth.

Clinical Case 46-1. *Chlamydia trachomatis* Pneumonia in Newborn Infants

Niida and associates described two female infants with *C. trachomatis* pneumonia. The first infant was born by vaginal delivery after 39 weeks gestation and the second by Caesarean section (because of fetal distress) at 40 weeks gestation. The infants were in good condition until fever and tachypnea developed at 3 and 13 days, respectively. Chest radiographs showed infiltrates over the whole lungs. Cultures of blood, urine, throat, feces, and CSF were negative, but antigen tests for *C. trachomatis* were positive from conjunctival and nasopharyngeal swabs. These cases illustrate the presentation of pneumonia in infants infected with *C. trachomatis* at or near birth, although the characteristic staccato cough was not described.

Figure 46—3. Mucopurulent cervicitis caused by *Chlamydia trachomatis*. (*From Cohen J, Powderly W: Infectious Diseases, 2nd ed. St Louis, Mosby, 2004. Photo by J. Paavonen.*)

Rhinitis is initially observed in such infants, after which a **distinctive staccato cough** develops. The child remains afebrile throughout the clinical illness, which can last for several weeks. Radiographic signs of infection can persist for months.

Ocular Lymphogranuloma Venereum

The LGV serotypes of *C. trachomatis* have been implicated in Parinaud oculoglandular conjunctivitis, a conjunctival inflammation associated with preauricular, submandibular, and cervical lymphadenopathy.

Urogenital Infections (Clinical Case 46-2)

Most genital tract infections in women are asymptomatic (as many as 80%) but can nevertheless become symptomatic. The clinical manifestations include bartholinitis, cervicitis, endometritis, perihepatitis, salpingitis, and urethritis. Asymptomatic patients with chlamydial infection are an important reservoir for the spread of *C. trachomatis*. A mucopurulent discharge (Figure 46-3) is seen in patients with symptomatic infection, whose specimens generally yield more organisms on

cultures than specimens from patients with asymptomatic infections. Urethritis caused by *C. trachomatis* may occur with or without a concurrent cervical infection.

Although most *C. trachomatis* genital infections in men are symptomatic, as many as 25% of the infections will be inapparent. Approximately 35% to 50% of cases of nongonococcal urethritis are caused by *C. trachomatis;* dual infections with both *C. trachomatis* and *Neisseria gonorrhoeae* are not uncommon. Symptoms of the chlamydial infection develop after successful treatment of the gonorrhea, because the incubation period is longer and the use of β-lactam antibiotics to treat gonorrhea would be ineffective against *C. trachomatis*. Although there is less purulent exudate in patients with chlamydial urethral infections, such infections cannot be differentiated reliably from gonorrhea, so specific diagnostic tests for both organisms should be performed.

It is believed that **Reiter syndrome** (urethritis, conjunctivitis, polyarthritis, and mucocutaneous lesions) is initiated by genital infection with *C. trachomatis*. Although chlamydiae have not been isolated from the synovial fluid of such patients, chlamydial elementary bodies have been observed in synovial fluid or tissue specimens from men with sexually acquired reactive arthritis. The disease usually occurs in young white men. Approximately 50% to 65% of patients with Reiter syndrome have a chlamydial genital infection at the onset of arthritis, and serologic studies indicate that more than 80% of men with Reiter syndrome have evidence of a preceding or concurrent infection with *C. trachomatis*.

Lymphogranuloma Venereum

After an incubation of 1 to 4 weeks, a primary lesion appears at the site of infection (e.g., penis, urethra, glans, scrotum, vaginal wall, cervix, and vulva) in patients with LGV. The lesion (either a papule or an ulcer) is often overlooked because it is small, painless, and heals rapidly. The absence of pain differentiates these ulcers from those observed in herpes simplex virus infections. The patient may experience fever, headache, and myalgia when the lesion is present.

Clinical Case 46-2. Reiter Syndrome and Pelvic Inflammatory Disease

Serwin, et al. (J Eur Acad Derm Vener 20:735-736, 2006) described a 30-year-old man who presented to a university hospital with complaints of dysuria for a 3-year duration, penile inflammation, joint swelling, and fever. Skin lesions and nail changes were also noted. High levels of *Chlamydia* antibodies were present, but antigen tests and nucleic acid amplification tests of the urethral exudates and conjunctiva were negative for *C. trachomatis*. A diagnosis of Reiter syndrome was made, and treatment with ofloxacin was initiated. Complete remission of the skin lesions and urethral symptoms was achieved. The patient's wife was also admitted to the hospital with a history of 2 years of lower abdominal pain and vaginal bleeding and discharge. The diagnosis of pelvic inflammatory disease (PID) was made, and *C. trachomatis* infection was confirmed by positive cervical and urethral antigen tests (DFA). The vaginal smear was also positive for *Trichomonas vaginalis*. These patients illustrate two complications of *C. trachomatis* urogenital infections: Reiter syndrome and PID.

The second stage of infection is marked by inflammation and swelling of the lymph nodes draining the site of initial infection. The inguinal nodes are most commonly involved, becoming painful, fluctuant **buboes** that gradually enlarge and can rupture, forming draining fistulas. Systemic manifestations include fever, chills, anorexia, headache, meningismus, myalgias, and arthralgia.

Proctitis is common in women with LGV, resulting from lymphatic spread from the cervix or the vagina. Proctitis develops in men after anal intercourse or as the result of lymphatic spread from the urethra. Untreated LGV may resolve at this stage or may progress to a chronic ulcerative phase, in which genital ulcers, fistulas, strictures, or genital elephantiasis develop.

Laboratory Diagnosis

C. trachomatis infection can be diagnosed (1) on the basis of cytologic, serologic, or culture findings, (2) through the direct detection of antigen in clinical specimens, and (3) through the use of molecular tests. The sensitivity of each method depends on the patient population examined, the site where the specimen is obtained, and the nature of the disease. For example, symptomatic infections are generally easier to diagnose than asymptomatic infections, because more chlamydiae are present in the specimen from a patient with symptoms. The quality of the specimen is also important. Because chlamydiae are obligate intracellular bacteria, specimens must be obtained from the involved site (e.g., urethra, cervix, rectum, oropharynx, and conjunctiva). A specimen of pus or a urethral exudate is inadequate. Chlamydiae infect columnar or squamocolumnar cells; therefore, endocervical and not vaginal specimens should be collected. It has been estimated that 30% of the specimens submitted for study in patients with suspected *Chlamydia* infection are inappropriate.

Cytology

Examination of Giemsa-stained cell scrapings for the presence of inclusions was the first method used for the diagnosis of *C. trachomatis* infection. However, this method is insensitive and is not recommended. Likewise, Papanicolaou staining of cervical material has been found to be an insensitive and nonspecific method.

Antigen Detection

Two general approaches have been used to detect chlamydial antigens in clinical specimens: **direct immunofluorescence staining** with fluorescein-conjugated monoclonal antibodies (Figure 46-4) and **enzyme-linked immunosorbent assays**. In both assays, antibodies that have been prepared against either the chlamydial MOMP or the cell wall LPS are used. Because antigenic determinants on LPS may be shared with other bacteria, particularly those in fecal specimens, tests that target the LPS antigen are less specific. The sensitivity of each assay method has been reported to vary enormously, but neither is considered as sensitive as

Figure 46—4. Fluorescent-stained elementary bodies (*arrows*) in a clinical sample. (*From Hart T, Shears P: Color Atlas of Medical Microbiology. London, Mosby-Wolfe, 2000.*)

cultur or nucleic-acid-based tests, particularly if male urethral specimens or specimens from asymptomatic patients are used. The latter pose a problem because they may contain relatively few chlamydiae.

Nucleic-Acid-Based Tests

Nucleic acid probe tests most commonly measure for the presence of a species-specific sequence of **16S ribosomal RNA**. The advantage of these tests is that the nucleic acid does not have to be amplified, making the tests rapid and relatively inexpensive; however, these tests are relatively insensitive for the detection of small numbers of chlamydiae. **Nucleic acid amplification tests (NAATs)** are more sensitive (generally reported to be 90% to 98% sensitive) and if properly monitored are very specific. These tests first amplify a specific sequence of genetic information and then detect it with a species-specific probe. First-voided urine from a patient with urethritis can be used, as well as urethral discharge. Care must be used to monitor for the presence of inhibitors (e.g., urine) to the amplification reaction and to prevent cross-contamination of specimens. Despite these cautions, NAATs are currently considered the tests of choice for the laboratory diagnosis of genital *C. trachomatis* infection.

Culture

The isolation of *C. trachomatis* in cell culture remains the most **specific** method of diagnosing *C. trachomatis* infections but is **relatively insensitive** compared with nucleic acid amplification techniques (Figure 46-5). The bacteria infect a restricted range of cell lines in vitro, similar to the narrow range of cells they infect in vivo. The sensitivity of culture is compromised if inadequate specimens are used and if chlamydial viability has been lost during transport of the specimen. It has been estimated that the sensitivity of the findings yielded by a single endocervical specimen may be only 70% to 85%.

Antibody Detection

Serologic testing is of limited value in the diagnosis of *C. trachomatis* urogenital infections in adults, because the

Figure 46–5. *Chlamydia trachomatis* is grown in cell cultures and detected by staining inclusion bodies *(arrows)* with either iodine or specific fluorescein-labeled antibodies.

test cannot differentiate between current and past infections. Demonstration of a significant increase in antibody levels can be useful; however, this increase may not be demonstrated for a month or longer, particularly in patients who receive antibiotic treatment. Testing for immunoglobulin (Ig)M antibodies is also usually not helpful, because these antibodies may not be detected in adolescents and adults. An exception is the detection of IgM antibodies in infants with chlamydial pneumonitis.

Antibody tests for the diagnosis of LGV can be helpful. Infected patients produce a vigorous antibody response that can be detected by complement fixation, microimmunofluorescence (MIF), or enzyme immunoassay (EIA). The CF test is directed against the genus-specific LPS antigen. Thus a positive result (i.e., fourfold increase in titer or a single titer ≥1:256) is highly suggestive of LGV. Confirmation is determined by the MIF test, which is directed against species- and serovar-specific antigens (the chlamydial MOMPs). Like the CF test, EIAs are genus specific. The advantage of these tests is that they are less technically cumbersome. However, the results must be confirmed by MIF.

Treatment, Prevention, and Control

It is recommended that patients with LGV be treated with doxycycline for 21 days. Treatment with erythromycin is recommended for children younger than 9 years, pregnant women, and patients unable to tolerate doxycycline. Ocular and genital infections in adults should be treated with a single dose of azithromycin or 7 days of doxycycline. Newborn conjunctivitis and pneumonia should be treated with erythromycin for 10 to 14 days.

It is difficult to prevent trachoma, because the population with endemic disease commonly has limited access to medical care. The blindness associated with advanced stages of trachoma can be prevented only by prompt treatment of early disease and prevention of reexposure. Although treatment can be successful in individuals living in areas where the disease is endemic, it is difficult to eradicate the disease within a population and to prevent reinfections unless sanitary conditions are improved. *Chlamydia* conjunctivitis and genital infections are prevented through the use of safe sex practices and the prompt treatment of symptomatic patients and their sexual partners.

Chlamydophila pneumoniae

C. pneumoniae was first isolated from the conjunctiva of a child in Taiwan. It was initially considered a psittacosis strain, because the morphology of the inclusions produced in cell culture was similar. However, it was subsequently shown that the Taiwan isolate (TW-183) was related serologically to a pharyngeal isolate, designated AR-39, and was unrelated to psittacosis strains. This new organism was initially called *TWAR*, then classified as *Chlamydia pneumoniae*, and finally placed in the new genus *Chlamydophila*. Only a single serotype (TWAR) has been identified. Respiratory secretions transmit infection; no animal reservoir has been identified.

C. pneumoniae is a **human pathogen** that causes sinusitis, pharyngitis, bronchitis, and pneumonia. Infections are believed to be transmitted person to person by respiratory secretions. The prevalence of infections is very controversial, with wide variations reported in the literature, in large part due to significant variation in diagnostic test methods. It is believed that most *C. pneumoniae* infections are asymptomatic or mild, causing a persistent cough and malaise; most patients do not require hospitalization. More severe respiratory tract infections typically involve a single lobe of the lungs. These infections cannot be differentiated from other atypical pneumonias, such as those caused by *Mycoplasma pneumoniae*, *Legionella pneumophila*, and respiratory viruses.

The role of *C. pneumoniae* in the pathogenesis of atherosclerosis remains to be defined. It is known that *C. pneumoniae* can infect and grow in smooth muscle cells, endothelial cells of the coronary artery, and macrophages. The organism has also been demonstrated in biopsy specimens of atherosclerotic lesions by means of culture, PCR amplification, immunohistologic staining, electron microscopy, and in situ hybridization. Thus the association of *C. pneumoniae* with atherosclerotic lesions is clear. What is not clear is the role of the organism in the development of atherosclerosis. It has been proposed that the disease results from an inflammatory response to chronic infection; however, this remains to be proven.

Diagnosis of *C. pneumoniae* infections is difficult. The organisms do not grow in the cell lines used for the isolation of *C. trachomatis*, and although *C. pneumoniae* will grow in the HEp-2 cell line, this cell line is not used in most clinical laboratories. Detection of *C. pneumoniae* by nucleic acid amplification tests has been successful; however, significant interlaboratory variation has been reported among laboratories with experience in the use of these assays. The microimmunofluorescence (MIF) test is the only acceptable test for serodiagnosis. The criteria for the diagnosis of acute

C. pneumoniae infection is a single IgM titer of >1:16 or a fourfold increase in IgG titer. A single elevated IgG titer cannot be used. Because IgG antibodies do not appear for 6 to 8 weeks after infection, serologic testing has limited value for the diagnosis of an acute infection.

Macrolides (erythromycin, azithromycin, and clarithromycin), doxycycline, or levofloxacin is recommended for treatment of *C. pneumoniae* infections, although evidence supporting their use is limited. Control of exposure to *C. pneumoniae* is likely to be difficult because the bacterium is ubiquitous.

Chlamydophila psittaci (Clinical Case 46-3)

C. psittaci is the cause of psittacosis (parrot fever), which can be transmitted to humans. The disease was first observed in parrots, thus the name **psittacosis** (*psittakos* is the Greek word for "parrot"). In reality, however, the natural reservoir of *C. psittaci* is virtually any species of bird, and the disease has been referred to more appropriately as **ornithosis** (derived from the Greek word *ornithos*, for "bird"). Other animals such as sheep, cows, and goats, as well as humans, can become infected. The organism is present in the blood, tissues, feces, and feathers of infected birds that may appear either ill or healthy.

Infection occurs by means of the respiratory tract, after which the bacteria spread to the reticuloendothelial cells of the liver and spleen. The organisms multiply in these sites, producing focal necrosis. The lung and other organs are then seeded as the result of hematogenous spread, which causes a predominantly lymphocytic inflammatory response in the alveolar and interstitial spaces. Edema, thickening of the alveolar wall, infiltration of macrophages, necrosis, and occasionally hemorrhage occur at these sites. Mucous plugs develop in the bronchioles, causing cyanosis and anoxia.

Fewer than 25 cases of the disease are reported annually in the United States, with most infections in adults.

Clinical Case 46-3. Psittacosis in a Previously Healthy Man

Scully, et al. (N Engl J Med 338:1527-1535, 1998) described a 24-year-old man who was admitted to a local hospital in acute respiratory distress. Several days before his hospitalization, he developed nasal congestion, myalgia, dry cough, mild dyspnea, and a headache. Immediately before admission, the cough became productive, and he developed pleuritic pain, fever, chills, and diarrhea. Radiographs demonstrated consolidation of the right upper lobe of the lungs and patchy infiltrates in the left lower lobe. Despite the fact his antibiotic treatment included erythromycin, doxycycline, ceftriaxone, and vancomycin, his pulmonary status did not begin to improve for 7 days, and he was not discharged from the hospital until a month after his admission. A careful history revealed the man had been exposed to parrots in a hotel lobby while vacationing. The diagnosis of *C. psittaci* pneumonia was made by serologic tests and growing the organism in cell culture.

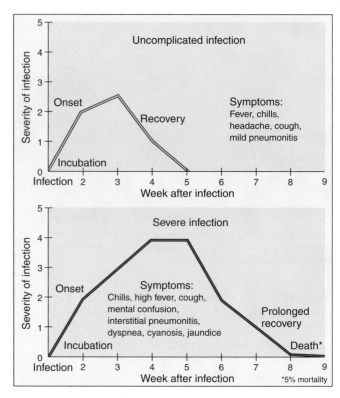

Figure 46—6. Time course of *Chlamydophila psittaci* infection.

This number certainly is an underestimation of the true prevalence of disease, however, because (1) human infections may be asymptomatic or mild, (2) exposure to an infected bird may not be suspected, (3) convalescent serum may not be collected to confirm the clinical diagnosis, and (4) antibiotic therapy may blunt the antibody response. Furthermore, because of the serologic cross-reactions with *C. pneumoniae*, specific estimates of the prevalence of disease will remain unreliable until a definitive diagnostic test is developed.

The bacterium is usually transmitted to humans through the inhalation of dried excrement, urine, or respiratory secretions from psittacine birds (e.g., parrots, parakeets, macaws, cockatiels). Person-to-person transmission is rare. Veterinarians, zookeepers, pet shop workers, and employees of poultry-processing plants are at increased risk for this infection.

The illness develops after an incubation of 5 to 14 days and usually manifests as headache, high fever, chills, malaise, and myalgias (Figure 46-6). Pulmonary signs include a nonproductive cough, rales, and consolidation. Central nervous system involvement is common, usually consisting of headache, but encephalitis, convulsions, coma, and death may occur in severe untreated cases. Patients may suffer gastrointestinal tract symptoms such as nausea, vomiting, and diarrhea. Other systemic symptoms include carditis, hepatomegaly, splenomegaly, and follicular keratoconjunctivitis.

Psittacosis is usually diagnosed on the basis of serologic findings. A fourfold increase in titer, shown by the CF testing of paired acute and convalescent phase sera, is suggestive of *C. psittaci* infection, but the species-specific MIF test must be performed to confirm the diagnosis. *C. psittaci* can be isolated in cell culture (e.g., with L cells) after 5 to 10 days of incubation, although this procedure is rarely performed in clinical laboratories.

Infections can be treated successfully with doxycycline or macrolides. Person-to-person transmission occurs rarely, so isolation of the patient and prophylactic treatment of contacts are not necessary. Psittacosis can be prevented only through the control of infections in domestic and imported pet birds. Such control can be achieved by treating birds with chlortetracycline hydrochloride for 45 days. No vaccine currently exists for this disease.

Case Study and Questions

A 22-year-old man came to the emergency department with a history of urethral pain and purulent discharge that developed after he had sexual contact with a prostitute. Gram stain of the discharge revealed abundant gram-negative diplococci resembling *Neisseria gonorrhoeae*. The patient was treated with penicillin and sent home. Two days later, the patient returned to the emergency room with a complaint of persistent, watery urethral discharge. Abundant white blood cells but no organisms were observed on Gram stain of the discharge. Culture of the discharge was negative for *N. gonorrhoeae* but positive for *C. trachomatis*.

1. Why is penicillin ineffective against *Chlamydia?* What antibiotic can be used to treat this patient?

2. Describe the growth cycle of *Chlamydia*. What structural features make the EBs and RBs well suited for their environment?

3. Describe the differences among the three species in the family Chlamydiaceae that cause human disease.

4. *C. trachomatis*, *C. pneumoniae*, and *C. psittaci* each cause respiratory tract infections. Describe the patient population most commonly infected and the epidemiology of these infections.

Bibliography

Arcari C, et al: Association between *Chlamydia pneumoniae* immunoglobulin A and acute myocardial infarction in young men in the United States military: Importance of timing of exposure measurements. Clin Infect Dis 40:1123-1130, 2005.

Boman J, Hammerschlag MR: *Chlamydia pneumoniae* and atherosclerosis: Critical assessment of diagnostic methods and relevance to treatment studies. Clin Microbiol Rev 15:1-20, 2002.

Centers for Disease Control and Prevention: Screening tests to detect *Chlamydia trachomatis* and *Neisseria gonorrhoeae* infections—2002. Morb Mortal Wkly Rep 51(RR-15):1-38, 2002.

Gambhir M, et al: Trachoma: Transmission, infection, and control. Lancet Infect Dis 7:420-427, 2007.

Kumar S, Hammerschlag M: Acute respiratory infection due to *Chlamydia pneumoniae*: Current status of diagnostic methods. Clin Infect Dis 44:568-576, 2007.

McLean C, et al: Treatment of lymphogranuloma venereum. Clin Infect Dis 44:S147-S152, 2007.

Morré S, et al: Urogenital *Chlamydia trachomatis* serovars in men and women with a symptomatic or asymptomatic infection: An association with clinical manifestations? J Clin Microbiol 38:2292-2296, 2000.

Van der Bij A, et al: Diagnostic and clinical implications of anorectal lymphogranuloma venereum in men who have sex with men: A retrospective case-control study. Clin Infect Dis 42:186-194, 2006.

Vanrompay D, et al: *Chlamydophila psittaci* transmission from pet birds to humans. Emerg Infect Dis 13:1109-1110, 2007.

Role of Bacteria in Disease

This chapter summarizes material presented in Chapters 21 to 46. The preceding chapters have focused on individual organisms and the diseases they cause. We believe this is an important process in understanding how individual organisms produce disease. However, when a patient develops an infection, a physician approaches diagnosis by assessing the clinical presentation and constructing a list of organisms that are most likely to cause the disease. The etiology in some diseases can be attributed to a single organism (e.g., tetanus—*Clostridium tetani*). More commonly, however, multiple organisms can produce a similar clinical picture (e.g., pneumonia, gastroenteritis, meningitis). The clinical management of infections is therefore predicated on the ability to develop an accurate differential diagnosis; that is, it is critical to know which organisms are most commonly associated with a particular infectious process.

The development of an infection depends on the complex interactions of (1) the host's susceptibility to infection,

(2) the organism's virulence potential, and (3) the opportunity for interaction between host and organism. It is impossible to summarize in a single chapter the complex interactions that lead to the development of disease in each organ system. That is the domain of comprehensive texts in infectious disease. Rather, this chapter is intended to serve as a very broad overview of the bacteria commonly associated with infections at specific body sites and with specific clinical manifestations (Tables 47-1 to 47-5). Because many factors influence the relative frequency with which specific organisms cause disease (e.g., age, underlying disease, epidemiologic factors, host immunity), no attempt is made to define all the factors associated with disease caused by specific organisms. That material is provided, in part, in the preceding chapters and in infectious disease texts. Furthermore, the roles of fungi, viruses, and parasites are not considered here but rather in the following sections of this book.

Table 47–1. Overview of Selected Bacterial Pathogens

Organism	Clinical Features	Epidemiologic Features	Virulence Factors	Treatment
Aerobic and Facultatively Anaerobic Gram-Positive Cocci				
Enterococcus faecalis and *E. faecium*	Bacteremia, intraabdominal abscess, urinary tract infection, endocarditis	Elderly patients and patients who have been hospitalized for extended periods receiving broad-spectrum antibiotics	Relatively avirulent	Penicillin/ampicillin or vancomycin; combined with gentamicin for endocarditis or severe infection
Staphylococcus aureus	Cutaneous infections: impetigo, folliculitis, furuncles, carbuncles, wounds; disseminated infections: pneumonia, empyema, osteomyelitis, septic arthritis; toxin-mediated infections: toxic shock syndrome, scalded skin syndrome, food poisoning; community-acquired infections	Colonize human skin and mucosal surfaces; survive on environmental surfaces; able to grow at temperature extremes and in high salt concentrations	Possess thick peptidoglycan layer, capsule, protein A, various toxins (cytotoxins, exfoliative toxins, enterotoxins, toxic shock syndrome toxin, Panton Valentine [PV] leukocidin) and hydrolytic enzymes	Oxacillin; vancomycin (for oxacillin-resistant strains)

Continued

Table 47–1. Overview of Selected Bacterial Pathogens—cont'd

Organism	Clinical Features	Epidemiologic Features	Virulence Factors	Treatment
Aerobic and Facultatively Anaerobic Gram-Positive Cocci				
Staphylococcus, coagulase negative	Opportunistic pathogen causing infections on foreign bodies (e.g., catheters, shunts, prosthetic joints, and heart valves); urinary tract infections (e.g., *S. saprophyticus*); native valve endocarditis (*S. lugdunensis*)	Colonize human skin and mucosal surfaces; survive on environmental surfaces; able to grow at temperature extremes	Possess thick peptidoglycan layer and loose polysaccharide slime layer; *S. saprophyticus* produces high concentrations of urease	Oxacillin; vancomycin (for oxacillin-resistant strains)
Streptococcus pyogenes (group A)	Suppurative infections: pharyngitis, scarlet fever, sinusitis, skin and soft-tissue infection (impetigo, erysipelas, cellulitis, necrotizing fasciitis), toxic shock–like syndrome; nonsuppurative infections: rheumatic fever; glomerulonephritis	Diverse populations	Capsule, M protein, M-like protein, F protein, pyrogenic exotoxins, streptolysin S and O, streptokinase, deoxyribonuclease (DNase); C5a peptidase	Penicillin, macrolides, cephalosporins, clindamycin, vancomycin; surgical débridement for necrotizing fasciitis
Streptococcus agalactiae (group B)	Neonatal disease (early onset, late onset; bacteremia, pneumonia, meningitis); urinary tract infections, bacteremia, pneumonia	Neonates; pregnant women; patients with diabetes, cancer, or alcoholism	Similar to group A but no capsule	Penicillin, macrolides, cephalosporins, clindamycin, vancomycin; penicillin and aminoglycoside for serious infections
Other β-hemolytic streptococci	Pharyngitis, otitis, sinusitis, skin and soft-tissue infection, impetigo, erysipelas, cellulitis, necrotizing fasciitis	Diverse populations	Similar to group A *Streptococcus*	Penicillin (drug of choice), macrolides, cephalosporins, clindamycin, vancomycin; surgical débridement for necrotizing fasciitis
Viridans streptococci	Abscess formation; septicemia in neutropenic patients; subacute endocarditis; odontogenic infections; dental caries	Patients with abnormal heart valves	Relatively avirulent	Penicillin; penicillin combined with aminoglycoside
Streptococcus pneumoniae	Pneumonia and other respiratory tract infections; meningitis; spontaneous bacterial peritonitis, endocarditis, septic arthritis; bacteremia	Diverse: neonates, children, adults with chronic diseases, elderly persons	Polysaccharide capsule; teichoic acid; immunoglobulin (Ig)A proteases; pneumolysin O	Penicillin; levofloxacin, cephalosporins, clindamycin
Aerobic or Facultatively Anaerobic Gram-Positive Rods				
Bacillus anthracis	Cutaneous anthrax, inhalation anthrax, gastrointestinal anthrax	Animal workers; microbiologic accidents; bioterrorism; eating contaminated meat	Capsule; edema toxin; lethal toxin; spore formation	Fluoroquinolones (ciprofloxacin); penicillin, doxycycline, erythromycin, or chloramphenicol as alternative therapy
Bacillus cereus	Gastroenteritis, ocular infections, bacteremia	Contaminated food; traumatic eye injury with introduction of soil; injection drug use	Heat-stable and heat-labile toxins, necrotic toxin	Symptomatic treatment for gastroenteritis; fluoroquinolones or vancomycin

ROLE OF BACTERIA IN DISEASE

Table 47–1. Overview of Selected Bacterial Pathogens—cont'd

Organism	Clinical Features	Epidemiologic Features	Virulence Factors	Treatment
Aerobic or Facultatively Anaerobic Gram-Positive Rods				
Corynebacterium diphtheriae	Diphtheria: respiratory, cutaneous	Spread by respiratory droplets to unimmunized individuals	Diphtheria toxin	Neutralizing exotoxin; penicillin or erythromycin to eliminate organism and terminate toxin production; immunization with diphtheria toxoid
Corynebacterium jeikeium	Septicemia, endocarditis; wound infections; foreign body infections	Immunocompromised patients at increased risk	Unknown	Vancomycin
Corynebacterium urealyticum	Urinary tract infections, including pyelonephritis with calculi; septicemia; endocarditis; wound infections	Risk factors include immunosuppression, underlying genitourinary disorders, antecedent urologic procedures, prior antibiotic therapy	Urease production	Vancomycin
Erysipelothrix rhusiopathiae	Erysipeloid (cellulitis characterized by painful, pruritic, inflammatory skin lesion)	Occupational disease of butchers, meat processors, farmers, poultry workers, fish handlers, and veterinarians	Unknown	Penicillin; cephalosporins, fluoroquinolones, erythromycin, or clindamycin as alternative therapy
Listeria monocytogenes	Early onset neonatal disease (granulomatosis infantiseptica); late-onset neonatal disease (meningitis with septicemia); flulike illness in adults; bacteremia or disseminated disease in pregnant women or patients with cell-mediated immune defects	Immunocompromised hosts, elderly persons, neonates, pregnant women; ingestion of contaminated food	Listeriolysin O; internalins; intracellular survival and growth; intracellular motility; growth at 4° C	Ampicillin (alone or in combination with gentamicin)
Mycobacteria				
Mycobacterium avium complex	Localized pulmonary disease; disseminated disease with multiorgan involvement	Localized disease in patients with chronic pulmonary disease; disseminated disease in AIDS and other immunocompromised patients	Intracellular replication	Clarithromycin or azithromycin combined with rifabutin or ethambutol
Mycobacterium leprae	Leprosy: range from tuberculoid form to lepromatous form	Close contact with infected individual most likely responsible for spread	Ability to survive and replicate in macrophages	Dapsone and rifampicin for tuberculoid form; add clofazimine for lepromatous form
Mycobacterium tuberculosis	Tuberculosis: pulmonary, extrapulmonary	All ages with HIV-infected patients at greatest risk for active disease	Ability to survive and replicate in macrophages	Multidrug therapy with isoniazid, rifampin, ethambutol, and pyrazinamide
Nocardia species	Bronchopulmonary disease; primary or secondary cutaneous infections; brain abscesses	Opportunistic pathogen in immunocompetent patients with chronic pulmonary disease or immunocompromised patients with T-cell deficiencies	Intracellular survival and growth; catalase and superoxide dismutase	Sulfonamides; amikacin, carbapenems, or broad-spectrum cephalosporins as alternative therapy if active

Continued

Table 47–1. Overview of Selected Bacterial Pathogens—cont'd

Organism	Clinical Features	Epidemiologic Features	Virulence Factors	Treatment
Mycobacteria				
Rhodococcus equi	Bronchopulmonary disease (lung abscesses); opportunistic infections in immunocompetent patients	Pathogen most commonly found in immunocompromised patients (e.g., AIDS patients, transplant recipients)	Intracellular survival and growth	Combination therapy with vancomycin, carbapenems, aminoglycosides, ciprofloxacin, rifampin, and/or erythromycin
Aerobic Gram-Negative Cocci				
Neisseria gonorrhoeae	Gonorrhea, pelvic inflammatory disease, arthritis	Sexual transmission, asymptomatic carriage	Pili, adhesins, IgA protease, transferrin-binding proteins, antigenic variation	Ceftriaxone, ciprofloxacin; cefoxitin plus doxycycline
Neisseria meningitidis	Meningitis, bacteremia (meningococcemia)	Carrier state, aerosol transmission, most common in children and young adults	Polysaccharide capsule, endotoxin, pili, adhesins, IgA protease, transferrin-binding proteins	Ceftriaxone, penicillin, chloramphenicol
Aerobic and Facultatively Anaerobic Gram-Negative Rods				
Acinetobacter	Pneumonia, septicemia, opportunistic infections	Nosocomial infections; common in military hospitals	Unknown	Imipenem or ceftazidime combined with aminoglycoside for serious infections; drug resistance common
Aeromonas	Wound infections; gastroenteritis	Healthy and immunocompromised patients	Unknown	Ciprofloxacin; sulfamethoxazole, gentamicin, or amikacin as alternative therapy
Bartonella henselae	Bacillary angiomatosis (BA); subacute endocarditis; cat-scratch disease (CSD)	Healthy (endocarditis, CSD) and immunocompromised patients (BA)	Unknown	Erythromycin or azithromycin; doxycycline
Bartonella quintana	Trench fever (TF); Recurrent fevers; bacillary angiomatosis (BA)	Healthy (TF) or immunocompromised patients (BA)	Unknown	As with *B. henselae*
Bordetella pertussis, Bordetella parapertussis	Pertussis (whooping cough)	Aerosol transmission; severe diseases in infants, milder in adults	Pertussis toxin, adenylate cyclase toxin, adhesins, tracheal cytotoxin	Supportive therapy, erythromycin (or other macrolides) to decrease infectivity and prophylaxis for contacts; fluoroquinolones
Brucella	Brucellosis	Exposure to infected goats, sheep, cattle, or other animals; bioterrorism	Ability to persist and replicate in macrophages	Doxycycline plus rifampin or gentamicin; trimethoprim-sulfamethoxazole
Burkholderia cepacia complex	Pulmonary infections; opportunistic infections	Compromised individuals, especially cystic fibrosis and chronic granulomatous disease patients	Unknown	Trimethoprim-sulfamethoxazole; piperacillin, ceftazidime, or ciprofloxacin as alternative therapy if trimethoprim-sulfamethoxazole resistant

Table 47–1. Overview of Selected Bacterial Pathogens—cont'd

Organism	Clinical Features	Epidemiologic Features	Virulence Factors	Treatment
Aerobic and Facultatively Anaerobic Gram-Negative Rods				
Burkholderia pseudomallei	Melioidosis (asymptomatic to severe pulmonary disease)	Opportunistic pathogen	Unknown	Trimethoprim-sulfamethoxazole combined with ceftazidime
Campylobacter jejuni, Campylobacter coli, Campylobacter upsaliensis	Gastroenteritis	Zoonotic infection following ingestion of contaminated food, milk, or water	Factors regulating adherence and invasion into intestinal mucosa	Self-limited; severe infections treated with erythromycin; tetracycline or fluoroquinolones used as alterative therapy
Campylobacter fetus	Septicemia; meningitis; gastroenteritis; spontaneous abortion	Infects elderly, immunocompromised patients	Unknown	Aminoglycosides, carbapenems, chloramphenicol
Cardiobacterium hominis	Subacute endocarditis	Opportunistic pathogen in patients with previously damaged heart valve	Unknown	Penicillin or ampicillin
Eikenella corrodens	Subacute endocarditis; wound infections	Human bite wounds; opportunistic pathogen in patients with previously damaged heart valve	Unknown	Penicillin, cephalosporins, tetracycline, or fluoroquinolones
Escherichia coli—enteropathogenic (EPEC)	Watery diarrhea and vomiting	Infants in developing countries	Bundle-forming pili, attaching and effacing	Unknown
E. coli—enterohemorrhagic (EHEC)	Watery diarrhea, hemorrhagic colitis, hemolytic uremic syndrome	Foodborne, waterborne outbreaks in developed countries	Shiga toxins, attaching and effacing	Antibiotics contraindicated
E. coli—enterotoxigenic (ETEC)	Watery diarrhea	Childhood diarrhea in developing countries, travelers' diarrhea	Pili, heat-labile and heat-stable enterotoxins	Ciprofloxacin shortens course (high level of resistance)
E. coli—enteroaggregative (EAEC)	Diarrhea with mucus	Childhood diarrhea	Pili, cytotoxins	Fluoroquinolones in AIDS patients
E. coli—enteroinvasive (EIEC)	Watery diarrhea, hemorrhagic colitis	Childhood diarrhea in developing countries	Invasion and destruction of colonic epithelial cells	Antibiotics reduce duration of disease and infectivity
E. coli—uropathogenic	Cystitis, pyelonephritis	Sexually active women	Adhesins (P pili, AAF/I, AAF/III, Dr), hemolysin, pathogenicity islands	Trimethoprim-sulfamethoxazole, fluoroquinolones
E. coli—meningitis associated	Acute meningitis	Neonates	K1 capsule, S fimbriae, cellular invasion	Extended-spectrum cephalosporins
Francisella tularensis	Tularemia: ulceroglandular, oculoglandular, pneumonic	Tick bites; skinning infected animals (rabbits); bioterrorism	Capsule	Streptomycin, gentamicin; fluoroquinolones
Haemophilus influenzae	Encapsulated type b strains: meningitis, septicemia, cellulitis, epiglottitis; unencapsulated strains: otitis media, sinusitis, bronchitis, pneumonia	Aerosol transmission in young, unimmunized children; spread from upper respiratory tract in elderly patients with chronic respiratory disease	Polysaccharide capsule, pili, adhesins, IgA protease	Broad-spectrum cephalosporin, azithromycin, or fluoroquinolone; many strains resistant to ampicillin

Continued

Table 47–1. Overview of Selected Bacterial Pathogens—cont'd

Organism	Clinical Features	Epidemiologic Features	Virulence Factors	Treatment
Aerobic and Facultatively Anaerobic Gram-Negative Rods				
Helicobacter pylori	Gastritis, peptic, and duodenal ulcers; gastric adenocarcinoma	Infections common, particularly in people in low socioeconomic class or in developing countries	Urease; heat-shock protein; acid-inhibitory protein adhesins; mucinase; phospholipases; vacuolating cytotoxin; other factors	Multidrug therapy: tetracycline, metronidazole, bismuth, and omeprazole
Kingella kingae	Subacute endocarditis	Opportunistic pathogen in patients with previously damaged heart valve	Unknown	β-Lactam with β-lactamase inhibitor, cephalosporins, macrolides, tetracycline, fluoroquinolones
Klebsiella pneumoniae	Pneumonia, urinary tract infections	Nosocomial infections; alcoholism	Capsule	Cephalosporins, fluoroquinolones
Legionella pneumophila	Legionnaires disease (pneumonia), Pontiac fever (flulike illness)	Waterborne; elderly and immunocompromised patients	C3b adhesin, cytotoxins, evasion of phagolysosome fusion	Macrolides (erythromycin, azithromycin, clarithromycin); fluoroquinolones (ciprofloxacin, levofloxacin) used as alternative therapy
Moraxella catarrhalis	Ear, eye, and respiratory infections	Children; patients with compromised pulmonary system	Unknown	Cephalosporins; amoxicillin/ clavulanic acid
Proteus	Urinary tract infections, wound infections	Structural abnormality in urinary tract	Urease, swarming motility	Amoxicillin, trimethoprim-sulfamethoxazole, cephalosporins, fluoroquinolones
Pseudomonas aeruginosa	Pulmonary; primary skin infection; urinary tract infection; ear or eye infections; bacteremia	Nosocomial infections	Capsule; exotoxin A; ExoS; phospholipase C; elastase	Combination therapy generally required (e.g., aminoglycoside with extended-spectrum cephalosporins, piperacillin-tazobactam, or carbapenem)
Salmonella enterica	Diarrhea, enteric fever (serovar Typhi)	Contaminated food; immunocompromised patients at higher risk for bacteremia	Type III secretion system; epithelial cell invasion; survival in macrophages	May prolong carrier state in simple diarrhea treatment; fluoroquinolones for enteric fever
Serratia, Enterobacter	Pneumonia, urinary tract infections, wound infections	Nosocomial infections	Unknown	Carbapenems; piperacillin-tazobactam
Shigella	Bacillary dysentery	Contaminated food or water; person-to-person spread	Type III secretion system; intracellular spread; induction of macrophage apoptosis	Ampicillin; trimethoprim-sulfamethoxazole; fluoroquinolones
Stenotrophomonas maltophilia	Wide variety of local and systemic infections	Nosocomial infections	Unknown	Trimethoprim-sulfamethoxazole
Streptobacillus moniliformis	Rat-bite fever; Haverhill fever	Bite of rat or other small rodents; ingestion of contaminated food or water	Unknown	Penicillin, doxycycline

Table 47—1. Overview of Selected Bacterial Pathogens—cont'd

Organism	Clinical Features	Epidemiologic Features	Virulence Factors	Treatment
Aerobic and Facultatively Anaerobic Gram-Negative Rods				
Vibrio cholerae	Severe watery diarrhea	Children and adults in developing countries	Cholera toxin; toxin-co-regulated pilus (TCP); other toxins; neuraminidase	Rehydration; doxycycline, trimethoprim-sulfamethoxazole, or furazolidone shortens course
Vibrio parahaemolyticus	Watery diarrhea	Seafood-borne outbreaks	Hemolysin/enterotoxin	Rehydration
Vibrio vulnificus	Wound infections; primary septicemia	Compromised individuals with preexisting hepatic or chronic diseases	Capsule; numerous degradative enzymes	Minocycline combined with a fluoroquinolone or cefotaxime; débridement
Anaerobes				
Actinomyces	Actinomycosis: cervicofacial, thoracic, abdominal, pelvic, central nervous system	Colonizes human mucosal surface (oropharynx, intestine, vagina)	Unknown	Penicillin; alternative drugs include erythromycin, clindamycin
Bacteroides fragilis	Polymicrobial infections of abdomen, female genital tract, cutaneous and soft tissues	Normal inhabitant of gastrointestinal tract	Polysaccharide capsule; short-chain fatty acids; catalase; superoxide dismutase; hydrolytic enzymes	Metronidazole
Clostridium botulinum	Botulism: foodborne, infant, wound	Found in environment (e.g., soil, water, sewage) and gastrointestinal tract of animals and humans	Spores; botulinum toxin blocks release of neurotransmitter acetylcholine	Ventilatory support; use of trivalent botulinum antitoxin
Clostridium difficile	Antibiotic-associated diarrhea; pseudomembranous colitis	Colonize human gastrointestinal tract and female genital tract; contaminates hospital environment; prior antibiotic use	Spores; enterotoxin; cytotoxin	Discontinue implicated antibiotic; metronidazole
Clostridium perfringens	Soft-tissue infections: cellulitis, fasciitis, myonecrosis; food poisoning; septicemia	Found in environment (e.g., soil, water, sewage) and gastrointestinal tract of animals and humans	Spores; production of many toxins and hemolytic enzymes	Surgical intervention and penicillin
Clostridium tetani	Tetanus: generalized, localized, neonatal	Found in environment (e.g., soil, water, sewage) and gastrointestinal tract of animals and humans	Spores; tetanospasmin blocks release of neurotransmitters for inhibitory synapses	Clean wound; passive immunization; vaccination with tetanus toxoid
Propionibacterium acne	Acne; opportunistic infections (e.g., of prosthetic devices)	Colonize human skin and mucosal surfaces	Opportunistic pathogen of relatively low virulence	Acne treated with benzoyl peroxide plus clindamycin or erythromycin
Anaplasma*, *Ehrlichia*, *Rickettsia*, *Coxiella*, *Mycoplasma*, *Chlamydia*, and *Chlamydophila				
Anaplasma phagocytophilum	Anaplasmosis (granulocytic ehrlichiosis)	Transmission by tick bite (*Ixodes*)	Intracellular survival and growth; oxidant-mediated cell injury	Doxycycline; rifampin used as alternative therapy
Chlamydophila pneumoniae	Pneumonia; cardiovascular disease (?)	Children, young adults	Unknown	Macrolides; fluoroquinolones; tetracyclines

Continued

Table 47–1. Overview of Selected Bacterial Pathogens—cont'd

Organism	Clinical Features	Epidemiologic Features	Virulence Factors	Treatment
Anaplasma, Ehrlichia, Rickettsia, Coxiella, Mycoplasma, Chlamydia, and *Chlamydophila*				
Chlamydophila psittaci	Pneumonia	Exposure to birds and their secretions	Unknown	Macrolides; tetracyclines
Chlamydia trachomatis	Trachoma; neonatal conjunctivitis and pneumonia; urethritis; cervicitis; salpingitis; lymphogranuloma venereum	Trachoma in developing countries; exposure to infected secretions during birth or sexual activities	Unknown	Tetracyclines; macrolides; fluoroquinolones
Coxiella burnetii	Q fever: acute (fever, headache, chills, myalgias, granulomatous hepatitis) and chronic (endocarditis, hepatic dysfunction)	Persons exposed to infected livestock; primarily acquired by inhalation; relatively uncommon in United States	Intracellular survival and replication; formation of endospore-like structures that enhance survival in the environment; formation of immune complexes in chronic disease	Doxycycline; rifampin with trimethoprim-sulfamethoxazole
Ehrlichia chaffeensis	Monocytic ehrlichiosis	Transmission by tick bite (*Amblyomma*)	Intracellular survival and replication; oxidant-mediated cell injury	Doxycycline; rifampin used as alternative therapy
Mycoplasma pneumoniae	Atypical pneumonia	Symptomatic disease more common in children than adults; severe disease in patients with hypogammaglobu-linemia	P1 adhesin protein	Macrolides; tetracycline; fluoroquinolones
Rickettsia rickettsii	Rocky Mountain spotted fever	Most prevalent in hikers and other individuals who spend a lot of time outdoors; transmission by tick bite (*Dermacentor* in United States)	Intracellular and rapid cell-to-cell spread; oxidant-spread; oxidant-mediated cell injury	Doxycycline; fluoroquinolones used as alternative therapy
Spirochetes				
Borrelia burgdorferi	Lyme disease: erythema migrans; cardiac, neurologic, or rheumatologic abnormalities	Transmission by ticks (*Ixodes*)	Surface-binding proteins	Oral penicillin; tetracyclines; ceftriaxone
Borrelia recurrentis	Epidemic relapsing fever	Transmission by human body louse; no animal host	Antigenic variation during infection causes relapses	Tetracyclines; erythromycin; chloramphenicol; penicillin
Borrelia species	Endemic relapsing fever	Transmission by tick bite (*Ornithodoros*); rodent and small mammal reservoir	Antigenic variation during infection causes relapses	Tetracyclines; erythromycin; chloramphenicol; penicillin
Leptospira interrogans	Leptospirosis: mild, viral-like illness to severe multiorgan illness (Weil syndrome)	Transmission by exposure to infected urine or tissues of rodents, dogs, farm animals, wild animals	Direct invasion through skin and replication in tissues; immune complex glomerulonephritis	Penicillin; doxycycline; vaccination of pets and herds
Treponema pallidum	Syphilis: primary, secondary, tertiary, congenital	Transmission congenitally or through sexual activity	Adherence to host cells; hyaluronidase; antiphagocytic coat; tissue destruction primarily mediated by host immune response	Penicillin; tetracyclines; erythromycin

Table 47—2. Summary of Bacteria Associated with Human Disease

System Affected	Pathogens
Upper Respiratory Infections	
Pharyngitis	*Streptococcus pyogenes*, Groups C *Streptococcus*, *Arcanobacterium haemolyticum*, *Chlamydophila pneumoniae*, *Neisseria gonorrhoeae*, *Corynebacterium diphtheriae*, *Corynebacterium ulcerans*, *Mycoplasma pneumoniae*, *Francisella tularensis*
Sinusitis	***Streptococcus pneumoniae, Haemophilus influenzae,* mixed anaerobes and aerobes, *Moraxella catarrhalis*,** *Staphylococcus aureus*, group A *Streptococcus*, *Chlamydophila pneumoniae*, *Pseudomonas aeruginosa* and other gram-negative rods
Epiglottitis	*Haemophilus influenzae, Streptococcus pneumoniae, Staphylococcus aureus*
Ear Infections	
Otitis externa	***Pseudomonas aeruginosa, Staphylococcus aureus,*** group A *Streptococcus*
Otitis media	***Streptococcus pneumoniae, Haemophilus influenzae, Moraxella catarrhalis,*** *Staphylococcus aureus*, group A *Streptococcus*, mixed anaerobes and aerobes
Eye Infections	
Conjunctivitis	***Staphylococcus aureus, Streptococcus pneumoniae, Haemophilus aegyptius,*** *Neisseria gonorrhoeae, Pseudomonas aeruginosa, Francisella tularensis, Chlamydia trachomatis*
Keratitis	***Staphylococcus aureus, Streptococcus pneumoniae, Pseudomonas aeruginosa,*** group A *Streptococcus, Proteus mirabilis* and other Enterobacteriaceae, *Bacillus* species, *Neisseria gonorrhoeae*
Endophthalmitis	***Bacillus cereus, Staphylococcus aureus, Pseudomonas aeruginosa,*** coagulase-negative *Staphylococcus, Propionibacterium* species, *Corynebacterium* species
Pleuropulmonary and Bronchial Infections	
Bronchitis	***Moraxella catarrhalis, Haemophilus influenzae, Streptococcus pneumoniae,*** *Bordetella pertussis, Mycoplasma pneumoniae, Chlamydophila pneumoniae*
Empyema	***Staphylococcus aureus, Streptococcus pneumoniae,* group A *Streptococcus,*** *Bacteroides fragilis, Klebsiella pneumoniae* and other Enterobacteriaceae, *Actinomyces* species, *Nocardia* species, *Mycobacterium tuberculosis* and other species
Pneumonia	***Streptococcus pneumoniae, Staphylococcus aureus, Klebsiella pneumoniae* and other Enterobacteriaceae,** *Moraxella catarrhalis, Haemophilus influenzae, Neisseria meningitidis, Mycoplasma pneumoniae, Chlamydia trachomatis, Chlamydophila pneumoniae, Chlamydophila psittaci, Pseudomonas aeruginosa, Burkholderia* species, *Legionella* species, *Francisella tularensis, Bacteroides fragilis, Nocardia* species, *Rhodococcus equi, Mycobacterium tuberculosis* and other species, *Coxiella burnetii, Rickettsia rickettsii*, and many other species
Urinary Tract Infections	
Cystitis and pyelonephritis	***Escherichia coli, Proteus mirabilis,* other Enterobacteriaceae,** *Pseudomonas aeruginosa, Staphylococcus saprophyticus, Staphylococcus aureus, Staphylococcus epidermidis*, group B *Streptococcus, Enterococcus* species, *Aerococcus urinae, Mycobacterium tuberculosis*
Renal calculi	***Proteus* species,** *Morganella morganii, Klebsiella pneumoniae, Corynebacterium urealyticum, Staphylococcus saprophyticus, Ureaplasma urealyticum*
Renal abscess	***Staphylococcus aureus,*** mixed anaerobes and aerobes, *Mycobacterium tuberculosis*
Prostatitis	***Escherichia coli,*** *Klebsiella pneumoniae*, other Enterobacteriaceae, *Enterococcus* species, *Neisseria gonorrhoeae, Mycobacterium tuberculosis* and other species
Intraabdominal Infections	
Peritonitis	***Escherichia coli, Bacteroides fragilis* and other species, *Enterococcus* species,** *Klebsiella pneumoniae*, other Enterobacteriaceae, *Pseudomonas aeruginosa, Streptococcus pneumoniae, Staphylococcus aureus, Fusobacterium* species, *Clostridium* species, mixed anaerobic cocci, *Neisseria gonorrhoeae, Chlamydia trachomatis, Mycobacterium tuberculosis*
Dialysis-associated peritonitis	**Coagulase-negative *Staphylococcus,*** *Staphylococcus aureus, Streptococcus* species, *Corynebacterium* species, *Propionibacterium* species, *Escherichia coli* and other Enterobacteriaceae, *Pseudomonas aeruginosa, Acinetobacter* species

Continued

Table 47–2. Summary of Bacteria Associated with Human Disease—cont'd

System Affected	Pathogens
Cardiovascular Infections	
Endocarditis	**Viridans *Streptococcus*, coagulase-negative *Staphylococcus*,** *Staphylococcus aureus*, HACEK organisms, *Streptococcus pneumoniae*, *Abiotrophia* species, *Rothia mucilaginosa*, *Enterococcus* species, *Bartonella* species, *Coxiella burnetii*, *Brucella* species, *Erysipelothrix rhusiopathiae*, Enterobacteriaceae, *Pseudomonas aeruginosa*, *Corynebacterium* species, *Propionibacterium* species
Myocarditis	*Corynebacterium diphtheriae*, *Clostridium perfringens*, group A *Streptococcus*, *Borrelia burgdorferi*, *Neisseria meningitidis*, *Staphylococcus aureus*, *Mycoplasma pneumoniae*, *Chlamydophila pneumoniae*, *Chlamydophila psittaci*, *Rickettsia rickettsii*, *Orientia tsutsugamushi*
Pericarditis	*Streptococcus pneumoniae*, *Staphylococcus aureus*, *Neisseria gonorrhoeae*, *Neisseria meningitidis*, *Mycoplasma pneumoniae*, *Mycobacterium tuberculosis* and other species
Sepsis	
General sepsis	***Staphylococcus aureus*, coagulase-negative *Staphylococcus*, *Escherichia coli*,** *Klebsiella* species, *Enterobacter* species, *Proteus mirabilis*, other Enterobacteriaceae, *Streptococcus pneumoniae* and other species, *Enterococcus* species, *Pseudomonas aeruginosa*, many other bacteria
Transfusion-associated sepsis	**Coagulase-negative *Staphylococcus*,** *Staphylococcus aureus*, *Yersinia enterocolitica*, *Pseudomonas fluorescens* group, *Salmonella* species, other Enterobacteriaceae, *Campylobacter jejuni* and other species, *Bacillus cereus* and other species
Septic thrombophlebitis	***Staphylococcus aureus*, *Bacteroides fragilis*,** *Klebsiella* species, *Enterobacter* species, *Pseudomonas aeruginosa*, *Fusobacterium* species
Central Nervous System Infections	
Meningitis	**Group B *Streptococcus*, *Streptococcus pneumoniae*, *Neisseria meningitidis*,** *Listeria monocytogenes*, *Haemophilus influenzae*, *Escherichia coli*, other Enterobacteriaceae, *Staphylococcus aureus*, coagulase-negative *Staphylococcus*, *Propionibacterium* species, *Nocardia* species, *Mycobacterium tuberculosis* and other species, *Borrelia burgdorferi*, *Leptospira* species, *Treponema pallidum*, *Brucella* species
Encephalitis	*Listeria monocytogenes*, *Treponema pallidum*, *Leptospira* species, *Actinomyces* species, *Nocardia* species, *Borrelia* species, *Rickettsia rickettsii*, *Coxiella burnetii*, *Mycoplasma pneumoniae*, *Mycobacterium tuberculosis* and other species
Brain abscess	***Staphylococcus aureus*, *Fusobacterium* species, *Peptostreptococcus* species, other anaerobic cocci,** Enterobacteriaceae, *Pseudomonas aeruginosa*, viridans streptococci, *Bacteroides* species, *Prevotella* species, *Porphyromonas* species, *Actinomyces* species, *Clostridium perfringens*, *Listeria monocytogenes*, *Nocardia* species, *Rhodococcus equi*, *Mycobacterium tuberculosis* and other species
Subdural empyema	***Staphylococcus aureus*, *Streptococcus pneumoniae*,** group B *Streptococcus*, *Neisseria meningitidis*, mixed anaerobes and aerobes
Skin and Soft-Tissue Infections	
Impetigo	**Group A *Streptococcus*, *Staphylococcus aureus***
Folliculitis	***Staphylococcus aureus*, *Pseudomonas aeruginosa***
Furuncles and carbuncles	***Staphylococcus aureus***
Paronychia	***Staphylococcus aureus*, group A *Streptococcus*,** *Pseudomonas aeruginosa*
Erysipelas	**Group A *Streptococcus***
Cellulitis	**Group A *Streptococcus*, *Staphylococcus aureus*,** *Haemophilus influenzae*, many other bacteria
Necrotizing cellulitis and fasciitis	**Group A *Streptococcus*, *Clostridium perfringens*** and other species, *Bacteroides fragilis*, other anaerobes, Enterobacteriaceae, *Pseudomonas aeruginosa*
Bacillary angiomatosis	***Bartonella henselae*, *Bartonella quintana***

Table 47–2. Summary of Bacteria Associated with Human Disease—cont'd

System Affected	Pathogens
Skin and Soft-Tissue Infections	
Infections of burns	***Pseudomonas aeruginosa***, *Enterobacter* species, *Enterococcus* species, *Staphylococcus aureus*, group A *Streptococcus*, many other bacteria
Bite wounds	***Eikenella corrodens, Pasteurella multocida***, *Pasteurella canis, Staphylococcus aureus*, group A *Streptococcus*, mixed anaerobes and aerobes, many gram-negative rods
Surgical wounds	***Staphylococcus aureus***, coagulase-negative *Staphylococcus*, groups A and B streptococci, *Clostridium perfringens*, *Corynebacterium* species, many other bacteria
Traumatic wounds	***Bacillus* species, *Staphylococcus aureus***, group A *Streptococcus*, many gram-negative rods, rapid-growing mycobacteria
Gastrointestinal Infections	
Gastritis	***Helicobacter pylori***
Gastroenteritis	***Salmonella* species, *Shigella* species, *Campylobacter jejuni* and other species**, *Vibrio cholerae*, *Vibrio parahaemolyticus*, other *Vibrio* species, *Yersinia enterocolitica*, *Escherichia coli* (ETEC, EIEC, EHEC, EPEC, others), *Edwardsiella tarda*, *Bacillus cereus*, *Pseudomonas aeruginosa*, *Aeromonas* species, *Plesiomonas shigelloides*, *Bacteroides fragilis*, *Clostridium botulinum*, *Clostridium perfringens*, *Clostridium difficile*
Food intoxication	***Staphylococcus aureus, Bacillus cereus***, *Clostridium botulinum*, *Clostridium perfringens*
Proctitis	***Neisseria gonorrhoeae***, *Chlamydia trachomatis*, *Treponema pallidum*
Bone and Joint Infections	
Osteomyelitis	***Staphylococcus aureus, Salmonella* species**, *Mycobacterium tuberculosis* and other species, β-hemolytic *Streptococcus*, *Streptococcus pneumoniae*, *Escherichia coli* and other Enterobacteriaceae, *Pseudomonas aeruginosa*, many less common bacteria
Arthritis	***Staphylococcus aureus, Neisseria gonorrhoeae***, *Streptococcus pneumoniae*, *Salmonella* species, *Pasteurella multocida*, *Mycobacterium* species
Prosthetic-associated infections	***Staphylococcus aureus*, coagulase-negative *Staphylococcus***, group A *Streptococcus*, viridans *streptococci*, *Corynebacterium* species, *Propionibacterium* species, *Peptostreptococcus* species, other anaerobic cocci
Genital Infections	
Genital ulcers	***Treponema pallidum, Haemophilus ducreyi***, *Chlamydia trachomatis*, *Francisella tularensis*, *Klebsiella granulomatis*, *Mycobacterium tuberculosis*
Urethritis	***Neisseria gonorrhoeae, Chlamydia trachomatis***, *Ureaplasma urealyticum*
Vaginitis	***Mycoplasma hominis, Mobiluncus* species, *Gardnerella vaginalis***
Cervicitis	***Neisseria gonorrhoeae, Chlamydia trachomatis***, *Neisseria meningitidis*, group B *Streptococcus*, *Mycobacterium tuberculosis*, *Actinomyces* species
Granulomatous Infections	
General	***Mycobacterium tuberculosis* and other species, *Nocardia* species, *Treponema pallidum***, *Treponema carateum*, *Brucella* species, *Francisella tularensis*, *Listeria monocytogenes*, *Burkholderia pseudomallei*, *Actinomyces* species, *Bartonella henselae*, *Tropheryma whippelii*, *Chlamydia trachomatis*, *Coxiella burnetii*

EHEC, enterohemorrhagic E. coli; *EIEC, enteroinvasive* E. coli; *EPEC, enteropathogenic* E. coli; *ETEC, enterotoxic* E. coli; *HACEK organisms,* Haemophilus influenzae, Actinobacillus actinomycetemcomitans, Cardiobacterium hominis, Eikenella corrodens, *and* Kingella kingae.
Organisms in bold are the most common pathogens.

Table 47—3. Selected Bacteria Associated with Foodborne Diseases

Organism	Implicated Food(s)
Aeromonas species	Meats, produce, dairy products
Bacillus cereus	Fried rice, meats, vegetables
Brucella species	Unpasteurized dairy products, meat
Campylobacter species	Poultry, unpasteurized dairy products
Clostridium botulinum	Vegetables, fruits, fish, honey
Clostridium perfringens	Beef, poultry, pork, gravy
Escherichia coli	
Enterohemorrhagic	Beef, unpasteurized milk, fruit juices
Enterotoxigenic	Lettuce, fruits, vegetables
Enteroinvasive	Lettuce, fruit, vegetables
Francisella tularensis	Rabbit meat
Listeria monocytogenes	Unpasteurized dairy products, coleslaw, poultry, cold cut meats
Plesiomonas shigelloides	Seafood
Salmonella species	Poultry, unpasteurized dairy products
Shigella species	Eggs, lettuce
Staphylococcus aureus	Ham, poultry, egg dishes, pastries
Streptococcus, group A	Egg dishes
Vibrio cholerae	Shellfish
Vibrio parahaemolyticus	Shellfish
Vibrio vulnificus	Shellfish
Yersinia enterocolitica	Unpasteurized dairy products, pork

Organisms in bold are the most common foodborne pathogens in the United States (Morb Mortal Wkly Rep 56:336-339, 2007).

Table 47—4. Selected Bacteria Associated with Waterborne Diseases

Organism	Disease
Aeromonas species	Gastroenteritis, wound infections, septicemia
Campylobacter species	Gastroenteritis
Escherichia coli	Gastroenteritis
Francisella tularensis	Tularemia
Legionella species	Respiratory disease
Leptospira species	Systemic disease
Mycobacterium marinum	Cutaneous infection
Plesiomonas shigelloides	Gastroenteritis
Pseudomonas species	Dermatitis
Salmonella species	Gastroenteritis
Shigella species	Gastroenteritis
Vibrio species	Gastroenteritis, wound infection, septicemia
Yersinia enterocolitica	Gastroenteritis

Organisms in bold are the most common waterborne pathogens in the United States (Morb Mortal Wkly Rep 55:1-30, 2006).

Table 47–5. Arthropod-Associated Diseases

Arthropod	Organism	Disease
Tick	*Anaplasma phagocytophilum*	Human anaplasmosis (formerly called *human granulocytic ehrlichiosis*)
	Borrelia burgdorferi	Lyme disease
	Borrelia garinii	Lyme disease
	Borrelia afzelii	Lyme disease
	Borrelia, other species	Endemic relapsing fever
	Coxiella burnetii	Q fever
	Ehrlichia chaffeensis	Human monocytic ehrlichiosis
	Ehrlichia ewingii	Canine (human) granulocytic ehrlichiosis
	Francisella tularensis	Tularemia
	Rickettsia rickettsii	Rocky Mountain spotted fever
Flea	*Rickettsia prowazekii*	Sporadic typhus
	Rickettsia typhi	Murine typhus
	Yersinia pestis	Plague
Lice	*Bartonella quintana*	Trench fever
	Borrelia recurrentis	Epidemic relapsing fever
	Rickettsia prowazekii	Epidemic typhus
Mite	*Rickettsia akari*	Rickettsialpox
	Orientia tsutsugamushi	Scrub typhus
Sandfly	*Bartonella bacilliformis*	Bartonellosis (Carrión disease)

Bibliography

Borriello P, Murray P, Funke G, (eds): Topley & Wilson's Microbiology and Microbial Infections: Bacteriology, 10th ed. London, Hodder, 2005.

Cohen J, Powderly WG: Infectious Diseases, 2nd ed. St Louis, Mosby, 2004.

Kasper D, et al. (eds): Harrison's Principles of Internal Medicine, 16th ed. New York, McGraw-Hill, 2004.

Mandell GL, Bennett JE, Dolin R (eds): Principles and Practice of Infectious Diseases, 6th ed. New York, Churchill Livingstone, 2005.

Murray P, Shea Y: Pocket Guide to Clinical Microbiology, 3rd ed. Washington, DC, ASM Press, 2004.

Murray PR, et al. (eds): Manual of Clinical Microbiology, 9th ed. Washington, DC, ASM Press, 2007.

Virology

Mechanisms of Viral Pathogenesis

Viruses cause disease after they break through the natural protective barriers of the body, evade immune control, and either kill cells of an important tissue (e.g., brain) or trigger a destructive immune and inflammatory response. The outcome of a viral infection is determined by the nature of the virus–host interaction and the host's response to the infection (Box 48-1). The immune response is the best treatment, but it often contributes to the pathogenesis of a viral infection. The tissue targeted by the virus defines the nature of the disease and its symptoms. Viral and host factors govern the severity of the disease; they include the strain of virus, the inoculum size, and the general health of the infected person. The ability of the infected person's immune response to control the infection determines the severity and duration of the disease.

A particular disease may be caused by several viruses that have a common tissue **tropism** (preference), such as hepatitis, liver; common cold, upper respiratory tract; encephalitis, central nervous system. On the other hand, a particular virus may cause several different diseases or no observable symptoms. For example, herpes simplex virus (HSV) type 1 (HSV-1) can cause gingivostomatitis, pharyngitis, herpes labialis (cold sores), genital herpes, encephalitis, or keratoconjunctivitis, depending on the affected tissue, or it can cause no disease at all. Although normally benign, this virus can be life threatening in a newborn or an immunocompromised person.

Many viruses encode activities (**virulence factors**) that promote the efficiency of viral replication, viral transmission, the access and binding of the virus to target tissue, or the escape of the virus from host defenses and immune resolution (see Chapter 12). These activities may not be essential for viral growth in tissue culture but are necessary for the pathogenicity or survival of the virus in the host. Loss of these virulence factors results in **attenuation** of the virus. Many live-virus vaccines are attenuated virus strains.

The discussion in this chapter focuses on viral disease at the cellular level (cytopathogenesis), the host level (mechanisms of disease), and the population level (epidemiology and control). The antiviral immune response is discussed here and in Chapter 12.

Basic Steps in Viral Disease

Viral disease in the body progresses through defined steps, just like viral replication in the cell (Figure 48-1A). These steps are noted in Box 48-2.

The incubation period may proceed without symptoms (**asymptomatic**) or may produce nonspecific early symptoms such as fever, head or body ache, or chills, termed the **prodrome**. The symptoms of the disease are caused by tissue damage and systemic effects caused by the virus and possibly the immune system. These symptoms may continue through **convalescence** while the body repairs the damage. The individual usually develops a memory immune response for future protection against a similar challenge with this virus.

Infection of the Target Tissue

The virus gains **entry into the body** through breaks in the skin (cuts, bites, injections) or across the mucoepithelial membranes that line the orifices of the body (eyes, respiratory tract, mouth, genitalia, and gastrointestinal tract). The skin is an excellent barrier to infection. Tears, mucus, ciliated epithelium, stomach acid, bile, and immunoglobulin A protect the orifices. *Inhalation is probably the most common route of viral infection.*

On entry into the body, the virus replicates in cells that express viral receptors and have the appropriate biosynthetic machinery. Many viruses initiate infection in the oral mucosa or upper respiratory tract. Disease signs may accompany viral replication at the primary site. The virus may replicate and remain at the primary site, may disseminate to other tissues via the bloodstream or the

Viral Pathogenesis

Cytopathogenesis

The three potential outcomes of a viral infection of a cell are as follows (Box 48-3 and Table 48-1):

1. Failed infection (abortive infection).
2. Cell death (lytic infection).
3. Replication without cell death (persistent infection).

Viral mutants, which cause abortive infections, do not multiply and therefore disappear. Persistent infections may be (1) **chronic** (nonlytic, productive), (2) **latent** (limited viral macromolecular but no virus synthesis), (3) **recurrent**, or (4) **transforming** (immortalizing).

The nature of the infection is determined by the characteristics of the virus and the target cell. A **nonpermissive cell** may lack a receptor, important enzyme pathway,

Table 48–1. Types of Viral Infections at the Cellular Level

Type	Virus Production	Fate of Cell
Abortive	–	No effect
Cytolytic	+	Death
Persistent		
Productive	+	Senescence
Latent	–	No effect
Transforming		
DNA viruses	–	Immortalization
RNA viruses	+	Immortalization

transcriptional activator, or expresses an antiviral mechanism that will not allow replication of a particular type or strain of virus. For example, neurons and nongrowing cells lack the machinery and substrates for replication of a DNA virus. These cells can also limit the amount of protein synthesis within the cells by phosphorylating eIF2α (elongation initiation factor 2 alpha) to prevent the assembly of ribosomes on mRNA, which shuts down protein synthesis. This protection can be triggered by the large amount of protein synthesis required for virus production or the activation of the interferon-α- (IFN-α) or interferon-β- (IFN-β) induced antiviral state by a double-stranded RNA replicative intermediate. Herpesviruses and some other viruses prevent this by inhibiting the phosphorylating enzyme (protein kinase R) or by activating a cellular protein phosphatase to remove the phosphate on eIF2α. Another example is APOBEC3, an enzyme that causes hypermutation inactivation of the cDNA of retroviruses. The viral infectivity factor (Vif) protein of human immunodeficiency virus overcomes this block by promoting the degradation of APOBEC3.

A **permissive cell** provides the biosynthetic machinery (e.g., transcription factors, posttranslational processing enzymes) to support the complete replicative cycle of the virus. Replication of the virus in a **semipermissive cell** may be very inefficient, or the cell may support some but not all the steps in viral replication.

Replication of the virus can initiate changes in cells that lead to cytolysis or to alterations in the cell's appearance, functional properties, or antigenicity. The effects on the cell may result from viral takeover of macromolecular synthesis, the accumulation of viral proteins or particles, modification or disruption of cellular structures, or manipulation of cellular functions (Table 48-2).

Lytic Infections

Lytic infection results when virus replication kills the target cell. Some viruses prevent cellular growth and repair by

---

Box 48–3. Determinants of Viral Pathogenesis

Interaction of Virus with Target Tissue

Access of virus to target tissue
Stability of virus in the body
   Temperature
   Acid and bile of the gastrointestinal tract
Ability to cross skin or mucous epithelial cells (e.g., cross
   the gastrointestinal tract into the bloodstream)
Ability to establish viremia
Ability to spread through the reticuloendothelial system
Target tissue
   Specificity of viral attachment proteins
   Tissue-specific expression of receptors

Cytopathologic Activity of the Virus

Efficiency of viral replication in the cell
   Optimum temperature for replication
   Permissiveness of cell for replication
Cytotoxic viral proteins
Inhibition of cell's macromolecular synthesis
Accumulation of viral proteins and structures (inclusion bodies)
Altered cell metabolism (e.g., cell immortalization)

Host Protective Responses

Antigen-nonspecific antiviral responses
   Interferon
   Natural killer cells and macrophages
Antigen-specific immune responses
   T-cell responses
   Antibody responses
Viral mechanisms of escape of immune responses

Immunopathology

Interferon: flulike systemic symptoms
T-cell responses: delayed-type hypersensitivity
Antibody: complement, antibody-dependent cellular
   cytotoxicity, immune complexes
Other inflammatory responses

Table 48–2. Mechanisms of Viral Cytopathogenesis

Mechanism	Examples
Inhibition of cellular protein synthesis	Polioviruses, herpes simplex virus, togaviruses, poxviruses
Inhibition and degradation of cellular DNA	Herpesviruses
Alteration of cell membrane structure	Enveloped viruses
Glycoprotein insertion	All enveloped viruses
Syncytia formation	Herpes simplex virus, varicella-zoster virus, paramyxoviruses, human immunodeficiency virus
Disruption of cytoskeleton	Nonenveloped viruses (accumulation), herpes simplex virus
Permeability	Togaviruses, herpesviruses
Inclusion Bodies	**Examples**
Negri bodies (intracytoplasmic)	Rabies
Owl's eye (intranuclear)	Cytomegalovirus
Cowdry type A (intranuclear)	Herpes simplex virus, subacute sclerosing panencephalitis (measles) virus
Intranuclear basophilic	Adenoviruses
Intracytoplasmic acidophilic	Poxviruses
Perinuclear cytoplasmic acidophilic	Reoviruses
Toxicity of virion components	Adenovirus fibers, reovirus NSP4 protein

change cell-to-cell interactions and the cell's appearance, making the cell a target for immune cytolysis.

Virus infection or cytolytic immune responses may induce **apoptosis** in the infected cell. Apoptosis is a preset cascade of events that, when triggered, leads to cellular suicide. This process may facilitate release of the virus from the cell, but it also limits the amount of virus that is produced by destroying the viral "factory." As a result, *many viruses (e.g., herpesviruses, adenoviruses, hepatitis C virus) encode methods for inhibiting apoptosis.*

Cell surface expression of the glycoproteins of some paramyxoviruses, herpesviruses, and retroviruses triggers the fusion of neighboring cells into multinucleated giant cells called **syncytia**. Cell-to-cell fusion may occur in the absence of new protein synthesis (fusion from without), as occurs in infections with Sendai virus and other paramyxoviruses, or may require new protein synthesis (fusion from within), as occurs in infection with HSV. Syncytia formation allows the virus to spread from cell to cell and escape antibody detection. Syncytia may be fragile and susceptible to lysis. The syncytia that occurs in infection with human immunodeficiency virus (HIV) also causes death of the cells.

Some viral infections cause characteristic changes in the appearance and properties of the target cells. For example, chromosomal aberrations and degradation may occur and can be detected with histologic staining (e.g., marginated chromatin ringing the nuclear membrane in HSV-infected and adenovirus-infected cells). In addition, new, stainable structures called **inclusion bodies** may appear within the nucleus or cytoplasm. These structures may result from virus-induced changes in the membrane or chromosomal structure or may represent the sites of viral replication or accumulations of viral capsids. Because the nature and location of these inclusion bodies are characteristic of particular viral infections, the presence of such bodies facilitates laboratory diagnosis (see Table 48-2). Viral infection may also cause vacuolization, or rounding of the cells, and other nonspecific histologic changes that are characteristics of sick cells.

Nonlytic Infections

A **persistent infection** occurs in an infected cell that is not killed by the virus. Some viruses cause a persistent productive infection because the virus is released gently from the cell through exocytosis or through budding (many enveloped viruses) from the plasma membrane.

A **latent infection** may result from DNA virus infection of a cell that restricts or lacks the machinery for transcribing all the viral genes. The specific transcription factors required by such a virus may be expressed only in specific tissues, in growing but not resting cells, or after hormone or cytokine induction. For example, HSV establishes a latent infection in neurons that lack the nuclear factors required to transcribe the immediate early viral genes, but stress and other stimuli can activate the cells to allow viral replication.

inhibiting the synthesis of cellular macromolecules or by producing degradative enzymes and toxic proteins. For example, HSV and other viruses produce proteins that inhibit the synthesis of cellular deoxyribonucleic acid (DNA) and messenger RNA (mRNA) and synthesize other proteins that degrade host DNA to provide substrates for viral genome replication. Cellular protein synthesis may be actively blocked (e.g., poliovirus inhibits translation of 5′-capped cellular mRNA) or passively blocked (e.g., through the production of much viral mRNA that successfully competes for ribosomes) (see Chapter 4).

Replication of the virus and the accumulation of viral components and progeny within the cell can disrupt the structure and function of the cell or disrupt lysosomes, causing cell death. The expression of viral antigens on the cell surface and disruption of the cytoskeleton can

Oncogenic Viruses

Some DNA viruses and retroviruses establish persistent infections that can also stimulate uncontrolled cell growth, causing the **transformation** or **immortalization** of the cell (Figure 48-2). Characteristics of transformed cells include continued growth without senescence, alterations in cell morphology and metabolism, increased cell growth rate and sugar transport, loss of cell-contact inhibition of growth, and ability to grow in a suspension or pileup into foci when grown in a semisolid agar.

Different **oncogenic** viruses have different mechanisms for immortalizing cells. Viruses immortalize cells by (1) activating or providing growth-stimulating genes, (2) removing the inherent braking mechanisms that limit DNA synthesis and cell growth, or (3) preventing apoptosis. Immortalization by DNA viruses occurs in semipermissive cells, which express only select viral genes but do not produce virus. The synthesis of viral DNA, late mRNA, late proteins, or virus leads to cell death, which precludes immortalization. Several oncogenic DNA viruses integrate into the host cell chromosome. Papillomavirus, SV40

virus, and adenovirus encode proteins that bind and inactivate cell growth-regulatory proteins, such as p53 and the retinoblastoma gene product (RB), thus releasing the brakes on cell growth. Loss of p53 also makes the cell more susceptible to mutation. Epstein-Barr virus immortalizes B cells by stimulating cell growth (as a B-cell mitogen) and by inducing expression of the cell's *bcl-2* oncogene, which prevents programmed cell death (apoptosis).

Retroviruses (RNA viruses) use two approaches to oncogenesis. Some oncoviruses encode **oncogene** proteins (e.g., *sis, ras, src, mos, myc, jun, fos*), which are almost identical to the cellular proteins involved in cellular growth control (e.g., components of a growth-factor signal cascade [receptors, G proteins, protein kinases], or growth-regulating transcription factors). The overproduction or altered function of these oncogene products stimulates cell growth. These oncogenic viruses *rapidly* cause tumors to form. *However, no human retrovirus of this type has been identified.*

Human T-cell lymphotropic virus type 1 (HTLV-1), the only human oncogenic retrovirus identified, uses more subtle mechanisms of leukemogenesis. It encodes a protein (**Tax**) that **transactivates** gene expression, including genes for growth-stimulating cytokines (e.g., interleukin-2). This constitutes the second approach to oncogenesis. The integration of the DNA copy of HTLV-1 near a cellular growth-stimulating gene can also cause the gene to be activated by the strong viral enhancer and promoter sequences encoded at each end of the viral genome (LTR sequences). *HTLV-1–associated leukemias **develop slowly**, occurring 20 to 30 years after infection.* Retroviruses continue to produce virus in immortalized or transformed cells.

Some viruses may initiate tumor formation indirectly. Hepatitis B virus (HBV) and hepatitis C virus (HCV) may have mechanisms for direct oncogenesis; however, both viruses establish persistent infections that require significant tissue repair. Continuous stimulation of liver cell growth and repair may promote mutations that lead to tumor formation. Human herpesvirus 8 (HHV8) promotes the development of Kaposi sarcoma by means of growth-promoting cytokines encoded by the virus; this disease occurs most often in immunosuppressed patients, such as those with acquired immune deficiency syndrome (AIDS).

Viral transformation is the first step but is generally not sufficient to cause oncogenesis and tumor formation. Instead, over time, immortalized cells are more likely than normal cells to accumulate other mutations or chromosomal rearrangements that promote development of tumor cells. Immortalized cells may also be more susceptible to cofactors and tumor promoters (e.g., phorbol esters, butyrate) that enhance tumor formation. Approximately 15% of human cancers can be related to oncogenic viruses such as HTLV-1, HBV and HCV, papillomaviruses 16 and 18, HHV8, and Epstein-Barr virus. HSV-2 may be a cofactor for human cervical cancer.

Figure 48—2. Mechanisms of viral transformation and immortalization. Cell growth is controlled (**A**) by the maintenance of a balance in the external and internal growth activators (accelerators) and by growth suppressors, such as p53 and the RB gene product (brakes). Oncogenic viruses alter the balance by removing the brakes (**B**) or by enhancing the effects of the accelerators (**C**). RB, retinoblastoma.

Host Defenses against Viral Infection

The ultimate goals of the host antiviral innate and immune responses are to prevent entry, prevent spread, and to eliminate the virus and the cells harboring or replicating the virus (resolution). The immune response is the best and in most cases the only means of controlling a viral infection. Both humoral and cellular immune responses are important for antiviral immunity. Interferon and cytotoxic T-cell responses may have evolved primarily as antiviral defense mechanisms. A detailed description of the antiviral immune response is presented in Chapter 12.

The skin is the best barrier to infection. The orifices of the body (e.g., mouth, eyes, nose, ears, and anus) are protected by mucous, ciliated epithelium, tears, and the gastric acid and bile of the gastrointestinal tract. After the virus penetrates these natural barriers, it activates the **antigen-nonspecific (innate) host defenses** (e.g., fever, interferon, macrophages, dendritic cells, natural killer [NK] cells), which attempt to limit and control local viral replication and spread. Viral molecules, including double-stranded RNA (which is the replicative intermediate of RNA viruses), certain forms of DNA and single-stranded RNA, and some viral glycoproteins, activate type I interferon production and innate cellular responses through interaction with cytoplasmic receptors or the Toll-like receptors (TLRs) on cell surfaces.

Antigen-specific immune responses take several days to be activated and become effective. The goal of these protective responses is to resolve the infection by eliminating all infectious virus and virus-infected cells from the body. **Antibody** is effective against extracellular virus and may be sufficient to control cytolytic viruses, because the virion factory within the infected cell is eliminated by viral replication. Antibody is essential to control virus spread to target tissue by viremia. **Cell-mediated immunity** is required for lysis of cells infected with a **noncytolytic virus** (e.g., hepatitis A virus) and infections caused by **enveloped viruses**.

The protection generated by prior immunity is provided by **memory B and T cells**, which can deliver a response much sooner and more effectively than during a primary infection. It may not prevent the initial stages of infection but in most cases does prevent disease progression. On rechallenge, cell-mediated responses are more effective at limiting the local spread of virus, and serum antibody can prevent viremic spread of the virus. Secondary responses develop much more rapidly and are more effective than primary responses; this is the basis for the development of vaccine programs.

Many viruses, especially the larger viruses, have the means to escape one or more aspects of immune control (see Chapter 12, Table 12-4). These mechanisms include preventing interferon action, changing virus antigens, spreading by cell-to-cell transmission to escape antibody, and suppressing antigen presentation and lymphocyte function. By preventing the consequences of the antiviral state induced by IFN-α and IFN-β, herpes simplex viral protein synthesis and replication can continue. Inhibition of major histocompatibility complex I expression by cytomegalovirus and adenoviruses prevents T-cell killing of the infected cell. Antigenic variation over the course of several years (antigenic shift and drift) by influenza or during the lifetime of the infected individual by HIV limits the antiviral efficacy of antibody. Failure to resolve the infection may lead to persistent infection, chronic disease, or death of the patient.

Immunopathology

The hypersensitivity and inflammatory reactions initiated by antiviral immunity can be the major cause of the pathologic manifestations and symptoms of viral disease (Table 48-3). Early responses to the virus and viral infection, such as interferon and cytokines, can initiate local inflammatory and systemic responses. For example, interferon and cytokines stimulate the **flulike systemic symptoms** that are usually associated with *respiratory viral infections and viremias (e.g.,*

Table 48—3. Viral Immunopathogenesis

Immunopathogenesis	Immune Mediators	Examples
Flulike symptoms	Interferon, cytokines	Respiratory viruses, arboviruses (viremia-inducing viruses)
Delayed-type hypersensitivity and inflammation	T cells, macrophages, and polymorphonuclear leukocytes	Enveloped viruses
Immune complex disease	Antibody, complement	Hepatitis B virus, rubella
Hemorrhagic disease	T cell, antibody, complement	Yellow fever, dengue, Lassa fever, Ebola viruses
Postinfection cytolysis	T cells	Enveloped viruses (e.g., postmeasles encephalitis)
Immunosuppression	—	Human immunodeficiency virus, cytomegalovirus, measles virus, influenza virus

fever, malaise, headache). These symptoms often precede (**prodrome**) the characteristic symptoms of the viral infection during the viremic stage. Later, immune complexes and complement activation (classic pathway), CD4 T-cell–induced delayed-type hypersensitivity, and CD8 cytolytic T-cell action may induce tissue damage. These actions often promote neutrophil infiltration and more cell damage.

The inflammatory response initiated by cell-mediated immunity is difficult to control and damages tissue. Infections by enveloped viruses, in particular, induce cell-mediated immune responses that usually produce more extensive immunopathologic conditions. For example, the classic symptoms of measles and mumps result from the T-cell–induced inflammatory and hypersensitivity responses rather than from cytopathologic effects of the virus. The presence of large amounts of antigen in blood during viremias or chronic infections (e.g., HBV infection) can initiate the **classic type III immune complex hypersensitivity reactions.** **Immune complexes** containing virus or viral antigen can activate the complement system, triggering inflammatory responses and tissue destruction. These immune complexes often accumulate in the kidney and cause renal problems.

In the case of dengue and measles viruses, partial immunity to a related or inactivated virus can result in a more severe host response and disease on subsequent challenge with a related or virulent virus. This is because antigen-specific T-cell and antibody responses are enhanced and induce significant inflammatory and hypersensitivity damage to infected endothelial cells (**dengue hemorrhagic fever**) or skin and the lung (**atypical measles**). In addition, a non-neutralizing antibody can facilitate the uptake of dengue and yellow fever viruses into macrophages through Fc receptors, where they can replicate.

Children generally have a less active cell-mediated immune response (e.g., NK cells) than adults and therefore usually have milder symptoms during infections by some viruses (e.g., measles, mumps, Epstein-Barr, and varicella-zoster viruses). However, in the case of hepatitis B virus, mild or no symptoms correlate with an inability to resolve the infection, resulting in chronic disease.

Viral Disease

The relative **susceptibility** of a person and the **severity** of the disease depend on the following factors:

1. The mechanism of exposure and site of infection.
2. The immune status, age, and general health of the person.
3. The viral dose.
4. The genetics of the virus and the host.

Once the host is infected, however, the host's immune status and competence are probably the major factors that determine whether a viral infection causes a life-threatening disease, a benign lesion, or no symptoms at all.

The stages of viral disease are shown in Figure 48-1C. During the **incubation period**, the virus is replicating but has not reached the target tissue or induced sufficient damage to cause the disease. *The incubation period is relatively short if the primary site of infection is the target tissue and produces the characteristic symptoms of the disease. Longer incubation periods occur when the virus must spread to other sites and be amplified before reaching the target tissue, or the symptoms are caused by immunopathology.* Nonspecific or flulike symptoms may precede the characteristic symptoms during the **prodrome**. The incubation periods for many common viral infections are listed in Table 48-4. Specific viral diseases are discussed in subsequent chapters and reviewed in Chapter 67.

Table 48—4. Incubation Periods of Common Viral Infections

Disease	Incubation Period (days)*
Influenza	1-2
Common cold	1-3
Herpes simplex	2-8
Bronchiolitis, croup	3-5
Acute respiratory disease (adenoviruses)	5-7
Dengue	5-8
Enteroviruses	6-12
Poliomyelitis	5-20
Measles	9-12
Smallpox	12-14
Chickenpox	13-17
Mumps	16-20
Rubella	17-20
Mononucleosis	30-50
Hepatitis A	15-40
Hepatitis B	50-150
Rabies	30-100
Papilloma (warts)	50-150
Human immunodeficiency virus (acquired immune deficiency syndrome)	1-10 years

Modified from White DO, Fenner F: Medical Virology, 3rd ed. New York, Academic, 1986.
*Until first appearance of prodromal symptoms. Diagnostic signs (e.g., rash, paralysis) may not appear until 2 to 4 days later.

The nature and severity of the symptoms of a viral disease are related to the function of the infected target tissue (e.g., liver, hepatitis; brain, encephalitis) and the extent of the immunopathologic responses triggered by the infection. **Inapparent infections** result if (1) the infected tissue is undamaged, (2) the infection is controlled before the virus reaches its target tissue, (3) the target tissue is expendable, (4) the damaged tissue is rapidly repaired, or (5) the extent of damage is below a functional threshold for that particular tissue. For example, many infections of the brain are inapparent or are below the threshold of severe loss of function, but encephalitis results if the loss of function becomes significant. Despite the lack of symptoms, virus-specific antibody will be produced. For example, although 97% of adults have antibody (seropositive) to varicella-zoster virus, less than half remember having had chickenpox. *Inapparent or asymptomatic infections are major sources of contagion.*

Viral infections may cause **acute** or **chronic disease** (**persistent infection**). The ability and speed with which a person's immune system controls and resolves a viral infection usually determine whether acute or chronic disease ensues, as well as the severity of the symptoms (Figure 48-3). The acute episode of a persistent infection may be asymptomatic (JC polyomavirus) or may later in life cause

symptoms similar to (varicella and zoster) or different from (HIV) those of the acute disease. **Slow viruses and prions** have long incubation periods, during which sufficient virus or tissue destruction accumulates before a rapid progression of symptoms.

Epidemiology

Epidemiology studies the spread of disease through a population. Infection of a population is similar to infection of a person in that the virus must spread through the population and is controlled by immunization of the population (Box 48-4). To endure, viruses must continue to infect new, immunologically naïve, susceptible hosts.

Exposure

People are exposed to viruses throughout their lives. However, some situations, vocations, lifestyles, and living arrangements increase the likelihood that a person will come in contact with certain viruses. In contrast, many viruses are ubiquitous. Exposure to HSV-1, HHV6, varicella-zoster virus, parvovirus B19, Epstein-Barr virus, and many respiratory and enteric viruses can be detected in most young children or by early adulthood by the presence of antibodies to the virus.

Poor hygiene and crowded living, school, and job conditions promote exposure to respiratory and enteric viruses. Daycare centers are consistent sources of viral infections, especially viruses spread by the respiratory and fecal-oral routes. Travel, summer camp, and vocations that bring people in contact with a virus vector (e.g., mosquitoes) put them at particular risk for infection by arboviruses and other zoonoses. Sexual promiscuity also promotes the spread and acquisition of several viruses. Health care workers, such as physicians, dentists, nurses, and technicians, are frequently exposed to respiratory and other viruses but are uniquely at risk for acquiring viruses from contaminated blood (HBV, HIV) or vesicle fluid (HSV).

Transmission of Viruses

Viruses are transmitted by direct contact (including sexual contact), injection with contaminated fluids or blood, the transplantation of organs, and the respiratory and fecal-oral routes (Table 48-5). *The route of transmission depends on the source of the virus (the tissue site of viral replication and secretion) and the ability of the virus to endure the hazards and barriers of the environment and the body en route to the target tissue.* For example, viruses that replicate in the respiratory tract (e.g., influenza A virus) are released in aerosol droplets, whereas enteric viruses (e.g., picornaviruses and reoviruses) are passed by the fecal-oral route. Cytomegalovirus is transmitted in most bodily secretions because it infects mucoepithelial, secretory, and other cells found in the skin, secretory glands, lungs, liver, and other organs.

The presence or absence of an envelope is the major structural determinant of the mode of viral transmission.

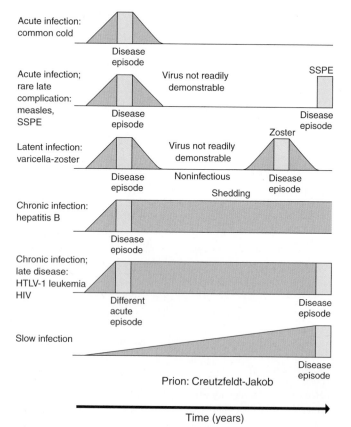

Figure 48—3. Acute infection and various types of persistent infection, as illustrated by the diseases indicated in the column at the left. *Blue* represents presence of virus; *green* indicates episode of disease. SSPE, subacute sclerosing panencephalitis. *(Modified from White DO, Fenner FJ: Medical Virology, 3rd ed. New York, Academic, 1986.)*

Box 48—4. Viral Epidemiology*

Mechanisms of Viral Transmission†

Aerosols
Food, water
Fomites (e.g., tissues, clothes)
Direct contact with secretions (e.g., saliva, semen)
Sexual contact, birth
Blood transfusion or organ transplant
Zoonoses (animals, insects [arboviruses])

Disease and Viral Factors That Promote Transmission

Stability of virion in response to the environment (e.g., drying, detergents, temperature)
Replication and secretion of virus into transmissible aerosols and secretions (e.g., saliva, semen)
Asymptomatic transmission
Transience or ineffectiveness of immune response to control reinfection or recurrence

Risk Factors

Age
Health
Immune status
Occupation: contact with agent or vector
Travel history
Lifestyle
Children in daycare centers
Sexual activity

Critical Community Size

Seronegative, susceptible people

Geography and Season

Presence of cofactors or vectors in the environment
Habitat and season for arthropod vectors (mosquitoes)
School session: close proximity and crowding
Home-heating season

Modes of Control

Quarantine
Elimination of the vector
Immunization
Vaccination
Treatment

*Infection of a population instead of a person.
†See also Table 48-5.

Table 48—5. Viral Transmission

Mode	Examples
Respiratory transmission	Paramyxoviruses, influenza viruses, picornaviruses, rhinoviruses, varicella-zoster virus, B19 virus
Fecal-oral transmission	Picornaviruses, rotavirus, reovirus, noroviruses, adenovirus
Contact (lesions, saliva, fomites)	Herpes simplex virus, rhinoviruses, poxviruses, adenovirus
Zoonoses (animals, insects)	Togaviruses (alpha), flaviviruses, bunyaviruses, orbiviruses, arenaviruses, hantaviruses, rabies virus, influenza A virus, orf (pox)
Transmission via blood	Human immunodeficiency virus, HTLV-1, hepatitis B virus, hepatitis C virus, hepatitis delta virus, cytomegalovirus
Sexual contact	Blood-borne viruses, herpes simplex virus, human papillomavirus, molluscum contagiosum
Maternal-neonatal transmission	Rubella virus, cytomegalovirus, B19 virus, echovirus, herpes simplex virus, varicella-zoster virus
Genetic	Prions, retroviruses

HTLV-1, human T-cell lymphotrophic virus type 1.

transmitted by the fecal-oral route and acquired from contaminated water, shellfish, and food. Rhinoviruses and many other nonenveloped viruses can be spread by contact with fomites such as handkerchiefs and toys.

Unlike the sturdy nonenveloped viruses, most **enveloped viruses** are comparatively fragile (see Chapter 4, Box 4-5). They require an intact envelope for infectivity. These viruses must remain wet and are spread (1) in respiratory droplets, blood, mucus, saliva, and semen; (2) by injection; or (3) in organ transplants. Most enveloped viruses are also labile to treatment with acid and detergents, a feature that precludes their being transmitted by the fecal-oral route. Exceptions are HBV and coronaviruses.

Animals can also act as **vectors** that spread viral disease to other animals and humans and even to other locales. They can also be **reservoirs** for the virus, which maintain and amplify the virus in the environment. Viral diseases that are shared by animals or insects and humans are called **zoonoses**. For example, raccoons, foxes, bats, dogs, and cats are vectors for the rabies virus. Arthropods, including mosquitoes, ticks, and sandflies, can act as vectors for togaviruses, flaviviruses, bunyaviruses, and reoviruses. These viruses are often referred to as **arboviruses** because they

Nonenveloped viruses (naked capsid viruses) can withstand drying, the effects of detergents, and extremes of pH and temperature, whereas enveloped viruses generally cannot (see Chapter 4, Box 4-4). Specifically, most nonenveloped viruses can withstand the acidic environment of the stomach and the detergent-like bile of the intestines and mild disinfection and insufficient sewage treatment. These viruses are generally transmitted by the respiratory and fecal-oral routes and can often be acquired from contaminated objects, termed **fomites**. For example, hepatitis A virus, a picornavirus, is a nonenveloped virus that is are *arthropod borne*. A more detailed discussion of arboviruses is presented in Chapter 62. Most arboviruses have a very broad host range, capable of replicating in specific insects, birds, amphibians, and mammals, in addition to humans. Also, the arboviruses must establish a viremia in the animal reservoir so that the insect can acquire the virus during its blood meal.

Other factors that can promote the transmission of viruses are the potential for asymptomatic infection, crowded living conditions, certain occupations, certain lifestyles, daycare centers, and travel. Virus transmission during an asymptomatic infection (e.g., HIV, varicella-zoster virus) occurs unknowingly and is difficult to restrict. This is an important characteristic of sexually transmitted diseases. Viruses that cause persistent productive infections (e.g., cytomegalovirus, HIV) are a particular problem, because the infected person is a continual source of virus that can be spread to immunologically naïve people. Viruses with many different serotypes (rhinoviruses), or viruses capable of changing their antigenicity (influenza and HIV), also readily find immunologically naïve populations.

Maintenance of a Virus in the Population

The persistence of a virus in a community depends on the availability of a critical number of immunologically naïve (seronegative), susceptible people. The efficiency of virus transmission determines the size of the susceptible population necessary for maintenance of the virus in the population. Immunization, produced by natural means or by vaccination, is the best way of reducing the number of such susceptible people.

Age

A person's age is an important factor in determining his or her susceptibility to viral infections. Infants, children, adults, and elderly persons are susceptible to different viruses and have different symptomatic responses to the infection. These differences may result from variations in body size, recuperative abilities, and most important, immune status in people in these age groups. Differences in lifestyles, habits, school environments, and job settings at different ages also determine when people are exposed to viruses.

Infants and children acquire a series of respiratory and exanthematous viral diseases at first exposure because they are immunologically naïve. Infants are especially prone to more serious presentations of paramyxovirus respiratory infections and viral gastroenteritis because of their small size and physiologic requirements (e.g., nutrients, water, electrolytes). However, children generally do not mount as severe an immunopathologic response as adults, and some diseases (herpesviruses) are more benign in children.

Elderly persons are especially susceptible to new viral infections and the reactivation of latent viruses. Because they are less able to initiate a new immune response, repair damaged tissue, and recover, elderly persons are therefore more susceptible to complications after infection and outbreaks of the new strains of the influenza A and B

viruses. Elderly persons are also more prone to zoster (shingles), a recurrence of varicella-zoster virus, as a result of a decline in this specific immune response with age.

Immune Status

The competence of a person's immune response and immune history determine how quickly and efficiently the infection is resolved and can also determine the severity of the symptoms. The rechallenge of a person with prior immunity usually results in asymptomatic or mild disease without transmission. People who are in an immunosuppressed state as a result of AIDS, cancer, or immunosuppressive therapy are at greater risk of suffering more serious disease on primary infection (measles, vaccinia) and are more prone to suffer recurrences of infections with latent viruses (e.g., herpesviruses, papovaviruses).

Other Host Factors

General health plays an important role in determining the competence and nature of the immune response and ability to repair diseased tissue. Poor nutrition can compromise a person's immune system and decrease his or her tissue regenerative capacity. Immunosuppressive diseases and therapies may allow viral replication or recurrence to proceed unchecked. Genetic makeup also plays an important role in determining the response of the immune system to viral infection. Specifically, genetic differences in immune response genes, genes for viral receptors, and other genetic loci affect susceptibility to a viral infection and the severity of disease.

Geographic and Seasonal Considerations

The geographic distribution of a virus is usually determined by whether the requisite cofactors or vectors are present or whether there is an immunologically naïve, susceptible population. For example, many of the arboviruses are limited to the ecologic niche of their arthropod vectors. Extensive global transportation is eliminating many of the geographically determined restrictions to virus distribution.

Seasonal differences in the occurrence of viral disease correspond with behaviors that promote the spread of the virus. For example, respiratory viruses are more prevalent in the winter, because crowding facilitates the spread of such viruses, and the temperature and humidity conditions stabilize them. Enteric viruses, on the other hand, are more prevalent during the summer, possibly because hygiene is more lax during this season. The seasonal differences in arboviral diseases reflect the life cycle of the arthropod vector or its reservoir (e.g., birds).

Outbreaks, Epidemics, and Pandemics

Outbreaks of a viral infection often result from the introduction of a virus (e.g., hepatitis A) into a new location. The outbreak originates from a **common source** (e.g., food preparation) and often can be stopped once the source is identified. **Epidemics** occur over a larger geographic area and generally result from the introduction of a new strain of virus into an immunologically naïve population. **Pandemics** are worldwide epidemics, usually resulting from the introduction of a new virus (e.g., HIV). Pandemics of influenza A used to occur approximately every 10 years as the result of the introduction of new strains of the virus.

Control of Viral Spread

The spread of a virus can be controlled by quarantine, good hygiene, changes in lifestyle, elimination of the vector, or immunization of the population. **Quarantine** was once the only means of limiting epidemics of viral infections and is most effective for limiting the spread of viruses that always cause symptomatic disease (e.g., smallpox). It is now used in hospitals to limit the **nosocomial spread** of viruses, especially to high-risk patients (e.g., immunosuppressed people). The proper sanitation of contaminated items and disinfection of the water supply are means of limiting the spread of enteric viruses. Changes in lifestyle have made a difference in the spread of sexually transmitted viruses such as HIV, HBV, and HSV. Elimination of an arthropod or its ecologic niche (e.g., drainage of the swamps it inhabits) has proved effective for controlling arboviruses.

The **best way to limit viral spread, however, is to immunize the population**. Immunization, whether produced by natural infection or by vaccination, protects individuals and reduces the size of the immunologically naïve, susceptible population necessary to promote the spread and maintenance of the virus.

Questions

1. What are the routes by which viruses gain entry into the body? For each route, list the barriers to infection and a virus that infects by it.

2. Describe or draw the disease path of a virus that is transmitted by an aerosol and causes lesions on the skin (similar to varicella).

3. Identify the structures that elicit a protective antibody response to adenovirus, influenza A virus, poliovirus, and rabies virus.

4. Describe the major roles of each of the following in promoting resolution of a viral infection: interferon, macrophage, natural killer cells, CD4 T cells, CD8 T cells, and antibody.

5. Why are interferon-α and interferon-β produced before interferon-γ?

6. How does the nucleoprotein of influenza virus become an antigen for cytolytic CD8 T cells?

7. What events occur during the prodromal periods of a respiratory virus disease (e.g., parainfluenza virus) and encephalitis (e.g., St. Louis encephalitis virus)?

8. List the viral characteristics (structure, replication, target tissue) that would promote transmission by the fecal-oral route, by arthropods, by fomites, by mother's milk, and by sexual activity.

9. What are the different mechanisms by which oncogenic viruses immortalize cells? Describe them.

Bibliography

Cann AJ: Principles of Molecular Virology. San Diego, Academic, 2005.
Carter J, Saunders V: Virology: Principles and Applications. Chichester, England, Wiley, 2007.
Cohen J, Powderly WG (eds): Infectious Diseases, 2nd ed. St Louis, Mosby, 2004.
Collier L, Oxford J: Human Virology, 3rd ed. Oxford, Oxford University Press, 2006.
Emond RT, Welsby PD, Rowland HAK: Color Atlas of Infectious Diseases, 4th ed. St Louis, Mosby, 2003.
Evans AS, Kaslow RA: Viral Infections of Humans: Epidemiology and Control, 4th ed. New York, Plenum, 1997.
Flint SJ, et al: Principles of Virology: Molecular Biology, Pathogenesis and Control of Animal Viruses, 2nd ed. Washington, DC, ASM Press, 2003.
Haller O, Kochs G, Weber F: The interferon response circuit: Induction and suppression by pathogenic viruses. Virology 344:119-130, 2006.
Hart CA, Broadhead RL: Color Atlas of Pediatric Infectious Diseases. St Louis, Mosby, 1992.
Hart CA, Shears P: Color Atlas of Medical Microbiology. London, Mosby, 2004.
Gershon AA, Hotez PJ, Katz SL: Krugman's Infectious Diseases of Children, 11th ed. St Louis, Mosby, 2004.
Knipe DM, Howley PM (eds): Fields' Virology, 4th ed. New York, Lippincott Williams & Wilkins, 2001.
Mandell GL, Bennet JE, Dolin R (eds): Principles and Practice of Infectious Diseases, 6th ed. Philadelphia, Churchill Livingstone, 2005.
Mims CA, et al: Medical Microbiology, 4th ed. Edinburgh, Mosby, 2007.
Mims CA, White DO: Viral Pathogenesis and Immunology. Oxford, Blackwell, 1984.
Rosenthal KS: Viruses: Microbial spies and saboteurs. Infect Dis Clin Pract 14:97-106, 2006.
Shulman ST, et al: The Biologic and Clinical Basis of Infectious Diseases, 5th ed. Philadelphia, WB Saunders, 1997.
Stark GR, et al: How cells respond to interferons. Ann Rev Biochem 67:227-264, 1998.
Strauss JM, Strauss EG: Viruses and Human Disease, 2nd ed. San Diego, Academic, 2007.
Voyles BA: The Biology of Viruses, 2nd ed. Boston, McGraw-Hill, 2002.
White DO, Fenner FJ: Medical Virology, 4th ed. San Diego, Academic, 1994.
Zuckerman AJ, Banatvala JE, Pattison JR: Principles and Practice of Clinical Virology, 5th ed. Chichester, England, Wiley, 2004.

Websites

Centers for Disease Control, Health topics A to Z: Available at www.cdc.gov/health/diseases.htm
National Center for Infectious Disease, Infectious disease information: Available at www.cdc.gov/ncidod/diseases/index.htm
National Center for Infectious Disease, Traveler's health: Available at www.cdc.gov/travel/diseases.htm
National Foundation for Infectious Diseases, Fact sheets on diseases: Available at www.nfid.org/factsheets/Default.html
Virology on the Internet and specific viruses: Available at www.virology.net/garryfavwebindex.html#C02.081.343
World Health Organization, Diseases and vaccines: Available at www.who.int/vaccines-diseases/index.html
World Health Organization, Infectious diseases: Available at www.who.int/health-topics/idindex.htm

Antiviral Agents

Unlike bacteria, viruses are obligate intracellular parasites that use the host cell's biosynthetic machinery and enzymes for replication (see Chapter 4). Hence it is more difficult to inhibit viral replication without also being toxic to the host. Most antiviral drugs are targeted toward viral-encoded enzymes or structures of the virus that are important for replication. Most of these compounds are classic biochemical inhibitors of viral-encoded enzymes. Some antiviral drugs are actually stimulators of host innate immune protective responses.

Unlike antibacterial drugs, the activity of most antiviral drugs is limited to a specific family of viruses. Antiviral drugs are available for viruses that cause significant morbidity and mortality, which also provide reasonable targets for drug action (Box 49-1). As has occurred with antibacterial drugs, however, resistance to antiviral drugs is becoming more of a problem because of the high rate of mutation for viruses and the long-term treatment of some patients, especially those who are immunocompromised (e.g., patients with the acquired immune deficiency syndrome [AIDS]).

Targets for Antiviral Drugs

The different targets for antiviral drugs (e.g., structures, enzymes, or processes important or essential for virus production) are discussed with respect to the steps of the viral replication cycle they inhibit. These targets and their respective antiviral agents are listed in Table 49-1 (see also Chapter 4, Figure 4-9).

Virion Disruption

Enveloped viruses are susceptible to certain lipid and detergent-like molecules that disperse or disrupt the envelope membrane, thereby preventing acquisition of the virus. Nonoxynol-9, a detergent-like component in birth control jellies, can inactivate herpes simplex virus (HSV) and

human immunodeficiency virus (HIV) and prevent sexual acquisition of the viruses. Rhinoviruses are susceptible to acid, and citric acid can be incorporated into facial tissues as a means of blocking virus transmission.

Attachment

The first step in viral replication is mediated by the interaction of a viral attachment protein with its cell surface receptor. This interaction can be blocked by **neutralizing antibodies**, which bind and coat the virion, or by **receptor antagonists**. The administration of specific antibodies (**passive immunization**) is the oldest form of antiviral therapy. Receptor antagonists include peptide or sugar analogues of the cell receptor or the viral attachment protein that competitively block the interaction of the virus with the cell. Specific peptides of the CCXCR5 molecule of T macrophages and T cells block the initial infection by HIV. Acidic polysaccharides, such as heparan and dextran sulfate, interfere with viral binding and have been suggested for the treatment of infection with HIV, HSV, and other viruses.

Penetration and Uncoating

Penetration and uncoating of the virus are required to deliver the viral genome into the cytoplasm of the host cell. Arildone, disoxaril, **pleconaril**, and other **methylisoxazole** compounds block uncoating of picornaviruses by fitting into a cleft in the receptor-binding canyon of the capsid and preventing disassembly of the capsid. For viruses that enter through endocytic vesicles, uncoating may be triggered by conformational changes in attachment proteins that promote fusion or by membrane disruption resulting from the acidic environment of the vesicle. **Amantadine, rimantadine**, and other hydrophobic amines (weak organic bases) are antiviral agents that can neutralize the pH of these compartments and inhibit virion uncoating. Amantadine and rimantadine have a more

BOX 49—1. Viruses Treatable with Antiviral Drugs

Herpes simplex virus
Varicella-zoster virus
Cytomegalovirus
Human immunodeficiency virus
Influenza A and B viruses
Respiratory syncytial virus
Hepatitis B and C viruses
Papillomavirus
Picornavirus

Table 49—1. Examples of Targets for Antiviral Drugs

Replication Step or Target	Agent	Targeted Virus*
Attachment	Peptide analogues of attachment protein	Human immunodeficiency virus (HIV) (gp120/CD4 receptor)
	Neutralizing antibodies	Most viruses
	Heparan and dextran sulfate	HIV; herpes simplex virus (HSV)
Penetration and uncoating	Amantadine, rimantadine	Influenza A virus
	Tromantadine	HSV
	Arildone, disoxaril, pleconaril	Picornaviruses
Transcription	Interferon	Hepatitis A, B, and C viruses; papillomavirus
	Antisense oligonucleotides	Papillomavirus
Protein synthesis	Interferon	Hepatitis A, B, and C viruses; papillomavirus
DNA replication (polymerase)	Nucleoside analogues	Herpesviruses; HIV; hepatitis B virus, poxviruses, etc.
	Phosphonoformate, phosphonoacetic acid	Herpesviruses
Nucleoside biosynthesis	Ribavirin	Respiratory syncytial virus; Lassa fever virus
Nucleoside scavenging (thymidine kinase)	Nucleoside analogues	HSV; varicella-zoster virus
Glycoprotein processing	—	HIV
Assembly (protease)	Hydrophobic substrate analogues	HIV
Virion integrity	Nonoxynol-9	HIV; HSV

*Therapies may not have received approval for human use.

specific activity against influenza A. These compounds bind to and block the H^+ channel formed by the viral M_2 protein. Without the influx of H^+, the M_1 matrix proteins do not dissociate from the nucleocapsid (uncoating), so movement of the nucleocapsid to the nucleus, transcription, and replication are prevented. Blockage of this proton pore also disrupts the proper processing of the hemagglutinin protein late in the replication cycle. In the absence of a functional M_2 proton pore, the hemagglutinin inopportunely changes its conformation into its "fusion form" and is inactivated as it traverses the normally acidic Golgi environment. **Tromantadine**, a derivative of amantadine, also inhibits penetration of HSV. Penetration and uncoating of HIV are blocked by a 33-amino acid peptide, T20 (**enfuvirtide [Fuzeon]**), which inhibits the action of the viral fusion protein gp41.

RNA Synthesis

Although messenger ribonucleic acid (mRNA) synthesis is essential for the production of virus, it is not a good target for antiviral drugs. It would be difficult to inhibit viral mRNA synthesis without affecting cellular mRNA synthesis. Deoxyribonucleic acid (DNA) viruses use the host cell's transcriptases for mRNA synthesis. The RNA polymerases encoded by RNA viruses may not be sufficiently different from host cell transcriptases to selectively inhibit this activity, and the high rate at which RNA viruses mutate results in the generation of many drug-resistant strains. **Guanidine** and 2-hydroxybenzylbenzimidine are two compounds that can block picornavirus RNA synthesis by binding to the 2C picornavirus protein, which is essential for RNA synthesis. **Ribavirin** resembles riboguanosine and inhibits nucleoside biosynthesis, mRNA capping, promotes hypermutation, and other processes (cellular and viral) important to the replication of many viruses.

The proper processing (splicing) and translation of viral mRNA can be inhibited by interferon and antisense oligonucleotides. **Isatin-β-thiosemicarbazone** induces mRNA degradation in poxvirus-infected cells and was used as a treatment for smallpox. Viral infection of an **interferon**-treated cell triggers a cascade of biochemical events that block viral replication. Specifically, the degradation of viral and cellular mRNA is enhanced, and ribosomal assembly is blocked, preventing protein synthesis and viral replication. Interferon is described further in Chapter 12. Interferon and artificial interferon inducers (**Ampligen, poly rI:rC**) have been approved for clinical use (papilloma, hepatitis B and C) or are in clinical trials.

Genome Replication

Most antiviral drugs are **nucleoside analogues**, which are nucleosides with modifications of the base, sugar, or both (Figure 49-1). The viral **DNA polymerases** of the herpesviruses and the **reverse transcriptases** of HIV and hepatitis B virus *are the prime targets for most antiviral drugs, because they are essential for virus replication and are different from host enzymes.* Before being used by the polymerase, the nucleoside analogues must be phosphorylated to the triphosphate form by viral enzymes (e.g., HSV thymidine kinase), cellular enzymes, or both. For example, the thymidine kinase of HSV and varicella-zoster virus (VZV) applies the first phosphate to **acyclovir (ACV)**, and the cellular enzymes apply the rest. HSV mutants lacking thymidine kinase activity are resistant to ACV.

Cellular enzymes phosphorylate **azidothymidine (AZT)** and many other nucleoside analogues.

Nucleoside analogues selectively inhibit viral polymerases because these enzymes are less accurate than host cell enzymes. The binding of a nucleoside analogue with modifications of the base, sugar, or both is several hundred times better than the host cell enzyme. These drugs either **prevent chain elongation**, as a result of the absence of a 3'-hydroxyl on the sugar, or **alter recognition and base pairing**, as a result of a base modification, and induce inactivating mutations (see Figure 49-1). Antiviral drugs that cause termination of the DNA chain by means of modified nucleoside sugar residues include ACV, ganciclovir (GCV), valacyclovir, penciclovir, famciclovir, adefovir, cidofovir, adenosine arabinoside (vidarabine, ara-A), zidovudine

Figure 49—1. Structure of the most common nucleoside analogues that are antiviral drugs. The chemical distinctions between the natural deoxynucleoside and the antiviral drug analogues are highlighted. Arrows indicate related drugs. Valacyclovir *(not shown)* is the L—valyl ester of acyclovir. Famciclovir *(not shown)* is the diacetyl 6-deoxyanalogue of penciclovir. Both of these drugs are metabolized to the active drug in the liver or intestinal wall.

(AZT), lamivudine (3TC), dideoxycytidine, and dideoxyinosine. Antiviral drugs that become incorporated into the viral genome and cause errors in replication (mutation) and transcription (inactive mRNA and proteins) because of modified nucleoside bases include **ribavirin, 5-iododeoxyuridine (idoxuridine)** and **trifluorothymidine (trifluridine)**. The rapid rate and large extent of nucleotide incorporation during viral replication make retrovirus and DNA virus replication especially susceptible to these drugs. A variety of other nucleoside analogues is also being developed as antiviral drugs.

Pyrophosphate analogues resembling the byproduct of the polymerase reaction, such as **phosphonoformic acid (foscarnet, PFA)** and **phosphonoacetic acid**, are classic inhibitors of the herpesvirus polymerases. **Nevirapine, delavirdine**, and other non-nucleoside reverse transcriptase inhibitors bind to sites on the enzyme other than the substrate site as noncompetitive inhibitors of the enzyme.

Deoxyribonucleotide scavenging enzymes (e.g., the thymidine kinase and ribonucleoside reductase of the herpesviruses) are also enzyme targets of antiviral drugs. Inhibition of these enzymes reduces the levels of deoxyribonucleotides necessary for the replication of the DNA virus genome preventing virus replication.

Integration of the cDNA of HIV into the host chromosome catalyzed by the viral integrase enzyme is essential for virus replication. An inhibitor of the integrase is now approved for anti-HIV therapy.

Protein Synthesis

Although bacterial protein synthesis is the target for several antibacterial compounds, viral protein synthesis is a poor target for antiviral drugs. The virus uses host cell ribosomes and synthetic mechanisms for replication, so selective inhibition is not possible. **Interferon-α (IFN-α)** and **interferon-β (IFN-β)** stop a virus by promoting the inhibition of viral protein synthesis in the infected cell. Inhibition of the posttranslational modification of proteins, such as the proteolysis of a viral polyprotein or glycoprotein processing (castanospermine, deoxynojirimycin), can inhibit virus replication.

Virion Assembly and Release

The **HIV protease** is unique and **essential** to the assembly of virions and the production of infectious virions. Computer-assisted molecular modeling was used to design inhibitors of the HIV protease, such as **saquinavir, ritonavir**, and **indinavir**, by modeling inhibitors that would fit into the active site of the enzyme. The enzyme structures were defined by x-ray crystallographic and molecular biologic studies. Proteases of other viruses are also targets for antiviral drugs.

The **neuraminidase of influenza** has also become a target for antiviral drugs. **Zanamivir (Relenza)** and **oseltamivir (Tamiflu)** act as enzyme inhibitors and, unlike amantadine

and rimantadine, can inhibit influenza A and B. Amantadine and rimantadine also inhibit release of influenza A.

Stimulators of Host Innate Immune Protective Responses

The best antiviral agents are those of the host's innate and immune antiviral response. Stimulation or supplementation of the natural response is an effective approach to limit or treat viral infections. Innate responses of dendritic cells, macrophages, and other cells can be stimulated by **imiquimod, resiquimod, and CpG oligodeoxynucleotides**, which bind to Toll-like receptors to stimulate release of protective cytokines, activation of natural killer cells and subsequent cell-mediated immune responses. **Interferon** and interferon inducers, including mismatched polynucleotides and double-stranded RNA (e.g., **Ampligen, poly rI:rC**), facilitate the treatment of chronic diseases of hepatitis C and papillomaviruses. **Antibodies**, acquired naturally or by passive immunization (see Chapters 12 and 13), prevent both the acquisition and the spread of the virus. For example, passive immunization is administered after exposure to rabies and hepatitis A and hepatitis B viruses.

Nucleoside Analogues

Most of the antiviral drugs approved by the U.S. Food and Drug Administration (FDA) (Table 49-2) are nucleoside analogues that inhibit viral polymerases. Resistance to the drug is usually caused by a mutation of the polymerase.

Acyclovir and Valacyclovir, Penciclovir and Famciclovir

Acyclovir (acycloguanosine) and its valyl derivative, valacyclovir, differ only in pharmacologic considerations. Acyclovir differs from the nucleoside guanosine by having an acyclic (hydroxyethoxymethyl) side chain instead of a ribose or deoxyribose sugar. ACV has selective action against HSV and VZV, the herpesviruses that encode a thymidine kinase (Figure 49-2). The viral thymidine kinase is required to activate the drug by phosphorylation, and host cell enzymes complete the progression to the diphosphate form and finally to the triphosphate form. Because there is no initial phosphorylation in uninfected cells, there is no active drug to inhibit cellular DNA synthesis or to cause toxicity. The ACV triphosphate competes with the guanosine triphosphate to inhibit the polymerase and cause termination of the growing viral DNA chain, because there is no 3′-hydroxyl group on the ACV molecule to allow chain elongation. This inactivates the DNA polymerase. The minimal toxicity of ACV is also a result of a 100-fold or greater use by the viral DNA polymerase than by cellular DNA polymerases. **Resistance to acyclovir** develops by mutation of either the thymidine kinase, so

Table 49—2. Some Antiviral Drug Therapies Approved by the U.S. Food and Drug Administration

Virus	Antiviral Drug	Trade Name	Virus	Antiviral Drug	Trade Name
Herpes simplex and varicella-zoster viruses	Acyclovir*	Zovirax	Human immunodeficiency virus		
	Valacyclovir*	Valtrex	Nucleoside analogue reverse transcriptase inhibitors	Azidothymidine (zidovudine)	Retrovir
	Penciclovir	Denavir		Dideoxyinosine (didanosine)	Videx
	Famciclovir*	Famvir		Dideoxycytidine (zalcitabine)	Hivid
	Iododeoxyuridine (idoxuridine)†	Stoxil		Stavudine (d4T)	Zerit
	Trifluridine	Viroptic		Lamivudine (3TC)	Epivir
Cytomegalovirus	Ganciclovir	Cytovene			
	Valganciclovir	Valcyte	Non-nucleoside reverse transcriptase inhibitors	Nevirapine	Viramune
	Cidofovir	Vistide		Delavirdine	Rescriptor
	Phosphonoformate (foscarnet)	Foscavir	Protease inhibitors	Saquinavir	Invirase
Influenza A virus	Amantadine	Symmetrel		Ritonavir	Norvir
	Rimantadine	Flumadine		Indinavir	Crixivan
Influenza A and B viruses	Zanamivir	Relenza		Nelfinavir	Viracept
	Oseltamivir	Tamiflu	CCR5 co-receptor antagonist	Maraviroc	Selzentry
Hepatitis B virus	Lamivudine	Epivir	Fusion inhibitor	Enfuvirtide	Fuzeon
	Adefovir dipivoxil	Hepsera			
Hepatitis C virus	Interferon-α, ribavirin	Various			
Papillomavirus	Interferon-α	Various			
Respiratory syncytial virus and Lassa virus	Ribavirin	Virazole			
Picornaviruses	Pleconaril	Picovir			

*Also active against varicella-zoster virus.
†Topical use only.

that activation of ACV cannot occur, or the DNA polymerase, to prevent ACV binding.

ACV is effective against all HSV infections, including encephalitis, disseminated herpes, and other serious herpes diseases. The fact that it is not toxic to uninfected cells allows its use as a prophylactic treatment to prevent recurrent outbreaks, especially in immunosuppressed people. A recurrent episode may be prevented if it is treated before the onset of inflammatory responses. ACV inhibits the replication of HSV but cannot resolve the latent HSV infection.

ACV can also be used for the treatment of VZV infection, although higher doses are required. VZV is less sensitive to the agent because ACV is phosphorylated less efficiently by the VZV thymidine kinase. **Valacyclovir**, the valyl ester derivative of ACV, is more efficiently absorbed after oral administration and rapidly converted into ACV, increasing the bioavailability of ACV for the treatment of HSV and serious VZV.

Penciclovir inhibits HSV and VZV in the same way ACV does but is concentrated and persists in the infected cells to a greater extent than ACV. Penciclovir also has some activity against the Epstein-Barr virus and cytomegalovirus (CMV). **Famciclovir** is a prodrug derivative of penciclovir that is well absorbed orally and then is converted to penciclovir in the liver or intestinal lining.

Acyclovir

ATP | Viral thymidine kinase

Acycloguanosine monophosphate (acyclo-GMP)

2 ATP

Cellular kinases

Acycloguanosine triphosphate (acyclo-GTP)

Figure 49–2. Activation of ACV (acycloguanosine) in herpes simplex virus–infected cells. ACV is converted to acycloguanosine monophosphate (acyclo-GMP) by herpes-specific viral thymidine kinase, then to acycloguanosine triphosphate (acyclo-GTP) by cellular kinases.

Resistance to penciclovir and famciclovir develops in the same manner as for acyclovir.

Ganciclovir

Ganciclovir (dihydroxypropoxymethyl guanine) (GCV) differs from ACV in having a single hydroxymethyl group in the acyclic side chain (see Figure 49-1). The remarkable result of this addition is that it confers considerable activity against CMV. CMV does not encode a thymidine kinase, but a viral-encoded protein kinase phosphorylates GCV. Once activated by phosphorylation, GCV inhibits all herpesvirus DNA polymerases. The viral DNA polymerases have nearly 30 times greater affinity for the drug than the cellular DNA polymerase. Similar to acyclovir, a valyl ester of GCV (**valganciclovir**) was developed to improve the pharmacologic properties of ganciclovir.

GCV is effective in the treatment of CMV retinitis and shows some efficacy in the treatment of CMV esophagitis, colitis, and pneumonia in patients with AIDS. The potential for bone marrow toxicity limits its use to the treatment of CMV infections in patients with AIDS.

Interestingly, this potential toxicity has been used as the basis for the development of an antitumor therapy. In one application, an HSV thymidine kinase gene was incorporated into the cells of a brain tumor with the use of a retrovirus vector. The retrovirus replicated only in the growing cells of the tumor, and the thymidine kinase was expressed only in the tumor cells, making the tumor cells susceptible to GCV.

Cidofovir and Adefovir

Cidofovir and **adefovir** are both nucleoside analogues that contain a phosphate attached to the sugar analogue. This obviates the need for the more difficult initial phosphorylation to become a nucleotide. Compounds with this type of sugar analogue are substrates for DNA polymerases or reverse transcriptases and have an expanded spectrum of susceptible viruses. Cidofovir, a cytidine analogue, inhibits replication of polyomavirus papillomavirus, and is effective against all of the herpesvirus, adenovirus, and poxvirus polymerases. Adefovir and adefovir dipivoxil (a diester prodrug) are analogues of adenosine and are approved for treatment of hepatitis B virus.

Azidothymidine

Originally developed as an anticancer drug, **azidothymidine** was the first useful therapy for HIV infection. AZT (Retrovir), a nucleoside analogue of thymidine, inhibits the reverse transcriptase of HIV (see Figure 49-1). Like other nucleosides, AZT must be phosphorylated by host cell enzymes. It lacks the 3′-hydroxyl necessary for DNA chain elongation and prevents complementary DNA synthesis. The selective therapeutic effect of AZT stems from the 100-fold lower sensitivity of the host cell DNA polymerase in comparison with the HIV reverse transcriptase.

Continuous oral AZT treatment is administered to HIV-infected people with depleted CD4 T-cell counts to prevent progression of disease. AZT treatment of pregnant HIV-infected women can reduce the likelihood of or prevent transmission of the virus to the baby. Side effects of AZT range from nausea to life-threatening bone marrow toxicity.

The high error rate of the HIV polymerase creates extensive mutations and promotes the development of antiviral-drug—resistant strains. This problem is being addressed by the administration of multiple-drug therapy as initial therapy (**highly active antiretroviral therapy**

[HAART]). It is more difficult for the HIV to develop resistance to multiple drugs with multiple target enzymes. Multiple-drug–resistant HIV strains are likely to be much weaker than the parent strains.

Dideoxyinosine, Dideoxycytidine, Stavudine, and Lamivudine

Several other nucleoside analogues have been approved as anti-HIV agents. **Dideoxyinosine** (didanosine) is a nucleoside analogue that is converted to dideoxyadenosine triphosphate (see Figure 49-1). Like AZT, dideoxyinosine, **dideoxycytidine**, and **stavudine** (d4T) lack a 3′-hydroxyl group. The modified sugar attached to **lamivudine** (2′-deoxy-3′-thiacytidine [3TC]) also inhibits the HIV reverse transcriptase by preventing DNA chain elongation and HIV replication. These drugs are available for the treatment of AIDS that is unresponsive to AZT therapy, or they can be given in combination with AZT. Lamivudine is also active on the reverse transcriptase-like polymerase of hepatitis B virus.

Ribavirin

Ribavirin is an analogue of the nucleoside guanosine (see Figure 49-1) but differs from guanosine in that its base ring is incomplete and open. Like other nucleoside analogues, ribavirin must be phosphorylated. The drug is active in vitro against a broad range of viruses.

Ribavirin monophosphate resembles guanosine monophosphate and inhibits nucleoside biosynthesis, mRNA capping, and other processes important to the replication of many viruses. Ribavirin depletes the cellular stores of guanine by inhibiting inosine monophosphate dehydrogenase, an enzyme important in the synthetic pathway of guanosine. It also prevents the synthesis of the mRNA 5′ cap by interfering with the guanylation and methylation of the nucleic acid base. In addition, ribavirin triphosphate inhibits RNA polymerases and promotes hypermutation of the viral genome. Its multiple sites of action may explain the lack of ribavirin-resistant mutants of respiratory syncytial virus and influenza A virus.

Ribavirin is administered in an aerosol to children with severe respiratory syncytial virus bronchopneumonia and potentially to adults with severe influenza or measles. The drug may be effective for the treatment of influenza B, as well as Lassa, Rift Valley, Crimean-Congo, Korean, and Argentine hemorrhagic fevers, for which it is administered orally or intravenously. Ribavirin is also active against hepatitis C virus, especially in combination with interferon-α.

Other Nucleoside Analogues

Idoxuridine, trifluorothymidine (see Figure 49-1), and **fluorouracil** are analogues of thymidine. These drugs either (1) inhibit the biosynthesis of thymidine, a nucleotide

essential for DNA synthesis, or (2) replace thymidine and become incorporated into the viral DNA. These actions inhibit further synthesis of the virus or cause extensive misreading of the genome, leading to mutation and inactivation of the virus. These drugs target cells in which extensive DNA replication is taking place, such as those infected with HSV, and spare nongrowing cells from harm.

Idoxuridine was the first anti-HSV drug approved for human use but has been replaced by trifluridine and other more effective, less toxic agents. Fluorouracil is an antineoplastic drug that kills rapidly growing cells but has also been used for the topical treatment of warts caused by human papillomaviruses.

Adenine arabinoside was the principal anti-HSV drug until ACV was introduced. Ara-A is a purine nucleoside analogue identical in structure to adenosine, except that arabinose is substituted for ribose as the sugar moiety (see Figure 49-1). This agent is phosphorylated by cellular enzymes (especially adenosine kinase), even in uninfected cells, and thus has a greater potential for causing toxicity than ACV. The viral enzyme is 6 to 12 times more sensitive than the cellular enzyme. Resistance can develop as a result of a mutation of the viral DNA polymerase.

Many other nucleoside analogues that have antiviral activity are being investigated for clinical use against the herpesviruses, hepatitis B virus, and HIV.

Non-Nucleoside Polymerase Inhibitors

Foscarnet (PFA) and the related phosphonoacetic acid (PAA) are simple compounds that resemble pyrophosphate (Figure 49-3). These drugs inhibit viral replication by binding to the pyrophosphate-binding site of the DNA

Figure 49–3. Structures of non-nucleoside antiviral drugs.

polymerase to block nucleotide binding. PFA and PAA do not inhibit cellular polymerases at pharmacologic concentrations, but they can cause renal and other problems because of their ability to chelate divalent metal ions (e.g., calcium) and become incorporated into bone. PFA inhibits the DNA polymerase of all herpesviruses and the HIV reverse transcriptase without having to be phosphorylated by nucleoside kinases (e.g., thymidine kinase). PFA has been approved for the treatment of CMV retinitis in patients with AIDS.

Nevirapine, delavirdine, efavirenz, and other non-nucleoside reverse transcriptase inhibitors bind to sites on the enzyme different from the substrate. Because these drugs' mechanisms of action differ from those of the nucleoside analogues, the mechanism of HIV resistance to the agents is also different. As a result, these drugs are very useful in combination with nucleoside analogues for the treatment of HIV infection.

Protease Inhibitors

The unique structure of the HIV protease and its essential role in the production of a functional virion have made this enzyme a good target for antiviral drugs. **Saquinavir, indinavir, ritonavir, nelfinavir, amprenavir**, and other agents work by slipping into the hydrophobic active site of the enzyme to inhibit its action. As occurs with the other anti-HIV drugs, drug-resistant strains arise through mutation of the protease. The combination of a protease inhibitor with AZT and a second nucleoside analogue (HAART) can reduce blood levels of HIV to undetectable levels. Development of resistance to a "cocktail" of anti-HIV drugs is also less likely than that to a single drug. Protease inhibitors are also being developed for hepatitis C and other viruses.

Anti-influenza Drugs

Amantadine and **rimantadine** are amphipathic amine compounds with clinical efficacy against the influenza A virus but not the influenza B or other viruses (see Figure 49-3). These drugs have several effects on influenza A replication. Both compounds are acidotrophic and concentrate in and buffer the contents of the endosomal vesicles involved in the uptake of the influenza virus. This effect can inhibit the acid-mediated change in conformation in the hemagglutinin protein that promotes the fusion of the viral envelope with cell membranes. However, the specificity for influenza A is a result of its ability to bind to and block the proton channel formed by the M_2 matrix protein of the influenza A virus. Resistance is the result of an altered M_2 matrix or hemagglutinin protein.

Amantadine and rimantadine may be useful in ameliorating an influenza A infection if either agent is taken within 48 hours of exposure. They are also useful as a prophylactic treatment in lieu of vaccination. In addition, amantadine is an alternative therapy for Parkinson disease. The principal toxic effect is on the central nervous system, with patients experiencing nervousness, irritability, and insomnia.

Zanamivir (Relenza) and **oseltamivir (Tamiflu)** inhibit influenza A and B as enzyme inhibitors of the neuraminidase of influenza. Without the neuraminidase, the hemagglutinin of the virus binds to sialic acid on other viral particles, forming clumps and preventing virus release. These drugs can be taken prophylactically as an alternative to vaccination or to reduce the length of illness if taken within the first 48 hours of infection.

Immunomodulators

Genetically engineered forms of IFN-α have been approved for human use. Interferons work by binding to cell surface receptors and initiating a cellular antiviral response. In addition, interferons stimulate the immune response and promote the immune clearance of viral infection.

IFN-α is active against many viral infections, including hepatitis A, B, and C, HSV, papillomavirus, and rhinovirus. It has been approved for the treatment of condyloma acuminatum (genital warts, a presentation of papillomavirus) and hepatitis C (especially with ribavirin). Attachment of polyethylene glycol to interferon alpha (pegylated interferon alfa) increases its potency. Pegylated interferon alfa is used with ribavirin to treat hepatitis C infections. Natural interferon causes the influenza-like symptoms observed during many viremic and respiratory tract infections, and the synthetic agent has similar side effects during treatment. Interferon is discussed further in Chapter 14.

Imiquimod, a Toll-like receptor ligand, stimulates innate responses to attack the virus infection. This therapeutic approach can activate local protective responses against papillomas, which generally escape immune control.

Questions

1. List the steps in viral replication that are poor targets for antiviral drugs. Why?

2. Which viruses can be treated with an antiviral drug? Distinguish the viruses treatable with an antiviral nucleoside analogue.

3. A mutation in the gene for which enzymes or proteins would confer resistance to the following antiviral drugs: ACV, ara-A, phosphonoformate, amantadine, AZT?

4. A patient has been exposed to influenza A virus and is in his third day of symptoms. He has heard that an anti-influenza drug is available and requests therapy. You tell him that therapy is not appropriate. To what therapeutic agents is the patient referring, and why did you decline to use the treatment?

Bibliography

Carter J, Saunders V. Virology: Principles and Applications. Chichester, England, Wiley, 2007.

Cohen J, Powderly WG (eds): Infectious Diseases, 2nd ed. St Louis, Mosby, 2004.

Collier L, Oxford J: Human Virology, 3rd ed. Oxford, Oxford University Press, 2006.

Flint SJ, et al: Principles of Virology: Molecular Biology, Pathogenesis and Control of Animal Viruses, 2nd ed. Washington, DC, ASM Press, 2003.

Galasso GJ, Whitley RJ, Merigan TC: Antiviral Agents and Human Viral Diseases, 4th ed. Philadelphia, Lippincott, 1997.

Hodinka RL: What clinicians need to know about antiviral drugs and viral resistance. Infect Dis Clin North Am 11:945-967, 1997.

Knipe DM, Howley PM (eds): Fields' Virology, 4th ed. New York, Lippincott Williams & Wilkins, 2001.

Richman DD, Whitley RJ, Hayden FG: Clinical Virology, 2nd ed. Washington, DC, ASM Press, 2004.

Richman DD: Antiviral drug resistance. Antiviral Res 71:117-121, 2006.

Strauss JM, Strauss EG: Viruses and Human Diseases, 2nd ed. San Diego, Academic, 2007.

Voyles BA: The Biology of Viruses, 2nd ed. Boston, McGraw-Hill, 2002.

Laboratory Diagnosis of Viral Diseases

There have been many new developments in laboratory viral diagnosis that provide more rapid and sensitive viral identification from clinical samples. These include better antibody reagents for direct analysis of samples and molecular genetic techniques for direct identification of viral genomes. Often, isolation of the organism is unnecessary and avoided to minimize the risk to laboratory and other personnel. The quicker turnaround allows a more rapid choice of the appropriate antiviral therapy.

The patient's history and symptoms provide the first clues to the diagnosis of a viral infection, often by excluding other types of infection (e.g., bacterial, fungal). Viral laboratory studies are performed to (1) confirm the diagnosis by identifying the viral agent of infection, (2) determine appropriate antiviral therapy, (3) define the course of the disease, (4) monitor the disease epidemiologically, and (5) educate physicians and patients.

The laboratory methods accomplish the following results:

1. Description of virus-induced **cytopathologic effects (CPEs)** on cells.
2. Electron microscopic detection of viral particles.
3. Isolation and growth of the virus.
4. Detection of viral components (e.g., proteins, enzymes, genomes).
5. Evaluation of the patient's immune response to the virus (**serology**).

The molecular and immunologic techniques used for many of these procedures are described in Chapters 16 and 17. Viruses, viral antigens, viral genomes, and CPEs can be detected by means of direct analysis of clinical specimens or after growth of the virus on tissue culture cells in the laboratory (Box 50-1).

Specimen Collection

The patient's symptoms and history, including recent travel, the season of the year, and a presumptive diagnosis,

help determine the appropriate procedures to be used to identify a viral agent (Table 50-1). For example, a focal encephalitis with a temporal lobe localization preceded by headaches and disorientation suggests herpes simplex virus (HSV) infection, for which cerebrospinal fluid is analyzed for viral deoxyribonucleic acid (DNA) sequences by polymerase chain reaction (PCR) amplification. The development of meningitis symptoms during the summer suggests an arbovirus, in which case cerebrospinal fluid (CSF) and blood should be collected, or an enterovirus, in which case CSF, throat swab, and stool specimens should be collected, for PCR analysis and possible virus isolation.

The selection of the appropriate specimen for viral culture is often complicated, because several viruses may cause the same clinical disease. For example, many agents can cause aseptic meningitis, so it may be necessary to obtain several types of specimens to identify the causal virus.

Specimens should be collected early in the acute phase of infection, before the virus ceases to be shed. For example, respiratory viruses may be shed for only 3 to 7 days, and shedding may lapse before the symptoms cease. HSV and varicella-zoster virus (VZV) may not be recoverable from lesions more than 5 days after the onset of symptoms. It may be possible to isolate an enterovirus from the cerebrospinal fluid for only 2 to 3 days after the onset of the central nervous system manifestations. In addition, antibody produced in response to the infection may block the detection of virus.

The shorter the interval between the collection of a specimen and its delivery to the laboratory, the greater the potential for isolating a virus. The reasons are that many viruses are labile, and the samples are susceptible to bacterial and fungal overgrowth. Viruses are best transported and stored on ice and in special media that contain antibiotics and proteins, such as serum albumin or gelatin. Significant losses in infectious titers occur when enveloped viruses (e.g., HSV, VZV, influenza virus) are kept at room temperature or frozen at −20° C. This is not a risk for nonenveloped viruses (e.g., adenoviruses, enteroviruses).

Box 50—1. Laboratory Procedures for Diagnosing Viral Infections

Cytologic examination
Electron microscopy
Virus isolation and growth
Detection of viral proteins (antigens and enzymes)
Detection of viral genomes
Serology

Cytology

Many viruses produce a characteristic CPE. Characteristic CPEs in the tissue sample or in cell culture include changes in cell morphology, cell lysis, vacuolation, syncytia (Figure 50-1), and inclusion bodies. **Syncytia** are multinucleated giant cells formed by viral fusion of individual cells. Paramyxoviruses, HSV, VZV, and HIV promote syncytia formation. **Inclusion bodies** are either histologic changes in the cells caused by viral components or virus-induced changes in cell structures. For example, nuclear owl's-eye

Table 50—1. Specimens for Viral Diagnosis

Common Pathogenic Viruses	Specimens for Culture	Comments
Respiratory Tract		
Adenovirus; influenza virus; enterovirus (picornavirus); rhinovirus; paramyxovirus; rubella virus; HSV	Nasal washing, throat swab, nasal swab, sputum	Enterovirus is also shed in stool
Gastrointestinal Tract		
Reovirus; rotavirus; adenovirus; Norwalk virus, calicivirus	Stool, rectal swab	Samples are analyzed by electron microscopy and antigen detection (ELISA); viruses are not cultured
Maculopapular Rash		
Adenovirus; enterovirus (picornavirus)	Throat swab, rectal swab	—
Rubella virus; measles virus	Urine	—
Vesicular Rash		
Coxsackievirus; echovirus; HSV; VZV	Vesicle fluid, scraping, or swab, enterovirus in stool	Initial diagnosis of HSV and VZV can be obtained from vesicle scraping (Tzanck smear)
Central Nervous System (Aseptic Meningitis, Encephalitis)		
Enterovirus (picornavirus)	Stool	PCR
Arboviruses (e.g., togaviruses, bunyavirus)	Rarely cultured	Diagnosis is by serologic tests
Rabies virus	Tissue, saliva, brain biopsy	Diagnosis is by immunofluorescence analysis for antigen
HSV; CMV; mumps virus; measles virus	Cerebrospinal fluid	PCR, virus isolation, and antigen are assayed
Urinary Tract		
Adenovirus; CMV	Urine	CMV may be shed without apparent disease
Blood		
HIV; human T-cell leukemia virus; hepatitis B, C, and D viruses	Blood	Serologic antigen or antibody detection (ELISA), PCR, and RT-PCR are performed

Data from Cherneskey MA, et al: Cumitech 15: Laboratory Diagnosis of Viral Infections. Washington, DC, ASM Press, 1982; and from Hsiung GD: Diagnostic Virology. New Haven, Conn, Yale, 1982.
CMV, cytomegalovirus; ELISA, enzyme-linked immunosorbent assay; HIV, human immunodeficiency virus; HSV, herpes simplex virus; PCR, polymerase chain reaction; RT-PCR, reverse transcriptase PCR; VZV, varicella-zoster virus.

Figure 50–1. Syncytium formation by measles virus. Multinucleated giant cell *(arrow)* visible in a histologic section of lung biopsy tissue from a measles virus–induced giant cell pneumonia in an immunocompromised child. *(From Hart C, Broadhead RL: A Color Atlas of Pediatric Infectious Diseases. London, Wolfe, 1992.)*

Figure 50–3. Negri bodies caused by rabies. **A,** A section of brain from a patient with rabies shows Negri bodies *(arrow)*. **B,** Higher magnification from another biopsy specimen. **(A** from Hart C, Broadhead RL: A Color Atlas of Pediatric Infectious Diseases. London, Wolfe, 1992.)

inclusion bodies found in the cells of tissues with cytomegalovirus (CMV) (see Chapter 53, Figure 53-17) or in the sediment of urine from patients with the infection are readily identifiable. Cowdry type A inclusions in single cells or in large syncytia (multiple cells fused together) are a characteristic finding in cells infected with HSV or VZV (Figure 50-2). Rabies may be detected through the finding of Negri bodies (rabies virus inclusions) in brain tissue (Figure 50-3).

Often the cytologic specimens will be examined for the presence of specific viral antigens by immunofluorescence or viral genomes by in situ hybridization or PCR for a rapid, definitive identification. These tests are specific for individual viruses and must be chosen based on the differential diagnosis. These methods are discussed in the following paragraphs.

Electron Microscopy

Electron microscopy is not a standard clinical laboratory technique, but it can be used to detect and identify some viruses if sufficient viral particles are present. The addition of virus-specific antibody to a sample can cause viral particles to clump, thereby facilitating the detection and simultaneous identification of the virus (immunoelectron microscopy). This method is useful for the detection of enteric viruses, such as rotavirus, that are produced in abundance and have a characteristic morphology. Appropriately processed tissue from a biopsy or clinical specimen can also be examined for the presence of viral structures.

Figure 50–2. HSV-induced CPE. A biopsy specimen of an HSV-infected liver shows an eosinophilic Cowdry type A intranuclear inclusion body *(A)* surrounded by a halo and a ring of marginated chromatin at the nuclear membrane. An infected cell *(B)* exhibits a smaller condensed nucleus (pyknotic). CPE, cytopathologic effect; HSV, herpes simplex virus. *(Courtesy Dr. J.I. Pugh, St. Albans; from Emond RT, Rowland HAK: A Color Atlas of Infectious Diseases, 3rd ed. London, Mosby, 1995.)*

Viral Isolation and Growth

A virus can be grown in tissue culture, embryonated eggs, and experimental animals (Box 50-2). Although embryonated eggs are still used for the growth of virus for some

Box 50–2. Systems for the Propagation of Viruses

People
Animals: cows (e.g., Jenner cowpox vaccine), chickens, mice, rats, suckling mice
Embryonated eggs
Organ culture
Tissue culture
- Primary
- Diploid cell line
- Tumor or immortalized cell line

Box 50–3. Viral Cytopathologic Effects

Cell death
- Cell rounding
- Degeneration
- Aggregation
- Loss of attachments to culture dish

Characteristic histologic changes: inclusion bodies in the nucleus or cytoplasm, margination of chromatin
Syncytia: multinucleated giant cells caused by virus-induced cell-cell fusion
Cell surface changes
- Viral antigen expression
- Hemadsorption (hemagglutinin expression)

vaccines (e.g., influenza), they have been replaced by cell cultures for routine virus isolation in clinical laboratories. Experimental animals are rarely used in clinical laboratories for the purpose of isolating viruses.

Cell Culture

Specific types of tissue culture cells are used to grow viruses. **Primary cell cultures** are obtained by dissociating specific animal organs with trypsin or collagenase. The cells yielded by this method are then grown as monolayers (fibroblast or epithelial) or in suspension (lymphocyte) in artificial media supplemented with bovine serum or another source of growth factors. Primary cells can be dissociated with trypsin, diluted, and allowed to grow into new monolayers (*passed*) to become secondary cell cultures. **Diploid cell lines** are cultures of a single cell type that are capable of being passed a large but finite number of times before they senesce, or undergo a significant change in their characteristics. **Tumor cell lines** and **immortalized cell lines**, which are initiated from patient tumors and by viruses or chemicals, consist of single cell types that can be passed continuously without senescing.

Primary monkey kidney cells are excellent for the recovery of influenza viruses, paramyxoviruses, many enteroviruses, and some adenoviruses. Human fetal diploid cells, which are generally fibroblastic cells, support the growth of a broad spectrum of viruses (e.g., HSV, VZV, CMV, adenoviruses, picornaviruses). HeLa cells, a continuous line of epithelial cells derived from a human cancer, are excellent for the recovery of respiratory syncytial virus, adenoviruses, and HSV. Many clinically significant viruses can be recovered in at least one of these cell cultures.

Viral Detection

A virus can be detected and initially identified through observation of the virus-induced CPE in the cell monolayer (Box 50-3; Figure 50-4) or by immunofluorescence or genome analysis of the infected cell culture. For example, a single virus infects, spreads, and kills surrounding cells (**plaque**). The type of cell culture, the characteristics of the CPE, and the rapidity of viral growth can be used to initially identify many clinically important viruses. This approach to identifying viruses is similar to that used in the identification of bacteria, which is based on the growth and morphology of colonies on selective differential media.

Some viruses grow slowly or not at all or do not readily cause a CPE in cell lines typically used in clinical virology laboratories. Some cause diseases that are hazardous to personnel. These viruses are most frequently diagnosed

Figure 50–4. CPE of HSV infection. **A,** Uninfected Vero cells, an African green monkey kidney cell line. **B,** HSV-1–infected Vero cells showing rounded cells, multinucleated cells, and loss of the monolayer. *Arrows* point to syncytia.

Figure 50—5. Hemadsorption of erythrocytes to cells infected with influenza viruses, mumps virus, parainfluenza viruses, or togaviruses. These viruses express a hemagglutinin on their surfaces, which bind erythrocytes of selected animal species.

Interpretation of Culture Results

In general, the detection of any virus in host tissues, cerebrospinal fluid, blood, or vesicular fluid can be considered a highly significant finding. However, viral shedding may also be induced by an underlying condition (e.g., another infection, an immunosuppressed state, stress) and may therefore be unrelated to the disease symptoms. Certain viruses can be intermittently shed without causing symptoms in the affected person for periods ranging from weeks (enteroviruses in feces) to many months or years (HSV or CMV in the oropharynx and vagina; adenoviruses in the oropharynx and intestinal tract). Also, virus may not be isolated from a sample if the sample is improperly handled, contains neutralizing antibody, or is acquired before or after viral shedding.

Detection of Viral Proteins

Enzymes and other proteins are produced during viral replication and can be detected by biochemical, immunologic, and molecular biologic means (Box 50-4). The viral proteins can be separated by electrophoresis and their patterns used to identify and distinguish different viruses. For example, the electrophoretically separated HSV-infected cell proteins and virion proteins exhibit different patterns for different types and strains of HSV-1 and HSV-2.

The detection and assay of characteristic enzymes or activities can identify and quantitate specific viruses. For example, the presence of reverse transcriptase in serum or cell culture indicates the presence of a retrovirus. Similarly, hemagglutination or hemadsorption can be used to easily assay the hemagglutinin produced by the influenza virus.

Antibodies can be used as sensitive and specific tools to detect, identify, and quantitate the virus and viral antigen in clinical specimens or cell cultures (immunohistochemistry). Specifically, monoclonal or monospecific antibodies

---

on the basis of serologic findings or through the detection of viral genomes or proteins.

Characteristic viral properties can also be used to identify viruses that do not have a classic CPE. For example, the rubella virus may not cause a CPE, but it does prevent (interfere with) the replication of picornaviruses in a process known as **heterologous interference**, which can be used to identify the rubella virus. Cells infected with the influenza virus, parainfluenza virus, mumps virus, and togavirus express a viral glycoprotein (hemagglutinin) that binds erythrocytes of defined animal species to the infected cell surface (**hemadsorption**) (Figure 50-5). When released into the cell culture medium, such viruses can be detected from the agglutination of erythrocytes, a process termed **hemagglutination**. The virus can then be identified from the specific antibody that blocks the hemagglutination, a process called **hemagglutination inhibition (HI)**. An innovative approach to detection of herpes simplex virus infection uses genetically modified tissue culture cells that express the β-galactosidase gene and can be stained blue when infected with HSV (enzyme-linked virus inducible system (ELVIS)).

One can quantitate a virus by determining the greatest dilution that retains the following properties (**titer**):

1. **Tissue culture dose (TCD_{50}):** titer of virus that causes cytopathologic effects in half the tissue culture cells.
2. **Lethal dose (LD_{50}):** titer of virus that kills 50% of a set of test animals.
3. **Infectious dose (ID_{50}):** titer of virus that initiates a detectable symptom, antibody, or other response in 50% of a set of test animals.

The number of infectious viruses can also be evaluated with a count of the plaques produced by tenfold dilutions of sample (**plaque-forming units**). The ratio of viral particles (from electron microscopy) to plaque-forming units is always greater than one, because numerous defective viral particles are produced during viral replication.

Box 50—4. Assays for Viral Proteins and Nucleic Acids

Proteins

Protein patterns (electrophoresis)
Enzyme activities (e.g., reverse transcriptase)
Hemagglutination and hemadsorption
Antigen detection (e.g., direct and indirect immunofluorescence, enzyme-linked immunosorbent assay, Western blot)

Nucleic Acids

Restriction endonuclease cleavage patterns
Size of RNA for segmented RNA viruses (electrophoresis)
DNA genome hybridization in situ (cytochemistry)
Southern, Northern, and dot blots
PCR (DNA)
Reverse transcriptase polymerase chain reaction (RNA)
Real-time PCR
Branched-chain DNA and related tests (DNA, RNA)
PCR, polymerase chain reaction

are useful for distinguishing viruses. Viral antigens on the cell surface or within the cell can be detected by **immunofluorescence** and enzyme immunoassay (EIA) (see Chapter 17, Figures 17-2 and 17-3). Virus or antigen released from infected cells can be detected by **enzyme-linked immunosorbent assay (ELISA)**, radioimmunoassay (RIA), and **latex agglutination (LA)** (see Chapter 17 for definitions). Tests for specific viral agents are commercially available.

The detection of CMV and other viruses can be enhanced through the use of a combination of cell culture and immunologic means. In this method the clinical sample is centrifuged onto cells grown on a coverslip on the bottom of a **shell vial** (glass tube). This step increases the efficiency and accelerates the progression of infection of the cells on the coverslip. The cells can then be analyzed with immunofluorescence (**direct fluorescence**) or EIA for early viral antigens, which are detectable within 24 hours, instead of the 7 to 14 days it takes for a CPE to become evident.

Detection of Viral Genetic Material

The genome structure and genetic sequence are major distinguishing characteristics of the family, type, and strain of virus (see Box 50-4). The electrophoretic patterns of ribonucleic acid (RNA) (influenza, reovirus) or restriction endonuclease fragment lengths from DNA viral genomes are like genetic fingerprints for these viruses. Different strains of HSV-1 and HSV-2 can be distinguished in this way by restriction fragment length polymorphism. Newer methods for viral genome detection use sequence-specific genetic probes and PCR-like DNA amplification approaches, which allow more rapid analysis with a minimum of risk from infectious virus.

DNA probes, with sequences complementary to specific regions of a viral genome, can be used like antibodies as sensitive and specific tools for detecting a virus. These probes can detect the virus even in the absence of viral replication. DNA probe analysis is especially useful for detecting slowly replicating or nonproductive viruses such as CMV and human papillomavirus, for which there is no CPE, or the viral antigen cannot be detected using immunologic tests (see Chapter 16, Figure 16-3). Specific viral genetic sequences in fixed, permeabilized tissue biopsy specimens can be detected by **in situ hybridization**.

Viral genomes can also be detected in clinical samples with the use of **dot blot** or **Southern blot analysis**. For the latter method, the viral genome or electrophoretically separated restriction endonuclease cleavage fragments of the genome are blotted onto nitrocellulose filters and then detected on the filter by their hybridization to DNA probes. Electrophoretically separated viral RNA (**Northern blot**—RNA:DNA probe hybridization) blotted onto a nitrocellulose filter can be detected in a similar manner. The DNA probes are detected with autoradiography or with

fluorescent or EIA-like methods. Many viral probes and kits for detecting viruses are now commercially available.

For many laboratories, detection of viral genomes by **PCR, reverse transcriptase PCR (RT-PCR)**, and related assays are becoming the primary tool for detection and identification of several viruses. Use of the appropriate primers for PCR can promote a millionfold amplification of a target sequence in a few hours. This technique is especially useful for detecting latent and integrated sequences of viruses, such as retroviruses, herpesviruses, papillomaviruses, and other papovaviruses, as well as evidence of viruses present in low concentrations and viruses that are difficult or too dangerous to isolate in cell culture. RT-PCR uses the retroviral reverse transcriptase to convert viral RNA to DNA and allow PCR amplification of the viral nucleic acid sequences. This approach was very useful for identifying and distinguishing the Hantaviruses that caused the outbreak in New Mexico in 1993.

Quantification of the amount of HIV within a patient (virus load) can be determined by **real-time PCR**. The concentration of HIV genome in a blood sample is proportional to the rate of PCR amplification of the genomic DNA.

PCR is the prototype for several other HIV genome amplification techniques. **Transcription-based amplification** uses reverse transcriptase and viral sequence specific primers to make a complementary DNA (cDNA) and attaches a sequence recognized by the DNA-dependent RNA polymerase from the T7 bacteriophage. The DNA is transcribed to RNA by the T7 RNA polymerase and the new RNA sequences are then cycled back into the reaction to amplify the relevant sequence. Unlike PCR, these reactions do not require special equipment.

Some other genome amplification and detection approaches are similar in concept to ELISA. These approaches use immobilized DNA sequences complementary to the relevant viral genomic sequence to capture the viral genome. This is followed by the binding of another complementary sequence that contains a detection system. The cDNA sequence may be attached to an extensively **branched chain of DNA** in which each of the branches elicits a reaction that amplifies the signal to detectable levels. Another variation of the theme uses an antibody that recognizes DNA-RNA complexes to capture viral DNA-RNA probe hybrids in the well of a plate, followed by an enzyme-labeled antibody and ELISA methods to detect the presence of the genome. Like ELISA, these methods can be automated and set up to analyze a panel of viruses.

Viral Serology

The humoral immune response provides a history of a patient's infections. Serologic studies are used for the identification of viruses that are difficult to isolate and grow in cell culture, as well as viruses that cause diseases of long duration (see Box 17-2). Serology can be used to identify the virus and its strain or serotype, whether it is acute or chronic disease, and determine whether it is a primary infection or a reinfection. The detection of **virus-specific immunoglobulin (Ig)M antibody**, which is present during the first 2 or 3 weeks of a primary infection, generally indicates a recent primary infection. **Seroconversion** is indicated by at least **a fourfold increase in the antibody titer** between the serum obtained during the acute phase of disease and that obtained at least 2 to 3 weeks later during the convalescent phase. Reinfection or recurrence later in life causes an anamnestic (secondary or booster) response. Antibody titers may remain high in patients who suffer frequent recurrence of a disease (e.g., herpesviruses).

Because of the inherent imprecision of serologic assays based on twofold serial dilutions, a fourfold increase in the antibody titer between acute and convalescent sera is required to indicate seroconversion. For example, samples with 512 and 1023 units of antibody would both give a signal on a 512-fold dilution but not on a 1024-fold dilution, and the titers of both would be reported as 512. On the other hand, samples with 1020 and 1030 units are not significantly different but would be reported as titers of 512 and 1024, respectively.

The course of a chronic infection can also be evaluated by a serologic profile. Specifically, the presence of antibodies to several key viral antigens and their titers can be used to identify the stage of disease caused by certain viruses. This approach is especially useful for the diagnosis of viral diseases with slow courses (e.g., hepatitis B, infectious mononucleosis caused by Epstein-Barr virus). In general, the first antibodies to be detected are directed against the antigens most available to the immune system (e.g., expressed on the virion or infected-cell surfaces). Later in the infection, when the infecting virus or the cellular immune response has lysed the cells, antibodies directed against the intracellular viral proteins and enzymes are detected. For example, antibodies to the envelope and capsid antigens of Epstein-Barr virus are detected first. Then during convalescence, antibodies to nuclear antigens, such as the Epstein-Barr virus nuclear antigen, are detected.

A serologic battery or panel consisting of assays for several viruses may be used for the diagnosis of certain diseases. Local epidemiologic factors, the time of year, and patient factors such as immunocompetence, travel history, and age influence the choice of virus assays to be included in a panel. For example, HSV and the viruses of mumps, western and eastern equine encephalitides, and St. Louis, West Nile, and California encephalitides might be included in a panel of tests for central nervous system diseases.

Serologic Test Methods

The serologic tests used in virology are listed in Chapter 17, Box 17-1, and described further in Chapter 1. **Neutralization** and **HI tests** assay antibody on the basis of

Figure 50–6. Neutralization, hemagglutination, and hemagglutination inhibition assays. In the assay shown, tenfold dilutions of serum were incubated with virus. Aliquots of the mixture were then added to cell cultures or erythrocytes. In the absence of antibody, the virus infected the monolayer (indicated by CPE) and caused hemagglutination (i.e., formed a gel-like suspension of erythrocytes). In the presence of the antibody, infection was blocked (neutralization), and hemagglutination was inhibited, allowing the erythrocytes to pellet. The titer of antibody in the serum was 100 pfu, plaque-forming units.

its recognition of and binding to virus. The antibody coating of the virus blocks its binding to indicator cells (Figure 50-6). Neutralization causes inhibition by the antibody of infection and cytopathologic effects of the virus in tissue culture cells. A neutralization antibody response is virus and strain specific. The presence of antibody often develops with the onset of symptoms and persists for long periods. HI is used for the identification of viruses that can selectively agglutinate erythrocytes of various animal species (e.g., chicken, guinea pig, human). Antibody in serum prevents a standardized amount of virus from binding to and agglutinating erythrocytes.

The indirect fluorescent antibody test and solid-phase immunoassays such as **LA, ELISA,** and **RIA** are commonly used to detect and quantitate viral antigen and antiviral antibody. The ELISA test is used to screen the blood supply to exclude individuals who are seropositive for hepatitis B and C viruses and HIV. **Western blot** analysis has become very important to confirm seroconversion and hence infection with HIV. The ability of the patient antibody to recognize specific viral proteins separated by electrophoresis, transferred (blotted) onto a

Figure 50–7. Western blot analysis of HIV antigens and antibody. HIV protein antigens are separated by electrophoresis and blotted onto nitrocellulose paper strips. The strip is incubated with patient antibody, washed to remove the unbound antibody, and then reacted with enzyme-conjugated antihuman antibody and chromophoric substrate. Serum from an HIV-infected person binds and identifies the major antigenic proteins of HIV. This data demonstrates the seroconversion of one HIV-infected individual with sera collected on day 0 (D0) to day 30 (D30) compared to a known positive control (PC) and negative control (NC). *(From Kuritzkes DR: Diagnostic tests for HIV infection and resistance assays. In Cohen J, Powderly WG: Infectious Diseases, 2nd ed. St Louis, Mosby, 2004.)*

filter paper (e.g., nitrocellulose, nylon), and visualized with an enzyme-conjugated antihuman antibody confirms the ELISA-indicated diagnosis of HIV infection (Figure 50-7).

Limitations of Serologic Methods

The presence of an antiviral antibody indicates previous infection but is not sufficient to indicate when the infection occurred. The finding of virus-specific IgM, a fourfold increase in the antibody titer between acute and convalescent sera, or specific antibody profiles is indicative of recent infection. False-positive or false-negative test results may confuse the diagnosis. In addition, patient antibody may be bound with viral antigen (as occurs in patients with hepatitis B) in immune complexes, thereby preventing antibody detection. Serologic cross-reactions between different viruses may also confuse the identity of the infecting agent (e.g., parainfluenza and mumps express related antigens). Conversely, the antibody used in the assay may be too specific (many monoclonal antibodies) and may not recognize other viruses from the same family, giving a false-negative result (e.g., rhinovirus). A good understanding of the clinical symptoms and a knowledge of the limitations and potential problems with serologic assays aid the diagnosis.

Questions

1. Brain tissue is obtained at autopsy from a person who died of rabies. What procedures could be used to confirm the presence of rabies virus—infected cells in the brain tissue?

2. A cervical Papanicolaou smear is taken from a woman with a vaginal papilloma (wart). Certain types of papilloma have been associated with cervical carcinoma. What method or methods would be used to detect and identify the type of papilloma in the cervical smear?

3. A legal case would be settled by identification of the source of an HSV infection. Serum and viral isolates are obtained from the infected person and two contacts. What methods could be used to determine whether the person is infected with HSV-1 or HSV-2? What methods could be used to compare the type and strain of HSV obtained from each of the three people?

4. A 50-year-old man experiences flulike symptoms. The figure below shows results of hemagglutination inhibition (HI) tests on serum specimens collected when the disease manifested (acute) and 3 weeks later. The HI data for the current strain of influenza A (H3N2) are presented at top right. Filled circles indicate hemagglutination. Is the patient infected with the current strain of influenza A?

Questions—cont'd

5. A policeman accidentally sticks his finger with a drug addict's syringe needle. He is concerned that he may be infected with HIV. Samples are taken from the policeman a month later for analysis. What assays would be appropriate to determine whether the man is infected with the virus? In this case, it may be too early to detect an antibody response to the virus. What procedures would be appropriate to assay for virus or viral components?

Bibliography

Carter J, Saunders V: Virology: Principles and Applications. Chichester, England, Wiley, 2007.

Cohen J, Powderly WG: Infectious Diseases, 2nd ed. St Louis, Mosby, 2004.

Collier L, Oxford J: Human Virology, 3rd ed. Oxford, Oxford University Press, 2006.

Flint SJ, et al: Principles of Virology: Molecular Biology, Pathogenesis and Control of Animal Viruses, 2nd ed. Washington, DC, ASM Press, 2003.

Forbes BA, Sahm DF, Weissfeld AS: Baily and Scott's Diagnostic Microbiology, 11th ed. St Louis, Mosby, 2007.

Hsiung GD: Diagnostic Virology, 3rd ed. New Haven, Conn, Yale, 1982.

Knipe DM, Howley PM: Fields' Virology, 4th ed. New York, Lippincott Williams & Wilkins, 2001.

Lennette EH: Laboratory Diagnosis of Viral Infections, 3rd ed. New York, Marcel Dekker, 1999.

Menegus MA: Diagnostic virology. In Belshe RB (ed): Textbook of Human Virology, 2nd ed. St Louis, Mosby, 1991.

Murray PR: Pocket Guide to Clinical Microbiology, 3rd ed. Washington, DC, ASM Press, 2004.

Murray PR, et al: Manual of Clinical Microbiology, 9th ed. Washington, DC, ASM Press, 2007.

Specter S, et al: Clinical Virology Manual, 3rd ed. Washington, DC, ASM Press, 2000.

Strauss JM, Strauss EG: Viruses and Human Disease, 2nd ed. San Diego, Academic, 2007.

Voyles BA: The Biology of Viruses, 2nd ed. Boston, McGraw-Hill, 2002.

Website

Viruses in cell culture: Available at www.uct.ac.za/depts/mmi/stannard/linda.html.

Papillomaviruses and Polyomaviruses

What used to be called the **papovavirus family** (Papovaviridae) has been divided into two families, Papillomaviridae and Polyomaviridae (Table 51-1). These viruses are capable of causing lytic, chronic, latent, and transforming infections, depending on the host cell. Human papillomaviruses (HPVs) cause **warts**, and several genotypes are associated with human cancer (e.g., **cervical carcinoma**). BK and JC viruses, members of the Polyomaviridae, usually cause asymptomatic infection but are associated with renal disease and **progressive multifocal leukoencephalopathy** (**PML**), respectively, in immunosuppressed people. Simian virus 40 (**SV40**) is the prototype polyomavirus.

The papillomaviruses and polyomaviruses are small, nonenveloped, icosahedral capsid viruses with double-stranded circular deoxyribonucleic acid (DNA) genomes (Box 51-1). They encode proteins that promote cell growth. The promotion of cell growth facilitates lytic viral replication in a permissive cell type but **may oncogenically transform a cell that is nonpermissive**. The polyomaviruses, especially SV40, have been studied extensively as model oncogenic viruses.

Human Papillomaviruses

Structure and Replication

Classification of the HPVs is based on DNA sequence homology. At least 100 types have been identified and classified into 16 (A through P) groups. HPV can be distinguished further as **cutaneous HPV** or **mucosal HPV** on the basis of the susceptible tissue. Within the mucosal HPV, there is a group associated with cervical cancer. Viruses in similar groups frequently cause similar types of warts.

The **icosahedral capsid** of HPV is 50 to 55 nm in diameter and consists of two structural proteins forming 72 capsomeres (Figure 51-1). The HPV genome is **circular** and has approximately 8000 base pairs. The HPV DNA encodes seven or eight early genes (E1 to E8), depending

on the virus, and two late or structural genes (L1 and L2). An upstream regulatory region contains the control sequences for transcription, the shared *N*-terminal sequence for the early proteins, and the origin of replication. All the genes are located on one strand (the plus strand) (Figure 51-2).

HPV replication is controlled by the host cell's transcriptional machinery, as determined by the differentiation of the skin or mucosal epithelium (Figure 51-3). The virus accesses the basal cell layer through breaks in the skin. The early genes of the virus stimulate cell growth, which facilitates replication of the viral genome by the host cell DNA polymerase when the cells divide. The virus-induced increase in cell number causes the basal and the prickle cell layer (stratum spinosum) to thicken (wart or papilloma). As the basal cell differentiates, the specific nuclear factors expressed in the different layers and types of skin and mucosa promote transcription of different viral genes. Expression of the viral genes correlates with the expression of specific keratins. The late genes encoding the structural proteins are expressed only in the terminally differentiated upper layer, and the virus assembles in the nucleus. As the infected skin cell matures and works its way to the surface, the virus matures and is shed with the dead cells of the upper layer.

Pathogenesis

Papillomaviruses infect and replicate in the squamous epithelium of skin (**warts**) and mucous membranes (**genital, oral**, and **conjunctival papillomas**) to induce epithelial proliferation. The HPV types are very tissue specific, causing different disease presentations. The wart develops as a result of virus stimulation of cell growth and thickening of the basal and prickle layers (stratum spinosum), as well as the stratum granulosum. **Koilocytes**, characteristic of papillomavirus infection, are enlarged keratinocytes with clear haloes around shrunken nuclei. It usually takes 3 to 4 months for the wart to develop

Table 51—1. Human Papillomaviruses and Polyomaviruses and Their Diseases

Virus	Disease
Papillomavirus	Warts
Polyomavirus	
BK virus	Renal disease*
JC virus	Progressive multifocal leukoencephalopathy*

Disease occurs in immunosuppressed patients.

Box 51—1. Unique Properties of Polyomaviruses and Papillomaviruses

Small icosahedral capsid virion
Double-stranded circular DNA genome is replicated and assembled in the nucleus
Papillomavirus: **HPV** types 1 to 58+ (as determined by genotype; types defined by DNA homology, tissue tropism, and association with oncogenesis)
Polyomavirus: SV40, **JC virus**, and **BK virus**
Viruses have defined tissue tropisms determined by receptor interactions and the transcriptional machinery of the cell
Viruses encode proteins that promote cell growth by binding to the cellular growth-suppressor proteins p53 and p105RB (p105 retinoblastoma gene product). Polyoma T antigen binds to p105RB and p53. **Papilloma E6 binds to p53, and E7 binds to p105RB**
Viruses can cause lytic infections in permissive cells but cause abortive, persistent, or latent infections or **immortalize (transform)** nonpermissive cells

(Figure 51-4). The viral infection remains local and generally regresses spontaneously but can recur. The HPV pathogenic mechanisms are summarized in Box 51-2.

Innate and cell-mediated immunity are important for control and resolution of HPV infections. HPV can suppress or hide from protective immune responses. In addition to very low levels of antigen expression (except in the "near-dead" terminally differentiated skin cell), the keratinocyte is an immunologically privileged site for replication. Inflammatory responses are required to activate protective cytolytic responses and promote resolution of warts. Immunosuppressed persons have recurrences and more severe presentations of papillomavirus infections.

The oncogenic potential of HPV has been extensively studied. Viral DNA is found in benign and malignant tumors, especially mucosal papillomas. HPV-16 and HPV-18 cause cervical papillomas and dysplasia, and **at least 85% of cervical carcinomas contain integrated HPV-DNA**. Breaking of the circular genome within the E1 or E2 genes to promote integration often causes these genes to be inactivated, thereby preventing viral replication without preventing the expression of other HPV genes, including the E6 and E7 genes (Figure 51-5). The E6 and E7 proteins of HPV-16 and HPV-18 have been identified as **oncogenes** because they bind and inactivate the cellular growth-suppressor (transformation-suppressor) proteins, p53 and p105 retinoblastoma gene product (p105RB). E6 binds the p53 protein and targets it for degradation, and E7 binds and inactivates p105RB. Without these brakes on cell growth, the cell is more susceptible to mutation, chromosomal aberrations, or the action of a cofactor and thereby develops into cancer.

Epidemiology

HPV resists inactivation and can be transmitted on fomites, such as the surfaces of countertops or furniture, bathroom floors, and towels (Box 51-3). Asymptomatic shedding may promote transmission. HPV infection is acquired (1) by direct contact through small breaks in the skin or mucosa, (2) during sexual intercourse, or (3) while an infant is passing through an infected birth canal.

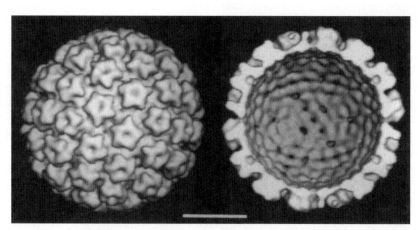

Figure 51—1. Computer reconstruction of cryoelectron micrographs of human papillomavirus (HPV). *Left,* View of the surface of HPV shows 72 capsomeres arranged in an icosadeltahedron. All the capsomeres (pentons and hexons) appear to form a regular five-point-star shape. *Right,* Computer cross-section of the capsid shows the interaction of the capsomeres and channels in the capsid. (*From Baker TS, et al: Biophys J 60:1445-1456, 1991.*)

Genome is a double-stranded circular molecule.

E1 protein binds DNA at ori and promotes viral DNA replication and has helicase activity (like T antigen of SV 40). E2 protein binds DNA, helps E1, and activates viral mRNA synthesis.

E5 oncoprotein activates the EGF receptor to promote growth.
E4 disrupts cytokeratins to promote release.
E6 and E7 of HPV-16 and HPV-18 can become immortalizing genes; HPV-16 and HPV-18 are associated with human cervical cancer.

L1 and L2 gene products are late structural (capsid) proteins.

| Enhancer promotor origin | Immortalize, growth promoting | Viral DNA replication | Transcriptional and replication regulator | | Minor capsid | Major capsid |

E7   E1   E5   L2

LCR   E6   E2   L1

E4

7906/1 1000 2000 3000 4000 5000 6000 7000

Figure 51–2. Genome of human papillomavirus type 16 (HPV-16). DNA is normally a double-stranded circular molecule, but it is shown here in a linear form. E6, oncogene protein that binds p53 and promotes its degradation; E7, oncogene protein that binds p105RB (p105 retinoblastoma gene product); L1, major capsid protein; L2, minor capsid protein; LCR (URR), long control region (upstream regulatory region); ori, origin of replication. (Courtesy Tom Broker, Baltimore.)

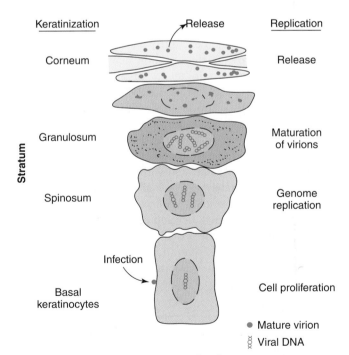

Keratinization   Release   Replication

Corneum   Release

Granulosum   Maturation of virions

Stratum

Spinosum   Genome replication

Infection

Basal keratinocytes   Cell proliferation

● Mature virion
⌇ Viral DNA

Figure 51–3. Development of papilloma (wart). Human papillomavirus (HPV) infection promotes the outgrowth of the basal layer, increasing the number of prickle cells (acanthosis). These changes cause the skin to thicken and promote the production of keratin (hyperkeratosis), thereby causing epithelial spikes to form (papillomatosis). Virus is produced in the granular cells close to the final keratin layer.

Figure 51–4. DNA probe analysis of an HPV-6—induced anogenital condyloma. A biotin-labeled DNA probe was localized by horseradish peroxidase—conjugated avidin conversion of a substrate to a chromogen precipitate. Dark staining is seen over the nuclei of koilocytotic cells. *(From Belshe RB: Textbook of Human Virology, 2nd ed. St Louis, Mosby, 1991.)*

Common, plantar, and flat warts are most common in children and young adults. Laryngeal papillomas occur in young children and middle-aged adults.

Human papillomavirus is possibly the most prevalent sexually transmitted infection in the world, with certain

Box 51–2. Disease Mechanisms of Papillomaviruses and Polyomaviruses

Papillomaviruses

Virus is acquired by **close contact** and infects the epithelial cells of the skin or mucous membranes.
Tissue tropism and disease presentation depend on the papillomavirus type.
Virus persists in the basal layer and then produces virus in terminally differentiated keratinocytes.
Viruses cause benign outgrowth of cells into **warts**.
HPV infection is hidden from immune responses and persists.
Warts resolve spontaneously, possibly as a result of immune response.
Certain types are associated with **dysplasia** that may become **cancerous** with the action of cofactors.
DNA of specific HPV types is present (integrated) in the tumor cell chromosomes.

Polyomaviruses (JC and BK Viruses)

Virus is probably acquired through the respiratory route and spread by viremia to the kidneys early in life.
Infections are **asymptomatic**.
Virus establishes **persistent** and **latent** infection in organs such as the kidneys and lungs.
In **immunocompromised** people, JC virus is activated, spreads to the brain, and causes progressive multifocal leukoencephalopathy (**PML**), a conventional slow virus disease.
In PML, JC virus partially transforms astrocytes and kills oligodendrocytes, causing characteristic lesions and sites of demyelination.
BK virus is ubiquitous but is not associated with serious disease.

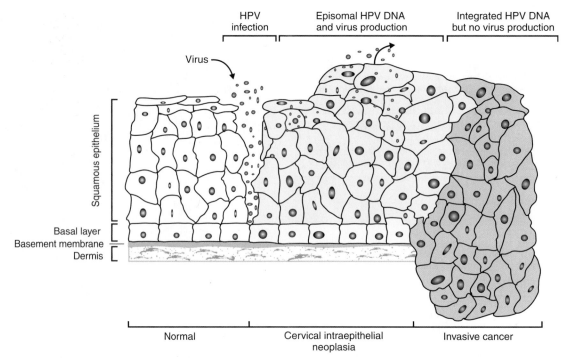

Figure 51—5. Progression of HPV-mediated cervical carcinoma. HPV infects and replicates in the epithelial cells of the cervix, maturing and releasing virus as the epithelial cells progress through terminal differentiation. Growth stimulation of the basal cells produces a wart. In some cells, the circular genome integrates into host chromosomes, inactivating the *E2* gene. Expression of the other genes without virus production stimulates growth of the cells and possible progression to neoplasia. (*Adapted from Woodman CBJ, Collins SI, Young LS: The natural history of cervical HPV infection: Unresolved issues. Nat Rev Cancer 7:11-22, 2007.*)

Box 51—3. Epidemiology of Polyomaviruses and Papillomaviruses

Disease/Viral Factors

Capsid virus is resistant to inactivation
Virus persists in host
Asymptomatic shedding is likely

Transmission

Papillomavirus: **direct contact, sexual contact** (sexually transmitted disease) for certain virus types, or passage through infected birth canal for laryngeal papillomas (types 6 and 11)
Polyomavirus: inhalation or contact with contaminated water

Who Is at Risk?

Papillomavirus: warts are common; sexually active people are at risk for infection with HPV types correlated with oral and genital cancers
Polyomavirus: ubiquitous; immunocompromised people at risk for progressive multifocal leukoencephalopathy

Geography/Season

Viruses are found worldwide
There is no seasonal incidence

Modes of Control

There are no modes of control

HPV types common among sexually active people. At least 20 million people in the United States are infected with HPV, with approximately 6 million new genital cases per year. HPV is present in 99.7% of all cervical cancers. HPV-16, HPV-18, HPV-31, and HPV-45 are high-risk and HPV-6 and HPV-11 are low-risk HPV types for cervical carcinoma, the second leading cause of cancer death in women (approximately 12,000 cases and 4000 deaths per year in the United States). Other types of HPV (including 52 and 58) are also associated with vaginal infections and cancer. Approximately 5% of all Pap smears contain HPV-infected cells, and 10% of women infected with the high-risk HPV types will develop cervical **dysplasia**, a precancerous state. Multiple sexual partners, smoking, a family history of cervical cancer, and immunosuppression are the major risk factors for infection and progression to cancer.

Clinical Syndromes

The clinical syndromes and the HPV types that cause them are summarized in Table 51-2.

Warts

A **wart** is a benign, self-limited proliferation of skin that regresses with time. Most people with HPV infection have the common types of the virus (HPV-1 through HPV-4)

enzyme-linked immunosorbent assays, and genome assays, including different variations of the polymerase chain reaction and DNA probe analysis, can be used to detect, type, and group the virus in clinical samples and tissue cultures. These approaches must be used for enteric adenovirus serotypes 40 to 42, which do not grow readily in available cell cultures. Serologic testing is rarely used, except for epidemiologic purposes or to confirm the significance of a fecal or upper respiratory tract isolate by identifying its serotype.

The isolation of most adenovirus types is best accomplished in cell cultures derived from epithelial cells (e.g., primary human embryonic kidney cells, continuous [transformed] lines such as HeLa and human epidermal carcinoma cells). Within 2 to 20 days, the virus causes a lytic infection with characteristic inclusion bodies. Recovery of virus from cell culture requires an average of 6 days. The characteristic intranuclear inclusions can be seen in infected tissue during histologic examination. However, such inclusions are rare and must be distinguished from those produced by cytomegalovirus.

Treatment, Prevention, and Control

Careful handwashing and chlorination of swimming pools can reduce transmission of adenovirus. There is no approved treatment for adenovirus infection. Live oral vaccines have been used to prevent infections with adenovirus types 4 and 7 in military recruits but are not used in civilian populations.

Gene Replacement Therapy

Adenoviruses have been used and are being considered for more applications of gene delivery for correction of several human diseases, including immune deficiencies (e.g., adenosine deaminase deficiency), cystic fibrosis, lysosomal storage diseases, and even cancer. The virus is inactivated by deletion or mutation of the *E1* and other viral genes (e.g., *E2, E4*). The appropriate gene is inserted into the genome, replacing this DNA, and is controlled by an appropriate promoter. The resultant virus vector must be grown in a cell that expresses the missing viral functions (E1, E4) and can complement the deficiency to allow production of virus. Adenovirus types 4 and 7 have been used most extensively since attenuated (vaccine) strains have been developed. Despite the genetically engineered attenuation, these viruses still can cause serious disease in people.

Case Study and Questions

A 7-year-old boy attending summer camp complains of sore throat, headache, cough, red eyes, and tiredness and is sent to the infirmary. His temperature is 40° C. Within hours, other campers and counselors visit the infirmary with similar symptoms. Symptoms last for 5 to 7 days. All the patients have gone swimming in the camp pond. More than 50% of the people in the camp complain of symptoms similar to those in the initial case. The Public Health Department identifies the agent as adenovirus serotype 3.

1. Toward which adenovirus syndrome do the symptoms point?
2. An outbreak as large as this indicates a common source of infection. What was the most likely source or sources? What were the most likely routes by which the virus was spread?
3. What physical properties of the virus facilitate its transmission?
4. What precautions should the camp owners take to prevent other outbreaks?
5. What sample or samples would have been used by the Public Health Department to identify the infectious agent, and what tests would be required to diagnose the infection?

Bibliography

Balows A, Hausler WJ Jr, Lennette EH: Laboratory Diagnosis of Infectious Diseases: Principles and Practice, vol 2. New York, Springer-Verlag, 1988.

Benihoud K, Yeh P, Perricaudet M: Adenovirus vectors for gene delivery. Curr Opin Biotechnol 10:440-447, 1999.

Carter J, Saunders V: Virology: Principles and Applications. Chichester, England, Wiley, 2007.

Cohen J, Powderly WG: Infectious Diseases, 2nd ed. St Louis, Mosby, 2004.

Collier L, Oxford J: Human Virology, 3rd ed. Oxford, Oxford University Press, 2006.

Doerfler W, Böhm P: Adenoviruses: Model and Vectors in Virus-Host Interactions. (Curr Top Microbiol Immunol, vols 272-273). New York: Springer, 2003.

Flint SJ, et al: Principles of Virology: Molecular Biology, Pathogenesis, and Control of Animal Viruses, 2nd ed. Washington, DC, ASM Press, 2003.

Ginsberg HS: The Adenoviruses. New York, Plenum, 1984.

Gorbach SL, Bartlett JG, Blacklow NR: Infectious Diseases, 3rd ed. Philadelphia, WB Saunders, 2004.

Knipe DM, Howley PM: Fields Virology, 4th ed. New York, Lippincott Williams & Wilkins, 2001.

Mandell GL, Bennet JE, Dolin R: Principles and Practice of Infectious Diseases, 6th ed. Philadelphia, Churchill Livingstone, 2005.

Robbins PD, Ghivizzani SC: Viral vectors for gene therapy. Pharmacol Ther 80:35-47, 1998.

Strauss JM, Strauss EG: Viruses and Human Disease, 2nd ed. San Diego, Academic, 2007.

Voyles BA: The Biology of Viruses, 2nd ed. Boston, McGraw-Hill, 2002.

Human Herpesviruses

The herpesviruses are an important group of large, deoxyribonucleic acid (DNA)—enveloped viruses with the following features in common: virion morphology, basic mode of replication, and capacity to establish latent and recurrent infections. Cell-mediated immunity is important for controlling infection with these viruses and causing symptoms. Herpesviruses encode proteins and enzymes that facilitate the replication and interaction of the virus with the host. The herpesviruses can cause lytic, persistent, and latent/recurrent infections, and Epstein-Barr virus (EBV) and HHV8 are associated with human cancers (Box 53-1).

The human herpesviruses are grouped into three subfamilies on the basis of differences in viral characteristics (genome structure, tissue tropism, cytopathologic effect, and site of latent infection), as well as the pathogenesis of the disease and disease manifestation (Table 53-1). The human herpesviruses are herpes simplex viruses types 1 and 2 (HSV-1 and HSV-2), varicella-zoster virus (VZV), Epstein-Barr virus, cytomegalovirus (CMV), human herpesviruses 6 and 7 (HHV6 and HHV7), and the more recently discovered human herpesvirus 8 (HHV8), associated with Kaposi sarcoma.

Herpesvirus infections are common, and the viruses are **ubiquitous**. Although these viruses usually cause benign disease, especially in children, they can also cause significant morbidity and mortality, especially in immunosuppressed people. Fortunately, some herpesviruses encode targets for antiviral agents, and there is a live-virus vaccine for VZV.

Structure of Herpesviruses

The herpesviruses are **large, enveloped** viruses that contain **double-stranded DNA**. The virion is approximately 150 nm in diameter and has the characteristic morphology shown in Figure 53-1. The DNA core is surrounded by an **icosadeltahedral capsid** containing 162 capsomeres.

This capsid is enclosed by a glycoprotein-containing envelope. Herpesviruses encode several glycoproteins for viral attachment, fusion, and for escaping immune control. Attached to the capsid and in the space between the envelope and the capsid (the **tegument**) are viral proteins and enzymes that help initiate replication. As enveloped viruses, the herpesviruses are sensitive to acid, solvents, detergents, and drying.

Herpesviral genomes are linear, double-stranded DNA, but they differ in size and gene orientation (Figure 53-2). Direct or inverted repeat sequences bracket unique regions of the genome (unique long [U_L], unique short [U_S]), allowing circularization and recombination within the genome. Recombination among inverted repeats of HSV, CMV, and VZV allows large portions of the genome to flip the orientation of their U_L and U_S gene segments, with respect to each other, to form isomeric genomes.

Herpesvirus Replication

Herpesvirus replication is initiated by the interaction of viral glycoproteins with cell surface receptors (see Chapter 4, Figure 4-12). The tropism of some herpesviruses (e.g., EBV) is restricted as a result of the tissue-specific expression of their receptors. The nucleocapsid is then released into the cytoplasm through fusion of the envelope with the plasma membrane. Enzymes and transcription factors are carried into the cell in the tegument of the virion. The nucleocapsid docks with the nuclear membrane and delivers the genome into the nucleus, where the genome is transcribed and replicated.

Transcription of the viral genome and viral protein synthesis proceeds in a coordinated and regulated manner in the following three phases:

1. **Immediate early proteins (α)**, consisting of proteins important for the regulation of gene transcription and takeover of the cell.

Box 53—1. Unique Features of Herpesviruses

Herpesviruses have large, enveloped icosadeltahedral capsids containing double-stranded DNA genomes.
Herpesviruses encode many proteins that manipulate the host cell and immune response.
Herpesviruses encode enzymes (**DNA polymerase**) that promote viral DNA replication and are good targets for **antiviral drugs**.
DNA replication and capsid assembly occurs in the nucleus.
Virus is released by exocytosis, cell lysis, and through cell-cell bridges.
Herpesviruses can cause **lytic, persistent, latent,** and (for Epstein-Barr virus) **immortalizing** infections.
Herpesviruses are ubiquitous.
Cell-mediated immunity is required for control.

2. **Early proteins (β)**, consisting of more transcription factors and enzymes, including the DNA polymerase.
3. **Late proteins (γ)**, consisting mainly of structural proteins, which are generated after viral genome replication has begun.

The viral genome is transcribed by the cellular DNA—dependent ribonucleic acid (RNA) polymerase and is regulated by viral-encoded and cellular nuclear factors. The interplay of these factors determines whether the proteins necessary for a lytic, persistent, or latent infection are produced. Cells that promote latent infection transcribe a special set of viral genes without genome replication. Progression to early and late gene expression results in cell death and lytic infection.

The viral-encoded DNA polymerase, which is a target of antiviral drugs, replicates the viral genome. Viral-encoded scavenging enzymes provide deoxyribonucleotide substrates for the polymerase. These and other viral enzymes facilitate replication of the virus in nongrowing cells that lack sufficient deoxyribonucleotides and enzymes for viral DNA synthesis (e.g., neurons).

Empty procapsids assemble in the nucleus, are filled with DNA, acquire an envelope at the nuclear or Golgi membrane, and exit the cell by exocytosis or by lysis of the cell. Transcription, protein synthesis, glycoprotein processing, and exocytotic release from the cell are performed by cellular machinery. The replication of HSV is discussed in more detail as the prototype of the herpesviruses.

Herpes Simplex Virus

HSV was the first human herpesvirus to be recognized. The name *herpes* is derived from a Greek word meaning "to creep." "Cold sores" were described in antiquity, and their viral etiology was established in 1919.

The two types of herpes simplex virus, HSV-1 and HSV-2, share many characteristics, including DNA homology, antigenic determinants, tissue tropism, and disease

Table 53—1. Properties Distinguishing the Herpesviruses

Subfamily	Virus	Primary Target Cell	Site of Latency	Means of Spread
Alphaherpesvirinae				
Human herpesvirus 1	Herpes simplex type 1	Mucoepithelial cells	Neuron	Close contact
Human herpesvirus 2	Herpes simplex type 2	Mucoepithelial cells	Neuron	Close contact (sexually transmitted disease)
Human herpesvirus 3	Varicella-zoster virus	Mucoepithelial and T cells	Neuron	Respiratory and close contact
Gammaherpesvirinae				
Human herpesvirus 4	Epstein-Barr virus	B cells and epithelial cells	B cell	Saliva (kissing disease)
Human herpesvirus 8	Kaposi sarcoma—related virus	Lymphocyte and other cells	B cell	Close contact (sexual), saliva?
Betaherpesvirinae				
Human herpesvirus 5	Cytomegalovirus	Monocyte, lymphocyte, and epithelial cells	Monocyte, lymphocyte, and ?	Close contact, transfusions, tissue transplant, and congenital
Human herpesvirus 6	Herpes lymphotropic virus	Like CMV, salivary glands, neurons	T cells and ?	Saliva
Human herpesvirus 7	Human herpesvirus 7	Like CMV	T cells and ?	Saliva

? Indicates that other cells may also be the primary target or site of latency.

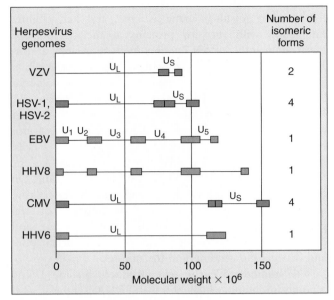

Figure 53—2. Herpesvirus genomes. The genomes of the herpesvirus are doubled-stranded DNA. The length and complexity of the genome differ for each virus. Inverted repeats in herpes simplex virus (HSV), varicella-zoster virus (VZV), and cytomegalovirus (CMV) allow the genome to recombine with itself to form isomers. Large genetic repeat sequences are boxed. The genomes of HSV and CMV have two sections, the unique long (U_L) and the unique short (U_S), each of which is bracketed by two sets of inverted repeats of DNA. The inverted repeats facilitate the replication of the genome but also allow the U_L and U_S regions to invert independently of each other to yield four different genomic configurations, or isomers. VZV has only one set of inverted repeats and can form two isomers. Epstein-Barr virus (EBV) exists in only one configuration, with several unique regions surrounded by direct repeats. Purple bars indicate direct repeat DNA sequences; green bars indicate inverted repeated DNA sequences. HHV6, human herpesvirus 6; HHV8, human herpesvirus 8.

Figure 53—1. Electron micrograph (A) and general structure (B) of the herpesviruses. The DNA genome of the herpesvirus in the core is surrounded by an icosadeltahedral capsid and an envelope. Glycoproteins are inserted into the envelope. (A from Armstrong D, Cohen J: Infectious Diseases. St Louis, Mosby, 1999.)

symptoms. However, they can still be distinguished by subtle but significant differences in these properties.

Structure

The HSV genome is large enough to encode approximately 80 proteins. Only half the proteins are required for viral replication; the others facilitate the HSV's interaction with different host cells and the immune response. The HSV genome encodes enzymes, including a DNA-dependent DNA polymerase and scavenging enzymes, such as deoxyribonuclease, thymidine kinase, ribonucleotide reductase, and protease. Ribonucleotide reductase converts ribonucleotides to deoxyribonucleotides, and thymidine kinase phosphorylates the deoxyribonucleosides to provide substrates for replication of the viral genome. The substrate specificities of these enzymes and the DNA polymerase differ significantly from those of their cellular analogues and thus represent potentially good targets for antiviral chemotherapy.

HSV encodes at least 10 glycoproteins that serve as viral attachment proteins (gB, gC, gD, gH, gE/gI), fusion proteins (gB), structural proteins, immune escape proteins (gC, gE, gI), and other functions. For example, the C3 component of the complement system binds to gC and is depleted from serum. The Fc portion of immunoglobulin G (IgG) binds to a gE/gI complex, thereby camouflaging the virus and virus-infected cells. These actions reduce the antiviral effectiveness of antibody.

Replication

HSV can infect most types of human cells and even cells of other species. The virus generally causes lytic infections of fibroblasts and epithelial cells and latent infections of neurons. (See Chapter 4, Figure 4-12, for a diagram.)

HSV-1 binds quickly and efficiently to cells through an initial interaction with heparan sulfate, a proteoglycan found on the outside of many cell types, and then a tighter interaction with receptor proteins at the cell surface. Penetration into the cell requires interaction with nectin-1 (HveC [herpesvirus entry mediator C]), an intercellular adhesion molecule that is a member of the immunoglobulin protein family and similar to the poliovirus receptor. Nectin-1 is found on most cells and neurons. Another receptor is HveA, a member of the tumor necrosis factor receptor family, which is expressed on activated T cells, neurons, and other cells. HSV penetrates the host cell by fusion of its envelope with the cell surface membrane. On fusion, the virion releases its capsid into the cytoplasm, along with a protein that promotes the initiation of viral gene transcription, a viral-encoded protein kinase, and cytotoxic proteins. The capsid docks with a nuclear pore and delivers the genome into the nucleus.

The **immediate early gene products** include DNA-binding proteins, which stimulate DNA synthesis and promote the transcription of the early viral genes. During a latent infection of neurons, the only region of the genome to be transcribed generates the **latency-associated transcripts (LATs)**, but these RNAs are not translated into protein.

The **early proteins** include the DNA-dependent DNA polymerase and a thymidine kinase. As catalytic proteins, relatively few copies of these enzymes are required to promote replication. Other early proteins inhibit the production and initiate the degradation of cellular messenger RNA (mRNA) and DNA. Expression of the early and late genes generally leads to cell death.

The genome is replicated as soon as the polymerase is synthesized. Circular, end-to-end concatameric forms of the genome are made initially. Later in the infection, the DNA is replicated by a rolling circle mechanism to produce a linear string of genomes that in concept resembles a roll of toilet paper. The concatamers are cleaved into individual genomes as the DNA is sucked into a procapsid.

Genome replication triggers transcription of the late genes from which structural and other proteins are encoded. Many copies of the structural proteins are required. The capsid proteins are then transported to the nucleus, where they are assembled into empty procapsids and filled with DNA. DNA-containing capsids associate with viral protein-disrupted nuclear membranes and bud into and then out of the endoplasmic reticulum into the cytoplasm. The viral glycoproteins are synthesized and processed like cellular glycoproteins. Tegument proteins associate with the viral capsid in the cytoplasm, and then the capsid buds into a portion of the trans-Golgi network to acquire their glycoprotein-containing envelope. The virus is released by exocytosis or cell lysis. Virus can also spread between cells through intracellular bridges, which allows the virus to escape antibody detection. Virus-induced syncytia formation also spreads the infection.

HSV infection of neurons may result in virus replication or establishment of latency, depending on which viral genes the neuron is capable of transcribing. Transcription of the LAT and no other viral gene will result in latency. If the cell can transcribe the immediate early genes of the virus, virus will replicate. As for other alphaherpesviruses, HSV encodes a thymidine kinase (scavenging enzyme) to facilitate replication in nondividing cells like neurons. HSV also encodes a protein, ICP34.5, which facilitates virus growth in neurons by removing a cellular block to protein synthesis activated in response to virus infection or as part of the response to interferon alpha.

Pathogenesis and Immunity

The mechanisms involved in the pathogenesis of HSV-1 and HSV-2 are very similar (Box 53-2). Both viruses initially infect, replicate in mucoepithelial cells, cause disease at the site of infection, and then establish latent infection of the innervating neurons. HSV-1 is usually associated with infections above the waist, and HSV-2 with infections below the waist (Figure 53-3), consistent with the means of spread for these viruses. HSV-1 and HSV-2 also differ in growth characteristics and antigenicity, and HSV-2 has a greater potential to cause viremia with associated systemic flulike symptoms.

HSV can cause **lytic** infections of most cells, **persistent** infections of lymphocytes and macrophages, and **latent** infection of neurons. Cytolysis generally results from the virus-induced inhibition of cellular macromolecular synthesis, the degradation of host cell DNA, membrane permeation, cytoskeletal disruption, and senescence of the cell. In addition, changes in the nuclear structure and margination of the chromatin occur, and **Cowdry type A acidophilic intranuclear inclusion bodies** are produced. Many strains of HSV also initiate **syncytia** formation. In tissue culture, HSV rapidly kills cells.

HSV initiates infection through mucosal membranes or breaks in the skin. The virus replicates in the cells at the base of the lesion and infects the innervating neuron, traveling by retrograde transport to the ganglion (the trigeminal ganglia for oral HSV and the sacral ganglia for genital HSV) (see Figure 53-5). CD8 T cells and interferon gamma are important to maintain HSV in latency.

Box 53–2. Disease Mechanisms for Herpes Simplex Viruses

Disease is initiated by direct contact and depends on infected tissue (e.g., oral, genital, brain).
Virus causes direct cytopathologic effects.
Virus avoids antibody by cell-to-cell spread and syncytia.
Virus establishes latency in neurons (hides from immune response).
Virus is reactivated from latency by stress or immune suppression.
Cell-mediated immunity is required for resolution, with limited role for antibody.
Cell-mediated immunopathologic effects contribute to symptoms.

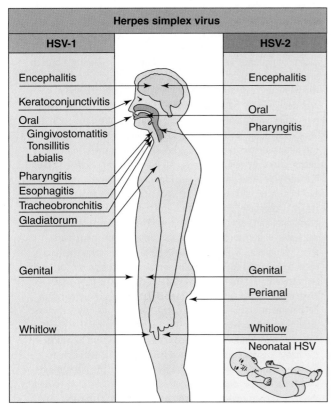

Herpes simplex virus		
HSV-1		**HSV-2**
Encephalitis		Encephalitis
Keratoconjunctivitis		
Oral		Oral
Gingivostomatitis		Pharyngitis
Tonsillitis		
Labialis		
Pharyngitis		
Esophagitis		
Tracheobronchitis		
Gladiatorum		
Genital		Genital
		Perianal
Whitlow		Whitlow
		Neonatal HSV

Figure 53–3. Disease syndromes of herpes simplex virus (HSV). HSV-1 and HSV-2 can infect the same tissues and cause similar diseases but have a predilection for the sites and diseases indicated.

Upon reactivation, the virus then returns to the initial site of infection, and the infection may be inapparent or may produce **vesicular lesions**. The vesicle fluid contains infectious virions. Tissue damage is caused by a combination of viral pathology and immunopathology. The lesion generally heals without producing a scar.

Innate protections, including interferon and natural killer cells, may be sufficient to limit the initial progression of the infection. *T-helper 1 (TH1)—associated and CD8 cytotoxic killer T-cell responses are required to kill infected cells and resolve the current disease.* The immunopathologic effects of the cell-mediated and inflammatory responses are also a major cause of the symptoms. Antibody directed against the glycoproteins of the virus neutralizes extracellular virus, limiting its spread, but is not sufficient to resolve the infection. In the absence of functional cell-mediated immunity, HSV infection is likely to recur, be more severe, and may disseminate to the vital organs and the brain.

HSV has several ways to escape host protective responses. The virus blocks the interferon-induced inhibition of viral protein synthesis and encodes a protein to plug the transporter associated with processing (TAP) channel, preventing delivery of peptides into the endoplasmic reticulum (ER), which blocks their association with class I major histocompatibility complex (MHC I) molecules and prevents CD8 T-cell recognition

of infected cells. The virus can escape antibody neutralization and clearance by direct cell-to-cell spread and by going into hiding during latent infection of the neuron. In addition, the virion and virus-infected cells express antibody (Fc) and complement receptors that weaken these humoral defenses.

Latent infection occurs in neurons and results in no detectable damage. A **recurrence** can be activated by various stimuli (e.g., stress, trauma, fever, sunlight [ultraviolet B]) (Box 53-3). These events trigger virus replication in an individual nerve cell within the bundle and allow the virus to travel back down the nerve to cause lesions to develop at the same dermatome and location each time. The stress triggers reactivation by promoting replication of the virus in the nerve, by transiently depressing cell-mediated immunity, or by inducing both processes. The virus can be reactivated despite the presence of antibody. However, recurrent infections are generally less severe, more localized, and of shorter duration than the primary episodes because of the nature of the spread and the existence of memory immune responses.

Epidemiology

Because HSV can establish latency with the potential for asymptomatic recurrence, the infected person is a lifelong source of contagion (Box 53-4). As an enveloped virus, HSV is transmitted in secretions and by close contact. The virus is very labile and is readily inactivated by drying, detergents, and the conditions of the gastrointestinal tract. Although HSV can infect animal cells, HSV infection is exclusively a human disease.

HSV is transmitted in vesicle fluid, saliva, and vaginal secretions (the **"mixing and matching of mucous membranes"**). The site of infection, and hence the disease, is determined primarily by which mucous membranes are mixed. Both types of HSV can cause oral and genital lesions.

HSV-1 is usually spread by oral contact (kissing) or through the sharing of drinking glasses, toothbrushes, or other saliva-contaminated items. HSV-1 infection of the fingers or body can result from lesion contact with skin, with the virus entering through a break in the skin. Autoinoculation may also cause infection of the eyes.

Box 53—3. Triggers of HSV Recurrences

UV-B radiation (skiing, tanning)
Fever (hence the name "fever blister")
Emotional stress (e.g., final examinations, big date)
Physical stress (irritation)
Menstruation
Foods: spicy, acidic, allergies
Immunosuppression:
    Transient (stress related)
    Chemotherapy, radiotherapy
    Human immunodeficiency virus

Box 53—4. Epidemiology of Herpes Simplex Virus (HSV)

Disease/Viral Factors

Virus causes lifelong infection
Recurrent disease is a source of contagion
Virus may cause asymptomatic shedding

Transmission

Virus is transmitted in saliva, in vaginal secretions, and by contact with lesion fluid (mixing and matching of mucous membranes)
Virus is transmitted orally and sexually and by placement into eyes and breaks in skin
HSV-1 is generally transmitted orally; HSV-2 is generally transmitted sexually

Who Is at Risk?

Children and sexually active people are at risk for classic presentations of HSV-1 and HSV-2, respectively
Physicians, nurses, dentists, and others in contact with oral and genital secretions are at risk for infections of fingers (herpetic whitlow)
Immunocompromised people and neonates are at risk for disseminated, life-threatening disease

Geography/Season

Virus is found worldwide
There is no seasonal incidence

Modes of Control

Antiviral drugs are available
No vaccine is available
Health care workers should wear gloves to prevent herpetic whitlow
People with active genital lesions should refrain from intercourse until lesions are completely reepithelialized

Clinical Case 53-1. Neonatal Herpes Simplex Virus

Parvey and Ch'ien (Pediatrics 65:1150-1153, 1980) reported a case of neonatal HSV contracted during birth. During a breech presentation, a fetal monitor was placed on the buttocks of the baby, and due to the greatly prolonged labor, the baby was delivered by cesarean section. The 5-pound boy had minor difficulties which were successfully treated, but on the sixth day, vesicles with an erythematous base appeared at the site where the fetal monitor had been placed. HSV was grown from the vesicle fluid, as well as from spinal fluid, cornea, saliva, and blood. The baby became moribund with frequent apneic episodes and seizures. Intravenous treatment with adenosine arabinoside (ara-A; vidarabine) was initiated. The baby also developed bradycardia and occasional vomiting. The vesicles spread to cover the lower extremities and were also on the back, palm, nares and right eyelid. Within 72 hours of ara-A treatment, the baby's condition started to improve. Treatment was continued for 11 days but discontinued due to a low platelet count. The baby was discharged on the 45th day after his birthday, and normal development was reported at 1 and 2 years of age. At 6 weeks after the birth, a herpes lesion was found on the mother's vulva. This was a fortunate case of neonatal HSV infection in which the baby was successfully treated with ara-A and was able to overcome the damage caused by the infection. The virus, most likely HSV-2, was probably acquired through an abrasion caused by the fetal monitor while the neonate was in the birth canal. Ara-A has since been replaced with the better, less toxic, and easier to administer antiviral drugs, acyclovir, valacyclovir and famciclovir.

amounts to approximately 45 million people with up to 1 million newly infected people per year.

Clinical Syndromes

HSV-1 and HSV-2 are common human pathogens that can cause painful but benign manifestations and recurrent disease. In the classic manifestation, the lesion is a clear vesicle on an erythematous base ("dewdrop on a rose petal") and then progresses to pustular lesions, ulcers, and crusted lesions (Figure 53-4). However, *both viruses can cause significant morbidity and mortality on infection of the eye or brain and on disseminated infection of an immunosuppressed person or a neonate.*

Oral herpes can be caused by HSV-1 or HSV-2. Primary herpes labialis or gingivostomatitis in toddlers and children is almost always caused by HSV-1, whereas young adults may be infected with HSV-1 or HSV-2. The lesions begin as clear vesicles that rapidly ulcerate. These whitish areas may be widely distributed around or throughout the mouth, involving the palate, pharynx, gingivae, buccal mucosa, and tongue (Figure 53-5). Many other conditions (e.g., Coxsackie virus, canker sores, acne) may resemble HSV lesions.

People may experience recurrent mucocutaneous HSV infection (**cold sores, fever blisters**) (Figure 53-6), even though they never had clinically apparent primary infection. The lesions usually occur at the corners of the mouth

HSV-1 infection is common. More than 90% of people living in underdeveloped areas have the antibody to HSV-1 by 2 years of age. This finding may result from crowded living conditions or poor hygiene.

HSV-2 is spread mainly by sexual contact or autoinoculation or from an infected mother to her infant at birth. Depending on a person's sexual practices and hygiene, HSV-2 may infect the genitalia, anorectal tissues, or oropharynx. The incidence of HSV-1 genital infection is approaching that of HSV-2. HSV may cause symptomatic or asymptomatic primary genital infection or recurrences. Neonatal infection usually results from the excretion of HSV-2 from the cervix during vaginal delivery (Clinical Case 53-1) but can occur from an ascending in utero infection during a primary infection of the mother. Neonatal infection results in disseminated and neurologic disease with severe consequences.

Initial infection with HSV-2 occurs later in life than infection with HSV-1 and correlates with increased sexual activity. The current statistics indicate that 22% of adults in the United States are infected with HSV-2, which

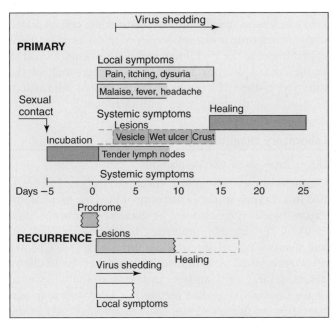

Figure 53—4. Clinical course of genital herpes infection. The time course and symptoms of primary and recurrent genital infection with herpes simplex virus type 2 (HSV-2) are compared. *Top,* Primary infection; *bottom,* recurrent disease. *(Data from Corey L, et al: Ann Intern Med 98:958-973, 1983.)*

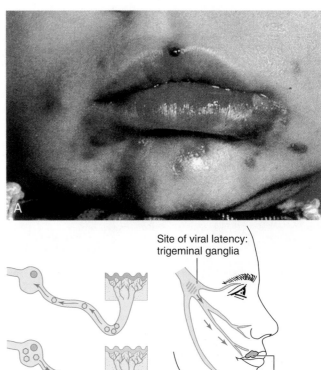

Figure 53—5. A, Primary herpes gingivostomatitis. **B,** Herpes simplex virus establishes latent infection and can recur from the trigeminal ganglia. *(**A** from Hart CA, Broadhead RL: A Color Atlas of Pediatric Infectious Diseases. London, Wolfe, 1992; **B** modified from Straus SE: Herpes simplex virus and its relatives. In Schaechter M, Eisenstein BI, Medoff G (eds): Mechanisms of Microbial Disease, 2nd ed. Baltimore, Williams & Wilkins, 1993.)*

or next to the lips. Recurrent facial herpes infections are generally activated from the trigeminal ganglia. As noted earlier, the symptoms of a recurrent episode are less severe, more localized, and of shorter duration than those of a primary episode. **Herpes pharyngitis** is becoming a prevalent diagnosis in young adults with sore throats. Severe HSV stomatitis, resembling a primary gingivostomatitis, may occur in immunosuppressed patients.

Herpetic keratitis is almost always limited to one eye. It can cause recurrent disease, leading to permanent scarring, corneal damage, and blindness.

Herpetic whitlow is an infection of the finger, and **herpes gladiatorum** is an infection of the body. The virus establishes infection through cuts or abrasions in the skin. Herpetic whitlow often occurs in nurses or physicians who attend patients with HSV infections, in thumb-sucking children (Figure 53-7), and in people who have genital HSV infections. Herpes gladiatorum is often acquired during wrestling or rugby.

Eczema herpeticum is acquired by children with active eczema. The underlying disease promotes the spread of the infection along the skin and potentially to the adrenal glands, liver, and other organs.

Genital herpes is usually caused by HSV-2 but can also be caused by HSV-1 (responsible for at least 10% of genital infections). In male patients, the lesions typically develop on the glans or shaft of the penis and occasionally in the urethra. In female patients, the lesions may be seen on the vulva, vagina, cervix, perianal area, or inner thigh and are frequently accompanied by itching and a mucoid vaginal discharge. The lesions are usually painful. In patients of

Figure 53—6. Cold sore of recurrent herpes labialis. It is less severe than that of primary disease. *(From Hart CA, Broadhead RL: A Color Atlas of Pediatric Infectious Diseases. London, Wolfe, 1992.)*

Figure 53—7. Herpetic whitlow. *(From Emond RTD, Rowland HAK: A Color Atlas of Infectious Diseases, 3rd ed. London, Mosby, 1995.)*

both sexes, a primary infection may be accompanied by fever, malaise, and myalgia, which are symptoms related to a transient viremia. HSV proctitis is a painful disease in which the lesions are found in the lower rectum and anus. The symptoms and time course of primary and recurrent genital herpes are compared in Figure 53-4.

Recurrent genital HSV disease is shorter in duration and less severe than the primary episode. In approximately 50% of patients, recurrences are preceded by a characteristic prodrome of burning or tingling in the area in which the lesions eventually erupt. Episodes of recurrence may be as frequent as every 2 to 3 weeks or may be infrequent. Unfortunately, any infected person may shed virus asymptomatically. Such individuals may be important vectors for spread of this virus.

Herpes encephalitis is usually caused by HSV-1. The lesions are generally limited to one of the temporal lobes. The viral pathology and immunopathology cause the destruction of the temporal lobe and give rise to erythrocytes in the cerebrospinal fluid, seizures, focal neurologic abnormalities, and other characteristics of viral encephalitis. HSV is the most common viral cause of sporadic encephalitis and results in significant morbidity and mortality, even in patients who receive appropriate treatment. The disease occurs at all ages and at any time of the year. **HSV meningitis** is most often a complication of genital HSV-2 infection; symptoms resolve by themselves.

HSV infection in the neonate is a devastating and often fatal disease caused most often by HSV-2. It may be acquired in utero but more commonly is contracted either during passage of the infant through the vaginal canal (possibly at the baby's scalp monitor site) because the mother is shedding herpesvirus at the time of delivery, or it is acquired postnatally from family members or hospital personnel. The baby initially appears septic, and

vesicular lesions may be present. Because the cell-mediated immune response is not yet developed in the neonate, HSV disseminates to the liver, lung, and other organs, as well as to the central nervous system (CNS). Progression of the infection to the CNS results in death, mental retardation, or neurologic disability, even with treatment.

Laboratory Diagnosis

Direct Analysis of Clinical Sample

Characteristic cytopathologic effects (CPEs) can be identified in a **Tzanck smear** (a scraping of the base of a lesion), Papanicolaou (Pap) smear, or biopsy specimen (Table 53-2). CPEs include syncytia, "ballooning" cytoplasm, and Cowdry type A intranuclear inclusions. (See Chapter 50, Figure 50-2.) A definitive diagnosis can be made by demonstrating viral antigen (using immunofluorescence or the immunoperoxidase method) or DNA (using in situ hybridization or polymerase chain reaction [PCR]) in the tissue sample or vesicle fluid. **PCR analysis** of cerebrospinal fluid has replaced immunofluorescence analysis of a brain biopsy in the diagnosis for herpes encephalitis.

Virus Isolation

Virus isolation is the most definitive assay for the diagnosis of HSV infection. Virus can be obtained from vesicles but not crusted lesions. Specimens are collected by aspiration of the lesion fluid or by application of a cotton swab to the vesicles and direct inoculation of the sample into cell cultures.

HSV produces CPEs within 1 to 3 days in HeLa cells, human embryonic fibroblasts, and rabbit kidney cells. Infected cells become enlarged and appear ballooned

Table 53—2. Laboratory Diagnosis of Herpes Simplex Virus (HSV) Infections

Approach	Test/Comment
Direct microscopic examination of cells from base of lesion	**Tzanck smear** shows **multinucleated giant cells** and **Cowdry type A inclusion bodies**
Cell culture	HSV replicates and causes identifiable cytopathologic effect in most cell cultures
Assay of tissue biopsy, smear, cerebrospinal fluid, or vesicular fluid for HSV antigen or genome	Enzyme immunoassay, immunofluorescent stain, in situ DNA probe analysis, and polymerase chain reaction (PCR)
HSV type distinction (HSV-1 vs. HSV-2)	Type-specific antibody, DNA maps of restriction enzyme fragments, sodium dodecyl sulfate—gel protein patterns, DNA probe analysis, and PCR
Serology	Serology is not useful except for epidemiology

(Chapter 51, Figure 51-4). Some isolates induce fusion of neighboring cells, giving rise to multinucleated giant cells (syncytia). A new, sensitive approach to isolation and identification uses a cell line that expresses β-galactosidase in HSV-infected cells (enzyme-linked viral inducible system [ELVIS]). Addition of the appropriate substrate produces color and allows detection of the enzyme in the infected cells.

HSV type-specific DNA probes, specific DNA primers for PCR, and antibodies are used to differentiate HSV-1 and HSV-2. The distinction between HSV-1 or HSV-2 and different strains of either virus can also be made by restriction endonuclease cleavage patterns of the viral DNA.

Serology

Serologic procedures are useful only for diagnosing a primary HSV infection and for epidemiologic studies. They are not useful for diagnosing recurrent disease, because a significant rise in antibody titers does not usually accompany recurrent disease.

Treatment, Prevention, and Control

HSV encodes several target enzymes for antiviral drugs (Box 53-5) (see Chapter 49). Most antiherpes drugs are nucleoside analogues and other inhibitors of the viral DNA polymerase, an enzyme essential for viral replication and the best antiviral drug target. Treatment prevents or shortens the course of primary or recurrent disease. None of the drug treatments can eliminate latent infection.

The prototype U.S. Food and Drug Administration (FDA)—approved anti-HSV drug is **acyclovir (ACV)**. **Valacyclovir** (the valyl ester of ACV), **penciclovir,** and **famciclovir** (a derivative of penciclovir) are related to ACV in their mechanisms of action but have different pharmacologic properties. Vidarabine (adenosine arabinoside [Ara A]), idoxuridine (iododeoxyuridine), and trifluridine, also FDA-approved for treatment of HSV, are less effective. Although **cidofovir** and **adefovir** are active against HSV, cidofovir is only approved for treatment of CMV.

ACV is the most prescribed anti-HSV drug. Phosphorylation of ACV and penciclovir by the viral **thymidine kinase** and cellular enzymes activates the drug as a substrate for the viral **DNA polymerase**. These drugs are then incorporated into and **prevent the elongation of the viral DNA**. (See Chapter 49, Figure 49-2.) ACV, valacyclovir, penciclovir, and famciclovir (1) are relatively nontoxic, (2) are effective in treating serious presentations of HSV disease and first episodes of genital herpes, and (3) are also used for prophylactic treatment.

The most prevalent form of resistance to these drugs results from mutations that inactivate the thymidine kinase, thereby preventing conversion of the drug to its active form. Mutation of the viral DNA polymerase also produces resistance. Fortunately, resistant strains appear to be less virulent.

Box 53–5. FDA-Approved Antiviral Treatments for Herpesvirus Infections

Herpes Simplex 1 and 2

Acyclovir
Penciclovir
Valacyclovir
Famciclovir
Adenosine arabinoside (ara-A)
Trifluridine

Varicella-Zoster Virus

Acyclovir
Famciclovir
Valacyclovir
Varicella-zoster immune globulin (VZIG)
Zoster immune plasma
Live vaccine

Epstein-Barr Virus

None

Cytomegalovirus

Ganciclovir*
Valganciclovir*
Iododeoxyuridine
Foscarnet*
Trifluridine
Cidofovir*

FDA, U.S. Food and Drug Administration.
*Also inhibits herpes simplex and varicella-zoster viruses.

Ara-A is less soluble, less potent, and more toxic than ACV. Trifluridine, penciclovir, and ACV have replaced iododeoxyuridine as topical agents for the treatment of herpetic keratitis. Tromantadine, an amantadine derivative, is approved for topical use in countries other than the United States. It works by inhibiting penetration and syncytia formation. Various nonprescription treatments may be effective for specific individuals.

HSV-1 is transmitted most often from an active mucocutaneous lesion, so avoidance of direct contact with lesions reduces the risk of infection. Unfortunately, the symptoms may be inapparent, and thus the virus can be transmitted unknowingly. Physicians, nurses, dentists, and technicians must be especially careful when handling potentially infected tissue or fluids. The wearing of gloves can prevent the acquisition of infections of the fingers (herpetic whitlow). People with recurrent herpetic whitlow disease are very contagious and can spread the infection to patients. Washing with soap readily disinfects the virus.

Patients who have a history of genital HSV infection must be instructed to refrain from sexual intercourse while they have prodromal symptoms or lesions and to resume sexual intercourse only after lesions are completely reepithelialized, because virus may be transmitted from lesions that have crusted over. Condoms may be useful and are undoubtedly better than nothing but may not be fully protective.

A pregnant woman who has active genital HSV infection or who is asymptomatically shedding the virus in the vagina at term may transmit HSV to the neonate if the infant is delivered vaginally. Such transmission can be prevented by cesarean section.

No vaccine is currently available for HSV. However, killed, subunit, vaccinia hybrid, and DNA vaccines are being developed to prevent acquisition of the virus or to treat infected people. The glycoprotein D is being used in several subunit vaccines.

Varicella-Zoster Virus

VZV causes **chickenpox (varicella)** and, upon recurrence, causes herpes **zoster, or shingles**. As an alphaherpesvirus, VZV shares many characteristics with HSV, including: (1) the ability to establish latent infection of neurons and recurrent disease, (2) the importance of cell-mediated immunity in controlling and preventing serious disease, and (3) the characteristic blister-like lesions. Like HSV, VZV encodes a **thymidine kinase** and is susceptible to **antiviral drugs.** Unlike HSV, VZV spreads predominantly by the **respiratory route.** Viremia occurs after local replication of the virus in the respiratory tract, leading to the formation of skin lesions over the entire body.

Structure and Replication

VZV has the smallest genome of the human herpesviruses. VZV replicates in a similar manner but slower and in fewer types of cells than HSV. Human diploid fibroblasts in vitro and activated T cells, epithelial cells, and epidermal cells in vivo support productive VZV replication. Like HSV, VZV establishes a latent infection of neurons, but unlike HSV, several viral RNAs and specific viral proteins can be detected in the cells.

Box 53—6. Disease Mechanisms of Varicella-Zoster Virus (VZV)

Initial replication is in the respiratory tract.
VZV infects epithelial cells, fibroblasts, T cells, and neurons.
VZV can form syncytia and spread directly from cell to cell.
Virus is spread by viremia to skin and causes lesions in
  successive crops.
VZV can escape antibody clearance, and cell-mediated
  immune response is essential to control infection.
  Disseminated, life-threatening disease can occur in
  immunocompromised people.
Virus establishes latent infection of neurons, usually dorsal root
  and cranial nerve ganglia.
Herpes zoster is a recurrent disease; it results from
  virus replication along the entire dermatome.
Herpes zoster may result from depression of cell-mediated
  immunity and other mechanisms of viral activation.

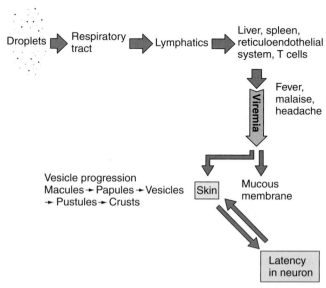

Figure 53—8. Mechanism of spread of varicella-zoster virus (VZV) within the body. VZV initially infects the respiratory tract and is spread to the reticuloendothelial system and T cells and then by cell-associated viremia to the skin.

Pathogenesis and Immunity

VZV is generally acquired by inhalation, and primary infection begins in the tonsils and mucosa of the respiratory tract. The virus then progresses via the bloodstream and lymphatic system to the cells of the reticuloendothelial system (Box 53-6; Figures 53-8 and 53-9). A secondary viremia occurs after 11 to 13 days and spreads the virus throughout the body and to the skin. The virus infects T cells, and these cells can home to the skin and transfer virus to skin epithelial cells. The virus overcomes inhibition by interferon alpha, and vesicles are produced in the skin. The virus remains cell associated and is transmitted on cell-cell interaction, except for terminally differentiated epithelial cells in the lungs and keratinocytes of skin lesions, which can release infectious virus. Virus replication in the lung is a major source of contagion. The virus causes

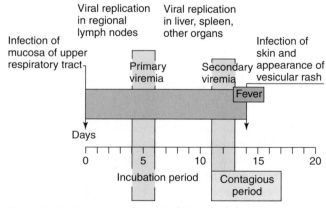

Figure 53—9. Time course of varicella (chickenpox). The course in young children, as presented in this figure, is generally shorter and less severe than that in adults.

a dermal vesiculopustular rash that develops over time in successive crops. Fever and systemic symptoms occur with the rash.

The virus becomes latent in the dorsal root or cranial nerve ganglia after the primary infection. The virus can be reactivated in older adults or in patients with impaired cellular immunity. On reactivation, the virus replicates and is released along the entire neural pathway to infect the skin, causing a vesicular rash along the entire dermatome, known as **herpes zoster**, or **shingles**.

Interferon alpha and interferon-stimulated protections limit the spread of the virus in tissue, but **antibody** is important for limiting the viremic spread of VZV. Passive immunization with varicella-zoster immune globulin (VZIG) within 4 days of infection is protective. Cell-mediated immunity is essential for resolving the disease. The virus causes more disseminated and more serious disease in the absence of cell-mediated immunity (e.g., in children with leukemia) and may recur on immunosuppression. Although important for protection, cell-mediated immune responses contribute to the symptomatology. An overzealous response in adults is responsible for causing more extensive cell damage and a more severe manifestation (especially in the lung) in primary infection than that seen in children. Waning of the immune response later in life is the major factor that allows VZV recurrence and herpes zoster.

Epidemiology

VZV is extremely communicable, with rates of infection exceeding 90% among susceptible household contacts (Box 53-7). The disease is spread principally by the respiratory route but may also be spread through contact with skin vesicles. Patients are contagious before and during symptoms. More than 90% of adults in developed countries have the VZV antibody. Herpes zoster results from the reactivation of a patient's latent virus. The disease develops in approximately 10% to 20% of the population infected with VZV, and the incidence rises with age. Herpes zoster lesions contain viable virus and therefore may be a source of varicella infection in a nonimmune person (child).

Clinical Syndromes

Varicella (chickenpox) is one of the five **classic childhood exanthems** (along with rubella, roseola, fifth disease, and measles). The disease results from a primary infection with VZV; it is usually a mild disease of childhood and is normally symptomatic, although asymptomatic infection can occur (see Figure 53-9). Varicella characteristics include fever and a maculopapular rash that appear after an incubation period of approximately 14 days (Figure 53-10). Within hours, each maculopapular lesion forms a thin-walled vesicle on an erythematous base ("dewdrop on a rose petal") that measures approximately 2 to 4 mm in

Box 53-7. Epidemiology of Varicella-Zoster Virus

Disease/Viral Factors

Virus causes lifelong infection.
Recurrent disease is a source of contagion.

Transmission

Virus is transmitted mainly by respiratory droplets but also by direct contact.

Who Is at Risk?

Children (ages 5 to 9) experience mild classic disease.
Teens and adults are at risk for more severe disease with potential pneumonia.
Immunocompromised people and newborns are at risk for life-threatening pneumonia, encephalitis, and progressive disseminated varicella.
Elderly and immunocompromised people are at risk for recurrent disease (herpes zoster [shingles]).

Geography/Season

Virus is found worldwide.
There is no seasonal incidence.

Modes of Control

Antiviral drugs are available.
Immunity may wane in the elderly population.
Varicella-zoster immunoglobulin is available for immunocompromised people and staff exposed to virus, as well as newborns of mothers showing symptoms within 5 days of birth.
Live vaccine (Oka strain) is available for children.

diameter. This vesicle is the hallmark of varicella. Within 12 hours, the vesicle becomes pustular and begins to crust, after which scabbed lesions appear. Successive crops of lesions appear for 3 to 5 days, and at any given time, all stages of skin lesions can be observed.

Figure 53–10. Characteristic rash of varicella in all stages of its evolution. *(From Hart CA, Broadhead RL: A Color Atlas of Pediatric Infectious Diseases. London, Wolfe, 1992.)*

Figure 53–11. Herpes zoster ("shingles") in a thoracic dermatome.

The rash spreads across the entire body but is more severe on the trunk than on the extremities. Its presence on the scalp distinguishes it from many other rashes. The lesions itch and cause scratching, which may lead to bacterial superinfection and scarring. Lesions on the mucous membrane typically occur in the mouth, conjunctivae, and vagina.

Primary infection is usually more severe in adults than in children. **Interstitial pneumonia** may occur in 20% to 30% of adult patients and may be fatal. The pneumonia results from inflammatory reactions at this primary site of infection.

As noted earlier, **herpes zoster** (*zoster* means "belt" or "girdle") is a recurrence of a latent varicella infection acquired earlier in the patient's life. Severe pain in the area innervated by the nerve usually precedes the appearance of the chickenpox-like lesions. The rash is usually limited to a dermatome and resembles varicella (Figure 53-11). A chronic pain syndrome called **postherpetic neuralgia**, which can persist for months to years, occurs in as many as 30% of patients older than 65 years in whom herpes zoster develops.

VZV infection in immunocompromised patients or neonates can result in serious, progressive, and potentially fatal disease. Defects of cell-mediated immunity in such patients increase the risk for dissemination of the virus to the lungs, brain, and liver, which may be fatal. The disease may occur in response to a primary exposure to varicella or because of recurrent disease.

Laboratory Diagnosis

Cytology

The CPEs in VZV-infected cells are similar to those seen in HSV-infected cells and include Cowdry type A intranuclear inclusions and syncytia. These cells may be seen in skin lesions, respiratory specimens, or organ biopsy specimens. Syncytia may also be seen in Tzanck smears of scrapings from a vesicle's base. A direct fluorescent antibody to membrane antigen (FAMA) test can also be used to examine skin lesion scrapings or biopsy specimens. Antigen detection and PCR are sensitive means of diagnosing VZV infection.

Virus Isolation

Isolation of VZV is not routinely done, because the virus is labile during transport to the laboratory and replicates poorly in vitro. Cultures of material from skin lesions that are crusted over (5 or more days after onset) are usually negative for the virus. Human diploid fibroblasts can support VZV replication and exhibit a CPE similar to that seen in HSV-infected cells but after a longer incubation period.

Serology

Serologic tests that detect antibodies to VZV are used to screen people for immunity to VZV. However, antibody levels are normally low, so sensitive tests such as immunofluorescence and enzyme-linked immunosorbent assay (ELISA) must be performed to detect the antibody. A significant increase in antibody level can be detected in people experiencing herpes zoster.

Treatment, Prevention, and Control

Treatment may be appropriate for adults and immunocompromised patients with VZV infections and for people with shingles, but no treatment is usually necessary for children with varicella. **ACV, famciclovir**, and **valacyclovir** have been approved for the treatment of VZV infections. The VZV DNA polymerase is much less sensitive to ACV treatment than the HSV enzyme, requiring large doses of ACV or the improved pharmacodynamics of famciclovir and valacyclovir (see Box 53-5). There is no good treatment, but analgesics and other painkillers, topical anesthetics, or capsaicin cream may provide some relief from the postherpetic neuralgia that follows zoster.

As with other respiratory viruses, it is difficult to limit the transmission of VZV. Because VZV infection in children is generally mild and induces lifelong immunity, exposure of children to VZV early in life is often encouraged. However, high-risk people (e.g., immunosuppressed children) should be protected from exposure to VZV.

Immunosuppressed patients susceptible to severe disease may be protected from serious disease through the administration of **varicella-zoster immunoglobulin (VZIG)**. VZIG is prepared through the pooling of plasma from seropositive people. VZIG prophylaxis can prevent viremic spread leading to disease but is ineffective as a therapy for patients already suffering from active varicella or herpes zoster disease.

A **live attenuated vaccine** for VZV (Oka strain) has been licensed for use in the United States and elsewhere and is administered after 2 years of age on the same schedule as the measles, mumps, and rubella vaccine.

The vaccine induces the production of protective antibody and cell-mediated immunity. It is effective as a prophylactic treatment in people, even after exposure to VZV. Most significantly, the vaccine promotes protection in immunodeficient children. A stronger version of this vaccine is available for older adults; it boosts antiviral responses to limit the onset of zoster.

Epstein-Barr Virus

EBV has developed into the ultimate B-lymphocyte parasite, and the diseases it causes reflect this association. EBV was discovered by electron-microscopic observation of characteristic herpes virions in biopsy specimens of a B-cell neoplasm, African Burkitt lymphoma (AfBL). Its association with infectious mononucleosis was discovered accidentally when serum collected from a laboratory technician convalescing from infectious mononucleosis was found to contain the antibody that recognized AfBL cells. This finding was later confirmed in a large serologic study performed on college students.

EBV causes *heterophile antibody-positive infectious mononucleosis* and has been causally associated with **AfBL (endemic Burkitt lymphoma)**, **Hodgkin disease**, and **nasopharyngeal carcinoma**. EBV has also been associated with B-cell lymphomas in patients with acquired or congenital immunodeficiencies. *EBV stimulates the growth and immortalizes B cells* in tissue culture.

Structure and Replication

EBV is a member of the subfamily Gammaherpesvirinae, with a very limited host range and a **tissue tropism** defined by the limited cellular expression of its receptor. The primary receptor for EBV is also *the receptor for the C3d component of the complement system (also called CR2 or CD21)*. It is expressed on B cells of humans and New World monkeys and on some epithelial cells of the oropharynx and nasopharynx.

EBV infection has the following three potential outcomes:

1. EBV can replicate in B cells or epithelial cells permissive for EBV replication.
2. EBV can cause latent infection of B cells in the presence of competent T cells.
3. EBV can stimulate and immortalize B cells.

EBV encodes more than 70 proteins, different groups of which are expressed for the different types of infections.

Permissive epithelial and B cells allow the transcription and translation of the ZEBRA (peptide encoded by the Z gene region) transcriptional activator protein, which activates the immediate early genes of the virus and the lytic cycle. After synthesis of the DNA polymerase and replication of DNA, the structural and other late proteins are synthesized. They include gp350/220 (related glycoproteins of 350,000 and 220,000Da), which is the viral attachment protein, and other glycoproteins. These glycoproteins bind to CD21 and MHC II molecules, receptors on B cells and epithelial cells, and also promote fusion of the envelope with cell membranes.

The viral proteins produced during a productive infection are serologically defined and grouped as **early antigen (EA)**, **viral capsid antigen (VCA)**, and the glycoproteins of the **membrane antigen (MA)** (Table 53-3).

During nonpermissive infection of B cells, the cells contain a small number of circular, plasmid-like EBV genomes that replicate only during cell division. Select viral genes are expressed, depending on the state of the B cell; they include **Epstein-Barr nuclear antigens (EBNAs)** 1, 2, 3A, 3B, and 3C; latent proteins (**LPs**); **latent membrane proteins (LMPs) 1 and 2;** and two small Epstein-Barr–encoded RNA (EBER) molecules, EBER-1 and EBER-2. The EBNAs and LPs are DNA-binding proteins that are essential for establishing and maintaining the infection (EBNA-1), immortalization (EBNA-2), and other purposes. The LMPs are membrane proteins with oncogene-like activity. These proteins stimulate the growth of and immortalize the B cell. EBV establishes latency in memory B cells in which only the EBNA-1 and LMP-2 are expressed, maintaining the genome in the cells but with minimal potential for immune recognition of the infected cell.

Pathogenesis and Immunity

EBV has adapted to the human B cell and manipulates and uses the different phases of B-cell development to establish lifelong infection of the individual and still promote its transmission. The diseases of EBV result from either an overactive immune response (infectious mononucleosis) or the lack of effective immune control (lymphoma and hairy cell leukoplakia).

The productive infection of B cells and epithelial cells of the oropharynx, such as in the tonsils (Box 53-8 and Figure 53-12), promotes virus shedding into saliva to transmit the virus to other hosts and establishes a viremia to spread the virus to other B cells in lymphatic tissue and blood.

EBV proteins activate B-cell growth and also prevent apoptosis (programmed cell death). T cells usually control the B-cell proliferation. In the absence of T cells (e.g., in tissue culture), EBV can immortalize B cells and promote the development of B-lymphoblastoid cell lines. In vivo, B-cell activation and proliferation occurs and is indicated by the spurious production of an IgM antibody to the Paul-Bunnell antigen, termed the **heterophile antibody** (see later discussion of serology). Continued B-cell proliferation in conjunction with the effects of other cofactors may result in the development of lymphoma.

During productive infection, antibody is first developed against the components of the virion, VCA and MA, and

Table 53—3. Markers of Epstein-Barr Virus (EBV) Infection

Name	Abbreviation	Characteristics	Biologic Association	Clinical Association
EBV nuclear antigens	EBNAs	Nuclear	EBNAs are nonstructural antigens and first antigens to appear; EBNAs seen in all infected and transformed cells and bind to cell DNA	Anti-EBNA develops late in infection
Early antigen	EA-R	Only cytoplasmic	EA-R appears before EA-D; appearance is first sign that infected cell has entered lytic cycle	Anti—EA-R seen in Burkitt lymphoma
	EA-D	Diffuse in cytoplasm and nucleus	—	Anti—EA-D seen in infectious mononucleosis
Viral capsid antigen	VCA	Cytoplasmic	VCA is a late antigen; found in virus producing cells	Anti-VCA IgM is transient; anti-VCA IgG is persistent
Membrane antigen	MA	Cell surface	MAs are envelope glycoproteins	Same as VCA
Heterophile antibody		Recognition of Paul-Bunnell antigen on sheep, horse, or bovine erythrocytes	EBV-induced B-cell proliferation promotes production of heterophile antibody	Early symptom occurs in more than 50% of patients

EA, early antigen; EBNA, Epstein-Barr nuclear antigen; MA, membrane antigen; VCA, viral capsid antigen.

later against the EA. After resolution of the infection (lysis of the productively infected cells), antibody against the nuclear antigens (EBNAs) is produced. T cells are essential for limiting the proliferation of EBV-infected B cells and controlling the disease (Figure 53-13). EBV counteracts some of the protective action of TH1 CD4 T-cell responses during productive infection by producing an interleukin-10 analogue (BCRF-1) that inhibits the protective TH1 CD4 T-cell responses and also stimulates B-cell growth.

Infectious mononucleosis *results from a "civil war" between the EBV-infected B cells and the protective T cells.* The T cells are surrounded by infected B cells and are activated by viral antigenic peptides presented on both the MHC I and II molecules. The classic **lymphocytosis** (increase in mononuclear cells), swelling of lymphoid

---

Box 53—8. Disease Mechanisms of Epstein-Barr Virus

Virus in saliva initiates infection of oral epithelia and spreads to B cells in lymphatic tissue.
There is productive infection of epithelial and B cells.
Virus promotes growth of B cells (immortalizes).
T cells kill and limit B-cell outgrowth. T cells are required for controlling infection. Antibody role is limited.
EBV establishes latency in memory B cells and is reactivated when the B cell is activated.
T-cell response (lymphocytosis) contributes to symptoms of **infectious mononucleosis**.
There is causative association with lymphoma in immunosuppressed people and African children living in malarial regions (African Burkitt lymphoma) and with nasopharyngeal carcinoma in China.

---

organs (lymph nodes, spleen, and liver), and malaise associated with infectious mononucleosis results mainly from the activation and proliferation of T cells. The T cells appear as **atypical lymphocytes** (also called **Downey cells**) (Figure 53-14). They increase in number in the peripheral blood during the second week of infection, accounting for 10% to 80% of the total white blood cell count at this time (hence the "mononucleosis"). Children have a less active immune response to EBV infection and therefore have very mild disease.

The virus persists in at least one memory B cell per milliliter of blood for the person's lifetime. EBV may be reactivated when the memory B cell is activated (especially in the tonsils or oropharynx) and may be shed in saliva.

Epidemiology

EBV is transmitted in saliva (Box 53-9). More than 90% of EBV-infected people intermittently shed the virus for life, even when totally asymptomatic. Children can acquire the virus at an early age by sharing contaminated drinking glasses. *Children generally have subclinical disease.* Saliva sharing between adolescents and young adults often occurs during kissing; thus EBV mononucleosis has earned the nickname "the kissing disease." Disease in these people may go unnoticed or may manifest in varying degrees of severity. At least 70% of the population of the United States is infected by age 30.

The geographic distribution of some EBV-associated neoplasms indicates a possible association with cofactors. The immunosuppressive potential of malaria has been

Figure 53—12. Progression of Epstein-Barr virus (EBV) infection. Infection may result in lytic, latent, or immortalizing infection, which can be distinguished on the basis of production of virus and expression of different viral proteins and antigens. T cells limit the outgrowth of the EBV-infected cells and maintain the latent infection. EA, early antigen; EBER, Epstein-Barr—encoded RNA; EBNA, Epstein-Barr nuclear antigen; LMP, latent membrane protein; LP, latent protein; MA, membrane antigen; VCA, viral capsid antigen; ZEBRA, peptide encoded by the Z gene region.

suggested as a cofactor in the progression of chronic or latent EBV infection to AfBL. The restriction of nasopharyngeal carcinoma to people living in certain regions of China indicates a possible genetic predisposition to the cancer or the presence of cofactors in the food or environment. More subtle mechanisms may facilitate the role of EBV in 30% to 50% of cases of Hodgkin disease.

Transplant recipients, patients with the acquired immune deficiency syndrome (AIDS), and genetically immunodeficient people are at high risk for lymphoproliferative disorders initiated by EBV. These disorders may appear as polyclonal and monoclonal B-cell lymphomas. Such people are also at high risk for a productive EBV infection in the form of **hairy oral leukoplakia**.

Clinical Syndromes (Clinical Case 53-2)

Heterophile Antibody—Positive Infectious Mononucleosis

The triad of classic symptoms for infectious mononucleosis is **lymphadenopathy** (swollen glands), **splenomegaly** (large spleen), and **exudative pharyngitis** accompanied by high fever, malaise, and often hepatosplenomegaly (large liver and spleen). A rash may occur, especially after ampicillin treatment (for the sore throat). The major complaint of people with infectious mononucleosis is fatigue

Figure 53—13. Pathogenesis of Epstein-Barr virus (EBV). EBV is acquired by close contact between persons through saliva and infects the B cells. The resolution of the EBV infection and many of the symptoms of infectious mononucleosis result from the activation of T cells in response to the infection.

Figure 53—14. Atypical T cell (Downey cell) characteristic of infectious mononucleosis. The cells have a more basophilic and vacuolated cytoplasm than normal lymphocytes, and the nucleus may be oval, kidney shaped, or lobulated. The cell margin may seem to be indented by neighboring red blood cells.

Box 53—9. Epidemiology of Epstein-Barr Virus

Disease/Viral Factors

Virus causes lifelong infection.
Recurrent disease is cause of contagion.
Virus may cause asymptomatic shedding.

Transmission

Transmission occurs via saliva, close oral contact ("kissing disease"), or sharing of items such as toothbrushes and cups.

Who Is at Risk?

Children experience asymptomatic disease or mild symptoms.
Teenagers and adults are at risk for infectious mononucleosis.
Immunocompromised people are at highest risk for life-threatening neoplastic disease.

Geography/Season

Infectious mononucleosis has worldwide distribution.
There is causative association with African Burkitt lymphoma in malarial belt of Africa.
There is no seasonal incidence.

Modes of Control

There are no modes of control.

Clinical Case 53-2. Epstein Barr Virus in the Immunocompromised Individual

Purtilo, et al (Ann Intern Med 101:180-186, 1984) reported on a boy with Duncan disease who presented with reduced levels of IgA, a history of thrush, and recurrent episodes of otitis media. This member of the Duncan family had an X-linked recessive progressive combined variable immunodeficiency disease caused by a mutation in the SH2D1A protein which prevents proper communication between B and T cells. Following exposure to EBV at age 11, the boy did not develop antibodies to EBV, but generic serum IgM levels increased, and EBNA-positive immortalized B-cell lines readily grew from his peripheral blood. Establishment of the B-cell lines is indicative of aberrant T-cell control of the virus-induced B-cell proliferation. At age 18, he was treated with packed red cells for red cell aplasia, and then 9 weeks later, he developed infectious mononucleosis (IM) with fever, generalized lymphadenomegaly, tender liver and swollen spleen, lymphocytosis with a predominance of atypical lymphocytes, and a positive monospot test. Within another 6 months, he was agammaglobulinemic with no detectable B cells and suffered from *Haemophilus influenzae* and *Mycobacterium tuberculosis* pneumonias. After an additional 5 months, B cells were again detected. The onset of IM at age 18 may have resulted from new infection or a reactivation of the earlier infection. This case illustrates the unusual nature of EBV and other virus infections when the immune response is compromised.

(Figure 53-15). The disease is rarely fatal in healthy people but can cause serious complications resulting from neurologic disorders, laryngeal obstruction, or rupture of the spleen. Neurologic complications include meningoencephalitis and the Guillain-Barré syndrome. Mononucleosis-like syndromes can also be caused by CMV, HHV6, *Toxoplasma gondii*, and human immunodeficiency virus (HIV). Like infections caused by other herpesviruses, EBV infection in a child is much milder than infection in an adolescent or adult. In fact, infection in children is usually subclinical.

Chronic Disease

EBV can cause cyclic recurrent disease in some people. These patients experience chronic tiredness and may also have low-grade fever, headaches, and sore throat. This disorder is different from chronic fatigue syndrome, which has an unknown etiology.

Epstein-Barr Virus—Induced Lymphoproliferative Diseases

On infection with EBV, people lacking T-cell immunity are likely to suffer life-threatening polyclonal leukemia-like B-cell proliferative disease and lymphoma instead of infectious mononucleosis. Men with congenital deficiencies of T-cell function are likely to suffer life-threatening X-linked lymphoproliferative disease. One such X-linked genetic defect in a T-cell gene (SLAM [signaling lymphocyte activation molecule]—associated protein) prevents the T cell from controlling B-cell growth during a normal immune

response to antigen or due to EBV. Transplant recipients undergoing immunosuppressive treatment are at high risk for **posttransplant lymphoproliferative** disease instead of infectious mononucleosis after exposure to the virus or on

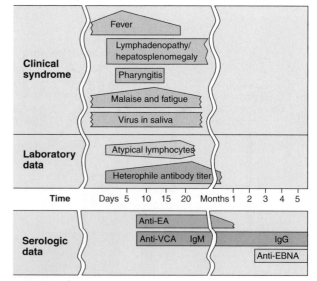

Figure 53—15. Clinical course of infectious mononucleosis and laboratory findings of those with the infection. Epstein-Barr virus (EBV) infection may be asymptomatic or may produce the symptoms of mononucleosis. The incubation period can last as long as 2 months. EA, early antigen; EBNA, Epstein-Barr nuclear antigen; VCA, viral capsid antigen.

reactivation of latent virus. Similar diseases are seen in patients with AIDS.

African Burkitt lymphoma (endemic lymphoma) is a poorly differentiated monoclonal B-cell lymphoma of the jaw and face that is endemic in children living in the malarial regions of Africa. The tumors contain EBV DNA sequences but express only the EBNA-1 viral antigen. Virions can occasionally be seen on electron micrographs of infected material. In addition to EBV DNA, the tumor cells contain chromosomal translocations that juxtapose the *C-myc* oncogene to a very active promoter, such as an immunoglobulin gene promoter [t(8;14), t(8;22), t(8;2)]. The tumor cells are also relatively invisible to immune control. It is not known how malaria acts to promote EBV involvement with AfBL. EBV is also associated with Burkitt lymphomas in people living in other parts of the world but to a much smaller extent. Many **Hodgkin lymphomas** can also be attributed to EBV.

As noted earlier, **nasopharyngeal carcinoma** is endemic in Asia, occurs in adults, and contains EBV DNA within the tumor cells. Unlike Burkitt lymphoma, in which the tumor cells are derived from lymphocytes, the tumor cells of nasopharyngeal carcinoma are of epithelial origin.

Hairy Oral Leukoplakia

Hairy oral leukoplakia is an unusual manifestation of a productive EBV infection of epithelial cells characterized by lesions of the tongue and mouth. It is an opportunistic manifestation that occurs in patients with AIDS.

Laboratory Diagnosis

EBV-induced infectious mononucleosis is diagnosed on the basis of the **symptoms** (Box 53-10), the finding of atypical lymphocytes, and the presence of **lymphocytosis** (mononuclear cells constituting 60% to 70% of the white blood

Box 53—10. Diagnosis of Epstein-Barr Virus

1. Symptoms
   a. Mild headache, fatigue, fever
   b. Triad: lymphadenopathy, splenomegaly, exudative pharyngitis
   c. Other: hepatitis, ampicillin-induced rash
2. Complete blood cell count
   a. Hyperplasia
   b. Atypical lymphocytes (Downey cells) (T cells)
3. Heterophile antibody (transient)
4. EBV-antigen specific antibody

cell count with 30% atypical lymphocytes), **heterophile antibody**, and antibody to viral antigens. Virus isolation is not practical. PCR and DNA probe analysis for the viral genome and immunofluorescent identification of viral antigens are used to detect evidence of infection.

Atypical lymphocytes are probably the earliest detectable indication of an EBV infection. These cells appear with the onset of symptoms and disappear with resolution of the disease.

Heterophile antibody results from the nonspecific, mitogen-like activation of B cells by EBV and the production of a wide repertoire of antibodies. These antibodies include an IgM heterophile antibody that recognizes the Paul-Bunnell antigen on sheep, horse, and bovine erythrocytes but not that on guinea pig kidney cells. The heterophile antibody response can usually be detected by the end of the first week of illness and lasts for as long as several months. It is an excellent indication of EBV infection in adults but is not as reliable in children or infants. The horse cell (Monospot) test and ELISA are rapid and widely used for the detection of the heterophile antibody.

Serologic tests for antibody to viral antigens are a more dependable method than heterophile antibody to confirm the diagnosis of EBV mononucleosis (Table 53-4; see Figure 53-15). EBV infection is indicated by the finding

Table 53—4. Serologic Profile for Epstein-Barr Virus (EBV) Infections

Patient's Clinical Status	Heterophile Antibodies		EBV-Specific Antibodies		Comment
	VCA-IgM	VCA-IgG	EA	EBNA	
Susceptible	−	−	−	−	−
Acute primary infection	+	+	+	±	−	−
Chronic primary infection	−	−	+	+	−	−
Past infection	−	−	+	−	+	−
Reactivation infection	−	−	+	+	+	EA restricted or diffuse
Burkitt lymphoma	−	−	+	+	+	EA restricted only
Nasopharyngeal carcinoma	−	−	+	+	+	EA diffuse only

Modified from Balows A, et al (eds): Laboratory Diagnosis of Infectious Diseases: Principles and Practices. New York, Springer-Verlag, 1988.
EA, early antigen; EBNA, Epstein-Barr nuclear antigen; Ig, immunoglobulin; VCA, viral capsid antigen.

of any of the following: (1) IgM antibody to the VCA, (2) the presence of VCA antibody and the absence of EBNA antibody, or (3) elevation of antibodies to VCA and early antigen. The finding of both VCA and EBNA antibodies in serum indicates that the person had a previous infection. Generation of antibody to EBNA requires lysis of the infected cell and usually indicates T-cell control of active disease.

Treatment, Prevention, and Control

No effective treatment or vaccine is available for EBV disease (see Box 53-5). The ubiquitous nature of the virus and the potential for asymptomatic shedding make control of infection difficult. However, infection elicits lifelong immunity. Therefore, the best means of preventing infectious mononucleosis is exposure to the virus early in life, because the disease is more benign in children.

Cytomegalovirus

CMV is a common human pathogen, infecting 0.5% to 2.5% of all newborns and approximately 40% of women visiting clinics for sexually transmitted diseases. It is the most common viral cause of **congenital defects**. Although usually causing mild or asymptomatic disease in children and adults, CMV is particularly important as an **opportunistic pathogen in immunocompromised patients**.

Structure and Replication

CMV is a member of the subfamily Betaherpesvirinae and is considered lymphotropic. It has the largest genome of the human herpesviruses. In contrast to the traditional definition of a virus, which states that a virion particle contains DNA or RNA, studies now indicate that CMV carries specific mRNAs into the cell in the virion particle to facilitate infection. Human CMV replicates only in human cells. Fibroblasts, epithelial cells, macrophages, and other cells are permissive for CMV replication. CMV establishes latent infection in mononuclear lymphocytes, the stromal cells of the bone marrow, and other cells.

Pathogenesis and Immunity

The pathogenesis of CMV is similar to that of other herpesviruses in many respects (Box 53-11). CMV is an excellent parasite and readily establishes persistent and latent infections rather than an extensive lytic infection. CMV is highly cell-associated and is spread throughout the body within infected cells, especially lymphocytes and leukocytes. The virus is reactivated by immunosuppression (e.g., corticosteroids, infection with HIV) and possibly by allogeneic stimulation (i.e., the host response to transfused or transplanted cells).

Box 53–11. Disease Mechanisms of Cytomegalovirus (CMV)

CMV is acquired from blood, tissue, and most body secretions.
CMV causes productive infection of epithelial and other cells.
CMV establishes latency in T cells, macrophages, and other cells.
Cell-mediated immunity is required for resolution and contributes to symptoms; role of antibody is limited.
Suppression of cell-mediated immunity allows recurrence and severe presentation.
CMV generally causes subclinical infection.

Cell-mediated immunity is essential for resolving and controlling the outgrowth of CMV infection. However, CMV has several means for evading the immune response. CMV infection alters the function of lymphocytes and leukocytes. The virus prevents antigen presentation to both CD8 cytotoxic T cells and CD4 T cells by preventing the expression of MHC I molecules on the cell surface and by interfering with cytokine-induced expression of MHC II molecules on antigen-presenting cells (including the infected cells). A viral protein also blocks natural-killer-cell attack of CMV-infected cells. Like EBV, CMV also encodes an interleukin-10 analogue that would inhibit TH1 protective immune responses.

Epidemiology and Clinical Syndromes

In most cases, CMV replicates and is shed without causing symptoms (Table 53-5). Activation and replication of CMV in the kidney and secretory glands promote its secretion in urine and bodily secretions. CMV can be isolated from urine, blood, throat washings, saliva, tears, breast milk, semen, stool, amniotic fluid, vaginal and cervical secretions, and tissues obtained for transplantation (Table 53-6 and Box 53-12). Virus can be transmitted to other individuals by means of blood transfusions and organ transplants. The congenital, oral, and sexual routes, blood transfusion, and tissue transplantation are the major means by which CMV is transmitted. CMV disease is an opportunistic disorder, rarely causing symptoms in the immunocompetent host but causing serious disease in an immunosuppressed or immunodeficient person, such as a patient with AIDS or a neonate (Figure 53-16).

Table 53–5. Sources of Cytomegalovirus Infection

Age Group	Source
Neonate	Transplacental transmission, intrauterine infections, cervical secretions
Baby or child	Body secretions: breast milk, saliva, tears, urine
Adult	Sexual transmission (semen), blood transfusion, organ graft

Table 53—6. Cytomegalovirus Syndromes

Tissue	Children/Adults	Immunosuppressed Patients
Predominant presentation	Asymptomatic	Disseminated disease, severe disease
Eyes	—	Chorioretinitis
Lungs	—	Pneumonia, pneumonitis
Gastrointestinal tract	—	Esophagitis, colitis
Nervous system	Polyneuritis, myelitis	Meningitis and encephalitis, myelitis
Lymphoid system	Mononucleosis syndrome, posttransfusion syndrome	Leukopenia, lymphocytosis
Major organs	Carditis,* hepatitis*	Hepatitis
Neonates	Deafness, intracerebral calcification, microcephaly, mental retardation	—

Complication of mononucleosis or posttransfusion syndrome.

Box 53—12. Epidemiology of Cytomegalovirus Infection

Disease/Viral Factors

Virus causes lifelong infection
Recurrent disease is source of contagion
Virus may cause asymptomatic shedding

Transmission

Transmission occurs via blood, organ transplants, and all secretions (urine, saliva, semen, cervical secretions, breast milk, and tears)
Virus is transmitted orally and sexually, in blood transfusions, in tissue transplants, in utero, at birth, and by nursing

Geography/Season

Virus is found worldwide
There is no seasonal incidence

Who Is at Risk?

Babies
Babies of mothers who experience seroconversion during term are at high risk for congenital defects
Sexually active people
Blood and organ recipients
Burn victims
Immunocompromised people: symptomatic and recurrent disease

Modes of Control

Antiviral drugs are available for patients with acquired immune deficiency syndrome.
Screening potential blood and organ donors for cytomegalovirus reduces transmission of virus.

Congenital Infection

CMV is the most prevalent viral cause of congenital disease. A significant percentage (0.5% to 2.5%) of all newborns in the United States are infected with CMV prior to birth, and a large percentage of babies are infected within the first months of life. Approximately 10% of affected newborns (4000 per year) show clinical evidence of disease. Disease signs include small size, thrombocytopenia, microcephaly, intracerebral calcification, jaundice, hepatosplenomegaly, and rash (**cytomegalic inclusion disease**). Unilateral or bilateral hearing loss and mental retardation are common consequences of congenital CMV infection. The risk for serious birth defects is extremely high for infants born to mothers who underwent primary CMV infections during their pregnancies.

Fetuses are infected by virus in the mother's blood (primary infection) or by virus ascending from the cervix (after a recurrence). The symptoms of congenital infection are less severe or can be prevented by the immune response of a seropositive mother. Congenital CMV infection is best documented by isolation of the virus from the infant's urine during the first week of life.

Perinatal Infection

In the United States, as many as 20% of pregnant women harbor CMV in the cervix at term and are likely to experience reactivation of the virus during pregnancy. Approximately half the neonates born through an infected cervix acquire CMV infection and become excreters of the virus at 3 to 4 weeks of age. Neonates may also acquire CMV from maternal milk or colostrum. Perinatal infection causes no clinically evident disease in healthy full-term infants.

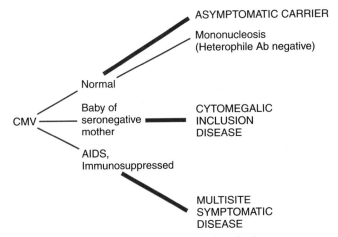

Figure 53—16. Outcomes of cytomegalovirus (CMV) infections. The outcome of CMV infection depends very heavily on the immune status of the patient.

Another means by which neonates can acquire CMV is through blood transfusions. Of the seronegative babies who are exposed to blood from seropositive donors, 13.5% acquire CMV infection in the immediate postnatal period. Significant clinical infection may occur in premature infants who acquire CMV from transfused blood, usually resulting in pneumonia and hepatitis.

Infection in Children and Adults

Only 10% to 15% of adolescents are infected with CMV, but this number increases to 50% to 85% of adults in the United States by the age of 40. CMV is more prevalent among people in low socioeconomic brackets living in crowded conditions and in people living in developing countries. CMV is a **sexually transmitted disease**. The titer of the CMV in semen is the highest of that in any body secretion. Approximately 40% of women seen at a venereal disease clinic had recently acquired the virus.

Although most CMV infections acquired in young adulthood are asymptomatic, patients may show a **heterophile-negative mononucleosis syndrome**. The symptoms of CMV disease are similar to those of EBV infection but with less severe pharyngitis and lymphadenopathy (see Figure 53-16). Although the presence of CMV-infected cells promotes a T-cell outgrowth (atypical lymphocytosis) similar to that seen in EBV infection, heterophile antibody is not present. The absence of this antibody reflects the differences in the target cell and the action of the viruses on the target cell. CMV disease should be suspected in a patient who has heterophile-negative mononucleosis or in whom there are signs of hepatitis, but results of tests for hepatitis A, B, and C are negative.

Transmission via Transfusion and Transplantation

Transmission of CMV by blood most often results in an asymptomatic infection; if symptoms are present, they typically resemble those of mononucleosis. Fever, splenomegaly, and atypical lymphocytosis usually begin 3 to 5 weeks after transfusion. Pneumonia and mild hepatitis may also occur. CMV may also be transmitted by organ transplantation (e.g., kidneys, bone marrow), and CMV infection is often reactivated in transplant recipients during periods of intense immunosuppression.

Infection in the Immunocompromised Host

CMV is a prominent opportunistic infectious agent. In immunocompromised people, it causes symptomatic primary or recurrent disease (see Table 53-6).

CMV disease of the lung (**pneumonia and pneumonitis**) is a common outcome in immunosuppressed patients and can be fatal if not treated. In addition, CMV often causes **retinitis** in patients who are severely immunodeficient (e.g., in as many as 10% to 15% of patients with AIDS). Interstitial pneumonia and encephalitis may also be caused by CMV but may be difficult to distinguish from infections caused by other opportunistic agents. CMV **colitis or esophagitis** may develop in as many as

Table 53—7. Laboratory Tests for Diagnosing Cytomegalovirus Infection

Test	Finding
Cytology and histology*	"Owl's-eye" inclusion body
	Antigen detection
	In situ DNA probe hybridization
	Polymerase chain reaction (PCR)
Cell culture	Cytologic effect in human diploid fibroblasts
	Immunofluorescence detection of early antigens (most common)
	PCR
Serology	Primary infection

*Samples taken for analysis include urine, saliva, blood, bronchoalveolar lavage specimens, and tissue biopsy specimens.

10% of patients with AIDS. CMV esophagitis may mimic candidal esophagitis. A smaller percentage of immunocompromised patients may experience CMV infection of the gastrointestinal tract. Patients with CMV colitis usually have diarrhea, weight loss, anorexia, and fever.

CMV is also responsible for the **failure of many kidney transplants**. This may be the result of virus replication in the graft after reactivation in the transplanted kidney or infection from the host.

Laboratory Diagnosis

Histology

The histologic hallmark of CMV infection is the **cytomegalic cell**, which is an **enlarged cell** (25 to 35 mm in diameter) that contains a dense, **central, "owl's eye," basophilic intranuclear inclusion body** (Table 53-7; Figure 53-17). Such infected cells may be found in any

Figure 53—17. Cytomegalovirus-infected cell with basophilic nuclear inclusion body.

tissue of the body and in urine and are thought to be epithelial in origin. The inclusions are readily seen with Papanicolaou or hematoxylin-eosin staining.

Immune and DNA Probe Techniques

A rapid, sensitive diagnosis can be obtained by detection of viral antigen using immunofluorescence or an ELISA or the viral genome using PCR and related techniques in cells of a biopsy, blood, bronchoalveolar lavage, or urine sample. (See Chapter 16, Figure 16-3.)

Culture

CMV is grown in diploid fibroblast cell cultures and normally must be maintained for at least 4 to 6 weeks, because the characteristic CPE develops very slowly in specimens with very low titers of the virus. Isolation of CMV is especially reliable in immunocompromised patients, who often have high titers of virus in their secretions. For example, in the semen of patients with AIDS, titers of viable virus may be greater than 10^6.

More rapid results are achieved by centrifuging a patient's sample onto cells grown on a coverslip within a shell vial. Specimens are examined after 1 to 2 days of incubation by indirect immunofluorescence for the presence of one or more of the immediate early viral antigens.

Serology

Seroconversion is usually an excellent marker for primary CMV infection. Titers of CMV-specific IgM antibody may be very high in patients with AIDS. However, CMV-specific IgM antibody may also develop during the reactivation of CMV and is therefore not a dependable indicator of primary infection.

Treatment, Prevention, and Control

Ganciclovir (dihydroxypropoxymethyl guanine), **valganciclovir** (valyl ester of ganciclovir), **cidofovir**, and **foscarnet** (phosphonoformic acid) have been approved by the FDA for the treatment of specific diseases resulting from CMV infections of immunosuppressed patients (see Box 53-5). Ganciclovir is structurally similar to ACV; it is phosphorylated and activated by a CMV-encoded protein kinase, inhibits the viral DNA polymerase, and causes DNA (see Chapter 49). Ganciclovir is more toxic than ACV. Ganciclovir can be used to treat severe CMV infections in immunocompromised patients. Valganciclovir is a prodrug of ganciclovir that can be taken orally, is converted to ganciclovir in the liver, and has better bioavailability than ganciclovir. Cidofovir is a phosphorylated cytidine nucleoside analogue that does not require a viral enzyme for activation. Foscarnet is a simple molecule that inhibits the viral DNA polymerase by mimicking the pyrophosphate portion of nucleotide triphosphates.

CMV spreads mainly by the sexual, tissue transplantation, and transfusion routes, and spread by these means is preventable. Semen is a major vector for the sexual spread of CMV to both heterosexual and homosexual contacts. The use of condoms or abstinence would limit viral spread. Transmission of the virus can also be reduced through the screening of potential blood and organ donors for CMV seronegativity. Screening is especially important for donors of blood transfusions to be given to infants. Although congenital and perinatal transmission of CMV cannot effectively be prevented, a seropositive mother is least likely to produce a baby with symptomatic CMV disease. No vaccine for CMV is available.

Human Herpesviruses 6 and 7

The two variants of HHV6, HHV6A and HHV6B, and HHV7, are members of the genus *Roseolovirus* of the subfamily Betaherpesvirinae. HHV6 was first isolated from the blood of patients with AIDS and grown in T-cell cultures. It was identified as a herpesvirus because of its characteristic morphology within infected cells. Like CMV, HHV6 is lymphotropic and ubiquitous. At least 45% of people are seropositive for HHV6 by age 2 years, and almost 100% by adulthood. In 1988, HHV6 was serologically associated with a common disease of children, **exanthem subitum**, commonly known as **roseola**. HHV7 was isolated in a similar manner from the T cells of a patient with AIDS who was also infected with HHV6, and later it was also shown to cause exanthem subitum.

Pathogenesis and Immunity

HHV6 infection occurs very early in life. The virus replicates in the salivary gland, is shed, and transmitted in saliva.

HHV6, like CMV, infects lymphocytes, monocytes, epithelial cells, endothelial cells, and neurons. HHV6 establishes a latent infection in T cells and monocytes but may replicate on activation of the cells. Cells in which the virus is replicating appear large and refractile and have occasional intranuclear and intracytoplasmic inclusion bodies.

Like the replication of CMV, the replication of HHV6 is controlled by cell-mediated immunity. Like CMV, the virus is likely to become activated in patients with AIDS or other lymphoproliferative and immunosuppressive disorders and cause opportunistic disease.

Clinical Syndromes (Box 53-13)

Exanthem subitum, or roseola, is caused by either HHV6B or HHV7 and is one of the five classic childhood exanthems previously mentioned (Figure 53-18). It is characterized by the rapid onset of high fever of a few days' duration, which is followed by a generalized rash that lasts only 24 to 48 hours. The presence of infected T cells or the activation of delayed-type hypersensitivity T cells in the

Box 53–13. Clinical Summaries

Primary oral herpes: A 5-year-old boy has an ulcerative rash with vesicles around the mouth. Vesicles and ulcers are also present within the mouth. Results of a Tzanck smear show multinucleated giant cells (syncytia) and Cowdry type A inclusion bodies. The lesions resolve after 18 days.

Recurrent oral herpes HSV: A 22-year-old medical student studying for examinations feels a twinge at the crimson border of his lip and 24 hours later has a single vesicular lesion at the site.

Recurrent genital HSV: A sexually active 32-year-old woman has a recurrence of ulcerative vaginal lesions with pain, itching, dysuria, and systemic symptoms 48 hours after being exposed to UVB light while skiing. The lesions resolve within 8 days. Results of a Papanicolaou smear shows multinucleated giant cells (syncytia) and Cowdry type A inclusion bodies.

Encephalitis HSV: A patient has focal neurologic symptoms and seizures. Magnetic resonance imaging results show destruction of a temporal lobe. Erythrocytes are present in the cerebrospinal fluid, and polymerase chain reaction is positive for viral DNA.

Varicella-Zoster Virus

Varicella (chickenpox): A 5-year-old boy develops a fever and a maculopapular rash on his abdomen 14 days after meeting with his cousin, who also developed the rash. Successive crops of lesions appeared for 3 to 5 days, and the rash spread peripherally.

Zoster (shingles): A 65-year-old woman has a belt of vesicles along the thoracic dermatome and experiences severe pain localized to the region.

Epstein-Barr Virus

Infectious mononucleosis: A 23-year-old college student develops malaise, fatigue, fever, swollen glands, and pharyngitis. After empirical treatment with ampicillin for sore throat, a rash appears. Heterophile antibody and atypical lymphocytes were detected from blood.

Cytomegalovirus

Congenital CMV disease: A neonate exhibits microcephaly, hepatosplenomegaly, and rash. Intracerebral calcification is noted on the radiograph. The mother had symptoms similar to mononucleosis during the third trimester of her pregnancy.

Human Herpesvirus 6

Roseola (exanthem subitum): A 4-year-old child experiences a rapid onset of high fever that lasts for 3 days and then suddenly returns to normal. Two days later, a maculopapular rash appears on the trunk and spreads to other parts of the body.

Figure 53–18. Time course of symptoms of exanthem subitum (roseola) caused by human herpesvirus 6 (HHV6). Compare these symptoms and this time course with those of fifth disease, which is caused by parvovirus B19 (see Chapter 56).

HHV6 may also cause a mononucleosis syndrome and lymphadenopathy in adults and may be a cofactor in the pathogenesis of AIDS. Like CMV, HHV6 may reactivate in transplant patients and contribute to the failure of the graft. HHV6 has also been associated with multiple sclerosis and chronic fatigue syndrome.

Other Human Herpesviruses

Human Herpesvirus 8 (Kaposi Sarcoma—Associated Herpesvirus)

HHV8 DNA sequences were discovered in biopsy specimens of **Kaposi sarcoma, primary effusion lymphoma** (a rare type of B-cell lymphoma), **and multicentric Castleman disease** through the use of PCR analysis. Kaposi sarcoma is one of the characteristic opportunistic diseases associated with AIDS. Genome sequence analysis showed that the virus was unique and a member of the subfamily Gammaherpesvirinae. Like EBV, the B cell is the primary target cell for HHV8, but the virus also infects a limited number of endothelial cells, monocytes, and epithelial and sensory nerve cells. Within the Kaposi sarcoma tumors, endothelial spindle cells contain the virus.

HHV8 encodes several proteins with homology to human proteins that promote the growth and prevent apoptosis of the infected and surrounding cells. These proteins include an interleukin-6 homologue (growth and antiapoptosis), a Bcl-2 analogue (antiapoptosis), chemokines, and a chemokine receptor. These proteins can promote the growth and development of polyclonal Kaposi sarcoma cells in AIDS patients and others. HHV8 DNA is present and is associated with peripheral blood lymphocytes, most likely B cells, in approximately 10% of immunocompetent people. HHV8 is limited to certain geographic areas (Italy, Greece, Africa) and to patients with AIDS. The virus is most likely a sexually transmitted disease but may be spread by other means.

Herpesvirus simiae (B virus) (subfamily Alphaherpesvirinae; the simian counterpart of HSV), is indigenous to Asian monkeys. The virus is transmitted to humans by monkey bites or saliva, or even by tissues and cells widely used in virology laboratories. Once infected, a human may have pain, localized redness, and vesicles at the site where the virus entered. An encephalopathy develops and is often fatal; most people who survive have serious brain damage. Virus isolation or serologic tests can be used to establish the diagnosis of B-virus infections.

skin may be the cause of the rash. The disease is effectively controlled and resolved by cell-mediated immunity, but the virus establishes a lifelong latent infection of T cells. Although usually benign, HHV-6 is the most common cause of febrile seizures in childhood (age 6 to 24 months).

Case Studies and Questions

A 2-year-old child with fever for 2 days has not been eating and has been crying often. On examination, the physician notes that the mucous membranes of the mouth are covered with numerous shallow, pale ulcerations. A few red papules and blisters are also observed around the border of the lips. The symptoms worsen over the next 5 days and then slowly resolve, with complete healing after 2 weeks.

1. The physician suspects that this is an HSV infection. How would the diagnosis be confirmed?

2. How could you determine whether this infection was caused by HSV-1 or HSV-2?

3. What immune responses were most helpful in resolving this infection, and when were they activated?

4. HSV escapes complete immune resolution by causing latent and recurrent infections. What was the site of latency in this child, and what might promote future recurrences?

5. What were the most probable means by which the child was infected with HSV?

6. Which antiviral drugs are available for the treatment of HSV infections? What are their targets? Were they indicated for this child? Why or why not?

A 17-year-old high school student has had low-grade fever and malaise for several days, followed by sore throat, swollen cervical lymph nodes, and increasing fatigue. The patient also notes some discomfort in the left upper quadrant of the abdomen. The sore throat, lymphadenopathy, and fever gradually resolve over the next 2 weeks, but the patient's full energy level does not return for another 6 weeks.

1. What laboratory tests would confirm the diagnosis of EBV-induced infectious mononucleosis and distinguish it from CMV infection?

2. To what characteristic diagnostic feature of the disease does *mononucleosis* refer?

3. What causes the swollen glands and fatigue?

4. Who is at greatest risk for a serious outcome of an EBV infection? What is the outcome? Why?

Bibliography

Boshoff C, Weiss RA (eds): Kaposi Sarcoma Herpesvirus: New Perspectives Series: Current Topics in Microbiology and Immunology, Vol. 312. New York, Springer-Verlag, 2007.

Cann AJ: Principles of Molecular Virology. San Diego, Academic, 2005.

Carter J, Saunders V: Virology: Principles and Applications, Chichester, England, Wiley, 2007.

Cohen J, Powderly WG: Infectious Diseases, 2nd ed. St Louis, Mosby, 2004.

Collier L, Oxford J: Human Virology, 3rd ed. Oxford, Oxford University Press, 2006.

Flint SJ, et al: Principles of Virology: Molecular Biology, Pathogenesis and Control of Animal Viruses, 2nd ed. Washington, DC, ASM Press, 2003.

Gorbach SL, Bartlett JG, Blacklow NR: Infectious Diseases, 3rd ed. Philadelphia, WB Saunders, 2004.

Knipe DM, Howley PM: Fields Virology, 4th ed. New York, Lippincott Williams & Wilkins, 2001.

Mandell GL, Bennet JE, Dolin R: Principles and Practice of Infectious Diseases, 6th ed. Philadelphia, Churchill Livingstone, 2004.

McGeoch DJ: The genomes of the human herpesviruses: Contents, relationships and evolution. Annu Rev Microbiol 43:235-265, 1989.

Richman DD, Whitley RJ, Hayden FG: Clinical Virology. Washington, DC, ASM Press, 2002.

Strauss JH, Strauss EG: Viruses and Human Disease, 2nd ed. San Diego, Academic, 2007.

Voyles BA: The Biology of Viruses, 2nd ed. Boston, McGraw-Hill, 2002.

White DO, Fenner FJ: Medical Virology, 4th ed. New York, Academic, 1994.

Herpes Simplex Virus

Arbesfeld DM, Thomas I: Cutaneous herpes simplex infections. Am Fam Physician 43:1655-1664, 1991.

Beauman JG: Genital herpes: A review. Am Fam Physician 72:1527-1534, 2005.

Cunningham AL, et al: The cycle of human herpes simplex virus infection: Virus transport and immune control. J Infect Dis 194(S1):S11-S18, 2006.

Dawkins BJ: Genital herpes simplex infections. Prim Care 17:95-113, 1990.

Kimberlin DW: Neonatal herpes simplex virus infection. Clin Microbiol Rev 17:1-13, 2004.

Landy HJ, Grossman JH III: Herpes simplex virus. Obstet Gynecol Clin North Am 16:495-515, 1989.

National Institute of Allergy and Infectious Diseases, Herpes simplex virus fact sheet: Available at www.niaid.nih.gov/factsheets/stdherp.htm

Rouse BT: Herpes simplex virus: Pathogenesis, immunobiology and control. Curr Top Microbiol Immunol 179:1-179, 1992.

Whitley RJ, Kimberlin DW, Roizman B: Herpes simplex virus: State of the art clinical article. Clin Infect Dis 26:541-555, 1998.

Varicella-Zoster Virus

Chia-Chi Ku V, Besser J, Abendroth A, et al: Varicella-zoster virus pathogenesis and immunobiology: New concepts emerging from investigations with the SCIDhu mouse model. J Virol 79:2651-2658, 2005.

Gnann JW Jr, Whitley RJ: Herpes zoster. New Engl J Med 347:340-346, 2002.

Ostrove JM: Molecular biology of varicella zoster virus. Adv Virus Res 38:45-98, 1990.

White CJ: Varicella-zoster virus vaccine. Clin Infect Dis 24:753-761; quiz 762-763, 1997.

Epstein-Barr Virus

Basgoz N, Preiksaitis JK: Post-transplant lymphoproliferative disorder. Infect Dis Clin North Am 9:901-923, 1995.

Cohen JI: The biology of Epstein-Barr virus: Lessons learned from the virus and the host. Curr Opin Immunol 11:365-370, 1999.

Faulkner GC, Krajewski AS, Crawford DH: The ins and outs of EBV infection. Trends Microbiol 8:185-189, 2000.

Hutt-Fletcher L: Epstein Barr virus entry. J Virol 81:7825-7832, 2007.

Sugden B: EBV's open sesame. Trends Biochem Sci 17:239-240, 1992.

Takada K: Epstein Barr Virus and Human Cancer (Curr Top Microbiol Immunol, vol 258). New York, Springer, 2001.

Thorley-Lawson DA: Epstein-Barr virus and the B cell: That's all it takes. Trends Microbiol 4:204-208, 1996.

Thorley-Lawson DA, Babcock GJ: A model for persistent infection with Epstein-Barr virus: The stealth virus of human B cells. Life Sci 65:1433-1453, 1999.

Cytomegalovirus and Human Herpesviruses 6, 7, and 8

Bigoni B, et al: Human herpesvirus 8 is present in the lymphoid system of healthy persons and can reactivate in the course of AIDS. J Infect Dis 173:542-549, 1996.

Campadelli-Fiume G, Mirandola P, Menotti L: Human herpesvirus 6: An emerging pathogen. Emerg Infect Dis, vol 5 (1999, online): Available at http://www.cdc.gov/ncidod/eid/vol5no3/campadelli

DeBolle L, Naesens L, De Clercq E: Update on human herpesvirus 6 biology, clinical features, and therapy. Clin Microbiol Rev 18: 217-245, 2005.

Gnann JW Jr, Pellett PE, Jaffe HW: Human herpesvirus 8 and Kaposi sarcoma in persons infected with human immunodeficiency virus. Clin Infect Dis 30:S72-S76, 2000.

McDougall JK: Cytomegalovirus. Curr Top Microbiol Immunol 154:1-279, 1990.

Miele PS, Smith MA: Human herpesvirus type 6 (2006, online): Available at http://www.emedicine.com/MED/topic1035.htm

Pellet PE, Black JB, Yamamoto Y: Human herpesvirus 6: The virus and the search for its role as a human pathogen. Adv Virus Res 41:1-52, 1992.

Plachter B, Sinzger C, Jahn G: Cell types involved in replication and distribution of human cytomegalovirus. Adv Virus Res 46:197-264, 1996.

Proceedings of a conference on pathogenesis of cytomegalovirus diseases. Transplant Proc 23(Suppl 3):1-182, 1991.

Shenk TE, Stinski MF (eds): Human Cytomegalovirus Series: Current Topics in Microbiology and Immunology, Vol. 325. New York, Springer-Verlag, 2008.

Stoeckle MY: The spectrum of human herpesvirus 6 infection: From roseola infantum to adult disease. Annu Rev Med 51:423-430, 2000.

Wyatt LS, Frenkel N: Human herpesvirus 7 is a constitutive inhabitant of adult human saliva. J Virol 66:3206-3209, 1992.

Yamanishi K, et al: Identification of human herpesvirus-6 as a causal agent for exanthema subitum. Lancet 1:1065-1067, 1988.

Poxviruses

The poxviruses include the human viruses **variola (smallpox)** (genus *Orthopoxvirus*) and **molluscum contagiosum** (genus *Molluscipoxvirus*), as well as some viruses that naturally infect animals but can cause incidental infection in humans (**zoonosis**). Many of these viruses share antigenic determinants with smallpox, allowing the use of an animal poxvirus for a human vaccine.

In eighteenth-century England, smallpox accounted for 7% to 12% of all deaths and the deaths of one third of children. However, the development of the first live vaccine in 1796 and the later worldwide distribution of this vaccine led to the eradication of smallpox by 1980. As a result, reference stocks of smallpox virus in two World Health Organization (WHO) laboratories were destroyed in 1996 after an international agreement to do so had been reached. Unfortunately, smallpox did not disappear. Stocks of the virus still exist in the United States and in Russia. While the world was successfully eliminating natural smallpox, the former U.S.S.R. (Union of Soviet Socialist Republics) was stockpiling immense amounts of weaponized smallpox virus for biowarfare. Smallpox is considered a *category A agent* by the U.S. Centers for Disease Control and Prevention (CDC), along with anthrax, plague, botulism, tularemia, and viral hemorrhagic fevers, because of their great potential as bioterrorism-biowarfare agents capable of large-scale dissemination and serious disease. The potential for these stocks of smallpox to be acquired and used by a terrorist has been the impetus to renew interest in developing new smallpox vaccine programs and antiviral drugs.

On a positive note, the vaccinia and canary pox viruses have found a beneficial use as gene delivery vectors and for the development of hybrid vaccines. These hybrid viruses contain and express the genes of other infectious agents, and infection results in immunization against both agents.

Structure and Replication

Poxviruses are the largest viruses, almost visible on light microscopy (Box 54-1). They measure 230 × 300 nm and are ovoid to brick shaped with a complex morphology. The poxvirus virion particle must carry many enzymes, including a deoxyribonucleic acid (DNA)–dependent ribonucleic acid (RNA) polymerase, to allow viral messenger RNA (mRNA) synthesis to occur in the cytoplasm. The viral genome consists of a large, double-stranded, linear DNA that is fused at both ends. The structure and replication of vaccinia virus is representative of the other poxviruses (Figure 54-1). The genome of vaccinia virus consists of approximately 189,000 base pairs.

The replication of poxviruses is unique among the DNA-containing viruses, in that the entire multiplication cycle takes place within the host cell cytoplasm (Figure 54-2). As a result, *poxviruses must encode the enzymes required for mRNA and DNA synthesis, as well as activities other DNA viruses normally obtain from the host cell.*

After binding to a cell surface receptor, the poxvirus outer envelope fuses with cellular membranes, either at the cell surface or within the cell. Early gene transcription is initiated on removal of the outer membrane. The virion core contains a specific transcriptional activator and all the enzymes necessary for transcription, including a multisubunit RNA polymerase, as well as enzymes for polyadenylate addition and capping mRNA. Among the early proteins produced is an uncoating protein (uncoatase) that removes the core membrane, thereby liberating viral DNA into the cell cytoplasm. Viral DNA then replicates in electron-dense cytoplasmic inclusions (Guarnieri inclusion bodies), referred to as **factories**. Late viral mRNA for structural, virion, and other proteins is produced after DNA replication. In poxviruses, unlike other viruses, the membranes assemble around the core factories. Approximately 10,000 viral particles are produced per infected cell. Different forms of virus are released by exocytosis or upon cell lysis, but both are infectious.

The vaccinia and canarypox viruses are being used as expression vectors to produce live recombinant/hybrid vaccines for more virulent infectious agents (Figure 54-3). For this process, a plasmid is constructed that contains the foreign gene that encodes the immunizing molecule, flanked by specific poxvirus gene sequences to promote recombination.

Box 54–1. Unique Properties of Poxviruses

Poxviruses are the largest, most complex viruses.

Poxviruses have complex, oval to brick-shaped morphology with internal structure.

Poxviruses have a linear, double-stranded DNA genome with fused ends.

Poxviruses are **DNA viruses that replicate in the cytoplasm**.

Virus encodes and carries all proteins necessary for mRNA synthesis.

Virus also encodes proteins for functions such as DNA synthesis, nucleotide scavenging, and immune escape mechanisms.

Virus is assembled in inclusion bodies (Guarnieri bodies), where it acquires its outer membranes.

This plasmid is inserted into a host cell, which is then infected with the poxvirus. The foreign gene is incorporated into the "rescuing" poxvirus genome because of the homologous viral sequences included on the plasmid. Immunization with the recombinant poxvirus results from expression of the foreign gene and its presentation to the immune response, almost as if by infection with the other agent. A vaccinia hybrid virus containing the G protein of rabies virus soaked onto a bait food and dropped into forests has been used successfully to immunize raccoons, foxes, and other mammals. Experimental vaccines for human immunodeficiency virus, hepatitis B, influenza, and other viruses have also been prepared using these techniques. The potential for producing other vaccines in this manner is unlimited.

Pathogenesis and Immunity

After being inhaled, smallpox virus replicates in the upper respiratory tract (Figure 54-4). Dissemination occurs via lymphatic and cell-associated viremic spread. Internal and dermal tissues are inoculated after a second, more intense viremia, causing the simultaneous eruption of the characteristic "pocks." Molluscum contagiosum and the

Figure 54–2. Replication of vaccinia virus. The core is released into the cytoplasm, where virion enzymes initiate transcription. A viral-encoded "uncoatase" enzyme then causes the release of DNA. Viral polymerase replicates the genome, and late transcription occurs. DNA and protein are assembled into cores with the core membrane. An outer membrane shrouds the core containing the lateral bodies and the enzymes required for infectivity. The virion buds through the plasma membrane or is released by cell lysis. mRNA, messenger RNA.

other poxviruses, however, are acquired through direct contact with lesions and do not spread extensively. Molluscum contagiosum causes a wartlike lesion rather than a lytic infection.

Figure 54–1. A, Structure of the vaccinia virus. Within the virion, the core assumes the shape of a dumbbell because of the large lateral bodies. Virions have a double membrane; the "outer membrane" assembles around the core in the cytoplasm, and the virus leaves the cell by exocytosis or upon cell lysis. **B,** Electron micrographs of orf virus. Note its complex structure.

Figure 54—3. Vaccinia virus as an expression vector for the production of live recombinant vaccines. *(Modified from Piccini A, Paoletti E: Adv Virus Res 34:43-64, 1988.)*

The poxviruses encode many proteins that facilitate their replication and pathogenesis in the host. They include proteins that initially stimulate host cell growth and then lead to cell lysis and viral spread.

Cell-mediated immunity is essential for resolving a poxvirus infection. However, poxviruses encode activities that help the virus evade immune control. These include the cell-to-cell spread of the virus to avoid antibody and proteins that impede the interferon, complement, and inflammatory, antibody, and cell-mediated protective responses. The disease mechanisms of poxviruses are summarized in Box 54-2.

Epidemiology

Smallpox and molluscum contagiosum are strictly human viruses. In contrast, the natural hosts for the other poxviruses important to humans are vertebrates other than humans (e.g., cow, sheep, and goats). The viruses infect humans only through accidental or occupational exposure (zoonosis). A recent outbreak of monkeypox in the United States is such an example. The infected individuals had purchased prairie dog pets that had been in contact with

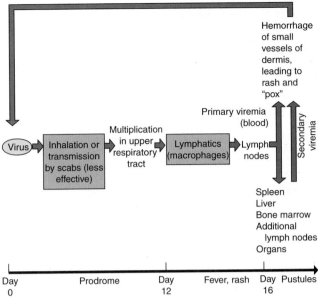

Figure 54—4. Spread of smallpox within the body. The virus enters and replicates in the respiratory tract without causing symptoms or contagion. The virus infects macrophages, which enter the lymphatic system and carry the virus to regional lymph nodes. The virus then replicates and initiates a viremia, causing the infection to spread to the spleen, bone marrow, lymph nodes, liver, and all organs, followed by the skin (rash). A secondary viremia causes the development of additional lesions throughout the host, followed by death or recovery with or without sequelae. Recovery from smallpox was associated with prolonged immunity and lifelong protection.

Gambian giant rats, which were the probable source of the virus. The revival of smallpox vaccination of military personnel has brought with it incidence of vaccine-mediated disease in contacts.

Smallpox (variola) was very contagious and, as just noted, was spread primarily by the respiratory route. It was also spread less efficiently through close contact with dried virus on clothes or other materials. Despite the severity of the disease and its tendency to spread, several factors contributed to its elimination, as listed in Box 54-3.

Clinical Syndromes

The diseases associated with poxviruses are listed in Table 54-1.

Box 54—2. Disease Mechanisms of Poxvirus

Smallpox is initiated by respiratory tract infection and is spread mainly by the lymphatic system and cell-associated viremia.
Molluscum contagiosum and **zoonoses** are transmitted by contact.
Virus may cause initial stimulation of cell growth and then cell lysis.
Virus encodes immune escape mechanisms.
Cell-mediated immunity and humoral immunity are important for resolution.
Most poxviruses share antigenic determinants allowing preparation of ''safe'' live vaccines from animal poxviruses.

Box 54—3. Properties of Natural Smallpox That Led to Its Eradication

Viral Characteristics

Exclusive human host range (no animal reservoirs or vectors)
Single serotype (immunization protected against all infections)

Disease Characteristics

Consistent disease presentation with visible pustules
(identification of sources of contagion allowed quarantine and vaccination of contacts)

Vaccine

Immunization with animal poxviruses protects against smallpox
Stable, inexpensive, and easy-to-administer vaccine
Presence of scar indicating successful vaccination

Public Health Service

Successful worldwide WHO program combining vaccination and quarantine

Figure 54—5. Child with smallpox. Note the characteristic rash.

Smallpox

The two variants of smallpox were variola major, which was associated with a mortality of 15% to 40%, and variola minor, which was associated with a mortality of 1%. Smallpox was usually initiated by infection of the respiratory tract, with subsequent involvement of local lymph glands, which in turn led to viremia.

The symptoms and course of the disease are presented in Figure 54-4, and the characteristic rash is shown in Figure 54-5. After a 5- to 17-day incubation period, the infected person experienced high fever, fatigue, severe headache, backache, and malaise, followed by the vesicular rash in the mouth and soon after on the body. Vomiting, diarrhea, and excessive bleeding would quickly follow. The simultaneous outbreak of the vesicular rash distinguishes smallpox from the vesicles of varicella-zoster, which erupt in successive crops.

Smallpox was usually diagnosed clinically but was confirmed by growth of the virus in embryonated eggs or cell cultures. Characteristic lesions (pocks) appeared on the chorioallantoic membrane of embryonated eggs. New polymerase chain reaction and rapid DNA sequencing techniques are available at the CDC.

Smallpox was the first disease to be controlled by immunization, and its eradication is one of the greatest triumphs of medical epidemiology. Eradication resulted from a massive WHO campaign to vaccinate all susceptible people, especially those exposed to anyone with the disease, and thereby interrupt the chain of human-to-human transmission. The campaign began in 1967 and succeeded. The last

Table 54—1. Diseases Associated with Poxviruses

Virus	Disease	Source	Location
Variola	Smallpox (now extinct)	Humans	Extinct
Vaccinia	Used for smallpox vaccination	Laboratory product	—
Orf	Localized lesion	Zoonosis—sheep, goats	Worldwide
Cowpox	Localized lesion	Zoonosis—rodents, cats, cows	Europe
Pseudocowpox	Milker's nodule	Zoonosis—dairy cows	Worldwide
Monkeypox	Generalized disease	Zoonosis—monkeys, squirrels	Africa
Bovine papular stomatitis virus	Localized lesion	Zoonosis—calves, beef cattle	Worldwide
Tanapox	Localized lesion	Rare zoonosis—monkeys	Africa
Yabapox	Localized lesion	Rare zoonosis—monkeys, baboons	Africa
Molluscum contagiosum	Many skin lesions	Humans	Worldwide

Modified from Balows A, et al (eds): Laboratory Diagnosis of Infectious Diseases: Principles and Practice, vol 2. New York, Springer-Verlag, 1988.

case of naturally acquired infection was reported in 1977, and eradication of the disease was acknowledged in 1980.

Variolation, an early approach to immunization, involved the inoculation of susceptible people with the virulent smallpox pus. It was first performed in the Far East and later in England. Cotton Mather introduced the practice to America. Variolation was associated with a fatality rate of approximately 1%, a better risk than that associated with smallpox itself. In 1796, Jenner developed and then popularized a vaccine using the less virulent cowpox virus, which shares antigenic determinants with smallpox.

As the eradication program neared its goal, it became apparent that the rate of serious reactions to vaccination (see the following discussion of vaccinia) exceeded the risk of infection in the developed world. Therefore, routine smallpox vaccination began to be discontinued in the 1970s and was totally discontinued after 1980. Newer, safer vaccines are being stockpiled in response to concerns regarding the use of smallpox in biowarfare.

Renewed interest is being paid to antiviral drugs that are effective against smallpox and other poxviruses. Cidofovir, a nucleotide analogue capable of inhibiting the viral DNA polymerase, is effective and approved for treatment of poxvirus infections.

Vaccinia and Vaccine-Related Disease
(Clinical Case 54-1)

Vaccinia is the virus used for the smallpox vaccine. Although thought to be derived from cowpox, it may be a hybrid or other poxvirus. The vaccination procedure consisted of scratching live virus into the patient's skin with a bifurcated needle and then observing for the development of vesicles and pustules to confirm a "take." As the incidence of smallpox waned, however, it became apparent that there were more complications related to vaccination than cases of smallpox. Several of these complications were severe and even fatal. They included encephalitis and progressive infection (vaccinia necrosum), the latter occurring occasionally in immunocompromised patients who were inadvertently vaccinated. Recent cases of vaccine-related disease have been noted in family members of immunized military personnel. These individuals are treated with vaccinia immune globulin and antiviral drugs.

Orf, Cowpox, and Monkeypox

Human infection with the orf (poxvirus of sheep and goat) or cowpox (vaccinia) virus is usually an occupational hazard resulting from direct contact with the lesions on the animal. A single nodular lesion usually forms on the point of contact, such as the fingers, hand, or forearm, and is hemorrhagic (cowpox) or granulomatous (orf or pseudocowpox) (Figure 54-6). Vesicular lesions frequently develop and then regress in 25 to 35 days, generally without scar formation. The lesions may be mistaken for anthrax. The virus can be grown in culture or seen directly with electron microscopy but is usually diagnosed from the symptoms and patient history.

The more than 100 cases of illnesses resembling smallpox have been attributed to the monkeypox virus. Except for the outbreak in Illinois, Indiana, and Wisconsin in 2003, they all have occurred in western and central Africa, especially Zaire. Monkeypox causes a milder version of smallpox disease, including the pocklike rash.

Clinical Case 54-1. Vaccinia Infection in Vaccinated Contacts

The CDC (Morb Mortal Wkly Rep 56(17):417-419, 2007) described the case of a woman who visited the public health clinic in Alaska because the pain from vaginal tears had increased over the course of 10 days. There was no fever, itching, or dysuria. Clinical examination showed two shallow ulcers, redness, and vaginal discharge. There was no inguinal lymphadenopathy. A viral specimen from the lesion was identified by the CDC as the vaccine strain of vaccinia virus. Presence of the virus was identified by a variation of a PCR test, which produces characteristic vaccinia DNA fragments from the genome. Although she routinely insists on using condoms during sex, a condom broke during vaginal intercourse with a new male sex partner. The male partner was in the U.S. Military and had been vaccinated for smallpox 3 days prior to initiating his relationship with the woman. Although routine smallpox immunization had been stopped due to elimination of the virus, increased numbers of military and other personnel are receiving vaccinia immunization for protection against weaponized smallpox. This increases the potential for unintentional transmission of the vaccinia vaccine virus. Other cases of vaccine-related vaccinia infection include infants and individuals with atopic dermatitis, who had more severe consequences.

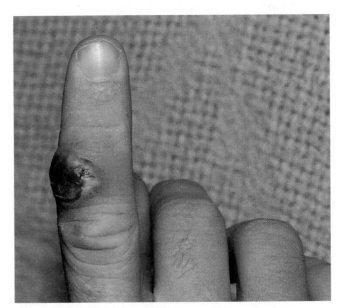

Figure 54–6. Orf lesion on the finger of a taxidermist. (*Courtesy Joe Meyers, MD, Akron, Ohio.*)

Box 54—4. Clinical Summaries

Molluscum contagiosum: A 5-year-old girl has a group of wartlike growths on her arm that exude white material on squeezing.

Molluscum Contagiosum (Box 54-4)

The lesions of molluscum contagiosum differ significantly from pox lesions in being nodular to wartlike (Figure 54-7A). They begin as papules and then become pearl-like, umbilicated nodules that are 2 to 10 mm in diameter and have a central caseous plug that can be squeezed out. They are most common on the trunk, genitalia, and proximal extremities and usually occur in a cluster of 5 to 20 nodules. The incubation period for molluscum contagiosum is 2 to 8 weeks, and the disease is spread by direct contact (e.g., sexual contact, wrestling) or fomites (e.g., towels). The disease is more common in children than adults, but its incidence is increasing in sexually active and immunocompromised individuals.

Figure 54—7. Molluscum contagiosum. **A,** Skin lesions. **B,** Microscopic view; epidermis is filled with molluscum bodies (Magnification 100×).

The diagnosis of molluscum contagiosum is confirmed histologically by the finding of characteristic large, eosinophilic, cytoplasmic inclusions (molluscum bodies) in epithelial cells (Figure 54-7B). These bodies can be seen in biopsy specimens or in the expressed caseous core of a nodule. The molluscum contagiosum virus cannot be grown in tissue culture or animal models.

Lesions of molluscum contagiosum disappear in 2 to 12 months, presumably as a result of immune responses. The nodules can be removed by curettage (scraping) or the application of liquid nitrogen or iodine solutions.

Questions

1. The structure of poxviruses is more complex than that of most other viruses. What problems does this complexity create for viral replication?

2. Poxviruses replicate in the cytoplasm. What problems does this feature create for viral replication?

3. How does the immune response to smallpox infection in an immunologically naïve person differ from that in a vaccinated person? When is antibody present in each case? What stage or stages of viral dissemination are blocked in each case?

4. What characteristics of smallpox facilitated its elimination?

5. Vaccinia virus is being used as a vector for the development of hybrid vaccines. Why is vaccinia virus well suited to this task? Which infectious agents would be appropriate for a vaccinia hybrid vaccine, and why?

Bibliography

Cann AJ: Principles of Molecular Virology. San Diego, Academic, 2005.

Carter J, Saunders V: Virology: Principles and Applications. Chichester, England,Wiley, 2007.

Cohen J, Powderly WG: Infectious Diseases, 2nd ed. St Louis, Mosby, 2004.

Collier L, Oxford J: Human Virology, 3rd ed. Oxford, Oxford University Press, 2006.

Fenner F: A successful eradication campaign: Global eradication of smallpox. Rev Infect Dis 4:916-930, 1982.

Flint SJ, et al: Principles of Virology: Molecular Biology, Pathogenesis, and Control of Animal Viruses, 2nd ed. Washington, DC, ASM Press, 2003.

Gorbach SL, Bartlett JG, Blacklow NR: Infectious Diseases, 2nd ed. Philadelphia, WB Saunders, 1997.

Knipe DM, Howley PM: Fields Virology, 4th ed. New York, Lippincott Williams & Wilkins, 2001.

Mandell GL, Bennet JE, Dolin R: Principles and Practice of Infectious Diseases, 6th ed. Philadelphia, Churchill Livingstone, 2004.

Moyer RW, Turner PC: Poxviruses. Curr Top Microbiol Immunol 163:1-211, 1990.

Piccini A, Paoletti E: Vaccinia: Virus, vector, vaccine. Adv Virus Res 34:43-64, 1988.

Poonawalla TA, Diven D, Kaufman HL, et al: Vaccinia (2006, online): Available at http://www.emedicine.com/med/byname/vaccinia.htm

Strauss JM, Strauss EG: Viruses and Human Disease. San Diego, Academic, 2002.

White DO, Fenner FJ: Medical Virology, 4th ed. New York, Academic, 1994.

Voyles BA: Biology of Viruses, 2nd ed. Boston, McGraw-Hill, 2002.

Parvoviruses

The Parvoviridae are the smallest of the deoxyribonucleic acid (DNA) viruses. Their small size and limited genetic repertoire make them more dependent than any other DNA virus on the host cell, or they require the presence of a helper virus to replicate. Only one member of the Parvoviridae, **B19**, a member of the genus *Parvovirus*, is known to cause human disease.

B19 normally causes **erythema infectiosum**, or **fifth disease**, a mild febrile exanthematous disease that occurs in children. It goes by the latter name because it was counted as one of five classical childhood exanthems (the first four being varicella, rubella, roseola, and measles). B19 is also responsible for episodes of **aplastic crisis in patients with chronic hemolytic anemia** and is associated with **acute polyarthritis** in adults. Intrauterine infection of a fetus may cause abortion.

Other parvoviruses, such as RA-1 (isolated from a person with rheumatoid arthritis) and fecal parvoviruses, have not been shown to cause human disease. Feline and canine parvoviruses do not cause human disease and are preventable with vaccination of the pet.

Adeno-associated viruses (**AAVs**) are members of the genus *Dependovirus* in the family Parvoviridae. They commonly infect humans but replicate only in association with a second "helper" virus, usually an adenovirus. Dependoviruses neither cause illness nor modify infection by their helper viruses. These properties and the propensity of AAVs to integrate into the host chromosome have made genetically modified AAVs candidates for use in **gene-replacement therapy**. A third genus of the family, *Densovirus*, infects only insects.

Structure and Replication

The parvoviruses are extremely small (18 to 26 nm in diameter) and have a nonenveloped, icosahedral capsid (Box 55-1 and Figure 55-1). The B19 virus genome contains one linear, single-stranded deoxyribonucleic acid (DNA) molecule with a molecular mass of 1.5 to 1.8×10^6 Da (5500 bases in length) (Box 55-2). Plus or minus DNA strands are packaged separately into virions. The genome encodes three structural and two major nonstructural proteins. Only one serotype of B19 is known to exist.

B19 virus replicates in mitotically active cells and prefers cells of the erythroid lineage, such as fresh human bone marrow cells, erythroid cells from fetal liver, and erythroid leukemia cells (Figure 55-2). After binding to the erythrocyte blood group P antigen (globoside) and its internalization, the virion is uncoated, and the single-stranded DNA genome is delivered to the nucleus. Factors available only during the S phase of the cell's growth cycle and cellular DNA polymerases are required to generate a complementary DNA strand.

The single-stranded DNA virion genome is converted to a double-stranded DNA version, which is required for transcription and replication. Inverted repeat sequences of DNA at both ends of the genome fold back and hybridize with the genome to create a primer for the cell's DNA polymerase. This creates the complementary strand and replicates the genome. The two major nonstructural proteins and the VP1 and VP2 structural capsid proteins are synthesized in the cytoplasm, and the structural proteins go to the nucleus, where the virion is assembled. The VP2 protein is cleaved later to produce VP3. The nuclear and cytoplasmic membrane degenerates, and the virus is released on cell lysis.

Pathogenesis and Immunity

B19 targets and is cytolytic for erythroid precursor cells (Box 55-3). B19 disease is determined by the direct killing of these cells and the subsequent immune response to the infection (rash and arthralgia).

Studies performed in volunteers suggest that B19 virus first replicates in the nasopharynx or upper respiratory tract then spreads by viremia to the bone marrow and elsewhere, where it replicates and kills erythroid precursor cells (Figure 55-3). The disease has a **biphasic course**.

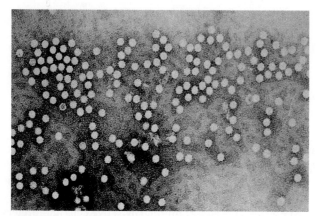

Figure 55–1. Electron micrograph of parvovirus. Parvoviruses are small (18 to 26 nm), nonenveloped viruses with single-stranded DNA. *(Courtesy Centers for Disease Control and Prevention, Atlanta.)*

The *initial febrile stage is the infectious stage.* During this time, erythrocyte production is stopped for approximately 1 week as a result of the viral killing of erythroid precursor cells. A large viremia occurs within 8 days of infection and is accompanied by nonspecific flulike symptoms. Large numbers of virus are also released into oral and respiratory secretions. Antibody stops the viremia and is important for resolution of the disease but contributes to the symptoms.

The *second, symptomatic, stage is immune mediated.* The rash and arthralgia seen in this stage coincide with the appearance of virus-specific antibody, the disappearance of detectable B19 virus, and the formation of immune complexes.

Hosts with chronic hemolytic anemia (e.g., sickle cell anemia) who are infected with B19 are at risk for a life-threatening reticulocytopenia, which is referred to as an **aplastic crisis**. The reticulocytopenia results from the combination of (1) B19 depletion of the red blood cell precursors and (2) shortened life span of the erythrocytes caused by the underlying anemia.

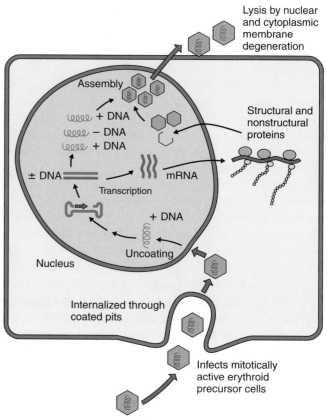

Figure 55–2. Postulated replication of parvovirus (B19) based on information from related viruses (minute virus of mice). The internalized parvovirus delivers its genome to the nucleus, where the single-stranded (plus or minus) DNA is converted to double-stranded DNA by host factors and DNA polymerases present only in growing cells. Transcription, replication, and assembly occur in the nucleus. Virus is released by cell lysis.

Epidemiology

Approximately 65% of the adult population has been infected with B19 by 40 years of age (Box 55-4). Erythema infectiosum is most common in children and adolescents ages 4 to 15 years, who are a source of contagion. Arthralgia and arthritis are

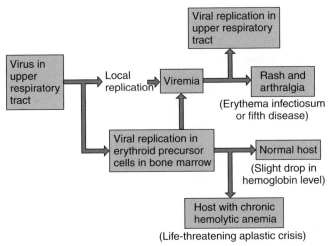

Figure 55—3. Mechanism of spread of parvovirus within the body.

likely to occur in adults. Respiratory droplets and oral secretions most probably transmit the virus. Disease usually occurs in late winter and spring. Parenteral transmission of the virus by blood-clotting-factor concentrate has also been described.

Clinical Syndromes (Clinical Case 55-1)

B19 virus, as stated earlier, is the cause of erythema infectiosum (fifth disease) (Box 55-5). Infection starts with an unremarkable prodromal period of 7 to 10 days, during which the person is contagious. Infection of a normal host may cause either no noticeable symptoms or fever and nonspecific symptoms such as sore throat, chills, malaise, and

myalgia, as well as a slight decrease in hemoglobin levels (Figure 55-4). This period is followed by a distinctive rash on the cheeks, which appear to have been slapped. The rash then usually spreads, especially to exposed skin such as the arms and legs (Figure 55-5), and then subsides over 1 to 2 weeks. Relapse of the rash is common.

B19 infection in adults causes polyarthritis, (with or without a rash) that can last for weeks, months, or longer. Arthritis of the hands, wrists, knees, and ankles predominates. The rash may precede the arthritis but often does not occur. B19 infection of immunocompromised people may result in chronic disease.

The most serious complication of parvovirus infection is the aplastic crisis that occurs in patients with chronic hemolytic anemia (e.g., sickle cell anemia). Infection in these people causes a transient reduction in erythropoiesis in the bone marrow. The reduction results in a transient reticulocytopenia that lasts 7 to 10 days and a decrease in hemoglobin level. An aplastic crisis is accompanied by fever and nonspecific symptoms such as malaise, myalgia, chills, and itching. A maculopapular rash with arthralgia and some joint swelling may also be present.

Box 55—4. Epidemiology of B19 Parvovirus Infection

Disease/Viral Factors

Capsid virus resistant to inactivation
Contagious period precedes symptoms
Virus crosses placenta and infects fetus

Transmission

Transmitted via respiratory droplets

Who Is at Risk?

Children, especially those in elementary school: erythema
    infectiosum (fifth disease)
Parents of children with B19 infection
Pregnant women: fetal infection and disease
People with chronic anemia: aplastic crisis

Geography/Season

Virus found worldwide
Fifth disease more common in late winter and spring

Modes of Control

No modes of control

Box 55—5. Clinical Consequences of Parvovirus (B19) Infection

Mild, flulike illness (fever, headache, chills, myalgia, malaise)
Erythema infectiosum (fifth disease)
Aplastic crisis in people with chronic anemia
Arthropathy (polyarthritis: symptoms in many joints)
Risk of fetal loss as a result of B19 virus crossing the placenta,
    causing anemia-related disease but not congenital anomalies

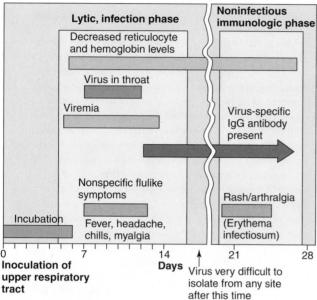

Lytic, infection phase	Noninfectious immunologic phase
Decreased reticulocyte and hemoglobin levels	
Virus in throat	
Viremia	Virus-specific IgG antibody present
Nonspecific flulike symptoms	Rash/arthralgia
Incubation	(Erythema infectiosum)
Fever, headache, chills, myalgia	

0   7   14   21   28

Inoculation of upper respiratory tract   **Days**   Virus very difficult to isolate from any site after this time

Figure 55—4. Time course of parvovirus (B19) infection. B19 causes biphasic disease: first, an initial lytic infection phase characterized by febrile, flulike symptoms and then a noninfectious immunologic phase characterized by a rash and arthralgia.

B19 infection of a seronegative mother increases the risk for fetal death. The virus can infect the fetus and kill erythrocyte precursors, causing anemia and congestive heart failure (**hydrops fetalis**). Infection of seropositive pregnant women often has no adverse effect on the fetus. There is no evidence that B19 causes congenital abnormalities (Box 55-6; see Box 55-5).

Laboratory Diagnosis

The diagnosis of erythema infectiosum is usually based on the clinical presentation. For B19 disease to be definitively

Figure 55—5. A "slapped-cheek" appearance is typical of the rash for erythema infectiosum. *(From Hart CA, Broadhead RL: A Color Atlas of Pediatric Infectious Diseases. London, Wolfe, 1992.)*

Box 55—6. Clinical Summaries

A 10-year-old patient has a 5-day history of a flulike illness (headache, fever, muscle pain, feels tired) then develops an intensely red rash over the cheeks and a fainter "lacy" rash over the trunk and extremities.

diagnosed, however, specific immunoglobulin M (IgM) or viral DNA must be detected (i.e., to distinguish the rash of B19 from that of rubella in a pregnant woman). Enzyme-linked immunosorbent assays for B19 IgM and IgG are available. The polymerase chain reaction test is a very sensitive method for detecting the B19 genome in clinical samples. Virus isolation is not performed.

Treatment, Prevention, and Control

No specific antiviral treatment or means of control is available. Vaccines are available for dog and cat parvoviruses.

Case Study and Questions

Mrs. Doe brought her daughter to the pediatrician with the complaint of a rash. The daughter's face appeared as if it had been slapped, but she had no fever or other notable symptoms. On questioning, Mrs. Doe reported that her daughter had had a mild cold within the previous 2 weeks and that she herself was currently having more joint pain than usual and felt very tired.

1. What features of this history indicate a parvovirus B19 etiology?

2. Was the child infectious at presentation? If not, when was she contagious?

3. What caused the symptoms?

4. Were the symptoms of the mother and daughter related?

5. What underlying condition would put the daughter at increased risk for serious disease after B19 infection? The mother?

6. Why is quarantine a poor means of limiting the spread of B19 parvovirus?

Bibliography

Anderson LJ: Human parvoviruses. J Infect Dis 161:603-608, 1990.
Anderson MJ: Parvoviruses. In Belshe RB (ed): Textbook of Human Virology, 2nd ed. St Louis, Mosby, 1991.
Berns KI: The Parvoviruses. New York, Plenum, 1984.
Berns KI: Parvovirus replication. Microbiol Rev 54:316-329, 1990.
Brown KE, Young NS: Parvovirus B19 in human disease. Annu Rev Med 48:59-67, 1997.
Cann AJ: Principles of Molecular Virology. San Diego, Academic, 2005.
Carter J, Saunders V: Virology: Principles and Applications. Chichester, England, Wiley, 2007.
Chorba T, et al: The role of parvovirus B19 in aplastic crisis and erythema infectiosum (fifth disease). J Infect Dis 154:383-393, 1986.
Cohen J, Powderly WG: Infectious Diseases, 2nd ed. St Louis, Mosby, 2004.
Collier L, Oxford J: Human Virology, 3rd ed. Oxford, Oxford University Press, 2006.

Cunningham D, Rennels MB: Parvovirus B19 (2006, online): Available at http://www.emedicine.com/ped/topic192.htm

Flint SJ, et al: Principles of Virology: Molecular Biology, Pathogenesis and Control of Animal Viruses, 2nd ed. Washington, DC, ASM Press, 2003.

Gorbach SL, Bartlett JG, Blacklow NR: Infectious Diseases, 3rd ed. Philadelphia, WB Saunders, 2004.

Knipe DM, Howley PM: Fields Virology, 4th ed. New York, Lippincott Williams & Wilkins, 2001.

Mandell GL, Bennet JE, Dolin R: Principles and Practice of Infectious Diseases, 6th ed. Philadelphia, Churchill Livingstone, 2005.

Naides SJ, et al: Rheumatologic manifestations of human parvovirus B19 infection in adults. Arthritis Rheum 33:1297-1309, 1990.

Törk TJ: Parvovirus B19 and human disease. Adv Intern Med 37:431-455, 1992.

Voyles BA: The Biology of Viruses, 2nd ed. Boston, McGraw-Hill, 2002.

Ware RE: Parvovirus infections. In Katz SL, Gerson AA, Lotez PJ (eds): Krugman's Infectious Diseases of Children, 10th ed. St. Louis, Mosby, 1998.

Young NS, Brown KE: Parvovirus B19. N Engl J Med 350(6):586-597, 2004.

Picornaviruses

Picornaviridae is one of the largest families of viruses and includes some of the most important human and animal viruses (Box 56-1). As the name indicates, these viruses are **small** *(pico)* **RNA** (ribonucleic acid) viruses that have a **naked capsid** structure. The family has more than 230 members divided into nine genera, including *Enterovirus, Rhinovirus, Hepatovirus, Cardiovirus,* and *Aphthovirus.* The enteroviruses are distinguished from the rhinoviruses by the stability of the capsid at pH 3, the optimum temperature for growth, the mode of transmission, and their diseases (Box 56-2).

At least 71 serotypes of human enteroviruses exist; they are members of the polioviruses, group A or B Coxsackie viruses, or echoviruses. Several different disease syndromes may be caused by a specific serotype of enterovirus. Likewise, several different serotypes may cause the same disease, depending on the target tissue affected. Hepatitis A virus was included in this group but has been reclassified as a *Hepatovirus* and is discussed separately in Chapter 65.

The capsids of enteroviruses are *very resistant to harsh environmental conditions* (sewage systems) and the conditions in the gastrointestinal tract, a fact that facilitates their transmission by the fecal-oral route. Although they may initiate infection in the gastrointestinal tract, the enteroviruses rarely cause enteric disease. In fact, most infections are usually asymptomatic. The best-known and most-studied picornavirus is poliovirus, of which there are three serotypes.

Coxsackieviruses are named after the town of Coxsackie, New York, where they were first isolated. They are divided into two groups, A and B, on the basis of certain biologic and antigenic differences, and are further subdivided into numeric serotypes on the basis of additional antigenic differences.

The name **echovirus** is derived from *e*nteric *c*ytopathic *h*uman *o*rphan, because these agents were not initially thought to be associated with clinical disease. Since 1967, newly isolated enteroviruses have been distinguished numerically.

The human rhinoviruses consist of at least 100 serotypes and are the major cause of the common cold. They are *sensitive to acidic pH and replicate poorly at temperatures above 33° C.* These properties usually limit rhinoviruses to causing upper respiratory tract infections.

Structure

The plus-strand RNA of the picornaviruses is surrounded by an **icosahedral capsid** approximately 30 nm in diameter. The icosahedral capsid has 12 pentameric vertices, each of which is composed of five protomeric units of proteins. The protomers are made of four virion polypeptides (VP1 to VP4). VP2 and VP4 are generated by the cleavage of a precursor, VP0. VP4 in the virion solidifies the structure, but it is not generated until the genome is incorporated into the capsid. This protein is released on binding of the virus to the cellular receptor. The capsids are stable in the presence of heat and detergent; with the exception of the rhinoviruses, they are also stable in acid. The capsid structure is so regular that paracrystals of virions often form in infected cells (Figures 56-1 and 56-2).

The **genome of the picornaviruses resembles a messenger RNA** (mRNA) (Figure 56-3). It is a single strand of plus-sense RNA of approximately 7200 to 8450 bases. It has a poly A at the 3′ end and a small protein, VPg (viral protein genome-linked; 22 to 24 amino acids), attached to the 5′ end. The poly A sequence enhances the infectivity of the RNA, and the VPg may be important in packaging the genome into the capsid and initiating viral RNA synthesis. *The naked picornavirus genome is sufficient to infect a cell.*

The genome encodes a polyprotein that is proteolytically cleaved to produce the enzymatic and structural proteins of the virus. In addition to the capsid proteins and VPg, the picornaviruses encode at least two proteases and an RNA-dependent RNA polymerase. Poliovirus also produces a protease that degrades the 200,000-Da cap-binding protein of eukaryotic ribosomes, thereby blocking the translation of most cellular mRNA.

Box 56–1. Picornaviridae

Enterovirus
  Poliovirus types 1, 2, and 3
  Coxsackie A virus types 1 to 22 and 24
  Coxsackie B virus types 1 to 6
  Echovirus (ECHO virus) types 1 to 9, 11 to 27, and 29 to 34
  Enterovirus 68 to 71
Rhinovirus types 1 to 100+
Cardiovirus
Aphthovirus
Heparnavirus
  Hepatitis A virus

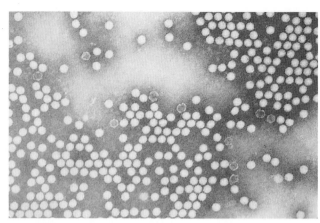

Figure 56–1. Electron micrograph of poliovirus. *(Courtesy Centers for Disease Control and Prevention, Atlanta.)*

Replication

The specificity of the picornavirus interaction for cellular receptors is the major determinant of the target tissue tropism and disease (see Chapter 4, Figure 4-13). The VP1 proteins at the vertices of the virion contain a canyon structure to which the receptor binds. The site of binding is protected from antibody neutralization. Pleconaril and related antiviral compounds contain a 3-methylisoxazole group that binds to the floor of this canyon and alters its conformation to prevent the uncoating of the virus.

The picornaviruses can be categorized according to their cell surface receptor specificity. The receptors for polioviruses, some coxsackieviruses, and rhinoviruses are members of the immunoglobulin superfamily of proteins. At least 80% of the rhinoviruses and several serotypes of coxsackievirus bind to the intercellular adhesion molecule-1 (ICAM-1) expressed on epithelial cells, fibroblasts, and endothelial cells. Several coxsackieviruses, echoviruses, and other enteroviruses bind to decay accelerating factor (CD55). Poliovirus binds to a different molecule (PVR/CD155) that is similar to the receptor for herpes simplex virus. The poliovirus receptor is present on many different human cells, but not all of these cells will replicate the virus.

On binding to the receptor, the VP4 is released and the virion weakened. The genome is then injected directly across the membrane through a channel created by the VP1 protein at one of the vertices of the virion. The genome binds directly to ribosomes, despite the lack of a 5′-cap structure. The ribosomes recognize a unique internal RNA loop in the genome that is also present in some cellular mRNAs. A polyprotein containing all the viral protein sequences is synthesized within 10 to 15 minutes of infection. This polyprotein is cleaved by viral proteases encoded in it. The viral RNA-dependent RNA polymerase generates a negative-strand RNA template from which the new mRNA/genome can be synthesized. The amount of viral mRNA increases rapidly in the cell, with the number of viral RNA molecules reaching as many as 400,000 per cell.

Most picornaviruses inhibit cellular RNA and protein synthesis during infection. For example, cleavage of the 200,000-Da cap-binding protein (EIF4-G) of the ribosome by a poliovirus protease prevents most cellular mRNA from binding to the ribosome. Inhibition of transcription factors decrease cellular mRNA synthesis, and permeability changes induced by picornaviruses reduce the ability of cellular mRNA to bind to the ribosome. In addition, viral mRNA can outcompete cellular mRNA for the factors required in protein synthesis. These activities contribute to the cytopathologic effect of the virus on the target cell.

As the viral genome is being replicated and translated, the structural proteins VP0, VP1, and VP3 are cleaved from the polyprotein by a viral-encoded protease and assembled into subunits. Five **subunits** associate into **pentamers**, and 12 **pentamers** associate to form the **procapsid**. After insertion of the genome, VP0 is cleaved into VP2 and VP4 to complete the **capsid**. As many as 100,000 virions per cell may be produced and released on cell lysis. The entire replication cycle may be as short as 3 to 4 hours.

Box 56–2. Unique Properties of Human Picornaviruses

Virion is a **naked, small** (25 to 30 nm) **icosahedral** capsid enclosing a single-stranded positive RNA genome.
Enteroviruses are resistant to pH 3 to pH 9, detergents, mild sewage treatment, and heat.
Rhinoviruses are labile at acidic pH; optimum growth temperature is 33° C.
Genome is an mRNA.
Naked genome is sufficient for infection.
Virus replicates in cytoplasm.
Viral RNA is translated into polyprotein, which is then cleaved into enzymatic and structural proteins.
Most viruses are **cytolytic.**

Enteroviruses

Pathogenesis and Immunity

Contrary to their name, enteroviruses do not usually cause enteric disease, but they do replicate within and are transmitted by the fecal-oral route. The diseases produced by the

Figure 56–2. **A,** Structure of the human rhinovirus and its interaction with ICAM-1 on the target cell. **B,** Cryoelectron microscopy computer-generated reconstruction of the human rhinovirus 16. **C,** Binding of the ICAM-1 molecule within the canyon of the virion triggers the opening of capsid for release of the genome into the cell. **D,** Cryoelectron microscopy reconstruction of the interaction of a soluble form of ICAM-1 with human rhinovirus 16. *Note:* There is one ICAM-1 per capsomere. ICAM-1, intercellular adhesion molecule-1. (***B** and **D** courtesy of Tim Baker, Purdue University, West Lafayette, Ind.)*

enteroviruses are determined mainly by differences in tissue tropism and the cytolytic capacity of the virus (Figure 56-4; Box 56-3). The upper respiratory tract, the oropharynx, and the intestinal tract are the portals of entry for enteroviruses. The virions are impervious to stomach acid, proteases, and bile. Viral replication is initiated in the mucosa and lymphoid tissue of the tonsils and pharynx, and the virus later infects lymphoid cells of Peyer patches underlying the intestinal mucosa. Primary viremia spreads the virus to receptor-bearing target tissues, including the

reticuloendothelial cells of the lymph nodes, spleen, and liver, to initiate a second phase of viral replication, resulting in a secondary viremia and symptoms.

Most enteroviruses are cytolytic, replicating rapidly and causing direct damage to the target cell. The hepatitis A virus is the exception because it is not very cytolytic. The kinetics of the immune response to hepatitis A correlate with the appearance of symptoms, indicating immunopathogenesis.

In the case of poliovirus, the virus gains access to the brain by infecting skeletal muscle and traveling up the innervating nerves to the brain, like the rabies virus (see Chapter 60). The virus is cytolytic for the motor neurons of the anterior horn and brain stem. The location and number of nerve cells destroyed by the virus govern the extent of paralysis and whether and when other neurons can reinnervate the muscle and restore activity. The combined loss of neurons to polio and to old age may result in paralysis later in life, termed **postpolio syndrome**.

Viral shedding from the oropharynx can be detected for a short time before symptoms begin, whereas viral production and shedding from the intestine may last for 30 days or longer, even in the presence of a humoral immune response.

Figure 56–3. Structure of the picornavirus genome. The genome (7200 to 8400 bases) is translated as a polyprotein, which is cleaved by viral-encoded proteases into individual proteins. g^r, guanidine resistance marker (a genetic locus involved in the initiation of RNA synthesis); Poly A, polyadenylate; •••, internal ribosomal entry site for initiation of protein synthesis.

Figure 56—4. Pathogenesis of enterovirus infection. The target tissue infected by the enterovirus determines the predominant disease caused by the virus. Coxsackie, coxsackievirus; echo, echovirus; HAV, hepatitis A virus; polio, poliovirus; rhino, rhinovirus.

Antibody is the major protective immune response to the enteroviruses. Secretory antibody can prevent the initial establishment of infection in the oropharynx and gastrointestinal tract, and serum antibody prevents viremic spread to the target tissue and therefore disease. The time course for antibody development after infection with a live vaccine is presented in Figure 56-10.

Cell-mediated immunity is not usually involved in protection but may play a role in pathogenesis. Hepatitis A virus is the exception, in that T cells are important for the resolution of the disease and are a major determinate of the pathogenesis.

Box 56—3. Disease Mechanisms of Picornaviruses

Enteroviruses enter via the oropharynx, intestinal mucosa, or upper respiratory tract and infect the underlying lymphatic tissue; rhinoviruses are restricted to the upper respiratory tract

In the absence of serum antibody, enterovirus spreads by viremia to cells of a receptor-bearing target tissue

Different picornaviruses bind to different receptors, many of which are members of the immunoglobulin superfamily (i.e., ICAM-1)

The infected target tissue determines the subsequent disease

Viral, rather than immune, pathologic effects are usually responsible for causing disease symptoms

The secretory antibody response is transitory but can prevent the initiation of infection

Serum antibody blocks viremic spread to target tissue, preventing symptoms

Enterovirus is shed in feces for long periods

Infection is often asymptomatic or causes mild, flulike or upper respiratory tract disease

---

T cells also appear to contribute to the pathogenesis of Coxsackie B virus—induced myocarditis in mice.

Epidemiology

The enteroviruses are exclusively human pathogens (Box 56-4). As the name implies, these viruses primarily spread via the **fecal-oral** route. **Asymptomatic shedding** can occur for up to a month, putting virus into the environment. Poor sanitation and crowded living conditions foster transmission of the viruses (Figure 56-5). Sewage contamination of water supplies can result in enterovirus epidemics. Outbreaks of enterovirus disease are seen in schools and daycare settings, and summer is the major season for such disease. The coxsackieviruses and echoviruses may also be spread in aerosol droplets and cause respiratory tract infections.

With the success of the polio vaccines, the wild-type poliovirus has been eliminated from the western hemisphere (Figure 56-6) and most, but not all, of the world. Paralytic polio is still prevalent in Africa and remains endemic in Afghanistan, Pakistan, India, and Nigeria. Wild-type polio also occurs in

---

Box 56—4. Epidemiology of Enterovirus Infections

Disease/Viral Factors

Nature of disease correlates with specific enterovirus and age of person
Infection often asymptomatic, with viral shedding
Virion resistant to environmental conditions (detergents, acid, drying, mild sewage treatment, and heat)

Transmission

Fecal-oral route: poor hygiene, dirty diapers (especially in daycare settings)
Ingestion via contaminated food and water
Contact with infected hands and fomites
Inhalation of infectious aerosols

Who Is at Risk?

Young children: at risk for polio (asymptomatic or mild disease)
Older children and adults: at risk for polio (asymptomatic to paralytic disease)
Newborns and neonates: at highest risk for serious coxsackievirus and enterovirus disease

Geography/Season

Viruses have worldwide distribution; wild-type polio virtually eradicated in developed countries because of vaccination programs
Disease more common in summer

Modes of Control

For polio, live oral polio vaccine (trivalent OPV) or inactivated trivalent polio vaccine (IPV) is administered
For other enteroviruses, no vaccine; good hygiene limits spread

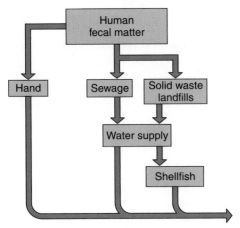

Figure 56—5. Transmission of enteroviruses. The capsid structure is resistant to mild sewage treatment, salt water, detergents, and temperature changes, allowing these viruses to be transmitted by fecal-oral routes, fomites, and on hands.

areas where the vaccine is not available and in communities where vaccination is contrary to religious beliefs or other teachings. A small but significant number of vaccine-related cases of polio result from the reversion of the live vaccine virus and its reestablishing neurovirulence. This development has prompted a change to promote the use of the inactivated polio vaccine. Polioviruses are spread most often during the summer and autumn.

Paralytic polio was once considered a middle class disease, because good hygiene would delay exposure of a person to the virus until late childhood, the adolescent years, or adulthood, when infection would produce the most severe symptoms. Infection during early childhood generally results in asymptomatic or very mild disease.

Like poliovirus infection, Coxsackie A virus disease is generally more severe in adults than in children. However, Coxsackie B virus and some of the echoviruses (especially echovirus 11) can be particularly harmful to infants.

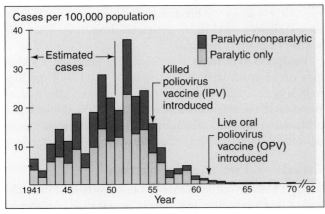

Figure 56—6. Incidence of polio in the United States. Killed (inactivated) poliovirus vaccine (IPV) was introduced in 1955, and live (oral) poliovirus vaccine (OPV) was introduced in 1961 and 1962. Wild-type polio has been eradicated in the United States. (*Courtesy Centers for Disease Control and Prevention: Immunization Against Disease: 1972. Washington, DC, U.S. Government Printing Office, 1973.*)

Clinical Syndromes

The clinical syndromes produced by the enteroviruses are determined by several factors, including: (1) viral serotype, (2) infecting dose, (3) tissue tropism, (4) portal of entry, (5) patient's age, gender, and state of health, and (6) pregnancy (Table 56-1). The incubation period for enterovirus disease varies from 1 to 35 days, depending on the virus, the target tissue, and the person's age. Viruses that affect oral and respiratory sites have the shortest incubation periods.

Poliovirus Infections

Wild-type polio infections are rare because of the success of the polio vaccines (see Figure 56-6). As noted earlier, however, vaccine-associated cases of polio do occur, and some populations remain unvaccinated, putting them at risk for infection. Poliovirus may cause one of the following four outcomes in unvaccinated people, depending on the progression of the infection (Figure 56-7):

1. **Asymptomatic illness** results if the viral infection is limited to the oropharynx and the gut. At least 90% of poliovirus infections are asymptomatic.
2. **Abortive poliomyelitis,** the **minor illness,** is a nonspecific febrile illness occurring in approximately 5% of infected people. Fever, headache, malaise, sore throat, and vomiting occur in such people within 3 to 4 days of exposure.
3. **Nonparalytic poliomyelitis** or **aseptic meningitis** occurs in 1% to 2% of patients with poliovirus infections. In this disease, the virus progresses into the central nervous system and the meninges, causing back pain and muscle spasms in addition to the symptoms of the minor illness.
4. **Paralytic polio,** the **major illness,** occurs in 0.1% to 2.0% of persons with poliovirus infections and is the most severe outcome. It appears 3 to 4 days after the minor illness has subsided, thereby producing a biphasic illness. In this disease, the virus spreads from the blood to the **anterior horn cells** of the spinal cord and to the motor cortex of the brain. The severity of paralysis is determined by the extent of the neuronal infection and by which neurons are affected. Spinal paralysis may involve one or more limbs, whereas bulbar (cranial) paralysis may involve a combination of cranial nerves and even the medullary respiratory center.

Paralytic poliomyelitis is characterized by an asymmetrical flaccid paralysis with no sensory loss. Poliovirus type 1 is responsible for 85% of the cases of paralytic polio. Reversion of the attenuated vaccine virus types 2 and 3 to virulence can cause vaccine-associated disease.

The degree of paralysis varies, in that it may involve only a few muscle groups (e.g., one leg) or there may be complete flaccid paralysis of all four extremities. The paralysis may then progress over the first few days and may result in

Table 56–1. Summary of Clinical Syndromes Associated with Major Enterovirus Groups

Syndrome	Occurrence	Polioviruses	Coxsackie A Viruses	Coxsackie B Viruses	Echoviruses
Paralytic disease	Sporadic	+	+	+	+
Encephalitis, meningitis	Outbreaks	+	+	+	+
Carditis	Sporadic		+	+	+
Neonatal disease	Outbreaks			+	+
Pleurodynia	Outbreaks			+	
Herpangina	Common		+		
Hand-foot-and-mouth disease	Common		+		
Rash disease	Common		+	+	+
Acute hemorrhagic conjunctivitis	Epidemics		+		
Respiratory tract infections	Common	+	+	+	+
Undifferentiated fever	Common	+	+	+	+
Diarrhea, gastrointestinal disease	Uncommon				+
Diabetes, pancreatitis	Uncommon			+	
Orchitis	Uncommon			+	
Disease in immunodeficient patients	—	+	+		+
Congenital anomalies	Uncommon		+	+	

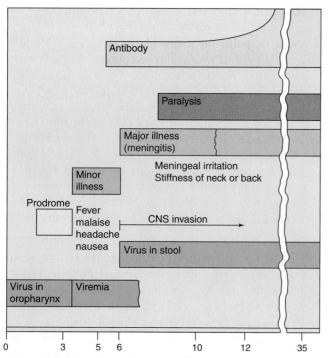

Figure 56–7. Progression of poliovirus infection. Infection may be asymptomatic or may progress to minor or major disease. CNS, central nervous system.

complete recovery, residual paralysis, or death. Most recoveries occur within 6 months, but as long as 2 years may be required for complete remission.

Bulbar poliomyelitis can be more severe, may involve the muscles of the pharynx, vocal cords, and respiration, and may result in death in 75% of patients. Iron lungs, chambers that provided external respiratory compression, were used during the 1950s to assist the breathing of patients with such polio disease. Before vaccination programs, iron lungs filled the wards of children's hospitals.

Postpolio syndrome is a sequela of poliomyelitis that may occur much later in life (30 to 40 years later) in 20% to 80% of the original victims. Affected people suffer a deterioration of the originally affected muscles. Poliovirus is not present, but the syndrome is believed to result from a loss of neurons in the initially affected nerves.

Coxsackievirus and Echovirus Infections

Several clinical syndromes may be caused by either a coxsackievirus or an echovirus (e.g., aseptic meningitis), but certain illnesses are specifically associated with coxsackieviruses. Coxsackie A viruses are associated with diseases involving vesicular lesions (e.g., herpangina), whereas Coxsackie B viruses (**B for *body***) are most frequently associated with myocarditis and pleurodynia. The coxsackieviruses can also cause

Figure 56–9. Hand-foot-and-mouth disease caused by Coxsackie A virus. Lesions initially appear in the oral cavity and then develop within 1 day on the palms and, as seen here, on soles. *(From Habif TP: Clinical Dermatology: A Color Guide to Diagnosis and Therapy, 3rd ed. St Louis, Mosby, 1996.)*

a polio-like paralytic disease (Clinical Case 56-1). The most common result of infection is lack of symptoms or a mild upper respiratory tract or flulike disease.

Herpangina is caused by several types of Coxsackie A virus and is not related to a herpesvirus infection. Fever, sore throat, pain on swallowing, anorexia, and vomiting characterize this disease. The classic finding is vesicular ulcerated lesions around the soft palate and uvula (Figure 56-8). Less typically, the lesions affect the hard palate. The virus can be recovered from the lesions or from feces. The disease is self-limited and requires only symptomatic management.

Hand-foot-and-mouth disease is a vesicular exanthem usually caused by coxsackievirus A16. The name is descriptive, because the main features of this infection consist of

Figure 56–8. Herpangina. Characteristic discrete vesicles are seen on the anterior tonsillar pillars. *(Courtesy Dr. GDW McKendrick. From Lambert HP, et al: Infectious Diseases Illustrated. London, Gower, 1982.)*

vesicular lesions on the hands, feet, mouth, and tongue (Figure 56-9). The patient is mildly febrile, and the illness subsides in a few days.

Pleurodynia (Bornholm disease), also known as the **devil's grip**, is an acute illness in which patients have a sudden onset of fever and unilateral low thoracic, pleuritic chest pain that may be excruciating. Abdominal pain and even vomiting may also occur, and muscles on the involved side may be extremely tender. Pleurodynia lasts an average of 4 days but may relapse after the condition has been asymptomatic for several days. Coxsackie B virus is the causative agent.

Myocardial and **pericardial infections** caused by Coxsackie B virus occur sporadically in older children and adults but are most threatening in newborns. Neonates with these infections have febrile illnesses and sudden and unexplained onset of heart failure. Cyanosis, tachycardia, cardiomegaly, and hepatomegaly occur. Electrocardiographic changes are found in patients with myocarditis. The mortality associated with the infection is high, and autopsy typically reveals the involvement of other organ systems, including the brain, liver, and pancreas. Acute benign pericarditis affects young adults but may be seen in older people. The symptoms resemble those of myocardial infarction with fever.

Viral (aseptic) meningitis is an acute febrile illness accompanied by headache and signs of meningeal irritation, including nuchal rigidity. Petechiae or a rash may occur in patients with enteroviral meningitis. Recovery is usually uneventful, unless the illness is associated with encephalitis (meningoencephalitis) or occurs in children younger than 1 year. Outbreaks of picornavirus meningitis (echovirus 11) occur each year during the summer and autumn.

Fever, rash, and **common coldlike symptoms** may occur in patients infected with echoviruses or coxsackieviruses. The rash is usually maculopapular but may occasionally be petechial or even vesicular. The petechial type of eruption must be differentiated from that of meningococcemia.

The symptoms of enteroviral infection are less intense for the child than meningococcemia. Coxsackieviruses A21 and A24 and echoviruses 11 and 20 can cause rhinovirus-like symptoms resembling the common cold.

Other Enterovirus Diseases

Enterovirus 70 and a variant of coxsackievirus A24 have been associated with an extremely contagious ocular disease, **acute hemorrhagic conjunctivitis**. The infection causes subconjunctival hemorrhages and conjunctivitis. The disease has a 24-hour incubation period and resolves within 1 or 2 weeks. Some strains of Coxsackie B virus and echovirus can be transmitted transplacentally to the fetus. Infection of the fetus or an infant by this or another route may produce severe disseminated disease. Coxsackie B virus infections of the pancreas have been suspected of causing insulin-dependent diabetes as a result of the destruction of the islets of Langerhans.

Laboratory Diagnosis

Clinical Chemistry

Cerebrospinal fluid (CSF) from poliovirus or enterovirus aseptic meningitis reveals a predominantly lymphocytic pleocytosis (presence of 25 to 500 cells/mm^3). In contrast with bacterial meningitis, the CSF in viral meningitis lacks neutrophils, and the glucose level is usually normal or slightly low. The CSF protein level is normal to slightly elevated. The CSF is rarely positive for the virus.

Culture

Polioviruses may be isolated from the patient's pharynx during the first few days of illness, from the feces for as long as 30 days, but only rarely from the CSF. The virus grows well in monkey kidney tissue culture. Coxsackieviruses and echoviruses can usually be isolated from the throat and stool during infection and often from the CSF in patients with meningitis. Virus is rarely isolated in patients with myocarditis, because the symptoms occur several weeks after the initial infection. The Coxsackie B viruses can be grown on primary monkey or human embryo kidney cells. Many strains of Coxsackie A virus do not grow in tissue culture, however, and must still be grown in suckling mice.

Genome and Serology Studies

The exact type of enterovirus can be determined through the use of specific antibody and antigen assays (e.g., neutralization, immunofluorescence, enzyme-linked immunosorbent assay) or reverse transcriptase polymerase chain reaction (RT-PCR) detection of specific viral RNA. RT-PCR of clinical samples has become a rapid and routine method for confirming a diagnosis of echovirus 11 meningitis in an infant, as well as other picornavirus diseases.

Serology is used to confirm an enterovirus infection through detection of specific immunoglobulin (Ig)M or the finding of a fourfold increase in the antibody titer between the time of the acute illness and the period of convalescence. Because of their many serotypes, this approach may not be practical for detection of echovirus and coxsackievirus unless a specific virus is suspected.

Treatment, Prevention, and Control

A new antiviral drug, pleconaril, is available on a limited basis. The drug inhibits the penetration of picornaviruses into the cell. It must be administered early in the course of the infection.

The prevention of paralytic poliomyelitis is one of the triumphs of modern medicine. By 1979, infections with the wild-type poliovirus disappeared from the United States, with the number of cases of polio decreasing from 21,000 per year in the prevaccine era to 18 in unvaccinated patients in 1977. Like smallpox, polio has been targeted for elimination. Health care delivery to underdeveloped countries is more difficult, and for this reason, wild-type viral disease still exists in Africa, the Middle East, and Asia. Misinformation, misunderstanding, and political unrest in Africa and other parts of the world have also limited acceptance of polio vaccination. New worldwide vaccination programs have been developed to reach the goal.

The two types of poliovirus vaccine are (1) **inactivated polio vaccine (IPV)**, developed by Jonas Salk, and (2) **live attenuated oral polio vaccine (OPV)**, developed by Albert Sabin. Both vaccines incorporate the three strains of polio, are stable, are relatively inexpensive, and induce a protective antibody response (Figure 56-10). The IPV was proven effective in 1955, but the oral vaccine took its place because it is inexpensive, easy to administer, and elicits lifelong immunity (Table 56-2).

The OPV was **attenuated** (i.e., rendered less virulent) by passage in human or monkey cell cultures. Attenuation yielded a virus that can replicate in the oropharynx and intestinal tract but cannot infect neuronal cells. A mixed blessing of the live vaccine strain is that it is shed in feces for weeks and may be spread to close contacts. The spread will immunize or reimmunize close contacts, thus promoting mass immunization. The major drawbacks of the live vaccine are that (1) the vaccine virus may infect an immunologically compromised individual and (2) there is a remote potential for the virus to revert to its virulent form and cause paralytic disease. The incidence of paralytic disease is estimated to be one per 4 million doses administered (versus one in 100 people infected with the wild-type poliovirus).

In the absence of wild-type poliovirus, new recommendations call for the use of the IPV for routine vaccination. Children should receive the IPV at 2 months, 4 months, and 15 months and then at 4 to 6 years of age. Alternatively, the first two doses of IPV can be followed by OPV.

There are no vaccines for coxsackieviruses or echoviruses. Transmission of these viruses can presumably be reduced by improvements in hygiene and living conditions.

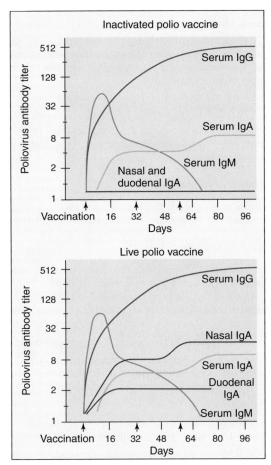

Figure 56—10. Serum and secretory antibody response to intramuscular inoculation of inactivated polio vaccine and to live attenuated oral polio vaccine. Note the presence of secretory IgA induced by the live polio vaccine. (*Redrawn from Ogra P, et al: Rev Infect Dis 2:352-369, 1980. Copyright 1980, University of Chicago Press.*)

Rhinoviruses

Rhinoviruses are the most important cause of the **common cold** and upper respiratory tract infections. Such infections are self-limited, however, and do not cause serious disease. More than 100 serotypes of rhinovirus have been identified. At least 80% of the rhinoviruses have a common receptor that is also used by some of the coxsackieviruses. This receptor has been identified as ICAM-1, a member of the immunoglobulin superfamily, which is expressed on epithelial, fibroblast, and B-lymphoblastoid cells.

Pathogenesis and Immunity

Unlike the enteroviruses, rhinoviruses are **unable to replicate in the gastrointestinal tract** (see Box 56-3). The rhinoviruses are **labile to acidic pH**. Also, they **grow best at 33° C**, a feature that may partly account for their predilection for the cooler environment of the nasal mucosa. Infection can be initiated by as little as one infectious viral particle. During the peak of illness, nasal secretions contain concentrations of 500 to 1000 infectious virions per milliliter. The virus enters through the nose, mouth, or eyes and initiates infection of the upper respiratory tract, including the throat. Most viral replication occurs in the nose, and the onset and the severity of the symptoms correlate with the time of viral shedding and the quantity (titer) of virus shed. Infected cells release bradykinin and histamine, which cause a "runny nose."

Interferon, which is generated in response to the infection, may limit the progression of the infection and contribute to the symptoms. Interestingly, the release of cytokines during inflammation can promote the spread of the virus by enhancing the expression of ICAM-1 viral receptors.

Immunity to rhinoviruses is transient and unlikely to prevent subsequent infection because of the numerous serotypes of the virus. Both nasal secretory IgA and serum IgG

Table 56—2. Advantages and Disadvantages of Polio Vaccines

Vaccine	Advantages	Disadvantages
Live (oral polio vaccine)	Effective Lifelong immunity Induction of secretory antibody response similar to that of natural infection Spread of attenuated virus circulating to contacts promotes indirect immunization (herd immunity) Inexpensive and easy to administer No need for repeated booster vaccine	Risk of vaccine-associated poliomyelitis in vaccine recipients or contacts; spread of vaccine to contacts without their consent Not safe for administration to immunodeficient patients
Inactivated polio vaccine	Effective Good stability during transport and in storage Safe administration in immunodeficient patients No risk of vaccine-related disease	Lack of induction of secretory antibody Booster vaccine needed for lifelong immunity Requires sterile syringes and needles Injection more painful than oral administration Higher community immunization levels needed than with live vaccine

antibody are induced by a primary rhinovirus infection and can be detected within a week of infection. The secretory IgA response dissipates quickly, and immunity begins to wane approximately 18 months after infection. Cell-mediated immunity is not likely to play an important role in controlling rhinovirus infections.

Epidemiology

Rhinoviruses cause at least half of all upper respiratory tract infections (Box 56-5). Other agents likely to cause the symptoms of the common cold are enteroviruses, coronaviruses, adenoviruses, and parainfluenza viruses. Rhinoviruses can be transmitted by two mechanisms: as aerosols and on fomites (e.g., by hands or on contaminated inanimate objects). Hands appear to be the major vector, and direct person-to-person contact is the predominant mode of spread. These nonenveloped viruses are extremely stable and can survive on such objects for many hours.

Rhinoviruses produce clinical illness in only half of the people infected. Asymptomatic people are also capable of spreading the virus, even though they may produce less of it.

Rhinovirus "colds" occur most often in early autumn and late spring in people living in temperate climates. This may reflect social patterns (e.g., return to school and daycare) rather than any change in the virus itself.

Rates of infection are highest in infants and children. Children younger than 2 years "share" their colds with their families. Secondary infections occur in approximately 50% of family members, especially other children.

Many different rhinovirus serotypes may be found in a given community during a specific cold season, but the

---

Box 56–5. Epidemiology of Rhinovirus Infections

Disease/Viral Factors

Virion is resistant to drying and detergents
Multiple serotypes preclude prior immunity
Replication occurs at optimum temperature of 33° C and cooler
 temperatures

Transmission

Direct contact via infected hands and fomites
Inhalation of infectious droplets

Who Is at Risk?

People of all ages

Geography/Season

Virus found worldwide
Disease more common in early autumn and late spring

Modes of Control

Washing hands and disinfecting contaminated objects help
 prevent spread

Box 56–6. Clinical Summaries

Polio: A 12-year-old girl from Kenya has headache, fever, nausea, and stiff neck. Symptoms improve and then recur several days later, with weakness and paralysis of her legs. She has no history of polio immunization

Coxsackie A Virus

Herpangina: Vesicular lesions on the tongue and roof of the mouth of a 7-year-old patient accompany fever, sore throat, and pain on swallowing

Coxsackie B (B for Body) Virus

Pleurodynia: A 13-year-old boy has fever and severe chest pain with headache, fatigue, and aching muscles lasting for 4 days

Coxsackie or Echovirus

Aseptic meningitis: A 7-month-old infant with fever and rash appears listless, with a stiff neck. A sample of his cerebrospinal fluid contains lymphocytes but has normal glucose and no bacteria. Full recovery occurs within 1 week

Common Cold (Rhinovirus)

A 25-year-old person develops runny nose, mild cough, and malaise with a low-grade fever. A co-worker in the office has had similar symptoms for the past few days

---

predominant strains are usually the newly categorized serotypes. This pattern indicates the existence of a gradual antigenic drift (mutation) similar to that seen for the influenza virus.

Clinical Syndromes (Box 56-6)

Common cold symptoms caused by rhinoviruses cannot readily be distinguished from those caused by other viral respiratory pathogens (e.g., enteroviruses, paramyxoviruses, coronaviruses). An upper respiratory tract infection usually begins with sneezing, which is soon followed by rhinorrhea (runny nose). The rhinorrhea increases and is then accompanied by symptoms of nasal obstruction. Mild sore throat also occurs, along with headache and malaise but usually without fever. The illness peaks in 3 to 4 days, but the cough and nasal symptoms may persist for 7 to 10 days or longer.

Laboratory Diagnosis

The clinical syndrome of the common cold is usually so characteristic that laboratory diagnosis is unnecessary. Virus can be obtained from nasal washings. Rhinoviruses are grown in human diploid fibroblast cells (e.g., WI-38) at 33° C. Virus is identified by the typical cytopathologic effect and the demonstration of acid lability. Serotyping is rarely necessary but can be performed with the use of pools of specific neutralizing sera. The performance of serologic testing to document rhinovirus infection is not practical.

Treatment, Prevention, and Control

There are many over-the-counter remedies for the common cold. Nasal vasoconstrictors may provide relief, but their use may be followed by rebound congestion and a worsening of symptoms. Inhaling hot, humidified air and even the steam from hot chicken soup may actually help by increasing nasal drainage.

No antiviral drugs are effective. Pleconaril and similar experimental antiviral drugs (e.g., arildone, rhodanine, disoxaril) contain a 3-methylisoxazole group that inserts into the base of the receptor-binding canyon and blocks uncoating of the virus. Enviroxime inhibits the viral RNA–dependent RNA polymerase. A polypeptide receptor analogue based on the ICAM-1 protein structure has also been evaluated as an antiviral drug. The intranasal administration of interferon can block infection for a short time after a known exposure, but its long-term use (e.g., throughout the "cold season") could cause symptoms at least as bad as those of the rhinovirus infection.

Rhinovirus is not a good candidate for a vaccine program. The multiple serotypes, the apparent antigenic drift in rhinoviral antigens, the requirement for secretory IgA production, and the transience of the antibody response pose major problems for the development of vaccines. In addition, the benefit-to-risk ratio would be very low because rhinoviruses do not cause significant disease.

Handwashing and the disinfection of contaminated objects are the best means of preventing the spread of the virus. Virucidal facial tissues impregnated with citric acid may also limit rhinovirus spread.

Bibliography

Ansardi D, et al: Poliovirus assembly and encapsidation of genomic RNA. Adv Virus Res 46:2-70, 1996.

Buenz EJ, Howe CL: Picornaviruses and cell death. Trends Microbiol 14:28-38, 2006.

Cann AJ: Principles of Molecular Virology. San Diego, Academic, 2005.

Carter J, Saunders V: Virology: Principles and Applications. Chichester, England, Wiley, 2007.

Centers for Disease Control and Prevention: Progress toward interruption of wild poliovirus transmission worldwide, January 2006-May 2007. Morb Mortal Wkly Rep 56(26):682-685, 2007.

Cohen J, Powderly WG: Infectious Diseases, 2nd ed. St Louis, Mosby, 2004.

Collier L, Oxford J: Human Virology, 3rd ed. Oxford, Oxford University Press, 2006.

Flint SJ, et al: Principles of Virology: Molecular Biology, Pathogenesis, and Control of Animal Viruses, 2nd ed. Washington, DC, ASM Press, 2003.

Knipe DM, Howley PM: Fields Virology, 4th ed. New York, Lippincott Williams & Wilkins, 2001.

Levandowski RA: Rhinoviruses. In Belshe RB (ed): Textbook of Human Virology, 2nd ed. St Louis, Mosby, 1991.

McKinlay MA, et al: Treatment of the picornavirus common cold by inhibitors of viral uncoating and attachment. Ann Rev Microbiol 46:635-654, 1992.

Moore M, Morens DM: Enteroviruses including polioviruses. In Belshe RB (ed): Textbook of Human Virology, 2nd ed. St Louis, Mosby, 1991.

Plotkin SA, Vidor E: Poliovirus vaccine—Inactive. In Plotkin SA, Orenstein WA (eds): Vaccines, 4th ed. Philadelphia, WB Saunders, 2004.

Racaniello VR: One hundred years of poliovirus pathogenesis. Virology 344:9-16, 2006.

Robbins FC: The history of polio vaccine development. In Plotkin SA, Orenstein WA (eds): Vaccines, 4th ed. Philadelphia, WB Saunders, 2004.

Strauss JM, Strauss EG: Viruses and Human Disease. San Diego, Academic, 2002.

Sutter RW, et al: Poliovirus vaccine—Live. In Plotkin SA, Orenstein WA (eds): Vaccines, 4th ed. Philadelphia, WB Saunders, 2004.

Tracy S, Chapman NM, Mahy BWJ: Coxsackie B Viruses (Curr Top Microbiol Immunol, vol 223. Berlin, Springer-Verlag, 1997.

Voyles BA: The Biology of Viruses, 2nd ed. Boston, McGraw-Hill, 2002.

Wilfert CM, et al: Enteroviruses and meningitis. Pediatr Infect Dis 2:333-341, 1983.

Websites

Hendrickson CS, Sloan SB, Alsina-Gibert M, Llambrich-Mañes A: Enteroviral infections (2006, online): Available at http://www.emedicine.com/derm/topic875.htm

Larry I, Lutwick LI, Bron Y: Picornavirus-overview (2006, online): Available at http://www.emedicine.com/med/topic1831.htm

Picornaviridae online: Available at http://www.picornaviridae.com

Tolan RW, Jr, Nguyen NM, Korb JD: Rhinovirus infection (2006, online): Available at http://www.emedicine.com/ped/topic2707.htm

Case Study and Questions

A 6-year-old girl was brought to the doctor's office at 4:30 PM because she had a sore throat, had been unusually tired, and was napping excessively. Her temperature was 39° C. She had a sore throat, enlarged tonsils, and a faint rash on her back. At 10:30 PM, the patient's mother reported that the child had vomited three times, continued to nap excessively, and complained of a headache when awake.

The doctor examined the child at 11:30 PM and noted that she was lethargic and aroused only when her head was turned, complaining that her back hurt. Her CSF contained no red blood cells, but there were 28 white blood cells/mm³, half polymorphonuclear neutrophils and half lymphocytes. The glucose and protein levels in the CSF were normal, and Gram stain of a specimen of CSF showed no bacteria.

1. What were the key signs and symptoms in this case?

2. What was the differential diagnosis?

3. What signs and symptoms suggested an enterovirus infection?

4. How would the diagnosis be confirmed?

5. What were the most likely sources and means of infection?

6. What were the target tissue and mechanism of pathogenesis?

Coronaviruses and Noroviruses

Coronaviruses

Coronaviruses are named for the solar corona–like appearance (the surface projections) of their virions when viewed with an electron microscope (Figure 57-1). Coronaviruses are the second most prevalent cause of the **common cold** (rhinoviruses are the first). In 2002, an outbreak of **severe acute respiratory syndrome (SARS)** in Guangdong Province, South China, spread to Hong Kong and then around the world. It was shown that the disease was caused by a coronavirus **(SARS-CoV)**. Electron microscopy findings have also linked coronaviruses to gastroenteritis in children and adults.

Structure and Replication

Coronaviruses are **enveloped virions** with the longest **positive (+) RNA** genome. Virions measure 80 to 160 nm in diameter (Box 57-1). The glycoproteins on the surface of the envelope appear as club-shaped projections that appear as a halo (corona) around the virus. Unlike most enveloped viruses, the "corona" formed by the glycoproteins allows the virus to endure the conditions in the gastrointestinal tract and be spread by the fecal-oral route.

The large, plus-stranded RNA genome (27,000 to 30,000 bases) associates with the N protein to form a helical nucleocapsid. Protein synthesis occurs in two phases, similar to that of the togaviruses. On infection, the genome is translated to produce a polyprotein that is cleaved to produce an RNA-dependent RNA polymerase (L [225,000Da]). The polymerase generates a negative-sense template RNA. The L protein then uses the template RNA to replicate new genomes and produce five to seven **individual messenger ribonucleic acids (mRNAs)** for the individual viral proteins. Generation of the individual mRNAs may also promote recombination events between viral genomes to promote genetic diversity.

Virions contain the glycoproteins E1 (20,000 to 30,000 Da) and E2 (160,000 to 200,000 Da) and a core nucleoprotein (N [47,000 to 55,000 Da]); some strains also contain a hemagglutinin-neuraminidase (E3 [120,000 to 140,000 Da]) (Table 57-1). The E2 glycoprotein is responsible for mediating viral attachment and membrane fusion and is the target of neutralizing antibodies. The E1 glycoprotein is a transmembrane matrix protein. The replication scheme for coronaviruses is shown in Figure 57-2.

Pathogenesis and Clinical Syndromes

Coronaviruses inoculated into the respiratory tracts of human volunteers have been found to infect epithelial cells. Infection remains localized to the upper respiratory tract because the *optimum temperature for viral growth is 33° C to 35° C* (Box 57-2). The virus is most likely spread by aerosols and in large droplets (e.g., sneezes). Most human coronaviruses cause an upper respiratory tract infection similar to the colds caused by rhinoviruses but with a longer incubation period (average, 3 days). The infection may exacerbate a preexisting chronic pulmonary disease, such as asthma or bronchitis, and on rare occasions may cause pneumonia.

Infections occur mainly in infants and children. Coronavirus disease appears either sporadically or in outbreaks in the winter and spring. Usually, one strain predominates in an outbreak. Findings from serologic studies show that coronaviruses cause approximately 10% to 15% of upper respiratory tract infections and pneumonias in humans. Antibodies to coronaviruses are uniformly present by adulthood, but reinfections are common, despite the preexisting serum antibodies.

Coronavirus-like particles have also been seen in electron micrographs of stool specimens obtained from adults and children with diarrhea and gastroenteritis and infants with neonatal necrotizing enterocolitis.

SARS is a form of atypical pneumonia characterized by high fever (>38° C), chills, rigors, headache, dizziness, malaise, myalgia, cough or breathing difficulty, and a history of exposure to a person or place associated with SARS within the previous 10 days. Up to 20% of patients will also develop diarrhea. Mortality is at least 10% of people with

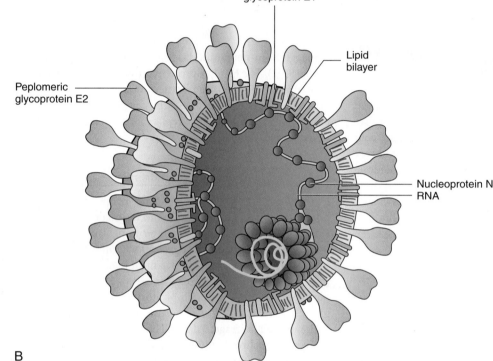

A

Transmembrane
glycoprotein E1

Lipid
bilayer

Peplomeric
glycoprotein E2

Nucleoprotein N
RNA

B

Figure 57–1. A, Electron micrograph of the human respiratory coronavirus (magnification 90,000×). **B,** Model of a coronavirus. The viral nucleocapsid is a long, flexible helix composed of the positive-strand genomic RNA and many molecules of the phosphorylated nucleocapsid protein N. The viral envelope consists of a lipid bilayer derived from the intracellular membranes of the host cell and two viral glycoproteins (E1 and E2). (*A courtesy of Centers for Disease Control and Prevention, Atlanta; B redrawn from Fields BF, Knipe DM: Virology. New York, Raven, 1985.*)

Box 57–1. Unique Features of Coronaviruses

Virus has medium-sized virions with a solar corona–like appearance.
Single-stranded, positive-sense RNA genome is enclosed in an envelope containing the E2 viral attachment protein, E1 matrix protein, and N nucleocapsid protein.
Translation of genome occurs in two phases: (1) the early phase produces an RNA polymerase (L), and (2) the late phase, from a negative-sense RNA template, yields structural and nonstructural proteins.
Virus assembles at the rough endoplasmic reticulum.
Virus is difficult to isolate and grow in routine cell culture.

---

indication of SARS infection. Although SARS-CoV is most likely transmitted in respiratory droplets, it is also present in sweat, urine, and feces.

As already mentioned, the outbreak of SARS started in November 2002 in South China's Guangdong Province, was brought to Hong Kong by a physician working within the original outbreak, and then was brought to Vietnam, Toronto, and other places by travelers. The virus was shown to be a coronavirus by its electron microscopic morphology and by reverse transcriptase polymerase chain reaction (RT-PCR). The virus apparently jumped to man from animals (masked-palm civets, raccoon dogs, and Chinese ferret badgers) raised for food. A World Health Organization WHO global alert prompted containment measures to limit the spread of the virus and controlled the outbreak to 8000 infected individuals but with at least 784 deaths. Travel restrictions and public concern resulted in a loss of hundreds of millions of dollars in travel and other business.

Table 57–1. Major Human Coronavirus Proteins

Proteins	Molecular Weight (kDa)	Location	Functions
E2 (peplomeric glycoprotein)	160-200	Envelope spikes (peplomer)	Binding to host cells; fusion activity
H1 (hemagglutinin protein)	60-66	Peplomer	Hemagglutination
N (nucleoprotein)	47-55	Core	Ribonucleoprotein
E1 (matrix glycoprotein)	20-30	Envelope	Transmembrane protein
L (polymerase)	225	Infected cell	Polymerase activity

Modified from Balows A, et al (eds): Laboratory Diagnosis of Infectious Diseases: Principles and Practice. New York, Springer-Verlag, 1988.

Laboratory Diagnosis

Laboratory tests are not routinely performed to diagnose coronavirus infections other than SARS. The method of choice for coronaviruses, including SARS-CoV, is detection of the viral RNA genome in respiratory and stool samples by RT-PCR. Virus isolation of the coronaviruses is difficult and for SARS-CoV requires stringent biosafety level 3 (BSL-3) conditions. Testing of samples suspected of containing SARS-CoV must be performed with appropriate BSL-2 precautions, attainable in many virology laboratories. Serology using enzyme-linked immunosorbent assay (ELISA) can be used to evaluate acute and convalescent sera. Electron microscopy has also been used to detect coronavirus-like particles in stool specimens.

Treatment, Prevention, and Control

Control of the respiratory transmission of the common cold form of coronavirus would be difficult and is probably unnecessary because of the mildness of the infection. Strict quarantine of individuals infected with SARS-CoV and screening for fever in travelers from a region with an outbreak of SARS are necessary to limit the spread of the virus. No vaccine or specific antiviral therapy is available.

Noroviruses

The noroviruses are members of the calicivirus family, which also includes astroviruses and other small, round gastroenteritis viruses. Norwalk virus, the prototypical Norovirus, was discovered on electron microscopic examination of stool samples from adults during an epidemic of acute gastroenteritis in Norwalk, Ohio. Many of the other viruses in this family also bear the names of the geographic locations where they were identified (Box 57-3).

Figure 57–2. Replication of human coronaviruses. The E2 glycoprotein interacts with receptors on epithelial cells, the virus fuses or is endocytosed into the cell, and the genome is released into the cytoplasm. Protein synthesis is divided into early and late phases, similar to that in the togaviruses. The genome binds to ribosomes, and an RNA-dependent RNA polymerase is translated. This enzyme generates a full-length, negative-sense RNA template for the production of new virion genomes and six individual mRNAs for the other coronavirus proteins. The genome associates with rough endoplasmic reticulum membranes modified by virion proteins and buds into the lumen of the rough endoplasmic reticulum. Vesicles that contain virus migrate to the cell membrane, and virus is released by exocytosis. *(Redrawn from Balows A, et al (eds): Laboratory Diagnosis of Infectious Diseases: Principles and Practice. New York, Springer-Verlag, 1988.)*

Box 57–2. Disease Mechanisms of Human Coronaviruses

Virus infects epithelial cells of upper respiratory tract.
Virus replicates best at 33° C to 35° C; therefore it prefers the upper respiratory tract.
Reinfection occurs in the presence of serum antibodies.
The glycoprotein "corona" helps this enveloped virus survive the gastrointestinal tract.
Severe acute respiratory syndrome infection is exacerbated by inflammatory responses.

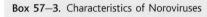

Structure and Replication

Noroviruses resemble and are approximately the same size as the picornaviruses. Their **positive-sense RNA genome** (approximately 7500 bases) has a VPg protein (viral protein genome-linked) and a 3′ terminal polyadenosine sequence similar to picornaviruses. The genome is contained in a 27-nm **naked capsid** consisting of 60,000-Da capsid proteins. Norwalk virions are round with a ragged outline, whereas other calicivirions have cup-shaped indentations or a six-point star shape. The virions of the astroviruses have a five- or six-point star shape on the surface but no indentations. Antibodies from seropositive people can also be used to distinguish these viruses.

Caliciviruses and astroviruses can be grown in cell culture, but the Norwalk viruses cannot. Expression of the structural protein genes of different Norwalk viruses in tissue culture cells produces Norwalk virus—like particles. These particles were used to show that Norwalk viruses bind to the carbohydrate of the A, B, or O blood group antigen on the cell surface. The noroviruses replicate like the picornaviruses, except for an early and late mRNA similar to the togaviruses and coronaviruses. The early mRNA encodes a polyprotein containing the RNA polymerase and other enzymes. The late mRNA encodes the capsid proteins.

Pathogenesis

As few as 10 virions will initiate disease in humans. Damage to the intestinal brush border prevents proper absorption of water and nutrients and causes a watery diarrhea. Although no histologic changes occur in the gastric mucosa, gastric emptying may be delayed, causing vomiting. Examination of jejunal biopsy specimens from human volunteers infected with noroviruses revealed the existence of blunted villi, cytoplasmic vacuolation, and infiltration with mononuclear cells. Shedding of the virus may continue for 2 weeks after symptoms have ceased.

Epidemiology

Norwalk and related viruses typically cause outbreaks of gastroenteritis as a result of a common source of contamination (e.g., water, shellfish, salad, food service). These viruses are transmitted mainly by the fecal-oral route. Outbreaks in developed countries may occur year-round and have been

Clinical Case 57-1. Norwalk Virus Outbreak

Brummer-Korvenkontio M, et al (Epidemiol Infect 129:335-360, 2002) described an outbreak of gastroenteritis in children who had attended a concert; infection was traced back to contamination of a specific seating area, bathrooms, and other areas by one individual. A male concert attendee was ill prior to attending a concert and then vomited four times in the concert hall: once in a waste bin in the corridor, into the toilets, onto the floor of the fire escape, and on a carpeted area in the walkway. His family members showed symptoms within 24 hours. A children's concert for several schools was held the next day. Children sitting in the same section as the incident case and those who traversed the contaminated carpet had the highest incidence of disease, characterized by watery diarrhea and vomiting for approximately 2 days. RT-PCR analysis of fecal samples from two ill children detected Norwalk virus genomic RNA. Infected vomit may have up to a million viruses per ml and only 10-100 viruses are required to transmit the disease. Contact with contaminated shoes, hands, clothing, or aerosols may have infected the children. The encapsidated nature of the Norwalk virus makes it resistant to routine cleansers; disinfection usually requires freshly prepared hypochlorite bleach—containing solutions or steam cleaning.

described in schools, resorts, hospitals, nursing homes, restaurants, and cruise ships. Common-source outbreaks can often be traced to a careless, infected food handler. The Centers for Disease Control and Prevention estimates that nearly 50% (23 million cases in the United States per year) of all foodborne outbreaks of gastroenteritis can be attributed to noroviruses, which is a tribute to the importance of this virus. Immunity is generally short lived at best and may not be protective. As many as 70% of children in the United States have antibodies to noroviruses by the age of 7.

Clinical Syndromes (Clinical Case 57-1; Box 57-4)

Norwalk and related viruses cause symptoms similar to those caused by the rotaviruses. Infection causes an acute onset of

Box 57—4. Clinical Summaries

Coronaviruses

Common cold: A 25-year-old person develops runny nose, mild cough, malaise, and a low-grade fever. A coworker in the office has had similar symptoms for the past few days.

SARS: A 45-year-old businessman returned from a 2-week trip to China. Five days after returning home to the United States, he developed a fever of 101.5° F (38.6° C) and cough. Now he observes that it is harder to catch his breath.

Norovirus

Norwalk virus: On the third day of a cruise (incubation period of 24 to 60 hours), a group of 45 passengers on a cruise ship experienced watery diarrhea, nausea, and vomiting for 12 to 60 hours, depending on the individual.

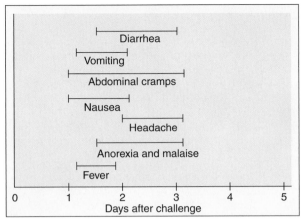

Figure 57—3. Response to ingestion of Norwalk virus. Symptoms vary in severity.

Case Study and Questions

Several adults complained of serious diarrhea, nausea, vomiting, and a mild fever 2 days after visiting Le Café Grease. The symptoms were too severe to result from food poisoning or a routine gastroenteritis but lasted only 24 hours.

1. What characteristics distinguished this disease from a rotavirus infection?
2. What was the most likely means of viral transmission?
3. What physical characteristics of the virus allowed it to be transmitted by these means?
4. What public health measures could be followed to prevent such outbreaks?

diarrhea, nausea, vomiting, and abdominal cramps, especially in children (Figure 57-3). Bloody stools do not occur. Fever may occur in as many as a third of patients. The incubation period is usually 24 to 48 hours, and the illness resolves within 12 to 60 hours without problems.

Laboratory Diagnosis

The use of RT-PCR for detection of the Norovirus genome in stool or emesis samples has enhanced the speed and detection of the virus during outbreaks. Immunoelectron microscopy can be used to concentrate and identify the virus from stool. The addition of an antibody directed against the suspected agent causes the virus to aggregate, thereby facilitating recognition. ELISA tests been developed to detect the virus and viral antigen. Serology can be used to confirm a diagnosis. RIA or ELISA can detect antibody to the Norwalk agent. Antibodies to the other calicivirus-like agents are more difficult to detect.

Treatment, Prevention, and Control

No specific treatment for infection with the calicivirus or other small, round gastroenteritis viruses is available. Bismuth subsalicylate may reduce the severity of the gastrointestinal symptoms. Outbreaks may be minimized by handling food carefully and by maintaining the purity of the water supply. More resistant than polioviruses or rotaviruses, Norwalk virus is resistant to heat (60° C), pH 3, detergent, and even the chlorine levels of drinking water.

Bibliography

Balows A, et al: Laboratory Diagnosis of Infectious Diseases: Principles and Practice. New York, Springer-Verlag, 1988.

Blacklow NR, Greenberg HB: Viral gastroenteritis. N Engl J Med 325:252-264, 1991.

Cann AJ: Principles of Molecular Virology. San Diego, Academic, 2005.

Carter J, Saunders V: Virology: Principles and Applications. Chichester, England, Wiley, 2007.

Christensen ML: Human viral gastroenteritis. Clin Microbiol Rev 2:51-89, 1989.

Cohen J, Powderly WG: Infectious Diseases, 2nd ed. St Louis, Mosby, 2004.

Collier L, Oxford J: Human Virology, 3rd ed. Oxford, Oxford University Press, 2006.

Flint SJ, et al: Principles of Virology: Molecular Biology, Pathogenesis and Control of Animal Viruses, 2nd ed. Washington, DC, ASM Press, 2003.

Knipe DM, Howley PM: Fields Virology, 4th ed. New York, Lippincott Williams & Wilkins, 2001.

Meulen V, Siddell S, Wege H: Biochemistry and Biology of Coronaviruses. New York, Plenum, 1981.

Strauss JM, Strauss EG: Viruses and Human Disease, 2nd ed. San Diego, Academic, 2007.

Tan M, et al: Mutations within the P2 domain of Norovirus capsid affect binding to human histo-blood group antigens: Evidence for a binding pocket. J Virol 77:12562-12571, 2003.

Voyles BA: The Biology of Viruses, 2nd ed. Boston, McGraw-Hill, 2002.

Xi JN, et al: Norwalk virus genome cloning and characterization. Science 250:1580-1583, 1990.

Websites

CDC Norovirus fact sheet (online): Available at http://www.cdc.gov/ncidod/dvrd/revb/gastro/norovirus.htm

Kamps BS, Hoffmann C: SARS reference (2003, online): Available at www.sarsreference.com/sarsref/preface.htm

National Institute of Allergy and Infectious Diseases research on SARS (online): Available at www.niaid.nih.gov/factsheets/sars.htm

Paramyxoviruses

The Paramyxoviridae include the following genera: *Morbillivirus, Paramyxovirus,* and *Pneumovirus* (Table 58-1). Human pathogens within the morbilliviruses include the **measles** virus; within the paramyxoviruses, the **parainfluenza** and **mumps** viruses; and within the pneumoviruses, the **respiratory syncytial virus (RSV)** and the newly discovered but relatively common **metapneumovirus.** Their virions have similar morphologies and protein components, and they share the capacity to induce **cell-cell fusion** (syncytia formation and multinucleated giant cells). A new group of highly pathogenic paramyxoviruses, including two zoonosis-causing viruses, **Nipah virus** and **Hendra virus,** was identified in 1998 after an outbreak of severe encephalitis in Malaysia and Singapore.

These agents cause some well-known major diseases. Measles virus causes a potentially serious generalized infection characterized by a maculopapular rash (**rubeola**). Parainfluenza viruses cause upper and lower respiratory tract infections, primarily in children, including pharyngitis, croup, bronchitis, bronchiolitis, and pneumonia. Mumps virus causes a systemic infection whose most prominent clinical manifestation is parotitis. RSV causes mild upper respiratory tract infections in children and adults but can cause life-threatening pneumonia in infants.

Measles and mumps viruses have only **one serotype**, and protection is provided by an effective **live vaccine**. In the United States and other developed countries, successful vaccination programs using the live attenuated measles and mumps vaccines have made measles and mumps rare. In particular, these programs have led to the virtual elimination of the serious sequelae of measles.

Structure and Replication

Paramyxoviruses consist of **negative-sense, single-stranded ribonucleic acid (RNA)** (5 to 8×10^6 Da) in a helical nucleocapsid surrounded by a pleomorphic **envelope** of approximately 156 to 300 nm (Figure 58-1). They are similar in many respects to orthomyxoviruses but are larger and do not have the segmented genome of the influenza viruses (Box 58-1). Although significant homology exists among paramyxovirus genomes, the order of the protein-coding regions differs for each genus. The gene products of the measles virus are listed in Table 58-2.

The nucleocapsid consists of the negative-sense, single-stranded RNA associated with the nucleoprotein (**NP**), polymerase phosphoprotein (**P**), and large (**L**) protein. The L protein is the RNA polymerase, the P protein facilitates RNA synthesis, and the NP protein helps maintain genomic structure. The nucleocapsid associates with the matrix (**M**) protein lining the inside of the virion envelope. The envelope contains two glycoproteins, a fusion (**F**) protein, which promotes fusion of the viral and host cell membranes, and a viral attachment protein (hemagglutinin-neuraminidase [**HN**], hemagglutinin [**H**], or **G** protein) (see Box 58-1). To express membrane-fusing activity, the F protein must be activated by proteolytic cleavage, which produces F_1 and F_2 glycopeptides held together by a disulfide bond.

Replication of the paramyxoviruses is initiated by the binding of the HN, H, or G protein on the virion envelope to sialic acid on the cell surface glycolipids. The measles virus can bind to the CD46 (membrane cofactor protein, MCP) present on most cell types and also CD150 SLAM (signaling lymphocyte-activation molecule) which is expressed on activated T and B cells. CD46 protects the cell from complement by regulating complement activation and is also the receptor for human herpes virus 6 and some strains of adenovirus. SLAM regulates TH1 and TH2 responses, and measles virus may upset this regulation. The F protein promotes fusion of the envelope with the plasma membrane. Paramyxoviruses are also able to induce cell—cell fusion, thereby creating multinucleated giant cells (syncytia).

The replication of the genome occurs in a manner similar to that of other negative-strand RNA viruses (i.e., rhabdoviruses). The RNA polymerase is carried into the cell as part of the nucleocapsid. Transcription, protein synthesis, and replication of the genome all occur in the host cell's cytoplasm.

Table 58—1. Paramyxoviridae

Genus	Human Pathogen
Morbillivirus	Measles virus
Paramyxovirus	Parainfluenza viruses 1 to 4
	Mumps virus
Pneumovirus	Respiratory syncytial virus
	Metapneumovirus

Box 58—1. Unique Features of the Paramyxoviridae

Large virion consists of a negative RNA genome in a helical nucleocapsid surrounded by an envelope containing a viral attachment protein (hemagglutinin-neuraminidase [HN], parainfluenza virus and mumps virus; hemagglutinin [H], measles virus; and glycoprotein [G], respiratory syncytial virus [RSV]) and a fusion glycoprotein (F).

The three genera can be distinguished by the activities of the viral attachment protein: HN of parainfluenza virus and mumps virus has hemagglutinin and neuraminidase, and H of measles virus has hemagglutinin activity, but G of RSV lacks these activities.

Virus replicates in the cytoplasm.

Virions penetrate the cell by fusion with the plasma membrane and exit by budding from the plasma membrane.

Viruses induce cell—cell fusion, causing multinucleated giant cells.

Paramyxoviridae are transmitted in respiratory droplets and initiate infection in the respiratory tract.

Cell-mediated immunity causes many of the symptoms but is essential for control of the infection.

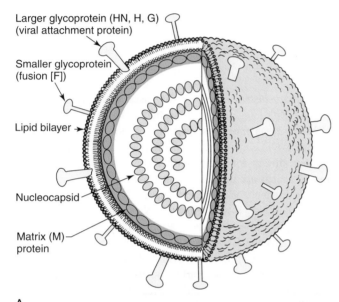

Larger glycoprotein (HN, H, G) (viral attachment protein)

Smaller glycoprotein (fusion [F])

Lipid bilayer

Nucleocapsid

Matrix (M) protein

A

B

Figure 58—1. A, Model of paramyxovirus. The helical nucleocapsid—consisting of negative-sense, single-stranded RNA and the P protein, nucleoprotein (NP), and large (L) protein—associates with the matrix (M) protein at the envelope membrane surface. The nucleocapsid contains RNA transcriptase activity. The envelope contains the viral attachment glycoprotein (hemagglutinin-neuraminidase [HN], hemagglutinin [H], or G protein [G]) and the fusion (F) protein. **B,** Electron micrograph of a disrupted paramyxovirus showing the helical nucleocapsid. (**A** redrawn from Jawetz E, Melnick JL, Adelberg EA: Review of Medical Microbiology, 17th ed. Norwalk, Conn, Appleton & Lange, 1987; **B** courtesy of Centers for Disease Control and Prevention, Atlanta.)

The genome is transcribed into individual messenger RNAs (mRNAs) and a full-length positive-sense RNA template. New genomes associate with the L, N, and NP proteins to form nucleocapsids, which associate with the M proteins on viral glycoprotein—modified plasma membranes. The glycoproteins are synthesized and processed like cellular glycoproteins. Mature virions then bud from the host cell plasma membrane and exit the cell. Replication of the paramyxoviruses is represented by the RSV infectious cycle shown in Figure 58-2.

Table 58—2. Viral-Encoded Proteins of Measles Virus

Gene Products*	Virion Location	Function
Nucleoprotein (NP)	Major internal protein	Protection of viral RNA
Polymerase phosphoprotein (P)	Association with nucleoprotein	Possible part of transcription complex
Matrix (M)	Inside virion envelope	Assembly of virions
Fusion protein (F)	Transmembranous envelope glycoprotein	Protein promotes fusion of cells, hemolysis, and viral entry
Hemagglutinin (H)	Transmembranous envelope glycoprotein	Viral attachment proteins
Large protein (L)	Association with nucleoprotein	Polymerase

Modified from Fields BN: Virology. New York, Raven, 1985.
*In order of transcription.

Figure 58—2. Replication of paramyxoviruses. The virus binds to glycolipids or proteins and fuses with the cell surface. Individual mRNAs for each protein and a full-length template are transcribed from the genome. Replication occurs in the cytoplasm. The nucleocapsid associates with matrix and glycoprotein-modified plasma membranes and leaves the cell by budding. (−), negative sense; (+), positive sense; ER, endoplasmic reticulum; RSV, respiratory syncytial virus. *(Redrawn from Balows A, et al: Laboratory Diagnosis of Infectious Diseases: Principles and Practice. New York, Springer-Verlag, 1988.)*

Measles Virus

Measles is one of the five classic childhood exanthems, along with rubella, roseola, fifth disease, and chickenpox. Historically, measles was one of the most common and unpleasant viral infections, with serious potential sequelae. Before 1960, more than 90% of the population younger than 20 years had experienced the rash, high fever, cough, conjunctivitis, and coryza of measles. Since the use of the live vaccine began in 1993, fewer than 1000 cases have been reported in the United States. Measles is still one of the most prominent causes of disease (45 million cases per year) and death (1 to 2 million per year) worldwide in unvaccinated populations.

Box 58—2. Disease Mechanisms of Measles Virus

Virus infects epithelial cells of respiratory tract.
Virus spreads systemically in lymphocytes and by **viremia**.
Virus replicates in cells of conjunctivae, respiratory tract, urinary tract, lymphatic system, blood vessels, and central nervous system.
Rash is caused by T-cell response to virus-infected epithelial cells lining capillaries.
Cell-mediated immunity is essential to control infection.
Sequelae in the central nervous system may result from immunopathogenesis (postinfectious measles encephalitis) or development of defective mutants (subacute sclerosing panencephalitis).

Pathogenesis and Immunity

Measles is known for its propensity to cause cell fusion, leading to the formation of giant cells (Box 58-2). As a result, the virus can pass directly from cell to cell and escape antibody control. Inclusions occur most commonly in the cytoplasm and are composed of incomplete viral particles. Infection usually leads to cell lysis, but persistent infections without lysis can occur in certain cell types (e.g., human brain cells).

Measles is **highly contagious** and is transmitted from person to person by **respiratory droplets** (Figure 58-3). Local replication of virus in the respiratory tract precedes its spread to the lymphatic system and cell-associated viremia. The wide dissemination of the virus causes infection of the conjunctiva, respiratory tract, urinary tract, small blood vessels, lymphatic system, and the central nervous system.

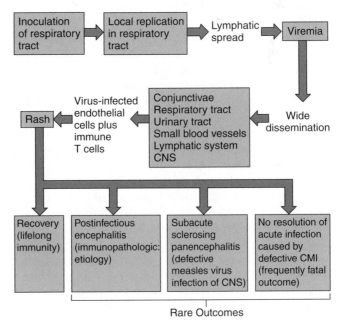

Figure 58—3. Mechanisms of spread of the measles virus within the body and the pathogenesis of measles. CMI, cell-mediated immunity; CNS, central nervous system.

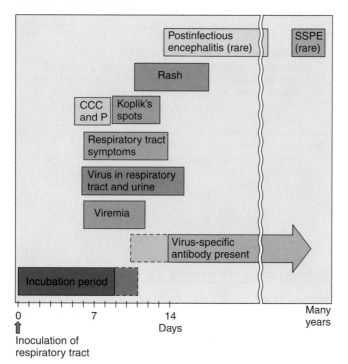

Figure 58—4. Time course of measles virus infection. Characteristic prodrome symptoms are cough, conjunctivitis, coryza, and photophobia (CCC and P), followed by the appearance of Koplik spots and rash. SSPE, subacute sclerosing panencephalitis.

*The characteristic **maculopapular** measles rash is caused by immune T cells targeted to measles-infected endothelial cells lining small blood vessels.* Recovery follows the rash in most patients, who then have **lifelong immunity** to the virus. The time course of measles infection is shown in Figure 58-4.

Measles can cause encephalitis in three ways: (1) direct infection of neurons, (2) a postinfectious encephalitis, which is believed to be immune mediated, and (3) subacute sclerosing panencephalitis (SSPE) caused by a defective variant of measles generated during the acute disease. The SSPE virus acts as a slow virus and causes symptoms and cytopathologic effect in neurons many years after acute disease.

Cell-mediated immunity is responsible for most of the symptoms and is essential for the control of measles infection. T-cell-deficient children who are infected with measles have an atypical presentation, consisting of **giant cell pneumonia without a rash**. During the incubation period, measles causes a decrease in eosinophils and lymphocytes, including B and T cells, and a depression of their response to activation (mitogens). The virus depresses the immune response by (1) directly infecting monocytes and T and B cells and (2) by promoting a switch from the TH1—associated interferon gamma and IL12 cytokines to the production of TH2-associated cytokines, especially interleukin 4 (IL4), IL5, IL10, and IL13. These cytokines reduce the host's ability to mount protective cell-mediated immune and DTH-type responses. This immunosuppression lasts throughout and for weeks after the infection, but protection from reinfection is lifelong.

Epidemiology

The development of effective vaccine programs has made measles a rare disease in the United States. In areas without a vaccine program, epidemics tend to occur in 1- to 3-year cycles, when a sufficient number of susceptible people have accumulated. Many of these cases occur in preschool-age children who have not been vaccinated and live in large urban areas. The incidence of infection peaks in the winter and spring. Measles is still common in people living in developing countries; it is the most significant cause of death in children 1 to 5 years of age in several countries. Immunocompromised and malnourished people with measles may not be able to resolve the infection, resulting in death.

Measles, which can be spread in respiratory secretions before and after the onset of characteristic symptoms, is one of the most contagious infections known (Box 58-3). In a household, approximately 85% of exposed susceptible people become infected, and 95% of these people develop clinical disease.

The measles virus has only one serotype, infects only humans, and infection usually manifests as symptoms. These properties facilitated the development of an effective vaccine program. Once vaccination was introduced, the yearly incidence of measles dropped dramatically in the United States, from 300 to 1.3 per 100,000 (U.S. statistics for 1981 to 1988). This change represented a 99.5% reduction in the incidence of infection from the prevaccination years of 1955 to 1962.

Box 58—3. Epidemiology of Measles

Disease/Viral Factors

Virus has large enveloped virion that is easily inactivated by dryness and acid.
Contagion period precedes symptoms.
Host range limited to humans.
Only one serotype exists.
Immunity is lifelong.

Transmission

Inhalation of large-droplet aerosols.

Who Is at Risk?

Unvaccinated people.
Immunocompromised people, who have more serious outcomes.

Geography/Season

Virus found worldwide.
Virus endemic from autumn to spring, possibly because of crowding indoors.

Modes of Control

Live attenuated vaccine (Schwartz or Moraten variants of Edmonston B strain) can be administered.
Immune serum globulin can be administered after exposure.

58

Despite the effectiveness of vaccination programs, poor compliance and the prevaccinated population (children under 2 years) continue to provide susceptible individuals. The virus may surface from within the community or can be imported by immigration from areas of the world lacking an effective vaccine program. Once again, outbreaks of measles are occuring more often in the US and England. An outbreak of measles in a daycare center (10 infants too young to have been vaccinated and two adults) was traced to an infant from the Philippines.

Clinical Syndromes

Measles is a serious febrile illness (Table 58-3). The incubation period lasts 7 to 13 days, and the prodrome starts with **high fever** and **'CCC and P'—cough, coryza, conjunctivitis**, and **photophobia.** The disease is most infectious during this time.

After 2 days of illness, the typical mucous membrane lesions known as **Koplik spots** (Figure 58-5) appear. They are seen most commonly on the buccal mucosa across from the molars, but they may appear on other mucous membranes as well, including the conjunctivae and the vagina. *The lesions, which last 24 to 48 hours, are usually small (1 to 2 mm) and are best described as grains of salt surrounded by a red halo.* Their appearance with the other disease signs establishes with certainty the diagnosis of measles.

Within 12 to 24 hours of the appearance of Koplik spots, the **exanthem** of measles starts below the ears and spreads over the body. The **rash is maculopapular,** usually very extensive, and often the lesions become confluent. The rash, which takes 1 or 2 days to cover the body, fades in the same order in which it appeared. The fever is highest and the patient is sickest on the day the rash appears (Figure 58-6).

Pneumonia, which can also be a serious complication, accounts for 60% of the deaths caused by measles. Like the

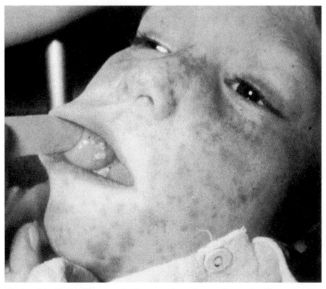

Figure 58—5. Koplik spots in the mouth and exanthem. Koplik spots usually precede the measles rash and may be seen for the first day or two after the rash appears. *(Courtesy Dr JI Pugh, St Albans; from Emond RTD, Rowland HAK: A Color Atlas of Infectious Diseases, 3rd ed. London, Mosby, 1995.)*

incidence of the other complications associated with measles, the mortality associated with pneumonia is higher in the malnourished and for the extremes of age. **Bacterial superinfection** is common in patients with pneumonia caused by the measles virus.

Figure 58—6. Measles rash. *(From Habif TP: Clinical Dermatology: Color Guide to Diagnosis and Therapy. St Louis, Mosby, 1985.)*

Table 58—3. Clinical Consequences of Measles Virus Infection

Disorder	Symptoms
Measles	Characteristic maculopapular rash, cough, conjunctivitis, coryza, photophobia, Koplik spots *Complications:* Otitis media, croup, bronchopneumonia, and encephalitis
Atypical measles	More intense rash (most prominent in distal areas); possible vesicles, petechiae, purpura, or urticaria
Subacute sclerosing panencephalitis	Central nervous system manifestations (e.g., personality, behavior, and memory changes; myoclonic jerks; spasticity; and blindness

One of the most feared complications of measles is **encephalitis**, which occurs in as few as 0.5% of those infected but carries a fatality rate of 15%. Encephalitis may rarely occur during acute disease but usually begins 7 to 10 days after the onset of illness. This **postinfectious encephalitis** is caused by immunopathologic reactions, is associated with demyelination of neurons, and occurs more often in older children and adults.

Atypical measles occurred in people who received the older inactivated measles vaccine and were subsequently exposed to the wild-type measles virus. It may also rarely occur in those vaccinated with the attenuated virus vaccine. Prior sensitization with insufficient protection can enhance the immunopathologic response to the challenge by wild measles virus. The illness begins abruptly and is a more intense presentation of measles.

Subacute sclerosing panencephalitis is an extremely serious, very late neurologic sequela of measles that afflicts approximately seven of every 1 million patients. The incidence of SSPE has decreased markedly as the result of measles vaccination programs.

This disease occurs when a defective measles virus persists in the brain and acts as a slow virus. The virus can replicate and spread directly from cell to cell but is not released. SSPE is most prevalent in children who were initially infected when younger than 2 years and occurs approximately 7 years after clinical measles. The patient demonstrates changes in personality, behavior, and memory, followed by myoclonic jerks, blindness, and spasticity. Unusually high levels of measles antibodies are found in the blood and cerebrospinal fluid of patients with SSPE.

The immunocompromised and malnourished child is at highest risk for severe outcome of measles (Clinical Case 58-1). **Giant cell pneumonia without rash** occurs in children lacking T-cell immunity. Severe bacterial superinfection and pneumonia occur in malnourished children, with up to 25% mortality.

Laboratory Diagnosis

The clinical manifestations of measles are usually so characteristic that it is rarely necessary to perform laboratory tests to establish the diagnosis. The measles virus is difficult to isolate and grow, although it can be grown in primary human- or monkey-cell cultures. Respiratory tract secretions, urine, blood, and brain tissue are the recommended specimens. It is best to collect respiratory and blood specimens during the prodromal stage and up until 1 to 2 days after the appearance of the rash.

Measles antigen can be detected in pharyngeal cells or urinary sediment with immunofluorescence; the measles genome can be identified by reverse transcriptase polymerase chain reaction (RT-PCR) in either of the aforementioned specimens. Characteristic cytopathologic effects, including multinucleated giant cells with cytoplasmic inclusion bodies, can be seen in Giemsa-stained cells taken from the upper respiratory tract and urinary sediment.

Clinical Case 58-1. Measles in the Immunocompromised Child

The lack of cell-mediated immune responses allows measles infection of immunocompromised individuals to progress to serious outcomes. In a case reported by Pullan, et al (Br Med J 1:1562-1565, 1976), within 3 days of exposure to measles, a child on chemotherapy for acute lymphoblastic leukemia (ALL) received pooled immunoglobulin. Despite the IgG therapy, 23 days after exposure, she developed an extensive measles rash, which became hemorrhagic. She had a fever of 39.5° C and bronchopneumonia. Measles was grown from nasopharyngeal secretions, and immunohistochemistry identified giant cells (syncytia) containing measles antigen within the secretions. Her chemotherapy was stopped, and she received several massive doses of immunoglobulin. She started to improve 1 month after the onset of the rash.

In another case, during the 2.5 years that a boy was under treatment for ALL, he suffered severe HSV infections around the mouth and herpes zoster on his trunk. During the third year on therapy, he was exposed to measles from his sister and received pooled IgG. After 19 days, he developed mild respiratory symptoms but no rash. After 29 days, he refused to go to school and misbehaved; behavior changes progressed. After 9 weeks, he developed focal motor seizures, increased drowsiness, slurring of speech, and confusion, which progressed to coma and death within 8 days of the onset of seizures. Serology indicated a lack of measles antibody. Autopsy indicated the presence of CMV but not measles in the lungs. The brain showed extensive degeneration, but no virus was isolated from the samples. Brain sections indicated large intranuclear and cytoplasmic inclusion bodies with tubular structures that resembled measles nucleocapsids in the cytoplasm. Immunofluorescence with antibody from individuals with subacute sclerosing panencephalitis (SSPE) or antimeasles antibody indicated the presence of measles antigen. These cases illustrate the excessive pathology that measles can cause in the absence of a competent T-cell response. The lack of immune control allowed the progression of the virus to the brain, where it or a variant (SSPE) caused pathology leading to encephalitis.

Antibody, especially immunoglobulin (Ig)M, can be detected when the rash is present. Measles infection can be confirmed by the finding of seroconversion or by a fourfold increase in the titer of measles-specific antibodies between sera obtained during the acute stage and the convalescent stage.

Treatment, Prevention, and Control

As stated previously, a live attenuated measles vaccine, in use in the United States since 1963, has been responsible for a significant reduction in the incidence of measles. The Schwartz or Moraten attenuated strains of the original Edmonston B vaccine are currently being used. Live attenuated vaccine is given to all children at 2 years of age, in combination with mumps and rubella (**MMR vaccine**) and the varicella vaccines (Box 58-4). Although early childhood immunization is successful in more than 95% of vaccines, revaccination before grade school or junior high school is required in many states. As noted earlier, a killed measles vaccine introduced in 1963 was not protective; its use was subsequently discontinued because recipients were at risk for the more serious atypical measles presentation on infection. Since it is strictly a human virus with only one serotype, measles is a good candidate for eradication, but this is prevented by difficulties in distributing the vaccine to regions that lack proper refrigeration facilities (e.g., Africa) and distribution networks.

Hospitals in areas experiencing endemic measles may wish to vaccinate or check the immune status of their employees to decrease the risk of nosocomial transmission. Exposed susceptible people who are immunocompromised should be given immune globulin to lessen the risk and severity of clinical illness. This product is most effective if given within 6 days of exposure. No specific antiviral treatment is available for measles.

Parainfluenza Viruses

Parainfluenza viruses, which were discovered in the late 1950s, are respiratory viruses that usually cause **mild coldlike symptoms** but can also cause **serious respiratory tract disease**. Four serologic types within the parainfluenza genus are human pathogens. Types 1, 2, and 3 are second only to RSV as important causes of severe lower respiratory tract infection in infants and young children. They are especially associated with **laryngotracheobronchitis (croup)**. Type 4 causes only mild upper respiratory tract infection in children and adults.

Pathogenesis and Immunity

Parainfluenza viruses infect epithelial cells of the upper respiratory tract (Box 58-5). The virus replicates more rapidly than measles and mumps viruses and can cause giant cell formation and cell lysis. Unlike measles and mumps viruses, the parainfluenza viruses rarely cause viremia. The viruses generally stay in the upper respiratory tract, causing only coldlike symptoms. In approximately 25% of cases, the virus spreads to the lower respiratory tract, and in 2% to 3%, disease may take the severe form of laryngotracheobronchitis.

The cell-mediated immune response both causes cell damage and confers protection. IgA responses are protective but short lived. Parainfluenza viruses manipulate cell-mediated immunity to limit development of memory. Multiple serotypes and the short duration of immunity after natural infection make reinfection common, but the reinfection disease is milder, suggesting at least partial immunity.

Epidemiology

Parainfluenza viruses are ubiquitous, and infection is common (Box 58-6). The virus is transmitted by person-to-person contact and respiratory droplets. Primary infections usually occur in infants and children younger than 5 years. Reinfections occur throughout life, indicating short-lived immunity. Infections with parainfluenza viruses 1 and 2, the major causes of croup, tend to occur in the autumn, whereas parainfluenza virus 3 infections occur throughout the year. All of these viruses spread readily within hospitals and can cause outbreaks in nurseries and pediatric wards.

Clinical Syndromes

Parainfluenza viruses 1, 2, and 3 may cause respiratory tract syndromes ranging from a **mild coldlike upper respiratory tract infection** (coryza, pharyngitis, mild bronchitis, wheezing, and fever) to **bronchiolitis** and **pneumonia.** Older children and adults generally experience milder infections than those seen in young children, although pneumonia may occur in the elderly.

A parainfluenza virus infection in infants may be more severe than infections in adults, causing bronchiolitis, pneumonia, and most notably croup (laryngotracheobronchitis). **Croup** results in subglottal swelling, which may close the airway. Hoarseness, a "seal bark" cough, tachypnea, tachycardia, and suprasternal retraction develop in infected patients after a 2- to 6-day incubation period. Most children recover within 48 hours. The principal differential diagnosis is epiglottitis caused by *Haemophilus influenzae.*

Laboratory Diagnosis

Parainfluenza virus is isolated from nasal washings and respiratory secretions and grows well in primary monkey kidney cells. Like other paramyxoviruses, the virions are labile during transit to the laboratory. The presence of virus-infected cells in aspirates or in cell culture is indicated by the finding of syncytia and is identified with immunofluorescence. Like the hemagglutinin of the influenza viruses, the hemagglutinin of the parainfluenza viruses promotes hemadsorption and hemagglutination. The serotype of the virus can be determined through the use of specific antibody to block hemadsorption or hemagglutination (hemagglutination inhibition). Rapid RT-PCR techniques are becoming the method of choice to detect and identify parainfluenza viruses from respiratory secretions.

Treatment, Prevention, and Control

Treatment of croup consists of the administration of nebulized cold or hot steam and careful monitoring of the upper airway. On rare occasions, intubation may become necessary. No specific antiviral agents are available.

Vaccination with killed vaccines is ineffective, possibly because they fail to induce local secretory antibody and appropriate cellular immunity. No live attenuated vaccine is available.

Mumps Virus

Mumps virus is the cause of acute, benign viral **parotitis** (painful swelling of the salivary glands). Mumps is rarely

Box 58-7. Disease Mechanisms of Mumps Virus

Virus infects epithelial cells of respiratory tract.
Virus spreads systemically by viremia.
Infection of parotid gland, testes, and central nervous system occurs.
Principal symptom is swelling of parotid glands caused by inflammation.
Cell-mediated immunity is essential for control of infection and responsible for causing some of the symptoms. Antibody is not sufficient because of virus's ability to spread cell to cell.

seen in countries that promote use of the live vaccine, which is administered with the measles and rubella live vaccines.

Mumps virus was isolated in embryonated eggs in 1945 and in cell culture in 1955. The virus is most closely related to parainfluenza virus 2, but there is no cross-immunity with the parainfluenza viruses.

Pathogenesis and Immunity

The mumps virus, of which only one serotype is known, causes a lytic infection of cells (Box 58-7). The virus initiates infection in the epithelial cells of the upper respiratory tract and infects the parotid gland, either by way of the Stensen duct or by means of a viremia. The virus is spread by the viremia throughout the body to the testes, ovary, pancreas, thyroid, and other organs. Infection of the central nervous system, especially the meninges, occurs in as many as 50% of those infected (Figure 58-7). Inflammatory responses are mainly responsible for the symptoms. The time course of human infection is shown in Figure 58-8. Immunity is lifelong.

Epidemiology

Mumps, like measles, is a very communicable disease with only one serotype, and it infects only humans (Box 58-8). In the absence of vaccination programs, infection occurs in 90% of people by the age of 15. The virus spreads by direct person-to-person contact and respiratory droplets. The virus is released in respiratory secretions from patients who are

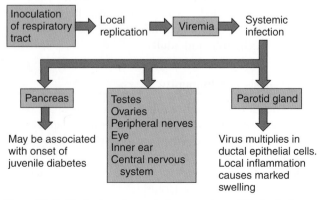

Figure 58-7. Mechanism of spread of mumps virus within the body.

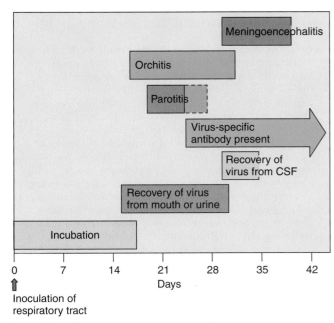

Figure 58—8. Time course of mumps virus infection.

accompanied by fever. Onset is sudden. Oral examination reveals redness and swelling of the ostium of the Stensen (parotid) duct. The swelling of other glands (epididymo-orchitis, oophoritis, mastitis, pancreatitis, and thyroiditis) and meningoencephalitis may occur a few days after the onset of the viral infection but can occur in the absence of parotitis. The swelling that results from mumps orchitis may cause sterility. Mumps virus involves the central nervous system in approximately 50% of patients; 10% of those affected may exhibit mild meningitis with 5 per 1000 cases of encephalitis.

Laboratory Diagnosis

Virus can be recovered from saliva, urine, the pharynx, secretions from the Stensen duct, and cerebrospinal fluid. Virus is present in saliva for approximately 5 days after the onset of symptoms and in urine for as long as 2 weeks. Mumps virus grows well in monkey kidney cells, causing the formation of multinucleated giant cells. The hemadsorption of guinea pig erythrocytes also occurs on virus-infected cells, due to the viral hemagglutinin.

A clinical diagnosis can be confirmed by serologic testing. A fourfold increase in the virus-specific antibody level or the detection of mumps-specific IgM antibody indicates active infection. Enzyme-linked immunosorbent assay, immunofluorescence tests, and hemagglutination inhibition can be used to detect the mumps virus, antigen, or antibody.

Treatment, Prevention, and Control

Vaccines provide the only effective means for preventing the spread of mumps infection. Since the introduction of the live attenuated vaccine (Jeryl Lynn vaccine) in the United States in 1967 and its administration as part of the MMR vaccine, the yearly incidence of the infection has declined from 76 to 2 per 100,000. Antiviral agents are not available.

asymptomatic and during the 7-day period before clinical illness, so it is virtually impossible to control the spread of the virus. Living or working in close quarters promotes the spread of the virus, and the incidence of the infection is greatest in the winter and spring.

Clinical Syndromes

Mumps infections are often asymptomatic. Clinical illness manifests as a parotitis that is almost always bilateral and

---

Box 58—8. Epidemiology of Mumps Virus

Disease/Viral Factors

Virus has large enveloped virion that is easily inactivated by dryness and acid.
Contagion period precedes symptoms.
Virus may cause asymptomatic shedding.
Host range is limited to humans.
Only one serotype exists.
Immunity is lifelong.

Transmission

Inhalation of large-droplet aerosols.

Who Is at Risk?

Unvaccinated people.
Immunocompromised people, who have more serious outcomes.

Geography/Season

Virus is found worldwide.
Virus is endemic in late winter and early spring.

Modes of Control

Live attenuated vaccine (Jeryl Lynn strain) is part of MMR vaccine.

Respiratory Syncytial Virus

RSV, first isolated from a chimpanzee in 1956, is a member of the *Pneumovirus* genus. Unlike the other paramyxoviruses, RSV lacks hemagglutinin and neuraminidase activities. It is the most common cause of **fatal acute respiratory tract infection** in infants and young children. It infects virtually everyone by 2 years of age, and reinfections occur throughout life, even among elderly persons.

Pathogenesis and Immunity

RSV produces an infection that is localized to the respiratory tract (Box 58-9). As the name suggests, RSV induces syncytia. The pathologic effect of RSV is mainly caused by direct viral invasion of the respiratory epithelium, which is followed by immunologically mediated cell injury. Necrosis of the bronchi and bronchioles leads to the formation of "plugs" of mucus,

Box 58–9. Disease Mechanisms of Respiratory Syncytial Virus

Virus causes localized infection of respiratory tract.
Virus does not cause viremia or systemic spread.
Pneumonia results from cytopathologic spread of virus (including syncytia).
Bronchiolitis is most likely mediated by host's immune response.
Narrow airways of young infants are readily obstructed by virus-induced pathologic effects.
Maternal antibody does not protect infant from infection.
Natural infection does not prevent reinfection.
Improper vaccination increases severity of disease.

fibrin, and necrotic material within smaller airways. The narrow airways of young infants are readily obstructed by such plugs. Natural immunity does not prevent reinfection, and vaccination with killed vaccine appears to enhance the severity of subsequent disease.

Epidemiology

RSV is very prevalent in young children; almost all children have been infected by 2 years of age (Box 58-10), with global annual infection rates of 64 million and mortality of 160,000. As many as 25% to 33% of these cases involve the lower respiratory tract, and 1% are severe enough to necessitate hospitalization (occurring in as many as 95,000 children in the United States each year).

Box 58–10. Epidemiology of Respiratory Syncytial Virus

Disease/Viral Factors

Virus has large enveloped virion that is easily inactivated by dryness and acid.
Contagion period precedes symptoms and may occur in absence of symptoms.
Host range is limited to humans.

Transmission

Inhalation of large-droplet aerosols.

Who Is at Risk?

Infants: lower respiratory tract infection (bronchiolitis and pneumonia).
Children: spectrum of disease mild to pneumonia.
Adults: reinfection with milder symptoms.

Geography/Season

Virus is ubiquitous and found worldwide.
Incidence is seasonal.

Modes of Control

Immune globulin is available for infants at high risk.
Aerosol ribavirin is available for infants with serious disease.

Box 58–11. Clinical Summaries

Measles: An 18-year-old woman had been home for 10 days after a trip to Haiti when she developed a fever, cough, runny nose, mild redness of her eyes; she now has a red, slightly raised rash over her face, trunk, and extremities. There are several 1-mm white lesions inside her mouth. She was never immunized for measles because of an "egg allergy."
Mumps: A 30-year-old man returning from a trip to Russia experienced a 1- to 2-day period of headache and decreased appetite, followed by swelling over both sides of his jaw. The swelling extended from the bottom of the jaw to in front of the ear. Five days after the jaw swelling appeared, the patient began complaining of nausea and lower abdominal and testicular pain.
Croup: A grumpy 2-year-old toddler with little appetite has a sore throat, fever, hoarse voice, and coughs with the sound of a barking seal. A high-pitched noise (stridor) is heard on inhalation. Flaring of the nostrils indicates difficulty breathing.

RSV infections almost always occur in the winter. Unlike influenza, which may occasionally skip a year, RSV epidemics occur every year.

The virus is very contagious, with an incubation period of 4 to 5 days. The introduction of the virus into a nursery, especially into an intensive care nursery, can be devastating. Virtually every infant becomes infected, and the infection is associated with considerable morbidity and occasionally death. The virus is transmitted on hands, by fomites, and to some degree by respiratory routes.

As already noted, RSV infects virtually all children by the age of 4 years, especially in urban centers. Outbreaks may also occur among the elderly population (e.g., in nursing homes). Virus is shed in respiratory secretions for many days, especially by infants.

Clinical Syndromes (Box 58-11)

RSV can cause any respiratory tract illness, from a **common cold** to **pneumonia** (Table 58-4). Upper respiratory tract infection with prominent rhinorrhea (runny nose) is most common in older children and adults. A more severe lower respiratory tract illness, **bronchiolitis**, may occur in infants. Because of inflammation at the level of the bronchiole, there is air trapping and decreased ventilation. Clinically, the patient usually has low-grade fever, tachypnea, tachycardia, and

Table 58–4. Clinical Consequences of Respiratory Syncytial Virus Infection

Disorder	Age Group Affected
Bronchiolitis, pneumonia, or both	Fever, cough, dyspnea, and cyanosis in children younger than 1 year
Febrile rhinitis and pharyngitis	Children
Common cold	Older children and adults

expiratory wheezes over the lungs. Bronchiolitis is usually self-limited, but it can be a frightening disease to observe in an infant. It may be fatal in premature infants, persons with underlying lung disease, and immunocompromised people.

Laboratory Diagnosis

RSV is difficult to isolate in cell culture. The presence of the viral genome in infected cells and nasal washings can be detected by RT-PCR techniques, and commercially available immunofluorescence and enzyme immunoassay tests are available for detection of the viral antigen. The finding of seroconversion or a fourfold or greater increase in the antibody titer can confirm the diagnosis for epidemiologic purposes.

Treatment, Prevention, and Control

In otherwise healthy infants, treatment is supportive, consisting of the administration of oxygen, intravenous fluids, and nebulized cold steam. **Ribavirin**, a guanosine analogue, is approved for the treatment of patients predisposed to a more severe course (e.g., premature or immunocompromised infants). It is administered by inhalation (nebulization).

Passive immunization with anti-RSV immunoglobulin is available for premature infants. Infected children must be isolated. Infection-control measures are required for hospital staff caring for infected children to avoid transmitting the virus to uninfected patients. These measures include handwashing and wearing gowns, goggles, and masks.

No vaccine is currently available for RSV prophylaxis. A previously available vaccine containing inactivated RSV caused recipients to have more severe RSV disease when subsequently exposed to the live virus. This development is thought to be the result of a heightened immunologic response at the time of exposure to the wild virus.

Human Metapneumovirus

Human metapneumovirus is a recently recognized member of the pneumovirus family. Use of RT-PCR methods was and remains the means of detecting the pneumoviruses and distinguishing them from other respiratory disease viruses. Its identity was unknown until recently, because it is difficult to grow in cell culture. The virus is ubiquitous and almost all 5-year-old children have experienced a virus infection and are seropositive.

As with its close cousin RSV, infections by human metapneumovirus may be asymptomatic, cause common cold–type disease or serious bronchiolitis and pneumonia. Seronegative children, the elderly and immunocompromised people are at risk to disease. Human metapneumovirus probably causes 15% of common colds in children, especially those which are complicated by otitis media. Signs of disease usually include cough, sore throat, runny nose, and high fever. Approximately 10% of patients with metapneumovirus will

experience wheezing, dyspnea, pneumonia, bronchitis, or bronchiolitis. As with other common cold agents, laboratory identification of the virus is not performed routinely but can be performed by RT-PCR. Supportive care is the only therapy available for these infections.

Nipah and Hendra Viruses

A new paramyxovirus, Nipah virus, was isolated from patients after an outbreak of severe encephalitis in Malaysia and Singapore in 1998. Nipah virus is more closely related to the Hendra virus, discovered in 1994 in Australia, than to other paramyxoviruses. Both viruses have broad host ranges, including pigs, man, dogs, horses, cats, and other mammals. For Nipah virus, the reservoir is a fruit bat (flying fox). The virus can be obtained from fruit contaminated by infected bats or amplified in pigs and then spread to humans. The human is an accidental host for these viruses, but the outcome of human infection is severe. Disease signs include flulike symptoms, seizures, and coma. Of the 269 cases occurring in 1999, 108 were fatal. Another epidemic in Bangladesh in 2004 had a higher mortality rate.

Case Studies and Questions

An 18-year-old college freshman complained of a cough, runny nose, and conjunctivitis. The physician in the campus health center noticed small white lesions inside the patient's mouth. The next day, a confluent red rash covered his face and neck.

1. What clinical characteristics of this case were diagnostic for measles?
2. Are any laboratory tests readily available to confirm the diagnosis? If so, what are they?
3. Is there a possible treatment for this patient?
4. When was this patient contagious?
5. Why is this disease not common in the United States?
6. Provide several possible reasons for this person's susceptibility to measles at 18 years of age.

A 13-month-old child had a runny nose, mild cough, and low-grade fever for several days. The cough got worse and sounded like "barking." The child made a wheezing sound when agitated. The child appeared well except for the cough. A lateral radiograph of the neck showed a subglottic narrowing.

1. What are the specific and common names for these symptoms?
2. What other agents would cause a similar clinical presentation (differential diagnosis)?
3. Are there readily available laboratory tests to confirm this diagnosis? If so, what are they?
4. Was there a possible treatment for this child?
5. When was this child contagious, and how was the virus transmitted?

Bibliography

Cann AJ: Principles of Molecular Virology. San Diego, Academic, 2005.

Carter J, Saunders V: Virology: Principles and Applications. Chichester, England, Wiley, 2007.

Centers for Disease Control and Prevention: Public-sector vaccination efforts in response to the resurgence of measles among preschool-aged children: United States, 1989-1991. Morb Mortal Wkly Rep 41:522-525, 1992.

Cohen J, Powderly WG: Infectious Diseases, 2nd ed. St Louis, Mosby, 2004.

Collier L, Oxford J: Human Virology, 3rd ed. Oxford, Oxford University Press, 2006.

Flint SJ, et al: Principles of Virology: Molecular Biology, Pathogenesis and Control of Animal Viruses, 2nd ed. Washington, DC, ASM Press, 2003.

Galinski MS: Paramyxoviridae: Transcription and replication. Adv Virus Res 40:129-163, 1991.

Griffin DE, Oldstone MB (Eds.): History and Basic Biology Series: Current Topics in Microbiology and Immunology, Vol. 329. New York, Springer-Verlag, 2009.

Griffin DE, Oldstone MB (Eds.): Pathogenesis and Control Series: Current Topics in Microbiology and Immunology, Vol. 330. New York, Springer-Verlag, 2009.

Hart CA, Broadhead RL: Color Atlas of Pediatric Infectious Diseases, St Louis, Mosby, 1992.

Hinman AR: Potential candidates for eradication. Rev Infect Dis 4: 933-939, 1982.

Gershon, et al: Krugman's Infectious Diseases of Children, 11th ed. St Louis, Mosby, 2004.

Knipe DM, Howley PM: Fields Virology, 4th ed. New York, Lippincott Williams & Wilkins, 2001.

Lennette EH: Laboratory Diagnosis of Viral Infections, 3rd ed. New York, Marcel Dekker, 1999.

Meulen V, Billeter MA: Measles virus. In Curr Top Microbiol Immunol, Vol. 191: Berlin, Springer-Verlag, pp 1-196.

Strauss JM, Strauss EG: Viruses and Human disease, 2nd ed. San Diego, Academic, 2007.

Voyles BA: The Biology of Viruses, 2nd ed. Boston, McGraw-Hill, 2002.

Websites

Burnett M, Krusinski P: Measles, Rubeola (2007, online): Available at http://www.emedicine.com/derm/topic259.htm#section~AuthorsandEditors

Demirci CS, Abuhammour W: Mumps (2006, online): Available at http://www.emedicine.com/ped/topic1503.htm

Fennelly GJ: Measles (2006, online): Available at http://www.emedicine.com/ped/topic1388.htm

Krilov LR: Respiratory Syncytial Virus Infection (2006, online): Available at http://www.emedicine.com/ped/topic2706.htm

expiratory wheezes over the lungs. Bronchiolitis is usually self-limited, but it can be a frightening disease to observe in an infant. It may be fatal in premature infants, persons with underlying lung disease, and immunocompromised people.

Laboratory Diagnosis

RSV is difficult to isolate in cell culture. The presence of the viral genome in infected cells and nasal washings can be detected by RT-PCR techniques, and commercially available immunofluorescence and enzyme immunoassay tests are available for detection of the viral antigen. The finding of seroconversion or a fourfold or greater increase in the antibody titer can confirm the diagnosis for epidemiologic purposes.

Treatment, Prevention, and Control

In otherwise healthy infants, treatment is supportive, consisting of the administration of oxygen, intravenous fluids, and nebulized cold steam. **Ribavirin**, a guanosine analogue, is approved for the treatment of patients predisposed to a more severe course (e.g., premature or immunocompromised infants). It is administered by inhalation (nebulization).

Passive immunization with anti-RSV immunoglobulin is available for premature infants. Infected children must be isolated. Infection-control measures are required for hospital staff caring for infected children to avoid transmitting the virus to uninfected patients. These measures include hand-washing and wearing gowns, goggles, and masks.

No vaccine is currently available for RSV prophylaxis. A previously available vaccine containing inactivated RSV caused recipients to have more severe RSV disease when subsequently exposed to the live virus. This development is thought to be the result of a heightened immunologic response at the time of exposure to the wild virus.

Human Metapneumovirus

Human metapneumovirus is a recently recognized member of the pneumovirus family. Use of RT-PCR methods was and remains the means of detecting the pneumoviruses and distinguishing them from other respiratory disease viruses. Its identity was unknown until recently, because it is difficult to grow in cell culture. The virus is ubiquitous and almost all 5-year-old children have experienced a virus infection and are seropositive.

As with its close cousin RSV, infections by human metapneumovirus may be asymptomatic, cause common cold–type disease or serious bronchiolitis and pneumonia. Seronegative children, the elderly and immunocompromised people are at risk to disease. Human metapneumovirus probably causes 15% of common colds in children, especially those which are complicated by otitis media. Signs of disease usually include cough, sore throat, runny nose, and high fever. Approximately 10% of patients with metapneumovirus will

experience wheezing, dyspnea, pneumonia, bronchitis, or bronchiolitis. As with other common cold agents, laboratory identification of the virus is not performed routinely but can be performed by RT-PCR. Supportive care is the only therapy available for these infections.

Nipah and Hendra Viruses

A new paramyxovirus, Nipah virus, was isolated from patients after an outbreak of severe encephalitis in Malaysia and Singapore in 1998. Nipah virus is more closely related to the Hendra virus, discovered in 1994 in Australia, than to other paramyxoviruses. Both viruses have broad host ranges, including pigs, man, dogs, horses, cats, and other mammals. For Nipah virus, the reservoir is a fruit bat (flying fox). The virus can be obtained from fruit contaminated by infected bats or amplified in pigs and then spread to humans. The human is an accidental host for these viruses, but the outcome of human infection is severe. Disease signs include flulike symptoms, seizures, and coma. Of the 269 cases occurring in 1999, 108 were fatal. Another epidemic in Bangladesh in 2004 had a higher mortality rate.

Case Studies and Questions

An 18-year-old college freshman complained of a cough, runny nose, and conjunctivitis. The physician in the campus health center noticed small white lesions inside the patient's mouth. The next day, a confluent red rash covered his face and neck.

1. What clinical characteristics of this case were diagnostic for measles?
2. Are any laboratory tests readily available to confirm the diagnosis? If so, what are they?
3. Is there a possible treatment for this patient?
4. When was this patient contagious?
5. Why is this disease not common in the United States?
6. Provide several possible reasons for this person's susceptibility to measles at 18 years of age.

A 13-month-old child had a runny nose, mild cough, and low-grade fever for several days. The cough got worse and sounded like "barking." The child made a wheezing sound when agitated. The child appeared well except for the cough. A lateral radiograph of the neck showed a subglottic narrowing.

1. What are the specific and common names for these symptoms?
2. What other agents would cause a similar clinical presentation (differential diagnosis)?
3. Are there readily available laboratory tests to confirm this diagnosis? If so, what are they?
4. Was there a possible treatment for this child?
5. When was this child contagious, and how was the virus transmitted?

Orthomyxoviruses

Influenza A, B, and C viruses are the only members of the Orthomyxoviridae family, and only influenza A and B viruses cause significant human disease. The orthomyxoviruses are **enveloped and have a segmented negative-sense RNA genome**. The segmented genome of these viruses facilitates the development of new strains through the mutation and reassortment of the gene segments among different human and animal (influenza A) strains of virus. This genetic instability is responsible for the annual **epidemics (mutation: drift)** and **periodic pandemics (reassortment: shift)** of influenza infection worldwide.

Influenza is one of the most prevalent and significant viral infections. There are even descriptions of influenza **epidemics (local dissemination)** that occurred in ancient times. Probably the most famous influenza **pandemic (worldwide)** is the Spanish influenza that swept the world in 1918 to 1919, killing 20 to 40 million people. In fact, more people died of influenza during that time than in the battles of World War I. Pandemics caused by novel influenza viruses occurred in 1918, 1947, 1957, 1968, and 1977, but fortunately none have occurred since. New virus strains have been detected since the last pandemic, including an outbreak of avian influenza first noted in Hong Kong in 1997, which has caused some human disease and fatalities. Fortunately, prophylaxis in the form of vaccines and antiviral drugs is now available for people at risk for serious outcomes.

Influenza viruses cause respiratory symptoms and the classic flulike symptoms of fever, malaise, headache, and myalgias (body aches). The term **flu,** however, has been mistakenly used to refer to many other respiratory and viral infections (e.g., "intestinal flu").

Structure and Replication

Influenza virions are pleomorphic, appearing spherical or tubular (Box 59-1 and Figure 59-1) and ranging in diameter from 80 to 120 nm. The envelope contains two glycoproteins, **hemagglutinin (HA)** and **neuraminidase (NA),** the **membrane (m_2) protein** and is internally lined by the **matrix (M_1)** protein. The genome of the influenza A and B viruses consists of **eight different helical nucleocapsid segments**, each of which contains a negative-sense RNA associated with the **nucleoprotein (NP)** and the **transcriptase (RNA polymerase components: PB1, PB2, PA)** (Table 59-1). Influenza C has only seven genomic segments.

The genomic segments in the influenza A virus range from 890 to 2340 bases. All the proteins are encoded on separate segments, with the exception of the nonstructural proteins (NS_1 and NS_2) and the M_1 and M_2 proteins, which are transcribed from one segment each.

The **HA** forms a spike-shaped trimer; each unit is activated by a protease and is cleaved into two subunits held together by a disulfide bond. (See Chapter 4, Figure 4-8.) The HA has several functions. It is the viral attachment protein, binding to sialic acid on epithelial cell surface receptors; it promotes fusion of the envelope to the cell membrane; it hemagglutinates (binds and aggregates) human, chicken, and guinea pig red blood cells; and it elicits the protective neutralizing antibody response. Mutation-derived changes in HA are responsible for the minor ("drift") and major ("shift") changes in antigenicity. *Shifts occur only with influenza A virus, and the different HAs are designated H1, H2, and so on.*

The **NA** glycoprotein forms a tetramer and has enzyme activity. The NA cleaves the sialic acid on glycoproteins, including the cell receptor. Cleavage of the sialic acid on virion proteins prevents clumping and facilitates the release of virus from infected cells, making NA a target for two antiviral drugs, **zanamivir (Relenza),** and **oseltamivir (Tamiflu)**. The NA of influenza A virus also undergoes antigenic changes, and major differences acquire the designations N1, N2, and so on.

The **M_1, M_2,** and **NP** proteins are type specific and are therefore used to differentiate influenza A from B or C viruses. The M_1 proteins line the inside of the virion and

Box 59–1. Unique Features of the Influenza A and B Viruses

Enveloped virion has a genome of **eight unique negative-sense RNA nucleocapsid segments.**

Hemagglutinin glycoprotein is the viral attachment protein and fusion protein; it elicits neutralizing, protective antibody responses.

Influenza transcribes and replicates its genome in the target cell nucleus but assembles and buds from the plasma membrane.

The antiviral drugs **amantadine** and **rimantadine** inhibit an uncoating step and target the M_2 (membrane) protein for influenza A *only.*

The antiviral drugs **zanamivir** and **oseltamivir** inhibit the NA protein of influenza A and B.

The segmented genome promotes **genetic diversity** caused by **mutation** and **reassortment** of segments on infection with two different strains.

Influenza A infects humans, mammals, and birds (zoonosis).

Figure 59–1. A, Model of influenza A virus. **B,** Electron micrographs of influenza A virus. (**A** *from Kaplan MM, Webster RG: The epidemiology of influenza. Sci Am 237:88-106, 1977;* **B** *from Balows A, et al (eds): Laboratory Diagnosis of Infectious Diseases: Principles and Practice, vol 2. Heidelberg, Germany, Springer-Verlag, 1988.)*

promote assembly. The M_2 protein forms a proton channel in membranes and promotes uncoating and viral release. The M_2 of influenza A is a target for the antiviral drugs **amantadine** and **rimantadine**.

Viral replication begins with the binding of HA to specific sialic acid structures on cell surface glycoproteins (Figure 59-2). The virus is then internalized into a coated vesicle and transferred to an endosome. Acidification of the endosome causes the HA to bend over and expose hydrophobic fusion-promoting regions of the protein. The viral envelope then fuses with the endosome membrane. The proton channel formed by the M_2 protein promotes acidification of the envelope contents to break the interaction between the M_1 protein and the NP, allowing uncoating and delivery of the nucleocapsid into the cytoplasm.

Unlike most RNA viruses, the influenza nucleocapsid travels to the nucleus, where it is transcribed into messenger ribonucleic acid (mRNA). The transcriptase (PA, PB1, and PB2) uses host cell mRNA as a primer for viral mRNA synthesis. In so doing, it steals the methylated cap region of the RNA, the sequence required for efficient binding to ribosomes. All the genomic segments are transcribed into 5′-capped, 3′-polyadenylated (poly A) mRNA for individual proteins except the segments for the M and NS proteins, which are each differentially spliced (using cellular enzymes) to produce two different mRNAs. The mRNAs are translated into protein in the cytoplasm. The HA and NA glycoproteins are processed by the endoplasmic reticulum and Golgi apparatus. The M_2 protein inserts into cellular membranes. Its proton channel prevents acidification of Golgi and other vesicles, thus preventing acid-induced folding and inactivation of the HA within the cell. The HA and NA are then transported to the cell surface.

Positive-sense RNA templates for each segment are produced, and the negative-sense RNA genome is replicated in the nucleus. The genomic segments associate with polymerase and NP proteins to form nucleocapsids, and the NS_2 protein facilitates the transport of ribonucleocapsids into the cytoplasm, where they interact with the M_1 protein lining plasma membrane sections containing M_2, HA, and NA. The genomic segments are enveloped in a random manner, with 8 to 11 segments per virion. This process produces a small number of virions with a complete set of the 8 genomic segments and numerous defective particles. The particles are antigenic and can also cause interference, which may limit the progression of the infection.

Table 59—1. Products of Influenza Gene Segments

Segment*	Protein	Function
1	PB2	Polymerase component
2	PB1	Polymerase component
3	PA	Polymerase component
4	HA	Hemagglutinin, viral attachment protein, fusion protein, target of neutralizing antibody
5	NP	Nucleocapsid
6	NA	Neuraminidase (cleaves sialic acid and promotes virus release)
7[†]	M_1	Matrix protein: viral structural protein (interacts with nucleocapsid and envelope, promotes assembly)
	M_2	Membrane protein (forms membrane channel and target for amantadine, facilitates uncoating and HA production)
8[†]	NS_1	Nonstructural protein (inhibits cellular messenger RNA translation)
	NS_2	Nonstructural protein (promotes export of nucleocapsid from nucleus)

*Listed in decreasing order of size.
[†]Encodes two messenger RNAs.

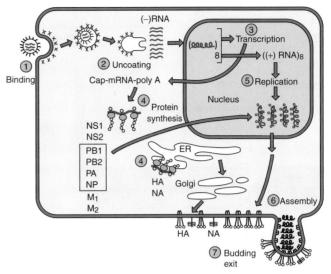

Figure 59—2. Replication of influenza A virus. After binding (1) to sialic acid—containing receptors, influenza is endocytosed and fuses (2) with the vesicle membrane. Unlike for most other RNA viruses, transcription (3) and replication (5) of the genome occur in the nucleus. Viral proteins are synthesized (4), helical nucleocapsid segments form and associate (6) with the M1 protein—lined membranes containing M2 and the HA and NA glycoproteins. The virus buds (7) from the plasma membrane with 8-11 nucleocapsid segments. (—), negative sense; (+), positive sense; ER, endoplasmic reticulum.

The virus buds selectively from the apical (airway) surface of the cell as a result of the preferential insertion of the HA in this membrane. Virus is released approximately 8 hours after infection.

Pathogenesis and Immunity

Influenza initially establishes a local upper respiratory tract infection (Box 59-2). To do so, the virus first targets and kills mucus-secreting, ciliated, and other epithelial cells, causing the loss of this primary defense system. NA facilitates the development of the infection by cleaving sialic acid residues of the mucus, thereby providing access to tissue. Preferential release of the virus at the apical surface of epithelial cells and into the lung promotes cell-to-cell spread and transmission to other hosts. If the virus spreads to the lower respiratory tract, the infection can cause severe desquamation (shedding) of bronchial or alveolar epithelium down to a single-cell basal layer or to the basement membrane.

In addition to compromising the natural defenses of the respiratory tract, influenza infection promotes bacterial adhesion to the epithelial cells. Pneumonia may result from a viral pathogenesis or from a secondary bacterial infection. Influenza may also cause a transient or low-level viremia but rarely involves tissues other than the lung.

Histologically, influenza infection leads to an inflammatory cell response of the mucosal membrane, which consists primarily of monocytes and lymphocytes and few neutrophils. Submucosal edema is present. Lung tissue

Box 59—2. Disease Mechanisms of Influenza A and B Viruses

Virus can establish infection of upper and lower respiratory tract.
Systemic symptoms are caused by the interferon and lymphokine response to the virus. Local symptoms result from epithelial cell damage, including ciliated and mucus-secreting cells.
Interferon and cell-mediated immune responses (NK [natural killer] and T cell) are important for immune resolution and immunopathogenesis.
Infected people are predisposed to bacterial superinfection because of the loss of natural barriers and exposure of binding sites on epithelial cells.
Antibody is important for future protection against infection and is specific for defined epitopes on HA and NA proteins.
The HA and NA of influenza A virus can undergo **major (reassortment: shift)** and **minor (mutation: drift)** antigenic changes to ensure the presence of immunologically naïve, susceptible people.
Influenza B virus undergoes only minor antigenic changes.

Key:

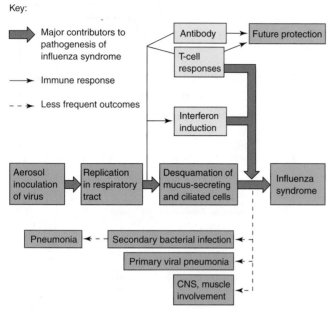

Figure 59—3. Pathogenesis of influenza A virus. The symptoms of influenza are caused by viral pathologic and immunopathologic effects, but the infection may promote secondary bacterial infection. CNS, central nervous system.

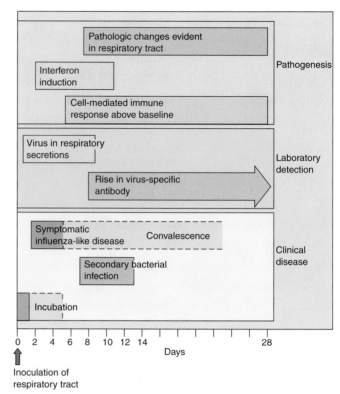

Figure 59—4. Time course of influenza A virus infection. The classic "flu syndrome" occurs early. Later, pneumonia may result from bacterial pathogenesis, viral pathogenesis, or immunopathogenesis.

may reveal hyaline membrane disease, alveolar emphysema, and necrosis of the alveolar walls (Figure 59-3).

Interferon and cytokine responses peak at almost the same time as virus in nasal washes and are concomitant with the febrile phase of disease. T-cell responses are important for effecting recovery and immunopathogenesis. However, influenza infection depresses macrophage and T-cell function, hindering immune resolution. Interestingly, recovery often precedes detection of antibody in serum or secretions.

Protection against reinfection is primarily associated with the development of antibodies to HA, but antibodies to NA are also protective. The antibody response is specific for each strain of influenza, but the cell-mediated immune response is more general and is capable of reacting to influenza strains of the same type (influenza A or B virus). Antigenic targets for T-cell responses include peptides from HA but also from the nucleocapsid proteins (NP, PB2) and M_1 protein. The NP, PB2, and M_1 proteins differ considerably for influenza A and B but not between strains of these viruses; hence T-cell memory may provide future protection against infection by different strains of either influenza A or B.

The symptoms and time course of the disease are determined by interferon and T-cell responses and the extent of epithelial tissue loss. Influenza is normally a self-limited disease that rarely involves organs other than the lung. *Many of the classic "flu" symptoms (e.g., fever, malaise, headache, and myalgia) are associated with interferon induction.* Repair of the compromised tissue is initiated within 3 to 5 days of the start of symptoms but may take as long as a month or more,

especially for elderly people. The time course of influenza virus infection is illustrated in Figure 59-4.

Epidemiology

Strains of influenza A virus are classified by the following four characteristics:

1. Type (A, B, and C)
2. Place of original isolation
3. Date of original isolation
4. Antigen (HA and NA)

For example, a current strain of influenza virus might be designated A/Bangkok/1/79 (H3N2), meaning that it is an influenza A virus that was first isolated in Bangkok in January 1979 and contains HA (H3) and NA (N2) antigens.

Strains of influenza B are designated by (1) type, (2) geography, and (3) date of isolation (e.g., B/Singapore/3/64), but without specific mention of HA or NA antigens, because influenza B does not undergo antigenic shift or pandemics like influenza A does.

New influenza A strains are generated through mutation and reassortment. The genetic diversity of influenza A is fostered by its segmented genomic structure and ability to infect and replicate in humans and many animal species (**zoonose**), including birds and pigs. Hybrid viruses are created by coinfection of a cell with different strains of

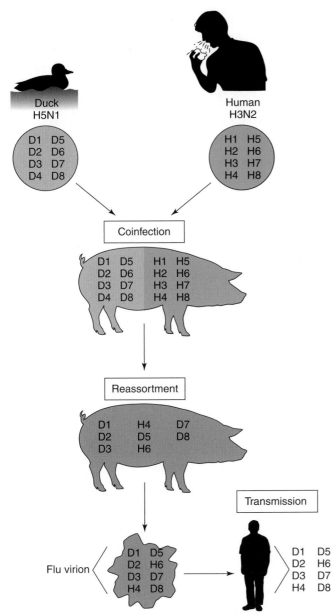

Figure 59–5. Example of reassortment of genomic fragments of influenza A virus. Diagram of the origin of a new human virus, with a shift from H3N2 to H5N1. Pigs were infected with a duck influenza virus, and another set of pigs with the human influenza virus. At some time, a pig underwent mixed infection with both viruses. The resulting virus created by reassortment of the viral gene segments could be transmitted to and infect humans.

is thought to be a breeding ground for new reassortant viruses and the source of many of the pandemic strains of influenza.

In 1997, a highly pathogenic avian influenza virus (HPAIV) (H5N1) strain was isolated from at least 18 humans and caused six deaths in Hong Kong (Clinical Case 59-1). Wild water fowl have become a reservoir for this virus and spread the virus around the world. Outbreaks of infection of poultry and isolated human cases continue to be reported in Africa, Europe, and Asia. Although relatively few humans were infected, this H5N1 virus is unusual because it is not a reassortant, it is very virulent, and it can pass directly from bird to man. A tropism for the lower lung requires inhalation of larger amounts of virus, and the virus and target tissue make human infection very lethal. Avian influenza is transmitted in bird feces, not by human-to-human transmission. Outbreaks of avian influenza require the destruction of all potentially infected birds, such as for the 1.6 million chickens in Hong Kong, to destroy the potential source of the virus. Concern that a reassortant with a human influenza virus might generate a pandemic has spearheaded an international drive for development and stockpiling of vaccines.

Clinical Case 59-1. H5N1 Avian Influenza

The first case of H5N1 avian influenza in a human was described by Ku and Chan (J Paediatr Child Health 35:207-208, 1999). After a 3-year-old boy from China developed a 40° C fever and abdominal pain, he was given antibiotics and aspirin. On the third day, he was hospitalized with sore throat, and his chest x-ray demonstrated bronchial inflammation. Blood studies showed a left shift with 9% band forms. On the 6th day, the boy was still febrile and fully conscious, but on the 7th day, his fever increased, he was hyperventilating, and his blood oxygen levels decreased. Chest x-ray indicated severe pneumonia. The patient was intubated. On the 8th day, the boy was diagnosed with fulminant sepsis and adult respiratory distress syndrome (ARDS). Therapy for ARDS and other attempts to improve oxygen uptake were unsuccessful. He was treated empirically for sepsis, herpes simplex virus (HSV) infection (acyclovir), methicillin-resistant *Staphylococcus aureus* (MRSA) (vancomycin), and fungal infection (amphotericin B), but his condition deteriorated further, with disseminated intravascular coagulation (DIC) and liver and renal failure. He died on the 11th day. Lab results indicated elevated Influenza A antibody on the 8th day, and influenza A was isolated from a tracheal isolate taken on the 9th day. The isolate was sent to the U.S. Centers for Disease Control and Prevention and elsewhere, where it was typed as H5N1 avian influenza and named *A/Hong Kong/156/97*. The child may have contracted the virus while playing with pet ducklings and chickens at his kindergarten. Although the H5N1 virus still has difficulty infecting humans, this case demonstrates the speed and severity of the respiratory and systemic manifestations of avian influenza H5N1 disease.

---

influenza A virus, allowing the genomic segments to randomly associate into new virions. An exchange of the HA glycoproteins may generate a new virus that can infect an immunologically naïve human population. For example, an H5N1 duck virus and an H3N2 human virus infected pigs, reassortants were isolated from the pig, and the resulting virus was able to infect humans (Figure 59-5). This type of reassortment is postulated to be the source of pathogenic human strains. Because of its high population density and proximity of humans, pigs, chickens, and ducks, China

Table 59—2. Influenza Pandemics Resulting from Antigenic Shift

Year of Pandemic	Influenza A Subtype
1918	$H_{SW}N1$; probable swine flu strain
1947	H1N1
1957	H2N2; Asian flu strain
1968	H3N2; Hong Kong flu strain
1977	H1N1

Minor antigenic changes resulting from mutation of the HA and NA genes are called **antigenic drift**. This process occurs every 2 to 3 years, causing local outbreaks of influenza A and B infection. **Major antigenic changes (antigenic shift)** result from the reassortment of genomes among different strains, including animal strains. *This process occurs only with the influenza A virus.* Such changes are often associated with the occurrence of pandemics.

Antigenic shifts occur infrequently but can be devastating (Table 59-2). For example, the prevalent influenza A virus in 1947 was the H1N1 subtype. In 1957, there was a shift in both antigens, resulting in an H2N2 subtype. H3N2 appeared in 1968, and H1N1 reappeared in 1977. The reappearance of H1N1 put the population younger than age 30 at risk to disease. Prior exposure and an anamnestic antibody response protected the members of the population older than 30 years. *In contrast to influenza A, influenza B is predominantly a human virus and does not undergo antigenic shift.*

The changing antigenic nature of influenza ensures a large proportion of immunologically naïve, susceptible people (especially children) in the population (Box 59-3). An influenza outbreak can be readily detected from the increased absenteeism in schools and work and the number of emergency department visits. During the winter, influenza outbreaks occur annually in temperate climates. Fortunately, influenza virus is present in a community for only a short time (4 to 6 weeks).

Influenza infection is spread readily via small airborne droplets expelled during talking, breathing, and coughing. The virus can also survive on countertops for as long as a day.

The most susceptible population is children, and school-age children are most likely to spread the infection. Contagion precedes symptoms and lasts for a long time, especially in children. Children, immunosuppressed people (including pregnant women), the elderly, and people with heart and lung ailments (including smokers) are at highest risk for more serious disease, pneumonia, or other complications of infection. More than 90% of mortalities occur in patients who are older than 65 years.

Box 59—3. Epidemiology of Influenza A and B Viruses

Disease/Viral Factors

Virus has a large, enveloped virion that is easily inactivated by dryness, acid, and detergents.
Segmented genome facilitates major genetic changes, especially on HA and NA proteins.
Influenza A infects many vertebrate species, including other mammals and birds.
Coinfection with animal and human strains of influenza can generate very different virus strains by genetic reassortment.
Transmission of virus often precedes symptoms.

Transmission

Virus is spread by inhalation of small aerosol droplets expelled during talking, breathing, and coughing.
Virus likes cool, less humid atmosphere (e.g., winter heating season).
Virus is extensively spread by school children.

Who Is at Risk?

Seronegative people.
Adults: classic flu syndrome.
Children: asymptomatic to severe respiratory tract infections.
High-risk groups: elderly and immunocompromised people, people in nursing homes or with underlying cardiac or respiratory problems (including asthma sufferers and smokers).

Geography/Season

There is worldwide occurrence. Epidemics are local; pandemics are worldwide.
Disease is more common in winter.

Modes of Control

Amantadine, rimantadine, zanamivir, and oseltamivir have been approved for prophylaxis or early treatment.
Killed and live vaccines contain predicted yearly strains of influenza A and B viruses.

Extensive surveillance of influenza A and B outbreaks is conducted to identify new strains that should be incorporated into new vaccines. The prevalence of a particular strain of influenza A or B virus changes each year and reflects the particular immunologic naïveté of the population at that time. Surveillance also extends into the animal populations because of the possible presence of recombinant animal influenza A strains that can cause human pandemics.

Clinical Syndromes (Box 59-4)

Depending on the degree of immunity to the infecting strain of virus and other factors, infection may range from asymptomatic to severe. Patients with underlying cardiorespiratory disease, people with immune deficiency

Box 59–4. Clinical Summaries

Influenza A: A 70-year-old woman has rapid onset of fever with headache, myalgia, sore throat, and nonproductive cough. The disease progresses to pneumonia with bacterial involvement. There is no history of recent immunization with influenza A vaccine. Her husband is treated with amantadine or a neuraminidase inhibitor.

(even that associated with pregnancy), the elderly, and smokers are more prone to have a severe case.

After an incubation period of 1 to 4 days, the "flu syndrome" begins with a brief prodrome of malaise and headache lasting a few hours. The prodrome is followed by the abrupt onset of fever, chills, severe myalgias, loss of appetite, weakness and fatigue, sore throat, and usually a nonproductive cough. The fever persists for 3 to 8 days, and unless a complication occurs, recovery is complete within 7 to 10 days. Influenza in young children (under 3 years) resembles other severe respiratory tract infections, causing bronchiolitis, croup, otitis media, vomiting, and abdominal pain, accompanied rarely by febrile convulsions (Table 59-3). Complications of influenza include bacterial pneumonia, myositis, and Reye syndrome. The central nervous system can also be involved. Influenza B disease is similar to influenza A disease.

Influenza may directly cause pneumonia, but it more commonly promotes a secondary bacterial superinfection that leads to bronchitis or pneumonia. The tissue damage caused by progressive influenza virus infection of alveoli can be extensive, leading to hypoxia and bilateral pneumonia. Secondary bacterial infection usually involves *Streptococcus pneumoniae*, *Haemophilus influenzae*, or *Staphylococcus aureus*. In these infections, sputum usually is produced and becomes purulent.

Although the infection generally is limited to the lung, some strains of influenza can spread to other sites in certain people. For example, myositis (inflammation of muscle) may occur in children. Encephalopathy, although rare, may accompany an acute influenza illness and can be fatal. Postinfluenza encephalitis occurs 2 to 3 weeks after recovery from influenza. It is associated with evidence of inflammation but is rarely fatal.

Reye syndrome is an acute encephalitis that affects children and occurs after a variety of acute febrile viral infections, including varicella and influenza B and A diseases. Children given salicylates (aspirin) are at increased risk for this syndrome. In addition to encephalopathy, hepatic dysfunction is present. The mortality rate may be as high as 40%.

Laboratory Diagnosis

The diagnosis of influenza is usually based on the characteristic symptoms, the season, and the presence of the virus in the community. Laboratory methods that distinguish influenza from other respiratory viruses and identify its type and strain confirm the diagnosis (Table 59-4).

Influenza viruses are obtained from respiratory secretions. The virus is generally isolated in primary monkey kidney cell cultures or the Madin-Darby canine kidney cell line. Nonspecific cytopathologic effects are often difficult to distinguish but may be noted within as few as 2 days (average, 4 days). Before the cytopathologic effects develop, the addition of guinea pig erythrocytes may reveal **hemadsorption** (the adherence of these erythrocytes to HA-expressing infected cells). (See Chapter 50, Figure 50-5.) The addition of influenza virus—containing media to erythrocytes promotes the formation of a gel-like aggregate due to **hemagglutination**. Hemagglutination and hemadsorption are not specific to influenza viruses, however; parainfluenza and other viruses also exhibit these properties.

More rapid techniques detect and identify the influenza genome or antigens of the virus. Rapid antigen assays (less than 30 min) can detect and distinguish influenza A and B. Reverse transcriptase polymerase chain reaction (RT-PCR) using generic influenza primers can be used to detect and distinguish influenza A and B, and more specific primers can be used to distinguish the different strains, such as H5N1. Enzyme immunoassay or immunofluorescence can be used to detect viral antigen in exfoliated cells, respiratory secretions, or cell culture and are more sensitive assays. Immunofluorescence or inhibition of hemadsorption or hemagglutination (hemagglutination inhibition [HI]) with

Table 59–3. Diseases Associated with Influenza Virus Infection

Disorder	Symptoms
Acute influenza infection in adults	Rapid onset of fever, malaise, myalgia, sore throat, and nonproductive cough
Acute influenza infection in children	Acute disease similar to that in adults but with higher fever, gastrointestinal tract symptoms (abdominal pain, vomiting), otitis media, myositis, and more frequent croup

Complications of influenza virus infection	Primary viral pneumonia
	Secondary bacterial pneumonia
	Myositis and cardiac involvement
	Neurologic syndromes:
	    Guillain-Barré syndrome
	    Encephalopathy
	    Encephalitis
	    Reye syndrome

Table 59–4. Laboratory Diagnosis of Influenza Virus Infection

Test	Detects
Cell culture in primary monkey kidney or Madin-Darby canine kidney cells	Presence of virus; limited cytopathologic effects
Hemadsorption to infected cells	Presence of HA protein on cell surface
Hemagglutination	Presence of virus in secretions
Hemagglutination inhibition	Type and strain of influenza virus or specificity of antibody
Antibody inhibition of hemadsorption	Identification of influenza type and strain
Immunofluorescence, ELISA	Influenza virus antigens in respiratory secretions or tissue culture
Serology: hemagglutination inhibition, hemadsorption inhibition, ELISA, immunofluorescence, complement fixation	Seroepidemiology
Genomics: RT-PCR	Identification of influenza type and strain

ELISA, enzyme-linked immunosorbent assay.

specific antibody (see Chapter 50) can also detect and distinguish different influenza strains. Laboratory studies are primarily used for epidemiologic purposes.

Treatment, Prevention, and Control

Hundreds of millions of dollars are spent on acetaminophen, antihistamines, and similar drugs to relieve the symptoms of influenza. The antiviral drug **amantadine** and its analogue **rimantadine** inhibit an uncoating step of the influenza A virus but do not affect the influenza B and C viruses. The target for their action is the M_2 protein. **Zanamivir** and **oseltamivir** inhibit both influenza A and B as enzyme inhibitors of neuraminidase. Without neuraminidase, the hemagglutinin of the virus binds to sialic acid on other viral particles to form clumps, thereby preventing virus release. Zanamivir is inhaled, whereas oseltamivir is taken orally as a pill. These drugs are effective for prophylaxis and for treatment during the first 24 to 48 hours after the onset of influenza A illness. Treatment cannot prevent the later host-induced immunopathogenic stages of the disease.

The airborne spread of influenza is almost impossible to limit. However, the best way to control the virus is through immunization. Natural immunization, which

results from prior exposure, is protective for long periods. A killed-virus vaccine representing the "strains of the year" and antiviral drug prophylaxis can also prevent infection.

The influenza vaccine is a mixture of extracts or purified HA and NA proteins from three different strains of virus. The vaccines are prepared from virus grown in embryonated eggs and then chemically inactivated. Killed (formalin-inactivated) virion preparations have also been used. Ideally the vaccine incorporates antigens of the A and B influenza strains that will be prevalent in the community during the upcoming winter. For instance, the trivalent influenza vaccine used for the 2006-2007 season included A/New Caledonia/20/1999 (H1N1)–like, A/Wisconsin/67/2005 (H3N2)–like, and B/Malaysia/2506/2004–like antigens. Vaccination is routinely recommended for persons older than 50, healthcare workers, pregnant women who will be in their second or third trimester during flu season, people living in a nursing home, people with chronic pulmonary heart disease, and others at high risk. As of 2008, all children aged 5-18 years should also be vaccinated. Persons with allergies to eggs should not get the vaccine.

A live vaccine is also available for administration as a nasal spray instead of a "flu shot." The trivalent vaccine consists of reassortants for the HA and NA gene segments of different influenza strains, with a master donor virus that is cold adapted to optimum growth at 25° C. This vaccine will elicit a more natural protection, including cell-mediated, antibody and mucosal-secretory immunoglobulin (Ig)A antibody. Currently the vaccine is recommended for people ages 5 to 50.

Case Study and Questions

In late December, a 22-year-old man suddenly experienced headache, myalgia, malaise, dry cough, and fever. He basically felt lousy. After a couple of days, he had a sore throat, his cough had worsened, he started to feel nauseated, and he began vomiting. Several of his family members had experienced similar symptoms during the previous 2 weeks.

1. In addition to influenza, what other agents could cause similar symptoms (differential diagnosis)?
2. How would the diagnosis of influenza be confirmed?
3. Amantadine is effective against influenza. What is its mechanism of action? Will it be effective for this patient? For uninfected family members or contacts?
4. When was the patient contagious, and how was the virus transmitted?
5. What family members were at greatest risk for serious disease and why?
6. Why is influenza so difficult to control, even when there is a national vaccination program?

Bibliography

Cann AJ: Principles of Molecular Virology. San Diego, Academic, 2005.

Carter J, Saunders V: Virology: Principles and Applications, Chichester, England, Wiley, 2007.

Cohen J, Powderly WG: Infectious Diseases, 2nd ed. St Louis, Mosby, 2004.

Collier L, Oxford J: Human Virology, 3rd ed. Oxford, Oxford University Press, 2006.

Cox NJ, Subbarao K: Global epidemiology of influenza: Past and present. Annu Rev Med 51:407-421, 2000.

Flint SJ, et al: Principles of Virology: Molecular Biology, Pathogenesis and Control of Animal Viruses, 2nd ed. Washington, DC, ASM Press, 2003.

Helenius A: Unpacking the incoming influenza virus. Cell 69:577-578, 1992.

Knipe DM, Howley PM: Fields Virology, 4th ed. New York, Lippincott Williams & Wilkins, 2001.

Laver WG, Bischofberger N, Webster RG: Disarming flu viruses. Sci Am 280:78-87, 1999.

Laver WG, Bischofberger N, Webster RG: The origin and control of pandemic influenza. Perspect Biol Med 43:173-192, 2000.

Poland GA, Jacobson RM, Targonski PV: Avian and pandemic influenza: An overview. Vaccine 25:3057-61, 2007.

Strauss JM, Strauss EG: Viruses and Human Disease, 2nd ed. San Diego, Academic, 2007.

Webster RG: Predictions for future human influenza pandemics. J Infect Dis 176(suppl 1):S14-S19, 1997.

Webster RG, et al: Evolution and ecology of influenza viruses. Microbiol Rev 56:152-179, 1992.

Webster RG, Govorkova EA: H5N1 Influenza, Continuing Evolution and Spread. N Engl J Med 355:2174-2177, 2006.

Voyles BA: The Biology of Viruses, 2nd ed. Boston, McGraw-Hill, 2002.

Websites

CDC information about influenza (online): Available at http://www.cdc.gov/flu/

Derlet R, Nguyen HH, Lawrence R: Influenza (2007, online): Available at http://www.emedicine.com/med/topic1170.htm

IFPMA Influenza Vaccine Supply International Task Force, Influenza fact sheets (online): Available at http://www.ifpma.org/Influenza/index.aspx?1

National Institute of Allergy and Infectious Disease, Influenza fact sheet available online at: www.niaid.nih.gov/publications/flu.htm

Webster RG: Influenza, an emerging disease. Centers for Disease Control, (1998, online): Available at http://www.cdc.gov/ncidod/EID/vol4no3/webster.htm

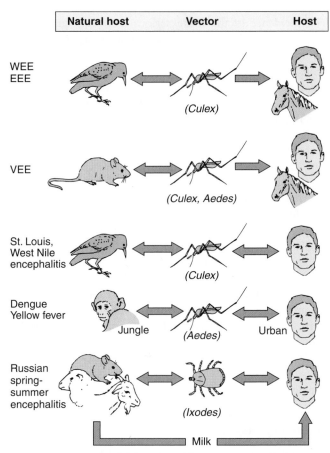

Figure 62—5. Patterns of alphavirus and flavivirus transmission. Birds and small mammals are the hosts that maintain and amplify an arbovirus, which is spread by the insect vector upon a blood meal. A double arrow indicates a cycle of replication in both host (including man) and vector. "Dead-end" infections with no transmission of the virus back to the vector are indicated by the single arrow. EEE, eastern equine encephalitis; VEE, Venezuelan equine encephalitis; WEE, western equine encephalitis.

maintain the virus. The virus may either (1) persist in arthropod larvae or eggs or in reptiles or amphibians that remain in the locale or (2) migrate with the birds and then return during the summer.

When humans travel into the ecologic niche of the mosquito vector, they risk being infected by the virus. Pools of standing water, drainage ditches, and trash dumps in cities can also provide breeding grounds for mosquitoes such as *Aedes aegypti*, the vector for yellow fever, dengue, and chikungunya. An increase in the population of these mosquitoes therefore puts the human population at risk for infection. Health departments in many areas monitor birds and mosquitoes caught in traps for arboviruses and initiate control measures, such as insecticide spraying, when necessary.

Urban outbreaks of arbovirus infections occur when the reservoirs for the virus are humans or urban animals. Humans can be reservoir hosts for yellow fever, dengue, and chikungunya viruses (see Figure 62-5). These viruses are maintained by *Aedes* mosquitoes in a **sylvatic** or **jungle cycle**, in which monkeys are the natural host, and also in an **urban cycle**, in which humans are the host. *A. aegypti*, a vector for each of these viruses, is a household mosquito. It breeds in pools of water, open sewers, and other accumulations of water in cities. The occurrence of numerous inapparent infections in high-density populations provides enough viremic human hosts for the continued spread of these viruses. St. Louis encephalitis and West Nile encephalitis viruses are maintained in an urban environment because their vectors, *Culex* mosquitoes, breed in stagnant water, including puddles and sewage, and the reservoir group includes common city birds (e.g., crows).

Clinical Syndromes

More humans are infected with alphaviruses and flaviviruses than show significant, characteristic symptoms. The incidence of arbovirus disease is sporadic. Alphavirus infections are usually asymptomatic or cause low-grade disease such as **flulike symptoms** (chills, fever, rash, and aches) that correlate with systemic infection during the initial viremia. Eastern equine encephalitis virus (EEEV), WEEV, and Venezuelan equine encephalitis virus (VEEV) infections can progress to **encephalitis** in humans. The equine encephalitis viruses are usually more of a problem to livestock than to humans. An affected human may experience fever, headache, and decreased consciousness 3 to 10 days after infection. Unlike herpes simplex virus encephalitis, the disease generally resolves without sequelae, but there is the possibility of paralysis, mental disability, seizures, and death. The name **chikungunya** (Swahili for "that which bends up") refers to the crippling arthritis associated with serious disease caused by infection with these viruses. Although predominant in South America and western Africa, this disease may spread to the United States because of the return of the *A. aegypti* mosquito, its vector.

outbreak in New York by the unusual deaths of captive birds at the Bronx Zoo. Reverse transcriptase—polymerase chain reaction (RT-PCR) analysis identified the virus as WNV. The virus is transmitted by *Culex pipiens* mosquitoes and crows, blue jays, and other wild birds are the reservoir. The virus spread throughout the United States, and by 2006 the virus and human disease had been noted in almost every state. WNV establishes a sufficient viremia in humans to be a risk factor for transmission through blood transfusions. Documentation of two such cases has led to screening blood donors for WNV and rejecting donors who have fever and headache during the week of blood donation.

Arbovirus diseases occur during the summer months and rainy seasons, when the arthropods breed and the arboviruses are cycled among a host reservoir (birds), an arthropod (e.g., mosquitoes), and human hosts. This cycle maintains and increases the amount of virus in the environment. In the winter, the vector is not present to

Most flavivirus infections are relatively benign, but serious **aseptic meningitis** and **encephalitic** or **hemorrhagic disease** can occur. The encephalitis viruses include St. Louis, **West Nile,** Japanese, Murray Valley, and Russian spring-summer viruses. Symptoms and outcomes are similar to those of the togavirus encephalitides. Hundreds to thousands of cases of St. Louis encephalitis virus disease are noted in the United States annually. Approximately 20% of individuals infected with WNV will develop West Nile fever, characterized by fever, headache, tiredness, and body aches, occasionally with a skin rash on the trunk of the body and swollen lymph glands usually lasting only a few days (Clinical Case 62-1). Encephalitis, meningitis, or meningoencephalitis occurs in approximately 1% of WNV-infected individuals.

The hemorrhagic viruses are dengue and yellow fever viruses. **Dengue virus** is a major worldwide problem, with up to 50 million cases of dengue fever and 300,000 cases of **dengue hemorrhagic fever (DHF)** occurring per year. Although not endemic in the United States, the virus and its vector are present in central and northern South America.

Clinical Case 62-1. West Nile Encephalitis Virus

Hirsch and Warner (N Engl J Med 348:2239-2247, 2003) described the case of a 38-year-old Massachusetts woman who presented with a progressively worsening headache, with photophobia and fever. It being August, she was on summer vacation and 10 days earlier (−10) had traveled to St. Louis and stayed for 8 days. While there, she walked in the woods and visited the zoo. A day before the onset of these symptoms (−1), she vacationed along the Atlantic shore and noted that she had been bitten by mosquitos and removed ticks from her dog. Four days later (+4), she was admitted with fever (40° C), chills, rapid heartbeat, confusion, lightheadedness, and lethargy. Although appearing alert, oriented, and only slightly ill, her neck was rigid and Kernig sign was present. The signs of meningitis prompted testing of CSF, which contained IgM to West Nile Virus (WNV) and low titers to St. Louis Encephalitis virus (SLE). Patient antibody neutralized WNV but not SLE virus infection of tissue culture cells, suggesting that the activity to SLE was due to cross reactivity between flaviviruses. Tests for other organisms were negative. She was treated empirically for meningitis and for HSV (acyclovir). Antibacterial and anti-HSV treatment for meningitis and encephalitis were necessary until the laboratory results were available. On day 5 post onset, she became more lethargic and had difficulty answering questions. An MRI indicated subtle changes in the brain. On day 6, she could not distinguish her right from her left hand, but her headache lessened, and she could respond to commands. On day 7, she had a tremor in her right arm, but her mental status was improving, and by day 8, she was alert and lucid. On day 9, a cranial MRI was normal, on day 10, she was recovered, and on day 11, she was released from the hospital. The season of the year, exposure to insects, and travel by this woman were suggestive of several different arboviral encephalitis diseases, in addition to West Nile encephalitis. Viruses in the differential diagnosis included eastern equine encephalitis, St. Louis encephalitis, Powassan virus (tick-borne flavivirus), HSV, and West Nile virus. Unlike HSV encephalitis, flavivirus meningoencephalitis usually resolves with limited sequelae.

The incidence of the more serious DHF has quadrupled since 1985. Dengue fever is also known as **break-bone fever**; the symptoms and signs consist of high fever, headache, rash, and back and bone pain that last 6 to 7 days. On rechallenge with another of the four related strains, dengue can also cause DHF and **dengue shock syndrome (DSS)**. Non-neutralizing antibody promotes uptake of the virus into macrophages, which causes memory T cells to become activated, release inflammatory cytokines, and initiate hypersensitivity reactions. These reactions and the virus result in weakening and rupture of the vasculature, internal bleeding, and loss of plasma, leading to shock symptoms and internal bleeding. In 1981 in Cuba, dengue-2 virus infected a population previously exposed to dengue-1 virus between 1977 and 1980, leading to an epidemic of more than 100,000 cases of DHF/DSS and 168 deaths.

Yellow fever infections are characterized by severe systemic disease, with degeneration of the liver, kidney, and heart, as well as hemorrhage. Liver involvement causes the jaundice from which the disease gets its name, but massive gastrointestinal hemorrhages ("black vomit") may also occur. The mortality rate associated with yellow fever during epidemics is as high as 50%.

Laboratory Diagnosis

The alphaviruses and flaviviruses can be grown in both vertebrate and mosquito cell lines, but most are difficult to isolate. Infection can be detected through the use of cytopathologic studies, immunofluorescence, and the hemadsorption of avian erythrocytes. Detection and characterization can be performed by RT-PCR testing of genomic RNA or viral mRNA in blood or other samples. After isolation, the viral RNA can also be distinguished by the finding of RNA "fingerprints" of the genomic RNA. Monoclonal antibodies to the individual viruses have become a useful tool for distinguishing the individual species and strains of viruses.

A variety of serologic methods can be used to diagnose infections, including hemagglutination inhibition, enzyme-linked immunosorbent assays, and latex agglutination. The presence of specific IgM or a fourfold increase in titer between acute and convalescent sera is used to indicate a recent infection. The serologic cross-reactivity among viruses limits distinction of the actual viral species in many cases.

Treatment, Prevention, and Control

No treatments exist for arbovirus diseases, other than supportive care. *The easiest means of preventing the spread of any arbovirus is elimination of its vector and breeding grounds.* After 1900, when Walter Reed and his colleagues discovered that yellow fever was spread by A. aegypti, the number of cases was reduced from 1400 to none within

2 years purely through control of the mosquito population. Many Public Health departments monitor the bird and mosquito populations in a region for arboviruses and periodically spray to reduce the mosquito population. Avoidance of the breeding grounds of a mosquito vector is also a good preventive measure.

A live vaccine against yellow fever virus and killed vaccines against EEEV, WEEV, Japanese, and Russian spring-summer encephalitis viruses are available. These vaccines are meant for people working with the virus or at risk for contact. A live vaccine against VEEV is available but only for use in domestic animals. A vaccine against dengue virus has not been developed because of the potential risk for immune enhancement of the disease on subsequent challenge.

The yellow fever vaccine is prepared from the 17D strain isolated from a patient in 1927 and grown for long periods in monkeys, mosquitoes, embryonic tissue culture, and embryonated eggs. The vaccine is administered intradermally and elicits lifelong immunity to yellow fever and possibly other cross-reacting flaviviruses.

Rubella Virus

Rubella virus has the same structural properties and mode of replication as the other togaviruses. However, unlike the other togaviruses, rubella is a **respiratory virus** and **does not cause readily detectable cytopathologic effects**.

Rubella is one of the five **classic childhood exanthems**, along with measles, roseola, fifth disease, and chickenpox. Rubella, meaning "little red" in Latin, was first distinguished from measles and other exanthems by German physicians; thus the common name for the disease, **German measles**. In 1941, an astute Australian ophthalmologist, Norman McAlister Gregg, recognized that maternal rubella infection was the cause of congenital cataracts. Maternal rubella infection has since been correlated with several other **severe congenital defects**. This finding prompted the development of a unique program to vaccinate children to prevent infection of pregnant women and neonates.

Pathogenesis and Immunity

Rubella virus is not cytolytic but does have limited cytopathologic effects in certain cell lines, such as Vero and RK13. The replication of rubella prevents (in a process known as **heterologous interference**) the replication of superinfecting picornaviruses. This property allowed the first isolations of rubella virus in 1962.

Rubella infects the upper respiratory tract and then spreads to local lymph nodes, which coincides with a period of lymphadenopathy (Figure 62-6). This stage is followed by establishment of viremia, which spreads the virus throughout the body. Infection of other tissues and the characteristic mild rash result. The prodromal period

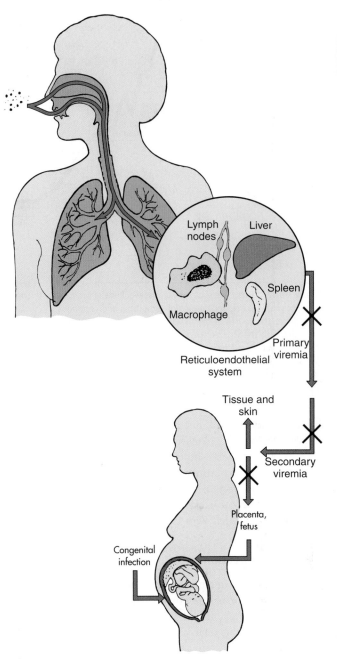

Figure 62—6. Spread of rubella virus within the host. Rubella enters and infects the nasopharynx and lung and then spreads to the lymph nodes and monocyte-macrophage system. The resulting viremia spreads the virus to other tissues and the skin. Circulating antibody can block the transfer of virus at the indicated points *(X)*. In an immunologically deficient pregnant woman, the virus can infect the placenta and spread to the fetus.

lasts approximately 2 weeks (Figure 62-7). The person can shed virus in respiratory droplets during the prodromal period and for as long as 2 weeks after the onset of the rash.

Immune Response

Antibody is generated after the viremia, and its appearance correlates with the appearance of the rash. The antibody

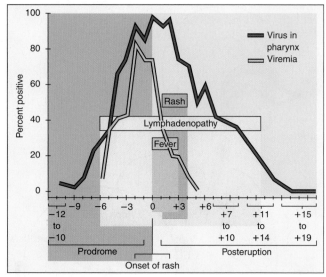

Figure 62–7. Time course of rubella disease. Rubella production in the pharynx precedes the appearance of symptoms and continues throughout the course of the disease. The onset of lymphadenopathy coincides with the viremia. Fever and rash occur later. The person is infectious as long as the virus is produced in the pharynx. *(Redrawn from Plotkin SA: Rubella vaccine. In Plotkin SA, Mortimer EA: Vaccines. Philadelphia, WB Saunders, 1988.)*

---

limits viremic spread, but cell-mediated immunity plays an important role in resolving the infection. Only one serotype of rubella exists, and natural infection produces lifelong protective immunity. Most important, serum antibody in a pregnant woman prevents spread of the virus to the fetus. *Immune complexes most likely cause the rash and arthralgia associated with rubella infection.*

Congenital Infection

Rubella infection in a pregnant woman can result in serious congenital abnormalities in the child. If the mother does not have antibody, the virus can replicate in the placenta and spread to the fetal blood supply and throughout the fetus. Rubella can replicate in most tissues of the fetus. The virus may not be cytolytic, but the normal growth, mitosis, and chromosomal structure of the cells of the fetus can be altered by the infection. The alterations can lead to improper development of the fetus, small size of the infected baby, and the **teratogenic effects** associated with congenital rubella infection. The nature of the disorder is determined by (1) the tissue affected and (2) the stage of development disrupted.

The virus may persist in tissues, such as the lens of the eye, for 3 to 4 years and may be shed up to a year after birth. The presence of the virus during the development of the baby's immune response may even have a tolerative effect on the system, preventing effective clearance of the virus after birth. Immune complexes that produce further clinical abnormalities may also form in the neonate or infant.

Box 62–4. Epidemiology of Rubella Virus

Disease/Viral Factors

Rubella infects only humans.
Virus can cause asymptomatic disease.
There is one serotype.

Transmission

Respiratory route.

Who Is at Risk?

Children: mild exanthematous disease.
Adults: more severe disease with arthritis or arthralgia.
Neonates younger than 20 weeks: congenital defects.

Modes of Control

Live attenuated vaccine is administered as part of measles, mumps, and rubella (MMR) vaccine.

Epidemiology

Humans are the only host for rubella (Box 62-4). The virus is spread in respiratory secretions and is generally acquired during childhood. Spread of virus, before or in the absence of symptoms, and crowded conditions, such as those in daycare centers, promote contagion.

Approximately 20% of women of childbearing age escape infection during childhood and are susceptible to infection unless vaccinated. Programs in many states in the United States test expectant mothers for antibodies to rubella.

Before the development and use of the rubella vaccine, cases of rubella in school children would be reported every spring, and major epidemics of rubella occurred at regular 6- to 9-year intervals. The severity of the 1964 to 1965 epidemic in the United States is indicated in Table 62-3. Congenital rubella occurred in as many as 1% of all the children born in cities such as Philadelphia during this epidemic. Since the development of the vaccine, however, the incidence of rubella and congenital rubella is now less than 1 and 0.1 per 100,000 pregnancies, respectively.

Clinical Syndromes

Rubella disease is normally benign in children. After a 14- to 21-day incubation period, the symptoms in children consist of a 3-day **maculopapular** or **macular rash** and swollen glands (Figure 62-8). Infection in adults, however, can be more severe and include problems such as bone and joint pain (arthralgia and arthritis) and (rarely) thrombocytopenia or postinfectious encephalopathy. Immunopathologic effects resulting from cell-mediated immunity and hypersensitivity reactions are a major cause of the more severe forms of rubella in adults.

Congenital disease is the most serious outcome of rubella infection. The fetus is at major risk until the

Table 62–3. Estimated Morbidity Associated with the 1964-1965 U.S. Rubella Epidemic

Clinical Events	Number Affected
Rubella cases	12,500,000
Arthritis-arthralgia	159,375
Encephalitis	2084
Deaths	
Excess neonatal deaths	2100
Other deaths	60
Total deaths	2160
Excess fetal wastage	6250
Congenital rubella syndrome	
Deaf children	8055
Deaf/blind children	3580
Mentally retarded children	1790
Other congenital rubella syndrome symptoms	6575
Total congenital rubella syndrome	20,000
Therapeutic abortions	5000

From National Communicable Disease Center: Rubella surveillance, U.S. Department of Health, Education and Welfare, No. 1, June 1969.

20th week of pregnancy. Maternal immunity to the virus resulting from prior exposure or vaccination prevents spread of the virus to the fetus. The most common manifestations of congenital rubella infection are cataracts, mental retardation, and deafness (Boxes 62-5 and 62-6; see Table 62-3). The mortality in utero and within the first year after birth is high for affected babies.

Figure 62–8. Close-up of the rubella rash. Small erythematous macules are visible. *(From Hart CA, Broadwell RL: A Color Atlas of Pediatric Infectious Disease. London, Wolfe, 1992.)*

Box 62–5. Prominent Clinical Findings in Congenital Rubella Syndrome

Cataracts and other ocular defects
Heart defects
Deafness
Intrauterine growth retardation
Failure to thrive
Mortality within the first year
Microcephaly
Mental retardation

Laboratory Diagnosis

Isolation of the rubella virus is difficult and rarely attempted. The presence of the virus can be detected by RT-PCR detection of viral RNA. The diagnosis is usually confirmed by the presence of antirubella-specific IgM. A fourfold increase in specific IgG antibody titer between acute and convalescent sera is also used to indicate a recent infection. Antibodies to rubella are assayed early in pregnancy to determine the immune status of the woman; this test is required in many states.

When isolation of the virus is necessary, the virus is usually obtained from urine and is detected as interference with replication of echovirus 11 in primary African green monkey kidney cell cultures.

Treatment, Prevention, and Control

No treatment has been found for rubella. The best means of preventing rubella is vaccination with the live cold-adapted RA27/3 vaccine strain of virus (Figure 62-9). The live rubella vaccine is usually administered with the measles and mumps vaccines (**MMR vaccine**) at 24 months of age.

Box 62–6. Clinical Summaries

West Nile Encephalitis: During August, a 70-year-old man from a swampy area of Louisiana develops fever, headache, muscle weakness, nausea, and vomiting. He has difficulty answering questions. He progresses into a coma. Magnetic resonance imaging results show no specific localization of lesions (unlike in herpes simplex virus encephalitis). His disease progresses to respiratory failure and death. His 25-year-old niece, living next door, complains of sudden onset of fever (39° C [102.2° F]), headache, and myalgias, with nausea and vomiting lasting 4 days. http://www.postgradmed.com/issues/2003/07_03/gelfand.shtml

Yellow fever: A 42-year-old man had fever (103° F), headache, vomiting, and backache, which started 3 days after returning from a trip to Central America. He appeared normal for a short time, but then his gums started to bleed, and he had bloody urine, vomited blood, and developed petechiae, jaundice, and a slower and weakened pulse. He started to improve 10 days after the onset of disease.

Rubella: A 6-year-old girl from Romania develops a faint rash on her face, accompanied by mild fever and lymphadenopathy. Over the next 3 days, the rash progresses to other parts of the body. She has no history of rubella immunization.

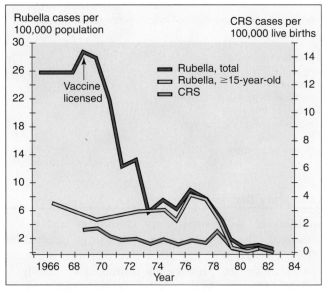

Figure 62–9. Effect of rubella virus vaccination on the incidence of rubella and congenital rubella syndrome (CRS). *(Redrawn from Williams MN, Preblud SR: Current trends: Rubella and congenital rubella—United States, 1983. Morb Mortal Wkly Rep 33:237-247, 1984.)*

The triple vaccine is included routinely in well-baby care. Vaccination promotes both humoral and cellular immunity.

The primary reason for the rubella vaccination program is to prevent congenital infection by decreasing the number of susceptible people in the population, especially children. As a result, there are fewer seronegative mothers and smaller chance that they will be exposed to the virus from contact with the children. Because only one serotype for rubella exists, and humans are the only reservoir, vaccination of a large proportion of the population can significantly reduce the likelihood of exposure to the virus.

Case Studies and Questions

A 27-year-old businessman experienced a high fever, serious retro-orbital headache, and severe joint and back pain 5 days after he and his family returned from a trip to Malaysia. The symptoms lasted for 4 days, and then a rash appeared on his palms and soles that lasted for 2 days.

At the same time, the man's 5-year-old son experienced mild flulike symptoms and then collapsed after 2 to 5 days. The boy's hands were cold and clammy, his face was flushed, and his body was warm. There were petechiae on his forehead and ecchymoses elsewhere. He bruised very easily. He was breathing rapidly and had a weak, rapid pulse. He then rapidly recovered after 24 hours.

1. What features of these cases pointed to the diagnosis of dengue virus infection?
2. Of what significance was the trip to Malaysia?

3. What was the source of infection in the father and son?
4. What were the significance of and the pathogenic basis for the petechiae and ecchymoses in the child?

   Two weeks after returning from a trip to Mexico, a 25-year-old man had arthralgia (joint aches) and a mild rash that started on his face and spread to his body. He recalled that he had felt as if he had the flu a few days before the onset of the rash. The rash disappeared in 4 days.

1. What features of this case pointed to the diagnosis of rubella infection?
2. Why is it significant that the symptoms started after a trip outside the United States?
3. What precaution could the man have taken to prevent this infection?
4. How was this infection transmitted?
5. Who was at risk for a serious outcome of this infection?
6. If this disease is normally mild in children, why is their immunization so important?

Bibliography

Chambers TJ, Monath TP: The Flaviviruses: Detection, Diagnosis, and Vaccine Development, vol 60, Pathogenesis and Immunity; vol 61, Advances in Virus Research. San Diego, Academic, 2003.

Cohen J, Powderly WG: Infectious Diseases, 2nd ed. St Louis, Mosby, 2004.

Flint SJ, et al: Principles of Virology: Molecular Biology, Pathogenesis, and Control of Animal Viruses, 2nd ed. Washington, DC, ASM Press, 2003.

Hahn CS, et al: Flavivirus genome organization, expression, and replication. Annu Rev Microbiol 44:663-688, 1990.

Johnson RT: Viral Infections of the Nervous System. Philadelphia, Lippincott-Raven, 1998.

Knipe DM, Howley PM: Fields Virology, 4th ed. New York, Lippincott Williams & Wilkins, 2001.

Koblet H: The "merry-go-round": Alphaviruses between vertebrate and invertebrate cells. Adv Virus Res 38:343-403, 1990.

Kuhn RJ, et al: Structure of dengue virus: Implications for flavivirus organization, maturation, and fusion. Cell 108:717-725, 2002.

Mackenzie JS, Barrett ADT, Deubel V: Japanese Encephalitis and West Nile Viruses. In Curr Top Microbiol Immunol, vol 267. Berlin, Springer-Verlag, 2002.

Monath TP: Yellow fever vaccine. In Plotkin SA, Orenstein WA (eds): Vaccines, 4th ed. Philadelphia, WB Saunders, 2004.

Mukhopadhyay S, Kim B-S, Chipman PR, et al: Structure of West Nile virus. Science 302(5643):248, 2003.

Nash, et al: The outbreak of West Nile virus infection in the New York City area in 1999. N Engl J Med 344:1807-1814, 2001.

Plotkin SA, Reef S: Rubella vaccine. In Plotkin SA, Orenstein WA (eds): Vaccines, 4th ed. Philadelphia, WB Saunders, 2004.

Strauss JH, Strauss EG: Viruses and Human Disease, 2nd ed. San Diego, Academic, 2007.

Tsai TF: Arboviral infections in the United States. Infect Dis Clin North Am 5:73-102, 1991.

Websites

Centers for Disease Control and Prevention, Arbovirus encephalitides facts (online): Available at http://www.cdc.gov/ncidod/dvbid/arbor/index.htm

Centers for Disease Control and Prevention, West Nile Virus facts (online): Available at http://www.cdc.gov/ncidod/dvbid/westnile/index.htm

Gelfand MS: West Nile virus infection. What you need to know about this emerging threat. Postgrad Med 114, 2003: Available at http://www.postgradmed.com/issues/2003/07_03/gelfand/shtml

Bunyaviridae and Arenaviridae

The Bunyaviridae and Arenaviridae share several similarities. The viruses of these families are negative-strand ribonucleic acid (RNA)—enveloped viruses with similar modes of replication. Both are zoonoses; most of the Bunyaviridae are arboviruses, but the Arenaviridae are not. Many of the viruses from these families cause encephalitis or hemorrhagic disease.

Bunyaviridae

The Bunyaviridae constitute a "supergroup" of at least **200 enveloped, segmented, negative-strand RNA viruses**. The supergroup of mammalian viruses is further broken down into genera on the basis of structural and biochemical features: *Bunyavirus, Phlebovirus, Nairovirus,* and *Hantavirus* (Table 63-1). Most of the Bunyaviridae are **arboviruses** (*ar*thropod-*bor*ne) that are spread by mosquitoes, ticks, or flies and are endemic to the environment of the vector. The **hantaviruses** are the exception; they are carried by **rodents**.

Structure

The bunyaviruses are roughly spherical particles 90 to 120 nm in diameter (Box 63-1). The envelope of the virus contains two glycoproteins (G1 and G2) and encloses three unique negative-strand RNAs, the large (**L**), medium (**M**), and small (**S**) RNAs that are associated with protein to form nucleocapsids (Table 63-2). The genome segments for the La Crosse and related California encephalitis viruses have complementary ends and form circles. The nucleocapsids include the RNA-dependent RNA polymerase (L protein) and two nonstructural proteins (NS_s, NS_m) (Figure 63-1). Unlike other negative-strand RNA viruses, the Bunyaviridae **do not have a matrix protein**. The genera of Bunyaviridae are distinguished by differences in (1) the number and sizes of the virion proteins, (2) the lengths of the L, M, and S strands of the genome, and (3) their transcription.

Replication

The Bunyaviridae replicate in the same way as other enveloped, negative-strand viruses. For most Bunyaviridae, the G1 glycoprotein interacts with β integrins on the cell surface, and the virus is internalized by endocytosis. After fusion of the envelope with endosomal membranes on acidification of the vesicle, the nucleocapsid is released into the cytoplasm, and messenger RNA (mRNA) and protein synthesis begin. Like influenza, the bunyaviruses steal the 5′-capped portion of mRNAs to prime the synthesis of viral mRNAs; but unlike influenza, this occurs in the cytoplasm.

The M strand encodes the NS_m nonstructural protein and the G1 (viral attachment) and G2 proteins, and the L strand encodes the L protein (polymerase) (see Table 63-2). The S strand of RNA encodes two nonstructural proteins, N and NS_s. For the *Phlebovirus* group, the S strand is ambisense, such that one protein is translated from the (+) strand and the other from the (−) RNA template.

Replication of the genome by the L protein also provides new templates for transcription, thereby increasing the rate of mRNA synthesis. The glycoproteins are then synthesized and glycosylated in the endoplasmic reticulum, after which they are transferred to the Golgi apparatus but not translocated to the plasma membrane. Virions are assembled by budding into the Golgi apparatus and are released by cell lysis or exocytosis.

Pathogenesis

Most of the Bunyaviridae are arboviruses and possess many of the same pathogenic mechanisms as the togaviruses and flaviviruses (Box 63-2). For example, the viruses are spread by an arthropod vector and are injected into the blood to initiate a viremia. Progression past this stage to secondary viremia and further dissemination of the virus can deliver the virus to target sites typically involved in that particular viral disease, such as the central nervous system, liver, kidney, and vascular endothelium.

Table 63–1. Notable Bunyaviridae Genera*

Genus	Members	Insect Vector	Pathologic Conditions	Vertebrate Hosts
Bunyavirus	Bunyamwera virus, California encephalitis virus, La Crosse virus, Oropouche virus; 150 members	Mosquito	Febrile illness, encephalitis, febrile rash	Rodents, small mammals, primates, marsupials, birds
Phlebovirus	Rift Valley fever virus, sandfly fever virus; 36 members	Fly	Sandfly fever, hemorrhagic fever, encephalitis, conjunctivitis, myositis	Sheep, cattle, domestic animals
Nairovirus	Crimean-Congo hemorrhagic fever virus; 6 members	Tick	Hemorrhagic fever	Hares, cattle, goats, seabirds
Uukuvirus	Uukuniemi virus; 7 members	Tick	—	Birds
Hantavirus	Hantaan virus	None	Hemorrhagic fever with renal syndrome, adult respiratory distress syndrome	Rodents
	Sin Nombre	None	Hantavirus pulmonary syndrome, shock, pulmonary edema	Deer mouse

An additional 35 viruses possess several common properties with Bunyaviridae but are as yet unclassified.

Many Bunyaviridae cause neuronal and glial damage and cerebral edema, leading to encephalitis. In certain viremic infections (e.g., Rift Valley fever), hepatic necrosis may occur. In others (e.g., Crimean-Congo hemorrhagic fever and Hantaan hemorrhagic disease), the primary lesion involves the leakage of plasma and erythrocytes through the vascular endothelium. In the latter infection, these changes are most prominent in the kidney and are accompanied by hemorrhagic necrosis of the kidney.

Unlike the other bunyaviruses, rodents are the reservoir and vector for hantaviruses, and humans acquire the virus by breathing aerosols contaminated with infected urine. The virus initiates infection and remains in the lung, where it causes hemorrhagic tissue destruction and lethal pulmonary disease.

Epidemiology

Most bunyaviruses are transmitted by infected mosquitoes, ticks, or *Phlebotomus* flies to rodents, birds, and larger animals (Box 63-3). The animals then become the **reservoirs** for the virus, thereby continuing the cycle of infection. Humans are infected when they enter the environment of the insect vector (Figure 63-2) but are usually dead-end hosts. Transmission occurs during the summer, but unlike many other arboviruses, many of the Bunyaviridae can survive a winter in the ova of the mosquito and remain in a locale.

Many of the members of this virus family are found in South America, southeastern Europe, southeast Asia, and Africa and bear the exotic names of their ecologic niches. Viruses of the **California encephalitis virus group** (e.g., La Crosse virus) are spread by mosquitoes found in the forests of North America (Figure 63-3). Up to 150 cases of encephalitis occur during the summer each year in the United States, but most infections are asymptomatic. These viruses are spread mainly by *Aedes triseriatus* and by *Culiseta*, which breeds in the water in tree holes and in discarded tires.

The hantaviruses do not have an arthropod vector but are maintained in a rodent species specific for each virus. Humans are infected by close contact with rodents or through the inhalation of aerosolized rodent urine. In May 1993, an outbreak of **hantavirus pulmonary syndrome** occurred in the Four Corners area of New Mexico. The outbreak is attributed to increased contact

---

Box 63–1. Unique Features of Bunyaviruses

There are at least 200 related viruses in five genera that share a common morphology and basic components.
Virion is enveloped with three (L, M, S) negative RNA nucleocapsids but no matrix proteins.
Virus replicates in the cytoplasm.
Virus can infect humans and arthropods.
Virus in an arthropod can be transmitted to its eggs.

Table 63–2. Genome and Proteins of California Encephalitis Virus

Genome*	Proteins
L	RNA polymerase, 170 kDa
M	Spike glycoprotein, 75 kDa
	Spike glycoprotein, 65 kDa
	Nonstructural protein, 15-17 kDa
S	Nucleocapsid protein, 25 kDa
	Nucleocapsid protein, 10 kDa

Negative-strand RNA.

Glycoprotein
(5–10 nm spikes)

Lipid
envelope

Nucleocapsids

1. L RNA
2. M RNA
3. S RNA
Ⓛ polymerase

Figure 63–1. A, Model of the bunyavirus particle. **B,** Electron micrograph of La Crosse variant of bunyavirus. Note the spike proteins at the surface of the virion envelope. (**A** *redrawn from Fraenkel-Conrat H, Wagner RR: Comprehensive Virology, vol 14. New York, Plenum, 1979;* **B** *courtesy of Centers for Disease Control and Prevention, Atlanta.)*

with the deer mouse vector during a season of unusually high rainfall, greater availability of food, and rise in the rodent population. Viruses of the Sin Nombre subfamily were isolated from the victims and rodents. Since this incident, viruses from this subfamily have been associated with outbreaks of respiratory tract disease in the eastern and western United States and Central and South America.

Clinical Syndromes (Clinical Case 63-1)

Bunyaviridae, which are mosquito-borne viruses, usually cause a nonspecific febrile, flulike, viremia-related illness (see Table 63-1) that is indistinguishable from illnesses caused by other viruses. The incubation period for these illnesses is approximately 48 hours, and the fevers typically last 3 days. Most patients with infections, even those infected by agents known to cause severe disease (e.g., Rift Valley fever virus, La Crosse virus), have mild illness.

Encephalitis illnesses (e.g., La Crosse virus) are sudden in onset after an incubation period of approximately 1 week, and symptoms at this time consist of fever, headache, lethargy, and vomiting. Seizures occur in 50% of patients with encephalitis, usually early in the illness. Signs of meningitis may also be present. The illness lasts 10-14 days. Death occurs in less than 1% of patients, but seizure disorders may occur as sequelae in as many as 20%.

Hemorrhagic fevers such as Rift Valley fever are characterized by petechial hemorrhages, ecchymosis, epistaxis, hematemesis, melena, and bleeding of the gums.

Death occurs in as many as half of patients with hemorrhagic phenomena. The **hantavirus pulmonary syndrome** is a terrible disease, manifesting initially as a prodrome of fever and muscle aches but followed rapidly by interstitial pulmonary edema, respiratory failure, and death within days.

Laboratory Diagnosis

Detection of viral RNA by reverse transcriptase polymerase chain reaction (RT-PCR) has become the accepted method for detecting and identifying bunyaviruses.

Box 63–3. Epidemiology of Bunyavirus Infections

Disease/Viral Factors

Virus is able to replicate in mammalian and arthropod cells.
Virus is able to pass into ovary and infect arthropod eggs, allowing virus to survive during winter.

Transmission

Via arthropods through break in skin; California encephalitis group: *Aedes* mosquito.
Aedes mosquitoes are daytime feeders and live in forests.
Aedes mosquitoes lay eggs in small pools of water trapped in places such as trees and tires.

Who is at Risk?

People in habitat of arthropod vector.
California encephalitis group: campers, forest rangers, woodsmen.

Geography/Season

Disease incidence correlates with distribution of vector.
Disease is more common in summer.

Modes of Control

Elimination of vector or vector's habitat.
Avoidance of vector's habitat.

Box 63–2. Disease Mechanisms for Bunyaviruses

Virus is acquired from an arthropod bite (e.g., mosquito).
Initial viremia may cause flulike symptoms.
Establishment of secondary viremia may allow virus access to specific target tissues, including the central nervous system, organs, and vascular endothelium.
Antibody is important in controlling viremia; interferon and cell-mediated immunity may prevent the outgrowth of infection.

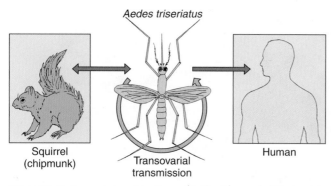

Figure 63—2. Transmission of La Crosse (California) encephalitis virus.

The Sin Nombre and Convict Creek hantaviruses were identified through the use of the RT-PCR test. Viral RNA from patient tissue was converted to complementary DNA with the use of the reverse transcriptase of a retrovirus, and then DNA primers representing conserved sequences of hantaviruses were used to promote synthesis of the characteristic hantavirus sequences.

Serologic tests are generally performed to confirm a diagnosis of bunyavirus infection. Virus neutralization assays can be used to identify the virus. Assays specific for immunoglobulin (Ig)M are useful in the documentation of acute infection. Seroconversion or a fourfold increase in the titer of the IgG antibody is used to document recent infection, but cross-reactions within viral genera are common. Enzyme-linked immunosorbent assay (ELISA) may detect antigen in clinical specimens from patients with an intense viremia (e.g., Rift Valley fever, hemorrhagic fever with renal syndrome, Crimean-Congo hemorrhagic fever). ELISAs that can detect viral antigen in mosquitoes have been developed.

the contact between humans and the vector, whether arthropod or mammal. Arthropod vectors are controlled by (1) eliminating the growth conditions for the vector, (2) spraying with insecticide, (3) installing netting or screening at windows and doors, (4) wearing protective clothing, and (5) controlling the tick infestation of animals. Rodent control minimizes the transmission of many viruses, especially hantaviruses. Rift Valley fever vaccines have been developed for use in humans and animals (sheep and cattle).

Treatment, Prevention, and Control

No specific therapy for infections of the Bunyaviridae is available. Human disease is prevented by interruption of

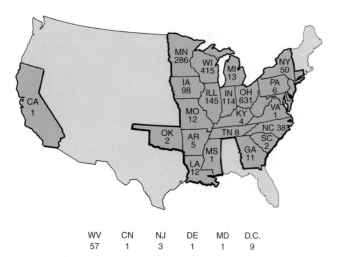

Figure 63—3. Distribution of California encephalitis, 1964 to 1989. *(Redrawn from Tsai TF: Infect Dis Clin North Am 5:73-102, 1991.)*

Arenaviruses

The arenaviruses include **lymphocytic choriomeningitis (LCM)** and **hemorrhagic fever viruses**, such as the **Lassa, Junin**, and **Machupo** viruses. These viruses cause persistent infections in specific rodents and can be transmitted to humans as **zoonoses**.

Structure and Replication

Arenaviruses are seen in electron micrographs as **pleomorphic, enveloped viruses** (diameter, 120 nm) that have a **sandy appearance** (the name comes from the Greek word **arenosa**, meaning "sandy") because of the **ribosomes in the virion** (Box 63-4). Although functional, the ribosomes do not seem to serve a purpose. Virions contain a beaded nucleocapsid with **two single-stranded RNA circles** (S, 3400 nucleotides; L, 7200 nucleotides) and a transcriptase. The L strand is a negative-sense RNA and encodes the polymerase. The S strand encodes the nucleoprotein (N protein) and the glycoproteins but is **ambisense**. Whereas the mRNA for the N protein is transcribed directly from the ambisense S strand, the mRNA for the glycoprotein is transcribed from a full-length template of the genome. As a result, the glycoproteins are produced as late proteins after genome replication. Arenaviruses replicate in the cytoplasm and acquire their envelope by budding from the host cell plasma membrane.

Arenaviruses readily cause persistent infections. This may result from inefficient transcription of the glycoprotein genes and thus poor virion assembly.

Pathogenesis

Arenaviruses are able to infect macrophages and possibly cause the release of mediators of cell and vascular damage. T-cell—induced immunopathologic effects significantly exacerbate tissue destruction. Persistent infection of rodents results from neonatal infection and the induction of immune tolerance. The incubation period for arenavirus infections averages 10 to 14 days.

Epidemiology

Most arenaviruses, except for the virus that causes LCM, are found in the tropics of Africa and South America. The arenaviruses, like the hantaviruses, infect specific rodents and are endemic to the rodents' habitats. Chronic asymptomatic infection is common in these animals and leads to a chronic viremia and long-term viral shedding in saliva, urine, and feces. Humans may become infected through the inhalation of aerosols, the consumption of contaminated food, or contact with fomites. Bites are not a usual mechanism of spread.

The virus that causes LCM infects hamsters and house mice *(Mus musculus)*. It was found in 20% of mice in Washington, DC. LCM disease in the United States is associated with contact with pet hamsters and with the animals in rodent-breeding facilities. Lassa fever virus infects *Mastomys natalensis*, an African rodent. The Lassa fever virus is spread from human to human through contact with infected secretions or body fluids, but the viruses that cause LCM or other hemorrhagic fevers are rarely, if ever, spread in this way.

During 1999 and 2000, three cases of fatal hemorrhagic disease in California were found to be caused by the Whitewater Arroyo arenavirus. This virus is normally found in the white-throated wood rat, so its occurrence in humans constitutes a newly emergent disease. The disease association was made by a special RT-PCR assay.

Clinical Syndromes (Box 63-5)

Lymphocytic Choriomeningitis

The name of this virus, **lymphocytic choriomeningitis**, suggests that meningitis is a typical clinical event, but actually, LCM causes a febrile illness with flulike myalgia more often than meningeal illness. Only about 10% of infected persons exhibit clinical evidence of a central nervous system infection. The meningeal illness, if it occurs, will start 10 days after the initial phase of illness, with full recovery. Perivascular mononuclear infiltrates may be seen in neurons of all sections of the brain and in the meninges of an affected patient.

Lassa and Other Hemorrhagic Fevers

Lassa fever, which is endemic to West Africa, is the best known of the hemorrhagic fevers caused by an arenavirus. Other agents, however, such as the Junin and Machupo viruses, cause similar syndromes in the inhabitants of different geographic areas (Argentina and Bolivia, respectively).

Clinical illness is characterized by fever, coagulopathy, petechiae, and occasional visceral hemorrhage, as well as liver and spleen necrosis, but not vasculitis. Hemorrhage and shock also occur, as does occasional cardiac and liver damage. In contrast to LCM, hemorrhagic fevers cause no lesions in the central nervous system. Pharyngitis, diarrhea, and vomiting may be prevalent, especially in patients with Lassa fever. Death occurs in as many as 50% of those with Lassa fever and in a smaller percentage of those infected with the other arenaviruses that cause hemorrhagic fevers. The diagnosis is suggested by recent travel to endemic areas.

Laboratory Diagnosis

An arenavirus infection is usually diagnosed on the basis of serologic and genomic (RT-PCR) findings. These viruses are too dangerous for routine isolation. Throat specimens can yield arenaviruses; urine is a source for the Lassa fever virus but not for the LCM virus. The risk of infection is substantial for laboratory workers handling body fluids. Therefore, if the diagnosis is suspected, laboratory personnel should be so warned and the specimens processed only in facilities that specialize in the isolation of contagious pathogens (**level 3 for LCM and level 4 for Lassa fever and other arenaviruses**).

Treatment, Prevention, and Control

The antiviral drug **ribavirin** has limited activity against arenaviruses and can be used to treat Lassa fever. However, supportive therapy is usually all that is available for patients with arenavirus infections.

These rodent-borne infections can be prevented by limiting contact with the vector. For example, improved hygiene to limit contact with mice reduced the incidence of LCM in Washington, DC. In the geographic areas where hemorrhagic fever occurs, trapping rodents and carefully storing food may decrease exposure to the virus.

The incidence of laboratory-acquired cases can be reduced if samples submitted for arenavirus isolation are processed in at least level 3 or 4 biosafety facilities and not in the usual clinical virology laboratory.

Case Studies and Questions

A 58-year-old woman complained of flulike symptoms, severe headache, stiff neck, and photophobia. She was lethargic and had a mild fever. The cerebrospinal fluid specimen contained 900 white blood cells per ml, mostly lymphocytes, and lymphocytic choriomeningitis virus. She recovered after a week. Her home was infested with gray mice (*Mus musculus*).

1. What were the significant symptoms of this disease?

2. How was the virus transmitted?

3. What type of immune response is most important in controlling this infection?

A 15-year-old summer camp counselor in Ohio suddenly complained of headache, nausea, and vomiting; she had a fever and experienced a stiff neck. She was admitted to the hospital, where a spinal tap and examination of cerebrospinal fluid revealed inflammatory cells. She became lethargic over the next day but became alert again after 4 to 5 days.

1. The physician suspected La Crosse encephalitis virus as the agent. What clues pointed to La Crosse virus?

2. What other agents would also be considered in the differential diagnosis?

3. How was the patient infected?

4. How would the transmission of this agent be prevented?

5. How could the local Public Health department determine the prevalence of La Crosse virus in the environment of the summer camp? What samples would they obtain, and how would they test them?

Bibliography

Bishop DHL, Shope RE: Bunyaviridae. In Fraenkel-Conrat H, Wagner RR (eds): Comprehensive Virology, vol 14. New York, Plenum, 1979.

Cohen J, Powderly WG: Infectious Diseases, 2nd ed. St Louis, Mosby, 2004.

Flint SJ, et al: Principles of Virology: Molecular Biology, Pathogenesis and Control of Animal Viruses, 2nd ed. Washington, DC, ASM Press, 2003.

Knipe DM, Howley PM: Fields Virology, 4th ed. New York, Lippincott Williams & Wilkins, 2001.

Kolakofsky D: Bunyaviridae. In Curr Top Microbiol Immunol, vol 169. Berlin, Springer-Verlag, 1991.

McKee KT, LeDuc JW, Peters CJ: Hantaviruses. In Belshe RB, (ed): Textbook of Human Virology, 2nd ed. St Louis, Mosby, 1991.

Oldstone MBA: Arenaviruses I and II. In Curr Top Microbiol Immunol, vols 262-263. Berlin, Springer-Verlag, 2002.

Peters CJ, LeDuc JW: Bunyaviruses, Phleboviruses and related viruses. In Belshe RB, (ed): Textbook of Human Virology, 2nd ed. St Louis, Mosby, 1991.

Peters CJ, Simpson GL, Levy H: Spectrum of hantavirus infection: Hemorrhagic fever with renal syndrome and hantavirus pulmonary syndrome. Annu Rev Med 50:531-545, 1999.

Schmaljohn CS, Nichol ST: Hantaviruses. In Curr Top Microbiol Immunol, vol 256. Berlin, Springer-Verlag, 2001.

Strauss JH, Strauss EG: Viruses and Human Disease, 2nd ed. San Diego, Academic, 2007.

Tsai TF: Arboviral infections in the United States. Infect Dis Clin North Am 5:73-102, 1991.

Wrobel S: Serendipity, science, and a new hantavirus. FASEB J 9:1247-1254, 1995.

Websites

Centers for Disease Control and Prevention, Lassa fever facts (online): Available at http://www.cdc.gov/ncidod/dvrd/spb/mnpages/dispages/lassaf.htm

Centers for Disease Control and Prevention, LCM virus facts (online): Available at http://www.cdc.gov/ncidod/dvrd/spb/mnpages/dispages/lcmv.htm

Centers for Disease Control and Prevention, Hantavirus facts (online): Available at http://www.cdc.gov/ncidod/diseases/hanta/hps/index.htm

Centers for Disease Control and Prevention, La Crosse virus facts (online): Available at http://www.cdc.gov/ncidod/dvbid/arbor/lacfact.htm

Mylonakis E, Emad Soliman E, Perez N, Gotuzzo E: California encephalitis (2006, online): Available at http://www.emedicine.com/med/topic3161.htm

Retroviruses

The retroviruses are probably the most studied group of viruses in molecular biology. These viruses are **enveloped, positive-strand ribonucleic acid (RNA)** viruses with a unique morphology and means of replication. In 1970, Baltimore and Temin showed that the retroviruses encode an **RNA-dependent deoxyribonucleic acid (DNA) polymerase (reverse transcriptase [RT])** and replicate through a DNA intermediate. The DNA copy of the viral genome is then integrated into the host chromosome to become a cellular gene. This discovery, which earned the Nobel Prize, contradicted what had been the central dogma of molecular biology—that genetic information passed from DNA to RNA and then to protein.

The first retrovirus to be isolated was the Rous sarcoma virus, shown by Peyton Rous to produce solid tumors (sarcomas) in chickens. Like most retroviruses, the Rous sarcoma virus proved to have a very limited host and species range. Cancer-causing retroviruses have since been isolated from other animal species and are classified as RNA tumor viruses or **oncornaviruses.** Many of these viruses alter cellular growth by expressing analogues of cellular growth—controlling genes (**oncogenes).** Not until 1981, however, when Robert Gallo and his associates isolated human T-lymphotropic virus (HTLV-1) from a person with adult human T-cell leukemia, was a human retrovirus associated with human disease.

In the late 1970s and early 1980s, an unusual number of young homosexual men, Haitians, heroin addicts, and hemophiliacs in the United States (the initial "4H club" of risk groups) were noted to be dying of normally benign opportunistic infections. Their symptoms defined a new disease, the **acquired immune deficiency syndrome (AIDS).** However, as is now known, AIDS is not limited to these groups but can occur in anyone exposed to the virus. Now approximately 40 million men, women, and children around the world are living with the virus that causes AIDS. Montagnier and associates in Paris, and Gallo and colleagues in the United States, reported the isolation of the human immunodeficiency virus (HIV-1) from patients with lymphadenopathy and

AIDS. A variant of HIV-1, designated **HIV-2**, was isolated later and is prevalent in West Africa. HIV appears to have evolved since the 1930s from a chimpanzee virus and then rapidly spread through Africa and the world by an increasingly mobile population. Although a devastating disease that cannot be completely cured, the development of antiviral drug cocktails (HAART, highly active antiretroviral therapy) has allowed many HIV patients to resume a normal life.

Our understanding of the retroviruses has paralleled progress in molecular biology. In turn, the retroviruses have provided a major tool for molecular biology, the reverse transcriptase enzyme, and through the study of viral oncogenes have also provided a means of advancing our understanding of cell growth, differentiation, and oncogenesis.

The three subfamilies of human retroviruses are the **Oncovirinae,** or oncovirus (HTLV-1, HTLV-2, HTLV-5); the **Lentivirinae** (HIV-1, HIV-2); and the **Spumavirinae** (Table 64-1). Although a spumavirus was the first human retrovirus to be isolated, no such virus has been associated with human disease. **Endogenous retroviruses**, the ultimate parasite, have integrated, are transmitted vertically, and may take up as much as 1% of the human chromosome. Although they may not produce virions, their gene sequences have been detected in many animal species and in humans.

Classification

The retroviruses are classified by the diseases they cause, tissue tropism and host range, virion morphology, and genetic complexity (see Table 64-1). The **oncoviruses** include the only retroviruses that can **immortalize or transform target cells**. These viruses are also categorized by the morphology of their core and capsid as type A, B, C, or D, as seen in electron micrographs (Figure 64-1; see Table 64-1). The **lentiviruses are slow viruses associated with neurologic and immunosuppressive diseases**. The spumaviruses, represented by a foamy virus, cause a distinct cytopathologic effect but, as already noted, do not seem to cause clinical disease.

Table 64–1. Classification of Retroviruses

Subfamily	Characteristics	Examples
Oncovirinae	Are associated with cancer and neurologic disorders	—
B	Have eccentric nucleocapsid core in mature virion	Mouse mammary tumor virus
C	Have centrally located nucleocapsid core in mature virion	Human T-lymphotropic virus* (HTLV-1, HTLV-2, HTLV-5), Rous sarcoma virus (chickens)
D	Have nucleocapsid core with cylindrical form	Mason-Pfizer monkey virus
Lentivirinae	Have slow onset of disease; cause neurologic disorders and immunosuppression; are viruses with D-type, cylindrical nucleocapsid core	Human immunodeficiency virus* (HIV-1, HIV-2), visna virus (sheep), caprine arthritis/encephalitis virus (goats)
Spumavirinae	Cause no clinical disease but have characteristic vacuolated "foamy" cytopathology	Human foamy virus*
Endogenous viruses	Have retrovirus sequences that are integrated into human genome	Human placental virus

Also classified as complex retroviruses because of the requirement for accessory proteins for replication.

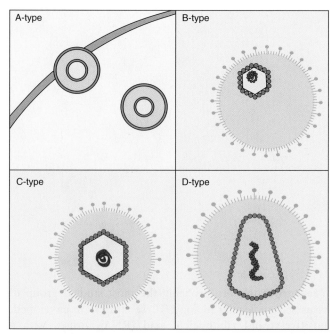

Figure 64–1. Morphologic distinction of retrovirions. The morphology and position of the nucleocapsid core are used to classify the viruses. A-type particles are immature intracytoplasmic forms that bud through the plasma membrane into mature B-type, C-type, and D-type particles.

Figure 64–2. Electron micrographs of two retroviruses. **A,** Human immunodeficiency virus. Note the cone-shaped nucleocapsid in several of the virions. **B,** Human T-leukemia virus. Note the C-type morphology characterized by a central symmetrical nucleocapsid. (*From Belshe RB: Textbook of Human Virology, 2nd ed. St Louis, Mosby, 1991.*)

Structure

The retroviruses are roughly spherical, enveloped, RNA viruses with a diameter of 80 to 120 nm (Figure 64-2 and Box 64-1). The envelope contains viral glycoproteins and is acquired by budding from the plasma membrane. The **envelope surrounds a capsid that contains two identical copies of the positive-strand RNA genome** inside an electron-dense core. The virion also contains 10 to 50 copies of the **reverse transcriptase and integrase enzymes** and **two cellular transfer RNA** (tRNAs). These tRNAs are base-paired to each copy of the genome to be used as a primer for the reverse transcriptase. The morphology of the core differs for different viruses and is used as a means of classifying the retroviruses (see Figure 64-1). The HIV virion core resembles a truncated cone (Figure 64-3).

The retrovirus genome has a 5′-cap and is polyadenylated at the 3′-end (Figure 64-4 and Table 64-2). Although the genome resembles a messenger RNA (mRNA), it is not

Box 64–1. Unique Characteristics of Retroviruses

Virus has an **enveloped** spherical virion that is 80 to 120 nm in diameter and encloses a capsid containing **two** copies of the **positive-strand RNA** genome (approximately 9 kilobases for HIV and HTLV).

RNA-dependent DNA polymerase (**reverse transcriptase**) and integrase enzymes are carried in the virion.

Virus receptor is the initial determinant of tissue tropism.

Replication proceeds through a DNA intermediate termed the *provirus*.

The provirus **integrates** randomly into the host chromosome and becomes a cellular gene.

Transcription of the genome is regulated by the interaction of host transcription factors with promoter and enhancer elements in the long-terminal repeat (LTR) portion of the genome.

Simple retroviruses encode *gag, pol,* and *env* genes. **Complex viruses** also encode accessory genes (e.g., *tat, rev, nef, vif,* and *vpu* for HIV).

Virus assembles and buds from the plasma membrane.

Final morphogenesis of HIV *requires* protease cleavage of gag and gag-pol polypeptides after envelopment.

HIV, human immunodeficiency virus; HTLV, human T-lymphotropic virus.

Figure 64–4. Genomic structure of human retroviruses. **A,** Human T-lymphotropic virus (HTLV-1). **B,** Human immunodeficiency virus (HIV-1). The genes are defined in Table 64-2 and Figure 64-7. Unlike the other genes of these viruses, production of the messenger RNA for *tax* and *rex* (HTLV-1) and *tat* and *rev* (HIV) requires excision of two intron units. HIV-2 has a similar genome map. The vpu for HIV-2 is termed vpx. LTR, long terminal repeat. Protein nomenclature for HIV: ca, capsid protein; in, integrase; ma, matrix protein; nc, nucleocapsid protein; pr, protease; rt, reverse transcriptase; su, surface glycoprotein component; tm, transmembrane glycoprotein component. *(Redrawn from Belshe RB: Textbook of Human Virology, 2nd ed. St Louis, Mosby, 1991.)*

infectious, because it does not encode a polymerase that can directly generate more mRNA. The genome of the **simple retroviruses** *consists of three major genes that encode polyproteins* for the following enzymatic and structural proteins of the virus: **gag** (group-specific antigen, *capsid, matrix and nucleic acid–binding proteins*), **pol**

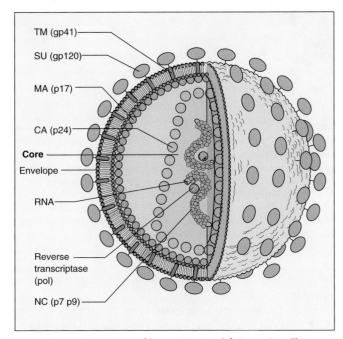

Figure 64–3. Cross section of human immunodeficiency virus. The enveloped virion contains two identical RNA strands, RNA polymerase, integrase, and two transfer RNAs (tRNAs) base-paired to the genome within the protein core. This is surrounded by proteins and a lipid bilayer. The envelope spikes are the glycoprotein (gp) 120 attachment protein and gp41 fusion protein. *(Redrawn from Gallo RC, Montagnier L: Sci Am 259:41-51, 1988.)*

(polymerase, protease, and *integrase),* and **env** (envelope, *glycoproteins).* At each end of the genome are **long-terminal repeat (LTR)** sequences. The LTR sequences contain promoters, enhancers, and other gene sequences used for binding different cellular transcription factors. Oncogenic viruses may also contain a growth-regulating **oncogene**. The **complex retroviruses**, HTLV, and the lentiviruses (including HIV) also *encode several virulence-enhancing proteins* that require more complex transcriptional processing (splicing) than the simple retroviruses.

The viral glycoproteins are produced by proteolytic cleavage of the polyprotein encoded by the *env* gene. The size of the glycoproteins differs for each group of viruses. For example, the (glycoprotein) gp62 of HTLV-1 is cleaved into gp46 and p21, and the *gp160 of HIV is cleaved into gp41 and gp120.* These glycoproteins form lollipop-like trimer spikes that are visible on the surface of the virion. The larger of the glycoproteins binds to cell surface receptors, initially determines the tissue tropism of the virus, and is recognized by neutralizing antibody. The smaller subunit (gp41 in HIV) forms the lollipop stick and promotes cell-cell fusion. The gp120 of HIV is extensively glycosylated, and *its antigenicity and receptor specificity can drift during the course of a chronic HIV infection.* These factors impede immune clearance of the virus.

Table 64–2. Retrovirus Genes and Their Function

Gene	Virus	Function
gag	All	Group-specific antigen: core and capsid proteins
int	All	Integrase
pol	All	Polymerase: reverse transcriptase, protease, integrase
pro	All	Protease
env	All	Envelope: glycoproteins
tax	HTLV	Transactivation of viral and cellular genes
tat	HIV-1	Transactivation of viral and cellular genes
rex	HTLV	Regulation of RNA splicing and promotion of export to cytoplasm
rev	HIV-1	Regulation of RNA splicing and promotion of export to cytoplasm
nef	HIV-1	Alteration of cell activation signals; progression to AIDS (essential)
vif	HIV-1	Virus infectivity, promotion of assembly, blocks a cellular antiviral protein
vpu	HIV-1	Facilitates virion assembly and release, decrease of cell surface CD4
vpr (vpx*)	HIV-1	Transport of complementary DNA to nucleus, arresting of cell growth
LTR	All	Promoter, enhancer elements

HIV, human immunodeficiency virus; HTLV, human T-lymphotropic virus; LTR, long-terminal repeat (sequence).
*In HIV-2.

Figure 64–5. The life cycle of human immunodeficiency virus (HIV). HIV binds to CD4 and chemokine co-receptors and enters by fusion. The genome is reverse transcribed into DNA in the cytoplasm and integrated into the nuclear DNA. Transcription and translation of the genome occur in a fashion similar to that of human T-lymphotropic virus (HTLV-1) (see Figure 64-7). The virus assembles at the plasma membrane and matures after budding from the cell. cDNA, complementary DNA. *(Redrawn from Fauci AS: Science 239:617-622, 1988.)*

Replication

Replication of the human retroviruses e.g., HIV starts with binding of the viral glycoprotein spikes (trimer of gp120 and gp41 molecules) to the primary receptor, **the CD4 protein**, and a second receptor, a 7-transmembrane G-protein-coupled chemokine receptor (Figure 64-5). The co-receptor is either **CCR5**, which is expressed on **macrophages, peripheral, and other T cells (macrophages, [M]-tropic)** or a different chemokine receptor (**CXCR4**), which is expressed primarily on T cells (**T-tropic**) (Figure 64-6). Chemokines are small peptides involved in promoting inflammatory responses and chemotaxis. A small percentage of people are resistant to infection because they have mutations in these co-receptors. Binding to the chemokine receptor brings the viral envelope and cell plasma membrane close together and allows the gp41 to interact with and promote the fusion of the two membranes. The fusion step is the target for an antiviral drug that interferes with the action of gp41. HIV can also bind to a cellular adhesion molecule, integrin alpha4beta 7, present on gut-associated lymphoid tissue.

Once the genome is released into the cytoplasm, the early phase of replication begins. The reverse transcriptase, encoded by the *pol* gene, uses the tRNA in the virion as a primer and synthesizes a **complementary**, negative-strand DNA (**cDNA**). The reverse transcriptase also acts as a ribonuclease H, degrades the RNA genome, and then synthesizes the positive strand of DNA (Figure 64-7). The reverse transcriptase is the major target for antiviral drugs.

Figure 64–6. Target cell binding of human immunodeficiency virus. *(Redrawn from Balter M: Science 274:1988, 1996.)*

The double-stranded cDNA is then delivered to the nucleus and spliced into the host chromosome with the aid of a virus-encoded, virion-carried enzyme, **integrase**. Integration requires cell growth, but the cDNA of HIV and other lentiviruses can remain in the nucleus and cytoplasm in a nonintegrated circular DNA form until the cell is activated.

Once integrated, the late phase begins, and viral DNA (termed the **provirus**) is transcribed as a cellular gene by the host RNA polymerase II. Transcription of the genome produces a full-length RNA, which for simple retroviruses is processed to produce several mRNAs that contain either the *gag*, *gag-pol*, or *env* gene sequences. The full-length transcripts of the genome can also be assembled into new virions.

Because the provirus acts as a cellular gene, its replication depends on the extent of methylation of the viral DNA and on the cell's growth rate, but mostly on the ability of the cell to recognize the enhancers and promoter sequences encoded in the LTR region. Stimulation of the cell in response to other infections (through the action of cytokines or mitogens) produces transcription factors that bind to the LTR and can activate transcription of the virus. If the virus encodes viral oncogenes, they can promote cell growth and stimulate transcription and hence viral replication. *The ability of a cell to transcribe the retroviral genome is the second major determinant of tissue tropism and host range for a retrovirus.*

HTLV and HIV are complex retroviruses and undergo two phases of transcription. During the early phase, HTLV-1 expresses two proteins, **tax** and **rex**, that regulate viral replication. Unlike the other viral mRNAs, the mRNA for tax and rex requires more than one splicing step. The *rex* gene encodes two proteins that bind to a structure on the viral mRNA and thereby prevents further splicing and promotes mRNA transport to the cytoplasm. The doubly spliced tax/rex mRNA is expressed early (at a low concentration of rex), and structural proteins are expressed late (high concentration of rex). Late in the infection, rex selectively enhances expression of the singly spliced structural genes, which are required in abundance. The tax protein is a **transcriptional activator** and enhances transcription of the viral genome from the promoter gene sequence in the 5′ LTR. Tax also activates other genes, including interleukin-2 (IL-2), IL-3, granulocyte-macrophage colony-stimulating factor, and the receptor for IL-2. Activation of these genes promotes the growth of the infected T cell.

HIV replication is regulated by as many as six "accessory" gene products (see Table 64-2). The **tat**, like tax, is a transactivator of the transcription of viral and cellular genes. The **rev** acts like the rex protein to regulate and promote transport of viral mRNA into the cytoplasm. The **nef** protein reduces cell surface expression of CD4 and major histocompatibility class I (MHC I) molecules, alters T-cell signaling pathways, regulates the cytotoxicity of the virus, and is required to maintain high viral loads.

During the synthesis of the virion DNA **(provirus)**, sequences from each end of the genome (U3 and U5) are duplicated, thus attaching the LTRs to both ends. This process creates sequences necessary for integration and *creates enhancer and promoter sequences within the LTR for the regulation of transcription*. The DNA copy of the genome is larger than the original RNA.

Reverse transcriptase is very error prone. For example, the error rate for the reverse transcriptase from HIV is one error per 2000 bases, or approximately five errors per genome (HIV, 9000 base pairs), the equivalent of at least one typo on every page of this text but different for every book. This genetic instability of HIV is responsible for promoting the generation of new strains of virus during a person's disease, a property that may alter the pathogenicity of the virus and promote immune escape.

Figure 64—7. Transcription and translation of human T-leukemia virus (HTLV-1). (A similar but more complex approach is used for human immunodeficiency virus [HIV].) All HTLV-1 and HIV messenger RNA (mRNA) include the 5' end of the genome. The mRNA for tax and rex requires excision of two sequences *(red X)*, the gag-pol and env sequences. The other mRNAs, including the env mRNA, require excision of one sequence. Translation of these mRNAs produces polyproteins, which are subsequently cleaved. Gene nomenclature: *env*, envelope glycoprotein; *gag*, group antigen gene; *pol*, polymerase; *rex*, regulator of splicing; *tax*, transactivator. Protein nomenclature: C, carboxyl terminus of peptide; CA, capsid; MA, matrix; N, amino terminus; NC, nucleocapsid; PR, protease; SU, surface component; TM, transmembrane component of envelope glycoprotein. Prefixes: gp, glycoprotein; gPr, glycosylated precursor polyprotein; p, protein; PR, precursor polyprotein.

The nef protein appears to be essential for causing the infection to progress to AIDS. The **vif** protein promotes assembly and maturation and binds to an antiviral cellular protein (APOBEC-3G) to prevent it from hypermutating the cDNA and helps the virus replicate in myeloid and other cells. The **vpu** reduces cell surface CD4 expression and enhances virion release. The **vpr** (vpx in HIV-2) is important for transport of the cDNA into the nucleus and for virus replication in nongrowing cells like macrophages. VPR also arrests the cell in the G2 phase of the growth cycle, which is likely to be optimal for HIV replication. The cell also controls HIV replication, and activation of the T cell by a cytokine, mitogen, or antigen also promotes virus replication.

The proteins translated from the gag, gag-pol, and env mRNAs are synthesized as polyproteins and are subsequently cleaved to functional proteins (see Figure 64-7). The viral glycoproteins are synthesized, glycosylated, and processed by the endoplasmic reticulum and Golgi apparatus. These glycoproteins are then cleaved into membrane-spanning and extracellular subunits of the viral attachment protein, which associate to form trimers and migrate to the plasma membrane.

The gag and the gag-pol polyproteins are acylated and then bind to the plasma membrane containing the envelope glycoprotein. The association of two copies of the genome and cellular transfer RNA molecules promotes budding of the virion. After envelopment and release from the cell, the viral protease cleaves the gag and gag-pol polyproteins to release the reverse transcriptase and form the virion core, thus ensuring the inclusion of these components into the virion. The protease step is required for the production of infectious virions and is a target for antiviral drugs.

The envelopment and release of retroviruses occur at the cell surface. The HIV envelope picks up cellular proteins, including MHC molecules, upon budding. Replication and budding of the retrovirus does not necessarily kill the cell. HIV can also spread from cell to cell through the production of multinucleated giant cells, or syncytia. Syncytia are fragile, and their formation enhances the cytolytic activity of the virus.

Human Immunodeficiency Virus

Pathogenesis and Immunity

The major determinant in the pathogenesis and disease caused by HIV is the **virus tropism for CD4-expressing T cells and macrophages** (Box 64-2 and Figure 64-8). HIV-induced immunosuppression (AIDS) results from a reduction in the number of CD4 T cells, which decimates the helper and delayed-type hypersensitivity (DTH) functions of the immune response.

During sexual transmission, HIV infects a mucosal surface, enters, and rapidly infects cells of the mucosal-associated lymphoid tissue (MALT). The initial stages of infection are

Box 64–2. Disease Mechanisms of HIV

Human immunodeficiency virus primarily infects CD4 T cells and cells of the macrophage lineage (e.g., monocytes, macrophages, alveolar macrophages of the lung, dendritic cells of the skin, and microglial cells of the brain).

Virus causes lytic infection of CD4 T cells and persistent low-level productive infection of macrophage lineage cells.

Virus causes syncytia formation, with cells expressing large amounts of CD4 antigen (T cells); subsequent lysis of the cells occurs.

Virus alters T-cell and macrophage cell function.

Virus reduces CD4 T cell numbers and helper-cell maintenance of CD8 T cell and macrophage function.

CD8 T cell numbers and macrophage function decrease.

mediated by M-tropic viruses, which bind to CD4 and the CCR5 chemokine receptor and infect dendritic and other monocyte-macrophage lineage cells, as well as peripheral blood T cells. Individuals who are deficient in the CCR5 receptor are also more resistant to HIV infection, and CCR5 binding is a target for an antiviral drug. HIV can also bind and remain on the surface of dendritic cells (including follicular DCs) through a lectin molecule, DC-SIGN, to promote infection of CD4 T cells. Macrophages and DCs are persistently infected with HIV and are probably the major reservoirs and means of distribution of HIV (Trojan Horse). Mutation in the

env gene for the gp120 shifts the tropism of the virus from M-tropic (R5) to T-tropic (X4 virus). The gp120 of the T-tropic virus binds to CD4 and the CXCR4 chemokine receptor. Some viruses may use both receptors (R5X4 viruses). The change in receptor preference to CXCR4 occurs late and correlates with progression of disease.

Reductions in the numbers of CD4 T cells may result from direct HIV-induced cytolysis, cytotoxic T-cell–induced immune cytolysis, or chronic activation in response to the large HIV antigen challenge, leading to a rapid terminal differentiation and death of T cells. Targeting of CCR5-expressing T cells depletes the gut-associated lymphoid tissue of CD4 T cells. Development of the symptoms of AIDS correlates with increased release of virus into the blood, an increase in T-tropic virus, and a decrease in CD4 T cells, with a subsequent decrease in total T cell numbers (CD3-bearing cells) due to the lack of helper function (Figure 64-9).

HIV induces several cytopathologic effects that may kill the infected T cell (Table 64-3). These include an accumulation of nonintegrated circular DNA copies of the genome, increased permeability of the plasma membrane, syncytia formation, and induction of apoptosis (programmed cell death). The relative ability of HIV to kill the target cell correlates with the

Figure 64–8. Pathogenesis of human immunodeficiency virus (HIV). HIV causes lytic and latent infection of CD4 T cells and persistent infection of cells of the monocyte macrophage family and disrupts neuron function. The outcomes of these actions are immunodeficiency and acquired immune deficiency syndrome (AIDS) dementia. DTH, delayed-type hypersensitivity. *(Redrawn from Fauci AS: Science 239:617-622, 1988.)*

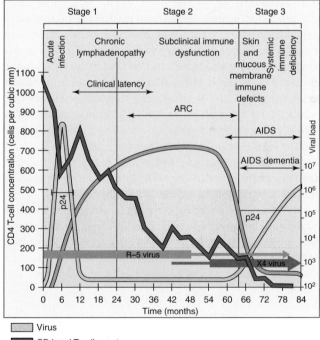

Figure 64–9. Time course and stages of human immunodeficiency virus (HIV) disease. A long clinical latency period follows the initial mononucleosis-like symptoms. Initial infection is with the R5-M-tropic virus, and later the X4-T-tropic virus arises. The progressive decrease in the number of CD4 T cells, even during the latency period, allows opportunistic infections to occur. The stages in HIV disease are defined by the CD4 T-cell levels and occurrence of opportunistic diseases. ARC, acquired immune deficiency syndrome (AIDS)-related complex. *(Redrawn from Redfield RR, Buske DS: Sci Am 259:90-98, 1988, updated 1996.)*

Table 64–3. Means of HIV Escape from the Immune System

Characteristic	Function
Infection of lymphocytes and macrophages	Inactivation of key element of immune defense
Inactivation of CD4 helper cells	Loss of activator of the immune system and delayed-type hypersensitivity
Antigenic drift of gp120	Evasion of antibody detection
Heavy glycosylation of gp120	Evasion of antibody detection

amount of CD4 expressed by the cell. Macrophages may be spared the cytolytic action of HIV because they express less CD4 than T cells. The accessory proteins of HIV are important for replication and virulence. The nef protein appears to be essential for promoting the progression of HIV infection to AIDS. Individuals infected with natural mutants of nef, and primates infected with mutants of the simian immunodeficiency virus, which lacks nef, have lived beyond their expected lifetimes (nonprogressors).

The immune response to HIV restricts viral infection but contributes to pathogenesis. Neutralizing antibodies are generated against gp120 and participate in antibody-dependent cellular cytotoxicity responses. Antibody-coated virus is infectious, however, and is taken up by macrophages. CD8 T cells are critical for controlling HIV disease progression. CD8 T cells can kill infected cells by direct cytotoxic action and by producing suppressive factors that restrict viral replication, including chemokines that also block the binding of virus to its co-receptor. However, CD8 T cells require activation by CD4 T cells, CD8 T-cell numbers decrease with CD4 T-cell number, and their reduction correlates with and is an indicator of disease progression to AIDS.

HIV has several ways of escaping immune control. Most significant is the virus's ability to undergo mutation and hence alter its antigenicity and escape antibody clearance. HIV compromises the entire immune system by targeting the CD4 T cell. Persistent infection of macrophages and resting CD4 T cells maintains the virus in an immune-privileged cell and cells in immune-privileged tissues (e.g., central nervous system and genital organs) (see Table 64-3).

The course of HIV disease parallels the reduction in CD4 T-cell numbers and the amount of virus in the blood (see Figure 64-9). Soon after sexual transmission, HIV infects and depletes CD4 T cells from the gut-associated lymphoid tissue (GALT). During the acute phase of the infection, there is a large burst of virus production (10^7 particles per ml of plasma). T cell proliferation and responses to the infected lymphoid and myeloid cells promotes a mononucleosis-like syndrome. Virus levels in the blood decrease during a clinically latent period, but viral replication continues in the lymph nodes. Virus also remains latent in macrophage and resting T cells. Late in the disease, virus levels in the blood increase, CD4 levels are significantly decreased, CD8 levels also decrease, T-tropic virus rises, the structure of the lymph nodes is destroyed, and the patient becomes immunosuppressed.

The central role of the CD4 helper T cells in the initiation of an immune response and DTH is indicated by the extent of the loss of immune responses caused by HIV infection (Figure 64-10). Activated CD4 T cells initiate immune responses by the release of cytokines required for the activation of macrophages, other T cells, B cells, and natural killer cells. When CD4 T cells are unavailable or not functional (CD4 numbers less than 200 per microliter), antigen-specific immune responses (especially cellular immune responses) are incapacitated, and humoral responses are uncontrolled. The loss of the CD4 T cells responsible for activating macrophages and DTH allows the outgrowth of many of the opportunistic intracellular infections characteristic of AIDS (e.g., fungi and intracellular bacteria). The decrease in number and the inability to activate CD8 T cells increases the potential for recurrence of latent viruses, including JC polyomavirus progressive multifocal leukoencephalopathy (PML), HSV, VZV, and CMV infections, and even EBV-associated lymphomas and HHV8-associated Kaposi sarcoma.

In addition to immunodepression, HIV can also cause neurologic abnormalities. The microglial cell and macrophage are the predominant HIV infected cell types in the brain. Infected monocytes and microglial cells release

Figure 64–10. CD4 T cells have a critical role in the regulation of the human immune response by mediating the release of soluble factors and the delayed-type hypersensitivity (DTH) response toward intracellular pathogens. Human immunodeficiency virus—induced loss of CD4 T cells results in loss of the functions shown, especially the DTH responses and the lymphokine control of immune responses.

neurotoxic substances or chemotactic factors that promote inflammatory responses and neuronal death in the brain. The immunosuppression also puts the individual at risk to opportunistic infections of the brain.

Epidemiology

AIDS was first noted in homosexual men in the United States but has spread in epidemic proportions throughout the population (Box 64-3). In 2006, it was estimated that 6.6 million new HIV infections occur per year, with 3.5 million deaths per year attributable to AIDS (according to Joint United Nations Programme on HIV/AIDS [UNAIDS] and World Health Organization [WHO] data) (Figures 64-11 and 64-12).

HIV is thought to be derived from a simian immunodeficiency virus and is genetically most similar to a chimpanzee virus. In fact, HIV-2 is similar to simian immunodeficiency virus. The initial human infection occurred in Africa in the 1930s but went unnoticed in rural areas. The migration of infected people to the cities after the 1960s brought the virus into population centers, and cultural acceptance of prostitution promoted its transmission throughout the population.

Box 64–3. Epidemiology of HIV Infections

Disease Viral Factors

Enveloped virus is easily inactivated and must be transmitted in body fluids.
Disease has a long prodromal period.
Virus can be shed before development of identifiable symptoms.

Transmission

Virus is present in blood, semen, and vaginal secretions.
See Table 64-4 for modes of transmission.

Who Is at Risk?

Intravenous drug abusers, sexually active people with many partners (homosexual and heterosexual), prostitutes, newborns of HIV-positive mothers.
Blood and organ transplant recipients and hemophiliacs before 1985 (before prescreening programs).

Geography/Season

There is an expanding epidemic worldwide.
There is no seasonal incidence.

Modes of Control

Antiviral drugs limit progression of disease.
Vaccines for prevention and treatment are in trials.
Safe, monogamous sex helps limit spread.
Sterile injection needles should be used.
Large-scale screening programs for blood for transfusions, organs for transplants, and clotting factors used by hemophiliacs.

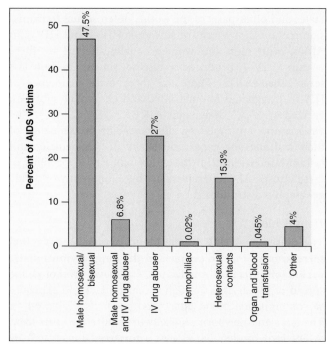

Figure 64–11. Acquired immune deficiency syndrome (AIDS) statistics for the United States as of December 2005. The percentages of AIDS cases are presented by exposure category for men, women, and children younger than 13 years. In the United States, unlike Africa and many other parts of the world, male homosexuals are the largest exposure category. However, intravenous (IV) drug abusers and heterosexual partners are becoming more prevalent. *(From the Centers for Disease Control and Prevention, HIV/AIDS surveillance report online: Available at http://www.cdc.gov/hiv/topics/surveillance/basic.htm#exposure)*

Clades and Geographic Distribution

HIV-1 infections are spreading worldwide, with the largest number of AIDS cases in sub-Saharan Africa but with a growing number of cases in Asia, the United States, and the rest of the world (see Figure 64-12). HIV-2 is more prevalent in Africa (especially West Africa) than in the United

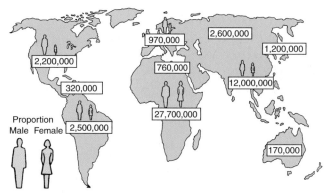

Figure 64–12. Upper estimates of numbers of people living with human immunodeficiency virus (HIV) infections as of the end of 2006. The estimated cumulative global total of HIV-infected adults in 2006 was approximately 47 million: new infections, 6.6 million; deaths, 3.5 million. Infection rates vary widely in different regions of the world. The highest rates are in sub-Saharan Africa. *(Modified from AIDS epidemic update [2006, online]: Available at http://data.unaids.org/pub/EpiReport/2006/12-Maps_2006_EpiUpdate_eng.pdf)*

States and other parts of the world. Heterosexual transmission is the major means of spread of HIV-1 and HIV-2 in Africa, with men and women equally affected by these viruses. HIV-2 produces a disease similar to but less severe than AIDS. There are three main genotypes of HIV-1, designated M (main), N, and O, and 11 subtypes, or **clades,** of M, designated A-K (for HIV-2, A-F). The designations are based on differences in the sequence of their *env* and *gag* genes and hence the antigenicity and immune recognition of the gp120 and capsid proteins of these viruses. The different clades have different worldwide geographic distributions.

Transmission

The presence of **HIV in the blood, semen, and vaginal secretions** of infected people and **the long, asymptomatic period of infection** are factors that have promoted the spread of the disease through sexual contact and exposure to contaminated blood and blood products (Table 64-4). The fetus and newborn are likely to acquire the virus from an infected mother. HIV is *not*, however, transmitted by casual contact, touching, hugging, kissing, coughing, sneezing, insect bites, water, food, utensils, toilets, swimming pools, or public baths.

Populations at Highest Risk

Sexually active people (homosexual and heterosexual), intravenous drug abusers and their sexual partners, and the newborns of HIV-positive mothers are at highest risk for HIV infections, with black and Hispanic persons disproportionately represented in the HIV-positive population.

As already noted, AIDS was initially described in young, promiscuous, homosexual men and is still prevalent in the gay community. Anal intercourse is an efficient means of viral transmission. However, heterosexual transmission by vaginal intercourse and intravenous drug abuse have become the major routes by which HIV is being spread in the larger population. The prevalence of HIV in drug abusers stems from sharing contaminated syringe needles, a common practice in "shooting galleries." In New York alone, more than 80% of intravenous drug abusers are positive for the HIV antibody, and these people are now the major source of heterosexual and congenital transmission of the virus. Tattoo needles and contaminated inks are other potential means by which HIV can be transmitted.

Before 1985, people receiving blood transfusions or organ transplants and hemophiliacs receiving clotting factors from pooled blood were at high risk for HIV infection. HIV was spread in many countries by health care workers using shared or improperly sterilized syringe needles or instruments. Proper screening of the blood supply and transplant tissue in the United States and elsewhere has practically eliminated the danger of HIV being transmitted in blood transfusions (see Figure 64-12). Hemophiliacs who receive pooled clotting factors are protected further by the proper handling of the factor (prolonged heating) to kill the virus or use of genetically engineered proteins.

Health care workers are at risk for HIV infection from accidental needle sticks or cuts or through the exposure of broken skin and mucosal membranes to contaminated blood. Fortunately, studies of needlestick victims have shown that seroconversion occurs in fewer than 1% of those exposed to HIV-positive blood.

Table 64-4. Transmission of HIV Infection

Routes	Specific Transmission
Known Routes of Transmission	
Inoculation in blood	Transfusion of blood and blood products
	Needle sharing among intravenous drug abusers
	Needlestick, open wound, and mucous membrane exposure in health care workers
	Tattoo needles
Sexual transmission	Anal and vaginal intercourse
Perinatal transmission	Intrauterine transmission
	Peripartum transmission
	Breast milk
Routes Not Involved in Transmission	
Close personal contact	Household members
	Health care workers not exposed to blood

Clinical Syndromes

AIDS is one of the most devastating epidemics ever recorded. Most HIV-infected people will become symptomatic, and the overwhelming majority of them will ultimately succumb to the disease without treatment. HIV disease progresses from an asymptomatic nonspecific disease to profound immunosuppression, referred to as **full-blown AIDS** (Clinical Case 64-1; see Figure 64-9). The diseases related to AIDS mainly consist of opportunistic infections, cancers, and the direct effects of HIV on the central nervous system (Table 64-5). Although rare, there are cases of long-term survivors. Some of these result from infection with HIV strains that lack a functional nef protein. Resistance to the virus correlates with a lack of expression of the chemokine co-receptor for the virus.

The initial symptoms following HIV infection (acute phase, 2 to 4 weeks after infection) may resemble those of influenza or infectious mononucleosis, with an "aseptic" meningitis or a rash occurring up to 3 months after

Clinical Case 64-1. An Early Case of HIV-AIDS

Elliott, et al (Ann Int Med 98:290-293, 1983) reported that in July 1981, a 27-year-old man complained of dysuria, fever, chills, night sweats, weakness, dyspnea, cough with white sputum, anorexia, and a 16-pound weight loss. For the past 7 years, he had been receiving up to 4 monthly infusions of factor VIII concentrate to correct his hemophilia. He did not have any other risk factors for HIV infection. In August, pulmonary infiltrates were visible by chest x-ray, and in September, blood test results were: hemoglobin 10.7 g/dL, leukocytes 4200/mm^3 with 50% polys, 2% band forms, 36% lymphocytes, and 12% monocytes. IgG antibody was present to CMV, EBV, toxoplasma, HBsAg and HBc. An immune deficiency was suggested by a lack of response in tuberculin, mumps and *Candida* skin tests. The presence of *Pneumocystis jirovecii* in a methenamine silver stain of a transbronchial lung biopsy specimen prompted oral treatment with trimethoprim/sulfamethoxazole. Episodes of thrush caused by *Candida albicans* prompted treatment with ketoconazole. In May of 1982, development of splenomegaly and lymphadenopathy prompted admission to the hospital with a leukocyte count of 2100/mm^3 and only 11% lymphocytes. At this time, *Mycobacterium avium-intracellulare* was detected in bone marrow, lymph nodes, and granulomas, and total lymphocyte counts were 448/mm^3, compared to a normal of 2668/mm^3; levels were not responsive to mitogen stimulation. In July 1982, total lymphocyte count fell to 220/mm^3 with 45/mm^3 CD3-positive T cells (normal 1725 and 64, respectively) and a CD4/CD8 ratio of 1:4 (normal 2.2:1). The patient continued to deteriorate and died at the end of September 1982. Cytomegalovirus was isolated from lung and liver and *M. avium-intracellulare* from most tissue samples. In 1981, AIDS was a newly described disease, and HIV had not been discovered. Monoclonal antibodies and immunophenotyping were new technology. The patient acquired HIV infection from the factor VIII concentrate in a time prior to routine screening of the blood supply.

Table 64—5. Indicator Diseases of AIDS*

Infection	Disease
Opportunistic infections	
Protozoal	Toxoplasmosis of the brain
	Cryptosporidiosis with diarrhea
	Isosporiasis with diarrhea
Fungal	Candidiasis of the esophagus, trachea, and lungs
	Pneumocystis jirovecii (previously called *Pneumocystis carinii*) pneumonia
	Cryptococcosis (extrapulmonary)
	Histoplasmosis (disseminated)
	Coccidioidomycosis (disseminated)
Viral	Cytomegalovirus disease
	Herpes simplex virus infection (persistent or disseminated)
	Progressive multifocal leukoencephalopathy
	Hairy leukoplakia caused by Epstein-Barr virus
Bacterial	*Mycobacterium avium-intracellulare* complex (disseminated)
	Any "atypical" mycobacterial disease
	Extrapulmonary tuberculosis
	Salmonella septicemia (recurrent)
	Pyogenic bacterial infections (multiple or recurrent)
Opportunistic neoplasias	Kaposi sarcoma
	Primary lymphoma of the brain
	Other non-Hodgkin lymphomas
Others	HIV wasting syndrome
	HIV encephalopathy
	Lymphoid interstitial pneumonia

Modified from Belshe RB: Textbook of Human Virology, 2nd ed. St Louis, Mosby, 1991.
HIV, human immunodeficiency virus.
*Manifestations of HIV infection—defining acquired immune deficiency syndrome according to criteria of Centers for Disease Control and Prevention.

infection (Box 64-4). As in mononucleosis, the symptoms stem from immune responses triggered by a widespread infection of lymphoid cells. These symptoms subside spontaneously after 2 to 3 weeks and are followed by a period of asymptomatic infection or a persistent generalized lymphadenopathy that may last for several years. During this period, the virus is replicating in the lymph nodes.

Deterioration of the immune response is indicated by increased susceptibility to opportunistic pathogens, especially those controlled by CD4 T cells, activated macrophages, CD8 T cells, and DTH responses (e.g., yeasts, herpes and other DNA viruses, or intracellular bacteria). The onset of symptoms correlates with a reduction in the number of CD4 T cells to less than 450/μl and increased levels of virus (as determined by polymerase chain reaction [PCR]-related techniques) and protein p24 in the blood. Full-blown AIDS occurs when the **CD4 T-cell counts are less than 200/μl** (oftentimes to 50/μl or undetectable), and virus load is greater than 75,000 copies per ml and involves

Box 64—4. Potential Antiviral Therapies for HIV Infection

Nucleoside Analogue Reverse Transcriptase Inhibitors (NRTI)

Azidothymidine (AZT) (Zidovudine/Retrovir)
Dideoxycytidine (ddC) (Zalcitabine)
Dideoxyinosine (ddI) (Didanosine)
d4T (Stavudine)
3TC (Lamivudine)
Tenofovir disoproxil fumarate (adenosine class) (Viread)
ABC (Abacavir)
FTC (Emtricitabine (Emtriva))

Non-nucleoside Reverse Transcriptase Inhibitors (NNRTI)

Nevirapine (Viramune)
Delavirdine (Rescriptor)
Efavirenz (Sustiva)

Protease Inhibitors (PI)

Saquinavir
Tipranavir
Darunavir
Ritonavir (Norvir)
Indinavir (Crixivan)
Lopinavir (Kaletra)
Nelfinavir (Viracept)
Amprenavir (Agenerase)
Fosamprenavir (Lexiva)
Atazanavir (Reyataz)
Tipranavir (Aptivus)

Binding and Fusion Inhibitors

CCR5 Inhibitor (maraviroc)
T-20 (enfuvirtide/Fuzeon)

Integrase Inhibitor

Raltegravir (isentress)

Examples of Highly Active Antiretroviral Therapy (HAART)*

Abacavir/zidovudine/lamivudine (Trizivir)
NNRTI + 2(NRTI)
Efavirenz+ tenofovir+ emtricitabine
Nevirapine+ abacavir + lamivudine
2PI + 2(NRTI)
Atazanavir + ritonavir + zidovudine + lamivudine
Efavirenz + emtricitabine + tenofovir disoproxil fumarate (Atripla)

*http://aidsinfo.nih.gov/contentfiles/AdultandAdolescentGL.pdf

the onset of more significant diseases, including HIV wasting syndrome (weight loss and diarrhea for more than 1 month) and the occurrence of indicator diseases such as **Kaposi sarcoma** or specific opportunistic diseases, especially **Pneumocystis pneumonia**, *Mycobacterium avium-intracellulare* **complex** infection, and **severe cytomegalovirus disease** (see Table 64-5).

AIDS may be manifested in several different ways, including lymphadenopathy and fever, opportunistic infections, malignancies, and AIDS-related dementia.

Lymphadenopathy and Fever

Lymphadenopathy and fever can occur, and this combination of clinical findings has been called the **AIDS-related complex (ARC)**. It is a process that develops insidiously and may be accompanied by weight loss and malaise. These findings may persist indefinitely or may progress. Symptoms may also include opportunistic infections, diarrhea, night sweats, and fatigue. The wasting disease is termed **slim disease** in Africa.

Opportunistic Infections

Normally benign infections caused by agents such as *Candida albicans* and other fungi, DNA viruses capable of recurrent disease, parasites, and intracellularly growing bacteria cause significant disease after the HIV depletion of CD4 T cells and subsequent reduction of CD8 T cells (see Table 64-5). *Pneumocystis jirovecii* (previously called *Pneumocystis carinii*)—**induced Pneumocystis (PCP) pneumonia** is a major sign of AIDS. Oral candidiasis (thrush), cerebral toxoplasmosis, and cryptococcal meningitis also often occur, as do prolonged and severe viral infections, including molluscum contagiosum poxvirus; papovaviruses (JC virus, causing progressive multifocal leukoencephalopathy); recurrences of the herpesviruses (e.g., herpes simplex virus; varicella-zoster virus; Epstein-Barr virus [EBV, hairy leukoplakia of the mouth, EBV-associated lymphomas]); and cytomegalovirus (especially retinitis, pneumonia, and bowel disease). Tuberculosis and other mycobacterial diseases and diarrhea caused by common pathogens (*Salmonella*, *Shigella*, and *Campylobacter* species) and uncommon agents (cryptosporidia, mycobacteria, and *Amoeba* species) are also common problems.

Malignancies

The most notable malignancy to develop in patients with AIDS is the human herpesvirus 8—associated Kaposi sarcoma, a rare and otherwise benign skin cancer that disseminates to involve visceral organs in immunodeficient patients. Non-Hodgkin lymphoma and EBV-related lymphomas are also prevalent.

Dementia Related to AIDS

AIDS-related dementia may result from opportunistic infection or HIV infection of the macrophages and microglial cells of the brain. Patients with this condition may undergo a slow deterioration of their intellectual abilities and exhibit other signs of a neurologic disorder, similar to the signs of the early stages of Alzheimer disease. Neurologic deterioration could also result from infection with one of the many opportunistic infections.

Laboratory Diagnosis

Tests for HIV infection are performed for one of four reasons: (1) to identify those with the infection so that antiviral drug therapy can be initiated, (2) to identify carriers who may transmit infection to others (specifically blood or organ

Table 64–6. Laboratory Analysis for HIV

Test	Purpose
Serology	
Enzyme-linked immunosorbent assay	Initial screening
Latex agglutination	Initial screening
Rapid oral antibody test	Initial screening
Western blot analysis	Confirmation test
Immunofluorescence	Confirmation test
Virion RNA RT-PCR	Detection of virus in blood
Real-time RT-PCR	Quantitation of virus in blood
Branched-chain DNA	Quantitation of virus in blood
p24 antigen	Early marker of infection
Isolation of virus	Test not readily available
CD4:CD8 T-cell ratio	Correlate of human immunodeficiency virus disease

RT-PCR, reverse transcriptase polymerase chain reaction.

donors, pregnant women, and sex partners), (3) to follow the course of disease and confirm the diagnosis of AIDS, or (4) to evaluate the efficacy of treatment (Table 64-6). The chronic nature of the disease allows the use of serologic tests to document HIV infection as supplemented by genomic detection and quantitation using PCR-related techniques. Unfortunately, serologic tests cannot identify recently infected people. HIV is very difficult to grow in tissue culture, and virus isolation is not performed. Recent infection or late-stage disease are indicated by the presence of large quantities of viral RNA in blood samples, the p24 viral antigen, or the reverse transcriptase enzyme, (see Figure 64-9). Viral RNA (in virions) in blood can be detected by the reverse transcriptase–polymerase chain reaction (RT-PCR), real-time PCR, and related methods. Blood levels of viral RNA are also useful as a monitor for the success of antiviral drug therapy.

Genomics

Newer methods for detection and quantitation of HIV genomes in blood have become a mainstay for following the course of an HIV infection and the efficacy of antiviral therapy. After converting viral RNA into DNA with a reverse transcriptase (laboratory provided), the cDNA of the genome can be detected by PCR and quantitated by real-time PCR, branched-chain DNA amplification, and other methods (see Chapter 16). Determination of the viral load (amount of genome in blood) is an excellent indicator of the course of disease and efficacy of therapy.

Serology

HIV antibody may develop slowly, taking 4 to 8 weeks in most patients; however, it may take 6 months or more in as many as 5% of those infected (see Figure 64-9). Enzyme-linked immunosorbent assays (ELISAs) or agglutination procedures are used for routine screening. The ELISA test, however, can yield false-positive results and will not detect a recent infection. More specific procedures, such as the Western blot analysis, are subsequently used to confirm seropositive results. The Western blot assay (see Chapter 50, Figure 50-7) demonstrates the presence of antibody to the viral antigens (p24 or p31) and glycoproteins (gp41 and gp120/160). Rapid screening tests are available that detect specific antibody in blood or oral fluid from a swab of the gums.

Immunologic Studies

The status of an HIV infection can be inferred from an analysis of the T-cell subsets. The absolute number of CD4 lymphocytes and the *ratio of CD4 to CD8 lymphocytes* are *abnormally low* in HIV-infected people. The particular concentration of CD4 lymphocytes identifies the stage of AIDS. The choice to initiate therapy is usually based on CD4 T-cell counts.

Treatment, Prevention, and Control

An extensive effort to develop antiviral drugs and vaccines effective against HIV has been initiated worldwide. The principal (as of 2007) anti-HIV therapies are listed in Box 64-5. The anti-HIV drugs approved by the U.S. Food and Drug Administration (FDA) can be classified as **binding, fusion-penetration, nucleoside analogue reverse transcriptase inhibitors, non-nucleoside reverse transcriptase inhibitors, integrase, or protease inhibitors**. The two newest targets approved by the FDA and added to the attack on HIV infection: are a CCR5 inhibitor (maraviroc) of binding and an integrase inhibitor (raltegravir).

Inhibition of binding to the CCR5 co-receptor (maraviroc) with a receptor agonist or fusion of the viral envelope and cell membrane with a peptide (T-20: enfuvirtide) that blocks the action of the gp41 molecule will prevent the initial infection event. Inhibition of the integrase prevents all subsequent events in the replication of the virus. Inhibition of the reverse transcriptase prevents the initiation of virus replication by blocking cDNA synthesis. Azidothymidine

Box 64–5. Clinical Summary

A 32-year-old ex-heroin addict had a mononucleosis-like illness for 2 weeks. He recalled experiencing occasional night sweats and fever for 3 years, and then presented with thrush, cytomegalovirus retinitis, and Pneumocystis pneumonia. His CD4 T-cell count is less than 200 per μl. He was started on highly active antiretroviral therapy treatment.

(AZT), dideoxyinosine (ddI), dideoxycytidine (ddC), and the other nucleotide analogues are phosphorylated by cellular enzymes and are incorporated into cDNA by the reverse transcriptase to cause DNA chain termination. Non-nucleoside reverse transcriptase inhibitors (nevirapine) inhibit the enzyme by other mechanisms. Protease inhibitors block the morphogenesis of the virion by inhibiting the cleavage of the gag and gag-pol polyproteins. The resulting virion is inactive. Most anti-HIV drugs have significant side effects, and the search continues for new anti-HIV drugs. Each of the replicative steps and all of the viral proteins are being targeted for development of new anti-HIV drugs.

AZT was the first successful anti-HIV therapy. Although still given to infants born to HIV positive mothers for 6 weeks postpartum, use of AZT by itself is decreasing. Anti-HIV therapy is currently given as a cocktail of several antiviral drugs termed **highly active antiretroviral treatment (HAART)** (see Box 64-4). The use of a mixture of drugs with different mechanisms of action has less potential to breed resistance. Multidrug therapy can reduce blood levels of virus to nearly zero and reduce morbidity and mortality in many patients with advanced AIDS. There are several different regimens, but which regimen depends upon the patient's level of tolerance to the side effects, cost, compliance, whether the female is of childbearing age, type of contraception, work schedules, type of co-infections, other drug interactions, etc. Some HAART are combined in a single pill, assisting compliance. Therapy should be initiated for individuals showing symptoms of AIDS, AIDS-defining illnesses, or if CD4 T cells drop below 200 per microliter. Therapy may also be considered if viral loads are high (>100,000), even if CD4 numbers are >350 per microliter. Therapy is also suggested for postexposure prophylaxis (e.g., needlestick) if HIV is detected in the individual. HAART is expensive and may require taking many pills during the day. These drugs are often difficult to tolerate, and each drug has its own side effects. Customization of the HAART for each patient can minimize the drug side effects, ease the pill-taking regimen, and allow the patient to return to nearly normal health and lifestyle.

Education

The principal way HIV infection can be controlled is by educating the population about the methods of transmission and the measures that may curtail viral spread. For instance, monogamous relationships, the practice of safe sex, and the use of condoms reduce the possibility of exposure. Because contaminated needles are a major source of HIV infection in intravenous drug abusers, people must be taught that needles must not be shared. The reuse of contaminated needles in clinics was the source of outbreaks of AIDS in the former Soviet bloc and other countries. In some places, efforts have been launched to provide sterile equipment to intravenous drug abusers. A successful anti-HIV education campaign in Uganda has been cited as more effective than antiviral drugs for saving lives.

Blood, Blood Product, and Organ Screening

Potential blood and organ donors are screened before they donate blood, tissue, and blood products. People testing positive for HIV must not donate blood. People who anticipate a future need for blood, such as those awaiting elective surgery, should consider donating blood beforehand. To limit the worldwide epidemic, blood screening must be initiated in developing nations as well.

Infection Control

The infection-control procedures for HIV infection are the same as those for hepatitis B virus. They include the use of universal blood and body fluid precautions, which are based on the assumption that all patients are infectious for HIV and other blood-borne pathogens. The precautions include wearing protective clothing (e.g., gloves, mask, gown) and using other barriers to prevent exposure to blood products. Syringes and surgical instruments should never be reused unless carefully disinfected. Contaminated surfaces should be disinfected with 10% household bleach, 70% ethanol or isopropanol, 2% glutaraldehyde, 4% formaldehyde, or 6% hydrogen peroxide. Washing laundry in hot water with detergent should be sufficient to inactivate HIV.

Vaccine Development

No vaccine against HIV is available, despite several trials. A successful vaccine would prevent acquisition of the virus by adults and transmission of the virus to infants of HIV-positive mothers; it would also block the progression of the disease.

Most HIV vaccines being investigated use gp120 or its precursor, gp160, as the immunogen to develop neutralizing antibody. The gene for this protein has been cloned, expressed in different eukaryotic cell systems (e.g., yeast, baculovirus), and developed as a subunit vaccine. The *env* gene has also been incorporated into the vaccinia canarypox and other carrier viruses to create hybrid vaccines. Specific epitopes and T-cell antigens from the *gag* gene product are also being investigated as possible peptide vaccines. Creating DNA vaccines consisting of eukaryotic expression vectors (plasmids) containing the gene for gp160 or other HIV genes is the newest approach to immunization. The hybrid and DNA vaccines have the potential to elicit both humoral and cellular protective immune responses.

The development of a vaccine against HIV is, however, fraught with several problems unique to the virus. For instance, initial protection would require the production of secretory antibody to prevent sexual transmission and acquisition of the virus. Both antibody and cell-mediated immunity are necessary to protect against and resolve an HIV infection. Although a live attenuated vaccine would be ideal (e.g., deletion of the *nef* gene), these viruses still have some virulence in tests on primates. Protective antibody is difficult to establish, because the antigenicity of the gp120 is different for virus in different HIV clades and changes readily through mutation during the infection of the individual. A further problem is that the virus can be spread through syncytia and remains latent, thereby hiding from antibody. HIV also infects and inactivates the cells required to initiate an immune response. Testing of the vaccine would be a problem because HIV is a human disease, and long-term follow-up is required to monitor the efficacy of the vaccine.

Human T-Leukemia Virus and Other Oncogenic Retroviruses

The Oncovirinae were originally called the **RNA tumor viruses** and have been associated with the development of leukemias, sarcomas, and lymphomas in many animals. These viruses are not cytolytic. The members of this family are distinguished by the mechanism of cell transformation and thus the length of the latency period between infection and the development of disease (Table 64-7).

The **sarcoma and acute leukemia viruses** have incorporated modified versions of cellular genes (proto-oncogenes) encoding growth-controlling factors into their genome (**v-onc**). These include genes that encode growth hormones, growth hormone receptors, protein kinases, guanosine triphosphate—binding proteins, and nuclear DNA-binding proteins. These viruses can cause transformation of cells relatively rapidly and are highly oncogenic. *No human virus of this type has been identified.*

At least 35 different viral oncogenes have been identified (Table 64-8). Transformation results from the overproduction or altered activity of the growth-stimulating oncogene product. Increased cell growth then promotes transcription, which also promotes viral replication. Incorporation of the oncogene into many of these viruses causes the coding sequences for the *gag, pol,* or *env* genes to be replaced, such that most of these viruses are defective and require helper viruses for replication. Many of these viruses remain endogenous and are transmitted vertically through the germ line of the animal.

The **leukemia viruses**, including HTLV-1, are competent in terms of replication but cannot transform cells in vitro. They cause cancer after a **long latency period** of at least 30 years. The leukemia viruses promote cell growth in more indirect ways than the oncogene-encoding viruses. For HTLV-1, a

transcriptional regulator, tax, is produced and is capable of activating promoters in the LTR region and specific cellular genes (including growth-controlling and cytokine genes such as IL-2 and granulocyte-macrophage colony-stimulating factor) to promote the outgrowth of that cell. Alternatively, by integrating near cellular growth—controlling genes, the enhancer and promoter gene sequences encoded in the viral LTR region can promote the expression of growth-stimulating proteins. Uncontrolled cell growth may be sufficient to transform the cell neoplastically or may promote other genetic aberrations over a long period. These viruses are also associated with nonneoplastic neurologic disorders and other diseases. For example, HTLV-1 causes **adult acute T-cell lymphocytic leukemia (ATLL)** and **HTLV 1—associated myelopathy (tropical spastic paraparesis)**, a nononcogenic neurologic disease.

The human oncoviruses include HTLV-1, HTLV-2, and HTLV-5, but only HTLV-1 has been definitively associated with disease (i.e., ATLL). HTLV-2 was isolated from atypical forms of hairy cell leukemia, and HTLV-5 was isolated from a malignant cutaneous lymphoma. HTLV-1 and HTLV-2 share as much as 50% homology.

Pathogenesis and Immunity

HTLV-1 is cell associated and is spread in cells after blood transfusion, sexual intercourse, or breastfeeding. The virus enters the bloodstream and infects the CD4 helper and DTH T cells. These T cells have a tendency to reside in the skin, thus contributing to the symptoms of ATLL. Neurons also express a receptor for HTLV-1.

HTLV is competent for replication, with the *gag, pol,* and *env* genes transcribed, translated, and processed as described earlier. In addition to its action on viral genes, the tax protein transactivates the cellular genes for the T-cell growth factor IL-2 and its receptor (IL-2R), which activates growth in the infected cell. A recently discovered gene and its protein, HBZ, limit tax activity, promoting cell survival. The virus may remain latent or may replicate slowly for many years but may also induce the clonal outgrowth of particular T-cell clones. There is a long latency period (approximately 30 years) before the onset of leukemia.

Although the virus can induce a polyclonal outgrowth of T cells, the HTLV 1—induced adult T-cell leukemia is usually monoclonal. Chromosomal aberrations and rearrangements in the T-cell antigen receptor β gene may accumulate in the HTLV growth-stimulated cells, and it may be this that causes the transition to leukemia.

Antibodies are elicited to the gp46 and other proteins of HTLV-1. HTLV-1 infection also causes immunosuppression.

Epidemiology

HTLV-1 is transmitted and acquired by the same routes as HIV. It is endemic in southern Japan, the Caribbean, Central Africa, and among African Americans in the southeastern United States. In the endemic regions of Japan,

Table 64–7. Mechanisms of Retrovirus Oncogenesis

Disease	Speed	Effect
Acute leukemia or sarcoma	Fast: oncogene	Direct effect Provision of growth-enhancing proteins
Leukemia	Slow: transactivation	Indirect effect Transactivation protein (tax) or long-terminal repeat promoter sequences that enhance expression of cellular growth genes

Table 64-8. Representative Examples of Oncogenes

Function	Oncogene	Virus
Tyrosine kinase	Src	Rous sarcoma virus
	Abl	Abelson murine leukemia virus
	Fes	ST feline sarcoma virus
Growth factor receptors	erb-B (EGF receptor)	Avian erythroblastosis virus
	erb-A (thyroid hormone receptor)	Avian erythroblastosis virus
Guanosine triphosphate—binding proteins	Ha-ras	Harvey murine sarcoma virus
	Ki-ras	Kirsten murine sarcoma virus
Nuclear proteins	Myc	Avian myelocytomatosis virus
	Myb	Avian myeloblastosis virus
	Fos	Murine osteosarcoma virus FBJ
	Jun	Avian sarcoma virus 17

Based on data from Jawetz E, et al: Medical Microbiology, 18th ed. Los Altos, Calif, Appleton & Lange, 1989.

the children acquire HTLV-1 in breast milk from their mothers, whereas the adults are infected sexually. The number of seropositive people in some regions of Japan may be as high as 35% (Okinawa), with twice the mortality rate from leukemia compared to other regions. Intravenous drug abuse and blood transfusion are becoming the most prominent means of transmitting the virus in the United States, where the high-risk groups for HTLV-1 infection are the same as those for HIV infection, and the seroprevalence of HTLV-1 is approaching that of HIV.

Clinical Syndromes

HTLV infection is usually asymptomatic but can progress to ATLL in approximately one in 20 persons over a 30- to 50-year period. ATLL caused by HTLV-1 is a neoplasia of the CD4 helper T cells that can be acute or chronic. The malignant cells have been termed "flower cells" because they are pleomorphic and contain lobulated nuclei. In addition to an elevated white blood cell count, this form of ATLL is characterized by skin lesions similar to those seen in another leukemia, Sézary syndrome. ATLL is usually fatal within a year of diagnosis, regardless of treatment. HTLV-1 can also cause other diseases, including uveitis, HTLV-associated infectious dermatitis, and other inflammatory disorders.

Laboratory Diagnosis

HTLV-1 infection is detected using ELISA to find virus-specific antigens in blood, using RT-PCR for viral RNA, or using ELISA to detect specific antiviral antibodies.

Treatment, Prevention, and Control

A combination of AZT and interferon-α has been effective in some patients with ATLL. However, no particular treatment has been approved for the management of HTLV-1 infection.

The measures used to limit the spread of HTLV-1 are the same as those used to limit the transmission of HIV. Sexual precautions, screening of the blood supply, and increased awareness of the potential risks and diseases all are ways to prevent transmission of the virus. Routine screening for HTLV-1, HIV, hepatitis B virus, and hepatitis C virus are performed to protect the blood supply. Maternal infection of children is very difficult to control, however.

Endogenous Retroviruses

Different retroviruses have integrated into and become a part of the chromosomes of humans and animals. In fact, retrovirus sequences may make up at least 1% of the human genome. Complete and partial provirus sequences with gene sequences similar to those of HTLV, mouse mammary tumor virus, and other retroviruses can be detected in humans. These endogenous viruses generally lack the ability to replicate because of deletions or the insertion of termination codons or because they are poorly transcribed. One such retrovirus can be detected in placental tissue and is activated by pregnancy. This virus may facilitate placental function.

Case Study and Questions

A 28-year-old man had several complaints. He had a bad case of thrush (oral candidiasis) and low-grade fever, had serious bouts of diarrhea, had lost 20 pounds in the past year without dieting, and most seriously, he complained of difficulty breathing. His lungs showed a bilateral infiltrate on radiographic examination, characteristic of *Pneumocystis carinii* pneumonia. A stool sample was positive for *Giardia* organisms. He was a heroin addict and admitted to sharing needles at a "shooting gallery."

1. What laboratory tests could be done to support and confirm a diagnosis of HIV infection and AIDS?

2. How did this man acquire the HIV infection? What are other high-risk behaviors for HIV infection?

3. What was the immunologic basis for the increased susceptibility of this patient to opportunistic infections?

4. What precautions should be taken in handling samples from this patient?

5. Several forms of HIV vaccines are being developed. What are possible components of an HIV vaccine? Who would be appropriate recipients of an HIV vaccine?

Bibliography

Antiretroviral therapy for HIV infection in 1996: Consensus statement. J Am Med Assoc 276:146-154, 1996.

Arts EJ, Wainberg MA: Human immunodeficiency virus type 1 reverse transcriptase and early events in reverse transcription. Adv Virus Res 46:99-166, 1996.

Caldwell JC, Caldwell P: The African AIDS epidemic. Sci Am 274:62-68, 1996.

Centers for Disease Control and Prevention: Updated U.S. Public Health Service guidelines for the management of exposures to HBV, HCV, and HIV and recommendations for postexposure prophylaxis. Morb Mortal Wkly Rep 50(RR11):1-42, 2001.

Christian Hoffmann C, Rockstroh JK, Kamps BS: HIV Medicine (2006, online): Available at www.HIVMedicine.com (a Flying Publisher website).

Cohen J, Powderly WG: Infectious Diseases, 2nd ed. St Louis, Mosby, 2004.

Flint SJ, et al: Principles of Virology: Molecular Biology, Pathogenesis, and Control of Animal Viruses, 2nd ed. Washington, DC, ASM Press, 2003.

Knipe DM, Howley PM: Virology, 4th ed, New York, Lippincott Williams & Wilkins, 2001.

Kräusslich HG: Morphogenesis and maturation of retroviruses. In Curr Top Microbiol Immunol, vol 214. Berlin, Springer-Verlag, 1996, pp 1-344.

Levy JA: HIV and the Pathogenesis of AIDS, 7th ed. Washington, DC, ASM Press, 2007.

Löwer R: The pathogenic potential of endogenous retroviruses: Facts and fantasies. Trends Microbiol 7:350-356, 1999.

Morse SA, et al: Atlas of Sexually Transmitted Diseases and AIDS, 3rd ed. St. Louis, Mosby, 2003.

Ng VL, McGrath MS: Human T-cell leukemia virus involvement in adult T-cell leukemia. Cancer Bull 40:276-280, 1988.

Oldstone MBA, Vitkovic L: HIV and dementia. In Curr Top Microbiol Immunol, vol 202. Berlin, Springer-Verlag, 1995, pp 1-279.

Stine GJ: AIDS Update 2008. New York, McGraw-Hill, 2008.

Strauss JM, Strauss EG: Viruses and Human disease, 2nd ed. San Diego, Academic, 2007.

Yeni G, et al: Antiretroviral therapy in adults: Updated recommendations of the International AIDS Society, USA Panel. J Am Med Assoc 292:251-265, 2004.

HIV/AIDS and HTLV Websites

AIDS Education Global Information System, general information (online): Available at www.aegis.com

HIV InSite (online): Available at http://hivinsite.ucsf.edu

National Institute of Allergy and Infectious Diseases (online): Available at http://www.niaid.nih.gov/spotlight/daids

NIAID fact sheet (online): Available at http://www.niaid.nih.gov/publications/aids.htm

Treatment options (online): Available at www.hivatis.org

CDC online: Available at http://www.cdc.gov/hiv/topics/surveillance/index.htm

UN AIDS (online): Available at http://www.unaids.org/en/HIV_data/default.asp

World Health Organization UNAIDS, HIV/AIDS information and data (online): Available at http://www.unaids.org/

Hoffmann C, Rockstroh JK, Kamps BS: HIV Medicine. Flying Publisher, 2006 (online book): Available at http://www.hivmedicine.com/

Wainscoat B, Salas C, Rich JD: Human T cell lymphotropic viruses. (2006, online): Available at http://www.emedicine.com/med/topic1038.htm

Bartlett's guide to medical management of HIV (online): Available at http://bartletthiv.com

DHHS guidelines for HIV therapy (online): Available at http://aidsinfo.nih.govOther sites: http://aids.about.com/and www.HIVMedicine.com

Unconventional Slow Viruses: Prions

The unconventional slow viruses cause spongiform encephalopathies, which are slow neurodegenerative diseases. These disorders include the human diseases kuru, Creutzfeldt-Jakob disease (CJD), variant CJD (vCJD), Gerstmann-Sträussler-Scheinker (GSS) syndrome, fatal familial insomnia (FFI), and sporadic fatal insomnia. The animal diseases include scrapie, bovine spongiform encephalopathy (BSE) (mad cow disease), chronic wasting disease (in mule, deer, and elk), and transmissible mink encephalopathy (Box 66-1). In the late 1990s, there were outbreaks of BSE and a rapid-progressing form of CJD (vCJD) affecting younger people (40 years) in the United Kingdom. CJD, FFI, and GSS syndrome are also genetic human disorders.

Slow virus agents are filterable and can transmit disease but otherwise do not conform to the standard definition of a virus (Table 66-1). Unlike conventional viruses, these agents have no virion structure or genome, elicit no immune response, and are extremely resistant to inactivation by heat, disinfectants, and radiation. The slow virus agent is a mutant or conformationally distinct form of a host protein known as a **prion (a small proteinaceous infectious particle)**, which can transmit the disease.

After long incubation periods, these agents cause damage to the central nervous system, leading to a subacute spongiform encephalopathy. The long incubation period, which can last 30 years in humans, has made study of these agents difficult. Carlton Gajdusek won the Nobel Prize for showing that kuru has an infectious etiology and for developing a method for analyzing the agent. Stanley Prusiner won the Nobel Prize in 1997 for developing a hamster infection model for the scrapie agent. He and his coworkers were able to purify, characterize, and then clone the genes for the scrapie and other prion agents and show that the prion protein (PrP) is sufficient to cause disease.

Structure and Physiology

The slow virus agents were originally suspected to be viruses, because they can pass through filters that block the passage of particles more than 100 nm in diameter and still transmit disease. Unlike viruses, the agents are resistant to a wide range of chemical and physical treatments, such as formaldehyde, ultraviolet radiation, and heat up to 80° C.

The prototype of these agents is scrapie, which has been adapted so that it can infect hamsters. Scrapie-infected hamsters have scrapie-associated fibrils in their brains. These fibrils are infectious and contain the prion. The prion, which lacks detectable nucleic acids, consists of aggregates of a protease-resistant, hydrophobic glycoprotein termed **PrP^{Sc}** (scrapie-like prion protein) (27,000 to 30,000 Da). Humans and other animals encode a protein **PrP^C** (cellular prion protein) of unknown function that is held in the cell membrane by a linkage between its terminal serine and a special lipid, glycophosphatidylinositol (GPI-linked protein). The PrP^C is closely related or can be identical to PrP^{Sc} in its protein sequence but differs in tertiary structure due to differences in the folding of the proteins (Table 66-2). PrP^{Sc} is protease resistant, aggregates into amyloid rods (fibrils), is found in cytoplasmic vesicles in the cell, and is secreted. The normal PrP^C, on the other hand, is protease sensitive and appears on the cell surface.

Many theories have been proposed to explain how an aberrant protein could cause disease. PrP^{Sc} binds to the normal PrP^C on the cell surface, causing it to refold and acquire the structure of PrP^{Sc}. The alpha helical structure of the PrP^C is changed to a more beta-pleated sheet structure of the PrP^{Sc}, which can be released from the cell and stack into aggregates as amyloid-like plaques in the brain. The cell then replenishes the PrP^C, and the cycle continues. The human version of the PrP^C is encoded on chromosome 20. The fact that these plaques consist of host protein may

Box 66–1. Slow Virus Diseases

Human

Kuru
Creutzfeldt-Jakob disease (CJD)
Variant CJD (vCJD)
Gerstmann-Sträussler-Scheinker (GSS syndrome)
Fatal familial insomnia (FFI)
Sporadic fatal insomnia

Animal

Scrapie (sheep and goats)
Transmissible mink encephalopathy
Bovine spongiform encephalopathy (BSE; mad cow disease)
Chronic wasting disease (mule, deer, and elk)

Table 66–2. Comparison of Scrapie Prion Protein (PrP^{Sc}) and (Normal) Cellular Prion Protein (Pr^{PC})

	PrP^{Sc}	PrP^{C}
Structure	Globular	Extended
Protease resistance	Yes	No
Presence in scrapie fibrils	Yes	No
Location in or on cells	Cytoplasmic vesicles and extracellular milieu	Plasma membrane
Turnover	Days	Hours

explain the lack of an immune response to these agents in patients with the spongiform encephalopathies.

Different strains of PrP^{Sc} occur because of mutations in the PrP^{C} or due to self-perpetuating alternative folding patterns of the protein. Specific mutations at codon 129 determine severity of vCJD disease. Conformational, rather than genetic, mutation is another property that distinguishes prions from viruses. When the PrP^{Sc} aggregates, the PrP^{Sc} acts as a template to transmit its conformation onto each new PrP^{Sc}, analogous to a genetic template (DNA or RNA) transmitting its sequence onto a new viral genome. The different conformational strains can have different properties and varying disease aspects (e.g., incubation period).

Pathogenesis

Spongiform encephalopathy describes the appearance of the vacuolated neurons, as well as their loss of function and the lack of an immune response or inflammation (Box 66-2). Vacuolation of the neurons, the formation of amyloid-containing plaques and fibrils, a proliferation and hypertrophy of astrocytes, and the fusion of neurons and adjacent glial cells are observed (Figure 66-1). The PrP^{Sc} is taken up by neurons and phagocytic cells but is difficult to degrade, a feature that may contribute to the vacuolation of the brain tissue. In addition, prions reach high concentrations in the brain, further contributing to the tissue damage. Prions can also be isolated from tissue other than the brain, but only the brain shows any disease. No inflammation or immune response to the agent is generated, distinguishing this disease from classic viral encephalitis. A protein marker (14-3-3 brain protein) can be detected in the cerebrospinal fluid of symptomatic persons.

The incubation period for CJD and kuru may be as long as 30 years, but once the symptoms become evident, the patient dies within a year.

Table 66–1. Comparison of Classic Viruses and Prions

	Virus	Prion
Filterable, infectious agents	Yes	Yes
Presence of nucleic acid	Yes	No
Defined morphology (electron microscopy)	Yes	No
Presence of protein	Yes	Yes
Disinfection by:		
Formaldehyde	Yes	No
Proteases	Some	No
Heat (80° C)	Most	No
Ionizing and ultraviolet radiation	Yes	No
Disease:		
Cytopathologic effect	Yes	No
Incubation period	Depends on virus	Long
Immune response	Yes	No
Interferon production	Yes	No
Inflammatory response	Yes	No

Box 66–2. Pathogenic Characteristics of Slow Viruses

No cytopathologic effect in vitro
Long doubling time of at least 5.2 days
Long incubation period
Cause vacuolation of neurons (spongiform), amyloid-like plaques, gliosis
Symptoms include loss of muscle control, shivering, tremors, dementia
Lack of antigenicity
Lack of inflammation
Lack of immune response
Lack of interferon production

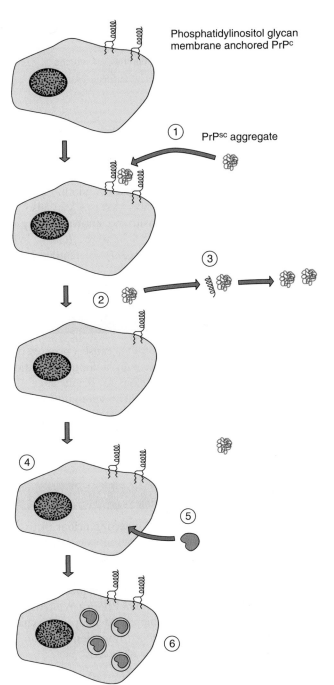

Figure 66—1. Model for proliferation of prions. PrP^c is a normal cellular protein that is anchored in the cell membrane by phosphatidylinositol glycan. PrPS^c is a hydrophobic globular protein that aggregates with itself and with PrP^c on the cell surface *(1)*. PrP^c acquires the conformation of PrPS^c, is released from the cell *(2)*, and is converted to PrPS^c *(3)*. The cell synthesizes new PrP^c *(4)*, and the cycle is repeated. A form of PrPS^c is internalized by neurons *(5)* and accumulates *(6)*, giving the cell a spongiform appearance. Other models have been proposed.

Epidemiology

CJD is transmitted predominantly by (1) injection, (2) transplantation of contaminated tissue (e.g., corneas), (3) contact with contaminated medical devices (e.g., brain electrodes), and (4) food (Box 66-3). CJD usually affects

---

Box 66—3. Epidemiology of Disease Caused by Slow Viruses

Disease/Viral Factors

Agents are impervious to standard viral disinfection procedures. Diseases have very long incubation periods, as long as 30 years.

Transmission

Transmission is via **infected tissue**, or syndrome **may be inherited**.
Infection occurs through cuts in skin, transplantation of contaminated tissues (e.g., cornea), use of contaminated medical devices (e.g., brain electrodes), and by ingestion of infected tissue.

Who Is at Risk?

Women and children of the Fore tribe in New Guinea were at risk for kuru.
Surgeons, transplant and brain-surgery patients, and others are at risk for CJD and GSS syndrome.

Geography/Season

GSS syndrome and CJD have sporadic occurrence worldwide. There is no seasonal incidence.

Modes of Control

No treatments are available.
Cessation of ritual cannibalism has led to the disappearance of kuru.
Elimination of animal products from livestock feed to prevent vCJD transmission.
For GSS syndrome and CJD, neurosurgical tools and electrodes should be disinfected in 5% hypochlorite solution or 1.0 M sodium hydroxide or autoclaved at 15 psi for 1 hour.

CJD, Creutzfeldt-Jakob disease; GSS, Gerstmann-Straüssler-Scheinker.

---

persons older than 50 years. CJD, FFI, and GSS syndrome are also inheritable, and families with genetic histories of these diseases have been identified. The diseases are rare but occur worldwide.

Kuru was limited to a very small area of the New Guinea highlands. The name of the disease means "shivering" or "trembling," and the disease was related to the cannibalistic practices of the Fore tribe of New Guinea. Before Gajdusek intervened, it was the custom of these people to eat the bodies of their deceased kinsmen. When Gajdusek began his study, he noted that women and children in particular were the most susceptible to the disease, and he deduced that the reasons were that the women and children prepared the food, and they were given the less desirable viscera and brains to eat. Their risk for infection was higher because they handled the contaminated tissue, making it possible for the agent to be introduced through the conjunctiva or cuts in the skin. In addition, they ingested the neural tissue, which contains the highest concentrations of the kuru agent. Cessation of this cannibalistic custom has stopped the spread of kuru.

Clinical Case 66-1. Transmission of Creutzfeld-Jakob Disease by Transfusion

In a case reported by Wroe, et al (Lancet 368:2061-2067, 2006), a 30-year-old man consulted his family doctor because of fatigue and inability to concentrate. The symptoms were attributed to a respiratory tract infection. Neurological exams for the patient at this time were normal. History was significant for the fact that during surgery 7 years earlier, the patient had received packed red cells, including blood from a donor who died 1 year later with variant Creutzfeldt-Jakob disease (vCJD). Within 6 months of his initial presentation, the patient had difficulty maintaining balance, a tendency to stagger, some memory problems, a tremor in his hands, and "searing pain" in his legs. At this time, there was no evidence of changes in vision or mental status. After another 6 weeks, his mental status and memory decreased, balance and walking became difficult and painful, MRI neuroimaging and electroencephalogram indicated changes, and a blood test showed the presence of the vCJD prion protein (PrP^{Sc}). The patient's mental status and physical ability continued to decline; he became mute, bedridden, poorly responsive, and he died 8 years and 8 months after the transfusion. Western immunoblot of autopsy samples from the brain and tonsils contained the PrP^{Sc} protein. PrP plaques and spongiform encephalopathy were noted in the brain.

Due to the long incubation period for prion diseases, prevention of transfusion transmission of CJD is difficult. Variant CJD has a more rapid onset of disease, and this case shows the classic progression through the five stages: (1) incubation (6 years); (2) prodromal fatigue and difficulty concentrating (18 months); (3) Progressive neurological decline (9 months); (4) late neurological phase (4 months); and (5) terminal phase. Immunoblot analysis of treated prion protein can now distinguish the PrP^{Sc} from the normal protein in samples which can be taken from the patient's tonsils (or at autopsy, from the brain).

An epidemic of BSE (mad cow disease) in 1980 in the United Kingdom and the unusual incidence of a more rapidly progressing CJD in younger people (younger than 45 years) in 1996 prompted concern that contaminated beef was the source of this new variant of CJD (vCJD). Infection of cattle is most likely caused by the use of contaminated animal byproducts (e.g., sheep entrails, brains) as a protein supplement in cattle feed. Ingestion of contaminated beef is likely to be the cause of 153 cases of vCJD, more than 98% of which have occurred in the United Kingdom.

In addition to infection, prion diseases can also be familial (genetic) or sporadic, with no known history of exposure. Gerstmann-Sträussler-Scheinker (GSS) syndrome and fatal familial insomnia (FFI) are familial prion diseases.

Figure 66–2. Progression of transmissible Creutzfeldt-Jakob disease.

Clinical Syndromes (Clinical Case 66-1, Box 66-4)

As already noted, the slow virus agents cause a progressive, degenerative neurologic disease with a long incubation period but with rapid progression to death after the onset of symptoms (Figure 66-2). The spongiform encephalopathies are characterized by a loss of muscle control, shivering, myoclonic jerks and tremors, loss of coordination, rapidly progressive dementia, and death.

Laboratory Diagnosis

There are no methods for directly detecting prions in tissue through the use of electron microscopy, antigen detection, or nucleic acid probes. Also, no serologic tests can detect antiprion antibody. The initial diagnosis must be made on clinical grounds. Confirmation of the diagnosis can be made by detection of a proteinase K—resistant form of PrP in a Western blot using antibody to PrP in a tonsil biopsy. At autopsy, the characteristic amyloid plaques, spongiform vacuoles, and immunohistologically detected PrP can be observed.

Treatment, Prevention, and Control

No treatment exists for kuru or CJD. The causative agents are also impervious to the disinfection procedures used for other viruses, including formaldehyde, detergents, and ionizing radiation. Autoclaving at 15 psi for 1 hour (instead of 20 minutes) or treatment with 5% hypochlorite solution or 1.0 M sodium hydroxide can be used for decontamination. Because these agents can be transmitted on instruments and brain electrodes, such items should be carefully disinfected before being reused.

The outbreak of BSE and vCJD in the United Kingdom promoted legislation to ban animal products in livestock feed and encouraged more careful monitoring of cattle.

Box 66—4. Clinical Summaries

CJD: A 63-year-old man complained of poor memory and difficulty with vision and muscle coordination. Over the course of the next year, he developed senile dementia and irregular jerking movements, progressively lost muscle function, and then died.

VCJD: A 25-year-old is seen by a psychiatrist for anxiety and depression. After 2 months, he has problems with balance and muscle control and has difficulty remembering. He develops myoclonus and dies within 12 months of onset.

Case Study and Questions

A 70-year-old woman complained of severe headaches, appeared dull and apathetic, and had a constant tremor in the right hand. One month later, she experienced memory loss and moments of confusion. The patient's condition continued to deteriorate, and at 2 months after onset of symptoms, an abnormal electroencephalograph tracing showing periodic biphasic and triphasic slow-wave complexes was obtained. By 3 months, the patient was in a coma-like state. She also had occasional spontaneous clonic twitching of the arms and legs and a startle myoclonic jerking response to a loud noise. The patient died of pneumonia 4 months after the onset of symptoms. No gross abnormalities were noted at autopsy. Astrocytic gliosis of the cerebral cortex, with fibrils and intracellular vacuolation throughout the cerebral cortex, were seen on microscopic examination. There was no swelling and no inflammation.

1. What viral neurologic diseases would have been considered in the differential diagnosis formulated on the basis of the symptoms described? What other diseases?

2. What key features of the postmortem findings were characteristic of the diseases caused by unconventional slow virus agents (e.g., spongiform encephalopathies, prions)?

3. What key features distinguish the unconventional slow virus diseases from more conventional neurologic viral diseases?

4. What precautions should the pathologist have taken for protection against infection during the postmortem examination?

Bibliography

Belay ED: Transmissible spongiform encephalopathies in humans. Annu Rev Microbiol 53:283-314, 1999.

Brown P, et al: Diagnosis of Creutzfeldt-Jakob disease by Western blot identification. N Engl J Med 314:547-551, 1986.

Cohen J, Powderly WG: Infectious diseases, 2nd ed. St Louis, Mosby, 2004.

Flint SJ, et al: Principles of Virology: Molecular Biology, Pathogenesis, and Control of Animal Viruses, 2nd ed. Washington, DC, ASM Press, 2003.

Hsich G, et al: The 14-3-3 brain protein in cerebrospinal fluid as a marker for transmissible spongiform encephalopathies. N Engl J Med 335:924-930, 1996.

Knipe DM, Howley PM: Fields' Virology, 4th ed. New York, Lippincott Williams & Wilkins, 2001.

Manson JC: Understanding transmission of the prion diseases. Trends Microbiol 7:465-467, 1999.

Prusiner SB: Molecular biology and genetics of neurodegenerative diseases caused by prions. Adv Virus Res 41:241-280, 1992.

Prusiner SB: Prions, Prions, Prions. In Curr Top Microbiol Immunol, vol 207. Berlin, Springer-Verlag, 1996.

Websites

Freudenrich CC: How mad cow disease works (online): Available at http://science.howstuffworks.com/mad-cow-disease6.htm

National Institutes of Health: Prion disease at NIH Genetics Home Reference (online): Available at http://ghr.nlm.nih.gov/condition=priondisease

Prion data (online): Available at http://www.priondata.org

Role of Viruses in Disease

Most viral infections cause mild or no symptoms and do not require extensive treatment. The common cold, influenza, flulike syndromes, and gastroenteritis are common viral diseases. Other viral infections that target essential tissues and organs are very cytolytic or induce immunopathologic effects and can cause serious and even life-threatening disease. In general, the symptoms and severity of a viral infection are determined by (1) the patient's ability to prevent or rapidly resolve the infection before the virus can reach important organs or cause significant damage, (2) the target tissue and virulence of the virus, and (3) the ability of the body to repair the damage.

Previous chapters stressed the viral characteristics that promote disease. In this chapter, viral diseases are discussed with respect to their symptoms, the organ system they target, and the host factors that influence their presentation.

Viral Diseases

The major sites of viral disease are the respiratory tract; the gastrointestinal tract; the epithelial, mucosal, and endothelial linings of the skin, mouth, and genitalia; the lymphoid tissue; the liver and other organs; and the central nervous system (CNS) (Figure 67-1). The examples given in this chapter represent more common causes of disease.

Oral and Respiratory Tract Infections

The oropharynx and respiratory tract are the **most common sites** of viral infection and disease (Table 67-1). The viruses are spread in respiratory droplets, aerosols, food, water, and saliva, as well as by close contact and on hands. Similar respiratory symptoms can be caused by several different viruses. For example, bronchiolitis may be caused by respiratory syncytial or parainfluenza virus. Alternatively, one virus may cause different symptoms in different people. Influenza virus can cause a mild upper respiratory tract infection in one person and life-threatening pneumonia in another.

Many viral infections start in the oropharynx or respiratory tract, infect the lung, and spread without causing significant respiratory symptoms. Varicella-zoster virus (VZV) and the measles virus initiate infection in the lung and can cause pneumonia but generally cause systemic infections resulting in an exanthem (rash). Other viruses that establish primary infection of the oropharynx or respiratory tract and then progress to other sites are rubella, mumps, enteroviruses, and several human herpesviruses—herpes simplex virus (HSV), Epstein-Barr virus (EBV), cytomegalovirus (CMV), and human herpesvirus 6 (HHV-6).

The symptoms and severity of a respiratory viral disease depend on the nature of the virus, the site of infection (upper or lower respiratory tract), and the immune status and age of the person. Conditions such as cystic fibrosis and smoking, which compromise the ciliated and mucoepithelial barriers to infection, increase the risk of serious disease.

Pharyngitis and oral disease are common viral presentations. Most enteroviruses infect the oropharynx and then progress by way of a viremia to other target tissues. For example, symptoms such as acute-onset pharyngitis, fever, and oral vesicular lesions are characteristic of Coxsackie A virus infections (herpangina, hand-foot-and-mouth disease) and some Coxsackie B virus and echovirus infections. Adenovirus and the early stages of EBV disease are characterized by sore throat and tonsillitis with exudative membranes; EBV goes on to infect B lymphocytes and cause infectious mononucleosis. HSV causes local primary infections of the oral mucosa and face (gingivostomatitis) and then establishes a latent neuronal infection that can recur in the form of herpes labialis (cold sores, fever blisters). HSV is also a common cause of pharyngitis. Vesicular lesions on the buccal mucosa (Koplik spots) are an early diagnostic feature of measles infection.

Upper respiratory tract viral infections, including the common cold and pharyngitis, account for at least 50% of absenteeism from schools and the workplace, despite being generally benign. Rhinoviruses and coronaviruses are the

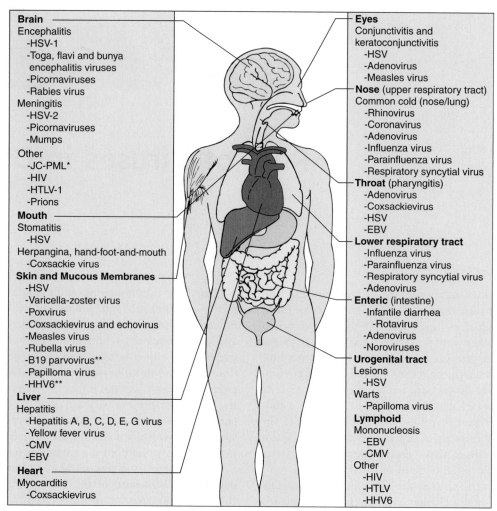

Brain
Encephalitis
- HSV-1
- Toga, flavi and bunya encephalitis viruses
- Picornaviruses
- Rabies virus
Meningitis
- HSV-2
- Picornaviruses
- Mumps
Other
- JC-PML*
- HIV
- HTLV-1
- Prions

Mouth
Stomatitis
- HSV
Herpangina, hand-foot-and-mouth
- Coxsackie virus

Skin and Mucous Membranes
- HSV
- Varicella-zoster virus
- Poxvirus
- Coxsackievirus and echovirus
- Measles virus
- Rubella virus
- B19 parvovirus**
- Papilloma virus
- HHV6**

Liver
Hepatitis
- Hepatitis A, B, C, D, E, G virus
- Yellow fever virus
- CMV
- EBV

Heart
Myocarditis
- Coxsackievirus

Eyes
Conjunctivitis and keratoconjunctivitis
- HSV
- Adenovirus
- Measles virus

Nose (upper respiratory tract)
Common cold (nose/lung)
- Rhinovirus
- Coronavirus
- Adenovirus
- Influenza virus
- Parainfluenza virus
- Respiratory syncytial virus

Throat (pharyngitis)
- Adenovirus
- Coxsackievirus
- HSV
- EBV

Lower respiratory tract
- Influenza virus
- Parainfluenza virus
- Respiratory syncytial virus
- Adenovirus

Enteric (intestine)
- Infantile diarrhea
- Rotavirus
- Adenovirus
- Noroviruses

Urogenital tract
Lesions
- HSV
Warts
- Papilloma virus

Lymphoid
Mononucleosis
- EBV
- CMV
Other
- HIV
- HTLV
- HHV6

Figure 67—1. Major target tissues of viral disease. (*) indicates progressive multifocal leukoencephalopathy. Infection by viruses indicated by (**) results in an immune-mediated rash.

predominant causes of upper respiratory tract infections. A runny nose (rhinitis) followed by congestion, cough, sneezing, conjunctivitis, headache, and sore throat are typical symptoms of the common cold. Other causes of the common cold and pharyngitis are specific serotypes of echoviruses and Coxsackie viruses, adenoviruses, influenza viruses, parainfluenza viruses, metapneumovirus, and respiratory syncytial virus.

Tonsillitis, laryngitis, and **croup** (laryngotracheobronchitis) may accompany certain respiratory tract viral infections. HSV and Coxsackie A viruses may also involve the tonsils, but with vesicular lesions. Inflammatory responses to viral infection cause the trachea to narrow below the vocal cords (subglottic area), resulting in laryngitis (adults) and croup (children). This narrowing causes loss of voice; a hoarse, barking cough; and the risk, especially in young children, for a blocked airway and choking. Children infected with parainfluenza viruses are especially at risk for croup.

Lower respiratory tract viral infections can also result in more serious disease. Symptoms of such infections include bronchiolitis (inflammation of the bronchioles), pneumonia, and related diseases. The parainfluenza, metapneumovirus, and respiratory syncytial viruses are major problems for infants and children but cause only asymptomatic infections or common cold symptoms in adults. Parainfluenza 3 virus and especially respiratory syncytial virus infections are major causes of life-threatening pneumonia or bronchiolitis in infants younger than 6 months. Infection with these viruses does not provide lifelong immunity.

Influenza virus is probably the best known and most feared of the common respiratory viruses, with the annual introduction of new strains of virus ensuring the presence of immunologically naïve victims. Children are universally susceptible to new strains of virus, whereas older people may have been immunized during a prior outbreak of the annual strain. Despite such immunization, the elderly are especially susceptible to pneumonia caused by new strains of virus, because they may not be able to mount a sufficient primary immune response to the new strain of influenza virus or to repair the tissue damage caused by the disease. Other possible viral agents of pneumonia are

Table 67–1. Oral and Respiratory Diseases

Disease	Etiologic Agent
Common cold (including pharyngitis)	Rhinovirus*
	Coronavirus*
	Influenza viruses
	Parainfluenza viruses
	Respiratory syncytial virus
	Metapneumovirus
	Adenovirus
	Enteroviruses
Pharyngitis	Herpes simplex virus
	Epstein-Barr virus
	Adenovirus*
	Coxsackie A virus* (herpangina, hand-foot-and-mouth disease) and other enteroviruses
Croup, tonsillitis, laryngitis, and bronchitis (children younger than 2 years)	Parainfluenza virus 1*
	Parainfluenza virus 2
	Influenza virus
	Adenovirus
	Epstein-Barr virus
Bronchiolitis	Respiratory syncytial virus* (infants)
	Metapneumovirus
	Parainfluenza virus 3* (infants and children)
	Parainfluenza viruses 1 and 2
Pneumonia	Respiratory syncytial virus* (infants)
	Metapneumovirus
	Parainfluenza virus* (infants)
	Influenza virus*
	Adenovirus
	Varicella-zoster virus (primary infection of adults or immunocompromised hosts)
	Cytomegalovirus (infection of immunocompromised host)
	Measles

Most common causal agents.

adenovirus, paramyxoviruses, and primary VZV infections of adults.

Flulike and Systemic Symptoms

Many viral infections cause classic **flulike symptoms** (e.g., fever, malaise, anorexia, headache, body aches), side effects caused by host responses to the infection. During the viremic phase, many viruses induce the release of interferon and cytokines. In addition to the respiratory viruses, flulike symptoms may accompany infections by arboencephalitis viruses, HSV type 2 (HSV-2), and other viruses.

Arthritis and other inflammatory diseases may result from immune hypersensitivity responses induced by the infection or immune complexes containing viral antigen. For example, B19 parvovirus infection of adults, rubella, and infection with several other togaviruses elicit arthritis. Immune complex disease that is associated with chronic hepatitis B virus (HBV) can result in various presentations, including arthritis and nephritis.

Gastrointestinal Tract Infections

Infections of the gastrointestinal tract can result in gastroenteritis, vomiting, diarrhea, or no symptoms (Box 67-1). Norwalk virus, caliciviruses, astroviruses, adenoviruses, reoviruses, and rotaviruses infect the small intestine but not the colon, altering the function or damaging the epithelial lining and the absorptive villi. This leads to the malabsorption of water and an electrolyte imbalance. The resultant diarrhea in older children and adults is generally self-limited and can be treated with rehydration and restoration of the electrolyte balance. These viruses, especially rotavirus, are major problems for adults and children in regions where there is drought and starvation.

Viral gastroenteritis has a more significant effect on infants and may necessitate hospitalization. The extent of tissue damage and consequent loss of fluids and electrolytes is a more significant problem for infants. Rotavirus and

Box 67–1. Gastrointestinal Viruses

Infants

Rotavirus A*
Adenovirus 40, 41
Coxsackie A24 virus

Infants, Children, and Adults

Norwalk virus*
Calicivirus
Astrovirus
Rotavirus B (outbreaks in China)
Reovirus

Most common cause.

adenovirus serotypes 40 and 41 are the major causes of infantile gastroenteritis.

Fecal-oral spread of the enteric viruses is promoted by poor hygiene and is especially prevalent in daycare centers. Norwalk virus and calicivirus outbreaks affecting older children and adults are generally linked to a common contaminated food or water source. Vomiting usually accompanies diarrhea in patients infected with the Norwalk virus and rotavirus. Although enteroviruses (picornaviruses) are spread by the fecal-oral route, they usually cause only mild or no gastrointestinal symptoms. Instead, these viruses establish a viremia, spread to other target organs, and then cause clinical disease.

Exanthems and Hemorrhagic Fevers

Virus-induced skin disease (Table 67-2) can result from infection through the mucosa or small cuts or abrasions in the skin (HSV), as a secondary infection after establishment of a viremia (VZV and smallpox), or as a result of the inflammatory response mounted against viral antigens (parvovirus B19). The major classifications of viral rashes are maculopapular, vesicular, nodular, and hemorrhagic. **Macules** are flat, colored spots. **Papules** are slightly raised areas of the skin that may result from immune or inflammatory responses rather than the direct effects of the virus. **Nodules** are larger, raised areas of the skin. **Vesicular lesions** are blisters and are likely to contain virus. Papillomaviruses cause warts, and molluscum contagiosum causes wartlike growths (nodules) by stimulating the growth of skin cells.

The classic childhood exanthems are roseola infantum (exanthem subitum [HHV-6]), fifth disease (erythema infectiosum [parvovirus B19]), and (in unvaccinated children) varicella, measles, and rubella. The rash follows a viremia and is accompanied by fever. Rashes are also caused by enterovirus infections, dengue, and other infections caused by flaviviruses or alphaviruses. They also are occasionally seen in patients with infectious mononucleosis.

The yellow fever virus, dengue virus, Ebola virus, Lassa fever, Sin Nombre virus, and other hemorrhagic fever viruses establish a viremia and infect the endothelial cell lining of the vasculature, possibly compromising the structure of the blood vessel. Viral or immune cytolysis can then lead to greater permeability or rupture of the vessel, producing a hemorrhagic rash with petechiae (pinpoint hemorrhages under the skin) and ecchymoses (massive bruises) and hence internal bleeding, the loss of electrolytes, and shock.

Infections of the Eye

Infections of the eye result from direct contact with a virus or from viremic spread (Box 67-2). Conjunctivitis (pinkeye) is a normal feature of many childhood infections and is a characteristic of infections caused by specific adenovirus serotypes (3, 4a, and 7), the measles virus, and the rubella virus. Keratoconjunctivitis caused by adenovirus (8, 19a, and 37), HSV, or VZV involves the cornea and can cause severe damage. HSV disease can recur, cause scarring and blindness. Enterovirus 70 and Coxsackie A24 virus can cause an acute hemorrhagic conjunctivitis. Cataracts are classic features of babies born with congenital rubella syndrome. Chorioretinitis is associated with CMV infection in newborns (congenital), as well as in immunosuppressed people (e.g., those with acquired immune deficiency syndrome [AIDS]).

Table 67–2. Viral Exanthems

Condition	Etiologic Agent
Rash	
Rubeola	Measles virus
German measles	Rubella virus
Roseola infantum	Human herpesvirus 6
Erythema infectiosum	Human parvovirus B19
Boston exanthem	Echovirus 16
Infectious mononucleosis	Epstein-Barr virus, cytomegalovirus
Vesicles	
Oral or genital herpes	Herpes simplex virus*
Chickenpox/shingles	Varicella-zoster virus*
Hand-foot-and-mouth disease, herpangina	Coxsackie A virus*
Papillomas	
Warts	Papillomavirus*
Molluscum	Molluscum contagiosum

Most common cause.

Infections of the Organs and Tissues

Infection of the major organs may cause significant disease or may result in further spread or secretion of the virus (see Box 67-2). The symptoms may arise from tissue damage or inflammatory responses.

The liver is a prominent target for many viruses that reach the liver by means of a viremia or the mononuclear phagocyte (reticuloendothelial) system. The liver acts as a source for a secondary viremia but can also be damaged by the infection. The classic symptoms of hepatitis result from infections with hepatitis A, B, C, G, D, and E viruses and yellow fever virus and are often associated with EBV

Box 67–2. Infections of the Organs and Tissues

Liver

Hepatitis A,* B,* C,* G, D, and E viruses
Yellow fever virus
Epstein-Barr virus
Hepatitis in the neonate or immunocompromised person:
    Cytomegalovirus
    Herpes simplex virus
    Varicella-zoster virus
    Rubella virus (congenital rubella syndrome)

Heart

Coxsackie B virus

Kidney

Cytomegalovirus

Muscle

Coxsackie B virus (pleurodynia)

Glands

Cytomegalovirus
Mumps virus

Eye

Herpes simplex virus
Adenovirus*
Measles virus
Rubella virus
Enterovirus 70
Coxsackie A24 virus

Most common cause.

Box 67–3. Central Nervous System Infections

Meningitis

Enteroviruses
    Echoviruses
    Coxsackie virus*
    Poliovirus
Herpes simplex virus 2
Adenovirus
Mumps virus
Lymphocytic choriomeningitis virus
Arboencephalitis viruses

Paralysis

Poliovirus
Enteroviruses 70 and 71
Coxsackie A7 virus

Encephalitis

Herpes simplex virus 1*
Varicella-zoster virus
Arboencephalitis viruses*
Rabies virus
Coxsackie A and B viruses
Polioviruses

Postinfectious Encephalitis (Immune Mediated)

Measles virus
Mumps virus
Rubella virus
Varicella-zoster virus
Influenza viruses

Other

JC virus (progressive multifocal leukoencephalopathy
    [in immunosuppressed people])
Measles variant (subacute sclerosing panencephalitis)
Prion (encephalopathy)
Human immunodeficiency virus (AIDS dementia)
Human T-cell lymphotrophic virus 1 (tropical spastic paraparesis)

Most common cause.

infectious mononucleosis and CMV infections. The liver is also a major target in disseminated HSV infection of neonates and infants.

The heart and other muscles are also susceptible to viral infection and damage. Coxsackie virus can cause myocarditis or pericarditis in newborns, children, and adults. Coxsackie B virus can infect muscle and cause pleurodynia (Bornholm disease). Other viruses (e.g., influenza virus, CMV) can also infect the heart.

Infection of the secretory glands, accessory sexual organs, and mammary glands results in contagious spread of CMV. An inflammatory response to the infection, as occurs in **mumps** (parotitis, orchitis), may be the cause of the symptoms. CMV infection of the kidney and reactivation are problems for immunosuppressed people and a predominant reason for kidney transplant failure.

Infections of the Central Nervous System

Viral infections of the brain and CNS may cause the most serious viral diseases because of the importance of the CNS and its very limited capacity to repair damage (Box 67-3).

Tissue damage is usually caused by a combination of viral pathogenesis and immunopathogenesis. Most neurotropic viral infections do not result in disease, however, because the virus does not reach the brain or does not cause sufficient tissue damage to produce symptoms.

Virus may spread to the CNS in blood (arboviruses) or in macrophages (human immunodeficiency virus [HIV]); it may spread from a peripheral infection of the neurons (olfactory), or it may first infect skin (HSV) or muscle (polio, rabies) and then progress to the innervating neurons. The virus may have a predilection for certain sites in the brain. For example, the temporal lobe is targeted in HSV encephalitis, Ammon's horn in rabies, and the anterior horn of the spinal cord and motor neurons for polio.

Viral infections of the CNS are usually distinguished from bacterial infections by the finding of mononuclear cells, low numbers of polymorphonuclear leukocytes, and normal or slightly reduced levels of glucose in the cerebrospinal fluid. Immunoassay detection of specific antigen, polymerase chain reaction detection of viral genomes or messenger RNA, or isolation of the virus from a cerebrospinal fluid or biopsy specimen confirms the diagnosis and identifies the viral agent. The season of the year also facilitates the diagnosis, in that enteroviral and arboviral diseases generally occur during the summer, whereas HSV encephalitis and other viral syndromes may be observed year-round.

Aseptic meningitis is caused by an inflammation and swelling of the meninges enveloping the brain and spinal cord in response to infection with enteroviruses (especially echoviruses and Coxsackie viruses), HSV-2, the mumps virus, or the lymphocytic choriomeningitis virus. The disease is usually self-limited and, unlike bacterial meningitis, resolves without sequelae unless the virus gains access to and infects neurons or the brain (**meningoencephalitis**). The viruses gain access to the meninges by means of a viremia.

Encephalitis and **myelitis** result from a combination of viral pathogenesis and immunopathogenesis in brain tissue and neurons and either are fatal or cause significant damage and permanent neurologic sequelae. HSV, VZV, rabies virus, California encephalitis viruses, West Nile and St. Louis encephalitis viruses, mumps, and measles virus are potential causes of encephalitis. Poliovirus and several other enteroviruses cause paralytic disease (myelitis).

HSV and VZV are ubiquitous and usually cause asymptomatic latent infections of the CNS but can also cause encephalitis. Most arboencephalitis virus infections result in flulike symptoms rather than encephalitis. Postmeasles encephalitis and subacute sclerosing panencephalitis were rare sequelae of measles in the prevaccine era.

Other virus-induced neurologic syndromes are HIV dementia, human T-leukemia virus type 1 (HTLV-1) tropical spastic paraparesis, JC papovavirus–induced progressive multifocal leukoencephalopathy in immunosuppressed people, and the prion-associated spongiform encephalopathies (kuru, Creutzfeldt-Jakob disease, Gerstmann-Sträussler-Scheinker disease). Progressive multifocal leukoencephalopathy and the spongiform encephalopathies have long incubation periods (conventional and unconventional slow viruses).

Hematologic Diseases

Lymphocytes and macrophages are not very permissive for viral replication but are targets for several viruses that establish persistent infections. Viral replication of EBV, HIV, or CMV during the acute phase of infection elicits a large T-cell response, resulting in **mononucleosis-like syndromes**. In addition, CMV, measles virus, and HIV infections of T cells are immunosuppressive. HIV reduces the numbers of CD4 helper and delayed-type hypersensitivity T cells, further compromising the immune system. HTLV-1 infection causes little disease on infection but may

Box 67—4. Viruses Transmitted in Blood

Hepatitis B, C, G, D
Human immunodeficiency virus
Human T-cell lymphotrophic virus 1
Cytomegalovirus
Epstein-Barr virus
West Nile encephalitis virus

lead to **adult T-cell leukemia** or tropical spastic paraparesis much later in life (Box 67-4).

Macrophages and cells of the macrophage lineage can be infected by many viruses. Macrophages act as vehicles for spreading the virus throughout the body because viruses replicate inefficiently in them, and the cells are generally not lysed by the infection. This process promotes persistent and chronic infections. The macrophage is the primary target cell for the dengue virus. Non-neutralizing antibody can promote uptake of dengue virus and HIV into the cell through Fc receptors. Macrophages and cells of the macrophage lineage are the initial cells infected with HIV and provide a reservoir for the virus and access to the brain. AIDS dementia is thought to result from the actions of HIV-infected macrophages and microglial cells in the brain.

Sexually Transmitted Viral Diseases

Sexual transmission is a major route for the spread of papillomavirus, HSV, CMV, HIV, HTLV-1, HBV, hepatitis C virus (HCV), and hepatitis D virus (HDV) (Box 67-5). Such viruses establish chronic and latent-recurrent infections, with asymptomatic shedding into the semen and vaginal secretions. These viral properties foster dissemination via a route of transmission that is used relatively infrequently and might be avoided during symptomatic disease. The viruses can also be transmitted neonatally or perinatally to infants. Papillomaviruses and HSV establish local primary infections with recurrent disease at the same site. Lesions and asymptomatic shedding are sources for sexual transmission and for perinatal transmission to the newborn. CMV and HIV enter the bloodstream and infect lymphoid cells, whereas the hepatitis viruses are delivered to the liver. CMV, HIV, and the hepatitis viruses are

Box 67—5. Sexually Transmitted Viruses

Human papillomavirus 6, 11, 42
Human papillomavirus 16 and 18 (associated with human cervical carcinoma)
Herpes simplex virus (predominantly HSV-2)
Cytomegalovirus
Hepatitis B, C, and D viruses
Human immunodeficiency virus
Human T-cell lymphotrophic virus 1

Human immunodeficiency syndrome
Hepatitis B
Hepatitis C
Human T-cell lymphotropic virus type I and II
West Nile encephalitis virus*
Syphilis

*Trial initiated in 2003 on 6 million units, with 818 positive units excluded from usage.

Table 67–3. Arboviruses and Zoonoses

Virus	Family	Reservoir/Vector
Eastern equine encephalitis	Toga	Birds/*Aedes* mosquito
Western equine encephalitis	Toga	Birds/*Culex* mosquito
West Nile encephalitis	Flavi	Birds/*Culex* mosquito
St. Louis encephalitis	Flavi	Birds/*Culex* mosquito
California encephalitis	Bunya	Small mammals/*Aedes* mosquito
La Crosse encephalitis	Bunya	Small mammals/*Aedes* mosquito
Yellow fever	Flavi	Birds/*Aedes* mosquito
Dengue	Flavi	Monkeys/*Aedes* mosquito
Colorado tick fever	Reo	Tick
Lymphocytic choriomeningitis	Arena	Small mammals
Lassa fever	Arena	Rats
Sin Nombre virus	Hanta	Deer mice
Ebola	Filo	unknown
Rabies	Rhabdo	Bats, foxes, raccoons, etc.

present in blood, semen, and vaginal secretions, which can transmit the virus to sexual partners and neonates.

Viruses Spread by Transfusion and Transplantation

HBV, HCV, HDV, HIV, HTLV-1, and CMV are transmitted by blood and organ transplants. These viruses are also present in semen and therefore are sexually transmitted. The chronic nature of the infection, the persistent asymptomatic release of the virus, or the infection of macrophages and lymphocytes promotes transmission by these routes. West Nile encephalitis virus establishes a sufficient viremia for a long enough period that transmission by transfusion has occurred. Screening of the blood supply for HBV, HCV, HIV, and HTLV has controlled transmission of these viruses in blood transfusions (Box 67-6). Large-scale procedures for screening the other viruses have not been developed, so the risk remains for the spread of CMV by these routes.

Viruses Spread by Arthropods and Animals

Many of the toga, flavi, bunya, and the Colorado tick fever reovirus establish sufficient viremia in birds or animals to allow their acquisition by mosquitos or ticks and subsequent transmission to humans. Arena, rhabdo, and hanta viruses are transmitted to humans in saliva, urine, feces or through the bite of an infected animal (Table 67-3).

Syndromes of Possible Viral Etiology

Several diseases either produce symptoms or have epidemiologic or other characteristics that resemble those of viral infections or may be the sequelae of viral infections (e.g., inflammatory responses to a persistent viral infection). They include **multiple sclerosis, Kawasaki disease, arthritis, diabetes**, and **chronic fatigue syndrome**.

Chronic and Potentially Oncogenic Infections

Chronic infections occur when the immune system has difficulty resolving the infection. The DNA viruses (except parvovirus and poxvirus) and the retroviruses cause latent infections with the potential for recurrence. CMV and other herpesviruses; hepatitis B, C, G, and D viruses; and retroviruses cause chronic, productive infections.

HBV, HCV, EBV, HHV-8, papillomavirus, and HTLV-1 are associated with **human cancers**. EBV, papillomavirus, and HTLV-1 can immortalize cells; after immortalization, cofactors, chromosomal aberrations, or both, enable a clone of virus-containing cells to grow into a cancer. EBV normally causes infectious mononucleosis but is also associated with African Burkitt lymphoma, Hodgkin lymphoma, lymphomas in immunosuppressed individuals, and nasopharyngeal carcinoma; HTLV-1 is associated with human adult T-cell leukemia. Many papillomaviruses induce a simple hyperplasia characterized by the development of a wart; however, several other strains of papillomaviruses have been associated with human cancers (e.g., type 16 and 18 associated with cervical carcinoma). Direct viral action or the chronic cell damage and repair in livers infected by HBV or HCV can result in a tumorigenic event leading to hepatocellular carcinoma. HSV-2 has been associated with human cervical carcinoma, most likely as a cofactor. Immunosuppression in patients who have AIDS, patients undergoing cancer chemotherapy, or transplant recipients also promotes the production of lymphoma by EBV. HHV-8 infection produces many cytokines to

Table 70—4. Mechanisms Involved in the Development of Resistance to Antifungal Agents in Pathogenic Fungi

Fungus	Amphotericin B	Flucytosine	Itraconazole	Fluconazole	Echinocandins
Aspergillus fumigatus			Altered target enzyme, 14α-demethylase Decreased azole accumulation		
Candida albicans	Decrease in ergosterol Replacement of polyene-binding sterols Masking of ergosterol	Loss of permease activity Loss of cytosine deaminase activity Loss of uracil phosphoribosyl-transferase activity		Overexpression or mutation of 14α-demethylase Overexpression of efflux pumps, *CDR* and *MDR* genes	Mutation in *FKS*1 gene
Candida glabrata	Alteration or decrease in ergosterol content	Loss of permease activity		Overexpression of efflux pumps (*CgCDR* genes)	Mutation in *FKS*1 gene
Candida krusei	Alteration or decrease in ergosterol content			Active efflux Reduced affinity for target enzyme, 14α-demethylase	Mutation in *FKS*1 gene
Candida lusitaniae	Alteration or decrease in ergosterol content Production of modified sterols				
Cryptococcus neoformans	Defects in sterol synthesis Decreased ergosterol Production of modified sterols			Alterations in target enzyme Overexpression of MDR efflux pump	

however, sterol analysis of resistant strains of *Candida* spp. and *Cryptococcus neoformans* suggest that they are defective in *ERG2* or *ERG3*, genes encoding for the C-8 sterol isomerase and C-5 sterol desaturase enzymes, respectively.

Azoles

The ubiquitous use of azoles, especially fluconazole, for the treatment and prevention of fungal infections has given rise to reports of emerging resistance to this class of antifungal agents. Fortunately, primary resistance to fluconazole is rare among most species of *Candida* causing bloodstream infection. Among the five most common species of *Candida* isolated from the blood of infected patients (*Candida albicans*, *Candida glabrata*, *Candida parapsilosis*, *Candida tropicalis*, and *Candida krusei*), only *Candida krusei* is considered intrinsically resistant to fluconazole. Among the remaining species, approximately 10% of *Candida glabrata* exhibit primary resistance to fluconazole, and less than 2% of *Candida albicans*, *Candida parapsilosis*, and *Candida tropicalis* are resistant to this agent. The new triazoles (voriconazole, posaconazole, and ravuconazole) are more potent than fluconazole against *Candida* spp.,

including activity against *Candida krusei* and some fluconazole-resistant strains of other *Candida* spp.; however, there is a strong positive correlation between the activity of fluconazole and that of the other triazoles, suggesting some degree of cross-resistance within the class.

Primary resistance to fluconazole is also rare among clinical isolates of *Cryptococcus neoformans*. Secondary resistance has been described in isolates obtained from individuals with AIDS and relapsing cryptococcal meningitis.

Only a small number of isolates of *Aspergillus* spp. have been shown to demonstrate resistance to itraconazole. In contrast to *Candida*, cross-resistance between itraconazole and the new triazoles is not complete among isolates of *Aspergillus* spp.; cross-resistance between itraconazole and posaconazole, but not voriconazole, has been reported.

Azole resistance in *Candida* spp. can be due to the following mechanisms: a modification in the quantity or quality of the target enzymes, reduced access of the drug to the target, or some combination of these mechanisms. Thus point mutations in the gene (*ERG*11) encoding the target enzyme, lanosterol 14α-demethylase, leads to an altered target with decreased affinity for azoles. Overexpression of *ERG*11 results in overproduction of the target enzyme, creating the need for higher concentrations of the drug within the cell to inactivate all the target enzyme molecules. Up-regulation of genes encoding for multidrug efflux pumps results in active efflux of the azole antifungal agents out of the cell. Up-regulation of genes encoding the **major facilitator type efflux pump (MDR)** leads to fluconazole resistance, and up-regulation of genes encoding the **ATP-binding cassette transporters (CDR)** leads to resistance to multiple azoles. These mechanisms may act individually, sequentially, or simultaneously, resulting in strains of *Candida* that exhibit progressively higher levels of azole resistance.

The mechanisms of azole resistance in *Aspergillus* spp. are poorly characterized, given the paucity of strains with documented resistance. It appears that both increased drug efflux and alterations in the 14α-demethylase target enzyme serve as mechanisms for resistance to itraconazole among isolates of *Aspergillus* spp.

Similarly, secondary resistance to fluconazole among isolates of *Cryptococcus neoformans* has been associated with overexpression of MDR efflux pumps and alteration of the target enzyme. *Cryptococcus neoformans* has also been shown to have a CDR-type efflux pump.

Echinocandins

Caspofungin, anidulafungin, and micafungin all demonstrate potent fungicidal activity against *Candida* spp., including azole-resistant strains. Clinical isolates of *Candida* spp. with reduced susceptibility to the echinocandins are very rare. Efforts to produce caspofungin-resistant mutants of *Candida albicans* in the laboratory have shown that the frequency with which these mutants arise is very low (1 in 10^8 cells), suggesting a low potential for the emergence of resistance in the clinical setting. Clinical isolates of *Aspergillus* spp. with reduced susceptibility to echinocandins are nonexistent at the present time, and efforts to produce resistance in the laboratory setting have been unsuccessful.

The mechanism of resistance to caspofungin that has been characterized in laboratory-derived mutants of *Candida albicans* is one of an altered glucan synthesis enzyme complex that shows a decreased sensitivity to inhibition by caspofungin. These strains have point mutations in the *FKS*1 gene that encodes for an integral membrane protein (*FKS*1), which is the catalytic subunit of the glucan synthesis enzyme complex. The *FKS*1 mutation results in strains that are resistant to all of the echinocandins but retain susceptibility to polyene and azole antifungal agents. Although the *FKS*1 gene is essential in *Aspergillus* species as well, similar mutations have not been demonstrated thus far.

Flucytosine

Primary resistance to flucytosine is uncommon among clinical isolates of *Candida* spp. and *Cryptococcus neoformans*. Secondary resistance, however, is well documented to occur among both *Candida* spp. and *Cryptococcus neoformans* during monotherapy with this agent.

Flucytosine resistance may develop due to decreased uptake of the drug (loss of permease activity) or by loss of enzymatic activity necessary to convert flucytosine to 5-FU (cytosine deaminase) and 5-fluorouridylic acid (FUMP pyrophosphorylase). Uracil phosphoribosyltransferase, another enzyme in the pyrimidine salvage pathway, is also important in the formation of FUMP (5-fluorouracilmonophosphate), and loss of its activity is sufficient to confer resistance to flucytosine.

Allylamines

Although clinical failures can occur during treatment of fungal infections with terbinafine and naftifine, they have not been shown to be due to resistance to these agents. It has been shown that the CDR1 multidrug efflux pump can use terbinafine as a substrate, suggesting that efflux-mediated resistance to allylamines is a possibility.

Clinical Factors Contributing to Resistance

Antifungal therapy may fail clinically, despite the fact that the drug employed is active against the infecting fungus. The complex interaction of the host, the drug, and the fungal pathogen may be influenced by a wide variety of factors, including the immune status of the host, the site and severity of the infection, presence of foreign body (e.g., catheter, vascular graft), the activity of the drug at the site of infection, the dose and duration of therapy, and patient compliance with the antifungal regimen. It must be recognized that the presence of neutrophils, use of immunomodulating drugs, concomitant infections (e.g., HIV), surgical procedures, age, and nutritional status of the host all may be more important in determining the outcome of the infection than the ability of the antifungal agent to inhibit or kill the infecting organism.

Antifungal Susceptibility Testing

In vitro susceptibility testing of antifungal agents is designed to determine the relative activity of one or more agents against the infecting pathogen in hopes of selecting the best option for treatment of the infection. Thus antifungal susceptibility tests are performed for the same reasons that tests with antibacterial agents are performed. Antifungal susceptibility tests will (1) provide a reliable estimate of the relative activity of two or more antifungal agents against the tested organism, (2) correlate with in vivo antifungal activity and predict the likely outcome of therapy, (3) provide a means with which to monitor the development of resistance among a normally susceptible population of organisms, and (4) predict the therapeutic potential of newly developed investigational agents.

Standardized methods for performing antifungal susceptibility testing are reproducible, accurate, and available for use in clinical laboratories. Antifungal susceptibility testing is now increasingly and appropriately used as a routine adjunct to the treatment of fungal infections. Guidelines for the use of antifungal testing as a complement to other laboratory studies have been developed. Selective application of antifungal susceptibility testing, coupled with broader identification of fungi to the species level, is especially useful in difficult to manage fungal infections. One must keep in mind, however, that the in vitro susceptibility of an infecting organism to the antimicrobial agent is only one of several factors that may influence the likelihood that therapy for an infection will be successful. (See previous page.)

Questions

1. What is the mechanism of action of the echinocandin antifungal agents? Why is this an advantage for this class of agents?

2. Describe the mechanisms of resistance to the azoles that are known for *Candida albicans*.

3. Why is combination therapy with antifungal agents attractive? Give an example of a mechanism that would likely produce synergy.

Bibliography

Arikan S, Rex JH: Antifungal agents. In Murray PR, et al (eds): Manual of Clinical Microbiology, 9th ed. Washington, DC, ASM Press, 2007.

Espinel-Ingroff A, Pfaller MA: Susceptibility test methods: Yeasts and filamentous fungi. In Murray PR, et al (eds): Manual of Clinical Microbiology, 9th ed. Washington, DC, ASM Press, 2007.

Ghannoum MA, Rice LB: Antifungal agents: Mode of action, mechanisms of resistance, and correlation of these mechanisms with bacterial resistance. Clin Microbiol Rev 12:501-517, 1999.

Johnson MD, et al: Combination antifungal therapy. Antimicrob Agents Chemother 48:693-715, 2004.

Rex JH, Pfaller MA: Has antifungal susceptibility come of age? Clin Infect Dis 35:982-989, 2002.

White TC: Mechanisms of resistance to antifungal agents. In Murray PR, et al. (eds): Manual of Clinical Microbiology, 9th ed. Washington, DC, ASM Press, 2007.

71

Superficial and Cutaneous Mycoses

Fungal infections of the skin and skin structures are extremely common. These infections are generally categorized by the structures that the fungi colonize or invade:

1. **Superficial mycoses**, limited to the outmost layers of the skin and hair.
2. **Cutaneous mycoses**, infections that involve the deeper layers of the epidermis and its integuments, the hair and nails.
3. **Subcutaneous mycoses**, involving the dermis, subcutaneous tissues, muscle, and fascia. The subcutaneous mycoses will be discussed separately in Chapter 72. This chapter will deal with the superficial and cutaneous mycoses.

Superficial Mycoses

Agents of superficial mycoses are fungi that colonize the keratinized outer layers of the skin, hair, and nails. Infections due to these organisms elicit little or no host immune response and are nondestructive and thus asymptomatic. They are usually of cosmetic concern only and are easy to diagnose and treat.

Pityriasis (Tinea) Versicolor

Pityriasis versicolor is a common superficial fungal infection that is seen worldwide. In certain tropical environments, it may affect up to 60% of the population. It is caused by the lipophilic yeast *Malassezia furfur*.

Morphology

When viewed in skin scrapings, *M. furfur* appears as clusters of spherical or oval, thick-walled yeastlike cells, 3 to 8 μm in diameter (Figure 71-1). The yeast cells may be mixed with short, infrequently branched hyphae that tend to orient end to end. The yeastlike cells represent phialoconidia and show polar bud formation with a "lip" or collarette around the point of bud initiation on the parent cell (Figure 71-2). In culture on standard media containing or overlaid with olive oil, *M. furfur* grows as cream-colored to tan yeastlike colonies composed of budding yeastlike cells; hyphae are infrequently produced.

Epidemiology

Pityriasis versicolor is a disease of healthy persons that occurs worldwide, but it is most prevalent in tropical and subtropical regions. Young adults are most commonly affected. *M. furfur* is not found as a saprophyte in nature, and pityriasis versicolor has not been documented in animals. Human infection is thought to result from the direct or indirect transfer of infected keratinous material from one person to another.

Clinical Syndromes

The lesions of pityriasis versicolor are small hypo- or hyperpigmented macules. The upper trunk, arms, chest, shoulders, face, and neck are most often involved, but any part of the body may be affected (Figure 71-3). The lesions are irregular, well-demarcated patches of discoloration that may be raised and covered by a fine scale. Because *M. furfur* tends to interfere with melanin production, lesions are hypopigmented in dark-skinned individuals. In light-skinned subjects, the lesions are pink to pale brown and become more obvious when they fail to tan after exposure to sunlight. Little or no host reaction occurs, and the lesions are asymptomatic, with the exception of mild pruritus in severe cases. Infection of the hair follicles, resulting in folliculitis, perifolliculitis, and dermal abscesses, is a rare complication of this disease.

Laboratory Diagnosis

The laboratory diagnosis of pityriasis versicolor is made by the direct visualization of the fungal elements on microscopic examination of epidermal scales in 10% KOH with or without calcofluor white. The organisms are

Figure 71–1. Pityriasis versicolor. PAS-stained skin scraping showing yeastlike cells and short, infrequently branched hyphae that are often oriented end to end (×100). (From Connor DH, et al: Pathology of Infectious Diseases. Stamford, Conn, Appleton & Lange, 1997.)

Figure 71–3. Pityriasis versicolor. Multiple, pale brown, hyperpigmented patches on chest and shoulders. (From Chandler FW, Watts JC: Pathologic Diagnosis of Fungal Infections. Chicago, ASCP, 1987.)

usually numerous and may also be visualized with H&E or PAS stains (see Figure 71-1). The lesions will also fluoresce with a yellowish color upon exposure to a Wood lamp.

Although not usually necessary for establishing the diagnosis, culture may be performed using synthetic mycologic media supplemented with olive oil as a source of lipid. Growth of yeastlike colonies appear following incubation at 30° C for 5 to 7 days. Microscopically, the colonies are comprised of budding yeastlike cells with occasional hyphae.

Treatment

Although spontaneous cure has been reported, the disease is generally chronic and persistent. Treatment consists of the use of topical azoles or selenium sulfide shampoo. For more widespread infection, oral ketoconazole or itraconazole may be used.

Tinea Nigra

Tinea nigra is a superficial phaeohyphomycosis caused by the black fungus *Hortaea werneckii* (formerly *Exophiala werneckii*).

Morphology

Microscopically, *H. werneckii* appears as dematiaceous, frequently branched, septate hyphae, 1.5 to 3.0 μm wide. Arthroconidia and elongate budding cells are also present (Figure 71-4). *H. werneckii* also grows in culture on standard mycologic media at 25° C, where it is a black mold producing annelloconidia (conidia possessing annelids or rings), which often slide down the sides of the conidiophore.

Epidemiology

Tinea nigra is a tropical or subtropical condition. It is likely contracted by traumatic inoculation of the fungus into the superficial layers of the epidermis. It is most prevalent in Africa, Asia, and Central and South America.

Figure 71–2. Scanning electron micrograph of *Malassezia furfur* demonstrating the liplike collarette around the point of bud initiation on the parent cell.

Figure 71–4. Tinea nigra. Dematiaceous hyphae of *Hortaea werneckii* (H&E, ×100). (From Connor DH, et al: Pathology of Infectious Diseases. Stamford, Conn, Appleton & Lange, 1997.)

Figure 71–5. Tinea nigra. Darkly pigmented macules with irregular edges present on the palm. *(From Chandler FW, Watts JC: Pathologic Diagnosis of Fungal Infections. Chicago, ASCP, 1987.)*

Figure 71–6. *Trichosporon* spp. Cornmeal agar showing hyphae and arthroconidia (×400). *(From Marler LM, et al: Mycology CD-ROM, Indiana Pathology Images, 2004.)*

Children and young adults are most often affected, with a higher incidence in females.

Clinical Syndromes

Tinea nigra appears as a solitary, irregular, pigmented (brown to black) macule, usually on the palms or soles (Figure 71-5). There is no scaling or invasion of hair follicles, and the infection is not contagious. Owing to its superficial location, there is little or no discomfort or host reaction. Because the lesion grossly may resemble a malignant melanoma, biopsy or local excision may be considered. Such invasive procedures may be avoided by a simple microscopic examination of skin scrapings of the affected area.

Laboratory Diagnosis

Tinea nigra is easily diagnosed by microscopic examination of skin scrapings placed in 10% to 20% KOH. The pigmented hyphae and yeast forms are confined to the outer layers of the stratum corneum and are easily detected on H&E stained (see Box 69-1) sections (see Figure 71-4). Once fungal elements are detected, skin scrapings should be placed on mycologic media with antibiotics. A dematiaceous yeastlike colony should appear within 3 weeks, becoming velvety with age. Microscopic examination reveals two-celled, cylindrical, yeastlike cells and, depending upon the age of the colony, toruloid hyphae.

Treatment

The infection responds well to topical therapy, including Whitfield ointment, azole creams, and terbinafine.

White Piedra

White piedra is a superficial infection of hair caused by yeastlike fungi of the genus *Trichosporon*: *T. inkin*, *T. asahii*, *T. beigelii*, or *T. mucoides*.

Morphology

Microscopic examination reveals hyphal elements, arthroconidia (rectangular cells resulting from the fragmentation of hyphal cells), and blastoconidia (budding yeast cells) (Figure 71-6).

Epidemiology

This condition occurs in tropical and subtropical regions and is related to poor hygiene.

Clinical Syndromes

White piedra affects the hairs of the groin and axillae. The fungus surrounds the hair shaft and forms a white to brown swelling along the hair strand. The swellings are soft and pasty and may be easily removed by running a section of the hair between the thumb and forefinger. The infection does not damage the hair shaft.

Laboratory Diagnosis

When microscopic examination reveals hyphal elements, arthroconidia, and/or budding yeast cells, infected hair should be placed on mycologic media without cycloheximide (cycloheximide will inhibit *Trichosporon* spp.). *Trichosporon* spp. will form cream-colored, dry, wrinkled colonies within 48 to 72 hours upon incubation at room temperature. The various species of *Trichosporon* can be identified in the same manner as other yeast isolates. Sugar assimilations, KNO$_3$ assimilation (negative), urease production (positive) and morphology on cornmeal agar (both arthroconidia and blastoconidia are present) should be determined.

Treatment

Treatment may be accomplished by the use of topical azoles; however, improved hygiene and shaving of the infected hair are also effective and usually negate the necessity of medical treatment.

Black Piedra

Another condition affecting the hair, primarily the scalp, is black piedra. The causative agent of black piedra is *Piedraia hortae*.

Morphology

The organism grows as pigmented (brown to reddish-black) mold. As the culture ages, asci-containing, spindle-shaped ascospores are formed within specialized structures. These structures (asci and ascospores) are also produced within the rock-hard hyphal mass that surrounds the hair shaft.

Epidemiology

Black piedra is uncommon and has been reported from tropical areas in Latin America and Central Africa. It is thought to be a condition of poor hygiene.

Clinical Syndromes

Black piedra presents as small, dark nodules that surround the hair shafts. It is asymptomatic and generally involves the scalp. The hyphal mass is held together by a cement-like substance and contains asci and ascospores, the sexual phase of the fungus.

Laboratory Diagnosis

Examination of the nodule reveals branched, pigmented, hyphae held together by a cement-like substance. *P. hortae* can be cultured on routine mycologic media. Very slow growth may be observed at 25° C and may begin as a yeast-like colony, later becoming velvety as hyphae develop. Asci may be observed microscopically, usually ranging from 4 to 30 μm and containing up to 8 ascospores.

Treatment

Treatment of black piedra is easily accomplished by a haircut and proper, regular washings.

Cutaneous Mycoses

The cutaneous mycoses include infections caused by dermatophytic fungi (dermatophytosis) and nondermatophytic fungi (dermatomycosis) (Table 71-1). Owing to the overwhelming importance of dermatophytes as etiologic agents of cutaneous mycoses, the majority of this section will deal with those fungi. The nondermatophytic fungi will be discussed regarding their role in onychomycosis. The superficial and cutaneous infections caused by *Candida* spp. will be discussed in Chapter 74.

Dermatophytoses (Clinical Cases 71-1 and 71-2)

The term **dermatophytosis** refers to a complex of diseases caused by any of several species of taxonomically related filamentous fungi in the genera *Trichophyton*, *Epidermophyton,* and *Microsporum* (Tables 71-1 through 71-3). These fungi are known collectively as **the dermatophytes,** and all possess the ability to cause disease in humans and/or animals. All have in common the ability to invade the skin, hair, or nails. In each case, these fungi are keratinophilic and keratinolytic and so are able to break down the keratin surfaces of these structures. In the case of skin infections, the dermatophytes invade only the upper, outermost layer of the epidermis, the stratum corneum. Penetration below the granular layer of the epidermis is rare. Likewise with hair and nails, being part of the skin, only the keratinized layers are invaded. The various forms of dermatophytosis are referred to as "tineas" or ringworm. Clinically the tineas are classified according to the anatomic site or structure affected: (1) tinea capitis of the scalp, eyebrows and eyelashes; (2) tinea barbae of the beard; (3) tinea corporis of the smooth or glabrous skin; (4) tinea cruris of the groin; (5) tinea pedis of the foot; (6) tinea unguium of the nails (also known as **onychomycosis**). The clinical signs and symptoms of dermatophytosis vary according to the etiologic agents, the host reaction, and the site of infection.

Morphology

Each genus of dermatophytic mold is characterized by a specific pattern of growth in culture and by the production of macroconidia and microconidia (see Table 71-2). Further identification to species level requires consideration of colony morphology, spore production, and nutritional requirements in vitro.

Microscopically, the genus *Microsporum* is identified by observation of its macroconidia, whereas microconidia are the characteristic structures of the genus *Trichophyton* (see Table 71-2). *Epidermophyton floccosum* does not produce microconidia, but its smooth-walled macroconidia borne in clusters of two or three are quite distinctive (Figure 71-7). *Microsporum canis* produces characteristic large, multicellular (5 to 8 cells per conidium), thick- and rough-walled macroconidia (Figure 71-8). *Trichophyton rubrum* produces microconidia that are teardrop or peg shaped and borne along the sides of hyphae (Figure 71-9), whereas *T. mentagrophytes* produces both single, cigar-shaped macroconidia and grapelike clusters of spherical microconidia (Figure 71-10). *T. tonsurans* produces variably sized and shaped microconidia, with relatively large spherical conidia often located right alongside small, parallel-walled conidia and other microconidia of various sizes and shapes (Figure 71-11).

In skin biopsies, all of the dermatophytes are morphologically similar and appear as hyaline septate hyphae, chains of arthroconidia, or dissociated chains of arthroconidia that invade the stratum corneum, hair follicles, and hairs. When the hair is infected, the pattern of fungal invasion can be either **ectothrix, endothrix**, or **favic** depending on the dermatophytic species (Figure 71-12). Septate hyphae may be seen within the hair shaft in all three patterns. In the **ectothrix** pattern, **arthroconidia** are formed on the outside of the hair (Figure 71-13; see Figure 71-12); in the **endothrix** pattern, arthroconidia are formed inside the hair (see Figure 71-12); and in the **favic** pattern, hyphae, arthroconidia, and empty spaces resembling air bubbles ("honeycomb" pattern) are formed inside the hair (see Figure 71-12). The dermatophytes can usually be seen on H&E stain; however,

Table 71–1. Common and Uncommon Agents of Superficial and Cutaneous Dermatomycoses and Dermatophytoses

Fungus	Type of Infection									
	TP	TCO	TCR	TCA	TBA	TVR	O	TN	BP	WP
Dermatophytic										
Trichophyton rubrum	X	X	X				X			
T. mentagrophytes	X	X	X	X			X			
T. tonsurans		X		X			X			
T. verrucosum		X		X	X					
T. equinum				X						
T. violaceum				X						
T. schoenleinii				X						
T. megnini							X			
Epidermophyton floccosum	X		X				X			
Microsporum canis		X		X						
M. audouinii				X						
Nondermatophytic										
Scopulariopsis brevicaulis							X			
Scytalidium spp.	X						X			
Malassezia spp.						X				
Candida albicans	X		X				X			
Aspergillus terreus							X			
Acremonium spp.							X			
Fusarium spp.							X			
Trichosporon spp.										X
Piedraia hortae									X	
Hortaea werneckii								X		

TP, tinea pedis; TCO, tinea corporis; TCR, tinea cruris; TCA, tinea capitis; TBA, tinea barbae;
TVR, tinea versicolor; O, onychomycosis; TN, tinea nigra; BP, black piedra; WP, white piedra;
X, etiologic agents of.

they are best visualized with special stains for fungi, such as GMS and PAS (see Figure 71-13 and Chapter 69).

Ecology and Epidemiology

Dermatophytes can be classified into three different categories based on their natural habitat (see Table 71-3): (1) geophilic, (2) zoophilic, and (3) anthropophilic. The geophilic dermatophytes live in the soil and are occasional pathogens of both animals and humans. Zoophilic dermatophytes normally parasitize the hair and skin of animals but

can be transmitted to humans. Anthropophilic dermatophytes generally infect humans and may be transmitted directly or indirectly from person to person. This classification is quite useful prognostically and emphasizes the importance of identifying the etiologic agent of dermatophytoses. Species of dermatophytes that are considered anthropophilic tend to cause chronic, relatively noninflammatory infections that are difficult to cure. In contrast, the zoophilic and geophilic dermatophytes tend to elicit a profound host reaction, causing lesions that are highly

---

Clinical Case 71-1. Dermatophytosis in an Immunocompromised Host

Squeo, et al. (J Am Acad Dermatol 39:379, 1998) describe a case of a 55-year-old renal transplant recipient with onychomycosis and chronic tinea pedis who presented with tender nodules on his left medial heel. He then developed papules and nodules on his right foot and calf. A skin biopsy demonstrated periodic acid–Schiff (PAS) positive, thick-walled, round cells, 2 to 6 microns in diameter in the dermis. Skin biopsy culture grew *Trichophyton rubrum*. *T. rubrum* has been described as an invasive pathogen in immunocompromised hosts. The clinical presentation, histopathology, and early fungal culture growth suggested *Blastomyces dermatitidis* in the differential diagnosis before the final identification of *T. rubrum*.

Clinical Case 71-2. Tinea Capitis in an Adult Woman

Martin and Elewski (J Am Acad Dermatol 49:S177, 2003) describe an 87-year-old woman with a 2-year history of a pruritic, painful, scaling scalp eruption and hair loss. Her previous treatment for this condition included numerous courses of systemic antibiotics and prednisone without success. Of interest in her social history was that she had recently acquired several stray cats that she kept inside her home. On physical exam, there were numerous pustules throughout the scalp, with diffuse erythema, crusting, and scale extending to the neck. There was extremely sparse scalp hair and prominent posterior cervical lymphadenopathy. She had no nail pitting. A Wood light examination of the scalp produced negative findings. A skin biopsy specimen and fungal, bacterial, and viral cultures were obtained. Bacterial culture grew rare *Enterococcus* species, whereas viral cultures showed no growth. The scalp biopsy specimen revealed an endothrix dermatophyte infection. Fungal culture grew *Trichophyton tonsurans*. The patient was treated with griseofulvin and Selsun shampoo. When seen at a 2-week follow-up visit, the patient demonstrated new hair growth and a resolution of her pustular eruption. With the brisk clinical response and culture growth of *T. tonsurans*, treatment with griseofulvin was continued for 8 weeks. The scalp hair grew back normally without permanent alopecia. Adults with alopecia require an evaluation for tinea capitis, including fungal cultures.

---

inflammatory and respond well to therapy. In some instances, these infections may heal spontaneously.

The dermatophytes are worldwide in distribution (see Table 71-3), and infection may be acquired from the transfer of arthroconidia or hyphae, or keratinous material containing these elements, from an infected host to a susceptible, uninfected host. Dermatophytes may remain viable in desquamated skin scales or hair for long periods, and infection may be either by direct contact or indirect via fomites. Individuals of both sexes and all ages are susceptible to dermatophytosis; however, tinea capitis is more common in prepubescent children, and tinea cruris and tinea pedis are primarily diseases of adult males. Although dermatophytoses occur worldwide, especially in tropical and subtropical regions, individual dermatophyte species may vary in their geographic distribution and in their virulence for humans (see Table 71-3). For example, *Trichophyton concentricum*, the cause of tinea imbricata, is confined to the islands of the South Pacific and Asia, whereas *T. tonsurans* has replaced *Microsporum audouinii* as the principal agent of tinea capitis in the United States. Infections due to dermatophytes are generally endemic but may assume epidemic proportions in selected settings (e.g., tinea capitis in school children). On a worldwide scale, *T. rubrum* and *T. mentagrophytes* account for 80% to 90% of all dermatophytoses.

Clinical Syndromes

Dermatophytoses manifest a wide range of clinical presentations, which may be affected by factors such as the species of dermatophytes, the inoculum size, the site of infection, and the immune status of the host. Any given disease manifestation may result from several different species of dermatophytes, as shown in Table 71-1.

The classic pattern of dermatophytosis is the "ringworm" pattern of a ring of inflammatory scaling with diminution of

---

Table 71–2. Characteristic In Vitro and In Vivo Features of Dermatophytes

| Genus | In vitro | | In vivo hair | |
	Macroconidia	Microconidia	Invasion	Fluorescence[a]
Epidermophyton	Smooth walled, borne in clusters of two or three	Absent	NA	NA
Microsporum	Numerous, large, thick and roughwalled[b]	Rare	Ectothrix	+/−[c]
Trichophyton	Rare, smooth, thin-walled	Numerous, spherical, teardrop or pegshaped[d]	Endothrix[e]	+/−[f]

[a]Fluorescence with a Wood lamp.
[b]Except M. audouinii.
[c]M. gypseum not fluorescent.
[d]Except T. schoenleinii.
[e]T. verrucosum, ectothrix; T. schoenleinii, favic.
[f]T. schoenleinii is fluorescent.
NA, not applicable.

Table 71–3. Classification of Dermatophytes According to Ecologic Niche

Ecologic Niche	Species	Principal Hosts	Geographic Distribution	Prevalence
Anthropophilic	*Epidermophyton floccosum*		Worldwide	Common
	Microsporum audouinii		Worldwide	Common
	M. ferrugineum		Africa, Asia	Endemic
	Trichophyton concentricum		Asia, Pacific Islands	Endemic
	T. megnini		Europe, Africa	Endemic
	T. mentagrophytes var. *interdigitale*		Worldwide	Common
	T. rubrum		Worldwide	Common
	T. schoenleinii		Europe, Africa	Endemic
	T. soudanese		Africa	Endemic
	T. tonsurans		Worldwide	Common
	T. violaceum		Europe, Africa, Asia	Common
Zoophilic	*Microsporum canis*	Cat, dog, horse	Worldwide	Common
	M. gallinae	Fowl	Worldwide	Rare
	M. nanum	Swine	Worldwide	Rare
	M. persicolor	Vole	Europe, USA	Rare
	Trichophyton equinum	Horse	Worldwide	Rare
	T. mentagrophytes var. *mentagrophytes*	Rodent	Worldwide	Common
	var. *erinacei*	Hedgehog	Europe, New Zealand, Africa	Occasional
	var. *quinckeanum*	Mouse	Worldwide	Rare
	T. sinii	Monkey	India	Occasional
	T. verrucosum	Cow	Worldwide	Common
	Microsporum gypseum		Worldwide	Occasional
	M. fulvum		Worldwide	Occasional

From Hiruma M, Yamaguchi H: Dermatophytes. In Anaissie EJ, McGinnis MR, Pfaller MA (eds): Clinical Mycology. New York, Churchill Livingstone, 2003.

inflammation toward the center of the lesion. Tineas of hair-bearing areas often present as raised, circular or ring-shaped patches of alopecia with erythema and scaling (Figure 71-14) or as more diffusely scattered papules, pustules, vesicles, and kerions (severe inflammation involving the hair shaft) (Figure 71-15). Hairs infected with certain species, such as *M. canis*, *M. audouinii*, and *T. schoenleinii*, often fluoresce yellow-green when exposed to a Wood light (see Table 71-2). Infections of smooth skin commonly present as erythematous and scaling patches that expand in a centripetal pattern with central

clearing. Dermatophytoses of the foot and hand may often become complicated by onychomycosis (Figure 71-16), in which the nail plate is invaded and destroyed by the fungus. Onychomycosis (tinea unguium) is caused by a variety of dermatophytes (see Table 71-1) and is estimated to affect approximately 3% of the population in most temperate countries. It is a disease seen mostly in adults, with toenails affected more commonly than fingernails. The infection is usually chronic, and the nails become thickened, discolored, raised, friable, and deformed (see Figure 71-16). *T. rubrum* is the

Figure 71—7. *Epidermophyton floccosum.* Lactophenol cotton blue showing smooth-walled macroconidia.

Figure 71—8. *Microsporum canis.* Lactophenol cotton blue showing rough-walled macroconidia *(black arrow)* and microconidia *(red arrow).*

Figure 71—9. *Trichophyton rubrum.* Lactophenol cotton blue showing multicelled macroconidia *(black arrow)* and teardrop- and peg-shaped microconidia *(red arrow).*

Figure 71—10. *Trichophyton mentagrophytes.* Lactophenol cotton blue showing cigar-shaped macroconidia *(black arrow)* and grapelike clusters of microconidia *(red arrow).*

most common etiologic agent in most countries. A rapidly progressive form of onychomycosis that originates from the proximal nailfold and involves the upper and underside of the nail is seen in AIDS patients.

Laboratory Diagnosis

The laboratory diagnosis of dermatophytoses relies on the demonstration of fungal hyphae by direct microscopy of skin, hair, or nail samples and the isolation of organisms in culture. Specimens are mounted in a drop of 10% to 20% KOH on a glass slide and examined microscopically. Filamentous, hyaline hyphal elements characteristic of dermatophytes may be seen in skin scrapings, nail scrapings, and hairs. In examining specimens for fungal elements, calcofluor white has been used with excellent results.

Cultures are always useful and can be obtained by scraping the affected areas and placing the skin, hair, or nail

Figure 71—11. *Trichophyton tonsurans.* Lactophenol cotton blue showing microconidia *(black arrow).*

A   Ectothrix

B   Endothrix

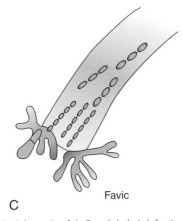

C   Favic

Figure 71–12. Schematic of **A,** Ectothrix hair infection. **B,** Endothrix hair infection. **C,** Favic hair infection.

clippings onto standard mycologic media such as Sabouraud agar, with and without antibiotics, or dermatophyte test medium. Colonies develop within 7 to 28 days. Their gross and microscopic appearance and nutritional requirements can be used in identification.

Treatment

Dermatophytic infections that are localized and that do not affect hair or nails can usually be treated effectively with topical agents; all others require oral therapy.

Figure 71–13. Arthroconidia surrounding a hair shaft. Ectothrix hair infection caused by *M. canis* (GMS-H&E, ×160). *(From Connor DH, et al: Pathology of Infectious Diseases. Stamford, Conn, Appleton & Lange, 1997.)*

Figure 71–14. Tinea capitis due to *M. canis*. *(From Hay RJ: Cutaneous and subcutaneous mycoses. In Anaissie EJ, McGinnis MR, Pfaller MA [eds]: Clinical Mycology. New York, Churchill Livingstone, 2003.)*

Figure 71–15. Tinea barbae caused by *T. verrucosum*. *(From Chandler FW, Watts JC: Pathologic Diagnosis of Fungal Infections. Chicago, ASCP, 1987.)*

Figure 71–16. Onychomycosis caused by *T. rubrum*. (From Hay RJ: *Cutaneous and subcutaneous mycoses. In Anaissie EJ, McGinnis MR, Pfaller MA [eds]: Clinical Mycology. New York, Churchill Livingstone, 2003.)*

Topical agents include azoles (miconazole, clotrimazole, econazole, tioconazole, and itraconazole), terbinafine, and haloprogin. Whitfield ointment (benzoic and salicylic acids) is an optional agent for dermatophytosis, but responses are usually slower than those seen with agents with specific antifungal activity.

Oral antifungal agents with systemic activity against dermatophytes include griseofulvin, itraconazole, fluconazole, and terbinafine. The azoles and terbinafine are more rapidly and broadly efficacious than griseofulvin, especially for the treatment of onychomycosis.

Onychomycosis Caused by Nondermatophytic Fungi

A number of nondermatophytic molds, as well as *Candida* species, have been associated with nail infections (see Table 71-1). These organisms include *Scopulariopsis brevicaulis*, *Scytalidium dimidiatum*, *S. hyalinum*, and a variety of others, including *Aspergillus*, *Fusarium*, and *Candida* species. Among these organisms, *S. brevicaulis* and *Scytalidium* spp. are proven nail pathogens. The other fungi certainly may be the cause of nail pathology; however, the interpretation of nail cultures with these organisms should be done with caution, as they may simply represent saprophytic colonization of abnormal nail material. Criteria used to determine an etiologic role for these fungi include isolation on multiple occasions and

the presence of abnormal hyphal or conidial structures on microscopic examination of nail material.

Infections due to *S. brevicaulis*, *S. dimidiatum*, and *S. hyalinum* are notoriously difficult to treat, because they are not usually susceptible to any antifungals. Partial surgical removal of infected nails, coupled with oral itraconazole or terbinafine or intensive treatment with 5% amorolfine nail lacquer or Whitfield ointment, may be useful in achieving a clinical response.

Case Study and Questions

Darrell, a 24-year-old medical student, just *loves* his new bulldog puppy, Delbert. He recently purchased Delbert from a local "backyard" breeder. Darrell has taken to giving Delbert frequent "smooches" on his muzzle, which Delbert loves, because he knows a treat is soon to follow. After about 3 months of proud puppy ownership and "smooching," Darrell noticed that his mustache began itching, and his upper lip was beginning to swell. Over a 1-week period, his upper lip became swollen and inflamed, and small pustular areas became apparent among the sparse hairs of his moustache. Similar changes were also becoming apparent on Delbert's muzzle. This concerned Darrell, so he promptly took Delbert to the vet. The vet took one look at the pair, wrote a prescription for Delbert, and told Darrell that he should make a visit to the dermatologist.

1. What was the likely cause of Darrell/Delbert's affliction? Be specific.
2. How would you go about making a diagnosis?
3. How would you go about treating this infection?
4. Who gave what to whom?

Bibliography

Chandler FW, Watts JC: Pathologic Diagnosis of Fungal Infections. Chicago, ASCP, 1987.

Hay RJ: Cutaneous and subcutaneous mycoses. In Anaissie EJ, McGinnis MR, Pfaller MA (eds): Clinical Mycology. New York, Churchill Livingstone, 2003.

Hiruma M, Yamaguchi H: Dermatophytes. In Anaissie EJ, McGinnis MR, Pfaller MA (eds): Clinical Mycology. New York, Churchill Livingstone, 2003.

Summerbell RC, et al: *Trichophyton, Microsporum, Epidermophyton*, and other agents of superficial mycoses. In Murray PR, et al (eds): Manual of Clinical Microbiology, 9th ed. Washington, DC, ASM Press, 2007.

Subcutaneous Mycoses

Many fungal pathogens can produce subcutaneous lesions as part of their disease process; however, certain fungi are commonly introduced traumatically through the skin and have a propensity to involve the deeper layers of the dermis, subcutaneous tissue, and bone. Although they may ultimately present clinically as lesions on the skin surface, they rarely spread to distant organs. In general, the clinical course is chronic and insidious; once established, the infections are refractory to most antifungal therapy. The main subcutaneous fungal infections include lymphocutaneous sporotrichosis, chromoblastomycosis, eumycotic mycetoma, subcutaneous zygomycosis, and subcutaneous phaeohyphomycosis. Two additional subcutaneous fungal or fungal-like processes, lobomycosis and rhinosporidiosis, are discussed separately in Chapter 75.

Although lymphocutaneous sporotrichosis is caused by a single fungal pathogen, *Sporothrix schenckii*, the other subcutaneous mycoses are clinical syndromes caused by multiple fungal etiologies (Table 72-1). The causative agents of subcutaneous mycoses are generally considered to have low pathogenic potential and are commonly isolated from soil, wood, or decaying vegetation. Exposure is largely occupational or related to hobbies (e.g., gardening, wood gathering). Infected patients generally have no underlying immune defect.

Lymphocutaneous Sporotrichosis
(Clinical Case 72-1)

Lymphocutaneous sporotrichosis is caused by *Sporothrix schenckii*, a dimorphic fungus that is ubiquitous in soil and decaying vegetation. Infection with this organism is chronic and is characterized by nodular and ulcerative lesions that develop along lymphatics that drain the primary site of inoculation (Figure 72-1). Dissemination to the other sites such as bones, eyes, lungs, and central nervous system is extremely rare (<1% of all cases) and will not be discussed further. At room temperature, *S. schenckii*

grows as a mold (Figure 72-2), and at 37° C and in tissue, it is a pleomorphic yeast (Figure 72-3; see Table 72-1).

Morphology

S. schenckii is thermally dimorphic. Mycelial form cultures grow rapidly and have a wrinkled membranous surface that gradually becomes tan, brown, or black. Microscopically, the mold form consists of narrow, hyaline, septate hyphae that produce abundant oval conidia (2×3 μm to 3×6 μm) borne on delicate sterigmata or in a rosette or "daisy petal" formation on conidiophores (see Figure 72-2). The yeast form consists of spherical, oval, or elongated ("cigar-shaped") yeastlike cells, 2 to 10 μm in diameter, with single or (rarely) multiple buds (see Table 72-1 and Figure 72-3). Although this is the "tissue phase" of *S. schenckii*, yeast forms are rarely seen on histopathologic examination of tissue.

Epidemiology

Sporotrichosis is usually sporadic and is most common in warmer climates. The major known areas of current endemicity are in Japan and in North and South America, especially Mexico, Brazil, Uruguay, Peru, and Colombia. Outbreaks of infection related to forest work, mining, and gardening have occurred. Classic infection is associated with traumatic inoculation of soil or vegetable or organic matter contaminated with the fungus. Zoonotic transmission has been reported in armadillo hunters and in association with infected cats. Between 1998 and 2001, a large outbreak of cat-transmitted sporotrichosis involving 178 patients was reported in Rio de Janeiro, Brazil.

Clinical Syndromes

Lymphangitic sporotrichosis classically appears following local trauma to an extremity. The initial site of infection appears as a small nodule, which may ulcerate. Secondary lymphatic nodules appear about 2 weeks after the appearance

Table 72–1. Common Agents of Subcutaneous Mycoses

Disease	Etiologic Agent(s)	Typical Morphology in Tissue	Usual Host Reaction
Sporotrichosis	*Sporothrix schenckii*	Pleomorphic, spherical to oval or cigar-shaped yeasts, 2-10 μm diameter with single or multiple (rare) buds See Figure 72-3	Mixed suppurative and granulomatous Splendore-Hoeppli material surrounds fungus (asteroid body) See Figure 72-4
Chromoblastomycosis	*Cladophialophora (Cladosporium) carrionii* *Fonsecaea compacta* *F. pedrosoi* *Phialophora verrucosa* *Rhinocladiella* *Exophiala* spp.	Large, 6-12 μm diameter, spherical, thick-walled, brown muriform cells (sclerotic bodies) with septations along one or two planes; pigmented hyphae may be present See Figure 72-6	Mixed suppurative and granulomatous Pseudoepitheliomatous hyperplasia
Eumycotic mycetoma	*Phaeoacremonium* spp. *Fusarium* spp. *Aspergillus nidulans* *Scedosporium apiospermum* *Madurella* spp. *Exophiala jeanselmei* among others	Granules, 0.2 to several mm diameter, composed of broad (2-6 μm), hyaline (pale granules) or dematiaceous (black granules), septate hyphae that branch and form chlamydoconidia	Suppurative with multiple abscesses, fibrosis, and sinus tracts; Splendore-Hoeppli material
Subcutaneous zygomycosis	*Basidiobolus ranarum (haptosporus)* *Conidiobolus coronatus*	Short, poorly stained hyphal fragments, 6-25 μm diameter, nonparallel sides, pauciseptate, random branches See Figure 72-10	Eosinophilic abscesses and granulation tissue, Splendore-Hoeppli material around hyphae
Subcutaneous phaeohyphomycosis	*Exophiala jeanselmei* *Wangiella dermatitidis* *Bipolaris* spp. *Alternaria* spp. *Chaetomium* spp. *Curvularia* spp. *Phialophora* spp. among others	Pigmented (brown) hyphae, 2-6 μm diameter, branched or unbranched, often constricted at prominent septations, yeast forms and chlamydoconidia may be present See Figure 72-11	Subcutaneous cystic or solid granulomas; overlying epidermis rarely affected

Adapted from Chandler FW, Watts JC: Pathologic Diagnosis of Fungal Infections. Chicago, ASCP, 1987.

of the primary lesion and consist of a linear chain of painless, subcutaneous nodules that extend proximally along the course of lymphatic drainage of the primary lesion (see Figure 72-1). With time, the nodules may ulcerate and discharge pus. Primary cutaneous lesions may remain "fixed" without lymphangitic spread. Clinically these lesions appear nodular, verrucous, or ulcerative and grossly may resemble a malignant process such as squamous cell carcinoma. Other infectious causes of lymphangitic and ulcerative lesions that must be ruled out include mycobacterial and nocardial infections.

Laboratory Diagnosis

Definitive diagnosis usually requires culture of infected pus or tissue. *S. schenckii* grows within 2 to 5 days on a variety of mycologic media and appears as a budding yeast at 35° C

and as a mold at 25° C (see Figures 72-2 and 72-3). Laboratory confirmation may be established by converting the mycelial growth to the yeast form by subculture at 37° C or immunologically through the use of the exoantigen test. In tissue, the organism appears as a 2 to 10 μm pleomorphic budding yeast (see Figure 72-3) but is rarely observed in human lesions. The appearance of Splendore-Hoeppli material surrounding yeast cells (asteroid body) may be helpful (Figure 72-4) but is also seen in other types of infection (see Table 72-1).

Treatment

The classic treatment for lymphocutaneous sporotrichosis is oral potassium iodide in saturated solution. The efficacy and low cost of this medication makes it a favored option,

Clinical Case 72-1. Sporotrichosis

Haddad and colleagues (Med Mycol 40:425, 2002) describe a case of lymphangitic sporotrichosis following injury with a fish spine. The patient was an 18-year-old male fisherman, resident in a rural area of Sao Paulo state, who wounded his third left finger on the dorsal spines of a fish that was netted during his work. Subsequently the area around the injury developed edema, ulceration, pain, and purulent secretion. The primary care physician interpreted the lesion as a pyogenic bacterial process and prescribed a 7-day course of oral tetracycline. No improvement was noted, and the therapy was changed to cephalexin, with similar results.

At examination 15 days after the accident, the patient presented with an oozing ulcer and nodules on the dorsum of the left hand and arm, forming an ascending nodular lymphangitic pattern. The diagnostic hypotheses considered were localized lymphangitic sporotrichosis, sporotrichoid leishmaniasis, and atypical mycobacteriosis (*Mycobacterium marinum*). A histopathologic examination of material from the lesion revealed a chronic ulcerated granulomatous pattern of inflammation, with intraepidermal microabscesses. No acid-fast bacilli or fungal elements were found. Culture of biopsy material on Sabouraud agar grew a mold characterized by septate, thin hyphae with conidia arranged in a rosette at the end of the conidiophores, consistent with *Sporothrix schenckii*. An intradermal reaction to sporotrichin was positive as well. The patient was treated with oral potassium iodide, with clinical resolution at 2 months of therapy.

The clinical presentation in this case was typical of sporotrichosis; however, the source of the infection (fish spine) was unusual. Despite the greater incidence of infection by *M. marinum* among fishermen and aquarists, sporotrichosis must be remembered when these workers show lesions in an ascending lymphangitic pattern after being injured by contact with fish.

Figure 72–2. Mold phase of *Sporothrix schenckii*.

used only if the patient cannot tolerate these other agents. Spontaneous remission is rare but was seen in 13 of the 178 cases in Brazil. The local application of heat has also been shown to be effective.

Chromoblastomycosis (Clinical Case 72-2)

Chromoblastomycosis (chromomycosis) is a chronic fungal infection affecting skin and subcutaneous tissues. It is characterized by the development of slow-growing verrucous nodules or plaques (Figure 72-5). Chromoblastomycosis is most commonly seen in the tropics, where the warm, moist environment, coupled with the lack of protective footwear and clothing, predisposes individuals to direct inoculation with infected soil or organic matter. The organisms most often associated with chromoblastomycosis are pigmented (dematiaceous) fungi of the genera *Fonsecaea*, *Cladosporium*, *Exophiala*, *Cladophialophora*, *Rhinocladiella*, and *Phialophora* (see Table 72-1).

especially in developing countries; however, it must be given daily over 3 to 4 weeks and has frequent adverse effects (nausea, salivary gland enlargement). Itraconazole has been shown to be safe and highly effective at low doses and is the current treatment of choice. Patients who do not respond may be given a higher dose of itraconazole, terbinafine, or potassium iodide. Fluconazole should be

Figure 72–1. Classic lymphocutaneous form of sporotrichosis, demonstrating a chain of subcutaneous nodules along the lymphatic drainage of the arm. *(From Chandler FW, Watts JC: Pathologic Diagnosis of Fungal Infections. Chicago, ASCP, 1987.)*

Figure 72–3. Yeast phase of *Sporothrix schenckii* in tissue (Gram stain, ×1000). *(From Marler LM, et al: Mycology CD-ROM, Indiana Pathology Images, 2004.)*

Figure 72—4. Asteroid body in sporotrichosis. The spherical yeastlike cells are surrounded by Splendore-Hoeppli material (H&E, ×160). *(From Connor DH, et al: Pathology of Infectious Diseases. Stamford, Conn, Appleton & Lange, 1997.)*

Figure 72—5. Chromoblastomycosis of the foot and leg. *(From Connor DH, et al: Pathology of Infectious Diseases. Stamford, Conn, Appleton & Lange, 1997.)*

Morphology

The fungi that cause chromoblastomycosis are all dematiaceous (naturally pigmented) molds but are morphologically diverse, and most are capable of producing several different forms when grown in culture. For example, *Exophiala* species may grow as molds and produce conidia-bearing cells called **annelids** and also as a yeastlike form that may appear in freshly isolated colonies. Although the basic form of these organisms is a pigmented septate mold, the different mechanisms of sporulation produced in culture makes specific identification difficult.

In contrast to the diverse morphology seen in culture, in tissue the fungi that cause chromoblastomycosis all characteristically form muriform cells (sclerotic bodies, Medlar bodies)

that are chestnut brown due to the melanin in their cell walls (Figure 72-6; see Table 72-1). Muriform cells divide by internal septation and appear as cells with vertical and horizontal lines within the same or different planes (see Figure 72-6). In addition to muriform cells, pigmented hyphae may also be present. The fungal cells may be free within the tissue but most often are contained within macrophages or giant cells.

Epidemiology

Chromoblastomycosis generally affects individuals working in rural areas of the tropics. The etiologic agents grow on woody plants and in the soil. Most infections have been in men and involve legs and arms, likely due to occupational exposure. Other body sites include shoulders, neck, trunk, buttocks, face, and ears. Local climatic factors may influence the distribution of different infections and different etiologic agents. For example, in Madagascar, infections caused by *Fonsecaea pedrosoi* are seen in areas of high

---

Clinical Case 72-2. Chromoblastomycosis

Marques, et al. (Med Mycol 42:261, 2004) describe a 52-year-old farmer from Brazil who presented with complaints of darkly pigmented pruritic skin lesions. The problem had appeared 2 years earlier and had progressed slowly since then. The patient was unaware of previous trauma but recalled an insect bite on his left arm. Initially the lesion that developed at this site was a small, raised, erythematous papule. Later, a new crop of lesions appeared on the left leg and, more recently, on the forehead and left side of the face. Physical examination revealed extensive lesions in scaly plaques situated at different sites on the face, arm, and leg. Direct KOH examination of biopsies of the lesions showed numerous pigmented, bilaterally dividing, rounded, sclerotic cells (Medlar bodies), thus confirming the clinical diagnosis of chromoblastomycosis. Cultures of the biopsies grew a darkly pigmented mould that was identified on the basis of characteristic conidiation as *Rhinocladiella aquaspersa*. The lesions improved with ketoconazole therapy, with decreasing pruritic symptoms. Unfortunately the patient was lost to follow-up. Chromoblastomycosis caused by *R. aquaspersa* is relatively uncommon. Furthermore, this case is unusual in that the lesions were dispersed over three different anatomical regions. Notably, the occurrence of facial lesions is very unusual.

Figure 72—6. Brown-pigmented muriform cell, or Medlar body, of chromoblastomycosis (H&E, ×250). *(From Connor DH, et al: Pathology of Infectious Diseases. Stamford, Conn, Appleton & Lange, 1997.)*

rainfall (200 to 300 cm annually), whereas in the same island, infections due to *Cladophialophora carrionii* occur in areas of low rainfall (50 to 60 cm annually). In the Americas, *F. pedrosoi* is the principal cause of chromoblastomycoses, and the lesions most often involve the lower extremities. In contrast, in Australia the most common cause is *C. carrionii*, and the lesions are most frequently on the upper limbs, especially the hands. There are no reports of person-to-person transmission.

Clinical Syndromes

Chromoblastomycosis tends to be chronic, pruritic, progressive, indolent, and resistant to treatment. In most instances, patients do not present until the infection is well established. Early lesions are small, warty papules and usually enlarge only slowly. There are different morphologic forms of the disease, ranging from verrucous lesions to flat plaques. Established infections appear as multiple, large, warty, "cauliflower-like" growths that are usually clustered within the same region (see Figure 72-5). Satellite lesions may occur secondary to autoinoculation. Plaquelike lesions often show central scarring as they enlarge. Ulceration and cyst formation may occur. Large lesions are hyperkeratotic, and the limb is grossly distorted due to fibrosis and secondary lymphedema (see Figure 72-5). Secondary bacterial infection may also occur and contribute to regional lymphadenitis, lymph stasis, and eventual elephantiasis.

Laboratory Diagnosis

The clinical presentation (see Figure 72-5), histopathologic findings of chestnut-brown, muriform cells (see Figure 72-6), and isolation in culture of one of the causal fungi (see Table 72-1) confirm the diagnosis. Scrapings obtained from the surface of the warty lesions where small dark dots are observed may result in the demonstration of the characteristic cells when mounted in 20% KOH. Biopsy specimens stained with H&E (see Chapter 69) will also show the organism present in the epidermis or in microabscesses containing macrophages and giant cells. The inflammatory reaction is both suppurative and granulomatous, with dermal fibrosis and pseudoepitheliomatous hyperplasia. The organisms are easily cultured from the lesions, although identification may be difficult. There are no serologic tests available for chromoblastomycosis.

Treatment

Treatment with specific antifungal therapy is often ineffective, owing to the advanced stage of infection upon presentation. The drugs that appear to be most effective are itraconazole and terbinafine. More recently, posaconazole has been used with modest success. These agents are often combined with flucytosine in refractory cases. In an effort to improve the response to treatment, attempts are often made

to shrink larger lesions with local heat or cryotherapy before administering antifungal agents. Because of the risk of recurrences developing within the scar, surgery is not indicated. Squamous cell carcinomas may develop in longstanding lesions, and those with atypical areas or fleshy outgrowths should be biopsied to rule out this complication.

Eumycotic Mycetoma

Eumycotic mycetomas are those caused by true fungi, as opposed to actinomycotic mycetomas, which are caused by aerobic actinomycetes (bacteria). This section will deal only with the eumycotic mycetomas.

As with chromoblastomycosis, most eumycotic mycetomas are seen in the tropics. A mycetoma is defined clinically as a localized, chronic, granulomatous, infectious process involving cutaneous and subcutaneous tissues. It is characterized by the formation of multiple granulomas and abscesses that contain large aggregates of fungal hyphae known as **granules** or **grains**. These grains contain cells that have marked modifications of internal and external structure, ranging from reduplications of the cell wall to the formation of a hard, cement-like extracellular matrix. The abscesses drain externally through the skin, often with extrusion of granules. The process may be quite extensive and deforming, with destruction of muscle, fascia, and bone. The etiologic agents of eumycotic mycetoma encompass a wide range of fungi, including *Phaeoacremonium*, *Curvularia*, *Fusarium*, *Madurella*, *Exophiala*, *Pyrenochaeta*, *Leptosphaeria*, and *Scedosporium* species (see Table 72-1).

Morphology

The granules of eumycotic mycetomas are composed of septate fungal hyphae that are 2 to 6 μm or greater in width and are either dematiaceous (black grain) or hyaline (pale or white grain), depending on the etiologic agent (Figure 72-7). The hyphae are frequently distorted and bizarre in form and size. Large, spherical, thick-walled chlamydoconidia are often present. The hyphae may be embedded in an amorphous cement-like substance. Splendore-Hoeppli material often interdigitates among the mycelial elements at the periphery of the granule. Eumycotic granules may be differentiated from actinomycotic granules based on morphologic (branched filaments versus septate hyphae and chlamydoconidia) and staining (gram-positive beaded rods vs. PAS- and GMS-positive hyphae) characteristics (see Chapter 69). Culture is usually necessary for definitive identification of the fungus (or actinomycete) involved.

Epidemiology

Mycetomas are primarily seen in tropical areas with low rainfall. Eumycotic mycetomas are more frequent in Africa

Figure 72–7. A, Mycetoma granule of *Curvularia geniculata*. **B,** Compact dematiaceous hyphae and chlamydoconidia embedded in cement-like substance.

and the Indian subcontinent but also may be seen in Brazil, Venezuela, and the Middle East. All patients are infected from sources in nature via traumatic percutaneous implantation of the etiologic agent into exposed parts of the body. The foot and hand are most common, but back, shoulders, and chest-wall infections are also seen. Men are more often affected than women. The fungi that cause eumycotic mycetomas differ from country to country, and the agents that are common in one region are rarely reported from others. Mycetomas are not contagious.

Clinical Syndromes

Similar to chromoblastomycosis, patients with eumycotic mycetoma most commonly present with longstanding infection. The earliest lesion is a small, painless, subcutaneous nodule or plaque that increases slowly but progressively in size. As the mycetoma develops, the affected area gradually enlarges and becomes disfigured as a result of chronic inflammation and fibrosis. With time, sinus tracts appear on the skin surface and drain serosanguineous fluid that often contains grossly visible granules. The infection commonly breaches tissue planes and destroys muscle and bone locally. Hematogenous or lymphatic spread from a primary focus to distant sites or viscera is extremely rare.

Laboratory Diagnosis

The key to the diagnosis of eumycotic mycetoma is the demonstration of grains or granules. Grains may be grossly visible in draining sinus tracts or may be expressed onto a glass slide. Material may also be obtained by deep surgical biopsy.

Grains can be visualized microscopically by mounting in 20% KOH. The hyphae are usually clearly visible, as is the presence or absence of pigmentation. Grains can be washed and then cultured or fixed and sectioned for histopathology.

Grains are easily visualized in tissue stained with H&E (see Figure 72-7). Special stains such as PAS and GMS may also be helpful. Although the color, shape, size, and microscopic morphology may be characteristic of a specific causal agent, culture is usually necessary for definitive identification of the organism. Most organisms will grow on standard mycologic medium; however, inclusion of an antibiotic such as penicillin may be useful to inhibit contaminating bacteria, which may overgrow the fungus.

Treatment

Treatment of eumycotic mycetoma is usually unsuccessful. Response of the various etiologic agents to amphotericin B, ketoconazole, or itraconazole is variable and often poor, although such therapy may slow the course of infection. Promising treatment responses have recently been reported for terbinafine, voriconazole, and posaconazole. Local excision is usually ineffective or not possible, and amputation is the only definitive treatment. Because these infections are usually slowly progressive and may be slowed further by specific antifungal therapy, the decision to amputate should take into account the rate of progression, the symptomatology, the availability of adequate prosthetics, and the individual circumstances of the patient. For all of these reasons, it is imperative to differentiate eumycotic mycetoma from actinomycotic mycetoma. Medical therapy is usually effective in cases of actinomycotic mycetoma.

Subcutaneous Zygomycosis

Subcutaneous zygomycosis, also known as **entomophthoromycosis**, is caused by Zygomycetes of the order Entomophthorales: *Conidiobolus coronatus* and *Basidiobolus ranarum (haptosporus)* (see Table 72-1). Both of these fungi cause a chronic subcutaneous form of zygomycosis

Figure 72—8. Subcutaneous zygomycosis caused by *Conidiobolus coronatus. (From Chandler FW, Watts JC: Pathologic Diagnosis of Fungal Infections. Chicago, ASCP, 1987.)*

that occurs sporadically as a result of traumatic implantation of the fungus present in plant debris in tropical environments. They differ in that they cause infections with different anatomic locations: *B. ranarum* causes subcutaneous infection of the proximal limbs in children, whereas *C. coronatus* infection is localized to the facial area, predominantly in adults (Figures 72-8 and 72-9).

Morphology

The appearance of the agents of subcutaneous zygomycosis in tissue differs from that of the mucoraceous Zygomycetes. The hyphal elements are sparse and often appear as hyphal fragments surrounded by intensely eosinophilic Splendore-Hoeppli material (Figure 72-10). The inflammatory response is granulomatous and rich in eosinophils. The hyphal fragments are thin-walled and poorly staining. Although septae are infrequent, they are more prominent than those seen with Mucoraceae. The hyphae of the Entomophthoraceae are not angioinvasive.

Epidemiology

Both types of subcutaneous zygomycosis are seen most commonly in Africa and to a lesser extent in India. Infection due to *B. ranarum* has also been reported from the Middle East, Asia, and Europe, whereas that due to *C. coronatus* has been reported from Latin America, as well as Africa and India. Both fungi are saprophytes that are present in leaf and plant debris. *B. ranarum* has also been found in the intestinal contents of small reptiles

and amphibians. Both are rare diseases without known predisposing factors (e.g., acidosis or immunodeficiency). Infection due to *B. ranarum* is thought to occur following traumatic implantation of the fungus into the subcutaneous tissues of the thighs, buttocks, and trunk. This form of subcutaneous zygomycosis occurs mainly in children (80% under the age of 20 years) with a male:female ratio of 3:1. *C. coronatus* infections occur following inhalation of the fungal spores, which then invade the tissues of the nasal cavity, the paranasal sinuses, and facial soft tissues. There is a 10:1 male:female ratio, and the disease is seen predominantly among young adults. Infection among children is rare.

Clinical Syndromes

Patients infected with *B. ranarum* have disk-shaped, rubbery, movable masses that may be quite large and are localized to the shoulder, pelvis, hips, and thighs (see Figure 72-9). The masses may expand locally and eventually ulcerate. Dissemination or involvement of deeper structures is rare. Gastrointestinal basidiobolomycosis has recently been reported in the southwestern United States.

C. coronatus infection is confined to the rhinofacial area and often does not come to medical attention until there is a noticeable swelling of the upper lip or face (see Figure 72-8). The swelling is firm and painless and may progress slowly to involve the nasal bridge and the upper and lower face, including the orbit. The facial deformity can be quite dramatic; however, owing to the lack of angioinvasion, intracranial extension does not occur.

Figure 72—9. Subcutaneous zygomycosis caused by *Basidiobolus ranarum.* The right thigh is extensively swollen and indurated. *(From Chandler FW, Watts JC: Pathologic Diagnosis of Fungal Infections. Chicago, ASCP, 1987.)*

Figure 72–10. Subcutaneous zygomycosis. Broad hyphal fragments surrounded by eosinophilic Splendore-Hoeppli material (H&E, ×160). *(From Chandler FW, Watts JC: Pathologic Diagnosis of Fungal Infections. Chicago, ASCP, 1987.)*

Laboratory Diagnosis

Both types of subcutaneous zygomycosis require biopsy for diagnosis, despite the characteristic clinical features of the infections. The histopathologic picture is the same for both organisms (see Figure 72-10) and is marked by focal clusters of inflammation, with eosinophils and typical zygomycotic hyphae often surrounded by eosinophilic Splendore-Hoeppli material. The organisms can be cultured from clinical material on standard mycologic medium.

Treatment

Both types of infection may be treated with itraconazole. Alternatively, oral potassium iodide in saturated solution has been used. Facial reconstructive surgery may be necessary in the case of *C. coronatus* infection; extensive fibrosis remains after eradication of the fungus.

Subcutaneous Phaeohyphomycosis
(Clinical Case 72-3)

Phaeohyphomycosis is a term used to describe a heterogeneous array of fungal infections caused by pigmented, or dematiaceous, fungi which are present in tissue as irregular hyphae (Figure 72-11) rather than the sclerotic muriform cells seen in chromoblastomycosis (see Table 72-1 and Figure 72-6). These infections may be caused by a wide range of fungi, all of which exist in nature as saprophytes of soil, wood, and decaying vegetation. Phaeohyphomycotic processes may be superficial, subcutaneous, or deeply invasive or disseminated. The superficial (see Chapter 71) and deeply invasive (see Chapter 74) forms are discussed in their respective chapters. The subcutaneous form is discussed in this section.

Clinical Case 72-3. Phaeohyphomycosis in a Renal Transplant Patient

Marques, et al (Med Mycol 44:671, 2006) describe a case of subcutaneous phaeohyphomycosis in a renal transplant recipient. The patient was a 49-year-old diabetic man, who for 5 years had been given immunosuppressive therapy with prednisone and cyclosporine A following a kidney transplantation He presented with a 1-year history of draining foot lesions. The patient denied any history of local trauma but had been working in rural activities at the time of the initial complaint. He had been treated for presumed bacterial infection, without response. Dermatologic examination revealed two confluent erythematous cystic tumors on the dorsum of the left foot, with drainage points emitting a serosanguineous secretion. A local CT scan showed only circumscribed hypodense lesions. A needle aspiration and a large biopsy were obtained to confirm the presumed diagnosis of phaeohyphomycosis. Histopathologic examination revealed intense inflammatory infiltrates and rare hyphal elements. Culture of the biopsy material revealed a slow-growing mould that eventually demonstrated a beige to gray-brown coloration. The organism was eventually identified as *Phaeoacremonium parasiticum* by a combination of morphology and molecular identification methods. The patient was treated with itraconazole coupled with local irrigation and a decrease in the dosing of cyclosporine A and achieved a satisfactory response.

This case illustrates an apparent trend for immunocompromised organ transplant patients with localized *P. parasiticum* infections to have acquired their infections without recognized trauma. It is unclear whether such infections are acquired via minor skin fissures or via inhalation or ingestion of an infectious particle, with subsequent translocation to subcutaneous capillary beds, where slightly diminished temperature or other local conditions may favor growth.

Morphology

The agents of subcutaneous phaeohyphomycosis are numerous and diverse (see Table 72-1), but all grow as black molds in culture and appear as dark-walled, irregular, hyphal and yeastlike forms in tissue (see Figure 72-11). The hyphae vary from 2 to 6 μm wide and may be branched or septate and are often constricted at the point of septation. Bizarre, thick-walled, vesicular swellings that may be as large as 25 μm in diameter may be present, as well as budding yeastlike structures. Cell wall pigmentation ranges from light to dark and may require special stains such as the Fontana-Masson melanin stain to confirm the dematiaceous nature of the fungus. In culture, the different fungi grow as black or brown molds and are identified by their characteristic mode of sporulation.

Epidemiology

More than 20 different dematiaceous fungi have been cited as causes of subcutaneous phaeohyphomycosis. The most frequent etiologic agents have been *Exophiala jeanselmei, Alternaria, Curvularia, Phaeoacremonium,* and *Bipolaris* spp. (see Table 72-1). Because these fungi are found in soil and

Figure 72–11. Subcutaneous phaeohyphomycosis. Dematiaceous yeastlike cells and septate hyphae of *Exophiala spinifera* (H&E, ×250). *(From Chandler FW, Watts JC: Pathologic Diagnosis of Fungal Infections. Chicago, ASCP, 1987.)*

plant debris, the route of infection is thought to be secondary to traumatic implantation of the fungus. Indeed, wood splinters have been found in histopathologic material, suggesting the mode of inoculation and possibly that the formation of the characteristic phaeohyphomycotic cyst is a reaction to implantation. There is no explanation for why some organisms produce phaeohyphomycotic cysts and others develop into mycetomas.

Clinical Syndromes

Most commonly, subcutaneous phaeohyphomycosis presents as a solitary inflammatory cyst. The lesions generally occur on the feet and legs, although the hands and other body sites may be involved. The lesions grow slowly and expand over a period of months or years. They may be firm or fluctuant and are usually painless. If located near a joint, they may be mistaken for a synovial cyst and may become large enough to interfere with movements. Other manifestations include the formation of pigmented plaquelike lesions that are indurated but nontender.

Laboratory Diagnosis

The diagnosis is made upon surgical excision of the cyst. On histopathologic examination, the appearance is of an inflammatory cyst with a fibrous capsule, granulomatous reaction, and central necrosis. Individual and clustered dematiaceous fungal elements are seen within giant cells and extracellularly amid the necrotic debris (Figure 72-11). Generally, the pigmentation is easily seen on examination

of H&E stained tissue. The organisms can be grown in culture and identified by their pattern of sporulation.

Treatment

The main treatment is surgical excision. Plaquelike lesions may not be amenable to this approach and generally respond to treatment with itraconazole with or without concomitant flucytosine. Posaconazole, voriconazole, and terbinafine may also be active against these groups of fungi.

Case Study and Questions

A 40-year-old "ecotourist" was on an extended trip to the jungles of Costa Rica. During this time, she camped, climbed trees, waded in streams, slogged through mud, and endured drenching rains. She lost her shoes about 2 weeks into the "adventure" and continued to hike about barefoot for another 2 weeks, during which time she sustained minor cuts and abrasions to both feet. Approximately 6 months after returning home, somewhere in the Midwest United States, she noticed mild swelling of her right foot. There was no pain, inflammation, or drainage from the foot. She comes to you for medical advice.

1. What is the differential diagnosis of this process?
2. What types of fungi might cause this infection?
3. How will you proceed with establishing the diagnosis?
4. What are the therapeutic options and the likelihood that they will be successful?

Bibliography

Basto de Lima Barros M, et al: Cat-transmitted sporotrichosis epidemic in Rio de Janeiro, Brazil: Description of a series of cases. Clin Infect Dis 38:529-535, 2004.

Chandler FW, Watts JC: Pathologic Diagnosis of Fungal Infections. Chicago, ASCP, 1987.

Connor DH, et al: Pathology of Infectious Diseases. Stamford, Conn, Appleton & Lange, 1997.

De Hoog GS, Vitale RG: *Bipolaris, Exophiala, Scedosporium, Sporothrix,* and other dematiaceous fungi. In Murray PR, et al (eds): Manual of Clinical Microbiology, 9th ed. Washington, DC, ASM Press, 2007.

De Hoog GS, et al: Fungi causing eumycotic mycetoma. In Murray PR, et al (eds): Manual of Clinical Microbiology, 9th ed. Washington, DC, ASM Press, 2007.

Hay RJ: Cutaneous and subcutaneous mycoses. In Anaissie EJ, McGinnis MR, Pfaller MA (eds): Clinical Mycology. New York, Churchill Livingstone, 2003.

Kauffman CA, et al: Clinical practice guidelines for the management of sporotrichosis: 2007 update by the Infectious Diseases Society of America. Clin Infect Dis 45:1255, 2007.

Systemic Mycoses Due to Dimorphic Fungi

The **dimorphic** fungal pathogens are organisms that exist in a mold form in nature or in the laboratory at 25° C to 30° C and in a yeast or spherule form in tissues or when grown on enriched medium in the laboratory at 37° C (Figure 73-1). The organisms in this group are considered primary **systemic** pathogens, owing to their ability to cause infection in both "normal" and immunocompromised hosts and for their propensity to involve the deep viscera after dissemination of the fungus from the lungs following its inhalation from nature. The dimorphic pathogens include *Blastomyces dermatitidis, Coccidioides immitis* and *C. posadasii, Histoplasma capsulatum* var. *capsulatum* and *H. capsulatum* var *duboisii, Paracoccidioides brasiliensis,* and *Penicillium marneffei* (Table 73-1). These organisms are also known as **endemic** pathogens, in that their natural habitat is delimited to specific geographic regions (Figure 73-2), and infection due to a particular fungus is acquired by inhalation of spores from that specific environment and geographic location (see Table 73-1). *H. capsulatum, C. immitis (C. posadasii),* and *P. marneffei* have emerged as major opportunistic pathogens in individuals with AIDS and other forms of immunosuppression. Recognition of these endemic mycoses may be complicated by the fact that they may become manifest only after the patient has left the area of endemicity. Often the infection may be quiescent, only to reactivate when the individual becomes immunosuppressed and is living in an area where the fungus is not endemic.

Blastomycosis (Clinical Case 73-1)

Blastomycosis is a systemic fungal infection caused by the dimorphic pathogen *Blastomyces dermatitidis.* Like other endemic mycoses, this infection is confined to specific geographic regions, with most infections originating in the Mississippi River basin, around the Great Lakes, and in the Southeast region of the United States (see Figure 73-2). Cases have also been diagnosed in other parts of the world, including Africa, Europe, and the Middle East.

Morphology

As a thermally dimorphic fungus, *B. dermatitidis* produces nonencapsulated yeastlike cells in tissue and in culture on enriched media at 37° C and white to tan, filamentous, mold colonies on standard mycologic media at 25° C. The mold form produces round to oval or pear-shaped conidia (2 to 10 μm) located on long or short terminal hyphal branches (Figure 73-3). Older cultures may also produce 7- to 18-μm diameter, thick-walled chlamydospores. This form of *B. dermatitidis* is not diagnostic and may not be distinguishable from the monomorphic *Chrysosporium* spp. or from an early culture of *H. capsulatum.*

The yeast form of *B. dermatitidis* is seen in tissue and in culture at 37° C. This form is quite distinctive (Figure 73-4). The yeast cells are spherical, hyaline, 8 to 15 μm in diameter, multinucleated, and have thick "double-contoured" walls. The cytoplasm is often retracted from the rigid cell wall as a result of shrinkage during the fixation process. The yeast cells reproduce by the formation of buds or **blastoconidia**. The buds are usually single and attached to the parent cell by broad bases (see Figure 73-4).

The yeast forms may be visualized in tissue stained with hematoxylin-eosin (H&E); however, the fungal stains, Gomori methenamine silver (GMS) and periodic acid–Schiff (PAS), help locate the organisms and delineate their morphology.

Epidemiology

The ecologic niche of *B. dermatitidis* appears to be in decaying organic matter. Studies in humans and animals indicate that infection is acquired following the inhalation of aerosolized

Saprobic phase (25° C)   Parasitic phase (37° C)

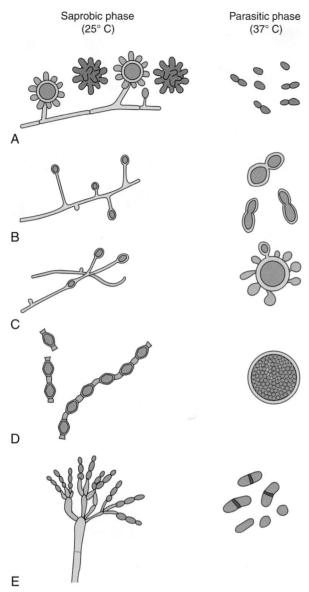

Figure 73—1. Saprobic and parasitic phases of endemic dimorphic fungi. **A,** *Histoplasma capsulatum.* **B,** *Blastomyces dermatitidis.* **C,** *Paracoccidioides brasiliensis.* **D,** *Coccidioides immitis.* **E,** *Penicillium marneffei.*

conidia produced by the fungus growing in soil and leaf litter (Figure 73-5). Outbreaks of infection have been associated with occupational or recreational contact with soil, and infected individuals include all ages and both genders. Blastomycosis is not transmitted from patient to patient; however, laboratory-acquired primary cutaneous and pulmonary blastomycosis has been reported.

In North America, the area of endemicity overlaps that of histoplasmosis (see Figure 73-2) and includes the southeastern and south central states, especially those bordering the Ohio and Mississippi River basins; the Midwest states and Canadian provinces bordering the Great Lakes; and an area in New York and Canada along the St. Lawrence River. Blastomycosis is also endemic in Africa. It is estimated that one to two cases of symptomatic blastomycosis requiring therapy occur per 100,000 population each year in areas with endemic disease.

Among animals, dogs are most susceptible; the infection rate is estimated to be 10 times that for humans.

Clinical Syndromes

The usual route of infection in blastomycosis is inhalation of conidia (see Figure 73-5). As with most of the endemic mycoses, the severity of symptoms and course of the disease is dependent on the extent of exposure and the immune status of the exposed individual. Based largely on studies of blastomycosis outbreaks, it appears that symptomatic disease occurs in less than half of infected individuals. Clinical illness caused by *B. dermatitidis* may present as pulmonary disease or an extrapulmonary disseminated disease. Among those patients with extrapulmonary dissemination, two thirds exhibit involvement of skin and bones. Other sites of hematogenous dissemination include prostate, liver, spleen, kidney, and central nervous system.

Pulmonary blastomycosis may be asymptomatic or present as a mild flulike illness. More severe infection resembles bacterial pneumonia with acute onset, high fever, lobar infiltrates, and cough. Progression to fulminant adult respiratory distress syndrome with high fever, diffuse infiltrates, and respiratory failure may occur. A more subacute or chronic respiratory form of blastomycosis may resemble tuberculosis or lung cancer, with radiographic presentation of pulmonary mass lesions or fibronodular infiltrates.

A classic form of blastomycosis is that of chronic cutaneous involvement. The cutaneous form of blastomycosis is almost always the result of hematogenous dissemination from the lung, in most instances without evident pulmonary lesions or systemic symptoms. The lesions may be papular, pustular, or indolent, ulcerative-nodular and verrucous with crusted surfaces and raised serpiginous borders. They are usually painless and are localized to exposed areas such as the face, scalp, neck, and hands. They may be mistaken for squamous cell carcinoma. Left untreated, cutaneous blastomycosis takes on a chronic course, with remissions and exacerbations and gradual increase in the size of lesions.

Blastomycosis is relatively uncommon among individuals with AIDS or other immunocompromising conditions. However, when it occurs in these individuals, it tends to be acute, involve the central nervous system, and have a much poorer prognosis.

Laboratory Diagnosis

The diagnosis of blastomycosis rests with microscopic detection of the fungus in tissue or other clinical material with confirmation by culture (Table 73-2). The most useful specimens for the diagnosis of pulmonary blastomycosis include sputum, bronchoalveolar lavage, or lung biopsy. Direct examination of material stained with GMS, PAS, Papanicolaou, or Giemsa stains should be performed. Likewise, fresh wet preparations of sputum, cerebrospinal fluid, urine, pus, skin scrapings, and tissue impression

Table 73–1. Characteristics of Endemic Dimorphic Mycoses

Mycosis	Etiology	Ecology	Geographic Distribution	Morphology in Tissue	Clinical Manifestation
Blastomycosis	*Blastomyces dermatitidis*	Decaying organic material	North America (Ohio and Mississippi River Valleys) Africa	Broad-based, budding yeasts (8-15 μm in diameter)	Pulmonary disease (<50%) Extrapulmonary: skin, bone, genitourinary, central nervous system Disseminated disease in immunocompromised patients
Coccidioidomycosis	*Coccidioides immitis* *C. posadasii*	Soil, dust	Southwestern United States, Mexico, Central and South America	Spherules (20-60 μm) containing endospores (2-4 μm)	Asymptomatic pulmonary infection (60%) in normal host Progressive pulmonary infection and dissemination (skin, bone, joints, meninges) in immunocompromised patients
Histoplasmosis capsulati	*Histoplasma capsulatum* var. *capsulatum*	Soil with high nitrogen content (bird/bat droppings)	North America (Ohio and Mississippi River valleys), Mexico, Central and South America	Small (2-4 μm), oval, narrow-based, budding yeasts (intracellular)	Asymptomatic pulmonary infection (90%) in normal host and low-intensity exposure Disseminated disease in immunocompromised host and in children
Histoplasmosis duboisii	*Histoplasma capsulatum* var. *duboisii*	Soil with high nitrogen content	Tropical areas of Africa	Larger (8-15 μm), thick-walled, budding yeast. Prominent isthmus and bud scar	Low rate of pulmonary disease. Higher frequency of skin and bone involvement
Paracoccidioidomycosis	*Paracoccidioides brasiliensis*	Likely soil-associated	South and Central America	Thin to moderately thick-walled, multiply budding yeast (15-30 μm; pilot wheel)	Self-limited pulmonary disease. Progressive pulmonary infection and dissemination (skin, mucosa, bones, lymph nodes, viscera, and meninges). More common in children and immunocompromised patients
Penicilliosis marneffei	*Penicillium marneffei*	Soil Bamboo rat	Southeast Asia	Globose to elongated sausage-shaped yeasts (3-5 μm) that are intracellular and divide by fission	Disseminated infection (skin, soft tissues, viscera) more common in AIDS Resembles histoplasmosis, cryptococcosis, or tuberculosis

Adapted from Perea S, Patterson TF: Endemic mycoses. In Anaissie EJ, McGinnis MR, Pfaller MA (eds): Clinical Mycology. New York, Churchill Livingstone, 2003.

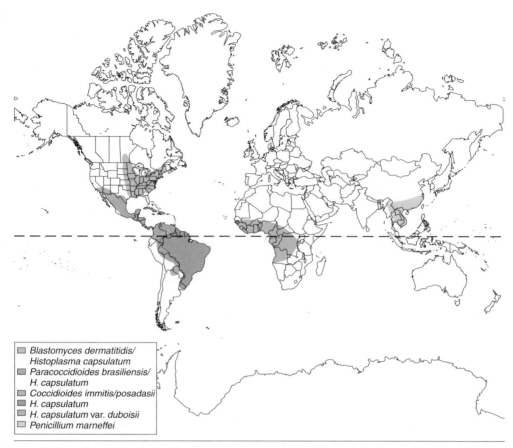

Figure 73—2. Major geographic regional distribution of the endemic mycoses.

smears may be examined directly using calcofluor white and fluorescence microscopy to detect the characteristic yeast forms. When typical broad-based budding yeast forms are present, a definitive diagnosis may be made.

Culture of clinical material on selective and nonselective mycologic media incubated at both 25° C to 30° C and at 37° C should be performed. The mycelial form of the fungus is easily cultured at 25° C to 30° C; however, growth is slow, often requiring 4 weeks or more. The mycelial form (see Figure 73-3) is not diagnostic, and the identity must be confirmed by conversion to the yeast form at 37° C, by exo-antigen testing (immunologic detection of cell-free antigen A), or by nucleic acid probe hybridization. Care should be taken to handle the culture in an appropriate biosafety cabinet, because the conidia are infectious.

Although serologic tests to detect antibodies directed at *B. dermatitidis* antigens are available (see Table 73-2), they are neither sensitive nor specific and are of little use in diagnosis. A test to detect antigen in serum and urine is commercially available, but its performance characteristics are not well described, and it is unclear what role it will play in diagnosis.

Treatment

The decision to treat patients with blastomycosis must take into consideration the clinical form and severity of disease, as well as the immune status of the patient and the toxicity of antifungal agents. Clearly, pulmonary blastomycosis in immunocompromised patients and those with progressive pulmonary disease should be treated. Likewise, all patients with evidence of hematogenous dissemination (e.g., skin, bone, all nonpulmonary sites) require antifungal therapy. Amphotericin B is the agent of choice for the treatment of life-threatening or meningeal disease. Mild or moderate disease may be treated with itraconazole. Fluconazole may be an alternative for those patients unable to tolerate itraconazole. Depending upon the severity of the disease and the status of the host, therapeutic success rates with amphotericin B or azole therapy range from 70% to 95%. Survival for AIDS patients and other immunocompromised patients is about half this figure. The latter patients may require long-term suppressive therapy with itraconazole in an effort to avoid relapses of the infection.

Coccidioidomycosis (Clinical Case 73-2)

Coccidioidomycosis is an endemic mycosis caused by either of two indistinguishable species, *Coccidioides immitis* and *C. posadasii*. The disease is caused by the inhalation of infectious arthroconidia (Figure 73-6) and may range from asymptomatic infection (in most people) to progressive infection and death. The two species differ in geographic distribution and genotype: *C. immitis* is localized to

Clinical Case 73-1. CNS Blastomycosis

Buhari and colleagues (Infect Med 24(Suppl 8):12-14, 2007) reported a case of central nervous system (CNS) blastomycosis. The patient was a 56-year-old homeless man from Detroit who presented with a 2-week history of left hemiparesis, aphasia, and generalized headache. There was no history of rash, respiratory symptoms, or fever. His medical history was significant for a left craniotomy 30 years ago for intracranial hemorrhage due to trauma. He lived in an abandoned building and was not taking any medications. On examination, he had expressive aphasia; new-onset left hemiparesis; and bilateral carotid bruits. The rest of the physical exam was unremarkable, as were routine serum chemistries and hematologic parameters. He was negative for antibodies to HIV. A chest x-ray was unremarkable. A contrast-enhanced CT scan of the head demonstrated multiple ring-enhancing lesions in the right cerebrum, with surrounding vasogenic edema and midline shift; significant encephalomalacia and generalized atrophy were present in the left cerebral hemisphere.

Serum and urine tests were negative for *Cryptococcus* (serum) and *Histoplasma* (serum and urine) antigens. Tuberculin skin tests were nonreactive, and imaging studies of the sinuses, chest, and abdomen were unremarkable. A brain biopsy was performed, and histopathologic examination revealed granulomatous inflammation and budding yeasts consistent with *Blastomyces dermatitidis*. Subsequent culture confirmed the diagnosis of CNS blastomycosis. The patient was treated with dexamethasone and amphotericin B but developed hypertension and bradycardia, with subsequent cardiopulmonary arrest and death.

This is an example of an unusual presentation of CNS blastomycosis without any other evidence of disseminated disease. The clinical syndrome of hypertension, bradycardia, and cardiopulmonary arrest suggest that the patient died of increased intracranial pressure, either as a complication of the infection or the diagnostic brain biopsy.

Figure 73—4. Giemsa stain of *Blastomyces dermatitidis* showing broad-based budding yeast.

Synonyms for coccidioidomycosis include **coccidioidal granuloma** and **San Joaquin Valley fever** among others.

Morphology

C. immitis (*C. posadasii*) is a dimorphic fungus that exists as a mold in nature and when cultured in the laboratory at 25° C and as an endosporulating spherule in tissue and under very specific conditions in vitro (Figures 73-7 and 73-8; see Table 73-2 and Figure 73-1). A variety of mold morphologies may be seen in culture at 25° C. Initial growth is white to gray, moist, and glabrous and occurs within 3 to 4 days. It rapidly develops abundant aerial mycelia, and the

California and *C. posadasii* accounts for the majority of infections outside of California. Aside from these differences, there does not appear to be any additional difference in phenotype or pathogenicity. As such, the more familiar name *C. immitis* will be used in this chapter.

Like syphilis and tuberculosis, coccidioidomycosis causes a wide variety of lesions and has been called "the great imitator."

Figure 73—3. *Blastomyces dermatitidis* mold phase.

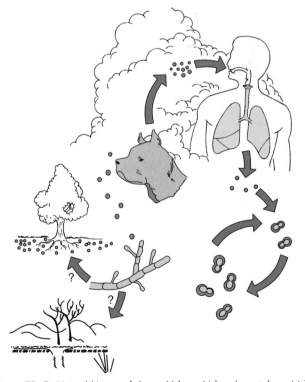

Figure 73—5. Natural history of the mold (saprobic) and yeast (parasitic) cycle of *Blastomyces dermatitidis*.

Table 73–2. Diagnosis of Endemic Dimorphic Mycoses

Mycosis	Culture	Morphology in Culture		Histopathology	Serology
		25° C	37° C		
Blastomycosis	Sputum, BAL, lung tissue, skin biopsy	Mold, round to oval or pear-shaped conidia (2-10 μm diameter)	Thick-walled, broad-based budding yeast (8-15 μm)	Broad-based, budding yeast	Antibody: CF, ID, EIA (poor sensitivity and specificity) Antigen: serum and urine (performance undefined)
Coccidioidomycosis	Sputum, BAL, tissue	Mold with barrel-shaped arthroconidia (3-6 μm)	NA	Spherules (20-60 μm) containing endospores	Antibody: TP, CF, ID, LP (diagnostic and prognostic) Antigen: urine (performance undefined)
Histoplasmosis capsulati	Sputum, BAL, blood, bone marrow, tissue	Mold with tuberculate macroconidia (8-15 μm) and small, oval microconidia (2-4 μm)	Small (2-4 μm), budding yeast	Intracellular budding yeast	Antibody: CF, ID Antigen: serum and urine (92% sensitive in disseminated disease)
Paracoccidioidomycoses	Sputum, BAL, tissue	Mold, round microconidia (2-3 μm) and intercalary chlamydospores	Large (15-30 μm), multiple, budding yeast	Large, multiply budding yeasts	Antibody: ID, CF (variable specificity; CF useful for monitoring response)
Penicilliosis Marneffei	Blood, bone marrow, tissue	Mold with diffusible red pigment Conidiophores terminating in conspicuous, penicillus-bearing, ellipsoidal, smooth conidia	Pleomorphic, elongated yeast (1-8 μm) with transverse septae	Intracellular elongated yeast with transverse septae	Under development

BAL, bronchoalveolar lavage; NA, not applicable; CF, complement fixation; ID, immunodiffusion; EIA, enzyme immunoassay; TP, tube precipitin; LP, latex particle agglutination.

Clinical Case 73-2. Coccidioidomycosis

Stafford, et al. (Infect Med 24(Suppl 8):23-25, 2007) describe a 31-year-old African American U.S. Army soldier who presented with fever, chills, night sweats and a nonproductive cough of 4 weeks duration. In addition, he had recently detected a painless right breast mass. His past medical history was unremarkable. He was stationed at Fort Irwin, California, where he was working as a telephone repairman. His physical exam was unremarkable, except for a firm, nontender, 3-cm subcutaneous mass overlying the right breast. Multiple small (less than 1cm), nontender lymph nodes were palpable in the axillae and groin. Laboratory studies revealed a white blood count of 11.9/microliter, with 30% eosinophils. Serum chemistries were notable for an elevated alkaline phosphatase level. Results of blood cultures, tests for serum *Cryptococcus* antigen, urinary *Histoplasma* antigen, and HIV antibody were negative, as was a tuberculin skin test. A chest x-ray showed bilateral interstitial micronodules in a miliary pattern, as well as a right-sided paratracheal fullness. A CT scan of the chest confirmed the presence of diffuse, 1- to 2-mm micronodules in all lobes. The CT scan also showed a lobular parenchymal mass lesion in the right middle lobe and a right chest wall mass. A fine-needle aspirate of the right breast mass revealed spherules filled with endospores, consistent with coccidioidomycosis. Culture of the material grew *Coccidioides immitis*. A serology panel for *C. immitis* was positive and revealed IgG compliment fixation titers at a dilution of greater than 1:256. CSF analysis was normal, but a bone scan revealed multiple regions of increased osteoblastic activity involving the left scapula, right anterior fifth rib, and midthoracic vertebral regions. Treatment was initiated with amphotericin B, but increasing neck pain prompted further imaging, which demonstrated a lytic lesion of the C1 vertebral body and a paravertebral mass. Despite antifungal therapy, progressive enlargement of the mass necessitated surgical debridement. The patient was continued on amphotericin B lipid formulation with plans for long-term, perhaps lifelong, antifungal therapy.

This is an example of the serious problems posed by coccidioidomycosis. Clues to the diagnosis of disseminated coccidioidomycosis in this patient included an infectious prodrome, peripheral eosinophilia, hilar lymphadenopathy, characteristic pattern of organ involvement (lungs, bones, soft tissues), residence in an endemic area, and African-American ethnicity (higher risk group for dissemination).

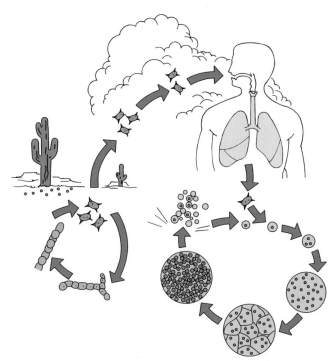

Figure 73—6. Natural history of the mold (saprobic) and spherule (parasitic) cycle of *Coccidioides immitis*.

pulmonary cavities associated with coccidioidomycosis, branched, septate hyphae and arthroconidia may be produced.

Epidemiology

Coccidioidomycosis is endemic to the desert southwestern United States, northern Mexico, and scattered areas of Central and South America (see Figure 73-2). *C. immitis* is found in soil, and the growth of the fungus in the environment is enhanced by bat and rodent droppings. Exposure to the infectious arthroconidia is greatest in late summer and fall when dusty conditions prevail. Cycles of

colony enlarges into a circular "bloom." Mature colonies usually become tan to brown or lavender.

Microscopically, the vegetative hyphae give rise to fertile hyphae which produce alternating (separated by disjunctor cells) hyaline arthroconidia (see Figure 73-7). When released, the infectious conidia are typically "barrel-shaped" and have an annular frill at both ends. As the culture ages, the vegetative hyphae also fragment into arthroconidia.

Upon inhalation, the arthroconidia (2.5 to 4 μm wide) become rounded as they convert to spherules in the lung (see Figure 73-8). At maturity, the spherules (20 to 60 μm in diameter) produce endospores by a process known as **progressive cleavage**. Rupture of the spherule walls releases the endospores, which in turn form new spherules (see Figure 73-6). In approximately 10% to 30% of

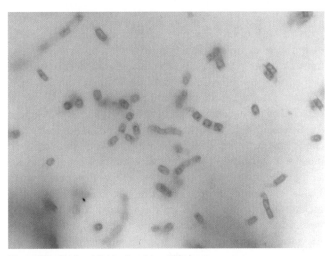

Figure 73—7. *Coccidioides immitis* mold phase.

Figure 73—8. *Coccidioides immitis* spherule filled with endospores.

Table 73—3. Risk Factors for Disseminated Coccidioidomycosis

Risk Factor	Highest Risk
Age	Infants and elderly
Sex	Male
Genetics	Filipino > African American > Native American > Hispanic > Asian
Serum CF antibody titer	> 1:32
Pregnancy	Late pregnancy and postpartum
Skin test	Negative
Depressed cell-mediated immunity	Malignancy, chemotherapy, steroid treatment, HIV infection

From Mitchell TG: Systemic fungi. In Cohen J, Powderly WG (eds): *Infectious Diseases*, 2nd ed. St Louis, Mosby, 2004.

drought and rain enhance dispersion of the organism, because heavy rains facilitate the growth of the organism in the nitrogenous soil wastes, and subsequent drought and windy conditions favor aerosolization of arthroconidia (see Figure 73-6). Acquisition of coccidioidomycosis occurs principally by inhalation of arthroconidia, and in endemic areas, infection rates may be 16% to 42% by early adulthood. The incidence of coccidioidomycosis is approximately 15 cases per 100,000 population annually in the endemic area; however, it is known to disproportionately affect persons aged ≥65 years (~36 per 100,000) and those with HIV infection (~20 per 100,000).

Clinical Syndromes

C. immitis is probably the most virulent of all human mycotic pathogens. The inhalation of only a few arthroconidia produces primary coccidioidomycosis, which may include asymptomatic pulmonary disease (~60% of patients) or a self-limited flulike illness marked by fever, cough, chest pain, and weight loss. Patients with primary coccidioidomycosis may have a variety of allergic reactions (~10%) as a result of immune complex formation, including an erythematous macular rash, erythema multiforme, and erythema nodosum.

Primary disease usually resolves without therapy and confers a strong, specific immunity to reinfection, which is detected by the coccidioidin skin test. In patients symptomatic for 6 weeks or longer, the disease progresses to secondary coccidioidomycosis, which may include nodules, cavitary disease, or progressive pulmonary disease (5% of cases); single or multisystem dissemination follows in approximately 1% of this population. Extrapulmonary sites of infection include skin, soft tissues, bones, joints, and meninges. Persons in certain ethnic groups (e.g., Filipino, African American, Native American, and Hispanic) run the highest risk of dissemination, with meningeal involvement a

common sequela (Table 73-3). In addition to ethnicity, males (9:1), women in the third trimester of pregnancy, individuals with a cellular immunodeficiency (including AIDS, organ transplantation recipients, and those treated with tumor necrosis factor [TNF] antagonists), and persons at the extremes of age are at high risk for disseminated disease (see Table 73-3). The mortality in disseminated disease exceeds 90% without treatment, and chronic infection is common.

Laboratory Diagnosis

The diagnosis of coccidioidomycosis includes the use of histopathologic examination of tissue or other clinical material, isolation of the fungus in the culture, and serologic testing (see Table 73-2). Direct microscopic visualization of endosporulating spherules in sputum, exudates, or tissue is sufficient to establish the diagnosis (see Figure 73-8) and is preferred over culture because of the highly infectious nature of the mold when grown in culture. Clinical exudates should be examined directly in 10% to 20% KOH with calcofluor white, and tissue from biopsy can be stained with H&E or specific fungal stains such as GMS or PAS (see Figure 73-8).

Clinical specimens may be cultured on routine mycologic media at 25° C. Colonies of *C. immitis* develop within 3 to 5 days, and typical sporulation may be seen in 5 to 10 days. Owing to the highly infectious nature of the fungus, all plates or tubes should be sealed using gas-permeable tape (plates) or screw caps (tubes) and only examined within a suitable biosafety cabinet. The identification of *C. immitis* from culture may be accomplished by using the exoantigen immunodiffusion test or nucleic acid hybridization. Conversion of the mold into spherules in vitro is not usually attempted outside of a research setting.

Several serologic procedures exist for initial screening, confirmation, or prognostic evaluation (see Table 73-2).

For initial diagnosis, the combined use of the immunodiffusion (ID) test and the latex particle agglutination (LP) test detects approximately 93% of cases. The complement fixation (CF) and tube precipitin (TP) tests may also be used for diagnosis, as well as prognosis. Prognostic studies frequently employ serial CF titers; rising titers are a bad prognostic sign, and falling titers indicate improvement. A test to detect antigen in urine is commercially available, but it is unclear what role it will play in diagnosis.

Treatment

Most individuals with primary coccidioidomycosis do not require specific antifungal therapy. For those with concurrent risk factors (see Table 73-3), such as organ transplant, HIV infection, high doses of corticosteroids, or when there is evidence of unusually severe infection, treatment is necessary. Primary coccidioidomycosis in the third trimester of pregnancy or during the immediate postpartum period requires treatment with amphotericin B.

Immunocompromised patients or others with diffuse pneumonia should be treated with amphotericin B followed by an azole (either fluconazole or itraconazole) as maintenance therapy. The total length of therapy should be at least 1 year. Immunocompromised patients should be maintained on an oral azole as secondary prophylaxis.

Chronic cavitary pneumonia should be treated with an oral azole for at least 1 year. In cases where the response is suboptimal, the alternatives are to switch to another azole (e.g., from itraconazole to fluconazole), increase the dose of the azole in the case of fluconazole, or switch to amphotericin B. Surgical treatment is required in the event of rupture of a cavity into the pleural space, hemoptysis, or for localized refractory lesions.

The treatment of nonmeningeal extrapulmonary disseminated infections is based on oral azole therapy with either fluconazole or itraconazole. In the case of vertebral involvement or inadequate clinical response, treatment with amphotericin B is recommended, along with appropriate surgical debridement and stabilization.

Meningeal coccidioidomycosis is managed with the administration of fluconazole or itraconazole (secondary choice because of poor CNS penetration) indefinitely. Intrathecal administration of amphotericin B is recommended only in the event of failure of azole therapy, owing to its toxicity when administered by this route.

Histoplasmosis (Clinical Case 73-3)

Histoplasmosis is caused by two varieties of *Histoplasma capsulatum*: *H. capsulatum* var. *capsulatum* and *H. capsulatum* var. *duboisii* (see Table 73-1). *H. capsulatum* var. *capsulatum* causes pulmonary and disseminated infections in the eastern half of the United States and most of Latin America, whereas *H. capsulatum* var. *duboisii* causes

---

Clinical Case 73-3. Disseminated Histoplasmosis

Mariani and Morris (Infect Med 24(Suppl 8):17-19, 2007) describe a case of disseminated histoplasmosis in a patient with AIDS. The patient was a 42-year-old El Salvadoran woman who was admitted to the hospital for evaluation of progressive dermatosis involving the right nostril, cheek, and lip, despite antibiotic therapy. She was HIV-positive (CD4 lymphocyte count 21/microliter) and had lived in Miami for the past 18 years. The lesion first appeared on the right nostril 3 months before admission. The patient sought medical attention and was treated unsuccessfully with oral antibiotics. Over the following 2 months, the lesion increased in size, involving the right nares and malar region, and was accompanied by fever, malaise, and a 50-pound weight loss. A necrotic area developed on the superior aspect of the right nostril, extending to the upper lip. A presumptive diagnosis of leishmaniasis was entertained, based in part on the patient's country of origin and a possible exposure to a sandfly bite.

Laboratory studies revealed anemia and lymphopenia. A chest x-ray was normal, and a CT scan of the head showed a soft-tissue mass in the right nasal cavity. Histopathologic evaluation of a skin biopsy showed chronic inflammation, with intracytoplasmic budding yeasts. Culture of the biopsy grew *Histoplasma capsulatum*, and results of a urine *Histoplasma* antigen test were positive. The patient was treated with amphotericin B followed by itraconazole with good results.

This case underscores the ability of *H. capsulatum* to remain clinically latent for many years, only to reactivate upon immunosuppression of the host. Cutaneous manifestations of histoplasmosis are usually a consequence of progression from primary (latent) to disseminated disease. Histoplasmosis is not endemic to South Florida but is endemic to much of Latin America, where the patient had lived prior to moving to Miami. A high index of suspicion and confirmation with skin biopsies, cultures, and testing for urinary antigen are crucial for timely and appropriate treatment of disseminated histoplasmosis.

---

predominately skin and bone lesions and is restricted to the tropical areas of Africa (see Figure 73-2).

Morphology

Both varieties of *H. capsulatum* are thermally dimorphic fungi existing as a hyaline mold in nature and in culture at 25° C and as an intracellular budding yeast in tissue and in culture at 37° C (Figures 73-9, 73-10, and 73-11; see Table 73-2). In culture, the mold forms of *H. capsulatum* var. *capsulatum* and var. *duboisii* are indistinguishable macroscopically and microscopically. The mold colonies grow slowly and develop as white or brown hyphal colonies after several days to a week. The mold form produces two types of conidia: (1) large (8 to 15 μm), thick-walled, spherical macroconidia with spikelike projections (tuberculate macroconidia) that arise from short conidiophores (see Figures 73-1 and 73-12) and (2) small, oval microconidia (2 to 4 μm) with smooth or slightly rough walls that are sessile or on short stalks (see Figures 73-1 and 73-12). The yeast cells are thin-walled, oval, and measure 2 to 4 μm (var. *capsulatum*) (see Figure 73-10) or thicker-walled and 8 to 15 μm (var. *duboisii*) (see Figure 73-11). The yeast cells of both

Figure 73—9. *Histoplasma capsulatum* mold phase showing tuberculate macroconidia.

Figure 73—11. H&E-stained tissue section showing intracellular yeast forms of *Histoplasma capsulatum* var. *duboisii*. *(From Connor DH, et al: Pathology of Infectious Diseases. Stamford, Conn, Appleton & Lange, 1997.)*

varieties of *H. capsulatum* are intracellular in vivo and are uninucleated (see Figures 73-10 and 73-11).

Epidemiology

Histoplasmosis capsulati is localized to the broad regions of the Ohio and Mississippi River valleys in the United States and occurs throughout Mexico and Central and South America (see Figure 73-2 and Table 73-1). Histoplasmosis duboisii, or African histoplasmosis, is confined to the tropical areas of Africa, including Gabon, Uganda, and Kenya (see Figure 73-2 and Table 73-1).

The natural habitat of the mycelial form of both varieties of *H. capsulatum* is soil with a high nitrogen content, such as that found in areas contaminated with bird or bat droppings. Outbreaks of histoplasmosis have been associated with exposure to bird roosts, caves, and decaying buildings or urban renewal projects involving excavation and demolition. Aerosolization of microconidia and hyphal fragments in the disturbed soil, with subsequent inhalation by exposed individuals, is considered to be the basis for

these outbreaks (Figure 73-12). Although attack rates may reach 100% in certain of these exposures, most cases remain asymptomatic and are detected only by skin testing. Immunocompromised individuals and children are more prone to develop symptomatic disease with either variety of *Histoplasma*. Reactivation of the disease and dissemination is common among immunosuppressed individuals, especially those with AIDS.

Clinical Syndromes

The usual route of infection for both varieties of histoplasmosis is via inhalation of microconidia, which in turn germinate into yeasts within the lung and may remain localized or disseminate hematogenously or by the lymphatic system (see Figure 73-12). The microconidia are rapidly phagocytosed by

Figure 73—10. Giemsa-stained preparation showing intracellular yeast forms of *Histoplasma capsulatum* var. *capsulatum*.

Figure 73—12. Natural history of the mold (saprobic) and yeast (parasitic) cycle of *Histoplasma capsulatum*.

pulmonary macrophages and neutrophils, and it is thought that conversion to the parasitic yeast form takes place intracellularly.

Histoplasmosis Capsulati

The clinical presentation of histoplasmosis caused by *H. capsulatum* var. *capsulatum* is dependent upon the intensity of exposure and immunologic status of the host. Asymptomatic infection occurs in 90% of individuals following a low-intensity exposure. In the event of an exposure to a heavy inoculum, however, most individuals exhibit some symptoms. The self-limited form of acute pulmonary histoplasmosis is marked by a flulike illness with fever, chills, headache, cough, myalgias, and chest pain. Radiographic evidence of hilar or mediastinal adenopathy and patchy pulmonary infiltrates may be seen. Most acute infections resolve with supportive care and do not require specific antifungal treatment. In rare instances, usually following very heavy exposure, acute respiratory distress syndrome may be seen. In approximately 10% of patients, inflammatory sequelae such as persistent lymphadenopathy with bronchial obstruction, arthritis, arthralgias, or pericarditis may be seen. Another rare complication of histoplasmosis is a condition known as **mediastinal fibrosis,** in which persistent host response to the organism may result in massive fibrosis and constriction of mediastinal structures, including the heart and great vessels.

Progressive pulmonary histoplasmosis may follow acute infection in approximately 1 in 100,000 cases per year. Chronic pulmonary symptoms are associated with apical cavities and fibrosis and are more likely to occur in patients with prior underlying pulmonary disease. These lesions generally do not heal spontaneously, and persistence of the organism leads to progressive destruction and fibrosis secondary to the immune response to the organism.

Disseminated histoplasmosis follows acute infection in 1 in 2000 adults and is much higher in children and immunocompromised adults. Disseminated disease may assume a chronic, subacute, or acute course. Chronic disseminated histoplasmosis is characterized by weight loss and fatigue, with or without fever. Oral ulcers and hepatosplenomegaly are common.

Subacute disseminated histoplasmosis is marked by fever, weight loss, and malaise. Oropharyngeal ulcers and hepatosplenomegaly are prominent. Bone marrow involvement may produce anemia, leukopenia, and thrombocytopenia. Other sites of involvement include the adrenals, cardiac valves, and the central nervous system. Untreated subacute disseminated histoplasmosis will result in death in 2 to 24 months.

Acute disseminated histoplasmosis is a fulminant process that is most commonly seen in severely immunosuppressed individuals, including those with AIDS, organ transplant recipients, and those receiving steroids or other immunosuppressive chemotherapy. In addition, children younger than 1 year and adults with debilitating medical conditions are also at risk, given sufficient exposure to the fungus. In contrast to the other forms of histoplasmosis, acute disseminated disease may present with a septic shock—like picture, with fever, hypotension, pulmonary infiltrates, and acute respiratory distress. Oral and gastrointestinal ulcerations and bleeding, adrenal insufficiency, meningitis, and endocarditis may also be seen. If untreated, acute disseminated histoplasmosis is fatal within days to weeks.

Histoplasmosis Duboisii

In contrast to classic histoplasmosis, pulmonary lesions are uncommon in African histoplasmosis. The localized form of histoplasmosis duboisii is a chronic disease characterized by regional lymphadenopathy, with lesions of skin and bone. Skin lesions are papular or nodular and eventually progress to abscesses, which then ulcerate. About one third of patients will exhibit osseous lesions characterized by osteolysis and involvement of contiguous joints. The cranium, sternum, ribs, vertebrae, and long bones are most frequently involved, often with overlying abscesses and draining sinuses.

A more fulminant disseminated form of histoplasmosis duboisii may be seen in profoundly immunodeficient individuals. Hematogenous and lymphatic dissemination to bone marrow, liver, spleen, and other organs occurs and is marked by fever, lymphadenopathy, anemia, weight loss, and organomegaly. This form of the disease is uniformly fatal unless promptly diagnosed and treated.

Laboratory Diagnosis

The diagnosis of histoplasmosis may be made by direct microscopy, culture of blood, bone marrow, or other clinical material, and by serology, including antigen detection in blood and urine (Table 73-4; see Table 73-2). The yeast phase of the organism can be detected in sputum,

Table 73—4. Laboratory Tests for Histoplasmosis

Test	Sensitivity (% True Positives) in Disease States		
	Disseminated	Chronic Pulmonary	Self-limited*
Antigen	92	21	39
Culture	85	85	15
Histopathology	43	17	9
Serology	71	100	98

From Wheat LJ: Endemic mycoses. In Cohen J, Powderly WG (eds): Infectious Diseases, 2nd ed. St Louis, Mosby, 2004.
*Includes acute pulmonary histoplasmosis, rheumatologic syndrome, and pericarditis.

bronchoalveolar lavage fluid, peripheral blood films, bone marrow, and tissue stained with Giemsa, GMS, or PAS stains (see Figure 73-10). In tissue sections, cells of *H. capsulatum* var. *capsulatum* are yeastlike, hyaline, spherical to oval, 2 to 4 µm in diameter, uninucleate, and have single buds attached by a narrow base. The cells are usually intracellular and clustered together. The cells of *H. capsulatum* var. *duboisii* are also intracellular, yeastlike, and uninucleate but are much larger (8 to 15 µm) and have thick "doubly-contoured" walls. They are usually in macrophages and giant cells (see Figure 73-11).

Because of the high organism burden in patients with disseminated disease, cultures of respiratory specimens, blood, bone marrow, and tissue are of value. They are less useful in self-limited or localized disease (see Table 73-4). Growth of the mycelial form in culture is slow, and once isolated, the identification must be confirmed by conversion to the yeast phase or by use of exoantigen testing or nucleic acid hybridization. As with the other dimorphic pathogens, cultures of *Histoplasma* must be handled with care in a biosafety cabinet.

Serologic diagnosis of histoplasmosis employs tests for both antigen and antibody detection (see Table 73-2). Antibody detection assays include a complement fixation (CF) assay and immunodiffusion (ID) test. These tests are usually used together to maximize sensitivity and specificity, but neither is useful in the acute setting; CF and ID are often negative in immunocompromised patients with disseminated infection.

Detection of *Histoplasma* antigen in serum and urine by enzyme immunoassay has become very useful, particularly in diagnosing disseminated disease (see Tables 73-2 and 73-4). The sensitivity of antigen detection is greater in urine specimens than in blood and ranges from 21% in chronic pulmonary disease to 92% in disseminated disease. Serial measurements of antigen may be used to assess response to therapy and for establishing relapse of the disease.

Treatment

Since most patients with histoplasmosis recover without therapy, the first decision must be whether specific antifungal therapy is necessary or not. Some immunocompetent patients with more severe infection may exhibit prolonged symptoms and may benefit from treatment with itraconazole. In cases of severe acute pulmonary histoplasmosis with hypoxemia and acute respiratory distress syndrome, amphotericin B should be administered acutely, followed by oral itraconazole to complete a 12-week course.

Chronic pulmonary histoplasmosis also warrants treatment, since it is known to progress if left untreated. Treatment with amphotericin B followed by itraconazole for 12 to 24 months is recommended.

Disseminated histoplasmosis usually responds well to amphotericin B therapy. Once stabilized, the patient may be switched to oral itraconazole to be administered over 6 to 18 months. Patients with AIDS may require lifelong therapy with itraconazole.

Histoplasmosis of the central nervous system is universally fatal if not treated. The therapy of choice is amphotericin B followed by fluconazole for 9 to 12 months.

Patients with severe obstructive mediastinal histoplasmosis require amphotericin B therapy. Itraconazole may be used for outpatient therapy.

Paracoccidioidomycosis

Paracoccidioidomycosis is a systemic fungal infection caused by the dimorphic pathogen *Paracoccidioides brasiliensis*. This infection is also known as **South American blastomycosis** and is the major dimorphic endemic fungal infection in Latin American countries. Primary paracoccidioidomycosis usually presents in young people as a self-limited pulmonary process. At this stage, it rarely displays a progressive acute or subacute course. Reactivation of a primary quiescent lesion may occur years later, resulting in chronic progressive pulmonary disease with or without involvement of other organs.

Morphology

The mold phase of *P. brasiliensis* grows slowly in vitro at 25° C. White colonies become apparent in 3 to 4 weeks, eventually taking on a velvety appearance. Glabrous, wrinkled, brownish colonies may also be seen. The mycelial form is nondescript and nondiagnostic: hyaline, septate, hyphae with intercalated chlamydoconidia. Specific identification requires conversion to the yeast form or by exoantigen testing.

The characteristic yeast form is seen in tissue and in culture at 37° C. Variable-sized (3 to 30 µm or more in diameter), oval to round, yeastlike cells with double refractile walls and single or multiple buds (blastoconidia) are characteristic of this fungus (Figure 73-13). The blastoconidia are connected to the parent cell by a narrow isthmus, and six or more of various sizes may be produced from a single cell: the so-called "mariner's" or "pilot-wheel" morphology. The variability in size and number of blastoconidia and their connection to the parent cell are identifying features (see Figure 73-13). These features are best disclosed by the GMS stain but may also be seen in H&E-stained tissues or in KOH mounts of clinical material.

Epidemiology

Paracoccidioidomycosis is endemic throughout Latin America but is more prevalent in South America than in Central America (see Figure 73-2). The highest incidence is

Figure 73–13. GMS-stained yeast form of *Paracoccidioides brasiliensis* showing multiple budding "pilot wheel" morphology. *(From Connor DH, et al: Pathology of Infectious Diseases. Stamford, Conn, Appleton & Lange, 1997.)*

seen in Brazil, followed by Colombia, Venezuela, Ecuador, and Argentina. All patients diagnosed outside of Latin America previously had lived in Latin America. The ecology of the endemic areas includes high humidity, rich vegetation, moderate temperatures, and acid soil. These conditions are found along rivers from the Amazon jungle to small indigenous forests in Uruguay. *P. brasiliensis* has been recovered from soil in these areas; however, its ecologic niche is not well established. The portal of entry is thought to be either by inhalation or traumatic inoculation (Figure 73-14), although even this is poorly understood. Natural infection has only been documented in armadillos.

Although infection occurs in children (peak incidence 10 to 19 years), overt disease is uncommon in both children and adolescents. In adults, disease is more common in men age 30 to 50 years. Most patients with clinically apparent

Figure 73–14. Natural history of the mold (saprobic) and yeast (parasitic) cycle of *Paracoccidioides brasiliensis*.

disease live in rural areas and have close contact with the soil. There are no reports of epidemics or human-to-human transmission. Depression of cell-mediated immunity correlates with the acute progressive form of the disease.

Clinical Syndromes

Paracoccidioidomycosis may be subclinical or progressive with acute or chronic pulmonary forms or acute, subacute, or chronic disseminated forms of the disease. Most primary infections are self-limited; however, the organism may become dormant for long periods of time and reactivate to cause clinical disease concomitant with impaired host defenses. A subacute disseminated form is seen in younger patients and immunocompromised individuals with marked lymphadenopathy, organomegaly, bone marrow involvement, and osteoarticular manifestations mimicking osteomyelitis. Recurrent fungemia results in dissemination and frequent skin lesions. Pulmonary and mucosal lesions are not seen in this form of the disease.

Adults most often present with a chronic pulmonary form of the disease marked by respiratory problems, often as the sole manifestation. The disease progresses slowly over months to years, with persistent cough, purulent sputum, chest pain, weight loss, dyspnea, and fever. Pulmonary lesions are nodular, infiltrative, fibrotic, and cavitary.

Although 25% of patients exhibit only pulmonary manifestations of the disease, the infection can disseminate to extrapulmonary sites in the absence of diagnosis and treatment. Prominent extrapulmonary locations include skin and mucosa, lymph nodes, adrenal glands, liver, spleen, central nervous system, and bones. The mucosal lesions are painful and ulcerated and usually are confined to the mouth, lips, gums, and palate. More than 90% of these individuals are male.

Laboratory Diagnosis

The diagnosis is established by the demonstration of the characteristic yeast forms on microscopic examination of sputum, bronchoalveolar lavage fluid, scrapings or biopsy of ulcers, pus draining from lymph nodes, cerebrospinal fluid, or tissue (see Table 73-2). The organism may be visualized by a variety of staining methods, including calcofluor fluorescence, H&E, GMS, PAS, or Papanicolaou stains (see Figure 73-13). The presence of multiple buds distinguishes *P. brasiliensis* from *Cryptococcus neoformans* and *Blastomyces dermatitidis*.

Isolation of the organism in culture requires confirmation by demonstration of thermal dimorphism or exoantigen testing (detection of exoantigen 1, 2, and 3). Cultures should be manipulated in a biosafety cabinet.

Serologic testing using either ID or CF to demonstrate antibody may be helpful in suggesting the diagnosis and in evaluating response to therapy (see Table 73-2).

Treatment

Itraconazole is the treatment of choice for most forms of the disease and generally must be given for at least 6 months. More severe or refractory infections may require amphotericin B therapy followed by either itraconazole or sulfonamide therapy. Relapses are common with sulfonamide therapy, and both dose and duration require adjustment based on clinical and mycologic parameters. Fluconazole has some activity against this organism, although frequent relapses have limited its use for the treatment of this disease.

Penicilliosis Marneffei

Penicilliosis marneffei is a disseminated mycosis caused by the dimorphic fungus *Penicillium marneffei*. This infection involves the mononuclear phagocytic system and occurs primarily in HIV-infected individuals in Thailand and Southern China (see Figure 73-2).

Morphology

P. marneffei is the only species of *Penicillium* that is a pathogenic dimorphic fungus. In its mold phase in culture at 25° C, it exhibits sporulating structures that are typical of the genus (see Figure 73-1). Identification is aided by the formation of a soluble red pigment that diffuses into the agar (see Table 73-3).

At 37° C in culture and in tissue, *P. marneffei* grows as a yeastlike organism that divides by fission and exhibits a transverse septum (Figure 73-15). The yeast form is intracellular in vivo and in this way resembles *H. capsulatum*, although it is somewhat more pleomorphic and elongated and does not bud (see Table 73-2 and Figures 73-10 and 73-15).

Epidemiology

P. marneffei has emerged as a prominent mycotic pathogen among HIV-infected individuals in Southeast Asia (see Figure 73-2). Imported cases have been reported in Europe and the United States. Although infection has been seen in immunocompetent hosts, the vast majority of infections since 1987 have been in patients with AIDS or other immunocompromised hosts residing in, or who have visited, Southeast Asia or Southern China. Penicilliosis marneffei has become an early indicator of HIV infection in that part of the world. *P. marneffei* has been isolated from bamboo rats and occasionally from soil. Laboratory-acquired infection has been reported in an immunocompromised individual exposed to the mycelial form in culture.

Clinical Syndromes

Penicilliosis marneffei is caused when a susceptible host inhales conidia of *P. marneffei* from the environment, and disseminated infection develops. The infection may mimic tuberculosis, leishmaniasis, and other AIDS-related opportunistic infections such as histoplasmosis and cryptococcosis. Patients present with fever, cough, pulmonary infiltrates, lymphadenopathy, organomegaly, anemia, leukopenia, and thrombocytopenia. Skin lesions reflect hematogenous dissemination and appear as molluscum contagiosum—like lesions on the face and trunk.

Laboratory Diagnosis

P. marneffei is readily recovered from clinical specimens, including blood, bone marrow, bronchoalveolar lavage specimens, and tissue. In culture at 25° C to 30° C, isolation of a mold that exhibits typical *Penicillium* morphology and a diffusible red pigment is highly suggestive. Conversion to the yeast phase at 37° C is confirmatory. Microscopic detection of the elliptical fission yeasts inside phagocytes in buffy coat preparations or smears of bone marrow, ulcerative skin lesions, or lymph nodes is diagnostic (see Figure 73-15). Serologic tests are under development.

Treatment

Amphotericin B with or without flucytosine is the treatment of choice. Administration of amphotericin B for 2 weeks should be followed by itraconazole for another 10 weeks. AIDS patients may require lifelong treatment with itraconazole to prevent relapses of the infection. Fluconazole therapy has been associated with a high rate of failure and is not recommended.

Figure 73-15. GMS-stained yeast forms of *Penicillium marneffei*, including forms with single, wide, transverse septa (center). *(From Connor DH, et al: Pathology of Infectious Diseases. Stamford, Conn, Appleton & Lange, 1997.)*

Case Study and Questions

Jane and Joan were two avid "outdoorspersons" in their mid-30s. In the past 5 years, they had been spelunking in southern Missouri, backpacking in northern Wisconsin, and camping in Arizona. Most recently, they had been renovating an old farmhouse in rural Iowa, and in the process had to tear down an old chicken coop that was attached to the back of the house. About 1 week into the process, they both suffered from a flulike illness, and Jane developed a cough and shortness of breath. They went to the family practice clinic to get "checked out." At the clinic, Joan appeared fine, but Jane was noted to be quite short of breath and appeared ill. The doctor thought it would be a good idea to get a chest x-ray on Jane. Joan got one too, just in case. Jane's chest x-ray showed a diffuse bilateral pneumonia. Although Joan's x-ray did not show pneumonia, it was noted that she had a solitary nodule in the right upper lobe.

1. What dimorphic fungal pathogens were Jane and Joan exposed to?

2. What constitutes a dimorphic fungus?

3. Aside from dimorphism, what feature is common to all of the endemic mycoses?

4. Describe the life cycles of the six dimorphic endemic pathogens.

5. What do you think is the cause of Jane's pneumonia? How would you make the diagnosis?

6. How would you treat her pneumonia?

7. What do you think accounts for Joan's lung nodule? How would you make the diagnosis? How would you treat her?

Bibliography

Brandt ME, Warnock DW: *Histoplasma, Blastomyces, Coccidioides*, and other dimorphic fungi causing systemic mycoses. In Murray PR, et al. (eds): Manual of Clinical Microbiology, 9th ed. Washington, DC, ASM Press, 2007.

Chu JH, et al: Hospitalization for endemic mycoses: A population-based national study. Clin Infect Dis 42:822, 2006.

Connor DH, et al: Pathology of Infectious Diseases. Stamford, Conn, Appleton & Lange, 1997.

Kauffman CA: Histoplasmosis: A clinical and laboratory update. Clin Microbiol Rev 20:115, 2007.

Mitchell TG: Systemic fungi. In Cohen J, Powderly WG (eds): Infectious Diseases, 2nd ed. St Louis, Mosby, 2004.

Perea S, Patterson TF: Endemic mycoses. In Anaissie EJ, Mc Ginnis MR, Pfaller MA (eds): Clinical Mycology, New York, Churchill Livingstone, 2003.

Vanittanakom N, et al: *Penicillium marneffei* infection and recent advances in the epidemiology and molecular biology aspects. Clin Microbiol Rev 19:95, 2006.

Wheat LJ: Endemic mycoses. In Cohen J, Powderly WG (eds): Infectious Diseases, 2nd ed. St Louis, Mosby, 2004.

Opportunistic Mycoses

The frequency of invasive mycoses due to opportunistic fungal pathogens has increased significantly over the past two decades. (See Chapter 5, Table 5-2.) This increase in infections is associated with excessive morbidity and mortality (see Chapter 5, Table 5-1) and is directly related to the increase in patient populations at risk for developing serous fungal infections. High-risk groups include individuals undergoing blood and marrow transplantation (BMT), solid organ transplantation, major surgery (especially gastrointestinal [GI] surgery), those with AIDS, neoplastic disease, immunosuppressive therapy, advanced age, and premature birth (Table 74-1). The most well-known causes of opportunistic mycoses include *Candida albicans*, *Cryptococcus neoformans*, and *Aspergillus fumigatus* (Box 74-1). The estimated annual incidence of invasive mycoses due to these pathogens is 72 to 290 infections per million population for *Candida*, 30 to 66 per million for *C. neoformans*, and 12 to 34 per million for *Aspergillus*. (See Chapter 5, Table 5-2.) In addition to these agents, of increasing importance is the growing list of "other" opportunistic fungi (see Box 74-1). New and emerging fungal pathogens include species *Candida* and *Aspergillus* other than *C. albicans* and *A. fumigatus*, opportunistic yeastlike fungi such as *Trichosporon* spp., *Malassezia* spp., *Rhodotorula* spp., and *Blastoschizomyces capitatus*, the Zygomycetes, hyaline molds such as *Fusarium*, *Acremonium*, *Scedosporium*, *Scopulariopsis*, *Paecilomyces*, and *Trichoderma* species, and a wide variety of dematiaceous fungi (see Box 74-1). Infections caused by these organisms range from catheter-related fungemia and peritonitis to more localized infections involving lung, skin, and paranasal sinuses to widespread hematogenous dissemination. Many of these fungi were previously thought to be nonpathogenic and now are recognized causes of invasive mycoses in compromised patients. Estimates of the annual incidence of the less common mycoses have been virtually nonexistent; however, data from a population-based survey conducted by the Centers for Disease Control (CDC) indicate that zygomycosis occurs at a rate

of 1.7 infections per million per year, hyalohyphomycosis (*Fusarium*, *Acremonium*, etc.) at 1.2 infections per million per year, and phaeohyphomycosis (dematiaceous molds) at 1.0 infection per million per year. (See Chapter 5, Table 5-1.)

Given the complexity of the patients at risk for infection and the diverse array of fungal pathogens, opportunistic mycoses pose a considerable diagnostic and therapeutic challenge. Diagnosis depends upon a heightened clinical suspicion (think **FUNGUS**) and obtaining appropriate material for culture and histopathology. Isolation and identification of the infecting organisms is very important in properly managing infections due to the less common opportunistic fungi. Some of these organisms are inherently nonsusceptible to standard azole, echinocandin, or polyene therapy (see Chapter 70) and may require the use of alternative antifungal agents in addition to surgical management and reversal of the underlying impairment of host defenses.

Candidiasis

It is clear that the most important group of opportunistic fungal pathogens is the *Candida* species. *Candida* spp. are the fourth most common cause of nosocomial bloodstream infections (BSI), exceeding that of any individual gram-negative pathogen (Table 74-2, Clinical Case 74-1). Between 1980 and the present, the frequency of *Candida* BSI has risen steadily in hospitals of all sizes and in all age groups. (See Chapter 5, Table 5-2.)

Although more than 100 species of *Candida* have been described, only a few have been implicated in clinical infections (see Box 74-1). *Candida albicans* is the species most commonly isolated from clinical material and generally accounts for 90% to 100% of mucosal isolates and 50% to 70% of isolates from bloodstream infections (BSI) (Table 74-3). Approximately 95% of all *Candida* BSI are accounted for by four species: *C. albicans*, *C. glabrata*, *C. parapsilosis*, and *C. tropicalis* (see Table 74-3). Among these common species, only *C. glabrata* can be

Table 74–1. Predisposing Factors for Opportunistic Mycoses

Factor	Possible Role in Infection	Major Opportunistic Pathogens
Antimicrobial agents (number and duration)	Promote fungal colonization Provide intravascular access	*Candida* spp., other yeastlike fungi
Adrenal corticosteroid	Immunosuppression	*Cryptococcus neoformans, Aspergillus* spp., Zygomycetes, other molds, *Pneumocystis*
Chemotherapy	Immunosuppression	*Candida* spp., *Aspergillus* spp., *Pneumocystis*
Hematologic/solid organ malignancy	Immunosuppression	*Candida* spp., *Aspergillus* spp., Zygomycetes, other molds and yeastlike fungi, *Pneumocystis*
Previous colonization	Translocation across mucosa	*Candida* spp.
Indwelling catheter (central venous, pressure transducer, Swan-Ganz)	Direct vascular access Contaminated product	*Candida* spp., other yeastlike fungi
Total parenteral nutrition	Direct vascular access Contamination of infusate	*Candida* spp., *Malassezia* spp., other yeastlike fungi
Neutropenia (WBC <500/mm^3)	Immunosuppression	*Aspergillus* spp., *Candida* spp., other molds and yeastlike fungi
Extensive surgery or burns	Route of infection Direct vascular access	*Candida* spp., *Fusarium* spp., Zygomycetes
Assisted ventilation	Route of infection	*Candida* spp., *Aspergillus* spp.
Hospitalization or intensive care unit stay	Exposure to pathogens Exposure to additional risk factors	*Candida* spp., other yeastlike fungi, *Aspergillus* spp.
Hemodialysis, peritoneal dialysis	Route of infection Immunosuppression	*Candida* spp., *Rhodotorula* spp., other yeastlike fungi
Malnutrition	Immunosuppression	*Pneumocystis, Candida* spp., *Cryptococcus neoformans*
HIV Infection/AIDS	Immunosuppression	*Cryptococcus neoformans, Pneumocystis, Candida* spp.
Extremes of age	Immunosuppression Numerous co-morbidities	*Candida* spp.

said to be truly "emerging" as a cause of BSI, owing in part to its intrinsic and acquired resistance to azoles and other commonly used antifungal agents. The remaining 5% of *Candida* BSI encompasses 12 to 14 different species, including *C. krusei, C. lusitaniae, C. dubliniensis,* and *C. rugosa* among others (see Box 74-1). Although these species must be considered "rare" causes of candidiasis, several have been observed to occur in nosocomial clusters and/or to exhibit innate or acquired resistance to one or more established antifungal agents.

Morphology

All *Candida* species exist as oval yeastlike forms (3 to 5 μm) that produce buds or blastoconidia. Species of *Candida* other than *C. glabrata* also produce pseudohyphae and true hyphae (Figure 74-1; also see Chapter 5, Figure 5-2A and Chapter 69, Figure 69-1). In addition, *C. albicans* forms germ tubes (Chapter 5, Figure 5-2) and terminal, thick-walled chlamydoconidia (Figure 74-2). *C. glabrata,* the second most common species of *Candida* in many settings, is incapable of forming pseudohyphae, germ tubes, or true hyphae under most conditions. In histologic sections, all *Candida* spp. stain poorly with H&E and well with the PAS, GMS, and Gridley fungus stains.

In culture, most *Candida* spp. form smooth, white, creamy, domed colonies. *C. albicans* and other species may also undergo **phenotypic switching** in which a single strain of *Candida* may change reversibly among several different morphotypes, ranging from the typical smooth, white colony composed of predominantly budding yeastlike cells to very "fuzzy" or "hairy" colonies composed

Box 74–1. Agents of Opportunistic Mycoses*

Candida spp.

C. albicans
C. glabrata
C. parapsilosis
C. tropicalis
C. krusei
C. lusitaniae
C. guilliermondii
C. dubliniensis
C. rugosa

Cryptococcus neoformans and Other Opportunistic Yeastlike Fungi

Cryptococcus neoformans
Malassezia spp.
Trichosporon spp.
Rhodotorula spp.
Blastoschizomyces capitatus

Aspergillus Species

A. fumigatus
A. flavus
A. niger
A. versicolor
A. terreus

Zygomycetes

Rhizopus spp.
Mucor spp.
Rhizomucor spp.
Absidia spp.
Cunninghamella spp.

Other Hyaline Molds

Fusarium spp.
Acremonium spp.
Scedosporium spp.
Paecilomyces spp.
Trichoderma spp.
Scopulariopsis spp.

Dematiaceous Molds

Alternaria spp.
Bipolaris spp.
Cladophialophora spp.
Curvularia spp.
Exophiala spp.
Exserohilum spp.
Wangiella spp.

Pneumocystis jirovecii

*List not all-inclusive.

Table 74–2. Nosocomial Bloodstream Infections: Most Frequent Associated Pathogens—SCOPE Surveillance Program

Rank	Pathogen	% of Isolates*
1	Coagulase-negative staphylococci	31.3
2	Staphylococcus aureus	20.2
3	Enterococcus spp.	9.4
4	Candida spp.	9.0
5	Escherichia coli	5.6
6	Klebsiella spp.	4.8
7	Pseudomonas aeruginosa	4.3
8	Enterobacter spp.	3.9
9	Serratia spp.	1.7
10	Acinetobacter baumannii	1.3

*Percent of a total of 20,978 infections.
Data from Wisplinghoff H, et al: Nosocomial bloodstream infections in U.S. hospitals: Analysis of 24,179 cases from a prospective nationwide surveillance study. Clin Infect Dis 39:309, 2004.

Clinical Case 74-1. Candidemia

Posteraro, et al. (J Clin Microbiol 44:3046-3047, 2006) describe a case of recurrent fungemia in a 35-year-old woman. The patient was seen at 5 weeks gestation following intrauterine insemination. She presented with fever, tachycardia, and hypotension. The white blood cell (WBC) count was 23,500 per microliter with 78% neutrophils. She experienced a spontaneous abortion. Severe chorioamnionitis was diagnosed, placental and fetal tissues were cultured, and blood cultures and vaginal swabs were obtained. The patient was treated with broad-spectrum antibacterial agents. Five days later, no clinical improvement was seen. The cultured blood and placental samples grew the yeast *Candida glabrata*, which was also isolated from the patient's vaginal cultures. On the basis of fluconazole minimal inhibitory concentrations (MICs) indicating that the organism was susceptible, the patient was placed on fluconazole. Four weeks later, she experienced complete resolution of her symptoms, with eradication of the fungus from her bloodstream. Antifungal treatment was discontinued, and the patient was sent home, where she did well. Six months later she was readmitted to the hospital with fever, chills, and fatigue. The WBC was elevated at 21,500 per microliter with 73% neutrophils. Consecutive blood cultures were again positive for *C. glabrata*, which was also found in cultures of vaginal fluid. All isolates were found to be resistant to fluconazole. On the basis of these findings, the patient was treated with amphotericin B. Within 1 week, the patient's clinical condition was improved. After 1 month of amphotericin B treatment, blood cultures were sterile, and she was discharged from the hospital. Three years later, she remained free of any evidence of infection.

This is an unusual case, in that the patient was not immunocompromised, yet experienced recurrent candidemia with *C. glabrata*. The use of fluconazole as initial therapy, although apparently successful, induced up-regulation of drug efflux pumps in the organism and allowed later isolates to become resistant to fluconazole and other azoles.

Table 74–3. Species Distribution of Clinical Isolates of *Candida* by Year: Data from the Global Antifungal Surveillance Program, 1997-2005

Species	% of Isolates by Year (No. Tested)					
	1997-2000	*2001*	*2002*	*2003*	*2004*	*2005*
Total cases	(55,229)	(21,809)	(24,680)	(33,002)	(33,406)	(28,387)
C. albicans	70.9	65.4	61.4	62.3	62.8	65.9
C. glabrata	10.2	11.1	10.7	12.0	11.7	11.2
C. tropicalis	5.4	7.5	7.4	7.5	7.5	7.6
C. parapsilosis	4.8	6.9	6.6	7.3	6.7	5.6
C. krusei	2.2	2.5	2.6	2.7	2.3	2.4
C. guilliermondii	0.7	0.7	1.0	0.8	0.7	0.7
C. lusitaniae	0.5	0.6	0.5	0.6	0.6	0.6

Adapted from Pfaller MA, et al: Results from the ARTEMIS DISK Global Antifungal Surveillance Study, 1997-2005: An 8.5-year analysis of susceptibilities of Candida *and other yeast species to fluconazole and voriconazole by CLSI standardized disk diffusion testing. J Clin Microbiol 45:1735, 2007.*

primarily of pseudohyphal and hyphal forms. The frequency of the switching phenomenon is too high to result from gene mutations and too low to be attributable to mass conversion, whereby all cells in the population change their phenotype in response to signals from the environment. It is likely that switching serves as some type of master system in *C. albicans*, and other species, for rapid response at the level of individual cells to changes in the local microenvironment. It has been postulated that phenotypic switching explains the ability of *C. albicans* to survive in many different environmental microniches within the human host.

Epidemiology

Candida spp. are known colonizers of humans and other warm-blooded animals. As such, they are found in humans and in nature worldwide. The primary site of colonization is the GI tract from mouth to rectum. They may also be found as commensals in the vagina and urethra, on the skin and under the finger- and toenails. *C. albicans*, the most common etiologic agent of human disease, has also been found apart from humans and animals in air, water, and soil.

It is estimated that 25% to 50% of healthy subjects carry *Candida* as part of the normal flora of the mouth, with *C. albicans* accounting for 70% to 80% of isolates. Oral carriage rates are increased substantially in hospitalized patients; those with HIV infection, dentures, and diabetes; patients receiving antineoplastic chemotherapy; those receiving antibiotics; and children. Virtually all humans may carry one or more *Candida* species throughout their GI tract, and the levels of carriage may increase to that detectable in illness or other circumstances in which the

Figure 74–1. *Candida tropicalis* blastoconidia and pseudohyphae (Gram stain, ×1000).

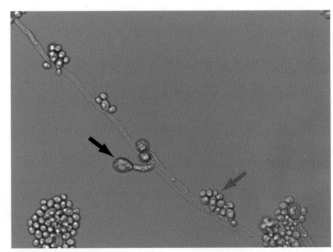

Figure 74–2. *Candida albicans*, microscopic morphology in cornmeal agar showing large chlamydospores (*black arrow*), blastoconidia (*red arrow*), hyphae, and pseudohyphae.

host's microbial suppression mechanisms become compromised.

The predominant source of infection due to *Candida* spp., from superficial mucosal and cutaneous disease to hematogenous dissemination, is the patient. That is, most types of candidiasis represent **endogenous** infection in which the normally commensal host flora take advantage of the "opportunity" to cause infection. In order to do so, there must be a lowering of the host's anti-*Candida* barrier. In the cases of *Candida* BSI, transfer of the organism from the GI mucosa to the bloodstream requires prior overgrowth of the numbers of yeasts in their commensal habitat coupled with a breach in the integrity of the GI mucosa.

Exogenous transmission of *Candida* may also account for a proportion of certain types of candidiasis. Examples include the use of contaminated irrigation solutions, parenteral nutrition fluids, vascular pressure transducers, cardiac valves, and corneas. Transmission of *Candida* spp. from healthcare workers to patients and from patient to patient has been well documented, especially in the intensive care unit environment. The hands of healthcare workers serve as potential reservoirs for nosocomial transmission of *Candida* spp.

Among the various species of *Candida* capable of causing human infection (see Box 74-1 and Table 74-3), *C. albicans* predominates in most types of infection. Infections of genital, cutaneous, and oral sites almost always involve *C. albicans*. A wider array of *Candida* spp. is seen causing BSI and other forms of invasive candidiasis, and although *C. albicans* usually predominates (see Table 74-3), the frequency with which this and other species of *Candida* are isolated from blood varies considerably according to the age of the patient (Figure 74-3) and the local, regional, or global setting (Table 74-4). Whereas *C albicans* and *C. parapsilosis* predominate as causes of BSI among infants and children, a decrease in *C. albicans*

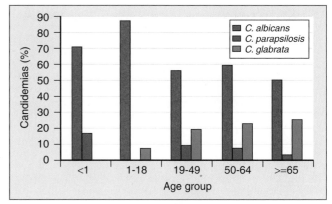

Figure 74–3. Percentage of all candidemias due to selected *Candida* species in each age group. Data are from the Emerging Infections and the Epidemiology of Iowa Organisms Survey, 1998 to 2001. *(Data from Pfaller MA, Diekema DJ: Epidemiology of invasive candidiasis: A persistent public health problem. Clin Microbiol Rev 20:133, 2007.)*

and *C. parapsilosis* infections and a prominent increase in *C. glabrata* infections is seen among older individuals (see Figure 74-3). Likewise, although *C. glabrata* is the second most common species causing BSI in North America, it is seen at a lower frequency in Latin America, where *C. parapsilosis* and *C. tropicalis* are more common (see Table 74-4). The differences in the number and types of *Candida* spp. causing infections may be influenced by numerous factors, including patient age, increased immunosuppression, antifungal drug exposure, or differences in infection-control practices. Each one of these factors, alone or in combination, may affect the prevalence of different *Candida* spp. in each institution. For example, the use of azoles (e.g., fluconazole) for antifungal prophylaxis may increase the likelihood of infections due to *C. glabrata* and *C. krusei*, two species with decreased susceptibility to this class of antifungals. Likewise, breaks

Table 74–4. Species Distribution of *Candida* Bloodstream Infection Isolates by Geographic Region

| Region | Number of Hospitals | Number of Isolates | % of Isolates by Species | | | | | |
			CA	CG	CP	CT	CK	Other
Asia-Pacific	17	441	73.5	10.2	8.4	3.9	3.2	0.8
Europe	40	775	57.6	12.9	14.1	7.5	3.4	4.5
Latin America	18	560	46.6	7.5	17.1	21.3	3.6	3.3
Canada	8	623	58.9	20.1	10.3	5.9	2.4	2.4
United States	167	3683	54.4	18.3	13.2	9.6	2.1	2.4
Total	250	6082	55.9	16.2	13.1	9.6	2.5	2.7

Adapted from Pfaller MA, Diekema DJ: Twelve years of fluconazole in clinical practice: Global trends in species distribution and fluconazole susceptibility of bloodstream isolates of Candida. *Clin Microbiol Infect 10(Suppl 1):11-23, 2004.*
CA, Candida albicans; CG, C. glabrata; CP, C. parapsilosis; CT, C. tropicalis; CK, C. krusei.

Table 74—5. Excess Mortality Attributable to Nosocomial Infections with *Candida* and *Aspergillus*

	Percent Mortality		
	Candida*		**Aspergillus†**
Type of Mortality Rate	1988	2001	1991
Crude mortality			
Cases	57	61	95
Controls	19	12	10
Attributable Mortality	38	49	85

*Patients with candidemia. Data from Wey SB, et al: Hospital-acquired candidemia: Attributable mortality and excess length of stay. Arch Intern Med 148:2642-2645, 1988; and Gudlagson O, et al: Attributable mortality of nosocomial candidemia, revisited. Clin Infect Dis 37:1172-1177, 2003.
†Bone marrow transplant patients with invasive pulmonary aspergillosis. Data from Pannuti CS, et al: Nosocomial pneumonia in adult patients undergoing bone marrow transplantation: A 9-year study. J Clin Oncol 9:1, 1991.

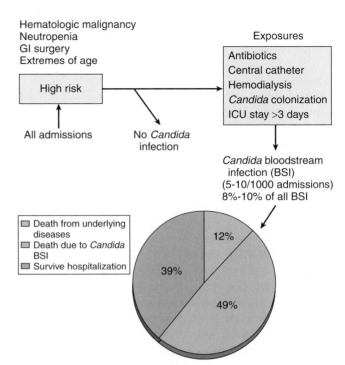

Figure 74—4. Global view of hospital-acquired candidemia. GI, gastrointestinal; ICU, intensive care unit. *(Adapted from Pfaller MA, Wenzel RP: The epidemiology of fungal infections. In Anaissie EJ, McGinnis MR, Pfaller MA (eds): Clinical Mycology. New York, Churchill Livingstone, 2003.)*

in infection-control precautions and in the proper care of vascular catheters may lead to more infections with *C. parapsilosis*, the predominant species isolated from the hands of healthcare workers and a frequent cause of catheter-related fungemia.

The consequences of *Candida* BSI in the hospitalized patient are severe. Hospitalized patients with candidemia have been shown to be at a twofold greater risk of death in hospital than those with noncandidal BSI. Among all patients with nosocomial (hospitalacquired) BSI, candidemia was found to be an independent predictor of death in hospital. Although estimates of mortality may be confounded by the serious nature of the underlying diseases in many of these patients, matched cohort studies have confirmed that the mortality directly attributable to the fungal infection is quite high (Table 74-5). Notably, the excess or attributable mortality due to candidemia has not decreased from that observed in the mid-1980s to that observed in the present day, despite the introduction of new antifungal agents with good activity against most species of *Candida*.

Clearly, more is known about the epidemiology of nosocomial candidemia than any other fungal infection. The accumulated evidence allows one to propose a general view of nosocomial candidemia (Figure 74-4). Certain hospitalized individuals are clearly at increased risk of acquiring candidemia during hospitalization as a result of their underlying medical condition: patients with hematologic malignancies and/or neutropenia, those undergoing GI surgery, premature infants, and patients greater than 70 years of age (see Table 74-1 and Figure 74-4). Compared to controls without the specific risk factors or exposures, the likelihood of these already high-risk patients contracting candidemia in hospital is approximately 2 times greater for each class of antibiotics they receive,

7 times greater if they have a central venous catheter, 10 times greater if *Candida* has been found to be colonizing other anatomic sites, and 18 times greater if the patient has undergone acute hemodialysis. Hospitalization in the intensive care unit setting provides the opportunity for transmission of *Candida* among patients and has been shown to be an additional independent risk factor.

The available epidemiologic data indicates that between 5 and 10 of every 1000 high-risk patients exposed to the above risk factors will contract BSI due to *Candida* spp. (8% to 10% of all nosocomial BSI; see Table 74-2). Approximately 49% of these patients will die as a result of their infection, 12% will die of their underlying disease, and 39% will survive hospitalization (see Figure 74-4). This picture has not changed, and may even be worse, from that seen in the mid-1980s. The outcome for almost half of those patients with candidemia could be improved by more effective means of prevention, diagnosis, and therapy. Clearly the most desirable of these is prevention, which is best approached by rigorous control of the exposures—especially limiting the use of broad-spectrum antibiotics, improving catheter care, and adhering to infection-control practices.

Clinical Syndromes

Given the right setting, *Candida* spp. can cause clinically apparent infection of virtually any organ system (Table 74-6). Infections range from superficial mucosal and cutaneous

Table 74–6. Types of *Candida* Infection and Associated Predisposing Factors

Type of Disease	Predisposing Factors	Type of Disease	Predisposing Factors
Oropharyngeal infection	Age extremes Denture wearers Diabetes mellitus Antibiotic use Radiotherapy for head and neck cancer Inhaled and systemic steroids Cytotoxic chemotherapy HIV infection Hematologic malignancies Stem-cell or solid-organ transplantation	Endocarditis	Major surgery Previous valvular disease Prosthetic valve Intravenous drug use Long-term central venous catheter
		Pericarditis	Thoracic surgery Immunosuppression
		Central nervous system (CNS) infection	CNS surgery Ventriculoperitoneal shunt Ocular surgery
Esophagitis	Systemic corticosteroids AIDS Cancer Stem cell or solid organ transplantation	Ocular infection	Trauma Surgery
		Bone and joint infection	Trauma Intraarticular injections Diabetic foot
Vulvovaginal infection	Oral contraceptives Pregnancy Diabetes mellitus Systemic corticosteroids HIV infection Antibiotic use	Abdominal infection	Perforation Abdominal surgery Anastomotic leaks Pancreatitis Continuous ambulatory peritoneal dialysis
Infections of the skin and nails	Local moisture and occlusion Immersion of hands in water Peripheral vascular disease	Hematogenous infection	Solid organ transplantation Colonization Prolonged antibiotic use Abdominal surgery Intensive care support Total parenteral nutrition Hemodialysis Immunosuppression Extremes of age Stem-cell transplantation
Chronic mucocutaneous candidiasis	T-lymphocyte defects		
Urinary tract infection	Indwelling urinary catheter Urinary obstruction Urinary procedures Diabetes mellitus		
Pneumonia	Aspiration		

Adapted from Dignani MC, Solomkin JS, Anaissie EJ: Candida. In Anaissie EJ, McGinnis MR, Pfaller MA (eds): Clinical Mycology. New York, Churchill Livingstone, 2003.

candidiasis to widespread hematogenous dissemination involving target organs such as the liver, spleen, kidney, heart, and brain. In the latter situation, the mortality directly attributable to the infectious process approaches 50% (see Table 74-5 and Figure 74-4).

Mucosal infections due to *Candida* spp. (known as "thrush") may be limited to the oropharynx or extend to the esophagus and the entire gastrointestinal tract. In women, the vaginal mucosa is also a common site of infection. These infections are generally seen in individuals with local or generalized immunosuppression or in those settings in which candidal overgrowth is favored (see Table 74-6). These infections usually present as white "cottage cheese"–like patches on the mucosal surface.

Other presentations include the **pseudomembranous** type, which reveals a raw bleeding surface when scraped; the **erythematous** type—flat, red, occasionally sore areas; candidal **leukoplakia**—non-removable white thickening of epithelium due to *Candida* spp.; and angular **cheilitis**—sore fissures at the corners of the mouth.

Candida spp. may cause localized skin infection in areas where the skin surface is occluded and moist (e.g., groin, axillae, toe webs, breast folds). These infections present as a pruritic rash with erythematous vesiculopustular lesions.

Onychomycosis and paronychia may occur in the setting of a mixed microbial flora including *Candida*. The species most commonly involved are *C. albicans*, *C. parapsilosis*, and *C. guilliermondii*.

Skin lesions may also appear during the course of hematogenous dissemination. These lesions are of major diagnostic importance; they can be directly biopsied and thus provide an etiologic diagnosis of a systemic process.

Chronic mucocutaneous candidiasis is a rare condition marked by a deficiency in T-lymphocyte responsiveness to *Candida* spp. These patients suffer from severe, unremitting mucocutaneous *Candida* lesions, including extensive nail involvement and vaginitis. The lesions may become quite large with a disfiguring granulomatous appearance.

Urinary tract involvement with *Candida* spp. ranges from asymptomatic bladder colonization to renal abscesses secondary to hematogenous seeding. Bladder colonization with *Candida* spp. is essentially not seen unless a patient requires an indwelling bladder catheter, has diabetes, suffers from urinary obstruction, or has had prior urinary procedures. Benign colonization of the bladder is most common in these settings, but urethritis and/or cystitis may occur. Hematogenous seeding of the kidney may result in renal abscess, papillary necrosis, or "fungus ball" of the ureter or renal pelvis.

Candida peritonitis may be seen in the setting of chronic ambulatory peritoneal dialysis or following GI surgery, anastomotic leak, or intestinal perforation. These infections may remain localized to the abdomen, involve adjacent organs, or lead to hematogenous candidiasis.

Hematogenous candidiasis may be acute or chronic and usually results in seeding of deep tissues, including the abdominal viscera, heart, eyes, bones and joints, and brain. Chronic hepatosplenic candidiasis may occur following either overt or occult fungemia and presents as an indolent process marked by fever, elevated alkaline phosphatase, and multiple lesions in the liver and spleen.

Central nervous system candidiasis may occur secondary to hematogenous disease or associated with neurosurgical procedures and ventriculoperitoneal shunts. This process may mimic bacterial meningitis, or the course may be indolent or chronic.

Most cardiac involvement with *Candida* spp. is the result of hematogenous seeding of a prosthetic or damaged heart valve, the myocardium, or pericardial space. Implantation of heart valves contaminated with *C. parapsilosis* has been reported. The clinical presentation resembles bacterial endocarditis, with fever and a new or changing heart murmur. The vegetations are classically large and friable, and embolic events are more common with endocarditis due to *Candida* spp. than with bacterial endocarditis.

The eye is frequently involved in patients with hematogenous candidiasis, presenting as chorioretinitis and endophthalmitis. For this reason, all patients at risk for candidemia should receive careful and frequent ophthalmologic examinations. Traumatic keratitis may also be seen.

Bone and joint infections due to *Candida* spp. are almost always sequelae of candidemia. Often these infections will present several months after successful treatment of candidemia. Similarly occult or "transient" candidemia may result in seeding of a skeletal focus that becomes clinically apparent at a later time. Vertebral osteomyelitis is a frequent presentation, with local pain and low-grade fever.

Although hematogenous candidiasis is most often an endogenous infection arising from the gastrointestinal or genitourinary tract, it may also result from the contamination of an indwelling catheter. Organisms transferred to the hub or lumen of the catheter may form a biofilm within the lumen of the catheter and subsequently spread into the circulation. Although such infections are no less serious than those arising from an endogenous source, they may be dealt with somewhat more successfully, since removal of the catheter essentially removes the nidus of infection. Of course, if the infected catheter resulted in the seeding of distant organs, the consequences and problems in treating the infection would be the same as those arising from an endogenous source.

Laboratory Diagnosis

The laboratory diagnosis of candidiasis involves the procurement of appropriate clinical material followed by direct microscopic examination and culture (see Chapter 69). Scrapings of mucosal or cutaneous lesions may be examined directly following treatment with 10% to 20% KOH containing calcofluor white. The budding yeastlike forms and pseudohyphae are easily detected upon examination with a fluorescence microscope (see Figure 69-1). Culture on standard mycologic medium will allow the isolation of the organism for subsequent identification to species. Increasingly, such specimens are plated directly on a selective chromogenic medium such as CHROMagar, which allows the detection of mixed species of *Candida* within the specimen and the rapid identification of *C. albicans* (green colonies) and *C. tropicalis* (blue colonies) based on their morphologic appearance (Figure 74-5).

All other types of infection require culture for diagnosis unless tissue can be obtained for histopathologic examination (see Chapter 69). Whenever possible, skin lesions should be biopsied and histologic sections stained with GMS or another fungal-specific stain. Visualization of characteristic budding yeasts and pseudohyphae is sufficient for the diagnosis of candidiasis (Figure 74-6). Cultures of blood, tissue, and normally sterile body fluids should also be performed. Identification of *Candida* isolates to species level is important, given the differences in response to the various antifungal agents (see Chapter 70). This can be accomplished as described in Chapter 69, using the germ-tube test (*C. albicans*), various chromogenic media/tests (see Figure 74-5), and commercially available sugar assimilation panels.

Immunologic, biochemical, and molecular markers for the diagnosis of candidiasis are described in Chapter 69. Unfortunately, these methods are not yet suitable for use in routine clinical diagnosis.

Figure 74–5. Differentiation of *Candida* species by isolates on CHROMagar *Candida*. The green colonies are *C. albicans*; the blue gray colonies are *C. tropicalis*, and the large, rough, pale pink colony is *C. krusei*. The smooth, pink or mauve colonies are another yeast species (only *C. albicans*, *C. tropicalis*, and *C. krusei* can be reliably recognized on this media; other species have colonies ranging from white, to pink, to mauve). *(From Anaissie EJ, McGinnis MR, Pfaller MA [eds]: Clinical Mycology. New York, Churchill Livingstone, 2003.)*

Treatment, Prevention, and Control

There are a wide variety of treatment options for candidiasis (see Chapter 70). Mucosal and cutaneous infections may be treated with a number of different topical creams, lotions, ointments, and suppositories containing various azole antifungal agents (see Table 70-1). Oral systemic therapy of these infections may also be accomplished with either fluconazole or itraconazole.

Bladder colonization or cystitis may be treated with either instillation of amphotericin B directly into the bladder (bladder wash) or by oral administration of fluconazole. Both of these measures will likely be unsuccessful if the bladder catheter cannot be removed.

Figure 74–6. *Candida* stained with GMS demonstrating budding yeasts and pseudohyphae. ×1000.

More deep-seated infections require systemic therapy, the choice of which depends upon the type of infection, the infecting species, and the overall status of the host. In many instances, oral fluconazole may be quite effective in treating candidiasis. It may be used in the treatment of peritonitis, as well as in more long-term maintenance therapy of invasive disease following an initial intravenous course of therapy. Fluconazole is efficacious when administered intravenously for the treatment of candidemia in non-neutropenic patients. Those patients who become candidemic while on fluconazole prophylaxis or those with documented infection due to *C. krusei* or fluconazole-resistant *C. glabrata* require treatment with either amphotericin B (conventional or lipid formulation) or an echinocandin (anidulafungin, caspofungin, or micafungin). In those clinical settings where *C. glabrata* or *C. krusei* are plausible etiologic agents (e.g., prior fluconazole therapy/prophylaxis or an endemic situation), initial therapy with either an echinocandin or an amphotericin B formulation is advised, with a switch to fluconazole (less toxic than amphotericin B, less expensive, and orally available vs. echinocandins) based upon final species identification and susceptibility test results. In every instance, care should be taken to remove the nidus of infection if possible. Thus vascular catheters should be removed or changed, abscesses should be drained, and other potentially infected implanted materials should be removed to the extent possible. Likewise, efforts should be directed towards immune reconstitution.

As in most infectious diseases, prevention is clearly preferable to the treatment of an established candidal infection. Avoidance of broad-spectrum antimicrobial agents, meticulous catheter care, and rigorous adherence to infection-control precautions are a must. Decreased colonization achieved by fluconazole prophylaxis has been shown to be efficacious when employed in **specific** high risk groups such as BMT patients and liver transplant patients. Such prophylaxis carries with it the potential for selecting for, or creating, strains or species that are resistant to the agent administered. This in fact has been seen with the emergence of fluconazole-resistant *C. glabrata* and *C. krusei* in certain institutions, but the overall benefit in the high-risk patient groups outweighs the risk. Transfer of this approach to other patient groups, however, is fraught with problems and should not be undertaken without careful study and risk-stratification to identify those individuals most likely to benefit from antifungal prophylaxis.

Opportunistic Mycoses Due to *Cryptococcus neoformans* and Other Noncandidal Yeastlike Fungi

In the same manner that *Candida* species have taken advantage of immunocompromising conditions, indwelling devices, and broad-spectrum antibiotic use, so too have a number of non-*Candida* yeastlike fungi found an "opportunity" to colonize and infect immunocompromised patients. These organisms may occupy environmental niches or be found in food and water and can be normal human microbial flora. The list of these opportunistic yeasts is long, but we will limit this discussion to one major pathogen, *Cryptococcus neoformans*, and four genera that pose particular problems as opportunistic pathogens: *Malassezia* spp., *Trichosporon* spp., *Rhodotorula* spp., and *Blastoschizomyces capitatus* (teleomorph, *Dipodascus capitatus*).

Cryptococcosis (Clinical Case 74-2)

Cryptococcosis is a systemic mycosis caused by the encapsulated, basidiomycetous, yeastlike fungus *Cryptococcus neoformans*. The fungus is worldwide in distribution and is found as a ubiquitous saprophyte of soil, especially that which is enriched with pigeon droppings. There are four main serotypes (A, B, C, and D) and three varieties of *C. neoformans*: *C. neoformans* var. *grubii* (serotype A), *C. neoformans* var. *neoformans* (serotype D), and *C. neoformans* var. *gattii* (serotypes B and C).

Clinical Case 74-2. Cryptococcosis

Pappas and colleagues (www.FrontlineFungus.org) describe a case of cryptococcosis in a heart transplant recipient. The 56-year-old patient, who underwent heart transplantation surgery 3 years prior, presented with new-onset cellulitis of his left leg and a mild headache of 2 weeks duration. The patient was on chronic immunosuppressive therapy with cyclosporine, azathioprine, and prednisone and was admitted for intravenous (IV) antibiotics. Despite 5 days of IV nafcillin, the patient failed to improve, and a skin biopsy of the cellulitic area was obtained for histopathologic studies and culture. Laboratory results revealed the presence of a yeast consistent with *Cryptococcus neoformans*. A lumbar puncture was also performed, and examination of the cerebrospinal fluid (CSF) disclosed cloudy fluid and an elevated opening pressure of 420 mm H_2O. Microscopic examination revealed encapsulated budding yeast forms. Cryptococcal antigen titers of CSF and blood were markedly elevated. Blood, CSF, and skin biopsy cultures grew *C. neoformans*. Systemic antifungal therapy with amphotericin B and flucytosine was initiated. Unfortunately, the patient suffered progressive mental status decline, despite aggressive management of intracranial pressure and maximizing doses of antifungals. He experienced slow, progressive decline, leading to death 13 days after initiation of antifungal therapy. CSF cultures obtained 2 days prior to death remained positive for *C. neoformans*.

The patient in this case was highly immunocompromised and presented with cellulitis and headache. Such a presentation should arouse suspicion of an atypical pathogen such as *C. neoformans*. Given the high mortality associated with cryptococcal infection, rapid and accurate diagnosis is important. Unfortunately, despite these efforts and use of aggressive therapy, many such patients will succumb to the infection.

Figure 74—7. *Cryptococcus neoformans*. Microscopic morphology, GMS stain.

Morphology

Microscopically, *C. neoformans* is a spherical to oval, encapsulated, yeastlike organism, 2 to 20 μm in diameter. Replication is by budding from a relatively narrow base. Single buds are usually formed, but multiple buds and chains of budding cells are sometimes present (Figure 74-7). Germ tubes, hyphae, and pseudohyphae are usually absent in clinical material.

In tissue and upon staining with India ink, the cells are variable in size, spherical, oval, or elliptical, and surrounded by optically clear, smoothly contoured, spherical zones or "halos" which represent the extracellular polysaccharide capsule (Figure 74-8). The capsule is a distinctive marker, which may have a diameter of up to five times that of the fungal cell and is readily detected with mucin stain such as Mayer mucicarmine (Figure 74-9). The organism stains poorly with H&E but is easily detected with PAS and GMS stains. The cell wall of *C. neoformans* contains melanin, which may be demonstrated by staining with the Fontana-Masson stain.

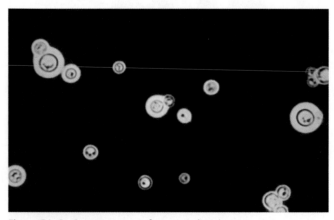

Figure 74—8. *Cryptococcus neoformans*. India ink preparation demonstrating the large capsule surrounding budding yeast cells (×1000).

Figure 74–9. *Cryptococcus neoformans* stained with mucicarmine (×1000).

Epidemiology

Cryptococcosis is usually acquired by inhaling aerosolized cells of *C. neoformans* from the environment (Figure 74-10). Subsequent dissemination from the lungs, usually to the central nervous system (CNS), produces clinical disease in susceptible individuals. Primary cutaneous cryptococcosis may occur following transcutaneous inoculation but is rare.

Although *C. neoformans* is pathogenic for immune competent individuals, it is most often encountered as an opportunistic pathogen. It is the most common cause of fungal meningitis and tends to occur in those patients with defective cellular immunity.

Whereas *C. neoformans* var. *neoformans* and var. *grubii* are found worldwide in association with soil contaminated with avian excreta, *C. neoformans* var. *gattii* is generally found in tropical and subtropical climates in association with *Eucalyptus* trees. Recently, however, an endemic focus of var. *gattii* has been identified in Vancouver Island, British Columbia, and in Washington state. All three varieties cause a similar disease, although var. *gattii* infection tends to occur in immunocompetent individuals and has a lower associated mortality but more severe neurologic sequelae, owing to CNS granuloma formation.

C. neoformans var. *neoformans* (and var. *grubii*) is a major opportunistic pathogen of patients with AIDS. Those individuals with CD4+ lymphocyte counts of less than 100/mm (usually <200/mm) are at high risk for CNS and disseminated cryptococcosis. The incidence of cryptococcosis seems to have peaked in the United States in the early 1990s (65.5 infections per million per year; see Chapter 5, Table 5-2) and has progressively declined since then due to the widespread use of fluconazole and, more importantly, successful treatment of the HIV infection with new antiretroviral drugs.

Clinical Syndromes

Cryptococcosis may present as a pneumonic process or, more commonly, as a CNS infection secondary to hematogenous and lymphatic spread from a primary pulmonary focus. Less often, a more widely disseminated infection may be seen with cutaneous, mucocutaneous, osseous, and visceral forms of the disease.

Pulmonary cryptococcosis is variable in presentation, from an asymptomatic process to a more fulminant bilateral pneumonia. Nodular infiltrates may be either unilateral or bilateral, becoming more diffuse in severe infections. Cavitation is rare.

C. neoformans is highly neurotropic, and the most common form of disease is cerebromeningeal. The course of disease is variable and may be quite chronic; however, it is inevitably fatal if untreated. Both meninges and the underlying brain tissue are involved, and the clinical presentation is that of fever, headache, meningismus, visual disturbances, abnormal mental status, and seizures. The clinical picture is highly dependent upon the patient's immune status and tends to be dramatically severe in AIDS patients and other severely compromised patients treated with steroids or other immunosuppressive agents.

Parenchymal lesions, or cryptococcomas, are uncommon in infections due to *C. neoformans* var. *neoformans* (and var. *grubii*) but are the most common presentation of CNS cryptococcosis in immunocompetent hosts infected with var. *gattii*.

Other manifestations of disseminated cryptococcosis include skin lesions, which occur in 10% to 15% of patients and may mimic those of molluscum contagiosum; ocular infections, including chorioretinitis, vitritis, and ocular nerve invasion; osseous lesions involving the vertebrae

Figure 74–10. Natural history of saprobic and parasitic cycle of *Cryptococcus neoformans*.

and bony prominences; and prostatic involvement, which may be an asymptomatic reservoir of infection.

Laboratory Diagnosis

The diagnosis of infection due to *C. neoformans* may be made by culture of blood, cerebrospinal fluid, or other clinical material (see Chapter 71). Microscopic examination of cerebrospinal fluid (CSF) may reveal the characteristic encapsulated budding yeast cells. The cells of *C. neoformans*, when present in CSF or other clinical material, may be visualized with Gram stain (see Chapter 69, Figure 69-2), as well as with India ink (see Figure 74-8) or other stains (see Figure 74-7). Culture of clinical material on routine mycologic media will produce mucoid colonies composed of round, encapsulated, budding yeast cells that are urease-positive within 3 to 5 days. Species identification may be accomplished by carbohydrate assimilation testing, by growth on niger seed agar (*C. neoformans* colonies become brown to black in color), or by directly testing for phenoloxidase activity (positive).

Most commonly, however, the diagnosis of cryptococcal meningitis is made by direct detection of the capsular polysaccharide antigen in serum or CSF (Table 74-7). Detection of cryptococcal antigen is accomplished by using one of several commercially available latex agglutination or enzyme immunoassay kits. These assays have been shown to be rapid, sensitive, and specific for the diagnosis of cryptococcal disease (see Table 74-7).

Treatment

Cryptococcal meningitis (and other disseminated forms of cryptococcosis) is universally fatal if left untreated. In addition to the prompt administration of appropriate antifungal therapy, effective management of central nervous system (CNS) pressure is key to the successful treatment of cryptococcal meningitis. All patients should receive amphotericin B plus flucytosine acutely for 2 weeks (induction therapy), followed by 8-week consolidation

Table 74–7. Sensitivity of Antigen Detection, India Ink Microscopy, and Culture of Cerebral Spinal Fluid in the Diagnosis of Cryptococcal Meningitis

Test	% Sensitivity	
	AIDS Patients	*Non-AIDS Patients*
Antigen	100	86-95
India ink	82	50
Culture	100	90

Adapted from Viviani MA, Tortorano AM, Ajello L: Cryptococcus. In Anaissie EJ, McGinnis MR, Pfaller MA (eds): Clinical Mycology. New York, Churchill Livingstone, 2003.

with either oral fluconazole (preferred) or itraconazole. AIDS patients generally require lifelong maintenance therapy with either fluconazole or itraconazole. In non-AIDS patients, treatment may be discontinued after the consolidation therapy; however, relapse may be seen in up to 26% of these patients within 3 to 6 months after discontinuation of therapy. Thus a prolonged consolidation treatment with an azole for up to 1 year may be advisable, even with patients without AIDS.

Treatment of these patients should be followed both clinically and mycologically. Mycologic follow-up requires repeat lumbar puncture to be performed (1) at the end of the 2-week induction therapy to ensure sterilization of the CSF; (2) at the end of the consolidation therapy; (3) whenever indicated by a change in clinical status during follow-up. *CSF samples collected during follow-up must be cultured.* Determination of CSF protein, glucose, cell count, and cryptococcal antigen titer are helpful in assessing the response to therapy but are not highly predictive of outcome. Failure to sterilize the CSF by day 14 of therapy is indicative of a much higher probability that the consolidation therapy will fail.

Other Mycoses Due to Yeastlike Fungi

Among the non-*Candida*, non-*Cryptococcus* yeastlike pathogens, nosocomial infections due to *Malassezia* spp., *Trichosporon* spp., *Rhodotorula* spp., and *Blastoschizomyces capitatus* are most prominent, either because they are difficult to detect or because they may pose particular problems with respect to antifungal resistance.

Infections due to *Malassezia* spp. (*M. furfur* and *M. pachydermatis*) are usually catheter-related and tend to occur in premature infants or in other patients receiving lipid infusions. Both of these organisms are budding yeasts (Figure 74-11; also see Chapter 71, Figure 71-2). *M. furfur* is a common skin colonizer and is the etiologic agent of tinea (pityriasis) versicolor (see Chapter 71), whereas *M. pachydermatis* is a frequent cause of otitis in dogs, as well as a human skin commensal.

Among the *Malassezia* spp., *M. furfur* is known for its requirement for exogenous lipid for growth. This growth requirement, plus its ecologic niche on skin, explains some of the epidemiology of *M. furfur*, because nosocomial infections due to this organism are directly related to the administration of intravenous lipid supplements through a central venous catheter. Although *M. pachydermatis* does not require exogenous lipids for growth, fatty acids do stimulate its growth, and infections due to this organism have been associated with parenteral nutrition and intravenous lipid administration. Although most infections with *Malassezia* spp. are sporadic, outbreaks of fungemia have been observed among infants receiving intravenous lipid supplementation. The growth of the organism is favored by the lipid-rich infusion, and the organism gains access to the bloodstream via the catheter. One notable outbreak of

Figure 74–11. Scanning electron micrograph of *Malassezia furfur* adhering to the lumen of a central venous catheter. *(Courtesy of S.A. Messer.)*

M. pachydermatis fungemia in a pediatric intensive care unit was linked to nurses who owned dogs with *M. pachydermatis* otitis. The outbreak strain was found on the hands of the nurses and at least one of the affected dogs.

Malassezia spp. should be considered when yeasts are seen microscopically in blood culture bottles or clinical material but no organisms are recovered on routine agar medium. To isolate *Malassezia* spp., especially *M. furfur*, on agar medium, the plates must be inoculated and then overlaid with sterile olive oil. Olive oil provides the lipid requirement, and growth should be detected in 3 to 5 days.

Treatment of fungemia due to *Malassezia* spp. does not usually require the administration of antifungal agents. The infection subsides once the lipid infusion is stopped and the intravascular lines are removed.

The genus *Trichosporon* currently consists of six species that are of clinical significance: *T. asahii* and *T. mucoides* are known to cause deep invasive infections; *T. asteroides* and *T. cutaneum* cause superficial skin infections; *T. ovoides* causes white piedra of the scalp, and *T. inkin* causes that of the pubic hair. Confusingly, most of the literature regarding deep-seated trichosporonosis refers to the older nomenclature of *T. beigelii*. Morphologically these organisms are similar and appear in clinical material as hyphae, arthroconidia, and budding yeast cells.

Trichosporon causes catheter-associated fungemia in neutropenic patients but also may gain entrance to the bloodstream via the respiratory or gastrointestinal tract. Widespread hematogenous dissemination may manifest as positive blood cultures and multiple cutaneous lesions. Chronic hepatic trichosporonosis may mimic hepatic candidiasis and is seen upon recovery from neutropenia. *Trichosporon* has been reported as the most common cause of noncandidal yeast infection in patients with hematologic malignancies and carries a mortality in excess of 80%. Susceptibility to amphotericin B is variable, and this agent lacks fungicidal activity against *Trichosporon*. Clinical failures with amphotericin B, fluconazole, and combinations of the two have been reported, and the outcome is generally dismal in the absence of neutrophil recovery. *Trichosporon* species are resistant to the echinocandins but appear to respond clinically to treatment with voriconazole.

Rhodotorula spp. are characterized by the production of carotenoid pigments (produce pink to red colonies) and variably encapsulated, multilateral, budding yeast cells. Species of *Rhodotorula* include *R. glutinis*, *R. mucilaginosa* (syn. *R. rubra*), and *R. minuta*. These yeastlike fungi are found as commensals on skin, nails, and mucous membranes, as well as in cheese and milk products and environmental sources including air, soil, shower curtains, bathtub grout, and toothbrushes. *Rhodotorula* species are emerging as important human pathogens in immunocompromised patients and those with indwelling devices. *Rhodotorula* has been implicated as a cause of central venous catheter infection and fungemia, ocular infections, peritonitis, and meningitis. Amphotericin B has excellent activity against *Rhodotorula* and, coupled with catheter removal, is an optimal approach to infections with this organism. Flucytosine has excellent activity as well but should not be considered for monotherapy. Neither fluconazole nor the echinocandins should be used to treat infections due to *Rhodotorula* species, and the role of the new extended-spectrum triazoles (e.g., voriconazole and posaconazole) is uncertain pending clinical data.

Among the emerging opportunistic yeastlike pathogens, *Blastoschizomyces capitatus* (teleomorph *Dipodascus capitatus*) is a rarely described fungus that produces severe systemic infection in immunocompromised patients, especially those with hematologic malignancies. This organism produces hyphae and arthroconidia, is widely distributed in nature, and may be found as part of the normal skin flora. Infection with *B. capitatus* presents similar to that with *Trichosporon* in neutropenic patients, with frequent fungemia and multiorgan (including brain) dissemination and a mortality rate of 60% to 80%. Blood cultures are usually positive. As with *Trichosporon*, a chronic disseminated form similar to chronic disseminated candidiasis may be seen upon resolution of neutropenia.

The optimal approach to therapy of infections due to *B. capitatus* is not yet defined. Some clinicians feel that *B. capitatus* has decreased susceptibility to amphotericin B. The excellent in vitro activity of voriconazole suggest that it may be a useful agent for treatment of infections due to this organism. Rapid removal of central venous catheters, adjuvant immunotherapy, and novel antifungal therapies (e.g., either voriconazole or high-dose fluconazole plus amphotericin B) are recommended for treatment of this rare but devastating infection.

Aspergillosis (Clinical Case 74-3)

Aspergillosis comprises a broad spectrum of diseases caused by members of the genus *Aspergillus* (Box 74-2).

Figure 74—12. *Aspergillus fumigatus*. Lactophenol cotton blue preparation showing conidial heads.

Figure 74—14. *Aspergillus* in tissue showing acute-angle branching, septate hyphae (GMS, ×1000).

Epidemiology

Aspergillus spp. are common throughout the world. Their conidia are ubiquitous in air, soil, and decaying matter. Within the hospital environment, *Aspergillus* spp. may be found in air, showerheads, hospital water storage tanks, and potted plants. As a result, they are constantly being inhaled. The type of host reaction, the associated pathologic findings, and the ultimate outcome of infection depend more on host factors than on the virulence or pathogenesis of the individual *Aspergillus* spp. The respiratory tract is the most frequent, and most important, portal of entry.

Clinical Syndromes

The allergic manifestations of aspergillosis constitute a spectrum of presentations based on the degree of hypersensitivity to *Aspergillus* antigens. In the broncho-

pulmonary form, asthma, pulmonary infiltrates, peripheral eosinophilia, elevated serum IgE, and evidence of hypersensitivity to *Aspergillus* antigens (skin test) may be seen. Allergic sinusitis shows laboratory evidence of hypersensitivity to go along with upper respiratory symptoms of nasal obstruction and discharge, headache, and facial pain.

Both the paranasal sinuses and the lower airways may become colonized with *Aspergillus* spp., resulting in obstructive bronchial aspergillosis and true aspergilloma ("fungus ball"). Obstructive bronchial aspergillosis usually occurs in the setting of underlying pulmonary disease such as cystic fibrosis, chronic bronchitis, or bronchiectasis. The condition is marked by the formation of bronchial casts or plugs composed of hyphal elements and mucinous material. The symptoms remain those of the underlying disease; no tissue injury results, and no treatment is necessary. An aspergilloma can form either in the paranasal sinuses or in a preformed pulmonary cavity secondary to old tuberculosis or other chronic cavitary lung disease. Aspergillomas may be seen on radiographic examination but usually are asymptomatic. Treatment is generally not warranted unless pulmonary hemorrhage occurs. In the event of pulmonary

Figure 74—13. *Aspergillus terreus*. Lactophenol cotton blue preparation showing conidial head.

Figure 74—15. *Aspergillus niger* in a cavitary lung lesion showing both hyphae and conidial head (GMS, ×1000).

Figure 74–16. *Aspergillus terreus* in tissue. Arrows point to aleurioconidia (GMS, ×1000). *(From Walsh et al: J Infect Dis 188: 305-310, 2003.)*

hemorrhage, which may be severe and life threatening, surgical excision of the cavity and fungus ball is indicated. Likewise, radical debridement of the paranasal sinuses may be necessary to alleviate any symptomatology or hemorrhage due to a fungus ball of the sinuses.

Forms of invasive aspergillosis run the gamut from superficially invasive disease that may occur in the setting of mild immunosuppression (e.g., low-dose steroid therapy, collagen vascular disease, or diabetes) to destructive, locally invasive pulmonary or disseminated aspergillosis. The more limited forms of invasion generally include necrotizing pseudomembranous bronchial aspergillosis and chronic necrotizing pulmonary aspergillosis. Bronchial aspergillosis may cause wheezing, dyspnea, and hemoptysis. Most patients with chronic necrotizing pulmonary aspergillosis have underlying structural pulmonary disease, which may be treated with low dose corticosteroids. This is a chronic infection that may be locally destructive, with the development of infiltrates and fungus balls seen on radiographic examination. It is not associated with vascular invasion or dissemination. Surgical resection of affected areas and administration of antifungal therapy are efficacious in treating this condition.

Invasive pulmonary aspergillosis (IPA) and disseminated aspergillosis are devastating infections seen in severely neutropenic and immunodeficient patients. The major predisposing factors for this infectious complication include neutrophil count less than 500/mm^3, cytotoxic chemotherapy, and corticosteroid therapy. Patients present with fever and pulmonary infiltrates, often accompanied by pleuritic chest pain and hemoptysis. Definitive diagnosis is often delayed, since sputum and blood cultures are usually negative. The mortality of this infection despite specific antifungal therapy is quite high, usually exceeding 70%

(see Table 74-5). Hematogenous dissemination of infection to extrapulmonary sites is common, owing to the angioinvasive nature of the fungus. Sites most often involved include brain, heart, kidneys, GI tract, liver, and spleen.

Laboratory Diagnosis

As with other ubiquitous fungi, the diagnosis of aspergillosis necessitates caution when evaluating the isolation of an *Aspergillus* species from clinical specimens. Recovery from surgically removed tissue or sterile sites, accompanied by positive histopathology (moniliaceous, septate, dichotomously branching hyphae) should always be considered significant; isolation from normally contaminated (e.g., respiratory) sites requires closer scrutiny.

Most etiologic agents of aspergillosis grow readily on routine mycologic media lacking cycloheximide. Species-level identification of the major human pathogens can be made by observing cultural and microscopic characteristics from growth on potato dextrose agar. Microscopic morphology (conidiophores, vesicles, metulae, phialides, and conidia) is best observed with a slide culture and is necessary for species identification.

Invasive aspergillosis caused by *A. fumigatus* and most other species is rarely documented by positive blood cultures. In fact, most bloodstream isolates of *Aspergillus* species have been shown to represent pseudofungemia or terminal events at autopsy. Notably, *A. terreus*, among all species of *Aspergillus*, has been shown to cause true aspergillemia. Similar to other angioinvasive filamentous fungi (e.g., *Fusarium*, *Scedosporium* spp.), *A. terreus* is capable of adventitious sporulation, in which yeastlike spores, or aleurioconidia, are formed in tissue and are more likely to be detected in blood obtained for culture (see Figure 74-16). Recognition of these aleurioconidia on microscopic examination of tissue, fine-needle aspirates, or bronchoscopy specimens can allow a rapid, presumptive identification of *A. terreus*.

The rapid diagnosis of invasive aspergillosis has been advanced by the development of immunoassays for the *Aspergillus* galactomannan antigen in serum. This test employs an enzyme immunoassay format and is available as a commercial kit or from reference laboratories. This test appears to be reasonably specific but exhibits variable sensitivity. It is best used on serial specimens from high-risk (primarily neutropenic and BMT patients) patients as an early indication to begin empiric or preemptive antifungal therapy and to more aggressively pursue a definitive diagnosis.

Treatment and Prevention

Prevention of aspergillosis in high-risk patients is paramount. Neutropenic and other high-risk patients are generally housed in facilities where the air is filtered so as to minimize exposure to *Aspergillus* conidia.

Specific antifungal therapy of aspergillosis usually involves the administration of amphotericin B or one of its lipid-based formulations. It is important to realize that *A. terreus* is considered resistant to amphotericin B and should be treated with an alternative agent such as voriconazole. The introduction of voriconazole provides a treatment option that is more efficacious and less toxic than amphotericin B (see Chapter 70). Concomitant efforts to decrease immunosuppression and/or reconstitute host immune defenses are important components of the treatment of aspergillosis. Likewise, surgical resection of involved areas, if possible, are recommended.

Figure 74–17. *Rhizopus* sp. showing sporangium and rhizoids.

Zygomycosis

Zygomycosis refers to diseases caused by fungi of the class Zygomycetes. The principal human pathogens in the class Zygomycetes are encompassed by two orders: the Mucorales and the Entomophthorales. The order Entomophthorales contains two pathogenic genera, *Conidiobolus* and *Basidiobolus*. These agents generally incite a chronic, granulomatous infection of subcutaneous tissues and are discussed in Chapter 72.

In the order Mucorales, pathogenic genera include *Rhizopus*, *Mucor*, *Absidia*, *Rhizomucor*, *Saksenaea*, *Cunninghamella*, *Syncephalastrum*, and *Apophysomyces*. Infections due to Zygomycetes are rare, occurring at an annual rate of 1.7 infections per million population in the United States. Unfortunately, when they do occur, infections due to these agents are generally acute and rapidly progressive, with mortality rates of 70% to 100%.

Morphology

Macroscopically, the pathogenic Mucorales grow rapidly, producing gray to brown wooly colonies within 12 to 18 hours. Further identification to the genus and species level is based upon microscopic morphology. Microscopically, the Zygomycetes are molds with broad, hyaline, sparsely septate, coenocytic hyphae. The asexual spores of the order Mucorales are contained within a sporangium and are referred to as **sporangiospores**. The sporangia are borne at the tips of stalklike sporangiophores that terminate in a bulbous swelling called the **columella** (Figure 74-17; also see Chapter 5, Figure 5-3A). The presence of rootlike structures, called **rhizoids,** is helpful in identifying specific genera within the Mucorales.

In tissue, Zygomycetes (order Mucorales) are seen as ribbon-like, aseptate or sparsely septate, moniliaceous (nonpigmented) hyphae (see Figure 74-18). In contrast to *Aspergillus* spp. and other hyaline molds, the diameter of the hyphae often exceeds 10 μm, and the hyphae are irregularly contoured and pleomorphic, often folding and twisting back upon themselves. The pattern of hyphal branching is haphazard and nonprogressive, and branches typically arise from the parent hyphae at right angles. The walls of the hyphae are thin, stain weakly with GMS and other fungal stains, and are often more easily detected with H&E (see Figure 74-18). The Zygomycetes are typically angioinvasive.

Epidemiology

Zygomycosis is a sporadic disease that occurs worldwide. *Rhizopus arrhizus* is the most common cause of human zygomycosis; however, additional species of *Rhizopus*, *Rhizomucor*, *Absidia*, and *Cunninghamella* are known to cause invasive disease in hospitalized individuals. The organisms are ubiquitous in soil and decaying vegetation, and infection may be acquired by inhalation, ingestion, or contamination of wounds with sporangiospores from the environment. As with *Aspergillus* spp., nosocomial spread of Zygomycetes may occur by way of air-conditioning systems, particularly during construction. Focal outbreaks of

Figure 74–18. *Rhizopus* sp. in tissue showing broad, ribbon-like, aseptate hyphae (H&E, ×1000).

zygomycosis have also been associated with the use of contaminated adhesive bandages or tape in surgical wound dressings, resulting in primary cutaneous zygomycosis.

Invasive zygomycosis occurs in immunocompromised patients and is similar clinically to aspergillosis. It is estimated that Zygomycetes may cause infection in 1% to 9% of solid organ transplants, especially those with underlying diabetes mellitus. Risk factors include corticosteroid and deferoxamine therapy, diabetic ketoacidosis, renal failure, hematologic malignancy, myelosuppression, and exposure to hospital construction activity. Recently, zygomycosis has been seen following blood and marrow transplantation (BMT) in patients receiving antifungal prophylaxis with voriconazole, an agent that is not active against the Zygomycetes.

Clinical Syndromes

There are several clinical forms of zygomycosis caused by members of the order Mucorales. Rhinocerebral zygomycosis is an acute invasive infection of the nasal cavity, paranasal sinuses, and orbit that involves the facial structures and extends into the CNS, involving the meninges and the brain. Most of these infections occur in patients with metabolic acidosis, particularly diabetic ketoacidosis, and those with hematologic malignancies.

Pulmonary zygomycosis occurs as a primary infection in neutropenic patients and may be misdiagnosed as invasive aspergillosis. The pulmonary lesions are infarctive as a result of hyphal invasion and subsequent thrombosis of large pulmonary vessels. Chest radiographs show a rapidly progressive bronchopneumonia, segmented or lobar consolidation, and signs of cavitation. Fungus-ball formation mimicking aspergilloma may be seen. Pulmonary hemorrhage with fatal hemoptysis may be seen as a result of vascular invasion by the fungus.

The angioinvasive nature of the mucoraceous zygomycetes often produces disseminated infection, with tissue infarction of various organs. Presenting symptoms point to neurologic, pulmonary, or gastrointestinal involvement. Involvement of the gastrointestinal tract often results in massive hemorrhage or perforation.

Cutaneous zygomycosis may be a sign of hematogenous dissemination. Lesions tend to be nodular with an ecchymotic center. Primary cutaneous zygomycosis may occur following traumatic injury, in surgical dressings, or as colonization of burn wounds. The infection may be superficial or extend rapidly into the subcutaneous tissues.

Laboratory Diagnosis

Because of the extremely poor prognosis of zygomycosis, every effort should be made to obtain tissue for direct microscopic examination, histologic study, and culture. The Zygomycetes are an extremely ubiquitous group of fungi, so demonstration of characteristic fungal elements in tissue merits considerably more importance than simple isolation in culture.

Appropriate specimens include scrapings of nasal mucosa, aspirates of sinus contents, bronchial alveolar lavage fluid, and biopsy of any and all necrotic infected tissue. Direct examination of material mounted in KOH with calcofluor white may reveal the broad, aseptate hyphae. Histopathologic sections stained with H&E or PAS are most useful (see Figure 74-18). Broad, irregularly branched, pauciseptate, twisted hyphae can be observed.

Tissue for culture should be minced, not homogenized, and placed on standard mycologic media without cycloheximide. Negative cultures are common, occurring about 40% of the time, despite the microscopic demonstration of hyphae in tissue. The diagnosis of zygomycosis cannot be established or rejected based on culture alone. It depends on a panel of evidence gathered by both the clinician and microbiologist. Unfortunately, there are no widely available serologic or molecular tests specific for the Zygomycetes yet available (see Chapter 69).

Treatment

Amphotericin B remains the first-line therapy for zygomycosis, often supplemented by surgical debridement and immune reconstitution. Most Zygomycetes appear quite susceptible to amphotericin B and are generally not susceptible to the azoles or echinocandins (see Chapter 70). Among the extended-spectrum triazoles, however, posaconazole stands out, in that it appears to be active against most of the Zygomycetes. Posaconazole has documented efficacy in murine models of zygomycosis and in limited experience in the treatment of infections in humans. In contrast, voriconazole is inactive against these agents, and breakthrough zygomycosis has been reported in BMT patients receiving voriconazole prophylaxis.

Mycoses Due to Other Hyaline Molds

The list of hyaline molds, also known as **hyalohyphomycetes**, is quite long, and it is well beyond the scope of this chapter to discuss them all (see Box 74-1). The taxonomically diverse agents of hyalohyphomycosis (infection due to nonpigmented molds) do share several characteristics, in that many exhibit decreased susceptibility to a number of antifungal agents and when present in tissue, they appear as hyaline (nonpigmented), septate, branching, filamentous fungi that may be indistinguishable from *Aspergillus*. Culture is necessary to identify these agents and may be critical in determining the most appropriate therapy.

Although infections caused by most of these fungi are relatively uncommon, they appear to be increasing in incidence. Most disseminated infections are thought to be acquired by the inhalation of spores or by the progression of previously localized cutaneous lesions. In this chapter, the discussion of specific genera is limited to selected clinically important hyaline molds: *Fusarium* spp., *Scedosporium* spp., *Acremonium* spp., *Paecilomyces* spp., *Trichoderma* spp., and *Scopulariopsis* spp. These organisms tend to cause infections in neutropenic patients, are often disseminated in nature, and are almost uniformly fatal in the absence of immune reconstitution. Several of these organisms are capable of adventitious conidiation (generation of spores in tissue) with concomitant hematogenous dissemination, positive blood cultures, and multiple cutaneous lesions.

Fusarium species have been recognized with increased frequency as causes of disseminated infection in immunocompromised patients. *Fusarium* is also an important cause of fungal keratitis, especially among contact lens wearers. The most common species isolated from clinical specimens include *Fusarium moniliforme*, *F. solani*, and *F. oxysporum*. The hallmark of disseminated fusariosis is the appearance of multiple purpuric cutaneous nodules with central necrosis (Clinical Case 74-4). Biopsy of these nodules generally reveals branching, hyaline, septate hyphae invading dermal blood vessels (Figure 74-19). Cultures of biopsy material and of blood are useful in establishing the diagnosis of *Fusarium* infection. Although blood cultures are virtually

Figure 74—19. *Fusarium* sp. in tissue showing acute-angle branching, septate hyphae that are indistinguishable from that of *Aspergillus* spp. *(From Chandler FW, Watts JC: Pathologic Diagnosis of Fungal Infections. Chicago, ASCP, 1987.)*

always negative in invasive infections due to *Aspergillus* spp., approximately 75% of patients with fusariosis will have positive blood cultures. In culture, colonies of *Fusarium* spp. are rapidly growing, cottony to wooly, flat, and spreading. Colors may include blue green, beige, salmon, lavender, red, violet, and purple. Microscopically, *Fusarium* spp. are characterized by the production of both macroconidia and microconidia. Microconidia are single- or double-celled, ovoid to cylindrical, and generally borne as mucous balls or short chains. Macroconidia are fusiform or sickle shaped and many celled (Figure 74-20). *Fusarium* spp. often appear resistant to amphotericin B in vitro, and breakthrough infections occur frequently in patients treated with this agent. Voriconazole and posaconazole have been used successfully in some patients with amphotericin B—refractory fusariosis. Primary therapy with either a lipid formulation of amphotericin B, voriconazole,

---

Clinical Case 74-4. Fusariosis

Badley, et al. (www.FrontlineFungus.org) describe a 38-year-old man, undergoing chemotherapy for recently diagnosed acute myeloid leukemia, who developed neutropenia and fever. He was placed on broad-spectrum antibacterial agents but remained febrile after 96 hours. A left internal jugular catheter was in place. Blood and urine cultures showed no growth. To combat a potential fungal infection, voriconazole was added to the therapeutic regimen. After 1 week of treatment, the patient was still febrile and neutropenic, and his antifungal therapy was changed to caspofungin. Four days later, the patient developed a mildly painful rash. Initially the rash developed on the upper extremities and consisted of papular, erythematous, plaquelike lesions with centers that became necrotic. Blood cultures and skin biopsy specimens were sent to the laboratory for analysis. The laboratory report indicated that the blood cultures were positive for "yeast" based on the presence of budding cells and pseudohyphae. The skin biopsy showed "mold" consistent with *Aspergillus*. However, serum galactomannan testing was negative. All cultures grew *Fusarium solani*. The patient's caspofungin was discontinued, and he was switched to a lipid preparation of amphotericin B and voriconazole. Despite the antifungal therapy, the lesions increased in number over the next 2 weeks and spread throughout his extremities, trunk, and face. The neutropenia and fever persisted, and he died approximately 3 weeks after the initial diagnosis.

The combination of skin lesions and positive blood cultures are typical findings in fusariosis. Although "yeast" was reported from the blood cultures, closer examination revealed the microconidia and hyphae of *Fusarium*. Likewise, the appearance of septate hyphae in the skin biopsy could represent a number of different hyaline molds, including *Fusarium*.

Figure 74—20. *Fusarium oxysporum*, lactophenol cotton blue preparation.

or posaconazole, plus vigorous efforts at immune reconstitution, are recommended for treatment of fusariosis.

Within the genus *Scedosporium*, *S. apiospermum* (teleomorph *Pseudallescheria boydii*) and *S. prolificans* represent two important antifungal-resistant opportunistic pathogens. *S. apiospermum* may be readily isolated from soil and is an occasional cause of mycetoma worldwide; however, it is also the cause of serious disseminated and localized infection in immunocompromised patients. In addition to widespread disseminated disease, *S. apiospermum* has been reported to cause corneal ulcers, endophthalmitis, sinusitis, pneumonia, endocarditis, meningitis, arthritis, and osteomyelitis. *S. apiospermum* is indistinguishable from *Aspergillus* spp. and other agents of hyalohyphomycosis on histopathologic examination. Such distinction is important clinically, because *S. apiospermum* is resistant to amphotericin B and susceptible to voriconazole and posaconazole. In culture, colonies are wooly to cottony and are initially white, becoming smoky brown to green. Microscopically, conidia are one-celled, elongate, and pale brown and are borne singly or in balls on either short or long conidiophores (Figure 74-21).

Scedosporium prolificans (formerly *S. inflatum*) is a potentially virulent and highly aggressive emerging agent of hyalohyphomycosis. Although far less important than *Fusarium* or *S. apiospermum,* infections due to *S. prolificans* are associated with soft-tissue trauma and are characterized by widespread local invasion, tissue necrosis, and osteomyelitis. *S. prolificans* resembles *S. apiospermum* in macroscopic and microscopic morphology. The formation by *S. prolificans* of annelloconidia in wet clumps at the apices of annellides with swollen bases is the most useful characteristic in differentiating this organism from *S. apiospermum*. *S. prolificans* is considered to be resistant to virtually all of the systemically active antifungal agents, including the extended spectrum triazoles and the

echinocandins. Surgical resection remains the only definitive therapy for infection by *S. prolificans*.

Invasive infections due to *Acremonium* spp. are almost exclusively seen in patients with neutropenia, transplantation, or other immunodeficiency and present in a manner similar to that of *Fusarium*, with hematogenously disseminated skin lesions and positive blood cultures. Species of *Acremonium* are commonly found in soil, decaying vegetation, and decaying food. Colonies of *Acremonium* spp. are whitish gray or rose, with a velvety to cottony surface. The conidia may be single-celled in chains or a conidial mass arising from short, unbranched, tapered phialides. The optimal treatment for infections due to *Acremonium* spp. has not been established. Resistance is seen to amphotericin B, itraconazole, and the echinocandins. A recent report of successful treatment of a pulmonary infection due to *Acremonium strictum* with posaconazole suggests that the new triazoles may be useful in treatment of *Acremonium* infections.

Although uncommon, *Paecilomyces* spp. may cause invasive disease in organ and hematopoietic stem cell recipients, individuals with AIDS, and other immunocompromised patients. The portal of infection is often through breaks in the skin or intravascular catheters. Dissemination of the infection may be aided by adventitious conidiation that takes place within the tissues. The two most common species are *P. lilacinus* and *P. variotti*. Microscopically, the *Paecilomyces* spp. conidia are unicellular, ovoid to fusiform, and form chains. Phialides have a swollen base and a long, tapered neck. Susceptibility to amphotericin B is variable, with resistance seen with *P. lilacinus*. Voriconazole has been used successfully to treat both severe cutaneous infection and disseminated disease.

Trichoderma spp. are excellent examples of fungi previously labeled as nonpathogenic that have emerged as important opportunistic pathogens in immunocompromised patients and in patients undergoing peritoneal dialysis. Fatal disseminated disease due to *T. longibrachiatum* occurs in patients with hematologic malignancies, following BMT or solid organ transplantation. Most *Trichoderma* spp. show decreased susceptibility to amphotericin B, itraconazole, fluconazole, and flucytosine. Voriconazole appears to be active against the few isolates tested.

Scopulariopsis spp. are ubiquitous soil saprobes that have been rarely implicated in invasive human disease. *Scopulariopsis brevicaulis* is the most frequently isolated species. Infection is usually confined to the nails; however, serious deep infection has been noted in neutropenic leukemia patients and following blood and marrow transplantation. Both local and disseminated infections have been described, with involvement of the nasal septum, skin and soft tissues, blood, lungs, and brain. Diagnosis is made by culture and histopathology. *Scopulariopsis* spp. grow moderately to rapidly on standard mycologic media. Colonies are initially smooth, becoming granular to powdery with age. Conidiophores are simple or branched;

Figure 74–21. *Scedosporium apiospermum (Pseudallescheria boydii).* Lactophenol cotton blue preparation showing conidia and septate hyphae.

the conidiogenous cells are annellides that form singly or in clusters or may form a broomlike structure, or *scopula*, similar to that seen with *Penicillium* spp. The annelloconidia are smooth initially, become rough at maturity, are shaped like light bulbs, and form basipetal chains. *Scopulariopsis* spp. are usually resistant to itraconazole and moderately susceptible to amphotericin B. Invasive infections may require surgical and medical treatment and are often fatal.

Phaeohyphomycosis

Phaeohyphomycosis is defined as tissue infection caused by dematiaceous (pigmented) hyphae and/or yeasts. Infections due to dematiaceous fungi constitute a significant and increasingly prevalent group of opportunistic fungal diseases and may take the form of disseminated disease or become localized to the lung, paranasal sinuses, or central nervous system. Primary inoculation, resulting in localized subcutaneous infection, occurs commonly in underdeveloped countries and has been discussed in Chapter 72.

The dematiaceous fungi that have been documented to cause human infection encompass a large number of different genera; however, the more common causes of human infection include *Alternaria*, *Bipolaris*, *Cladosporium*, *Curvularia*, and *Exserohilum* species. Additionally, several of the dematiaceous fungi appear to be neurotropic: *Cladophialophora bantiana*, *Bipolaris spicifera*, *Exophiala* spp., *Wangiella dermatitidis*, *Ramichloridium obovoideum* and *Chaetomium atrobrunneum*. Brain abscess is the most common CNS presentation. *Bipolaris* spp. and *Exserohilum* spp. infections may present initially as sinusitis, which then extends into the CNS.

In tissue, hyphae with or without yeast forms are present. Most often, the pale brown to dark melanin-like pigment within the cell wall is apparent in H&E- or Papanicolaou-stained tissue (Figure 74-22). Staining with the Fontana-Masson technique (a melanin-specific stain) may help visualize the dematiaceous elements.

The dematiaceous fungi differ considerably in the clinical spectrum of infection and response to therapy. Furthermore, the different genera are not readily distinguished on histopathologic examination. Thus, an accurate microbiologic diagnosis based on culture of the infected tissue is important for optimal clinical management of infections due to these fungi.

Alternaria spp. are important causes of paranasal sinusitis in both healthy and immunocompromised individuals. Other sites of infection include skin and soft tissue, cornea, lower respiratory tract, and peritoneum. *Alternaria alternata* is the best-documented human pathogen in this genus. In culture, *Alternaria* colonies are rapidly growing, cottony, and gray to black. The conidiophores are usually solitary and simple or branched. The conidia develop in branching chains and are dematiaceous, muriform, and smooth or rough and taper toward the distal end with a short beak at their apices (Figure 74-23).

Cladosporium spp. usually cause superficial cutaneous infections but may cause deep infections as well. These fungi are rapidly growing with a velvety, olive gray to black colony. The conidiophores arise from the hyphae and are dematiaceous, tall, and branching. The conidia may be smooth or rough and single- to several-celled and form branching chains at the apex of the conidiophore.

Curvularia spp. are ubiquitous inhabitants of the soil and have been implicated in both disseminated and local infections. Sites of infection include endocarditis, local catheter-site infections, nasal septum and paranasal sinuses, lower respiratory tract, skin and subcutaneous tissues, bones, and cornea. In tissue, the hyphae may appear nonpigmented. Common species found to be etiologic agents of human infection include *C. geniculata*, *C. lunata*, *C. pallescens*, and *C. senegalensis*. In culture, colonies are rapidly growing,

Figure 74–22. *Cladophialophora bantiana* in tissue showing pigmented hyphae (H&E, ×400). *(From Marler LM et al: Mycology CD-ROM, Indiana Pathology Images, 2004.)*

Figure 74–23. *Alternaria* sp. Lactophenol cotton blue preparation showing darkly pigmented chains of muriform conidia.

Figure 74–24. *Bipolaris* sp. Lactophenol cotton blue preparation showing pigmented conidia *(black arrow)* borne on geniculate conidiophores *(red arrow)*.

Figure 74–25. *Pneumocystis jirovecii* in bronchoalveolar lavage fluid. Giemsa stain shows intracystic forms (×1000).

wooly, and gray to grayish black. Microscopically, the conidia are dematiaceous, solitary or in groups, septate, simple or branched, sympodial, and geniculate.

Infections caused by the genera *Bipolaris* and *Exserohilum* present similarly to those of *Aspergillus* spp., except that the disease progresses more slowly. Clinical presentations include dissemination with vascular invasion and tissue necrosis, involvement of the central nervous system and paranasal sinuses, and association with allergic bronchopulmonary disease. These organisms cause sinusitis in "normal" (atopic or asthmatic) hosts and more invasive disease in immunocompromised hosts. In culture, both *Bipolaris* and *Exserohilum* form rapidly growing, wooly, gray to black colonies. Microscopically, the conidiophores are sympodial and geniculate. The conidia are dematiaceous, oblong to cylindrical, and multicelled (Figure 74-24).

The optimal treatment of deep-seated phaeohyphomycosis has not yet been established, although it most often includes early administration of amphotericin B and aggressive surgical excision. Despite these efforts, phaeohyphomycosis does not respond well to treatment and relapses are common. Posaconazole has been used successfully to treat disseminated infection due to *Exophiala spinifera*. In those patients with brain abscesses, complete excision of the lesion has been associated with improved survival. Long-term triazole (posaconazole or voriconazole) therapy coupled with repeated surgical excision may prevent recurrences.

Pneumocystosis

Pneumocystis jirovecii (formerly *P. carinii*) is an organism that causes infection almost exclusively in debilitated and immunosuppressed patients, especially those with HIV

infection. It is the most common opportunistic infection among individuals with AIDS; however, the incidence has decreased considerably in recent years with the use of highly active antiretroviral therapy (HAART). Although previously considered to be a protozoan parasite, recent molecular and genetic evidence place it among the fungi (see Chapter 5).

The life cycle of *P. jirovecii* includes both sexual and asexual components. During the course of human infection, *P. jirovecii* may exist as free trophic forms (1.5 to 5 μm in diameter), as a uninucleate sporocyst (4 to 5 μm), or as a cyst (5 μm) containing up to 8 ovoid to fusiform intracystic bodies (Figure 74-25). Following rupture of the cyst, the cyst wall may be seen as an empty, collapsed structure (Figure 74-26).

Figure 74–26. *Pneumocystis jirovecii* in bronchoalveolar lavage fluid. GMS stain shows typical intact and collapsed cysts (×1000).

The reservoir for *P. jirovecii* in nature is unknown. Although airborne transmission has been documented experimentally among rodents, the rodent strains are genetically distinct from those of humans, making it unlikely that rodents serve as a zoonotic reservoir for human disease.

The respiratory tract is the main portal of entry for *P. jirovecii* in humans. Pneumonia is clearly the most common presentation of pneumocystosis, although extrapulmonary manifestations may be seen among AIDS patients. Involvement of lymph nodes, spleen, bone marrow, liver, small bowel, genitourinary tract, eyes, ears, skin, bone, and thyroid have been reported. Recent evidence suggests that both reactivation of quiescent old infection and primary infection can occur. Malnourished, debilitated, and immunosuppressed patients, especially AIDS patients with low CD4 counts (<200/μl), are at high risk of infection.

The hallmark of *P. jirovecii* infection is an interstitial pneumonitis with a mononuclear infiltrate composed predominantly of plasma cells. The onset of disease is insidious, with signs and symptoms including dyspnea, cyanosis, tachypnea, nonproductive cough, and fever. The radiographic appearance is typically one of diffuse interstitial infiltrates with a ground-glass appearance extending from the hilar region, but x-rays may appear normal or show nodules or cavitation. The mortality rate is high among untreated patients, and death is due to respiratory failure.

Histologically, a foamy exudate is seen within the alveolar spaces, with an intense interstitial infiltrate composed predominantly of plasma cells. Other patterns, including diffuse alveolar damage, noncaseating granulomatous inflammation, and infarct-like coagulative necrosis may also be seen.

The diagnosis of *P. jirovecii* infection is almost entirely based upon microscopic examination of clinical material, including bronchoalveolar lavage (BAL) fluid, bronchial brushing, induced sputum, and transbronchial or open-lung biopsy specimens. Examination of BAL fluid has been shown to have a sensitivity of 90% to 100% and usually precludes the need for transbronchial or open-lung biopsy. Microscopic examination of induced sputum may be useful in AIDS patients with a very high organism load; however, it has a 20% to 25% false-negative rate. A variety of histologic and cytologic stains have been used to detect *P. jirovecii*: GMS, Giemsa, PAS, toluidine blue, calcofluor, and immunofluorescence. The Giemsa stain demonstrates the trophic forms but does not stain the cyst wall (see Figure 74-25), whereas the GMS stain is specific for the cyst wall (see Figure 74-26). Immunofluorescent techniques stain both trophic forms and the cyst wall.

The cornerstone for both prophylaxis and treatment is trimethoprim-sulfamethoxazole. Alternative therapies have been used in AIDS patients; they include pentamidine, trimethoprim-dapsone, clindamycin-primaquine, atovaquone, and trimetrexate.

Case Study and Questions

George is a 45-year-old man who underwent an allogeneic stem cell transplant as part of his treatment for acute leukemia. The transplant went well, and following engraftment George was discharged from the hospital. During the course of his transplant, George's physicians placed him on antifungal prophylaxis with voriconazole, owing to concerns regarding aspergillosis, which had been a problem in the hospital over the past few years. Following discharge George did well, and his antifungal prophylaxis was continued; however, on a clinical visit on day 140 posttransplant, he was noted to have a rash and elevated liver function studies. About 1 week later, he began having bloody diarrhea, and his physician became concerned about graft versus host disease (GVHD). A rectal biopsy was performed, confirming GVHD, and George's immunosuppressive regimen was increased, as was his daily dose of voriconazole. The signs and symptoms of GVHD continued, and eventually George was readmitted to the hospital, where he was found to be confused, febrile, and short of breath. A chest x-ray showed a wedge-shaped infiltrate in the right lower lung field, and imaging studies of his sinuses showed bilateral opacification.

1. What is the differential diagnosis of this process?

2. What fungal pathogens would you be concerned about in an immunosuppressed individual receiving voriconazole prophylaxis?

3. How would you go about making a diagnosis?

4. What course of therapy would you undertake?

Bibliography

Anaissie EJ, McGinnis MR, Pfaller MA (eds): Clinical Mycology. New York, Churchill Livingstone, 2003.

Chandler FW, Watts JC: Pathologic Diagnosis of Fungal Infections. Chicago, ASCP, 1987.

Cohen J, Powderly WG: Infectious Diseases, 2nd ed. St Louis, Mosby, 2004.

Connor DH, et al: Pathology of Infectious Diseases. Stamford, Conn, Appleton & Lange, 1997.

Dignani MC, Solomkin JS, Anaissie EJ: *Candida*. In Anaissie EJ, McGinnis MR, Pfaller MA (eds): Clinical Mycology. New York, Churchill Livingstone, 2003.

Gudlagson O, et al: Attributable mortality of nosocomial candidemia, revisited. Clin Infect Dis 37:1172-1177, 2003.

Pannuti CS, et al: Nosocomial pneumonia in adult patients undergoing bone marrow transplantation: A 9-year study. J Clin Oncol 9:1, 1991.

Pfaller MA, Wenzel RP: The epidemiology of fungal infections. In Anaissie EJ, McGinnis MR, Pfaller MA (eds): Clinical Mycology. New York, Churchill Livingstone, 2003.

Pfaller MA, Diekema DJ: Twelve years of fluconazole in clinical practice: Global trends in species distribution and fluconazole susceptibility of bloodstream isolates of *Candida*. Clin Microbiol Infect 10(Suppl 1):11-23, 2004.

Pfaller MA, Diekema DJ: Rare and emerging opportunistic fungal pathogens: Concern for resistance beyond *Candida albicans* and *Aspergillus fumigatus*. J Clin Microbiol 42:4419, 2004.

Pfaller MA, Diekema DJ: Epidemiology of invasive candidiasis: A persistent public health problem. Clin Microbiol Rev 20:133, 2007.

Pfaller MA, et al: Results from the ARTEMIS DISK Global Antifungal Surveillance Study, 1997-2005: An 8.5 year analysis of susceptibilities of *Candida* and other yeast species to fluconazole and voriconazole by CLSI standardized disk diffusion testing. J Clin Microbiol 45:1735, 2007.

Pfaller MA, et al: Infections due to emerging non-*Candida,* non-*Cryptococcus* opportunistic yeast pathogens. Curr Fungal Infect Rep 1:53, 2007.

Viviani MA, Tortorano AM, Ajello L: *Cryptococcus.* In Anaissie EJ, McGinnis MR, Pfaller MA (eds): Clinical Mycology, New York, Churchill Livingstone, 2003.

Wey SB, et al: Hospital-acquired candidemia: Attributable mortality and excess length of stay. Arch Intern Med 148:2642-2645, 1988.

Wisplinghoff H, et al: Nosocomial bloodstream infections in U.S. hospitals: Analysis of 24,179 cases from a prospective nationwide surveillance study. Clin Infect Dis 39:309, 2004.

Fungal and Fungal-Like Infections of Unusual or Uncertain Etiology

Thus far we have discussed mycotic processes caused by reasonably well characterized fungi that may serve as colonizers, opportunistic pathogens, or true pathogens. Although many of these organisms have undergone minor taxonomic reclassification over time, they all share the characteristics of the Kingdom Fungi (see Chapter 5). One notable exception to this statement is *Pneumocystis jirovecii* (*carinii*), an organism formerly considered to be a protozoan and now classified as a fungus of the class Archiascomycetes based on molecular evidence (see Chapters 5 and 74). The fact that *P. jirovecii* cannot be grown on artificial media has complicated its characterization and assignment to the proper taxonomic category. In this chapter, we will discuss several infections that historically have been considered to represent fungal or "fungal-like" processes based on clinical and histopathologic presentation but, similar to *P. jirovecii*, have been difficult to classify because they cannot be grown on artificial media. In one instance, recent molecular evidence has suggested that an organism previously thought to be a fungus (*Rhinosporidium seeberi*) is in fact a protistan parasite. We also discuss two algal infections and an unusual infection due to the oomycete *Pythium insidiosum*. In addition to being unusual, as well as uncommon, these infections are all diagnosed based on detection of characteristic structures on histopathologic examination of tissue. A listing of the infections, the etiologic agents, and the typical morphology in tissue is provided in Table 75-1.

Adiaspiromycosis

In humans, adiaspiromycosis is a rare, self-limited, pulmonary infection caused by inhalation of the asexual conidia of the soil saprophytes *Emmonsia crescens* and *E. parva*. Synonyms include **haplomycosis** or **adiasporosis**.

Morphology

The fungi, *E. crescens* and *E. parva*, grow as molds in culture at room temperature and in nature. The hyphae are septate and branched. The small (2-4 μm) aleurioconidia are borne on conidiophores that arise at right angles to the vegetative hyphae. Upon incubation at 40° C in vitro, or when introduced into the lungs, the conidia transform into spherical adiaconidia which then undergo massive enlargement but show no evidence of replication (e.g., budding, endospore formation).

When mature, the adiaconidia are thick-walled spherules measuring 200 to 400 μm or more in diameter (Figure 75-1; see Table 75-1). The walls of the spherule are refractile, 20 to 70 μm thick, and when stained with hematoxylin-eosin (H&E) stain, comprise two layers: a narrow, outer, eosinophilic layer containing periodic fenestrations; and a broad, hyaline, inner layer composed predominantly of chitin (see Figure 75-1). The conidial walls stain with Gomori methenamine silver (GMS), periodic acid–Schiff (PAS), and the Gridley fungus stains but not with mucicarmine (Table 75-2). In human lung tissue, the adiaconidia are usually empty but may contain small eosinophilic globules along the inner surface of the walls (see Figure 75-1).

Epidemiology

Although human adiaspiromycosis is uncommon, the infection is prevalent in rodents worldwide. Likewise, the fungus may be found in nature, predominantly in temperate zones. Human disease has been reported from France, Czechoslovakia, Russia, Honduras, Guatemala, Venezuela, and Brazil. Rodents may serve as a zoonotic reservoir for the disease. The likely mode of infection is by inhalation of fungal conidia aerosolized by contaminated soil.

Table 75—1. Morphologic Features of Fungal and Fungal-Like Infections of Unusual or Uncertain Etiology

Disease	Etiologic Agent(s)	Typical Morphology in Tissue	Usual Host Reaction
Adiaspiromycosis	*Emmonsia* spp.	Large adiaconidia, 200-400 μm diameter with thick (20-70 μm) walls; see Figure 75-1	Granulomatous fibrotic and noncaseating
Chlorellosis	*Chlorella* sp. (chlorophyllous green algae)	Unicellular, endosporulating, round organisms, 4-15 μm diameter, containing multiple cytoplasmic granules (chloroplasts); lesions are green pigmented; see Figure 75-2	Pyogranulomatous
Lacaziosis (Lobomycosis)	*Lacazia loboi (Loboa loboi)*	Spherical, budding yeasts, 5-12 μm diameter, that form chains of cells connected by tubelike structures; secondary budding may be present; see Figure 75-3	Granulomatous
Protothecosis	*Prototheca wickerhamii, P. zopfii* (achlorophyllous green algae)	Spherical, oval, or polyhedral spherules, 2-25 μm diameter, containing 2-20 endospores when mature; see Figure 75-5	Variable; no reaction to granulomatous
Pythiosis insidiosi	*Pythium insidiosum* (not a true fungus; belongs to Class Oomycetes)	Hyphae and short hyphal fragments that are hyaline, thin-walled, pauciseptate, irregularly branched, 5-7 μm wide with nonparallel contours; angioinvasive; see Fig. 75-6	Granulomatous, necrotizing, suppurative, arteritis
Rhinosporidiosis	*Rhinosporidium seeberi* (aquatic protistan parasite of the Mesomycetozoa clade)	Large sporangia (100-350 μm diameter) with thin walls (3-5 μm) that enclose numerous endospores (6-8 μm diameter) with a zonal distribution; see Figures 75-7 and 75-8	Nonspecific chronic inflammatory or granulomatous

Data from Chandler FW, Watts JC: Pathologic Diagnosis of Fungal Infections. Chicago, ASCP, 1987; Connor DH, et al: Pathology of Infectious Diseases, vol 2. Stamford, Conn, Appleton & Lange, 1997.

Clinical Syndromes

As with many fungal infections, most cases of documented adiaspiromycosis have been asymptomatic. Pulmonary nodules may be detected radiographically or incidentally at autopsy or in surgical specimens of lung removed for another reason.

Figure 75—1. Pulmonary adiaspiromycosis. The hematoxylin-eosin (H&E) stain defines three layers in the wall of the adiaconidium. Each adiaconidium has evoked a fibrogranulomatous response (H&E, ×40). *(From Connor DH, et al: Pathology of Infectious Diseases, vol 2. Stamford, Conn., Appleton & Lange, 1997.)*

Three forms of human adiaspiromycosis have been recognized: solitary granuloma, localized granulomatous disease, and diffuse, disseminated granulomatous disease. Patients with the disseminated granulomatous form of pulmonary adiaspiromycosis may experience fever, cough, and progressive dyspnea due to compression and displacement of distal airways and alveolar parenchyma by the expanding granulomas. Fungal replication in the lungs does not occur, and dissemination to extrapulmonary sites has not been reported. The severity of the disease appears to be entirely commensurate with the number of conidia inhaled.

Laboratory Diagnosis

The diagnosis of adiaspiromycosis is established by histopathologic examination of affected lung and identification of the characteristic adiaconidia. Each adiaconidium is surrounded by an epithelioid and giant-cell granulomatous response, which is further encompassed by a dense capsule of fibrous tissue (see Figure 75-1). All of the granulomas are at a similar stage of development, reflecting a one-time exposure without subsequent replication within the lung.

The spherules represented by the adiaconidia should not be confused with those of *Coccidioides immitis* or

Table 75–2. Comparative Morphologic Features of Fungi and Fungal-Like Organisms That Appear as Large Spherules in Tissue

Feature	Organisms		
	Coccidioides immitis	*Rhinosporidium seeberi*[a]	*Emmonsia* spp.[b]
External diameter of spherule (μm)	20-200	10-350	200-400
Thickness of spherule wall (μm)	1-2	3-5	20-70
Diameter of endospores (μm)	2-5	6-10[c]	None
Pigmentation	None	None	None
Hyphae or arthroconidia	Rare	None	None
Host reaction	**Necrotic granulomas**	**Mucosal polyps with acute and chronic inflammation**	**Fibrotic granulomas**
Growth in culture	+	−	±[d]
Special stain reactions			
GMS	+	+	+
PAS	+	+	+
Mucicarmine	−	+	−

Adapted from Chandler FW, Watts JC: Pathologic Diagnosis of Fungal Infections. Chicago, ASCP, 1987.
[a]*Not a fungus. Newly classified as an aquatic protistan parasite of the Mesomycetozoa clade.*
[b]*Adiaconidia.*
[c]*Endospores arranged in characteristic zonal distribution. Mature endospores contain distinctive eosinophilic globules.*
[d]*Grows as a mold on agar medium. Organism not recoverable from tissue.*

Rhinosporidium seeberi, two other organisms that produce large spherules in tissue (see Table 75-2). In contrast to *C. immitis*, the adiaconidia of *Emmonsia* spp. are much larger, have a thicker wall, and do not contain endospores. The sporangia of *R. seeberi* are distinguished by the zonation of the sporangiospores and the distinctive eosinophilic globules seen within the mature sporangiospores (see Table 75-2). No other fungus of medical importance has walls as thick as those of the adiaconidia of *Emmonsia* spp. Culture of infected tissue is not useful, since the adiaconidia do not represent a replicative form of the fungus.

Treatment

Human pulmonary adiaspiromycosis is a self-limited infection. Specific antifungal therapy is not necessary.

Chlorellosis

Chlorellosis is an infection of humans and animals caused by a unicellular green algae of the genus *Chlorella*. In contrast to *Prototheca*, another algae that causes human infection, *Chlorella* contains chloroplasts, which give the lesions of chlorellosis a distinct green color. Most infections with this organism occur in sheep and cattle. A single human infection has been reported thus far.

Morphology

Chlorella spp. are unicellular, ovoid, spherical, or polygonal, 4 to 5 μm in diameter, and reproduce by endosporulation. The organisms contain numerous green chloroplasts, which appear as cytoplasmic granules. The chloroplasts contain starch granules, which stain intensely with GMS, PAS, and Gridley fungal stains. The cell walls may appear doubly contoured (Figure 75-2; see Table 75-1). *Chlorella* spp. reproduce asexually by internal septation and cytoplasmic cleavage,

Figure 75–2. *Chlorella* sp. showing intracellular chloroplasts and doubly contoured cell wall (GMS, ×400). *(From Connor DH, et al: Pathology of Infectious Diseases, vol 2. Stamford, Conn, Appleton & Lange, 1997.)*

producing up to 20 daughter cells (sporangiospores) within the sporangium (parent cell). Upon maturation, the outer wall of the sporangium ruptures, releasing the sporangiospores, each of which goes on to produce sporangiospores of its own.

Epidemiology

The single human case took place in Nebraska and resulted from exposure of a surgical wound to river water. Infections in domestic (sheep and cattle) and wild animals (beaver) range from lymph node and deep organ involvement to cutaneous and subcutaneous lesions, presumably related to exposure to water containing the organism.

Clinical Syndromes

As noted above, the human case of chlorellosis involved a healing surgical wound contaminated with river water. The wound subsequently drained a greenish yellow exudate. The infection was cured by repeated surgical débridement over a 10-month period. In animals, fresh lesions in liver, lymph nodes, and subcutaneous tissue are green on gross examination, and smears reveal organisms that contain green refractile granules (chloroplasts).

Laboratory Diagnosis

Infections due to *Chlorella* spp. may be diagnosed by culture and by histopathologic examination of infected tissue. The organism grows well on most solid media, producing bright green colonies. Wet mounts of wound exudate or touch preparations of infected tissue reveal ovoid, endosporulating cells with characteristic green cytoplasmic granules representing chloroplasts. In tissue, the cells stain well with GMS and PAS but not H&E stains. They may be distinguished histopathologically from *Prototheca* by the intracellular chloroplasts.

Treatment

Treatment in the only human case of chlorellosis consisted of repeat débridement, irrigation with Dakin solution, and gauze packing and removal for drainage and granulation. Alternatively, amphotericin B therapy combined with administration of tetracycline has proven efficacious in the treatment of protothecosis and may be useful for chlorellosis as well.

Lacaziosis (Lobomycosis) Clinical Case 75-1

Lacaziosis is a chronic fungal infection of the skin caused by *Lacazia loboi* (formerly *Loboa loboi*). *L. loboi* is currently classified as an ascomycete fungus in the order Onygenales

Clinical Case 75-1. Lacaziosis

Elsayed, et al. (Emerg Infect Dis 10:715-718, 2004) described a case of lacaziosis (lobomycosis) in a Canadian geologist. The patient presented to her dermatologist with a slowly growing, 1.5-cm diameter, dusky red, nontender, plaquelike lesion surrounded by keloidal scar on the posterior aspect of her right upper arm. It was located at the site of a scar from a previous excision attempt of a similar lesion 2 years earlier. The original lesion was first noticed while the patient was visiting Southeast Asia in 1996, although she did not seek medical attention until returning to Canada 1 year later. At that time, coccidioidomycosis was diagnosed, based on a history of travel to an endemic region and on the presence of oval, yeastlike organisms in histologic sections. However, *Coccidioides immitis* was never cultured from the lesion, and serologic studies for this infection remained negative. She remained well until a new lesion reappeared at the site of the scar and gradually increased in size. The patient had an extensive travel history, including prolonged stays in Mexico, Costa Rica, South America, Indonesia, and the Philippines. During her travels, she generally lived in rural camps and had extensive exposure to freshwater, soil, and underground caves. Her medical history included episodes of amoebic dysentery, dengue fever, and intestinal helminthiasis but was otherwise unremarkable. Biopsied specimens of the new lesion were obtained and submitted for pathologic and microbiologic examination. The hematoxylin- and eosin-stained sections showed a diffuse, superficial and deep, granulomatous dermatitis with multinucleated giant cells. Intracellular and extracellular unstained fungal cells with thick refractile walls were seen. The fungal cells stained strongly with periodic acid–Schiff and GMS stains; cells were spherical or lemon shaped, approximately 10 microns in diameter, and uniform in size. They were arranged as single cells or in short, budding chains joined by narrow, tubelike bridges. The organisms were not cultivatable. Fungal morphology was consistent with *Lacazia (Loboa) loboi*. The lesion was completely excised, with no subsequent recurrence. This disease should be suspected in patients with single or multiple keloidal skin lesions, particularly if they have traveled to remote areas of Latin America.

and the family Ajellomycetaceae. The disease is seen primarily in the South- and Central-American tropics. Natural infection occurs only in humans and dolphins, although it has been reproduced experimentally by injecting infected tissue into hamsters and armadillos. The organism has never been cultured in vitro.

Morphology

L. loboi is spherical to oval and yeastlike in appearance. The fungi are 6 to 12 μm in diameter and have a thick, double-refractile cell wall. *L. loboi* reproduces by sequential budding and usually forms chains of cells connected by narrow, tubelike bridges (Figure 75-3). Some of the cells may have one or two secondary buds and may be mistaken for the "pilot's wheel" form of *Paracoccidioides brasiliensis*. *L. loboi* is usually intracellular, although extracellular forms may be seen.

Figure 75—3. *Lacazia loboi.* The fungi form a single chain with individual cells joined by tubelike bridges (Gridley, ×400). *(From Chandler FW, Watts JC: Pathologic Diagnosis of Fungal Infections. Chicago, ASCP, 1987.)*

Figure 75—4. Multiple keloid-like lesions of lacaziosis. *(From Chandler FW, Watts JC: Pathologic Diagnosis of Fungal Infections. Chicago, ASCP, 1987.)*

Epidemiology

The human disease is endemic in the tropical regions of Central and South America and has been reported in central and western Brazil, Bolivia, Columbia, Costa Rica, Ecuador, Guyana, French Guiana, Mexico, Panama, Peru, Surinam, and Venezuela. Isolated cases have been reported from Holland, and a single case has been reported recently in the United States in a patient with a history of travel to Venezuela.

L. loboi is believed to be a saprophyte of soil or vegetation, and lacaziosis predominates in tropical regions with thick vegetation, such as the Amazon rain forests. Cutaneous trauma is believed to be the mode of infection. A plant reservoir has not been identified.

Given the fact that lacaziosis occurs in marine dolphins and marine freshwater dolphins, an aquatic habitat is likely as well. Infection among dolphins has been reported for Florida, the Texas coast, the Spanish-French coast, the South Brazilian coast, and the Surinam River estuary. One instance of dolphin-to-human transmission has been reported; however, there is no evidence of human-to-human transmission.

Lacaziosis occurs primarily in men, or in women who are involved in farming and jungle clearing. Farmers, miners, hunters, and rubber plant workers have an increased incidence of disease. There is no racial predilection, and lobomycosis affects all age groups, with the peak age of onset being 20 to 40 years.

Clinical Syndromes

Lacaziosis is characterized by slowly developing cutaneous nodules of varying size and shape (Figure 75-4). The dermal lesions are polymorphic, ranging from macules, papules, keloidal nodules, and plaques to verrucous and ulcerated lesions, all of which may be present in a single patient (see Figure 75-4). The nodular keloid-like lesion is the most common. The disease is characterized by a long dormancy period of months to years. The increase in the number and size of lesions is also a slow process, progressing over a period of 40 to 50 years. Lesions tend to arise on traumatized areas of skin, such as the face, ears, arms, legs, and feet. The disease does not involve mucous membranes or internal organs. Local cutaneous spread may occur through autoinoculation. Aside from occasional pruritus and hypesthesia or anesthesia of the affected area, patients are asymptomatic. There are no systemic manifestations of the disease.

Laboratory Diagnosis

Diagnosis is based on demonstrating the presence of the characteristic yeast cells in lesion exudate or tissue sections. Biopsy reveals a dispersed granulomatous infiltrate, along with numerous fungal forms in the dermis and subcutaneous tissue. The granuloma consists primarily of giant cells, macrophages, and epithelioid cells. Both the giant cells and macrophages contain fungi that have been phagocytosed.

L. loboi stains intensely with both GMS and PAS stains. H&E stain reveals the thick, doubly contoured, hyaline cell wall and one or more hematoxylinophilic nuclei.

Although grossly the lesions of lacaziosis resemble keloids, microscopically, keloids have marked fibrosis, which is not the case with lacaziosis. Similarly, keloids lack granulomas and fungal elements. The morphology and pattern of budding of *L. loboi* are distinctive and should not be confused with that of *P. brasiliensis* (multiple buds, variable size), *Blastomyces dermatitidis* and *Histoplasma capsulatum* var. *duboisii* (no chains of cells) or *Sporothrix schenckii* and *H. capsulatum* var. *capsulatum* (both smaller, 2 to 8 μm vs. 5 to 12 μm). The latter fungi will also grow in culture, whereas *L. loboi* has never been cultured in vitro.

Treatment

Surgical excision of localized lesions is the optimal therapy. More widespread disease usually recurs when treated surgically and does not respond to antifungal therapy. Clofazimine has been used in these situations, but at this time medical treatment of lacaziosis is not satisfactory.

Protothecosis

Protothecosis is an infection of humans and animals caused by achlorophyllous algae of the genus *Prototheca*. These organisms belong to the same family as the green algae of the genus *Chlorella*. Two species, *P. wickerhamii* and *P. zopfii*, are known to cause infection. Three forms of human protothecosis have been described: (1) cutaneous, (2) olecranon bursitis, and (3) disseminated.

Morphology

The prototheciae are unicellular, oval, or spherical organisms that reproduce asexually by internal septation and irregular cleavage within hyaline sporangia. Each sporangium contains between 2 and 20 sporangiospores arranged in a "morula" configuration (Figure 75-5). The sporangiospores are released following rupture of the sporangium and in turn develop into mature endosporulating forms. The cells measure 3 to 30 μm in diameter and differ from those of *Chlorella* by the lack of chloroplasts. Prototheciae differ from fungi by the lack of glucosamine in their cell walls. The two species of *Prototheca* that cause human disease differ from one another in size: *P. wickerhamii* measures 3 to 15 μm in diameter, whereas *P. zopfii* measures 7 to 30 μm in diameter. Both species are readily stained with PAS, GMS, and the Gridley fungus stain (see Figure 75-5) and are gram-positive organisms.

Figure 75—5. *Prototheca wickerhamii.* Single and endosporulating algal cells that are readily demonstrated with the PAS stain. A classic "morula" form is present (×1000).

Epidemiology

Prototheca spp. are ubiquitous environmental saprobes that have been isolated from grass, soil, water, and both wild and domestic animals. Human protothecosis has been reported on all continents with the exception of Antarctica.

Clinical Syndromes

At least half of all cases of protothecosis are simple cutaneous infections. For the most part, these infections occur in patients who are immunocompromised because of immunosuppressive therapy, AIDS, malnutrition, renal or hepatic disease, cancer, or autoimmune disorders. Lesions usually arise in areas exposed to traumatic implantation and present in an indolent fashion as nodules, papules, or as an eczematoid eruption.

Those individuals presenting with olecranon bursitis are usually not immunocompromised, but most report some sort of penetrating or nonpenetrating trauma to the affected elbow. Signs and symptoms of olecranon bursitis usually occur several weeks after the trauma and include mild induration of the bursa, tenderness, erythema, and production of a variable amount of serosanguineous fluid.

Disseminated protothecosis is rare but has been reported in individuals with no known immunologic deficiency. One patient with visceral protothecosis presented with abdominal pain and abnormal liver function studies that were initially considered to be due to cholangitis. The patient had multiple peritoneal nodules that resembled metastatic cancer but were in fact manifestations of protothecosis. Another patient presented with prototheca lesions on the forehead and nose.

Laboratory Diagnosis

Prototheca spp. grow easily on a wide variety of solid media at 30° C to 37° C. Colonies are yeastlike, white, and creamy in appearance and consistency. A wet mount of the culture material may be stained with lactophenol cotton blue to reveal the characteristic sporangia and sporangiospores. The organisms are quite metabolically active and may be identified to species using one of several commercially available yeast identification panels to determine the carbohydrate assimilation profile.

On histopathologic examination of infected tissue, *Prototheca* spp. appear as sporangiospores that are wedge shaped and arranged in a radial or "morula" pattern within the sporangium (see Figure 75-5). The organisms are best visualized by stains used to demonstrate fungi in tissue: the GMS, PAS, and Gridley fungus procedures. In addition to the size differences noted above, the two species of *Prototheca* differ in that *P. wickerhamii* tends to form very symmetrical morula forms, whereas these forms are rare with *P. zopfii*, which exhibits more random internal divisions. The inflammatory response in protothecosis is predominantly granulomatous.

Treatment

Treatment of olecranon bursitis usually involves bursectomy. Repeated drainage has failed; however, drainage coupled with local instillation of amphotericin B was curative in one patient. Treatment of cutaneous protothecosis with a variety of topical and systemic antibacterial, antifungal, and anti-protozoal agents has been unsuccessful. Local excision coupled with topical amphotericin B, systemic tetracycline, and systemic ketoconazole has proven useful, despite keto-conazole-related hepatotoxicity. Disseminated protothecosis has been treated with systemic antifungal agents; both amphotericin B and ketoconazole have been used.

Pythiosis Insidiosi (Clinical Case 75-2)

Pythiosis insidiosi is a "fungal-like" infection of humans and animals caused by the Oomycete *Pythium insidiosum*. Although described as an "aquatic fungus" this organism is not a true fungus. It belongs to the Kingdom Stramenopila, Phylum Oomycota, Class Oomycetes, and Family Pythiaceae. In humans, pythiosis is a cutaneous and subcutaneous vascular process marked by rapidly developing granulomatous lesions leading to progressive arterial insufficiency, tissue infarction, aneurysms, and occasionally death. In animals (cats, dogs, horses, cattle), it is an osseous, subcutaneous, or pulmonary infection. Dogs and horses may also present with intestinal infection.

Morphology

P. insidiosum grows as white colonies with submerged vegetative hyphae and short aerial hyphae on solid culture medium. As this organism is a plant pathogen, it requires water cultures containing the appropriate leaves in order to produce zoosporangia and zoospores in vitro. In nature, it produces biflagellate zoospores that attach and penetrate the leaves of various grasses and water lilies. The zoospores have a strong tropism for skin and hair, as well as water lily and grass leaves. If zoospores contact injured tissue, they encyst, form germ tubes that produce hyphae, and cause invasive disease.

In tissue, *P. insidiosum* exists as hyaline, pauciseptate, thin-walled hyphae or hyphal fragments that branch infrequently. The hyphal elements are 5 to 7 µm wide with nonparallel contours and superficially resemble those of Zygomycetes (Figure 75-6). Like the Zygomycetes, *P. insidiosum* is angioinvasive and stains poorly with GMS and other special stains for fungi.

Epidemiology

P. insidiosum grows in aquatic to wet environments in tropical to subtropical regions. Reports of pythiosis have come from Australia, Costa Rica, India, Japan, New Guinea, Thailand, and the United States.

Clinical Case 75-2. Pythiosis

Bosco, et al. (Emerg Infect Dis 11:715-718, 2005) describe a case of pythiosis in a 49-year-old Brazilian man. The patient was admitted to the hospital for the treatment of a skin lesion on his leg, initially diagnosed as cutaneous zygomycosis. The patient stated that a small pustule developed on his left leg 3 months earlier, 1 week after he fished in a lake with standing water. The pustule was initially diagnosed as bacterial cellulitis; it was treated with intravenous antibiotics, with no improvement. A biopsy of the lesion showed a suppurative granulomatous inflammation associated with several nonseptate hyphae (shown by GMS stain), a finding that led to the diagnosis of zygomycosis. The treatment was changed to amphotericin B. After receiving 575 mg (cumulative dosage) of amphotericin B plus 2 surgical débridements, the patient showed only slight improvement; he was then transferred to another hospital. At admission, the physical exam showed a pre-tibial ulcer 15 cm in diameter with an infiltrating and nodular proximal border. Serum chemistries showed azotemia, hypokalemia, and anemia as adverse effects of the amphotericin B treatment. His white blood cell count was 4,200/cubic mm with 9% eosinophils. His blood glucose was normal and an HIV serology was negative. Results of a second biopsy again suggested zygomycosis. The patient received itraconazole and potassium iodide with no significant improvement. Attempts to isolate the organism in the laboratory failed. With progression of the disease, an extensive surgical débridement was considered. A course of amphotericin B was begun, and the lesion was débrided down to and including the fascia lata. A skin graft was placed and produced an acceptable recovery. Tissue was submitted for culture and molecular testing, using the generic primers for fungal internal transcribed spacer (ITS) regions of rDNA. Cultures grew colorless colonies which on microscopic examination showed broad, branched, and sparsely septate hyphae without fruiting bodies, which were later identified as *Pythium insidiosum*. PCR followed by sequencing of the ITS amplicons gave results showing 100% identity with *Pythium insidiosum*. This case illustrates the clinical and diagnostic issues surrounding human pythiosis.

Figure 75–6. *Pythium insidiosum* invading an arterial wall. Infrequently septate, weakly stained hyphae and hyphal fragments resemble those of Zygomycetes (GMS, ×160). *(From Connor DH, et al: Pathology of Infectious Diseases, vol 2. Stamford, Conn, Appleton & Lange, 1997.)*

Clinical Syndromes

Human disease due to *P. insidiosum* has occurred in patients with thalassemia who developed pythiosis insidiosi of the lower limbs. The disease process was marked by progressive ischemia of the lower limbs, necrosis, thrombosis of major arteries due to fungal invasion, gangrene, aneurism formation, and ultimately fatal hemorrhage. Orbital pythiosis has been misdiagnosed as a zygomycotic fungal infection. Less serious forms of the infection include keratitis and localized cutaneous infections following injury.

In horses, pythiosis presents as localized inflammation and necrotic sores of the legs and lower abdomen with necrotic cores. Septic arthritis, osteitis, and tenosynovitis are also common.

Laboratory Diagnosis

The organism may be isolated from fresh clinical material seeded onto mycologic medium such as Sabouraud glucose agar. Demonstration of biflagellate zoospores may be accomplished using water cultures with grass or lily bait incubated at 37° C for 1 hour.

Histopathologic examination of infected tissue shows a necrotizing arteritis and thrombosis. Vascular invasion by sparsely septate, irregularly branched hyphae is seen (see Figure 75-6). The acute perivascular inflammatory reaction is eventually replaced by granulomas that contain sparse hyphae and hyphal fragments. The hyphal elements of *P. insidiosum* may be surrounded by the eosinophilic Splendore-Hoeppli phenomenon. Pythiosis insidiosi in humans must be differentiated from cutaneous and subcutaneous zygomycosis, sporotrichosis, mycetoma, and neoplasms.

Treatment

Although potassium iodide has been used to treat cutaneous infections, medical treatment of pythiosis insidiosi is generally not effective. Surgical débridement and excision of infected tissue has been used with some success. There is some evidence that azole antifungal agents such as fluconazole, ketoconazole, itraconazole, and miconazole exhibit in vitro activity against this organism. A case of orbital pythiosis responded well to a combination of itraconazole and terbinafine, although this combination has not been useful in other cases of pythiosis. Immunotherapy has been useful in the treatment of equine pythiosis and has a 55% cure rate in human disease.

Rhinosporidiosis (Clinical Case 75-3)

Rhinosporidiosis is a granulomatous disease of humans and animals that is characterized by the development of polyps that primarily affect the nasopharynx and the ocular conjunctiva of infected individuals. The disease is

---

Clinical Case 75-3. Rhinosporidiosis

Gaines and Clay (South Med J 89:65-67, 1996) describe three cases of rhinosporidiosis in young boys who had not traveled outside of the United States. In fact, there was no history of their having traveled outside of the state of Georgia. All of the patients lived in rural areas in the northeast portion of the state. One had a polypoid conjunctival lesion, and the other 2 had nasal polyps. In each case, the lesions were excised, and histopathologic examination revealed structures morphologically typical of *Rhinosporidium seeberi*. No other treatment was given, and follow-up showed no evidence of recurrence. Despite the very rare nature of these cases, the distinctive appearance of the developmental forms of *R. seeberi* in histopathologic sections is diagnostic.

---

caused by *Rhinosporidium seeberi*, an organism with a confusing taxonomic history. This organism has been considered to be a protozoan, a fungus, and most recently has been placed in a novel clade of aquatic protistan parasites, the Mesomycetozoa. Since *R. seeberi* will not grow in synthetic media, this reclassification was based on sequence analysis of the 18S small-subunit ribosomal DNA (rDNA) of this organism. This analysis placed *R. seeberi* among the Mesomycetozoa (formerly DRIP: *Dermocystidium*, Rosette agent, *Ichthyophonus*, and *Psorospermium*), a clade of fish parasites that form a branch of the evolutionary tree near the animal-fungal divergence.

Morphology

Given the fact that *R. seeberi* will not grow on artificial media, the morphologic descriptions are entirely based on the organism as it appears in infected tissue. Two developmental forms of *R. seeberi* are seen in tissue: the large spherical form, or sporangia, and the smaller trophocyte. The sporangium is considered the mature form of the organism and measures 100 to 350 μm in diameter. The sporangial wall is 3 to 5 μm thick and is composed of an inner hyaline layer and thin outer eosinophilic layer. The sporangium contains numerous sporangiospores (endospores) arranged in a characteristic zonal formation whereby the small, flattened, uninucleate immature sporangiospores (1 to 2 μm) form a crescentic mass at the periphery of one wall of the sporangiospore, with the larger maturing and mature sporangiospores arranged sequentially toward the center (Figure 75-7). The mature sporangiospores range in size from 5 to 10 μm in diameter and contain multiple refractile cytoplasmic globules. This zonal arrangement of immature, maturing, and fully mature sporangiospores is diagnostic of this pathogen and distinguishes it from other spherical endosporulating organisms in the tissue (see Table 75-2).

The trophocytes are considered to develop directly from sporangiospores that have been released from the sporangium. The trophocytes range in size from 10 to 100 μm in diameter and have refractile eosinophilic walls (2 to 3 μm thick), granular cytoplasm, and a round, pale nucleus with

Figure 75—7. Mature sporangium of *Rhinosporidium seeberi* showing the zonal arrangement of immature, maturing, and fully mature sporangiospores (H&E, ×480). *(From Chandler FW, Watts JC: Pathologic Diagnosis of Fungal Infections. Chicago, ASCP, 1987.)*

a prominent nucleolus. Ultimately, the trophocytes enlarge and transform into mature sporangia through a process of endosporulation.

The walls of both the sporangia and sporangiospores stain with both GMS and PAS fungal stains. In addition, the walls of the sporangiospores and the inner wall of the sporangium stain positively with the mucin stain, mucicarmine (Figure 75-8; see Table 75-2).

Epidemiology

Approximately 90% of all known cases of rhinosporidiosis occur in India and Sri Lanka. The disease also occurs in the Americas, Europe, and Africa. The natural habitat and the extent of distribution of *R. seeberi* in nature are unknown. The disease occurs primarily in young men 20 to 40 years old and appears to be associated with both rural and aquatic environments. There is no evidence that rhinosporidiosis is contagious.

Figure 75—8. Mature sporangium of R. *seeberi*. The walls of the mature sporangiospores are carminophilic, (Mayer mucicarmine, ×100). *(From Connor DH, et al: Pathology of Infectious Diseases, vol 2. Stamford, Conn, Appleton & Lange, 1997.)*

Clinical Syndrome

Rhinosporidiosis manifests as slow-growing polypoid or tumor-like masses, usually of the nasal mucosa or conjunctiva. Lesions may also be seen in the paranasal sinuses, larynx, and external genitalia. Secondary spread to surrounding skin is thought to result from autoinoculation by scratching. In most patients, the disease remains localized, and symptoms are primarily nasal obstruction and bleeding due to polyp formation. Limited systemic dissemination has been reported but is rare.

Laboratory Diagnosis

The diagnosis of rhinosporidiosis is made by histopathologic examination of the affected tissue. The distinctive appearance of the trophocytes and sporangia in routine H&E stained sections is diagnostic (see Figure 75-7). Although other organisms that occur in tissue in the form of large spherules may be mistaken for *R. seeberi*, they are usually easily differentiated from this organism by consideration of the tissue involved and the morphologic and staining characteristics of the spherule and the endospores (see Table 75-2).

Treatment

The only effective form of treatment is surgical excision of the lesions. Recurrences are common, especially in mucosal sites such as the oropharynx and paranasal sinuses, where complete excision is often difficult to achieve.

Case Study and Questions

Jim is a 50-year-old ex-smoker who went to his family physician for an annual physical examination. In the process, a chest x-ray was performed, which revealed a nodule in the left upper lobe of the lung. Because of his age and prior smoking history, Jim underwent a thoracotomy, and the nodule was excised. Pathologic examination revealed fibrosis and several large spherical structures but no evidence of cancer.

1. What is the differential diagnosis of a solitary lung nodule?

2. Describe how one can differentiate the spherules of *Rhinosporidium seeberi* from those of *Coccidioides immitis* and *Emmonsia* spp.

3. Describe the disease process of adiaspiromycosis.

4. Which of the following agents can be identified using commercially available yeast identification systems?

    a. *Lacazia loboi*

    b. *Pythium insidiosum*

    c. *Rhinosporidium seeberi*

    d. *Prototheca wickerhamii*

5. How are the agents of chlorellosis and protothecosis different from one another? How are they similar?

Bibliography

Burns RA, et al: Report of the first human case of lobomycosis in the United States. J Clin Microbiol 38:1283-1285, 2000.

Chandler FW, Watts JC: Pathologic Diagnosis of Fungal Infections. Chicago, ASCP, 1987.

Connor DH, et al: Pathology of Infectious Diseases, vol 2. Stamford, Conn, Appleton & Lange, 1997.

Fredericks DN, et al: *Rhinosporidium seeberi*: A human pathogen from a novel group of aquatic protistan parasites. Emerg Infect Dis 6:273-282, 2000.

Herr RA, et al: Phylogenetic analysis of *Rhinosporidium seeberi*'s 18S small-subunit ribosomal DNA groups this pathogen among members of the protoctistan Mesomycetozoa clade. J Clin Microbiol 37:2750-2754, 1999.

Krajaejun T, et al: Clinical and epidemiological analysis of human pythiosis in Thailand. Clin Infect Dis 43:569, 2006.

Mendoza L, et al: Orbital pythiosis: A nonfungal disease mimicking orbital mycotic infections, with a retrospective review of the literature. Mycoses 47:14, 2004.

Mendoza L: *Lacazia*, *Pythium*, and *Rhinosporidium*. In Murray PR, et al. (eds): Manual of Clinical Microbiology, 9th ed. Washington, DC, ASM Press, 2007.

Taborda PR, et al: *Lacazia loboi* gen. nov., comb. nov., the etiologic agent of lobomycosis. J Clin Microbiol 37:2031-2033, 1999.

Mycotoxins and Mycotoxicoses

In addition to their role as opportunistic pathogens, filamentous fungi can produce toxins that have been implicated in a variety of illnesses and clinical syndromes in humans and in animals. These mycotoxins are secondary fungal metabolites that cause diseases, known collectively as *mycotoxicoses*, following ingestion, inhalation, or direct contact with the toxin (Figure 76-1). Mycotoxicoses may manifest as acute or chronic disease, ranging from rapid death to tumor formation. In this regard, mycotoxicoses are analogous to the pathologies caused by other "poisons" such as pesticides or heavy metal residues. The presenting symptoms and severity of a mycotoxicosis depend on the type of mycotoxin; the amount and duration of exposure; the route of exposure; and the age, sex, and health of the exposed individual. In addition, a variety of other circumstances, such as malnutrition, alcohol abuse, infectious disease status, and other toxin exposures, may act synergistically to compound the effect and severity of mycotoxin poisoning.

There are more than 100 toxigenic fungi and over 300 compounds now recognized as mycotoxins. The number of people affected by mycotoxicoses, however, is unknown. The majority of mycotoxicoses result from eating contaminated foods. The occurrence of mycotoxins in foods is most commonly due to preharvest contamination of the material by toxigenic fungi that are plant pathogens. In addition, stored grains may be damaged by insects or moisture, providing a portal of entry for toxigenic fungi present in the storage environment. Mycotoxicoses are more common in undeveloped countries where methods of food handling and storage are inadequate, where malnutrition is prevalent, and where there are few regulations designed to protect exposed populations.

Some mycotoxins are dermonecrotic, and cutaneous or mucosal contact with mold-infected substrates may result in disease. Likewise, inhalation of spore-borne toxins also constitutes an important form of exposure. Aside from supportive therapy, there are almost no treatments for mycotoxin exposure. Fortunately, mycotoxicoses are not communicable from person to person.

Among fungal plant pathogens, the elaboration of mycotoxins plays a role in causing or exacerbating the plant disease. Despite the fact that mycotoxins may be poisonous to humans, and some may have potent immunosuppressive properties, there is very little evidence that mycotoxins enhance the ability of the fungus to grow and cause disease in vertebrate hosts. Those fungi, such as *Aspergillus fumigatus*, which are both important opportunistic pathogens and are capable of producing gliotoxins (inhibitors of T-cell activation and proliferation) generally do not produce the toxin in significant amounts during the course of human disease to have an effect on the disease process. Whereas an opportunistic fungus must be able to grow at human body temperature (37° C) in order to cause disease, the optimum temperature for biosynthesis of most mycotoxins is much lower (20° C to 30° C). For these and other reasons, the importance of mycotoxin exposure during the course of a mycotic infection with a toxigenic fungus is largely unknown.

In the remainder of this chapter, we will discuss those mycotoxins that have been implicated in human disease, as well as metabolites that are produced by molds that may be associated with human foods or living/working environments. Although mushroom poisoning is a form of mycotoxicosis, it will not be discussed herein. A listing of mycotoxicoses where there is considerable evidence for the involvement of a specific mycotoxin is provided in Table 76-1.

Aflatoxins (Clinical Case 76-1)

The aflatoxins are produced primarily by *Aspergillus flavus* and *A. parasiticus*, but many other species of *Aspergillus* produce aflatoxins as well. *A. flavus* is the most common aflatoxin-producing species found in agriculture and may produce as much as 10^6 mg/kg. The commodities most often affected in the United States are corn, cottonseed, peanuts, and certain tree nuts. Aflatoxin B_1 is the most

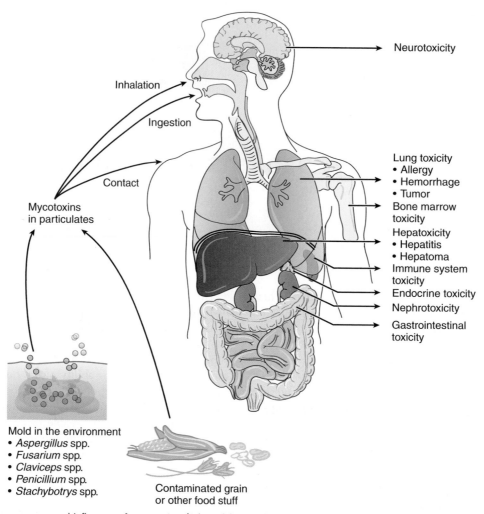

Neurotoxicity

Inhalation

Ingestion

Contact

Mycotoxins
in particulates

Lung toxicity
• Allergy
• Hemorrhage
• Tumor
Bone marrow
toxicity
Hepatoxicity
• Hepatitis
• Hepatoma
Immune system
toxicity
Endocrine toxicity
Nephrotoxicity
Gastrointestinal
toxicity

Mold in the environment
• *Aspergillus* spp.
• *Fusarium* spp.
• *Claviceps* spp.
• *Penicillium* spp.
• *Stachybotrys* spp.

Contaminated grain
or other food stuff

Figure 76–1. Various exposures and influences of mycotoxins. *(Adapted from Richard JL: Mycotoxins and human disease. In Anaissie EJ, McGinnis MR, Pfaller MA [eds]: Clinical Mycology. New York, Churchill Livingstone, 2003.)*

potent natural carcinogen known and is the major aflatoxin produced by toxigenic strains; however, there are more than a dozen other aflatoxins that have been described.

Aflatoxin is associated with both toxicity and carcinogenicity in human and animal populations. Acute aflatoxicosis results in death, whereas chronic aflatoxicosis results in more prolonged pathologic changes, including cancer and immunosuppression. The liver is the primary target organ, and liver damage has been documented in rodents, poultry, and nonhuman primates following ingestion of aflatoxin B1. Acute aflatoxicosis has been manifested in humans as an acute hepatitis. In India in 1974, an outbreak of hepatitis occurred in which 100 people died following consumption of maize that was heavily contaminated with aflatoxin. Aflatoxin B1 was detected in high concentration in the livers of those individuals who died.

It has been hypothesized that both kwashiorkor, a severe malnutrition disease, and Reye syndrome, marked by encephalopathy and fatty degeneration of the viscera, represent forms of pediatric aflatoxicosis. Although aflatoxins have been found in the livers of children with kwashiorkor and in Reye syndrome patients, a strong cause-and-effect relationship between aflatoxin exposure and these disease states has not been established.

Chronic low-level exposure to aflatoxins in the diet is considered a risk factor for the development of hepatocellular carcinoma. Such exposure has been shown experimentally to produce cancer in many animal species. Hepatocellular carcinoma is one of the leading causes of cancer mortality in Asia and Africa, and several epidemiologic investigations have shown that increased aflatoxin ingestion correlates with increased risk.

The primary mode of human exposure to aflatoxins is the consumption of contaminated foods such as peanuts and cereal grains. Aflatoxins can be aerosolized and have been detected in air near farm sources, as well as in dust. Aflatoxin is a pulmonary carcinogen in experimental animals; however, the evidence that airborne aflatoxin exposure leads to cancer in humans is generally weak.

The mechanism of aflatoxin-induced carcinogenesis is thought to involve tumor promotion or progression. There is evidence that aflatoxin is involved in the activation of proto-oncogenes (C-*myc*, C-Ha-*ras*, Ki-*ras*, and N-*ras*) and

Table 76–1. Mycotoxin-Related Illnesses Postulated to Affect Humans, Based on Analytic or Epidemiologic Data

Disease	Toxin	Substrate	Fungus	Clinical Presentation
Akakabi-byo (red mold disease)	*Fusarium* metabolites	Wheat, barley, oats, rice	*Fusarium* spp.	Headaches, vomiting, diarrhea
Alimentary toxic aleukia (ATA)	Trichothecenes (T-2 toxin, DAS)	Cereal grains (toxic bread)	*Fusarium* spp.	Vomiting, diarrhea, angina, skin inflammation
Balkan endemic nephropathy (BEN)	Ochratoxin	Cereal grains	*Aspergillus* spp. *Penicillium* spp.	Chronic nephritis
Cardiac beriberi	Citreoviridin	Rice	*Penicillium* spp.	Palpitations, vomiting, mania, respiratory failure
Ergotism (gangrenous and convulsive)	Ergot alkaloids	Rye, cereal grains	*Claviceps purpurea* *C. fusiformis*	Gangrenous: vasoconstriction, edema, pruritus, and necrosis of extremities Convulsive: numbness, tingling, pruritus, cramps, seizures, hallucinations
Esophageal cancer	Fumonisins	Corn	*Fusarium moniliforme*	Dysphagia, pain, hemorrhage
Hepatitis and hepatic cancer	Aflatoxins	Cereal grains, peanuts	*Aspergillus flavus* *A. parasiticus*	Acute and chronic hepatitis, liver failure
Kodua poisoning	Cyclopiazonic acid	Millet	*Penicillium* spp. *Aspergillus* spp.	Somnolence, tremors, giddiness
Moldy sugarcane poisoning	3-Nitropropionic acid	Sugarcane	*Arthrinium* spp.	Dystonia, seizures, carpopedal spasms, coma
Onyalai disease	*Fusarium* metabolites	Millet	*Fusarium* spp.	Thrombocytopenia, purpura
Stachybotryotoxicosis	Trichothecenes (T-2 toxin, DAS)	Hay, cereal grains, fodder (skin contact, inhaled hay dust)	*Stachybotrys, Fusarium, Myrothecium, Trichoderma, Cephalosporium* spp.	Tremors, loss of vision, dermonecrosis, gastrointestinal bleeding (horses and cattle), nasal inflammation, dermatitis, headache, fatigue, respiratory symptoms (humans), idiopathic pulmonary hemorrhage of infants (?)
Yellow rice disease	Citrinin	Wheat, oats, barley, rice	*Penicillium* spp. *Aspergillus* spp.	Nephropathy

Data from Kuhn DM, Ghannoum MA: Indoor mold, toxigenic fungi, and Stachybotrys chartarum: Infectious disease perspective. Clin Microbiol Dis 16:144-172, 2003; Richard JL: Mycotoxins and human disease. In Anaissie EJ, McGinnis MR, Pfaller MA (eds): Clinical Mycology. New York, Churchill Livingstone, 2003; Bennett JW, Klich M: Mycotoxins. Clin Microbiol Rev 16:497-516, 2003.

also may cause mutations in the tumor suppressor gene *p53*. Aflatoxin exposure and *p53* mutations have been tightly linked in epidemiologic studies in Africa and China. Specifically, aflatoxin has been linked to a *p53* mutation whereby there occurs a G-to-T transversion at codon 249. This particular mutation has been called the first example of a "carcinogen-specific" biomarker that remains fixed in the human tissue. This biomarker has been used in epidemiologic studies to establish the link between aflatoxins and hepatic cancer and also to show that cofactors such as infection with hepatitis

B virus increase the risk of hepatocellular cancer substantially.

Significant aflatoxin exposure is uncommon among those living in developed countries where sufficient amounts of food is available and regulations exist to monitor the level of aflatoxin in those foods. Notably, liver cancer incidence rates are 2 to 10 times higher in developing countries than in developed countries. In those countries where food supplies are limited and people are facing starvation, or where regulations are nonexistent or not enforced, routine ingestion of aflatoxin may occur.

Citrinin

Citrinin is produced by several species of *Penicillium* and *Aspergillus*, including strains used to produce cheese (*P. camemberti*) and sake (*A. oryzae*). Citrinin acts as a potent nephrotoxin in all animal species tested and has been associated with yellow rice disease in Japan (see Table 76-1). Citrinin may act synergistically with another nephrotoxin, Ochratoxin A. Citrinin is regularly associated with human foods, including wheat, oats, rye, corn, barley, and rice; however, its significance as a cause of human disease is unknown.

Ergot Alkaloids

The ergot alkaloids constitute a family of compounds that are derived from a tetracyclic ergoline ring system. Lysergic acid is a structure common to all ergot alkaloids, and the hallucinogen lysergic acid diethylamide (LSD) was discovered as a result of research with these compounds.

Mixtures of these alkaloids are produced within the sclerotia, or ergots, of common grass pathogens of the genus *Claviceps*. The ergots are hardened masses of fungal tissue (sclerotia) that are formed when the fungus invades the floret and replaces the grain of wheat, barley, or rye. The ergots are ingested when the contaminated grain is used to make bread or in cereals. The two forms of ergotism, convulsive and gangrenous (see Table 76-1), are thought to be due to different modes of action of the various alkaloids produced by different species of *Claviceps*. The gangrenous form, marked by peripheral vasoconstriction and necrosis of the distal extremities, is associated primarily with the ingestion of wheat and rye contaminated with *Claviceps purpurea* and containing alkaloids of the ergotamine group. In addition to tissue infarction and necrosis, the gangrenous form of ergotism is associated with edema, pruritus, and sensations varying from pricking to severe muscle pain.

Convulsive ergotism has been associated with the ingestion of millet contaminated by *C. fusiformis*. Neurologic or convulsive ergotism is marked by muscle spasms, seizures, and hallucinations. The ergot of pearl millet implicated in an outbreak of convulsive ergotism in India in 1974 contained alkaloids of the clavine group.

Apparently, different species of *Claviceps* produce different alkaloids, although it is likely that the substrate also plays a role in the composition of the secondary metabolites. Although modern methods of grain cleaning have virtually eliminated ergotism as a human disease, it is still an important veterinary problem. Cattle, pigs, sheep, and poultry are the animals at highest risk. Clinical symptoms of ergotism among these animals include gangrene, abortion, seizures, and ataxia.

Fumonisins

Fumonisins are produced by a number of *Fusarium* species. The major species of economic importance is *F. moniliforme* (*F. verticilloides*), a corn pathogen. Fumonisins, especially fumonisin B1, interfere with sphingolipid metabolism and cause leukoencephalomalacia (severe necrotizing brain disease) in horses, pulmonary edema and hydrothorax in pigs, and hepatotoxic and carcinogenic effects in the liver of rats. Fumonisin B1 has been associated with a higher incidence of esophageal cancer in people living in South Africa, China, and Italy. It may be isolated in high concentrations in cornmeal and corn grits. Although this evidence is intriguing, multiple factors, including other mycotoxins, have been implicated in the etiology of human esophageal cancer.

Acute intoxication with fumonisin B1 has been observed in India, where consumption of unleavened bread made from moldy corn caused transient abdominal pain and diarrhea. Fumonisins have also been shown to cause neural tube defects in experimental animals and may have a role in human cases. Fumonisins have been classified as group 2B carcinogens (probably carcinogenic) by the International Agency for Research on Cancer.

Ochratoxin

Ochratoxin belongs to a group of secondary metabolites produced by *Aspergillus* and *Penicillium* species found on cereals, coffee, bread, and foods of animal origin (e.g., pork). Ochratoxin A (OA) is the most common and most toxic chemical in its class. OA is nephrotoxic, teratogenic, and carcinogenic in all animals tested. It has been implicated in porcine nephropathy, as well as urinary tract tumors, and may cause cholinergic responses such as bronchospasm, vasodilation, and smooth muscle contraction.

Ochratoxin has been linked to a disease known as **Balkan Endemic Nephropathy (BEN)**, which is a chronic, progressive nephritis seen in populations living in areas bordering the Danube River in parts of Romania, Bulgaria, and the former Yugoslavia. In addition, individuals with BEN also suffer from a high frequency of renal tumors. Ochratoxin contamination of food and the presence of OA in human serum have been shown to be more common in families with BEN and those with urinary tract tumors than in unaffected families. Despite this evidence, a number of other factors such as genetics, heavy metals, and possible occult infectious agents may also contribute to this disease. Although much of the evidence for the cause of BEN leans toward ochratoxin, the evidence is not conclusive. Regardless, its acute nephrotoxicity, immunosuppressive action, and teratogenic effects in animals, coupled with its propensity to be carried through the food chain, merit concern and further investigation.

Trichothecenes (Clinical Case 76-2)

The trichothecenes are all tricyclic sesquiterpinoid metabolites that are produced by a number of fungi, including *Fusarium*, *Myrothecium*, *Stachybotrys*, *Trichoderma*, and *Cephalosporium* spp. (see Table 76-1). There are more than 148 natural trichothecenes, of which at least 40 are mycotoxins. Trichothecenes act by inhibiting various aspects of protein synthesis in eukaryotic cells. The most potent of these mycotoxins are T-2 toxin, diacetoxyscirpenol (DAS), deoxynivalenol (vomitoxin) and fusarenon-X. These mycotoxins are commonly found as food and feed contaminants, the consumption of which can result in gastrointestinal hemorrhage and vomiting; direct contact causes dermatitis.

So-called **moldy grain intoxication** of humans and animals is well documented in Japan. Such intoxications have been attributed to *Fusarium* mycotoxins. Akakabi-byo toxicosis, or red mold disease, is believed to be caused by ingestion of grain contaminated with *Fusarium graminearum* (see Table 76-1).

T-2 toxin, DAS, and deoxynivalenol are the most widely studied of the fusarial trichothecenes. The symptoms produced by these agents include effects on almost every system of the vertebrate body. T-2 toxin and DAS appear to be the most potent and exhibit both cytotoxic and immunosuppressive activity. They cause a wide range of gastrointestinal, dermatologic, and neurologic symptoms and

also decrease host resistance to infection with various microbes. Deoxynivalenol is a common contaminant of grains used in animal feed. When ingested in high doses, it causes vomiting and diarrhea; at lower doses, farm animals exhibit weight loss and food refusal.

Both T-2 toxin and DAS have been implicated in a human disease known as **alimentary toxic aleukia (ATA)**. The most important outbreak of ATA occurred in Russia during World War II. Thousands of people became sick after eating over-wintered grain contaminated with *Fusarium sporotrichioides* and *F. poae*. The disease was characterized by several stages, with initial oral mucosal ulceration and gastroenteritis followed by pancytopenia, bleeding from the nose, mouth, and vagina, hypotension, and vertigo. The high acute mortality rate was augmented

---

Clinical Case 76-2. *Stachybotrys* and Acute Idiopathic Pulmonary Hemorrhage

Colin and colleagues (Morb Mortal Wkly Rep 53:817-820, 2004) described an investigation of acute idiopathic pulmonary hemorrhage (AIPH) in infants in Massachusetts. During 1993 to 1996, investigation of cases of AIPH among infants in Cleveland, Ohio, suggested an association between AIPH and being male, exposure to molds (notably *Stachybotrys chartarum*), exposure to tobacco smoke, and lack of breast feeding. However, reviews of that investigation by CDC identified shortcomings in the methodology and determined that no association between AIPH and exposure to molds had been established. It was recommended that CDC collaborate with state and local public health officials to investigate future cases of AIPH, particularly when clusters are identified. During December 2002 to June 2003, four cases of AIPH among full-term infants were reported in the Boston, Massachusetts, area. In a 4-month period, three of the infants were patients at the same hospital, which typically has one case of AIPH among infants per year. CDC, in collaboration with the Massachusetts Department of Public Health, investigated this cluster and determined that two of the infants had von Willebrand disease (vWD), an inherited bleeding disorder, and one had borderline test results for vWD. The findings suggest that the infants with AIPH might have an underlying acquired or genetic susceptibility that predisposed them to pulmonary bleeding.

All the infants in this cluster also were exposed to certain environmental factors that might have affected their lungs, including environmental tobacco smoke, particulate matter (e.g., construction dust), and mold. *Cladosporium* and *Penicillium*, the molds most commonly identified in each of the homes, typically are the most abundant fungal genera in indoor air. Total fungal spore counts in two of the homes were at concentrations that have been associated with increased risk for lower respiratory illness, and all four infants were treated presumptively for respiratory infections before their hemorrhagic episodes. Only seven spores of *S. chartarum* were found in one home and a single spore was found in another. Although the full significance of spore counts is not known, toxic and other non-IgE—mediated health effects that have been hypothesized to occur with exposure to *S. chartarum* appear unlikely to have contributed to these AIPH cases.

by opportunistic bacterial infections during the later neutropenic stages of the disease. Despite the fact that the two species of *Fusarium* that were isolated from the moldy grain were subsequently shown to be able to produce T-2 toxin and other trichothecenes, no attempt was made to document the presence of these mycotoxins in the grain or the affected people. Almost all signs of ATA have been documented in animals given T-2 toxin; however, the association between the toxin and human disease remains merely speculative.

Stachybotryotoxicosis is a well-described disease among horses and cattle consuming moldy straw and hay contaminated with *Stachybotrys*. Equine stachybotryotoxicosis is characterized by acute neurologic signs, such as tremors, incoordination, and loss of vision, and more chronic manifestations such as dermonecrosis, leukopenia, and gastrointestinal bleeding. Humans handling moldy hay have exhibited contact dermatitis, as well as mucosal inflammation, fever, chest pain, and leukopenia secondary to inhalation of dust from the hay. Macrocyclic trichothecenes were isolated from the contaminated hay.

Given these findings, and because *Stachybotrys* grows well on wet building materials such as ceiling tiles, wood fiber boards, and dust-lined air conditioning ducts, toxins from this fungus have become suspect in illnesses of humans living or working in *Stachybotrys*-contaminated buildings. Complaints of pulmonary irritation, headaches, fatigue, malaise, and diarrhea have been registered by residents and workers in buildings contaminated with *S. chartarum*. *Stachybotrys* has also been associated with idiopathic pulmonary hemorrhage of infants; however, a cause-and-effect relationship has not been proven. Critical evaluation of the available literature has failed to find supportive evidence for serious human illness due to *Stachybotrys* exposure in the contemporary human environment.

Other Mycotoxins and Purported Mycotoxicoses

Given the wide variety of environmental molds that have been shown to be capable of producing mycotoxins, it is not surprising that there is a vast literature describing the potential role of these agents in human and animal disease states. Unfortunately, much of this literature is quite flawed, and critical review almost always finds it to be lacking in rigorous proof of a cause-and-effect relationship between mycotoxins and human disease.

Cyclopiazonic acid is an indole tetramic acid that is a specific inhibitor of calcium-dependent ATPase and induces alterations in ion transport across cell membranes. It is produced by many species of *Penicillium* and *Aspergillus*, including *A. flavus*. Consumption of millet that was heavily contaminated with molds and contained high levels of cyclopiazonic acid produced a condition known as **Kodua poisoning**, characterized by giddiness and nausea (see Table 76-1).

Cardiac beriberi, a condition seen in Japan and other Asian countries in the early twentieth century, has been associated with the yellow rice toxins, citreoviridin, citrinin, and related compounds. This disease is characterized by palpitations, nausea, vomiting, respiratory distress, hypotension, and violent mania leading to respiratory failure and death. The neurologic symptoms and respiratory failure have been reproduced in animals given citreoviridin.

Several rare and obscure diseases have been purported to be mycotoxicosis, often with minimal objective evidence. These include Kashin-Beck disease in Russia, Onyalai disease in Africa, and moldy sugar cane disease in China (see Table 76-1).

It is difficult to prove that a disease is a mycotoxicosis. Even known toxigenic molds may be present in foods or the environment and not produce toxin. The mere isolation of mold from cultures of a given substrate is not the same as detection of a specific mycotoxin. Likewise, even when mycotoxins are detected, it is difficult to prove conclusively that they are the cause of specific acute or chronic disease states. Regardless, valid concerns do exist with respect to the relationship between mycotoxins and human disease. Examples of certain fungus-disease associations are reasonably well documented in the literature, including ATA from *Fusarium*, liver disease from *Aspergillus*, and ergotism from *Claviceps* spp. Beyond these examples, the evidence is tenuous. It is likely that mycotoxins do pose an important danger to the health of humans and animals, the extent of which can only be determined by rigorous well-designed clinical and laboratory studies.

Questions

1. Which of the following mycotoxins is the most potent natural carcinogen?
   a. Ochratoxin A
   b. Fumonisin
   c. Cyclopiazonic acid
   d. Aflatoxin B1
2. Describe the different mycotoxicoses caused by aflatoxin.
3. Describe the different presentations of ergotism.
4. What is the relationship between *Stachybotrys chartarum* and idiopathic pulmonary hemorrhage of infancy?

Bibliography

Bennett JW, Klich M: Mycotoxins. Clin Microbial Rev 16:497-516, 2003.

Halsall WJ, et al: Mycotoxins. In Murray PR, et al. (eds): Manual of Clinical Microbiology, 9th ed. Washington, DC, ASM Press, 2007.

Kuhn DM, Ghannoum MA: Indoor mold, toxigenic fungi, and *Stachybotrys chartarum*: Infectious disease perspective. Clin Microbiol Dis 16:144-172, 2003.

Richard JL: Mycotoxins and human disease. In Anaissie EJ, McGinnis MR, Pfaller MA (eds): Clinical Mycology. New York, Churchill Livingstone, 2003.

77

Role of Fungi in Disease

A summary of fungi (yeasts and molds) most commonly associated with human disease is presented in this chapter. Mycotic diseases in humans develop as pathogenic processes in one or more organ systems. The affected systems may be as superficial as the outer layers of the skin or as deep as the heart, central nervous system, or abdominal viscera. Although a single fungus may be more commonly associated with infection involving a single organ system (e.g., *Cryptococcus neoformans* and the central nervous system), more often several different organisms may produce a similar disease syndrome. Because the management of a given infection may differ according to the etiologic agent, to guide subsequent diagnostic and therapeutic efforts, it is useful to develop a differential diagnosis, which includes the most likely fungal pathogens.

Because the development of a fungal infection depends on factors that often outweigh the virulence potential of the infecting organism, one must take into account numerous factors, such as the immune status of the host, the opportunity for interaction between host and fungus (e.g., Is the fungus **endogenous** to the patient or **exogenous?**), and the potential infectious dose (e.g., in the case of

an endemic dimorphic fungus), in determining the possibility of a fungal infection, the significance of the microbiologic data (e.g., culture results), and the necessity to treat and with what agent. Fungal infections often occur in very sick patients, and it is not possible to summarize here the incredibly complex interactions that ultimately lead to the establishment of infection and disease in each organ system. Instead, this chapter provides a very broad listing of the various fungi commonly associated with infections at specific body sites and/or specific clinical manifestations (Table 77-1). This information is meant to be used in conjunction with that in Chapter 69, Table 69-1, as an aid in establishing a differential diagnosis and for the selection of the most likely clinical specimens that will help establish a specific etiologic diagnosis. Other factors that may be important in determining the relative frequency with which specific fungi cause disease (e.g., age, co-morbidities, host immunity, epidemiologic exposures and risk factors) are covered in the individual chapters in this text or in the more comprehensive infectious disease texts cited in this and other chapters.

Table 77–1. Summary of Fungi Associated with Human Disease

System Affected	Pathogens
Upper Respiratory Infections	
Oropharyngeal	*Candida* spp., *Cryptococcus neoformans, Histoplasma capsulatum, Blastomyces dermatitidis, Paracoccidioides brasiliensis, Penicillium marneffei, Geotrichum candidum*
Sinusitis	*Aspergillus* spp., Zygomycetes, *Fusarium* spp., dematiaceous molds (e.g., *Alternaria, Bipolaris, Exophiala* spp.)
Laryngeal	*Histoplasma capsulatum, Sporothrix schenckii, Blastomyces dermatitidis*
Esophageal	*Candida* spp.
Ear Infections	
External Otitis	*Aspergillus niger, Candida* spp.

Table 77–1. Summary of Fungi Associated with Human Disease—cont'd

System Affected	Pathogens
Eye Infections	
Endophthalmitis	*Candida* spp., *Aspergillus* spp., *Blastomyces dermatitidis*, *Coccidioides immitis/posadasii*, *Fusarium* spp., *Histoplasma capsulatum*, *Cryptococcus neoformans*
Keratitis	*Candida* spp., *Fusarium* spp., dematiaceous molds, *Scedosporium* spp., *Paecilomyces lilacinus*
Sino-orbital	Zygomycetes, *Aspergillus* spp.
Dacryocystitis and canaliculitis	*Candida albicans*, *Aspergillus niger*
Pleuropulmonary and Bronchial Infections	
Bronchitis	*Aspergillus* spp., *Cryptococcus neoformans*
Pneumonia	*Aspergillus* spp., Zygomycetes, *Fusarium* spp., *Scedosporium apiospermum*, *Trichosporon* spp., dematiaceous molds, *Cryptococcus neoformans*, *Histoplasma capsulatum*, *Blastomyces dermatitidis*, *Coccidioides immitis/posadasii*, *Paracoccidioides brasiliensis*, *Penicillium marneffei*, *Pneumocystis jirovecii*, *Candida* spp. (rare)
Fungus ball	*Aspergillus* spp., Zygomycetes, *Scedosporium apiospermum*, *Fusarium* spp., *Candida* spp.
Empyema	*Aspergillus* spp., Zygomycetes, *Scedosporium apiospermum*, *Fusarium* spp., *Candida* spp., *Coccidioides immitis/posadasii*
Genitourinary Tract Infections	
Vulvovaginal	*Candida* spp., *Saccharomyces cerevisiae*
Cystitis and pyelonephritis	*Candida* spp. (most common), *Cryptococcus neoformans*, *Aspergillus* spp., *Coccidioides immitis/posadasii*, *Histoplasma capsulatum*, *Blastomyces dermatitidis* (rare), *Trichosporon* spp. (rare), *Blastoschizomyces capitatus* (rare), *Rhodotorula* spp. (rare)
Epididymitis and orchitis	*Candida* spp., *Cryptococcus neoformans*, *Aspergillus* spp., *Coccidioides immitis/posadasii*, *Histoplasma capsulatum*, *Blastomyces dermatitidis* (all rare)
Prostatitis	*Candida* spp. (common), *Cryptococcus neoformans* (common), *Blastomyces dermatitidis* (common), *Histoplasma capsulatum*, *Aspergillus* spp. (rare), *Coccidioides immitis/posadasii* (rare)
Intraabdominal Infections	
Peritonitis	*Candida* spp., *Rhodotorula* spp., *Trichosporon* spp., *Aspergillus* spp. (rare)
Visceral abscesses	*Candida* spp., *Trichosporon* spp., *Blastoschizomyces capitatus*
Cardiovascular Infections	
Endocarditis	*Candida* spp., *Trichosporon* spp., *Rhodotorula* spp., *Aspergillus* spp., other hyaline hyphomycetes (e.g., *Fusarium*, *Acremonium*), dematiaceous molds
Pericarditis	*Candida* spp., *Aspergillus* spp., *Histoplasma capsulatum*, *Coccidioides immitis/posadasii*
Central Nervous System	
Meningitis	*Candida* spp., *Cryptococcus neoformans*, *Aspergillus* spp., Zygomycetes (rare), *Coccidioides immitis/posadasii*, *Histoplasma capsulatum*, *Blastomyces dermatitidis* (rare), *Rhodotorula* spp., *Blastoschizomyces capitatus*, *Penicillium marneffei*
Brain abscess	*Candida* spp., *Cryptococcus neoformans*, *C. gattii*, *Aspergillus* spp., Zygomycetes, *Scedosporium apiospermum*, *Trichosporon* spp., *Trichoderma* spp., dematiaceous molds (especially *Cladophialophora bantiana* and *Bipolaris hawaiiensis*), endemic dimorphic fungi (rare)
Skin and Soft-Tissue Infections	
Superficial and cutaneous	Dermatophytes, *Candida* spp., *Scytalidium* spp., *Scopulariopsis* spp., *Aspergillus* spp., *Malassezia* spp., *Paecilomyces lilacinus*

Continued

Table 77–1. Summary of Fungi Associated with Human Disease—cont'd

System Affected	Pathogens
Skin and Soft-Tissue Infections	
Subcutaneous	Dematiaceous molds, *Fusarium* spp., *Acremonium* spp., *Scedosporium apiospermum*, *Sporothrix schenckii*, *Basidiobolus* sp., *Conidiobolus* sp.
Wounds (surgical or traumatic)	*Candida* spp., Zygomycetes, *Aspergillus* spp., *Fusarium* spp., *Trichosporon* spp., *Rhodotorula* spp., *Scedosporium prolificans*
Cutaneous nodules (hematogenous)	*Candida* spp., *Aspergillus* spp., Zygomycetes, *Cryptococcus neoformans*, *Trichosporon* spp., *Blastomyces dermatitidis*, *Coccidioides immitis/posadasii*, *Penicillium marneffei*, *Fusarium* spp., *Acremonium* spp., dematiaceous molds (rare), *Histoplasma capsulatum* var. *duboisii*
Bone and Joint Infections	
Osteomyelitis	*Blastomyces dermatitidis*, *Coccidioides immitis/posadasii*, *Candida* spp., *Cryptococcus neoformans*, *Aspergillus* spp., Zygomycetes, dematiaceous molds (mycetoma), other hyaline hyphomycetes (e.g., *Scedosporium* spp., *Trichosporon*), *Histoplasma capsulatum* var. *duboisii*
Arthritis	*Coccidioides immitis/posadasii*, *Blastomyces dermatitidis*, *Cryptococcus neoformans*, *Candida* spp., *Aspergillus* spp., dematiaceous molds (mycetoma; rare), *Histoplasma capsulatum* (rare), *Paracoccidioides brasiliensis* (rare), *Sporothrix schenckii* (rare)
Other Infections	
Prosthetic joint	*Candida* spp., all others very rare
Hematogenous dissemination	*Candida* spp., *Histoplasma capsulatum*, *Blastomyces dermatitidis*, *Coccidioides immitis/posadasii*, *Cryptococcus neoformans*, *Paracoccidioides brasiliensis*, *Sporothrix schenckii*, *Aspergillus* spp., *Fusarium* spp., *Trichosporon* spp., *Malassezia* spp., *Blastoschizomyces capitatus*, *Penicillium marneffei*, others (e.g., *Rhodotorula*, *Acremonium*, *Saccharomyces* spp. in neutropenic or transplant patients)

Bibliography

Anaisse EJ, McGinnis MR, Pfaller MA (eds): Clinical Mycology. New York, Churchill Livingstone, 2003.

Chandler FW, Watts JC: Pathologic Diagnosis of Fungal Infections. Chicago, ASCP, 1987.

Cohen J, Powderly WG: Infectious Diseases, 2nd ed. St Louis, Mosby, 2004.

Connor DH, et al: Pathology of Infectious Diseases. Stamford, Conn, Appleton & Lange, 1997.

Murray PR, et al: Manual of Clinical Microbiology, 9th ed. Washington, DC, ASM Press, 2007.

Pfaller MA, Diekema DJ: Rare and emerging opportunistic fungal pathogens: Concern for resistance beyond *Candida albicans* and *Aspergillus fumigatus*. J Clin Microbiol 42:4419, 2004.

Pfaller MA, et al: Invasive fungal pathogens: Current epidemiological trends. Clin Infect Dis 43(Suppl 1):S3, 2006.

Table 77–1. Summary of Fungi Associated with Human Disease—cont'd

System Affected	Pathogens
Skin and Soft-Tissue Infections	
Subcutaneous	Dematiaceous molds, *Fusarium* spp., *Acremonium* spp., *Scedosporium apiospermum*, *Sporothrix schenckii*, *Basidiobolus* sp., *Conidiobolus* sp.
Wounds (surgical or traumatic)	*Candida* spp., Zygomycetes, *Aspergillus* spp., *Fusarium* spp., *Trichosporon* spp., *Rhodotorula* spp., *Scedosporium prolificans*
Cutaneous nodules (hematogenous)	*Candida* spp., *Aspergillus* spp., Zygomycetes, *Cryptococcus neoformans*, *Trichosporon* spp., *Blastomyces dermatitidis*, *Coccidioides immitis/posadasii*, *Penicillium marneffei*, *Fusarium* spp., *Acremonium* spp., dematiaceous molds (rare), *Histoplasma capsulatum* var. *duboisii*
Bone and Joint Infections	
Osteomyelitis	*Blastomyces dermatitidis*, *Coccidioides immitis/posadasii*, *Candida* spp., *Cryptococcus neoformans*, *Aspergillus* spp., Zygomycetes, dematiaceous molds (mycetoma), other hyaline hyphomycetes (e.g., *Scedosporium* spp., *Trichosporon*), *Histoplasma capsulatum* var. *duboisii*
Arthritis	*Coccidioides immitis/posadasii*, *Blastomyces dermatitidis*, *Cryptococcus neoformans*, *Candida* spp., *Aspergillus* spp., dematiaceous molds (mycetoma; rare), *Histoplasma capsulatum* (rare), *Paracoccidioides brasiliensis* (rare), *Sporothrix schenckii* (rare)
Other Infections	
Prosthetic joint	*Candida* spp., all others very rare
Hematogenous dissemination	*Candida* spp., *Histoplasma capsulatum*, *Blastomyces dermatitidis*, *Coccidioides immitis/posadasii*, *Cryptococcus neoformans*, *Paracoccidioides brasiliensis*, *Sporothrix schenckii*, *Aspergillus* spp., *Fusarium* spp., *Trichosporon* spp., *Malassezia* spp., *Blastoschizomyces capitatus*, *Penicillium marneffei*, others (e.g., *Rhodotorula*, *Acremonium*, *Saccharomyces* spp. in neutropenic or transplant patients)

Bibliography

Anaisse EJ, McGinnis MR, Pfaller MA (eds): Clinical Mycology. New York, Churchill Livingstone, 2003.

Chandler FW, Watts JC: Pathologic Diagnosis of Fungal Infections. Chicago, ASCP, 1987.

Cohen J, Powderly WG: Infectious Diseases, 2nd ed. St Louis, Mosby, 2004.

Connor DH, et al: Pathology of Infectious Diseases. Stamford, Conn, Appleton & Lange, 1997.

Murray PR, et al: Manual of Clinical Microbiology, 9th ed. Washington, DC, ASM Press, 2007.

Pfaller MA, Diekema DJ: Rare and emerging opportunistic fungal pathogens: Concern for resistance beyond *Candida albicans* and *Aspergillus fumigatus*. J Clin Microbiol 42:4419, 2004.

Pfaller MA, et al: Invasive fungal pathogens: Current epidemiological trends. Clin Infect Dis 43(Suppl 1):S3, 2006.

Parasitology

Pathogenesis of Parasitic Diseases

Given the wide diversity that exists among human parasites, it is not surprising that the pathogenesis of protozoan and helminthic disease is highly variable. Although the various human parasites exhibit a wide range of direct pathogenic mechanisms, in most instances the organisms themselves are not highly virulent, are unable to replicate within the host, or have both reactions. Thus the severity of illness caused by many parasites is related to the infecting dose and the number of organisms acquired over time. Unlike many bacterial and viral infections, parasitic infections are often chronic, lasting months to years. Repeated exposures result in an ever-increasing parasite burden. When infection with a particular organism is associated with a strong immune response, there is undoubtedly a considerable immunopathologic contribution to the disease manifestations attributed to the infection.

Important factors to consider when discussing parasite pathogenicity are listed in Box 78-1. Parasites are almost always exogenous to the human host and thus must enter the body through ingestion or direct penetration of anatomical barriers. Inoculum size and duration of exposure greatly influence the disease-causing potential of an organism. Likewise, the route of exposure is critical for most organisms. For example, pathogenic strains of *Entamoeba histolytica* are unlikely to cause disease on exposure to intact skin but may cause severe dysentery after oral ingestion. Many parasites have active, self-directed means of invading the human host. Once they have invaded, parasites attach to specific host cells or organs, avoid immune detection, replicate (most protozoa and some helminths), produce toxic substances that destroy tissue, and cause disease secondary to the host's own immunologic response (see Box 78-1). In addition, some parasites physically obstruct and damage organs and tissues because of their size alone. This chapter discusses factors that are important for parasite pathogenicity and provides examples of organisms and disease processes related to each factor.

Exposure and Entry

Although many infectious diseases are caused by **endogenous** organisms that are part of the normal flora of the human host, this is not the case with most diseases caused by protozoan and helminthic parasites. These organisms are virtually always acquired from an **exogenous** source and as such have evolved numerous ways to enter the body of the human host. The most common modes of entry are oral ingestion or direct penetration through the skin or other surfaces (Table 78-1). Transmission of parasitic diseases is frequently facilitated by environmental contamination with human and animal wastes. This is most applicable to diseases transmitted by the fecal-oral route but also applies to helminthic infections such as hookworm disease and strongyloidiasis, which rely on larval penetration of the skin.

Many parasitic diseases are acquired via the bites of **arthropod** vectors. Transmission of disease in this manner is extraordinarily effective, as evidenced by the widespread distribution of diseases such as malaria, trypanosomiasis, and filariasis. Examples of parasites and their ports of entry are listed in Table 78-1. This compilation should not be considered exhaustive; rather, the list provides examples of some of the more common parasites and the means by which they enter the human body.

Additional factors that determine the outcome of the interaction between parasite and host are route of **exposure** and **inoculum** size. Most human parasites have a limited range of organs or tissues in which they can replicate or survive. For example, simple skin contact with most intestinal protozoa does not result in disease; rather, the organisms must be ingested for the disease process to be initiated. Likewise, a minimum number of organisms is required to establish infection. Although some parasitic diseases may be acquired by the ingestion or inoculation of only a few organisms, a sizable inoculum is usually required. Whereas an individual may acquire malaria by a single bite of an infected female mosquito, large inocula are usually necessary to produce diseases such as amebiasis in humans.

Box 78—1. Factors Associated with Parasite Pathogenicity

Infective dose and exposure
Penetration of anatomic barriers
Attachment
Replication
Cell and tissue damage
Disruption, evasion, and inactivation of host defenses

Adherence and Replication

Most infections are initiated by the attachment of the organism to host tissues, followed by replication to establish colonization. The life cycle of a parasite is based on species and **tissue tropisms**, which determine the organs or tissues of the host in which a parasite can survive. The attachment of the parasite to host cells or tissue can be relatively nonspecific, can be mediated by mechanical or biting mouthparts, or can result from the interaction between structures on the parasite surface known as *adhesins* and specific glycoprotein or glycolipid receptors found on some cell types but not on others. Specific surface structures that facilitate parasite adhesion include surface **glycoproteins** such as glycophorin A and B, complement receptors, adsorbed components of the complement cascade, fibronectin and *N*-acetylglucosamine conjugates. Examples of some of the adherence mechanisms identified in human parasites are listed in Table 78-2.

E. histolytica is a good model for the importance of **adhesins** in virulence. The pathogenesis of invasive amebiasis requires adherence of amoebae to the colonic mucosal layer, parasite attachment to and lysis of colonic epithelium and acute inflammatory cells, and resistance of the amoebic trophozoites to host humoral and cell-mediated immune defense mechanisms. Amoebic adherence to colonic mucins, epithelial cells, and leukocytes is mediated by a surface lectin inhibitable by galactose (gal) or *N*-acetyl-D-galactosamine (GalNAc). Binding of the galactose-inhibitable adherence lectin to carbohydrates on the host cell surface is required for *E. histolytica* trophozoites to exert their cytolytic activity. The presence of the galactose-inhibitable adherence lectin is one feature that distinguishes pathogenic from nonpathogenic strains of *E. histolytica*.

Various attachment mechanisms have been associated with specific infections. For example, the **Duffy blood group antigen** acts as an attachment site for *Plasmodium vivax*. Red blood cells from most West Africans, in contrast to those from Europeans, lack the Duffy antigen. Accordingly, malaria resulting from *P. vivax* is almost unknown in West Africa. The physical structures of parasites may act with adhesion molecules to promote attachment to host cells. *Giardia lamblia* is a protozoan parasite that uses a ventral disk to attach to the intestinal epithelium by a clasping or suction-like mechanism. Two recently identified adhesins, trypsin-activated *G. lamblia* lectin (taglin) and *G. lamblia* adherence molecule-1 (GLAM-1), may also be important in attachment to enterocytes. It is believed that initial contact of the parasite with the intestinal surface is facilitated by taglin, which is distributed over the surface of the parasite, and that the disk-specific GLAM-1 is responsible for the avid attachment of the disk to the enterocyte surface.

After attachment to the specific cell or tissue type, the parasite may undergo replication as the next step in establishing infection. Most protozoan parasites replicate intracellularly or extracellularly in the human host, whereas replication is generally not observed with the helminths capable of establishing human infection.

Temperature may also play an important role in the ability of parasites to infect a host and cause disease. This is well illustrated by the *Leishmania* species. *Leishmania donovani* replicates well at 37° C and causes visceral leishmaniasis involving the bone marrow, liver, and spleen. In contrast, *L. tropica* grows well at 25° C to 30° C but poorly at 37° C and causes an infection of the skin without involvement of deeper organs.

Cell and Tissue Damage

Although some microorganisms may cause disease by localized multiplication and elaboration of potent microbial **toxins**, most organisms initiate the disease process by invading normally sterile tissue with subsequent replication and destruction. Parasitic protozoa and helminths are generally not known to produce toxins with potencies comparable to those of classic bacterial toxins such as anthrax toxin and botulinum toxin; however, parasitic disease can be established by the elaboration of toxic products, mechanical tissue damage, and immunopathologic reactions (Table 78-3).

Numerous authors have suggested that toxic products elaborated by parasitic protozoa are responsible for at least

Table 78—1. Parasite Ports of Entry

Route	Examples
Ingestion	*Giardia* species, *E. histolytica*, *Cryptosporidium* species, cestodes, nematodes
Direct penetration	
Arthropod bite	Malaria, *Babesia* species, filaria, *Leishmania* species, trypanosomes
Transplacental penetration	*Toxoplasma gondii*
Organism-directed penetration	Hookworm, *Strongyloides* species, schistosomes

Table 78–2. Examples of Parasitic Adherence Mechanisms

Organism	Disease	Target	Mechanism of Attachment and Receptor
Plasmodium vivax	Malaria	Red blood cell	Merozoite (noncomplement-mediated attachment), Duffy antigen
Plasmodium falciparum	Malaria	Red blood cell	Merozoite and glycophorin A and B
Babesia species	Babesiosis	Red blood cell	Complement-mediated C3b receptor
Giardia lamblia	Diarrhea	Duodenal and jejunal epithelium	Trypsin-activated *G. lamblia* lectin and mannose-6-phosphate. *G. lamblia* adherence molecule—1 on disk
Entamoeba histolytica	Dysentery	Colonic epithelium	Lectin and *N*-acetylglucosamine conjugates
Trypanosoma cruzi	Chagas' disease	Fibroblast	Penetrin, fibronectin, and fibronectin receptor
Leishmania major	Leishmaniasis	Macrophage	Adsorbed C3bi and CR3
Leishmania mexicana	Leishmaniasis	Macrophage	Surface glycoprotein (gp63) and CR2
Necator americanus *Ancylostoma duodenale*	Hookworm	Intestinal epithelium	Mechanical and biting mouthparts

Table 78–3. Some Pathologic Mechanisms in Parasitic Diseases

Mechanism	Examples
Toxic Parasite Products	
Hydrolytic enzymes, proteinases, collagenase, elastase	Schistosomes (cercariae), *Strongyloides* species, hookworm, *Entamoeba histolytica*, African trypanosomes, *Plasmodium falciparum*
Amoebic ionophore	*E. histolytica*
Endotoxins	African trypanosomes, *Plasmodium falciparum*
Indole catabolites	Trypanosomes
Mechanical Tissue Damage	
Blockage of internal organs	*Ascaris* species, tapeworms, schistosomes, filaria
Pressure atrophy	*Echinococcus* species, *Cysticercus* species
Migration through tissue	Helminthic larvae
Immunopathology	
Hypersensitivity	See Table 78-4
Autoimmunity	See Table 78-4
Protein-losing enteropathies	Hookworm, tapeworm, *Giardia* species, *Strongyloides* species
Metaplastic changes	*Opisthorchis* species (liver flukes), schistosomes

some aspects of pathology (see Table 78-3). **Proteases** and **phospholipases** may be secreted and are released on the destruction of the parasites. These enzymes can cause host cell destruction, inflammatory responses, and gross tissue pathology. For example, the intestinal parasite *E. histolytica* produces proteinases that can degrade epithelial basement membrane and cell-anchoring proteins, disrupting epithelial cell layers. Furthermore, the amoebae produce phospholipases and an ionophore-like protein that lyse the responding host neutrophils, resulting in the release of neutrophil constituents that are toxic to host tissues. The expression of certain proteinases increases relative to the virulence of the strain of *E. histolytica*. In contrast to the protozoan parasites, many of the pathogenic consequences of helminthic infections are related to the size, movement, and longevity of the parasites. The host is exposed to long-term damage and immune stimulation, as well as the sheer physical consequences of being inhabited by large foreign bodies. The most obvious forms of direct damage from helminthic parasites are those resulting from mechanical blockage of internal organs or from the effects of pressure exerted by growing parasites. Large adult *Ascaris* organisms can physically block the intestine and the bile ducts. Likewise, blockage of lymph flow, leading to elephantiasis, is associated with the presence of adult *Wuchereria* organisms in the lymphatic system. Some neurologic manifestations of cysticercosis are due to the pressure exerted by the slowly expanding larval cysts of *Taenia solium* on the central nervous system (CNS) and eyes. Migration of helminths (usually larval forms) through body tissues such as the skin, lungs, liver, intestines, eyes, and CNS can damage the tissues directly and initiate hypersensitivity reactions.

Table 78–5. Microbial Interference with or Avoidance of Immune Defenses

Type of Interference or Avoidance	Mechanism	Examples
Antigenic variation	Variation of surface antigens within the host	African trypanosomes, *Plasmodium* species, *Babesia* species, *Giardia* species
Molecular mimicry	Microbial antigens mimicking host antigens, leading to poor antibody response	*Plasmodium* species, trypanosomes, schistosomes
Concealment of antigenic site (masking)	Acquisition of coating of host molecules	Hydatid cyst, filaria, schistosomes, trypanosomes
Intracellular location	Failure to display microbial antigen on host cell surface Inhibition of phagolysosomal fusion Escape from phagosome into cytoplasm, with subsequent replication	*Plasmodium* species (RBC), trypanosomes, *Leishmania* species, *Toxoplasma* species *Toxoplasma* species *Leishmania* species, *Trypanosoma cruzi*
Immunosuppression	Suppression of parasite-specific B- and T-cell responses Degradation of immunoglobulins	Trypanosomes, *Plasmodium* species Schistosomes

Questions

1. What are the most common modes of entry of parasites into the human host?
2. Name two factors that determine the outcome of the interaction between parasite and host.
3. Give an example of an adhesin that is directly related to the virulence of a parasite.
4. Name three pathologic mechanisms thought to be important in parasitic diseases.
5. How can parasites resist immunologic clearance? Give at least one example of each mechanism.
6. Name the four types of immunopathologic reactions that occur in parasitic diseases and provide examples of each.

Bibliography

Choi BI, Han JK, Hong ST, Lee KH: Clonorchiasis and cholangiocarcinoma: Etiologic relationship and imaging diagnosis. Clin Microbiol Rev 17:540-552, 2004.
Clark IA, et al: Pathogenesis of malaria and clinically similar conditions. Clin Microbiol Rev 17:509-539, 2004.
Conway DJ: Molecular epidemiology of malaria. Clin Microbiol Rev 20:188-204, 2007.
Cunningham MW, Fujinami RS: Molecular Mimicry, Microbes, and Autoimmunity. Washington, DC, ASM Press, 2000.
Espinosa-Cantellano M, Martinez-Palomo A: Pathogenesis of intestinal amebiasis: From molecules to disease. Clin Microbiol Rev 13:318-331, 2000.
Girones N, Cuervo H, Fresno M: *Trypanosoma cruzi*–induced molecular mimicry and Chagas disease (Curr Top Microbiol Immunol, vol 296). Berlin, Springer-Verlag, 2005.
Graczyk TK, Knight R, Tamang L: Mechanical transmission of human protozoan parasites by insects. Clin Microbiol Rev 18:128-132, 2005.
Hotez PJ, Brooker S, Bethony JM, et al: Hookworm infection. N Engl J Med 351:799-807, 2004.

Laboratory Diagnosis of Parasitic Disease

The diagnosis of parasitic infections may be very difficult, particularly in the nonendemic setting. The clinical manifestations of parasitic diseases are seldom specific enough to raise the possibility of these processes in the mind of the clinician, and routine laboratory tests are seldom helpful. Although peripheral eosinophilia is widely recognized as a useful indicator of parasitic disease, this phenomenon is characteristic only of helminthic infection and even in these cases is frequently absent. Thus the physician must maintain a heightened index of suspicion and must rely on detailed travel, food intake, transfusion, and socioeconomic history to raise the possibility of parasitic disease. Proper diagnosis requires that (1) the physician consider the possibility of parasitic infection, (2) appropriate specimens be obtained and transported to the laboratory in a timely fashion, (3) the laboratory competently performs the appropriate procedures for the recovery and identification of the etiologic agent, (4) the laboratory results be effectively communicated to the physician, and (5) the results be correctly interpreted by the physician and applied to the care of the patient. In addition, for most parasitic diseases, appropriate test selection and interpretation is based on an understanding of the **life cycle** of the parasite, as well as the **pathogenesis** of the disease process in humans.

Numerous methods for diagnosing parasitic diseases have been described (Box 79-1). Some are useful in detecting a wide variety of parasites, and others are particularly useful for one or a few parasites. Although the mainstay of diagnostic clinical microbiology is the isolation of the causative pathogen in culture, the diagnosis of parasitic diseases is accomplished almost entirely by morphologic (usually microscopic) demonstration of parasites in clinical material. Occasionally, demonstration of a specific antibody response (serodiagnosis) helps in establishing the diagnosis. The detection of parasite antigens in serum, urine, or stool now provides a rapid and sensitive means of diagnosing infection with certain organisms. Likewise, the development of nucleic-acid-based assays may prove to be an excellent means of detecting and identifying a number of parasites in biologic samples such as blood, stool, urine, sputum, and tissue biopsies obtained from infected patients. In general, it is better for the laboratory to offer a limited number of competently performed procedures than to offer a wide variety of infrequently and poorly performed tests.

This chapter provides a general description of the principles of specimen collection and processing necessary to diagnose most parasitic infections. Specific details of these and other procedures of general and limited usefulness may be found in several reference texts listed in the Bibliography.

Parasite Life Cycle as an Aid in Diagnosis

Parasites may have complex life cycles involving single or multiple hosts. Understanding the life cycle of parasitic organisms is a key to understanding important features of geographical distribution, transmission, and pathogenesis of many parasitic diseases. The life cycles of parasites often suggest useful clues for diagnosis as well. For example, in the life cycle of filariae that infect humans, certain species such as *Wuchereria bancrofti* have a **"nocturnal periodicity"** in which greater numbers of microfilariae are found in the peripheral blood at night. Sampling the blood of such patients during daytime hours may fail to detect the microfilariae, whereas blood specimens collected between 10 PM and 4 AM may demonstrate many microfilariae. Likewise, intestinal nematodes such as *Ascaris lumbricoides* and hookworm, which reside in the lumen of the intestine, produce large numbers of eggs that can be detected easily in the stool of an infected patient. In contrast, another intestinal nematode, *Strongyloides stercoralis*, lays its eggs in the bowel wall rather than in the intestinal lumen. As a result, the eggs are rarely seen on stool examination; to make the diagnosis, the parasitologist must be alert for the presence of larvae. Finally, parasites may cause clinical symptoms at a time when diagnostic forms are not yet present in the usual site. For example, in certain intestinal nematode infections, the **migration** of larvae through the tissues may cause intense symptomatology weeks before the characteristic eggs are present in the feces.

General Diagnostic Considerations

The importance of appropriate specimen collection, the number and timing of specimens, timely transport to the laboratory, and prompt examination by an experienced microscopist cannot be overemphasized. Because the majority of parasitologic examinations and identifications are based entirely on recognizing the characteristic morphology of the organisms, any condition that may obscure or distort the morphologic appearance of the parasite may result in an erroneous identification or missed diagnosis. As noted previously and in Box 79-1, there may be alternatives to microscopy for the detection and identification of certain parasites. These tests (e.g., antigen detection, nucleic acid amplification/detection), although presently uncommon, may become more widely applied in the future. They offer the promise of more rapid, sensitive, and specific diagnostic testing for parasitic diseases. These diagnostic test options may expand the testing capabilities of many laboratories, allowing laboratories with limited proficiency in parasitology to offer diagnostic testing for certain parasitic diseases. A list of common and uncommon diagnostic procedures and specimens to be collected for selected parasitic infections is provided in Table 79-1.

Parasitic Infections of the Intestinal and Urogenital Tracts

Protozoa and helminths may colonize or infect the intestinal and urogenital tracts of humans. Most commonly, these parasites are amoebae, flagellates, or nematodes (Table 79-2).

However, infection with trematodes, cestodes, ciliate, coccidian, or microsporidian parasites may also be encountered.

In intestinal and urogenital infections, a simple wet mount or stained smear is often inadequate. Repeated specimen collection and testing are often necessary to optimize the detection of organisms that are shed intermittently or in fluctuating numbers. Concentration of specimens by sedimentation or flotation techniques may be required to detect low numbers of ova (of worms) or cysts (of protozoa) in fecal specimens.

Occasionally, specimens other than stool or urine must be examined (see Table 79-1). Optimal detection of small bowel pathogens such as *Giardia lamblia* and *S. stercoralis* may require the aspiration of duodenal contents or even small-bowel biopsy. Likewise, the detection of colonic parasites such as *Entamoeba histolytica* and *Schistosoma mansoni* may necessitate proctoscopic or sigmoidoscopic examination with aspiration or biopsy of mucosal lesions. Sampling of the perianal skin is a useful means of recovering the eggs of *Enterobius vermicularis* (pinworm) or *Taenia* species (tapeworm).

Fecal Specimen Collection

Patients, clinicians, and laboratory personnel must be properly instructed on collection and handling of specimens. Fecal specimens should be collected in clean, wide-mouthed, waterproof containers with a tight-fitting lid to ensure and maintain adequate moisture. Specimens must not be contaminated with water, soil, or urine, because water and soil may contain free-living organisms that can be mistaken for human parasites, and urine can destroy motile trophozoites and may cause helminth eggs to hatch. Stool specimens should not contain barium, bismuth, or medications containing mineral oil, antibiotics, antimalarials, or other chemical substances, because such specimens compromise the detection of intestinal parasites. Specimen collection should be delayed for 5 to 10 days to allow barium to clear and for at least 2 weeks after antibiotics such as tetracycline to allow intestinal parasites to recover from the toxic (but not curative) effects of the drugs.

Purged specimens may be collected when organisms are not detected in normally passed fecal specimens; however, only certain purgatives (sodium sulfate and buffered sodium biphosphate [Phospho-Soda]) are satisfactory. One series of purged specimens may be examined in place of, or in addition to, a series of normally passed specimens.

Unpreserved formed fecal specimens should arrive in the laboratory within 2 hours after passage. If the stool is liquid and thus more likely to contain trophozoites, it should reach the laboratory for examination within 30 minutes. Soft or loose stools should be examined within 1 hour of passage. If examination is not possible within the recommended time limits, all fresh fecal samples should be placed into preservatives such as 10% formalin, polyvinyl alcohol

Table 79–1. Body Sites, Specimen Collection, and Diagnostic Procedures for Selected Parasitic Infections

Infecting Organism	Specimen Options	Collection Methods	Diagnostic Procedure
Blood			
Plasmodium species, *Babesia* species, filaria, *Leishmania*, *Toxoplasma*, *Trypanosoma* species	Whole blood, anticoagulated	Venipuncture	Microscopic examination (Giemsa stain) or acridine orange fluorescent stain Thin film Thick film Blood concentration (filaria) Serology Antibody Antigen PCR
Bone Marrow			
Leishmania species, *Trypanosoma cruzi*	Aspirate Serum	Sterile Venipuncture	Microscopic examination (Giemsa stain) Culture Serology (antibody) PCR
Central Nervous System			
Acanthamoeba species, *Naegleria* species, trypanosomes, *Toxoplasma gondii*	Spinal fluid Serum	Sterile Venipuncture	Microscopic examination Wet mount Permanent stain Culture Serology (antibody) PCR
Cutaneous Ulcers			
Leishmania species, *Acanthamoeba* species	Aspirate Biopsy Serum	Sterile plus smears Sterile, nonsterile to histology Venipuncture	Microscopic examination (Giemsa stain) Culture Serology (antibody) PCR
Eye			
Acanthamoeba species, *Loa loa*	Corneal scrapings Corneal biopsy	Sterile saline, air-dried smear Sterile saline	Microscopic examination Wet mount Permanent stain Culture
Intestinal Tract			
Entamoeba histolytica	Fresh stool Preserved stool Sigmoidoscopy material Serum	Waxed container Formalin, PVA Fresh, PVA Schaudinn smears Venipuncture	Microscopic examination Wet mount Permanent stains Serology Antigen (stool) Antibody (serum) Culture PCR
Giardia species	Fresh stool Preserved stool Duodenal contents	Waxed container Formalin, PVA Entero-Test or aspirate	Microscopic examination Wet mount Permanent stains Antigen IFA EIA Culture
Cryptosporidium species	Fresh stool Preserved stool Biopsy	Waxed container Formalin, PVA Saline	Microscopic examination (acid-fast) Antigen IFA EIA

Continued

Table 79–1. Body Sites, Specimen Collection, and Diagnostic Procedures for Selected Parasitic Infections—cont'd

Infecting Organism	Specimen Options	Collection Methods	Diagnostic Procedure

Microsporidia	Fresh stool
	Preserved stool
	Duodenal contents
	Biopsy
		Waxed container
		Formalin, PVA
		Aspirate
		Saline
			Microscopic
			  Giemsa stain
			  Gram stain
			  Chromotrope stain

Pinworm	Anal impression smear	Cellophane tape	Macroscopic examination Microscopic examination (eggs)
Helminths	Fresh stool Preserved stool Serum	Waxed container Formalin, PVA Venipuncture	Macroscopic examination (adults) Microscopic examination (larvae and eggs) Serology (antibody) Culture (*Strongyloides*)
Liver, Spleen			

E. histolytica, Leishmania species	Aspirates
	
	Biopsy
	
	Serum
		Sterile, collected in four
		  separate aliquots (liver)
		Sterile; nonsterile to
		  histology
		Venipuncture
			Microscopic examination
			  Wet mount
			  Permanent stains
			Serology
			  Antigen
			  Antibody
			Culture

Lung			

Rarely: amoebae, (*E. histolytica*),
  trematodes (*P. westermani*), larvae
  (*S. stercoralis*), or cestode hooklets
	Sputum
	Lavage
	Transbronchial
	  aspirate
	Brush biopsy
	Open lung biopsy
		Induced, no preservative
		No preservative
		Air dried smears
		
		Same as above
		Fresh squash preparation;
		  nonsterile to histology
			Microscopic examination
			  Giemsa stain
			  Gram stain
			  Hematoxylin and eosin
			Antigen
			  IFA
			  EIA
			Serum (antibody)

Muscle			

Trichinella spiralis,
Trypanosoma cruzi
	Biopsy
	Serum
		Nonsterile to histology
		Venipuncture
			Microscopic examination (permanent stains)
			Serology
			  Antibody
			  Antigen

Skin			

Onchocerca volvulus, Leishmania species
Cutaneous larval migrans
	Scrapings
	Skin snip
	Biopsy
	Serum
		Aseptic, smear, or vial
		No preservative
		Nonsterile to histology
		Venipuncture
			Microscopic examination
			  Wet mount
			  Permanent stains
			Serology (antibody)
			Culture (*Leishmania* species)

Urogenital System			

Trichomonas vaginalis	Vaginal discharge
	Prostatic secretions
	Urethral discharge
		Saline swab, culture medium
		Same as above
			Microscopic examination
			  Wet mount
			  Permanent stains
			Antigen (IFA)
			Culture (*T. vaginalis*)
			Serology (antibody)
			Nucleic acid probes (*T. vaginalis*)

Schistosoma haematobium	Urine Biopsy	Single unpreserved specimen Nonsterile to histology	Microscopic examination

EIA, enzyme immunoassay; IFA, immunofluorescent assay; PCR, polymerase chain reaction; PVA, polyvinyl alcohol.

Table 79–1. Body Sites, Specimen Collection, and Diagnostic Procedures for Selected Parasitic Infections

Infecting Organism	Specimen Options	Collection Methods	Diagnostic Procedure
Blood			
Plasmodium species, *Babesia* species, filaria, *Leishmania*, *Toxoplasma*, *Trypanosoma* species	Whole blood, anticoagulated	Venipuncture	Microscopic examination (Giemsa stain) or acridine orange fluorescent stain Thin film Thick film Blood concentration (filaria) Serology Antibody Antigen PCR
Bone Marrow			
Leishmania species, *Trypanosoma cruzi*	Aspirate Serum	Sterile Venipuncture	Microscopic examination (Giemsa stain) Culture Serology (antibody) PCR
Central Nervous System			
Acanthamoeba species, *Naegleria* species, trypanosomes, *Toxoplasma gondii*	Spinal fluid Serum	Sterile Venipuncture	Microscopic examination Wet mount Permanent stain Culture Serology (antibody) PCR
Cutaneous Ulcers			
Leishmania species, *Acanthamoeba* species	Aspirate Biopsy Serum	Sterile plus smears Sterile, nonsterile to histology Venipuncture	Microscopic examination (Giemsa stain) Culture Serology (antibody) PCR
Eye			
Acanthamoeba species, *Loa loa*	Corneal scrapings Corneal biopsy	Sterile saline, air-dried smear Sterile saline	Microscopic examination Wet mount Permanent stain Culture
Intestinal Tract			
Entamoeba histolytica	Fresh stool Preserved stool Sigmoidoscopy material Serum	Waxed container Formalin, PVA Fresh, PVA Schaudinn smears Venipuncture	Microscopic examination Wet mount Permanent stains Serology Antigen (stool) Antibody (serum) Culture PCR
Giardia species	Fresh stool Preserved stool Duodenal contents	Waxed container Formalin, PVA Entero-Test or aspirate	Microscopic examination Wet mount Permanent stains Antigen IFA EIA Culture
Cryptosporidium species	Fresh stool Preserved stool Biopsy	Waxed container Formalin, PVA Saline	Microscopic examination (acid-fast) Antigen IFA EIA

Continued

Table 79–2. Most Commonly Identified Intestinal Parasites in U.S. Laboratories

Organism	% of Total Positive Specimens (n = 2453)
Giardia lamblia	37
Blastocystis hominis	27
Cryptosporidium parvum	10
Dientamoeba fragilis	5
Entamoeba histolytica/E. dispar	5
Ascaris lumbricoides	4
Trichuris trichiura	2
Hookworm	2
Enterobius vermicularis	2
Strongyloides stercoralis	2
Hymenolepis nana	1
Isospora species	<1
Microsporidia	<1
Clonorchis/Opisthorchis species	<1
Other helminths	1

Data compiled from Valenstein, et al: The use and abuse of routine stool microbiology: A College of American Pathologists Q-Probes study of 601 institutions. Arch Pathol Lab Med 120:206-211, 1996; Amin OM: Seasonal prevalence of intestinal parasites in the United States during 2000. Am J Trop Med Hyg 66:799-803, 2002.

Table 79–3. Number of Specimens Required to Detect Intestinal Parasites

Number of Specimens per Patient	Percentage of Infected Patients Detected*
1	71.5
2	86.9
3	100

*n = 130
Data compiled from Branda, et al: A rational approach to the stool ova and parasite examination. Clin Infect Dis 42:972-978, 2006.

(PVA), merthiolate-iodine-formalin (MIF), or sodium acetate formalin (SAF). Fecal specimens may be stored at 4° C but should not be incubated or frozen.

The number of specimens required to demonstrate intestinal parasites varies, depending on the quality of the specimen submitted, the accuracy of the examination performed, the severity of the infection, and the purpose for which the examination is made. If the physician is interested only in determining the presence or absence of helminths, one or two examinations may suffice, provided that concentration methods are used. For a routine parasitic examination, a total of three fecal specimens is recommended. The examination of three specimens using a combination of techniques ensures detection of more than 99% of infections. In a survey conducted in the United States, examination of three specimens was required to detect 100% of infected patients (Table 79-3).

It is inappropriate for multiple specimens to be collected on the same patient on the same day. It is also not recommended for the three specimens to be submitted one each day for 3 consecutive days. The series of three specimens should be collected within no more than 10 days. Many parasites do not appear in fecal specimens in consistent numbers on a daily basis; therefore collection of specimens on alternate days tends to yield a higher percentage of positive findings.

It has become apparent that in the United States, submission of stool for parasitologic examination from patients with hospital-acquired diarrhea (onset more than 3 days after admission) is usually inappropriate. This is because the frequency of acquisition of protozoan or helminthic parasites in a hospital is vanishingly rare. A request for stool examination for ova and parasites in a hospitalized patient should be accompanied by a clear statement of clinical indications and only after the more common causes of hospital-acquired diarrhea (e.g., antibiotic induced) have been ruled out.

Techniques of Stool Examination

Specimens should be examined systematically by a competent microscopist for helminth eggs and larvae, as well as intestinal protozoa. For optimal detection of these various infectious agents, a combination of several techniques of examination is required.

Macroscopic Examination

The fecal specimen should be examined for consistency and for the presence of blood, mucus, worms, and proglottids.

Direct Wet Mount

Fresh stools should be examined under the microscope using the saline and iodine wet-mount technique to detect motile trophozoites or larvae (*Strongyloides*). The saline and iodine wet mounts are also used to detect helminth eggs, protozoan cysts, and host cells such as leukocytes and red blood cells. This approach is also useful in examining material from sputum, urine, vaginal swabs, duodenal aspirates, sigmoidoscopy, abscesses, and tissue biopsies.

Concentration

All fecal specimens should be placed in 10% formalin to preserve parasite morphology and should be concentrated using a procedure such as formalin ethyl acetate (or formalin ether), sedimentation, or zinc sulfate flotation. These methods separate protozoan cysts and helminth eggs from the bulk of fecal material and thus enhance the ability to detect small numbers of organisms usually missed by the use of only a direct smear. After concentration, the material is stained with iodine and examined microscopically.

Permanently Stained Slides

The detection and correct identification of intestinal protozoa often depend on the examination of the permanently stained smear. These slides provide a permanent record of the protozoan organisms that are identified. The cytologic detail revealed by one of the permanent staining methods is essential for accurate identification, and most identification should be considered tentative until confirmed by the permanently stained slide. The common permanent stains used are trichrome, iron hematoxylin, and phosphotungstic acid–hematoxylin. Slides are made either by preparing smears of fresh fecal material and placing them in Schaudinn fixative solution or by fixing a small amount of fecal material in PVA fixative.

Collection and Examination of Specimens Other Than Stool

Frequently, specimens other than fecal material must be collected and examined to diagnose infections caused by intestinal pathogens. These specimens include perianal samples, sigmoidoscopic material, aspirates of duodenal contents, and liver abscesses, sputum, urine, and urogenital specimens.

Perianal Specimens

The collection of perianal specimens is frequently necessary to diagnose pinworm (*E. vermicularis*) and occasionally *Taenia* (tapeworm) infections. The methods include the preparation of a clear cellulose tape slide or an anal swab. The cellulose tape slide preparation is the method of choice for the detection of pinworm eggs. Specimens collected by either method should be obtained in the morning before the patient bathes or goes to the bathroom. The tape method requires that the adhesive surface of the tape be pressed firmly against the right and left perianal folds and then spread onto the surface of a microscope slide. Likewise, the anal swab should be rubbed gently over the perianal area and transported to the laboratory for microscopic examination. With either collection method, the slides or swabs should be kept at 4° C if transport to the laboratory is to be delayed.

Sigmoidoscopic Material

Material from sigmoidoscopy can be helpful in the diagnosis of *E. histolytica* infection that has not been detected by routine fecal examinations. The specimens consist of scraped or aspirated material from the mucosal surface.

At least six areas should be sampled. After collection, the material should be placed in a tube containing 0.85% saline and should be kept warm during transport to the laboratory. The specimens should be examined immediately for motile trophozoites.

Duodenal Aspirates

Sampling and examination of duodenal contents is a means of recovering *Strongyloides* larvae; the eggs of *Clonorchis*, *Opisthorchis*, and *Fasciola* species; and other small bowel parasites such as *Giardia*, *Isospora*, and *Cryptosporidium* organisms. Specimens may be obtained by endoscopic intubation or by the use of the enteric capsule or string test (Entero-Test). Endoscopic biopsy of the small intestinal mucosa may reveal *Giardia* organisms, *Cryptosporidium* organisms, and microsporidia, as well as *Strongyloides* larvae. Specimens should be collected in saline and transported directly to the laboratory for microscopic examination.

Liver Abscess Aspirate

Suppurative lesions of the liver and subphrenic spaces may be caused by *E. histolytica* (extraintestinal amebiasis). Extraintestinal amebiasis may occur in the absence of any history of symptomatic intestinal infection. The specimen should be collected from the liver abscess margin instead of the necrotic center. The first portion removed is usually yellowish white in appearance and seldom contains amoebae. Later portions, which are reddish, are more likely to contain organisms. A minimum of two separate portions of exudative material should be removed. After aspiration, the collapse of the abscess and the subsequent inflowing of blood often release amoebae from the tissue. Subsequent aspirations may have a greater chance of revealing organisms. The aspirated material should be transported immediately to the laboratory.

Sputum

Occasionally, intestinal parasites may be detected in sputum. These organisms include the larvae of *Ascaris*, *Strongyloides*, and hookworm; cestode hooklets; and intestinal protozoa such as *E. histolytica* and *Cryptosporidium* species. The specimen should be a deep sputum rather than primarily saliva, and it should be delivered immediately to the laboratory. Microscopic examination should include saline wet-mount and permanent stain preparations.

Urine

Examination of urine specimens may be useful in diagnosing infections caused by *Schistosoma haematobium* (occasionally other species as well) and *Trichomonas vaginalis*. Detection of eggs in urine can be accomplished using direct detection or concentration using the sedimentation centrifugation technique. Eggs may be trapped in mucus or pus and are more frequently present in the last few drops of the specimen rather than the first portion. The production of *Schistosoma* eggs fluctuates; therefore examinations should be performed over several days. *T. vaginalis* may be found in the urinary sediment of male and female patients.

Urogenital Specimens

Urogenital specimens are collected if infection with *T. vaginalis* is suspected. Identification is based on wet-mount preparation examinations of vaginal and urethral discharges, prostatic secretions, or urine sediment. Specimens should be placed in a container with a small amount of 0.85% saline and sent immediately to the laboratory for examination. If no organisms are detected by direct wet mounts, culture may be used.

Parasitic Infections of Blood and Tissue

Parasites localized within the blood or tissues of the host are more difficult to detect than intestinal and urogenital parasites. Microscopic examination of blood films is a direct and useful means of detecting malarial parasites, trypanosomes, and microfilariae. Unfortunately, the concentration of organisms often fluctuates; thus the collection of multiple specimens over several days is required. The preparation of both wet mounts (microfilariae and trypanosomes) and permanently stained thick and thin blood films is the mainstay of diagnosis. Examination of sputum may reveal helminth ova (lung flukes) or larvae (*Ascaris* and *Strongyloides* species) after appropriate concentration techniques. Biopsy of skin (onchocerciasis) or muscle (trichinosis) may be required for the diagnosis of certain nematode infections (see Table 79-1).

Blood Films

The clinical diagnosis of parasitic diseases such as malaria, leishmaniasis, trypanosomiasis, and filariasis largely rests on the collection of appropriately timed blood samples and the expert microscopic examination of properly prepared and stained thick and thin blood films. The optimal time for obtaining blood for parasitologic examination varies with the particular parasite expected.

Because malaria is one of the few parasitic infections that can be acutely life threatening, blood collection and examination of blood films should be performed immediately if the diagnosis is suspected. Laboratories offering this service should be prepared to do so on a 24-hour basis, 7 days a week. Because the levels of parasitemia may be low or fluctuating, it is recommended that repeat blood films be obtained and examined at 6, 12, and 24 hours after the initial sample. Detection of trypanosomes in blood is occasionally possible during the early acute phase of the disease. *Trypanosoma cruzi* (Chagas' disease) may also be detected during subsequent febrile periods. After several months to a year, the trypomastigotes of African trypanosomiasis (*Trypanosoma brucei rhodesiense* and *T. b. gambiense*) are

better demonstrated in spinal fluid than blood. Blood samples for the detection of nocturnal microfilariae (*W. bancrofti* and *Brugia malayi*) should be obtained between 10 PM and 4 AM, whereas for the diurnal *Loa loa*, samples are obtained around noon.

Two types of blood films are prepared for the diagnosis of blood parasite infections: thin films and thick films. Although wet-mount preparations of blood films can be examined for motile parasites (microfilariae and trypanosomes), most laboratories proceed directly to the preparation of thick and thin films for staining. In the thin film, the blood is spread over the slide in a thin (single cell) layer, and the red blood cells remain intact after staining. In the thick film, the red cells are lysed before staining, and only the white blood cells, platelets, and parasites (if present) are visible. Thick films allow a larger amount of blood to be examined, which increases the possibility of detecting light infections. Unfortunately, increased distortion of the parasites makes species identification using the thick film particularly difficult. Proper use of this technique usually requires a great deal of expertise and experience.

Occasionally, other blood-concentration procedures may be used to detect light infections. Alternative concentration methods for detecting blood parasites include the use of microhematocrit centrifugation, the examination of buffy coat preparations, a triple centrifugation technique for the detection of low numbers of trypanosomes, and a membrane filtration technique for the detection of microfilariae.

Once prepared, blood films must be stained. The most dependable staining of blood parasites is obtained with Giemsa stain buffered to pH 7.0 to 7.2, although special stains may be occasionally used to identify species of microfilariae. Giemsa stain is particularly useful for the staining of protozoa (malaria and trypanosomes); however, the sheath of microfilariae may not always stain with Giemsa. In this case, hematoxylin-based stains may be used.

Specimens Other Than Blood

Examination of tissue and body fluids other than blood may be necessary, based on clinical presentation and epidemiologic considerations. Smears and concentrates of cerebrospinal fluid are necessary to detect trophozoites of *Naegleria fowleri*, trypanosomes, and larvae of the nematode *Angiostrongylus cantonensis* within the central nervous system. Cerebrospinal fluid must be promptly examined, because the trophozoite forms of these parasites are very labile (trypanosomes) or tend to round up and become nonmotile (*Naegleria fowleri*). Examination of tissue impression smears of lymph nodes, liver biopsy material, spleen, or bone marrow stained with Giemsa stain is very useful in detecting **intracellular** parasites such as *Leishmania* species and *Toxoplasma gondii*. Likewise, biopsies of various tissues are an excellent means of detecting localized or disseminated infections caused by protozoan and helminthic parasites. Saline mounts of superficial skin snips are very useful in detecting the microfilariae of *Onchocerca volvulus.* Examination of sputum (induced) is indicated when there is a question of pulmonary paragonimiasis (lung fluke) or abscess formation with *E. histolytica. Strongyloides* larvae may be detected in sputum in hyperinfection syndrome.

Alternatives to Microscopy

In the majority of cases, the diagnosis of parasitic disease is made in the laboratory by microscopic detection and morphologic identification of the parasite in clinical specimens. In some cases, the parasite cannot be detected despite a careful search because of low or absent levels of organisms in readily available clinical material. In such cases, the clinician may need to rely on alternative methods based on the detection of parasite-derived material (antigens or nucleic acids) or by the host response to parasitic invasion (antibodies). Additional approaches used in selected infections include culture, animal inoculation, and xenodiagnosis.

Immunodiagnostics

Immunodiagnostic methods have long been used as aids in the diagnosis of parasitic diseases. The majority of these serologic tests are based on the detection of specific antibody responses to the presence of the parasite. The analytical approaches include the use of classical agglutination, complement fixation, and gel diffusion methods, as well as the more modern immunofluorescence, enzyme immunoassay (EIA), and Western blot assays. Antibody detection is useful and indicated in the diagnosis of many protozoan diseases (e.g., extraintestinal amebiasis, South American trypanosomiasis, leishmaniasis, transfusion-acquired malaria, and toxoplasmosis) and helminthic diseases (e.g., clonorchiasis, cysticercosis, hydatidosis, lymphatic filariasis, schistosomiasis, trichinellosis, and toxocariasis). There is a problem with the detection of antibody as a means of diagnosis: because of the persistence of antibody for months to years after the acute infection, demonstration of antibody can rarely differentiate between acute and chronic infection.

In contrast to antibody detection, the measurement of circulating parasite antigen in serum, urine, or feces may provide a more appropriate marker for the presence of active infection and may also indicate parasite load. Likewise, demonstrations of specific **parasite antigen** in lesion fluid, such as material from an amoebic abscess or fluid from a hydatid cyst, may provide a definitive diagnosis of the infecting organism. Most common antigen-detection assays use an EIA format; however, immunofluorescence, radioimmunoassay, and immunoblot methods have also proved useful. Several commercial assays for the detection of parasite antigens are now available in kits. These include EIA and immunochromatographic assays for the detection of *Giardia, E. histolytica, E. dispar,* and *Cryptosporidium* species in stool, EIA for the detection of *T. vaginalis* in

urogenital specimens, and immunofluorescent assays (IFA) for the detection of *Giardia, Cryptosporidium,* and *Trichomonas* species. Several antigen detection tests are also available for detection of blood parasites (malaria, filariasis) in conjunction with microscopic examination of thick and thin blood smears. Most of the kits are not available in the United States. The reported sensitivity and specificity for most of these kits are quite good. The advantages to these approaches are labor savings and a potential increase in sensitivity. The disadvantages are the loss of parasitologic expertise and the fact that in some instances, the available assay tests for only a single organism, whereas conventional microscopic examination provides the opportunity to recognize many different parasites. Although antigen-detection assays have been described for many other parasites, they are not widely available. The availability of a broad panel of antigen-detection assays potentially would make the use of an antigen screen a viable alternative to tedious microscopic examination.

Molecular Diagnostic Approaches

In addition to immunodiagnostic methods, the diagnosis of parasitic diseases has been enhanced considerably by the application of molecular diagnostic methods based on **nucleic acid hybridization**. This approach takes advantage of the fact that all organisms contain nucleic acid sequences that may be used in a hybridization assay to distinguish among strains, species, and genera. Thus parasites may be simultaneously detected and identified in clinical material, depending on the specificity of the nucleic acid probe used. Another advantage of nucleic-acid-based detection systems is that they are independent of the patient's immunologic status or previous infection history, thereby identifying active infection. Finally, the development of target amplification techniques such as the polymerase chain reaction provides exquisite sensitivity, allowing the detection of as little as one organism in a biologic sample (Table 79-4).

Nucleic-acid-based methods can be used to detect parasites not only in clinical samples of blood, stool, or tissue from infected patients but also in their natural vector. The application of DNA "fingerprinting" allows precise identification of the parasite to the subspecies or strain level and has considerable value in epidemiologic studies. Assay formats using nucleic acid probes range from dot blot and Southern hybridization methods to in situ hybridization in tissue to polymerase chain reaction (PCR) amplification coupled with solid or solution phase hybridization. The use of nonisotopic DNA labeling techniques greatly expands the potential applicability of these assays worldwide. Diagnostic kits based on these methods are not widely available; however, several are under development and may be available for clinical use in the near future. A simple nucleic acid probe assay for *T. vaginalis* in urogenital specimens is now available commercially in kit form for use in clinics and physicians' offices.

Table 79—4. Examples of Techniques for Detection of Parasitic Infections Based on Polymerase Chain Reaction (PCR) Analysis

Organism	Gene	Target Sensitivity (%)	Comment
Plasmodium vivax	Circumsporozoite gene	91-96	Dried blood—spotted filter paper samples are used.
Leishmania species	kDNA minicircle sequence	87-100	Results are compared to culture and microscopy of biopsy specimens.
Trypanosoma cruzi	kDNA minicircle sequence	100	Results are compared to serology and xenodiagnosis of blood samples.
Toxoplasma gondii	B1 repetitive gene P30 major surface antigen Recombinant DNA sequences	46-99	PCR of BAL, blood, cerebrospinal fluid, and amniotic fluid show great potential for diagnosis of toxoplasmosis.
Entamoeba histolytica	P145 tandem repeat sequence SSU rRNA	96 >90	Results are compared to microscopic diagnosis of stool samples. Test may distinguish pathogenic from nonpathogenic strains.

PCR, Polymerase chain reaction; BAL, bronchoalveolar lavage; SSU rRNA, small subunit ribosomal RNA.

Irrespective of the assay format, nucleic acid probes and amplification techniques are now being used on a research basis for the detection and identification of numerous species and strains, including *Plasmodium* species, *Leishmania* species, *T. cruzi*, *E. histolytica*, and *Toxoplasma gondii* (see Table 79-4). It must be understood that the application of nucleic acid hybridization methods to the diagnosis of parasitic diseases is still in its infancy. The widespread use of these techniques requires further development of simple procedures for sample handling and preparation and will require extensive clinical and field testing before they can be applied broadly to aid in clinical diagnosis.

Culture

Although culture is the standard for the diagnosis of most infectious diseases, it is not commonly used in the parasitology laboratory. Certain protozoan parasites such as *T. vaginalis*, *E. histolytica*, *Acanthamoeba* species, *Naegleria fowleri*, *Leishmania* species, *T. cruzi*, and *Toxoplasma gondii* can be cultured with relative ease. However, culture of other parasites has not been successful or is too difficult or cumbersome to be of practical value in routine diagnostic efforts.

Animal Inoculation

Animal inoculation is a sensitive means of detecting infection caused by blood and tissue parasites such as *T. b. gambiense*, *T. b. rhodesiense*, *T. cruzi*, *Leishmania* species, and *T. gondii*. Although useful, this approach is not practical for most diagnostic laboratories and is largely confined to research settings.

Xenodiagnosis

The technique of xenodiagnosis employs the use of laboratory-raised arthropod vectors to detect low levels of parasites in infected individuals. Classically, this approach was used to diagnose Chagas' disease by allowing an uninfected reduviid bug to feed on an individual suspected of having the disease. Subsequently, the bug was dissected and examined microscopically for evidence of developmental stages of *T. cruzi*. Although this technique may be used in endemic areas, it is obviously not practical for most diagnostic laboratories.

Questions

1. Why is it important to understand the life cycle of parasites when diagnosing parasitic diseases?
2. What factors may confound the use of microscopy in the diagnosis of parasitic disease?
3. Describe the important considerations in collecting and submitting a fecal specimen for parasitologic examination.
4. Which parasites can be detected in blood?
5. What are the alternatives to microscopy for the diagnosis of parasitic infections?

Bibliography

Amin OM: Seasonal prevalence of intestinal parasites in the United States during 2000. Am J Trop Med Hyg 66:799-803, 2002.
Branda JA, et al: A rational approach to the stool ova and parasite examination. Clin Infect Dis 42:972-978, 2006.

Deplazes P, Garcia LS, Shimizu R: Specimen collection, transport, and processing: Parasitology. In Murray PR, et al (eds): Manual of Clinical Microbiology, 9th ed. Washington, DC, ASM Press, 2007.

Fotedar R, et al: Laboratory diagnostic techniques for *Entamoeba* species. Clin Microbiol Rev 20:511-532, 2007.

Garcia LS, Schimizu RY, Bernard CN: Detection of *Giardia lamblia*, *Entamoeba histolytica/Entamoeba dispar*, and *Cryptosporidium parvum* antigens in human fecal specimens using the Triage Parasite Panel enzyme immunoassay. J Clin Microbiol 38:3337-3340, 2000.

Garcia LS, Shimizu RY, Paltridge GP: Algorithms for detection and identification of parasites. In Murray PR, et al (eds): Manual of Clinical Microbiology, 9th ed. Washington, DC, ASM Press, 2007.

Moody A: Rapid diagnostic tests for malaria parasites. Clin Microbiol Rev 15:66-78, 2002.

Rosenblatt JE: Clinical importance of adequately performed stool ova and parasite examinations. Clin Infect Dis 42:979-980, 2006.

Valenstein P, Pfaller M, Yungbluth M: The use and abuse of routine stool microbiology: A College of American Pathologists Q-Probes study of 601 institutions. Arch Pathol Lab Med 120:206-211, 1996.

80

Antiparasitic Agents

The chemotherapeutic approach to the management of infectious diseases has clearly changed the face of medicine. Unfortunately, few of the anti-infective agents that have proved so successful against bacterial pathogens have been effective against parasites. In many instances, clinicians continue to rely on antiparasitic agents from the pre-antibiotic era. These and some newer agents remain limited in effectiveness and are relatively toxic. Many antiparasitic agents require prolonged or parenteral administration and may be effective only in certain disease states. Fortunately, in the last 5 to 10 years, several new agents have appeared that constitute significant advances in the treatment of parasitic diseases. In each case, the previously available drugs were toxic and often ineffective.

In large part, the difficulties in the treatment of parasitic diseases stem from the fact that parasites are **eukaryotic** organisms and thus are more similar to the human host than the more successfully treated prokaryotic bacterial pathogens. Furthermore, the chronic and prolonged course of infection, the complex life cycles, and multiple developmental stages of many parasites add to the difficulties of effective chemotherapeutic intervention. Additional complicating factors in developing countries, where the majority of parasitic diseases occur, include (1) the presence of multiple infections and the high probability of reinfection, (2) the large number of persons immunocompromised by malnutrition and human immunodeficiency virus infection, and (3) the overwhelming influence of poverty and poor sanitation, which facilitate the transmission of many parasitic infections. Although chemotherapeutic approaches may be used effectively to treat and prevent many parasitic infections, some agents have adverse effects or eventually meet with resistance (microbial and social). Most antiparasitic agents are too expensive for widespread use in developing countries. Thus the global approach to the prevention and treatment of parasitic diseases must involve several strategies, including improved hygiene and sanitation, control of the disease vector, use of **vaccinations** if available (largely unavailable for parasitic diseases), and prophylactic and therapeutic administration of safe and effective chemotherapy. Notably large-scale chemotherapy administered one to three times per year in endemic regions has reduced transmission of, and morbidity and mortality from, certain infections, including lymphatic filariasis, onchocerciasis, schistosomiasis, and intestinal nematodes. These strategies now must also include efforts to decrease the transmission of infection by the human immunodeficiency virus.

Targets for Antiparasite Drug Action

As mentioned previously, parasites are eukaryotic organisms and thus have more similarities than differences with the human host. Consequently, many antiparasitic agents act on pathways (nucleic acid synthesis, carbohydrate metabolism) or targets (neuromuscular function) shared by both the parasite and the host. For this reason, developing safe and effective antiparasitic drugs based on biochemical **differences** between the parasite and host has been difficult. **Differential toxicity** is commonly achieved by preferential uptake, metabolic alteration of the drug by the parasite, or differences in the susceptibility of functionally equivalent sites in the parasite and host. Fortunately, as our understanding of the basic biology and biochemistry of parasites and the mechanism of action of antimicrobial agents has improved, so has our recognition of potential parasite-specific targets for chemotherapeutic attack. Increasingly, investigators are exploiting newly completed genome projects for protozoan parasites to identify potential drug targets for high-throughput screening. Examples of the chemotherapeutic strategies that exploit the differences between parasite and host are provided in Table 80-1. These are discussed in greater detail as we deal with the specific agents.

Table 80–1. Chemotherapeutic Strategies That Exploit Differences Between Parasite and Host

Unique Site of Attack	Drug	Organism
Drug-concentrating mechanism unique to parasite	Chloroquine	*Plasmodium* species
Folic acid pathway (parasite unable to use exogenous folate)	Pyrimethamine or trimethoprim-sulfamethoxazole	*Plasmodium* or *Toxoplasma* species
Inhibitor of trypanothione-dependent mechanisms for reducing oxidized thiol groups	Arsenicals, difluoromethylornithine	Trypanosomes
Interference with neuromediators unique to parasites	Pyrantel pamoate, diethylcarbamazine	*Ascaris* species
Interacts with chloride channels, resulting in hyperpolarization of cells, paralysis, and death of parasites	Ivermectin	Filaria
Interaction with tubulin unique to parasites	Benzimidazoles	Many helminths
Inhibition of topoisomerase II	Pentamidine	Trypanosomes
Inhibition of pyruvate ferredoxin oxidoreductase	Nitazoxanide	*Cryptosporidium* and *Giardia*

Drug Resistance

Resistance to antimicrobial agents is an important consideration in the treatment of infections resulting from bacteria and fungal pathogens and certainly plays a role in the chemotherapy of parasitic diseases. Unfortunately, our understanding of the molecular and genetic basis for resistance to most antiparasitic agents is quite limited. Greater understanding of the epidemiology and mechanisms of drug resistance can provide valuable guidance for a better use of existing compounds and for the development of novel agents. Much of the information regarding the molecular mechanisms of drug resistance in parasites has come from studies in plasmodia. Resistance to chloroquine, a major antimalarial agent, is most likely due to the presence of an active chloroquine efflux mechanism similar to that producing the rapid efflux of anticancer drugs observed in multidrug-resistant mammalian cancer cells. In addition, the development of plasmodial resistance to antifolate compounds such as pyrimethamine is due to a series of mutations in the parasite's combined dihydrofolate reductase–thymidylate synthetase enzyme. These efforts have led to further studies and improved understanding of mechanisms of drug resistance in *Trichomonas* (metronidazole), *Leishmania* (pentavalent antimonials), African trypanosomes (melarsoprol, pentamidine), and schistosomes (oxamniquine). Further insights into the mechanisms of action and resistance to antiparasitic agents are necessary to optimize the effectiveness of antiparasite chemotherapy.

Antiparasitic Agents

Although the number of effective antiparasitic agents is small relative to the vast array of antibacterial agents, the list is expanding (Table 80-2). Certainly in many cases, the goal of antiparasitic therapy is similar to that of antibacterial therapy: to eradicate the organism rapidly and completely. In many cases, however, the agents and treatment regimens used for parasitic diseases are designed simply to decrease the parasite burden, to prevent the systemic complications of chronic infection, or both actions. Thus the goals of antiparasitic therapy, particularly as applied in endemic areas, may be quite different from those usually considered for therapy of microbial infection in the United States or other developed countries. Given the significant toxicity of many of these agents, in every case the need for treatment must be weighed against the toxicity of the drug. A decision to withhold therapy may often be correct, particularly when the drug can cause severe adverse effects.

Immunocompromised individuals pose a particular problem with respect to antiparasitic chemotherapy. On the one hand, **prophylaxis**, such as that administered for toxoplasmosis, may be effective in preventing infection. However, once infection is established, radical cure may not be possible, and long-term **suppressive therapy** may be indicated. In some diseases, such as cryptosporidiosis and microsporidiosis, effective (curative) therapy is not available, and care must be taken to avoid unnecessary toxicity while providing supportive care for the patient.

The remainder of this chapter provides an overview of the major classes of antiprotozoal and anthelmintic agents. These and additional antiparasitic agents, their mechanisms of action, and their clinical indications are listed in Table 80-2. Treatment of specific infections is discussed in the chapters that deal with the parasites. The Bibliography lists several excellent reviews for more complete information and for discussions of the antiparasitic agents that are available.

Table 80–2. Mechanisms of Action and Clinical Indications for the Major Antiparasitic Agents

Drug Class	Mechanism of Action	Examples	Clinical Indications
Antiprotozoal Agents			
Heavy metals: arsenicals and antimonials	Inactivate sulfhydryl groups	Melarsoprol, sodium stibogluconate, meglumine antimonate	Trypanosomiasis, leishmaniasis
Aminoquinoline analogues	Accumulate in parasitized cells. Interfere with DNA replication. Bind to ferriprotoporphyrin IX. Raise intravesicular pH. Interfere with hemoglobin digestion	Chloroquine, mefloquine, quinine, primaquine	Malaria prophylaxis and therapy Radical cure (exoerythrocytic-primaquine only)
Folic acid antagonists	Inhibit dihydropteroate synthetase and dihydrofolate reductase	Sulfonamides, pyrimethamine, trimethoprim	Toxoplasmosis, malaria, cyclosporiasis
Inhibitors of protein synthesis	Block peptide synthesis at level of ribosome	Clindamycin, spiramycin, paromomycin, tetracycline, doxycycline	Malaria, babesiosis, amebiasis, cryptosporidiosis
Diamidines	Bind DNA Interfere with uptake and function of polyamines	Pentamidine	Pneumocystosis, leishmaniasis, trypanosomiasis
Nitroimidazoles	Unclear Interact with DNA Inhibit metabolism of glucose and interfere with mitochondrial function	Metronidazole, benzimidazole, tinidazole	Amebiasis, giardiasis, trichomoniasis
Quinolones	Inhibit DNA gyrase	Ciprofloxacin	Malaria
Sesquiterpenes	React with heme, causing free-radical damage to parasite membranes	Artemisinin	Malaria
Ornithine analogue	Inhibits ornithine decarboxylase Interferes with polyamine metabolism	Difluoromethylornithine	African trypanosomiasis
Inhibitors of nucleic acid synthesis	Inhibit enzymes in purine salvage pathway	Allopurinol	Leishmaniasis
Acetanilide	Unknown	Diloxanide furoate	Intestinal amebiasis
Sulfated naphthylamine	Inhibits *sn*-glycerol phosphate oxidase and glycerol 3-phosphate dehydrogenase, causing decreased ATP synthesis	Suramin	African trypanosomiasis
Phenanthrenemethanols	Bind to ferriprotoporphyrin IX Affect mitochondria	Halofantrine	Malaria
Anthelmintic Agents			
Benzimidazoles	Inhibit fumarate reductase. Inhibit glucose transport. Disrupt microtubular function	Mebendazole, thiabendazole, albendazole	Broad-spectrum anthelmintic: nematodes, cestodes
Tetrahydropyrimidine	Blocks neuromuscular action Inhibits fumarate reductase	Pyrantel pamoate	Ascariasis, pinworm, hookworm
Piperazines	Cause neuromuscular paralysis. Stimulate phagocytic cells	Piperazine, diethylcarbamazine	*Ascaris* and pinworm infections
Avermectins	Block neuromuscular action Hyperpolarize nerve and muscle cells Inhibit filarial reproduction	Ivermectin	Filarial infections

Continued

Table 80—2. Mechanisms of Action and Clinical Indications for the Major Antiparasitic Agents—cont'd

Drug Class	Mechanism of Action	Examples	Clinical Indications
Pyrazinoisoquinoline	Calcium agonist Causes tetanic muscular contractions Causes tegumental disruption Provides synergy with host defenses	Praziquantel	Broad-spectrum anthelmintic: cestodes, trematodes
Phenol	Uncouples oxidative phosphorylation	Niclosamide	Intestinal tapeworm
Quinolone	Alkylates DNA Inhibits DNA, RNA, and protein synthesis	Bithionol, oxamniquine	Paragonimiasis, schistosomiasis
Organophosphate	Anticholinesterase Blocks neuromuscular action	Metrifonate	Schistosomiasis
Sulfated naphthylamidine	Inhibits glycerophosphate oxidase and dehydrogenase	Suramin	Onchocerciasis

ATP, Adenosine triphosphate.

Antiprotozoal Agents

Similar to antibacterial and antifungal agents, the antiprotozoal agents are generally targeted at relatively rapidly proliferating, young, growing cells. Most commonly these agents target nucleic acid synthesis, protein synthesis, or specific metabolic pathways (e.g., folate metabolism) unique to the protozoan parasites.

Heavy Metals

The heavy metals used for the treatment of parasitic infections include arsenical (melarsoprol) and antimonial compounds (sodium stibogluconate, meglumine antimonate). These agents are thought to oxidize sulfhydryl groups of enzymes, which are essential catalysts in carbohydrate metabolism. Melarsoprol inhibits parasite pyruvate kinase, causing decreased concentrations of adenosine triphosphate (ATP), pyruvate, and phosphoenolpyruvate. Arsenicals also inhibit *sn*-glycerol 3-phosphate oxidase, which is needed for the regeneration of nicotinamide adenine dinucleotide in trypanosomes but is not found in mammalian cells. The antimonials, sodium stibogluconate and meglumine antimonate, inhibit the glycolytic enzyme phosphofructokinase and certain Krebs cycle enzymes in *Leishmania* organisms. They have also been shown to interfere with the metabolism of glutathione and trypanothione, resulting in an increased sensitivity of the organisms to oxidant stress. In each instance, the inhibition of parasite metabolism is **parasiticidal**. Unfortunately, the heavy metal compounds are toxic to the host, as well as the parasite. The toxicity is greatest on cells that are most metabolically active, such as neuronal, renal tubular, intestinal, and bone marrow stem cells. Their differential toxicity and therapeutic value are largely related to enhanced uptake by the parasite and its intense metabolic activity.

Melarsoprol is the drug of choice for trypanosomiasis involving the central nervous system. It can penetrate the blood-brain barrier and is effective in all stages of trypanosomiasis. The antimonial compounds are restricted to the management of leishmaniasis. Meglumine antimonate and sodium stibogluconate are important agents for the treatment of leishmaniasis and are active against all forms of the disease. Prolonged therapy is usually required for disseminated leishmaniasis, and relapses are common. Despite the use of antimonials worldwide for the treatment of leishmaniasis for over six decades with little evidence of resistance, acquired resistance has become a clinical threat within the past 10 years. This resistance is so far unique to *Leishmania donovani* causing visceral leishmaniasis in the hyperendemic region of Bihar, India. The mechanism of resistance is not completely understood but likely involves activation of an efflux pump in the plasma membrane of the organism with transport of the drug out of the cells.

Quinoline Derivatives

The quinoline derivatives include the 4-aminoquinolines (chloroquine), the cinchona alkaloids (quinine, quinidine), the 8-aminoquinolines (primaquine), and the synthetic quinoline compounds (mefloquine, halofantrine). These compounds all have antimalarial activity and accumulate preferentially in parasitized red blood cells. Several potential mechanisms of action have been proposed, including (1) binding to DNA and interfering with DNA replication; (2) binding to ferriprotoporphyrin IX released from hemoglobin in infected erythrocytes, producing a toxic complex; and (3) raising the pH of the parasite's intracellular acid vesicles, thus interfering with its ability to degrade hemoglobin. Quinine, quinidine, the 4-aminoquinolines, and the synthetic quinolines rapidly destroy the erythrocytic stage of malaria and thus may be used **prophylactically** to suppress clinical illness or **therapeutically** to terminate an acute attack. The 8-aminoquinolines (e.g., primaquine) accumulate in tissue cells and destroy the extraerythrocytic (hepatic) stages of malaria, resulting in a radical cure of the infection.

Chloroquine remains the drug of choice for the prophylaxis and treatment of susceptible malaria strains. Chloroquine is active against all four *Plasmodium* species that infect humans (*P. falciparum, P. vivax, P. ovale, P. malariae*) and is well tolerated, inexpensive, and effective orally. Unfortunately, resistance of *P. falciparum* to chloroquine is widespread in Asia, Africa, and South America, greatly limiting the use of this agent. Resistance of *P. vivax* to chloroquine has also been reported from Papua New Guinea, the Solomon Islands, Indonesia, and Brazil.

Quinine and quinidine are used primarily to treat chloroquine-resistant *P. falciparum* infection. Presumably, they are active against the rare chloroquine-resistant strains of *P. vivax* as well. Quinine is used orally only to treat mild attacks and by the intravenous route to treat acute attacks of multidrug-resistant *P. falciparum*. Both quinine and quinidine are quite toxic and not rapidly parasiticidal; thus they should not be used alone but rather in combination with a sulfonamide or tetracycline antibiotic with antimalarial activity.

Mefloquine is a 4-quinolinemethanol antimalarial agent used for the prophylaxis and treatment of falciparum malaria. It displays a high level of activity against most chloroquine-resistant parasites. Unfortunately, mefloquine-resistant strains of falciparum malaria have been reported from Southeast Asia and Africa.

Halofantrine is a synthetic phenanthrene-methanol compound with proven efficacy in the treatment of *P. vivax* and *P. falciparum* malaria. It is not recommended for prophylaxis of malaria because of toxicity. Halofantrine is more active than mefloquine; however, cross-resistance between these drugs occurs. It is considered a second-line agent for the treatment of malaria due to its expense and toxicity.

Folic Acid Antagonists

Similar to other organisms, protozoan parasites require folic acid for the synthesis of nucleic acids and ultimately DNA. Protozoa are unable to absorb exogenous folate and thus are susceptible to drugs that inhibit folate synthesis. The folic acid **antagonists** that are useful in treating protozoan infections include the diaminopyrimidines (pyrimethamine and trimethoprim) and the sulfonamides. These compounds block separate steps in the folic acid pathway. The sulfonamides inhibit the conversion of aminobenzoic acid to dihydropteroic acid. The diaminopyrimidines inhibit dihydrofolate reductase, which effectively blocks the synthesis of tetrahydrofolate, a precursor necessary for the formation of purines, pyrimidines, and certain amino acids. These agents are effective at concentrations far below those needed to inhibit the mammalian enzyme, so selectivity can be attained. When a diaminopyrimidine is used with a sulfonamide, a **synergistic effect** is achieved via the blockade of two steps in the same metabolic pathway, resulting in very effective inhibition of protozoan growth.

The diaminopyrimidine trimethoprim is used with sulfamethoxazole to treat toxoplasmosis. Another diaminopyrimidine, pyrimethamine, has a high affinity for sporozoan dihydrofolate reductase and has been very effective when combined with a sulfonamide in the treatment of malaria and toxoplasmosis. Resistance to antifolates is due to specific point mutations at the active site of the parasite's dihydrofolate reductase and has been largely confined to species of plasmodia.

Inhibitors of Protein Synthesis

Several antibiotics that inhibit protein synthesis in bacteria also exhibit antiparasitic activity in vitro and in vivo. These agents include clindamycin, spiramycin, tetracycline, and doxycycline.

Clindamycin and the tetracyclines are active against *Plasmodium* species, *Babesia* species, and amoebae. Doxycycline is used for the chemoprophylaxis of chloroquine-resistant *P. falciparum* malaria, and tetracycline may be used with quinine for the treatment of chloroquine-resistant *P. falciparum* infection. Clindamycin may be useful in the treatment of central nervous system toxoplasmosis. Spiramycin is recommended as an alternative to the antifolates in the treatment of toxoplasmosis. Although spiramycin appears active against *Cryptosporidium* species in vitro, it has not been shown to be effective clinically for human cryptosporidiosis. Recent studies suggest that paromomycin, an older aminoglycoside, may be at least partially effective in treating cryptosporidiosis. Paromomycin, which is not systemically absorbed, is also used as a secondary drug in amebiasis and giardiasis.

Diamidines

Pentamidine, a diamidine, is a relatively toxic agent. Pentamidine is a polycation and may interact with DNA, or it may interfere with the uptake and function of polyamines.

Pentamidine is effective in treating the tissue forms of leishmania and the early (pre–central nervous system) forms of African trypanosomiasis. Pentamidine does not penetrate the central nervous system and therefore is not useful in the late stages of infection with *Trypanosoma brucei gambiense*. Pentamidine may also inhibit kinetoplast topoisomerase II activity and may act against trypanosomes in part by this mechanism.

Nitroimidazoles

The nitroimidazoles include the well-known antibacterial agent metronidazole, as well as benzimidazole and tinidazole. The mechanism of action of these compounds is unclear. It has been suggested that they inhibit DNA and RNA synthesis and also inhibit the metabolism of glucose and interfere with mitochondrial function. Metronidazole binds to parasite guanine and cytosine residues, causing the loss of helical structure and breakage of DNA strands.

The nitroimidazoles have excellent penetration into body tissues and therefore are particularly effective for the treatment of disseminated amebiasis. Metronidazole is the drug of choice for trichomoniasis and is effective in the treatment of giardiasis. Tinidazole appears to be more effective and less mutagenic than metronidazole; however, it is not yet available for use in the United States.

Sesquiterpenes

The sesquiterpenes are antimicrobial agents that are represented by the artemisinins, artemether and artesunate. These agents react with the heme moiety, causing **free-radical damage** to parasite membranes. The artemisinins are the most active of the available antimalarial compounds and produce a fractional reduction in parasite biomass of approximately 10^4 per asexual cycle. Artemisinins have efficacy against small-ring forms, as well as maturing schizonts of both *P. vivax* and *P. falciparum*, stages that are less susceptible to quinolines or quinine. The earlier stage ring forms are immediately cleared (within 6 to 12 hours) after exposure to artemisinins. The artemisinin derivatives also have the advantage of reducing gametocyte carriage and thus transmission. These agents are highly effective when used in combination with mefloquine, halofantrine, or lumefantrine in the treatment of severe malaria, including that due to multidrug-resistant *P. falciparum*. Artemisinin-based combination treatments are now considered the best therapy for falciparum malaria, combining unrelated compounds with different molecular targets (and thus different potential mechanisms of resistance), thereby delaying the emergence of resistances.

Atovaquone-Proguanil (Malarone)

Atovaquone is a hydroxynaphthoquinone, and proguanil is an antifolate. The combination of these two agents, Malarone, is used for the prophylaxis and treatment of malaria. Atovaquone inhibits the electron transport system in the mitochondria of parasites, thus blocking nucleic acid synthesis and inhibiting replication. Proguanil selectively inhibits plasmodial dihydrofolate reductase; however, in combination with atovaquone it directly lowers the effective concentration at which atovaquone causes collapse of the mitochondrial membrane potential. Malarone is effective against all stages of development of *P. falciparum* and is recommended for prophylaxis and treatment of falciparum malaria. It is also active against the erythrocytic stages of *P. vivax* and *P. ovale* and shows good efficacy in the treatment of *P. malariae* infections. There are a few reports of clinical failure and resistance of *P. falciparum* isolates to Malarone associated with a single gene mutation.

Miltefosine

Miltefosine is an oral phosphocholine analogue used for the treatment of visceral leishmaniasis. It is becoming increasingly important because of the growing resistance of *Leishmania* strains to the pentavalent antimonials.

Miltefosine has direct antiparasitic activity and appears to act on key enzymes involved in the metabolism of ether lipids present on the surface of parasites, but the exact mechanisms of its parasiticidal activity are unknown. Miltefosine is active against both pentavalent antimonial—resistant and susceptible strains of *L. donovani* and has been found to have a cure rate of 94% to 97% at 6 months in patients with visceral leishmaniasis. Resistance is due to decreased uptake of the drug. In addition to *Leishmania* spp., miltefosine has activity against *Trypanosoma cruzi*, *T. brucei*, *Entamoeba histolytica*, and *Acanthamoeba* spp.

Nitazoxanide

Nitazoxanide (NTZ) is a novel 5-nitrothiazole derivative with broad-spectrum activity against numerous intestinal protozoa and helminths. Nitazoxanide inhibits pyruvate ferredoxin oxidoreductase, an enzyme essential to anaerobic energy metabolism in protozoa, as well as anaerobic bacteria. The mechanism of action of this agent against helminths is unknown. Nitazoxanide is licensed in the United States for the treatment of cryptosporidiosis in children and giardiasis in children and adults. It also has been shown to be effective in vitro and/or in vivo against infections caused by many enteric protozoa and helminths, including *Ascaris lumbricoides*, *Balantidium coli*, *Blastocystis hominis*, *Cyclospora cayetanensis*, *Echinococcus* spp., *Entamoeba histolytica*, *Fasciola hepatica*, hookworms, *Hymenolepis nana*, *Isospora belli*, microsporidial species, *Taenia saginata*, *Trichomonas vaginalis*, and *Trichuris trichiura*.

Other Antiprotozoal Agents

A number of additional agents used in therapy, their mechanisms of action (if known), and clinical use are listed in Table 80-2.

Anthelmintic Agents

The strategy for the use of anthelmintic drugs is quite different from that for the use of drugs for treating most protozoal infections. Most anthelmintic drugs are targeted at **nonproliferating** adult organisms, whereas with protozoa the targets are generally younger, more rapidly proliferating cells. The helminthic life cycle is frequently quite complex, and the adaptation to survival in the human host depends strongly on (1) neuromuscular coordination for feeding movements and for maintenance of a favorable location of the worm within the host; (2) carbohydrate metabolism as the major source of energy, with glucose the primary substrate; and (3) microtubular integrity, since egg laying and hatching, larval development, glucose transport, and enzyme activity and secretion are impaired when microtubules are modified. Most anthelmintic agents are targeted at one of these biochemical functions in the adult organism.

The mechanisms of action and clinical indications for common anthelmintic agents are listed in Table 80-2.

Benzimidazoles

The benzimidazoles are broad-spectrum anthelmintic agents and include mebendazole, triclabendazole, and albendazole. The basic structure of these agents consists of linked imidazole and benzene rings. Three mechanisms of action have been proposed for the benzimidazoles: (1) inhibition of fumarate reductase; (2) inhibition of glucose transport, resulting in glycogen depletion, cessation of ATP formation, and paralysis or death; and (3) disruption of microtubular function. Benzimidazoles block the assembly of tubulin dimers into tubulin polymers in a process mimicked by colchicine, a powerful antimitotic and embryotoxic drug. Because tubulin is important for parasite motility, drugs such as the benzimidazoles, which bind to parasite tubulin, are thought to act against nematode parasites by reducing or eliminating their motility.

The benzimidazoles have a wide spectrum of activity, including intestinal nematodes (*Ascaris*, *Trichuris*, *Necator*, and *Ancylostoma* species; *Enterobius vermicularis*), as well as a number of cestodes (*Taenia*, *Hymenolepis*, and *Echinococcus* species). Triclabendazole is the agent of choice for fascioliasis and is an alternative to praziquantel for therapy of paragonimiasis and intestinal flukes. Mebendazole is active against the intestinal nematodes and the cestodes previously listed. Albendazole has a spectrum similar to that of mebendazole and may have greater activity against *Echinococcus* species. In addition to its broad-spectrum antihelminth activity, albendazole also has activity against *Giardia* species and appears promising in the treatment of intestinal microsporidiosis in patients with acquired immunodeficiency syndrome. Albendazole is being increasingly used in combination with either diethylcarbamazine or ivermectin for treatment of filariasis and loiasis; it is especially useful for these infections as part of a single-dose regimen for mass chemotherapy programs.

Tetrahydropyrimidines

Pyrantel pamoate, a tetrahydropyrimidine, is a cholinergic agonist that has a powerful effect on nematode muscle cells by binding to cholinergic receptors, which results in cell depolarization and muscle contraction. This **paralytic action** on intestinal nematodes leads to expulsion of the worm from the host intestinal tract.

Pyrantel pamoate is not readily absorbed from the intestine and is active against *Ascaris* species, pinworm, and hookworm. An analogue of pyrantel, oxantel, may be used with pyrantel to provide effective therapy for the three major soil-transmitted nematodes: *Ascaris* species, hookworm, and *Trichuris* species.

Piperazines

The piperazine anthelmintic used most commonly is diethylcarbamazine. Diethylcarbamazine (DEC) is predominantly a microfilaricidal agent that is thought to act by stimulating cholinergic receptors and depolarizing muscle cells, with subsequent paralysis of the worms. However, additional evidence suggests that it enhances the adherence of leukocytes to microfilariae and thus may act by altering the parasite surface membrane or by directly stimulating phagocytic cells.

DEC is active against the filariae that produce river blindness (*Onchocerca volvulus*) and lymphatic filariasis (*Wuchereria bancrofti* and *Brugia malayi*). Unfortunately, destruction of the microfilariae in the tissues may increase the pathology because of the host inflammatory response to the parasite antigens released on exposure to DEC. Recent information suggests that single-dose treatment with DEC may produce antiparasitic effects similar to those obtained with 14- to 21-day courses, without the severe side effects observed with the multidose regimens. In addition to its use as individual therapy for filarial infections, DEC is also used for mass community chemotherapy programs either alone or in combination with ivermectin or albendazole.

Avermectins

Ivermectin, an avermectin, acts by interacting with the chloride channel in nerve and muscle cell membranes, resulting in hyperpolarization of the affected cells and consequent paralysis and death of the parasites. The drug also inhibits the reproductive function of the adult female *O. volvulus* and alters the ability of the *O. volvulus* microfilariae to evade the host immune system.

Although ivermectin is used extensively to control gut-dwelling nematode infections in domestic and farm animals, its use in humans is limited primarily to treating ocular and lymphatic filariasis. Ivermectin is effective in the treatment of strongyloidiasis, as well as several common intestinal parasitic nematodes, including *Ascaris*, *Trichuris*, and *Enterobius* species. When used to treat filariasis, ivermectin has fewer side effects than diethylcarbamazine, and a single dose can eliminate microfilariae for up to 6 months. Ivermectin has a dramatic effect on the tissue-dwelling microfilariae of *O. volvulus* and reduces the severity of the ocular pathology seen in onchocerciasis. Because of its ability to markedly reduce the number of microfilariae in the skin of people with onchocerciasis, ivermectin has been effective in reducing the transmission of onchocerciasis in endemic areas.

Pyrazinoisoquinolines

Praziquantel, a pyrazinoisoquinoline, is an anthelmintic active against a broad spectrum of trematodes and cestodes. The drug is rapidly taken up by susceptible helminths, in which it acts as a **calcium agonist**. The entry of calcium into various cells results in elevated intracellular calcium levels, tetanic muscular contraction, and destruction of the tegument. Praziquantel appears to act with the host immune system to produce a synergistic anthelmintic effect. The drug causes disruption of the parasite surface and tegument, allowing antibodies to attack parasite antigens not normally exposed on the surface (Figure 80-1). Irreversible damage to the parasite probably occurs when

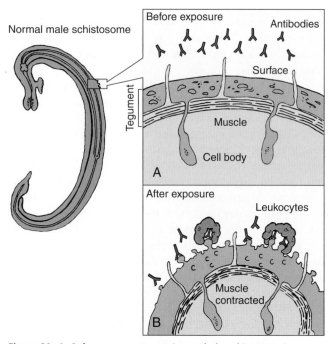

Figure 80—1. Before exposure to praziquantel, the schistosome is capable of avoiding the numerous antibodies directed toward surface and internally located antigens. **A,** Cross section of the dorsal surface of a normal male schistosome. Within 1 to 2 seconds after exposure to praziquantel, the muscles of the schistosome contract because of a drug-induced influx of calcium ions into the schistosome tegument. **B,** The change in permeability of the schistosome surface toward external ions initiates the appearance of small holes and balloon-like structures, making the parasite vulnerable to antibody-mediated adherence of host leukocytes that kill the helminth. *(From Wingard LB Jr, et al: Human Pharmacology: Molecular to Clinical. St Louis, Mosby, 1991.)*

complement or host leukocytes are recruited to the sites where antibody is bound.

Praziquantel has extremely broad-spectrum activity against trematodes, including *Fasciolopsis, Clonorchis, Opisthorchis, Paragonimus,* and *Schistosoma* species. It is also active against cestodes, including *Echinococcus, Taenia,* and *Dipylidium* species. Praziquantel is the drug of choice for the treatment of schistosomiasis, clonorchiasis, opisthorchiasis, and intestinal fluke infections. There is now reliable evidence that praziquantel reduces hepatosplenomegaly and portal hypertension in schistosomiasis. Most tapeworm infections respond to praziquantel. Praziquantel is also used in the treatment of neurocysticercosis and echinococcal infections, either alone or in combination with albendazole.

Phenols

Niclosamide, a phenol, is a nonabsorbable anthelmintic with selective activity against intestinal tapeworms. The drug is absorbed by gut-dwelling cestodes but not by nematodes. It acts by uncoupling oxidative phosphorylation in mitochondria, resulting in a loss of helminth ATP that ultimately immobilizes the parasite so that it is expelled with the feces. Niclosamide is effective in the treatment of intestinal tapeworms in humans and animals.

Other Anthelmintic Agents

Additional anthelmintic agents, including oxamniquine, metrifonate, and suramin, are described in Table 80-2. These agents are generally considered secondary agents for the treatment of trematode (oxamniquine and metrifonate) and filarial (suramin) infections.

Questions

1. What are the obstacles to effective treatment and prophylaxis of parasitic diseases in developing countries?
2. What are the goals of antiparasitic therapy, and how are they different from antibacterial therapy?
3. What is the importance of aminoquinoline analogues?
4. How does the strategy for the use of anthelmintic agents differ from that for the use of drugs for protozoal infections?

Bibliography

Ali V, Nozaki T: Current therapeutics, their problems, and sulfur containing amino acid metabolism as a novel target against infections by "amitochondriate" protozoan parasites. Clin Microbiol Rev 20:164-187, 2007.

Baird JK: Effectiveness of antimalarial drugs. N Engl J Med 352:1565-1577, 2005.

Croft SL, Sundar S, Fairlamb AH: Drug resistance in leishmaniasis. Clin Microbiol Rev 19:111-126, 2006.

Doenhoff MJ, Kusel JR, Coles GC, Cioli D: Resistance of *Schistosoma mansoni* to praziquantel: Is there a problem? Trans R Soc Trop Med Hyg 96:465-469, 2002.

Edwards G, Krishna S: Pharmacokinetic and pharmacodynamic issues in the treatment of parasitic infections. Eur J Clin Microbiol Infect Dis 23:233-242, 2004.

Gardner TB, Hill DR: Treatment of giardiasis. Clin Microbiol Rev 14:114-128, 2001.

Geertz S, Gryseels B: Drug resistance in human helminths: Current situation and lessons from livestock. Clin Microbiol Rev 13(2):207-222, 2000.

Hotez PJ, Molyneux DH, Fenwick A: Control of neglected tropical diseases. N Engl J Med 357:1018-1027, 2007.

Leder K, Weller PF: Antiparasitic agents. In Murray PR, et al (eds): Manual of Clinical Microbiology, 9th ed. Washington, DC, ASM Press, 2007.

Secor WE, Nguyen-Dinh P: Mechanisms of resistance to antiparasitic agents. In Murray PR, et al (eds): Manual of Clinical Microbiology, 9th ed. Washington, DC, ASM Press, 2007.

Talisuna AO, Bloland P, D'Alessandro U: History, dynamics, and public health importance of malaria parasite resistance. Clin Microbiol Rev 178:235-254, 2004.

Wingard LB Jr, et al (eds): Human Pharmacology: Molecular to Clinical, St Louis, Mosby, 1991.

Intestinal and Urogenital Protozoa

Protozoa may colonize and infect the oropharynx, duodenum and small bowel, colon, and urogenital tract of humans. The majority of these parasites belong to the amoebae and flagellates; however, infection with ciliate, coccidian, or microsporidian parasites may also be encountered (Table 81-1). These organisms are transmitted by the **fecal-oral route**. In the United States, transmission of intestinal protozoa is particularly problematic in daycare centers, where several outbreaks of diarrhea caused by *Giardia* or *Cryptosporidium* species have been documented. In other parts of the world, the spread of enteric protozoal infections may be controlled in part by improved sanitation and by chlorination and filtration of water supplies; however, this may be difficult or impossible in many developing countries.

Amoebae

The amoebae are primitive **unicellular** microorganisms. Their life cycle is relatively simple and divided into two stages: the actively motile feeding stage (trophozoite) and the quiescent, resistant, infective stage (cyst). Replication is accomplished by binary fission (splitting the trophozoite) or by the development of numerous trophozoites within the mature multinucleated cyst. Motility is accomplished by extension of a **pseudopod** ("false foot") with extrusion of the cellular ectoplasm and then drawing up of the rest of the cell in a snail-like movement to meet this pseudopod. The amoebic trophozoites remain actively motile as long as the environment is favorable. The cyst form develops when the environmental temperature or moisture level drops.

Most amoebae found in humans are **commensal** organisms (*Entamoeba coli, Entamoeba hartmanni, Entamoeba dispar, Entamoeba moshkovskii, Entamoeba gingivalis, Endolimax nana, Iodamoeba bütschlii*). However, *Entamoeba histolytica* is an important human pathogen. Other amoebae, particularly *Entamoeba polecki*, can cause human disease but are rarely isolated. The pathogenicity of *Blastocystis hominis* is still controversial. Some free-living amoebae (*Naegleria fowleri, Acanthamoeba* species) are present in soil and in warm freshwater ponds or swimming pools and can be opportunistic human pathogens, causing meningoencephalitis or keratitis.

Entamoeba histolytica

Physiology and Structure

Cyst and trophozoite forms of *E. histolytica* are detected in fecal specimens from infected patients (Figure 81-1). Trophozoites can also be found in the crypts of the large intestine. In freshly passed stools, actively motile trophozoites can be seen, whereas in formed stools, the cysts are usually the only form recognized. For the diagnosis of amebiasis, distinguishing between the *E. histolytica* trophozoites and cysts and those of commensal amoebae is important.

Pathogenesis

After ingestion, the cysts pass through the stomach, where exposure to gastric acid stimulates the release of the pathogenic trophozoite in the duodenum. The trophozoites divide and produce extensive local necrosis in the large intestine. The basis for this tissue destruction is incompletely understood, although it is attributed to production of a **cytotoxin**. Attachment of *E. histolytica* trophozoites to host cells via a galactose-inhibitable adherence protein is required for cytolysis and tissue necrosis to occur. The lysis of colonic epithelial cells, human neutrophils, lymphocytes, and monocytes by trophozoites is associated with a lethal alteration of host cell membrane permeability, resulting in an irreversible increase in intracellular calcium levels. The release of toxic neutrophil constituents after the lysis of neutrophils may contribute to the tissue destruction. Flask-shaped ulcerations of the intestinal mucosa are present with inflammation, hemorrhage, and secondary bacterial infection. Invasion into the deeper mucosa with extension into the peritoneal cavity may occur. This can lead to secondary involvement of other organs, primarily the liver but also the lungs, brain, and heart. Extraintestinal amebiasis is associated with

Table 81—1. Morphologic Identification of *Entamoeba histolytica* and *Entamoeba coli*

	*E. histolytica**	*E. coli*
Size (diameter, μm)		
Trophozoite	12-50 μm	20-30 μm
Cyst	10-20 μm	10-30 μm
Pattern of peripheral nuclear chromatin	Fine, dispersed ring	Coarse, clumped
Karyosome	Central, sharp	Eccentric, coarse
Ingested erythrocytes	Present	Absent
Cyst structure		
No. of nuclei	1-4	1-8
Chromatoidal bars	Rounded ends	Splintered, frayed ends

E. histolytica is morphologically indistinguishable from the commensal species *E. dispar* and *E. moshkovskii*.

trophozoites. Amoebae are found only in environments that have a low oxygen pressure because the protozoa are killed by ambient oxygen concentrations.

Recently, lectin binding, zymodeme analysis, genome DNA analysis, and staining with specific monoclonal antibodies have been used as markers to identify invasive strains of *E. histolytica*. It is now recognized that the

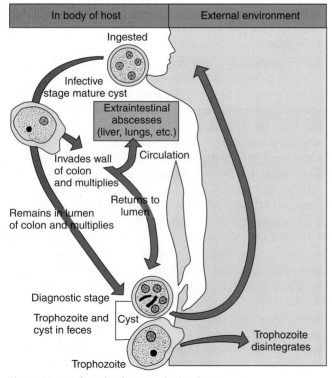

Figure 81—1. Life cycle of *Entamoeba histolytica*.

amoeba morphologically identified as *E. histolytica* is actually three distinct species. The pathogenic species is *E. histolytica*, and the nonpathogenic species are *E. dispar* and *E. moshkovskii*. The zymodeme profiles and biochemical, molecular, and immunologic differences are stable and support the existence of three species. Notably, these three species are morphologically indistinguishable from one another.

Epidemiology

E. histolytica has a worldwide distribution. Although it is found in cold areas such as Alaska, Canada, and Eastern Europe, its incidence is highest in tropical and subtropical regions that have poor sanitation and contaminated water. The average prevalence of infection in these areas is 10% to 15%, with as many as 50% of the population infected in some areas. Many of the infected individuals are asymptomatic carriers, who represent a reservoir for the spread of *E. histolytica* to others. The prevalence of infection in the United States is 1% to 2%.

Patients infected with *E. histolytica* pass noninfectious trophozoites and the infectious cysts in their stools. The trophozoites cannot survive in the external environment or in transport through the stomach if ingested. Therefore the main source of water and food contamination is the asymptomatic carrier who passes cysts. This is a particular problem in hospitals for the mentally ill, military and refugee camps, prisons, and crowded daycare centers. Flies and cockroaches can also serve as vectors for the transmission of *E. histolytica* cysts. Sewage containing cysts can contaminate water systems, wells, springs, and agricultural areas where human waste is used as fertilizer. Finally, cysts can be transmitted by oral-anal sexual practices, with amebiasis prevalent in homosexual populations. Direct trophozoite transmission in sexual encounters can produce cutaneous amebiasis.

Clinical Syndromes

The outcome of infection may result in a carrier state, intestinal amebiasis, or extraintestinal amebiasis. If the strain of *E. histolytica* has a low virulence, if the inoculum is low, or if the patient's immune system is intact, the organisms may reproduce, and cysts may be passed in stool specimens with no clinical symptoms. Although infections with *E. histolytica* may be asymptomatic, most asymptomatic individuals are infected with the noninvasive *E. dispar* or *E. moshkovskii*, as characterized by specific isoenzyme profiles (zymodemes), DNA-based assays, their susceptibility to complement-mediated lysis, and their failure to agglutinate in the presence of the lectin concanavalin A. Detection of carriers of *E. histolytica* in areas with a low endemicity is important for epidemiologic purposes.

Patients with intestinal amebiasis develop clinical symptoms related to the localized tissue destruction in the large intestine. These include abdominal pain, cramping, and colitis with diarrhea. More severe disease is characterized by numerous bloody stools per day. Systemic signs of infection (fever, leukocytosis, rigors) are present in patients with extraintestinal amebiasis. The liver is primarily involved because trophozoites in the blood are removed as they pass through this organ. Abscess formation is common (Clinical Case 81-1). The right lobe is most commonly involved. Pain over the liver with hepatomegaly and elevation of the diaphragm is observed.

Laboratory Diagnosis

The identification of *E. histolytica* trophozoites (Figure 81-2) and cysts in stools and trophozoites in tissue is diagnostic of amoebic infection. Care must be taken to distinguish between these amoebae and commensal amoebae, as well as between these amoebae and polymorphonuclear leukocytes. Microscopic examination of stool specimens is inherently insensitive, because the protozoa are not usually distributed homogeneously in the specimen, and the parasites are concentrated in the intestinal ulcers and at the margins of the abscess, not in the stool or the necrotic center of the abscess. For this reason, multiple stool specimens should be collected. Extraintestinal amebiasis is

---

Clinical Case 81-1. HIV and Amoebic Liver Abscess

Liu and colleagues (J Clin Gastroenterol 33:64-68, 2001) described a 45-year-old homosexual man who developed intestinal and hepatic amebiasis. The patient initially presented with intermittent fever followed by right upper quadrant pain and diarrhea. On admission to the hospital, he was afebrile with an elevated white blood count and abnormal liver function tests. Stool examinations were positive for occult blood and white blood cells. He underwent colonoscopy, and multiple discrete ulcers were detected in the rectum and colon. The diagnosis of amoebic colitis was confirmed by the demonstration of numerous trophozoites on histopathologic examination of colon biopsy specimens. Ultrasonic examination of the abdomen revealed a large heterogeneous mass within the liver, consistent with an abscess. Percutaneous drainage of the abscess obtained chocolate-like pus, and examination of a biopsy from the margin of the abscess revealed only necrotic material without evidence of amoebae. PCR amplification of amoebic 16S ribosomal RNA from the aspirate was positive, indicating infection with *Entamoeba histolytica*. The patient was treated with metronidazole followed by iodoquinol to eradicate the luminal amoebas. Subsequent history revealed a history of travel to Thailand 2 months prior to the onset of the present illness. HIV serology was positive as well. The patient improved rapidly on antiamoebic therapy and was discharged on antiretroviral therapy.

Although amoebic cysts are frequently detected in the stools of homosexual men, previous studies in Western countries suggested that almost all isolates belonged to the nonpathogenic species, *E. dispar*, and invasive amebiasis was considered rare in HIV-positive individuals. This case illustrates that invasive amebiasis, such as amoebic liver abscess and colitis, can accompany HIV infection. The possible association of invasive amebiasis with HIV infection should be kept in mind in patients living in, or with a history of travel to, areas endemic with *E. histolytica*.

Figure 81—2. *Entamoeba histolytica* trophozoite (**A**) and cyst (**B**). Trophozoites are motile and vary in size from 12 to 60 μm (average, 15 to 30 μm). The single nucleus in the cell is round with a central dot (karyosome) and an even distribution of chromatin granules around the nuclear membrane. Ingested erythrocytes may be in the cytoplasm. The cysts are smaller (10 to 20 μm with an average size of 15 to 20 μm) and contain one to four nuclei (usually four). Round chromatoidal bars may be in the cytoplasm. *(From Marler LM, et al: Parasitology CD-ROM, Indiana Pathology Images, 2003.)*

sometimes diagnosed using scanning procedures for the liver and other organs. Specific serologic tests, together with microscopic examination of the abscess material, can confirm the diagnosis. Virtually all patients with hepatic amebiasis and most patients (more than 80%) with intestinal disease have positive serologic findings at the time of clinical presentation. This may be less useful in endemic areas where the prevalence of positive serologic results is higher. Examinations of stool specimens are frequently negative in extraintestinal disease. In addition to conventional microscopic and serologic tests, researchers have developed several immunologic tests for the detection of fecal antigen, as well as polymerase chain reaction and DNA-probe assays for the detection of pathogenic strains of *E. histolytica* (versus nonpathogenic *E. dispar* and *E. moshkovskii*). These newer diagnostic approaches are promising and are now commercially available.

Treatment, Prevention, and Control

Acute, fulminating amebiasis is treated with metronidazole followed by iodoquinol. Asymptomatic carriage can be eradicated with iodoquinol, diloxanide furoate, or paromomycin. As already noted, human infection results from the ingestion of food or water contaminated with human feces or as a result of specific sexual practices. The elimination of the cycle of infection requires the introduction of adequate sanitation measures and education about the routes of transmission. The chlorination and filtration of water supplies may limit the spread of these and other enteric protozoal infections but are not possible in many developing countries. Physicians should alert travelers to developing countries of the risks associated with the consumption of water (including ice cubes), unpeeled fruits, and raw vegetables. Water should be boiled and fruits and vegetables thoroughly cleaned before consumption.

Other Intestinal Amoebae

Other amoebae that can parasitize the human gastrointestinal tract include *E. coli*, *E. hartmanni*, *E. polecki*, *E. nana*, *I. bütschlii*, and *Blastocystis hominis*. *E. polecki*, which is primarily a parasite of pigs and monkeys, can cause human disease, a mild, transient diarrhea. The diagnosis of *E. polecki* infection is confirmed by the microscopic detection of cysts in stool specimens. Treatment is the same as for *E. histolytica* infections.

Blastocystis hominis, previously regarded as a nonpathogenic yeast, is now the center of considerable controversy concerning its taxonomic position and its pathogenicity. *B. hominis* has recently been placed in the kingdom Chromista, based on analysis of 18S rRNA and other molecular evidence. It is the first Chromist known to parasitize humans. The organism is found in stool specimens from asymptomatic individuals, as well as from persons with persistent diarrhea. It has been suggested that the presence of large numbers of these parasites (five or more per oil-immersion microscopic field) in the absence of other intestinal pathogens indicates disease. Other investigators have concluded that "symptomatic blastocystosis" is attributable to an undetected pathogen or functional bowel problems. The organism may be detected in wet mounts or trichrome-stained smears of fecal specimens. Treatment with iodoquinol or metronidazole has been successful in eradicating the organisms from the intestine and alleviating symptoms. However, the definitive role of this organism in disease remains to be demonstrated.

The nonpathogenic intestinal amoebae are important because they must be differentiated from *E. histolytica*, *E. polecki*, and *B. hominis*. This is particularly true for *E. coli*, which is frequently detected in stool specimens collected from patients exposed to contaminated food or water. Accurate identification of intestinal amoebae requires careful microscopic examination of the cyst and trophozoite forms present in stained and unstained stool specimens (Table 81-1). Likewise, differentiation of *E. dispar* and *E. moshkovskii* from *E. histolytica* is now possible using specific immunologic reagents.

Flagellates

The flagellates of clinical significance include *Giardia lamblia* (*duodenalis/intestinalis*), *Dientamoeba fragilis*, and *Trichomonas vaginalis*. Nonpathogenic commensal flagellates such as *Chilomastix mesnili* (enteric) and *Trichomonas tenax* (oral) may also be observed. *Giardia* organisms, like *E. histolytica*, have cyst and trophozoite stages in their life cycles. In contrast, no cyst stage has been observed for *Trichomonas* or *Dientamoeba* species. Unlike the amoebae, most flagellates move by the lashing of flagella that pull the organisms through fluid environments. Diseases produced by flagellates are primarily the result of mechanical irritation and inflammation. For example, *G. lamblia* (*duodenalis/intestinalis*) attaches to the intestinal villi with an adhesive disk, resulting in localized tissue damage. The tissue invasion with extensive tissue destruction, as seen with *E. histolytica*, is rare with flagellates.

Giardia lamblia (*G. duodenalis*; *G. intestinalis*)

The literature refers to this organism as *G. lamblia*, *G. duodenalis*, and *G. intestinalis*, reflecting the ambiguity surrounding the classification and nomenclature of this flagellate. Further studies are necessary to determine species designations or groupings; however, *G. lamblia* is the name predominantly used in the United States and will be used in this chapter.

Physiology and Structure

Both cyst and trophozoite forms of *G. lamblia* are detected in fecal specimens from infected patients (Figure 81-3).

Pathogenesis

Infection with *G. lamblia* is initiated by ingestion of cysts (Figure 81-4). The minimum infective dose for humans is estimated to be 10 to 25 cysts. Gastric acid stimulates excystation with the release of trophozoites in the duodenum and jejunum, where the organisms multiply by **binary fission**. The trophozoites can attach to the intestinal villi by a prominent ventral sucking disk. Although the tips of the villi may appear flattened, and inflammation of the mucosa with hyperplasia of lymphoid follicles may be observed, frank tissue necrosis does not occur. In addition, metastatic spread of disease beyond the gastrointestinal tract is very rare.

Epidemiology

Giardia species has a worldwide distribution, and this flagellate has a sylvatic or "wilderness" distribution in many streams, lakes, and mountain resorts. This sylvatic distribution is maintained in reservoir animals such as beavers and muskrats. Giardiasis is acquired by the consumption of inadequately treated contaminated water, ingestion of contaminated uncooked vegetables or fruits, or person-to-person spread by the fecal-oral or oral-anal route. The cyst stage is resistant to chlorine concentrations (1 to 2 parts per million)

Figure 81—3. *Giardia lamblia* trophozoite (**A**) and cyst (**B**). Trophozoites are 9 to 12 μm long and 5 to 15 μm wide. Flagella are present, as are two nuclei with large central karyosomes, a large ventral sucking disk for attachment of the flagellate to the intestinal villi, and two oblong parabasal bodies below the nuclei. The morphology gives the appearance that the trophozoites are looking back at the viewer. Cysts are smaller—8 to 12 μm long and 7 to 10 μm wide. Four nuclei and four parabasal bodies are present. *(From Marler LM, et al: Parasitology CD-ROM, Indiana Pathology Images, 2003.)*

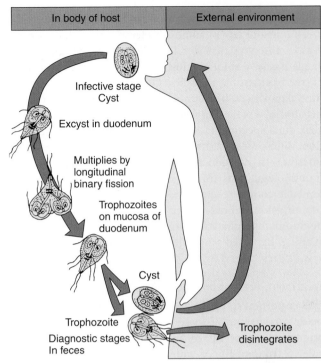

Figure 81—4. Life cycle of *Giardia lamblia*.

used in most water-treatment facilities. Thus adequate water treatment should include chemicals with filtration.

Risk factors associated with *Giardia* infections include poor sanitary conditions, travel to known endemic areas, consumption of inadequately treated water (e.g., from contaminated mountain streams), daycare centers, and oral-anal sexual practices. Infections may occur in outbreak and endemic forms within daycare centers and other institutional settings and among family members of infected children. Scrupulous attention to handwashing and treatment of all infected individuals are important in controlling the spread of infection in these settings.

Clinical Syndromes

Giardia infection can result in either asymptomatic carriage (observed in approximately 50% of infected individuals) or symptomatic disease ranging from mild diarrhea to a severe malabsorption syndrome (Clinical Case 81-2). The incubation period before symptomatic disease develops ranges from 1 to 4 weeks (average, 10 days). The onset of disease is sudden, with foul-smelling, watery diarrhea,

abdominal cramps, flatulence, and steatorrhea. Blood and pus are rarely present in stool specimens, which is consistent with the absence of tissue destruction. Spontaneous recovery generally occurs after 10 to 14 days, although a more chronic disease with multiple relapses may develop. This is particularly a problem for patients with immunoglobulin A deficiency or intestinal diverticula.

Laboratory Diagnosis

With the onset of diarrhea and abdominal discomfort, stool specimens should be examined for cysts and trophozoites (see Figure 81-3). *Giardia* species may occur in

---

Clinical Case 81-2. Drug-Resistant Giardiasis

Abboud and colleagues (Clin Infect Dis 32:1792-1794, 2001) described a case of metronidazole-and albendazole-resistant giardiasis that was successfully treated with nitazoxanide. The patient was a 32-year-old homosexual man with AIDS who was admitted to the hospital because of intractable diarrhea. Examination of stool revealed the presence of numerous cysts of *Giardia duodenalis* (*G. lamblia*). The patient was treated unsuccessfully five times with metronidazole and albendazole without improvement in diarrhea or cyst shedding. Although combined antiretroviral therapy was also administered, it was ineffective, and viral genotypic analysis found mutations associated with high resistance to most antiretroviral drugs. The patient was subsequently treated for giardiasis with nitazoxanide, which resulted in resolution of the diarrhea and negative results of tests for stool cyst shedding. Resistance of the infecting strain of *G. lamblia* to both metronidazole and albendazole was confirmed by in vivo and in vitro studies. Nitazoxanide may be considered a useful alternative therapy for resistant giardiasis.

"showers," with many organisms present in the stool on a given day and few or none detected the next day. For this reason, the physician should never accept the results of a single negative stool specimen as evidence that the patient is free of intestinal parasites. One stool specimen per day for 3 days should be examined. If stools remain persistently negative in a patient in whom giardiasis is highly suspected, additional specimens can be collected by duodenal aspiration, Entero-Test or string test, or biopsy of the upper small intestine. In addition to conventional microscopy, several immunologic tests for the detection of **fecal antigen** are available commercially. These tests include countercurrent immunoelectrophoresis, enzyme immunoassay, an immunochromatographic assay, and indirect immunofluorescent staining. Reported sensitivities range from 88% to 98% and specificities from 87% to 100%.

Treatment, Prevention, and Control

It is important to eradicate *Giardia* species from asymptomatic carriers and diseased patients. The drug of choice is metronidazole or nitazoxanide with furazolidone, tinidazole, paromomycin or quinacrine all acceptable alternatives. The prevention and control of giardiasis involves the avoidance of contaminated water and food, especially by the traveler and outdoorsman. Protection is afforded by boiling drinking water from streams and lakes or in countries with a high incidence of endemic disease. Maintenance of properly functioning filtration systems in municipal water supplies is also required, because cysts are resistant to standard chlorination procedures. Public health efforts should be made to identify the reservoir of infection to prevent spread of disease. In addition, high-risk sexual behavior should be avoided.

Dientamoeba fragilis

Physiology and Structure

Dientamoeba fragilis was initially classified as an amoeba; however, the internal structures of the trophozoite are typical of a flagellate. No cyst stage has been described.

Epidemiology

D. fragilis has a worldwide distribution. The transmission of the delicate trophozoite is not completely understood. Some observers believe the organism can be transported from person to person inside the protective shell of worm eggs such as *E. vermicularis*, the pinworm. Transmission by the fecal-oral and oral-anal routes does occur.

Clinical Syndromes

Most infections with *D. fragilis* are asymptomatic, with colonization of the cecum and upper colon. However, some patients may develop symptomatic disease with abdominal discomfort, flatulence, intermittent diarrhea, anorexia, and weight loss. There is no evidence of tissue invasion with this flagellate, although irritation of the intestinal mucosa occurs.

Laboratory Diagnosis

Infection is confirmed by the microscopic examination of stool specimens in which typical trophozoites can be seen. The trophozoite is small (5 to 12 μm), with one or two nuclei. The central karyosome consists of four to six discrete granules. The excretion of the parasite may fluctuate markedly from day to day, and thus collection of several stool samples may be necessary. Examination of a purged stool sample may also be useful.

Treatment, Prevention, and Control

The therapy of choice for *D. fragilis* infection is iodoquinol, with tetracycline and paromomycin acceptable alternatives. The reservoir for this flagellate and the organism's life cycle are unknown. Thus specific recommendations for prevention and control are difficult. However, infections can be avoided by maintaining adequate sanitary conditions. The eradication of infections with *Enterobius* organisms may also reduce the transmission of *Dientamoeba* infection.

Trichomonas vaginalis

Physiology and Structure

T. vaginalis is not an intestinal protozoan but rather the cause of urogenital infections. The flagellate's four flagella and short, undulating membrane are responsible for motility. *T. vaginalis* exists only as a trophozoite and is found in the urethras and vaginas of women and the urethras and prostate glands of men.

Epidemiology

This parasite has worldwide distribution, with sexual intercourse as the primary mode of transmission (Figure 81-5). Occasionally, infections have been transmitted by fomites (toilet articles, clothing), although this transmission is limited by the lability of the trophozoite form. Infants may be infected by passage through the mother's infected birth canal. The prevalence of this flagellate in developed countries is reported to be 5% to 20% in women and 2% to 10% in men.

Clinical Syndromes

Most infected women are asymptomatic or have a scant, watery vaginal discharge. Vaginitis may occur with more extensive inflammation and erosion of the epithelial lining that is associated with itching, burning, and painful urination. Men are primarily asymptomatic carriers who serve as a reservoir for infections in women. However, men occasionally experience urethritis, prostatitis, and other urinary tract problems.

Laboratory Diagnosis

The microscopic examination of vaginal or urethral discharge for characteristic trophozoites is the diagnostic method of choice (Figure 81-6). Stained (Giemsa, Papanicolaou) or unstained smears can be examined. The diagnostic yield

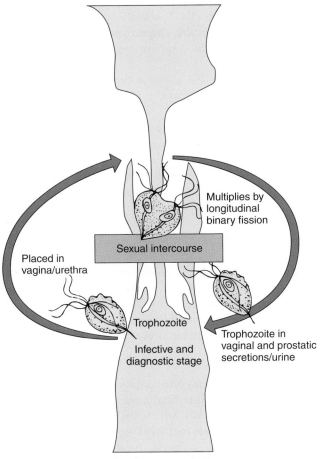

Figure 81—5. Life cycle of *Trichomonas vaginalis*.

may be improved by culturing the organism (93% sensitivity) or using monoclonal fluorescent antibody staining (86% sensitivity). A nucleic acid probe assay is also available commercially. Serologic tests may be useful in epidemiologic surveillance.

Figure 81—6. *Trichomonas vaginalis* trophozoite. The trophozoite is 7 to 23 μm long and 6 to 8 μm wide (average, 13 × 7 μm). The flagella and a short, undulating membrane are present at one side, and an axostyle extends through the center of the parasite.

Treatment, Prevention, and Control

The drug of choice is metronidazole. Both male and female sex partners must be treated to avoid reinfection. Resistance to metronidazole has been reported and may require retreatment with higher doses. More recently, tinidazole has received U.S. Food and Drug Administration (FDA) approval for treatment of trichomoniasis in adults and may be used as first-line agent or for cases refractory to metronidazole. Personal hygiene, avoidance of shared toilet articles and clothing, and safe sexual practices are important preventive actions. Elimination of carriage in men is critical for the eradication of disease.

Ciliates

The intestinal protozoan *Balantidium coli* is the only member of the ciliate group that is pathogenic for humans. Disease produced by *B. coli* is similar to amebiasis, because the organisms elaborate proteolytic and cytotoxic substances that mediate tissue invasion and intestinal ulceration.

Balantidium coli

Physiology and Structure

The life cycle of *B. coli* is simple, involving ingestion of infectious cysts, excystation, and invasion of trophozoites into the mucosal lining of the large intestine, cecum, and terminal ileum (Figure 81-7). The trophozoite is covered with rows of hairlike cilia that aid in motility. Morphologically more

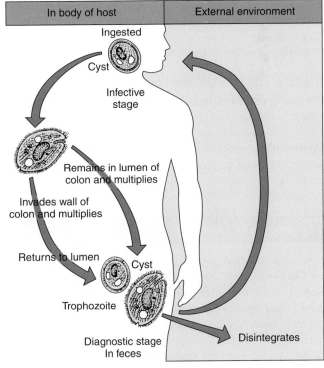

Figure 81—7. Life cycle of *Balantidium coli*.

Laboratory Diagnosis

Careful examination of concentrated stool sediment and special staining with iodine or a modified acid-fast procedure reveal the parasite (Figure 81-9). Small bowel biopsy has been used to establish the diagnosis when the results of tests on stool specimens are negative.

Treatment, Prevention, and Control

The drug of choice is trimethoprim-sulfamethoxazole, with the combination of pyrimethamine and sulfadiazine an acceptable alternative. Prevention and control are effected by maintaining personal hygiene and highly sanitary conditions and by avoiding oral-anal sexual contact.

Sarcocystis Species

Physician awareness of the genus *Sarcocystis* is important only in recognizing that it can be detected in stool specimens. *Sarcocystis* species can be isolated from pigs and cattle and are identical in all aspects to *Isospora* species with one exception: *Sarcocystis* oocysts rupture before passage in stool specimens, and only sporocysts are present. Intestinal disease may occur following ingestion of infected meat and is characterized by nausea, abdominal pain, and diarrhea. Some individuals can be infected and show no clinical signs. Muscular *Sarcocystis* infections in humans may occur if sporocysts are ingested but are usually mild or subclinical. There is no known treatment for intestinal or muscular sarcocystosis in humans.

Cryptosporidium Species

Physiology and Structure

The life cycle of *Cryptosporidium* species is typical of coccidians, as is the intestinal disease, but this species differs in the intracellular location of the organism in the epithelial cells (Figure 81-10). In contrast to the deep intracellular invasion observed with *Isospora* species, *Cryptosporidium* organisms are found just within the brush border of the intestinal epithelium. The coccidia attach to the surface of the cells and replicate by a series of processes (merogony, gametogony, sporogony) leading to the production of new infectious oocysts. After sporogony, the mature oocysts may either excyst within the digestive tract of the host, leading to the infection of new cells, or may be excreted into the environment.

Epidemiology

Cryptosporidium species are distributed worldwide. Infection is reported in a wide variety of animals, including mammals, reptiles, and fish. There are at least 16 different species of *Cryptosporidium*; however, *C. hominis* and *C. parvum* are the species most commonly infecting humans. Waterborne transmission of cryptosporidiosis is now well documented as an important route of infection. The massive outbreak of

Figure 81—9. Oocyst of *Isospora belli* containing two sporoblasts. **A,** Wet mount. **B,** Acid-fast stain. Oocysts are ovoid (approximately 25 μm long and 15 μm wide) with tapering ends.

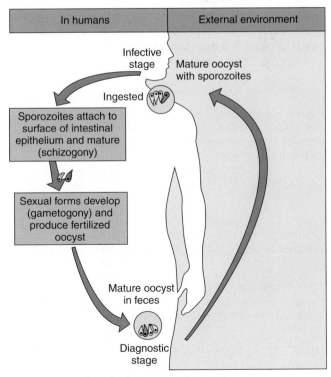

Figure 81—10. Life cycle of *Cryptosporidium* species.

cryptosporidiosis in Milwaukee in 1993 (approximately 300,000 individuals infected) was linked to contamination of the municipal water supply. Cryptosporidia are resistant to the usual water-purification procedures (chlorination and ozone), and it is believed that runoff of local waste and surface water into municipal water supplies is an important source of contamination. Zoonotic spread from animal reservoirs to humans, as well as person-to-person spread by fecal-oral and oral-anal routes, is also common means of infection. Veterinary personnel, animal handlers, and homosexuals are at particularly high risk for infection. Many outbreaks have now been described in daycare centers, where fecal-oral transmission is common.

Clinical Syndromes (Clinical Case 81-3)

As with other protozoan infections, exposure to *Cryptosporidium* organisms may result in asymptomatic carriage. Disease in previously healthy individuals is usually a mild, self-limiting **enterocolitis** characterized by watery diarrhea without blood. Spontaneous remission after an average of 10 days is characteristic. In contrast, disease in immunocompromised patients (e.g., patients with AIDS), characterized by 50 or more stools per day and tremendous fluid loss, can be severe and last for months to years. In some patients with AIDS, disseminated *Cryptosporidium* infections have been reported.

Laboratory Diagnosis

Cryptosporidium may be detected in large numbers in unconcentrated stool specimens obtained from immunocompromised individuals with diarrhea. Oocysts generally measure 5 to 7 microns and may be concentrated with the modified zinc sulfate centrifugal flotation technique or by Sheather sugar flotation procedure. Specimens may be stained using the modified **acid-fast** method (Figure 81-11) or by

Figure 81–11. Acid-fast stained *Cryptosporidium* oocysts (approximately 5 to 7 μm in diameter). *(From Marler LM, et al: Parasitology CD-ROM, Indiana Pathology Images, 2003.)*

an indirect immunofluorescence assay. Both an enzyme immunoassay and an immunochromatographic assay for detecting fecal antigen are commercially available. The number of oocysts shed in stool may fluctuate; therefore a minimum of three specimens should be examined. Serologic procedures are used in epidemiologic and seroprevalence studies but are not yet widely available for diagnosing and monitoring infections.

Treatment, Prevention, and Control

Unfortunately, no broadly effective therapy has been developed for managing *Cryptosporidium* infections in immunocompromised patients. Therapeutic information is largely based on isolated reports and anecdotal information. Spiramycin may help control the diarrhea in some patients in the early stages of AIDS who have cryptosporidiosis, but it is ineffective in patients who have progressed to the later stages of AIDS. Spiramycin was no more effective than placebo in treating cryptosporidial diarrhea in infants. Nitazoxanide is approved by the FDA for the treatment of cryptosporidiosis in children ages 1 to 11 years, but it is not yet approved for treatment of cryptosporidiosis in immunocompromised individuals. Reports concerning efficacy of azithromycin and paromomycin are promising, but these need confirmation. Therapy consists primarily of supportive measures to restore the tremendous fluid loss from the watery diarrhea.

Because of the widespread distribution of this organism in humans and other animals, preventing infection is difficult. The same methods of improved personal hygiene and sanitation used for other intestinal protozoa should be maintained for this disease. Contaminated water supplies should be treated with chlorination and filtration. In addition, avoidance of high-risk sexual activities is critical.

Cyclospora Species

Physiology and Structure

Cyclospora is a coccidian parasite that is taxonomically related to *Isospora* species, *Cryptosporidium parvum*, and

---

Clinical Case 81-3. Cryptosporidiosis

Quiroz and colleagues (J Infect Dis 181:685-700, 2000) described an outbreak of cryptosporidiosis that was linked to a food handler. In the fall of 1998, an outbreak of gastroenteritis among university students was reported to the Department of Health. Preliminary findings suggested that the illness was associated with eating at one of the campus cafeterias; four employees of this cafeteria had similar illness. The outbreak was thought to be due to a viral agent until *Cryptosporidium parvum* was detected in the stool specimen of several cafeteria employees. In a case-control study of 88 case patients and 67 control subjects, eating in one of two cafeterias was associated with diarrheal illness. *C. parvum* was detected in stool samples of 16 (70%) of 23 ill students and 2 of 4 ill employees. One ill food handler with laboratory-confirmed cryptosporidiosis prepared raw produce on the days surrounding the outbreak. All 25 *C. parvum* isolates submitted for DNA analysis, including three from the ill food handler, were genotype 1. This outbreak illustrates the potential for cryptosporidiosis to cause foodborne illness. Epidemiologic and molecular evidence indicate that an ill food handler was the likely outbreak source.

Toxoplasma gondii. A single species infecting humans, *C. cayetanensis*, has been identified thus far.

Although the details of its life cycle have yet to be determined, *Cyclospora* organisms are similar to *Isospora* in that oocysts are excreted unsporulated and require a period of time outside the host for maturation to occur. The pathogenic mechanisms by which *Cyclospora* species cause clinical illness are unknown; however, the organism usually infects the upper small bowel and causes pronounced histopathologic changes. The organism is found within vacuoles in the cytoplasm of jejunal epithelial cells, and its presence is associated with inflammatory changes, villous atrophy, and crypt hyperplasia.

The morphologic characteristics of *Cyclospora* species are similar to those of *Isospora* species and *C. parvum* with a few exceptions. The oocysts of *Cyclospora* species are spherical and are 8 to 10 μm in diameter, as opposed to the smaller oocysts of *C. parvum* (5 to 7 μm) and the much larger elliptical oocysts of *Isospora* species (15 to 25 μm). The oocysts of *Cyclospora* species contain two sporocysts, each of which contain two sporozoites, which in turn contain a membrane-bound nucleus and micronemes characteristic of the sporozoans. In contrast, the *Cryptosporidium* oocyst contains four naked, or nonencysted, sporozoites, whereas the *Isospora* oocyst contains two sporocysts, each containing four sporozoites.

Epidemiology

As with *Cryptosporidium*, *Cyclospora* is widely distributed throughout the world and infects a variety of reptiles, birds, and mammals. Although direct animal-to-human or person-to-person transmission has not been documented, there is now compelling evidence that *Cyclospora* infection is acquired through contaminated water. In areas of endemicity, such as Nepal, studies have documented an annual surge of cyclosporiasis that coincides with the rainy season. The prevalence of infection (symptomatic and asymptomatic) ranges from 2% to 18% in endemic areas and is estimated at 0.1% to 0.5% in developed countries. Outbreaks in the United States have occurred during the summer months and have been correlated with the consumption of contaminated fruits and vegetables; transmission via contaminated water has also been suggested. Like *Cryptosporidium*, *Cyclospora* species is resistant to chlorination and is not readily detected by methods used currently to ensure the safety of supplies of drinking water.

Clinical Syndromes

The clinical manifestations of cyclosporiasis resemble those of cryptosporidiosis and include mild nausea, anorexia, abdominal cramping, and watery diarrhea. Fatigue, malaise, flatulence, and bloating have also been reported. In immunocompetent hosts, diarrhea is self-limited but may be prolonged and last for weeks. Among immunocompromised people, specifically patients infected with the human immunodeficiency virus (HIV), clinical illness is typically prolonged and severe and is associated with a high rate of recurrence. Biliary tract infection with *Cyclospora* infection has been reported in two patients with AIDS.

Laboratory Diagnosis

The diagnosis of cyclosporiasis is based on the microscopic detection of oocysts in stool. Oocysts may be detected by light microscopic examination of unstained fecal material (wet mount), where they appear as nonrefractile, spherical to oval, slightly wrinkled bodies measuring 8 to 10 μm in diameter; they have an internal cluster of membrane-bound globules (Figure 81-12). In fresh specimens, *Cyclospora* organisms fluoresce when examined with an ultraviolet fluorescence microscope fitted with a 365-nm excitation filter.

Cyclospora oocysts may be concentrated with the modified zinc sulfate centrifugal flotation technique or by Sheather sugar flotation procedure. Organisms are acid-fast and thus can be detected using one of the many acid-fast staining techniques, including the modified Ziehl-Neelsen stain or the Kinyoun acid-fast stain (Figure 81-13). A distinguishing feature of *Cyclospora* species is its variable appearance on acid-fast staining, which ranges from unstained to mottled pink to deep red.

The relative sensitivity, specificity, and predictive value of the various methods for diagnosing *Cyclospora* infection are not known. Currently there are no immunodiagnostic techniques to aid in the diagnosis and monitoring of these infections. The rudimentary nature of the available diagnostic techniques and the incomplete understanding of the disease process may contribute to under-recognition of *Cyclospora* infection.

Treatment, Prevention, and Control

The effectiveness of trimethoprim-sulfamethoxazole has been demonstrated in anecdotal reports, in a large, open-label study of patients infected with HIV, and in a

Figure 81—12. Sporulated oocyst of *Cyclospora cayetanensis*. The oocysts measure 8 to 10 μm in diameter and contain two sporocysts with two sporozoites. (Saline wet mount; ×900.) *(Courtesy Mr J Williams; from Peters W, Giles HM: Color Atlas of Tropical Medicine and Parasitology, 4th ed. London, Mosby, 1995.)*

Figure 81–13. Oocysts of *Cryptosporidium parvum (lower left)* and *Cyclospora cayetanensis (upper right)*. Both parasites stain red with Ziehl-Neelsen stain; however, *Cyclospora* organisms typically take up variable amounts of the stain, and the oocysts are larger (8 to 10 μm compared with 5 to 7 μm). *(Courtesy Mr J Williams; from Peters W, Giles HM: Color Atlas of Tropical Medicine and Parasitology, 4th ed. London, Mosby, 1995.)*

placebo-controlled trial. In HIV-infected patients, it appears that the high rate of recurrence can be attenuated with long-term suppressive therapy with trimethoprim-sulfamethoxazole. Although numerous additional agents, including metronidazole, nitazoxanide, norfloxacin, quinacrine, nalidixic acid, tinidazole, and diloxanide furoate, have been used in various trials, the effectiveness of any one of these agents has not been proved.

As with *Cryptosporidium* species, prevention of *Cyclospora* infection is difficult. Although *Cyclospora* organisms appear resistant to chlorination, the treatment of water supplies with chlorination and filtration remains a reasonable practice. In addition, the same methods of improved personal hygiene and sanitation used for other intestinal protozoa should be used as preventive measures for this disease.

Microsporidia

Physiology and Structure

Microsporidia are obligate intracellular pathogens belonging to the kingdom Fungi, phylum Microspora. They are considered to be primitive eukaryotic organisms, because they lack mitochondria, peroxisomes, Golgi membranes, and other typically eukaryotic organelles. The organisms are characterized by the structure of their spores, which have a complex tubular extrusion mechanism used for injecting the infective material (sporoplasm) into cells. Microsporidia have been detected in human tissues and implicated as participants in human disease. To date, seven genera of Microsporidia (*Encephalitozoon, Pleistophora, Nosema, Vittaforma, Trachipleistophora, Brachiola,* and *Enterocytozoon*) and unclassified *Microsporidium* species have been reported in humans.

Pathogenesis

Infection with Microsporidia is initiated by the ingestion of spores. After ingestion, the spores pass into the duodenum, where the sporoplasm with its nuclear material is injected into an adjacent cell in the small intestine. Once inside a suitable host cell, the Microsporidia multiply extensively, either within a **parasitophorous vacuole** or free within the cytoplasm. The intracellular multiplication includes a phase of repeated divisions by binary fission (**merogony**) and a phase culminating in spore formation (**sporogony**). The parasites spread from cell to cell, causing cell death and local inflammation. Although some species are highly selective in the cell type they invade, collectively the Microspora are capable of infecting every organ of the body, and disseminated infections have been described in severely immunocompromised individuals. After sporogony the mature spores containing the infective sporoplasm may be excreted into the environment, thus continuing the cycle.

Epidemiology

Microsporidia are distributed worldwide and have a wide host range among invertebrate and vertebrate animals. *Enterocytozoon bieneusi* and *Encephalitozoon (Septata) intestinalis* have gained increasing attention as causes of chronic diarrhea in patients with AIDS. Both *Encephalitozoon*-like and *Enterocytozoon*-like organisms have been reported in the tissues of AIDS patients with hepatitis and peritonitis. *Trachipleistophora* and *Nosema* are known to cause myositis in immunocompromised patients. *Nosema* species has caused localized keratitis, as well as disseminated infection in a child with severe combined immunodeficiency. *Microsporidium* species and *Encephalitozoon hellem* have caused infection of the human cornea.

Although the reservoir for human infection is unknown, transmission is likely accomplished by ingestion of spores that have been shed in the urine and feces of infected animals or individuals. As with cryptosporidial infection, individuals with AIDS and other cellular immune defects appear to be at increased risk for infection with microsporidia.

Clinical Syndromes

Clinical signs and symptoms of microsporidiosis are quite variable in the human cases reported (Clinical Case 81-4). Intestinal infection caused by *E. bieneusi* in patients with AIDS is marked by persistent and debilitating diarrhea similar to that seen in patients with cryptosporidiosis, cyclosporiasis, and isosporiasis. The clinical presentation of infection with other species of Microspora depends on the organ system involved and ranges from localized ocular pain and loss of vision (*Microsporidium* and *Nosema* species) to neurologic disturbances and hepatitis (*Encephalitozoon cuniculi*) to a more generalized picture of

Clinical Case 81-4. Microsporidia

Coyle and colleagues (N Engl J Med 351:42-47, 2004) described a case of fatal myositis due to the microsporidian *Brachiola algerae*. The patient was a 57-year-old woman with rheumatoid arthritis and diabetes who presented with a 6-week history of increasing fatigue, generalized muscle and joint pain, profound weakness, and fever. She was taking immunosuppressive agents (prednisone, methotrexate, leflunomide) for rheumatoid arthritis and had no evidence of HIV infection. In the 6 months before admission, she began taking infliximab, a monoclonal antibody with high binding affinity for tumor necrosis factor α (TNF-α). The patient resided in a small town in northeastern Pennsylvania and had no recent travel history. She had no contact with animals. On admission, her serum creatine kinase was elevated, and a test for HIV was negative. A muscle biopsy from the left anterior thigh contained microorganisms that were consistent with microsporidia. The morphologic appearance suggested *Brachiola* species, and the identity was confirmed by PCR with the use of primers specific for *Brachiola algerae*, a mosquito pathogen.

The muscle pain worsened, and the patient became increasingly debilitated, requiring mechanical ventilation after respiratory insufficiency developed. Despite the administration of albendazole and itraconazole, a repeat muscle biopsy from the right quadriceps muscle revealed microsporidia. Four weeks after admission, the patient died from a massive cerebrovascular infarction. A postmortem muscle biopsy revealed necrosis and persistent organisms.

B. algerae is a well-known microsporidian pathogen of mosquitoes but has not been reported previously to cause myositis in humans. The present case report illustrates that insect pathogens such as *B. algerae* are capable of causing disseminated disease in humans. Anti—TNF-α therapy (infliximab) may have an adverse effect on microsporidiosis.

Figure 81—14. Gram-positive spores of *Encephalitozoon* species. *(From Marler LM, et al: Parasitology CD-ROM, Indiana Pathology Images, 2003.)*

These techniques are not yet considered reliable enough for routine diagnosis.

Treatment, Prevention, and Control

There is no completely effective treatment for microsporidian infections. Treatment with albendazole has resulted in clinical cure of HIV-associated encephalitozoonosis. Likewise, some patients treated with sulfa drugs have survived. Oral fumagillin administration has resulted in transient improvement in a small study of HIV-associated diarrhea due to *E. bieneusi*. Albendazole is the current drug of choice for ocular (*Encephalitozoon hellem*, *E. cuniculi*, *Vittaforma corneae* [*Nosema corneum*]), intestinal (*Encephalitozoon* [*Septata*] *intestinalis*) and disseminated (*E. hellem*, *E. cuniculi*, *E. intestinalis*, *Pleistophora* spp.) microsporidiosis. Notably, albendazole is not effective for *Enterocytozoon* infection.

As with *Cryptosporidium*, preventing microsporidian infection is difficult. The same methods of improved personal hygiene and sanitation used for other intestinal protozoa should be maintained with this disease.

dissemination with fever, vomiting, diarrhea, and malabsorption (*Nosema* species). In a report of disseminated infection with *Nosema connori*, the organism was observed involving the muscles of the stomach, bowel, arteries, diaphragm, and heart and the parenchymal cells of the liver, lungs, and adrenal glands.

Laboratory Diagnosis

Diagnosis of microsporidia infection may be made by detection of the organisms in biopsy material and by light microscopic examination of cerebrospinal fluid and urine. Spores measuring between 1.0 and 2.0 μm may be visualized by Gram (gram-positive), acid-fast, periodic acid—Schiff, immunochemical, and Giemsa staining techniques (Figure 81-14). A chromotrope-based staining technique for light-microscopic detection of *E. bieneusi* and *Encephalitozoon* (*Septata*) *intestinalis* spores in stool and duodenal aspirates has also been described (Figure 81-15). Electron microscopy is considered the gold standard for diagnostic confirmation of microsporidiosis; however, its sensitivity is unknown. Additional diagnostic techniques, including polymerase chain reaction, culture, and serologic testing, are under investigation.

Figure 81—15. Smear of formalin-fixed stool specimen showing pinkish red—stained microsporidia spores. Bacteria are stained a faint green. (Chromotrope-based stain; ×1000.) *(From Marler LM, et al: Parasitology CD-ROM, Indiana Pathology Images, 2003.)*

Case Study and Questions

A 31-year-old female veterinarian complained of diarrhea that she had experienced for 2 weeks. The diarrhea was described as thin, watery, and nonbloody. The patient described 10 to 14 diarrheal stools per day, the frequency of which was not influenced by a variety of over-the-counter antidiarrheal medications.

Physical examination revealed a well-developed, well-nourished woman who appeared somewhat fatigued and mildly dehydrated. The workup included a negative HIV serologic test, a normal flexible sigmoidoscope examination, and a negative stool culture for bacterial pathogens. A microscopic examination of the stool for white blood cells was negative, as was a test for *Clostridium difficile* toxin. A stool specimen was sent for ova and parasite examination and, after appropriate concentration measures, demonstrated acid-fast oocysts.

1. Which parasite was found in the patient's stool?

2. What was the likely source of this individual's infection?

3. If this individual were HIV positive, what other intestinal pathogens would have been considered?

4. Other than conventional microscopy, what other methods could have been used to diagnose this infection?

5. Should this patient have received specific antimicrobial therapy? If so, what would have been prescribed? If not, why not?

Bibliography

Adam RD: Biology of *Giardia lamblia*. Clin Microbiol Rev 14:447-475, 2001.

Cama VA, Ross JM, Crawford S, et al: Differences in clinical manifestations among *Cryptosporidium* species and subtypes in HIV-infected person. J Infect Dis 196:684-691, 2007.

Connor DH, et al: Pathology of Infectious Diseases, vol 2. Stamford, Conn, Appleton & Lange, 1997.

Espinosa-Cantellano M, Martinez-Palomo A: Pathogenesis of intestinal amebiasis: From molecules to disease. Clin Microbiol Rev 13:318-331, 2000.

Fayer R: *Sarcocystis* spp. in humans. Clin Microbiol Rev 17:894-902, 2004.

Fotedar R, et al: Laboratory diagnostic techniques for *Entamoeba* species. Clin Microbiol Rev 20:511-532, 2007.

Gardner TB, Hill DR: Treatment of giardiasis. Clin Microbiol Rev 14:114-128, 2001.

Herwaldt BL: *Cyclospora cayetanensis*: A review, focusing on the outbreaks of cyclosporiasis in the 1990s. Clin Infect Dis 31:1040-1057, 2000.

Hunter PR, Nichols G: Epidemiology and clinical features of *Cryptosporidium* infection in immunocompromised patients. Clin Microbiol Rev 15:145-154, 2002.

Leber AL, Novak SM: Intestinal and urogenital amebae, flagellates, and ciliates. In Murray PR, et al (eds): Manual of Clinical Microbiology, 9th ed. Washington, DC, ASM Press, 2007.

Lindsay DS, Upton SJ, Weiss LM: *Isospora, Cyclospora*, and *Sarcocystis*. In Murray PR, et al. (eds): Manual of Clinical Microbiology, 9th ed. Washington, DC, ASM Press, 2007.

Mathis A, Weber R, Deplazes P: Zoonotic potential of microsporidia. Clin Microbiol Rev 18:423-445, 2005.

Peters W, Giles HM: Color Atlas of Tropical Medicine and Parasitology, 4th ed. London, Mosby, 1995.

Weber R, Mathis A, Deplazes P: Microsporidia. In Murray PR, et al (eds): Manual of Clinical Microbiology, 9th ed. Washington, DC, ASM Press, 2007.

Xiao L, et al: *Cryptosporidium* taxonomy: Recent advances and implications for public health. Clin Microbiol Rev 17:72-97, 2004.

Xiao L, Cama V: *Cryptosporidium*. In Murray PR, et al (eds): Manual of Clinical Microbiology, 9th ed. Washington, DC, ASM Press, 2007.

Blood and Tissue Protozoa

The protozoa of blood and tissues are closely related to the intestinal protozoan parasites in practically all aspects, except for their sites of infection (Box 82-1). The malaria parasites (*Plasmodium* species) infect both blood and tissues.

Plasmodium Species

Plasmodia are coccidian or sporozoan parasites of blood cells, and as seen with other coccidia, they require two hosts: the mosquito for the sexual reproductive stages and humans and other animals for the asexual reproductive stages. Infection with *Plasmodium* spp. (i.e., malaria) accounts for 1 to 5 billion febrile episodes and 1 to 3 million deaths annually, 85% of which are in Africa (Clinical Case 82-1).

The four species of plasmodia that infect humans are *P. vivax*, *P. ovale*, *P. malariae*, and *P. falciparum* (Table 82-1). These species share a common life cycle, as illustrated in Figure 82-1. Human infection is initiated by the bite of an *Anopheles* mosquito, which introduces infectious plasmodia **sporozoites** via its saliva into the circulatory system. The sporozoites are carried to the parenchymal cells of the liver, where asexual reproduction **(schizogony)** occurs. This phase of growth is termed the **exoerythrocytic cycle** and lasts 8 to 25 days, depending on the plasmodial species. Some species (e.g., *P. vivax*, *P. ovale*) can establish a dormant hepatic phase in which the sporozoites (called **hypnozoites** or **sleeping forms**) do not divide. The presence of these viable plasmodia can lead to the relapse of infections months to years after the initial clinical disease (relapsing malaria). The hepatocytes eventually rupture, liberating the plasmodia (termed **merozoites** at this stage), which in turn attach to specific receptors on the surface of erythrocytes and enter the cells, thus initiating the erythrocytic cycle.

Asexual replication progresses through a series of stages (ring, trophozoite, schizont) that culminates in the rupture of the erythrocyte, releasing up to 24 merozoites, which initiates another cycle of replication by infecting other erythrocytes. Some merozoites also develop within erythrocytes into male and female **gametocytes**. If a mosquito ingests mature male and female gametocytes during a blood meal, the sexual reproductive cycle of malaria can be initiated, with the eventual production of sporozoites infectious for humans. This sexual reproductive stage within the mosquito is necessary for the maintenance of malaria within a population.

Most malaria seen in the United States is acquired by visitors or residents of countries with endemic disease **(imported malaria)**. However, the appropriate vector *Anopheles* mosquito is found in several sections of the United States, and domestic transmission of disease has been observed **(introduced malaria)**. In addition to transmission by mosquitos, malaria can also be acquired by blood transfusions from an infected donor **(transfusion malaria)**. This type of transmission can also occur among narcotic addicts who share needles and syringes **("mainline" malaria)**. Congenital acquisition, although rare, is also a possible mode of transmission **(congenital malaria)**.

Plasmodium vivax

Physiology and Structure

P. vivax (Figure 82-2) is selective in that it invades only young, immature erythrocytes containing the **Duffy blood group antigen** on the cell surface (see Chapter 78). In infections caused by *P. vivax*, infected red blood cells are usually enlarged and contain numerous pink granules or **Schüffner dots**, the trophozoite is ring shaped but amoeboid in appearance, more mature trophozoites and erythrocytic schizonts containing up to 24 merozoites are present, and the gametocytes are round. The mature schizonts often contain golden-brown **hemozoin** pigment granules **(malarial pigment)**. These characteristics are helpful in identifying the specific plasmodial species, which is important for the treatment of malaria.

Box 82–1. Medically Important Blood and Tissue Protozoa

Plasmodium species
Babesia species
Toxoplasma species
Sarcocystis species
Acanthamoeba species
Balamuthia species
Naegleria species
Leishmania species
Trypanosoma species

Table 82–1. Human Malarial Parasites

Parasite	Disease
Plasmodium vivax	Benign tertian malaria
P. ovale	Benign tertian or ovale malaria
P. malariae	Quartan or malarial malaria
P. falciparum	Malignant tertian malaria

Epidemiology

P. vivax is the most prevalent of the human plasmodia, with the widest geographical distribution, including the tropics, subtropics, and temperate regions.

Clinical Syndromes

After an incubation period (usually 10 to 17 days), the patient experiences vague influenza-like symptoms with headache, muscle pains, photophobia, anorexia, nausea, and vomiting.

As the infection progresses, increased numbers of rupturing erythrocytes liberate merozoites, as well as toxic cellular debris and hemoglobin, into the circulation. Together these produce the **typical pattern of chills, fever, and malarial rigors**. These **paroxysms** usually reappear periodically

Clinical Case 82-1. Malaria

Mohin and Gupta (Infect Dis Clin Pract 15:209-212, 2007) describe a case of severe malaria due to *Plasmodium vivax*. The patient was a 59-year-old man who presented with a 1-day history of high-grade fever after recently returning from Guyana in South America. He did not take any medications before, during, or after the trip. He noted that his symptoms were similar to those of a previous malaria infection (5 years ago), also acquired in Guyana. A peripheral blood smear as part of the initial workup showed numerous red blood cells with schizonts, consistent with *Plasmodium* infection, with more than 5% parasitemia. Several blood tests, including a DNA polymerase chain reaction (PCR), were sent for parasite species determination. The patient was started on quinine and doxycycline oral therapy because of concerns regarding chloroquine-resistant malaria. Subsequently, during the next 4 days, the patient developed severe thrombocytopenia, non-oliguric renal, acute respiratory, and circulatory failure, despite a decrease in parasitemia to less than 0.5%. He received intravenous quinidine and an exchange transfusion to treat *P. falciparum* infection, suspected at the time because of the severity of his symptoms. The next day, however, the results of the PCR of the blood revealed the parasite to be *P. vivax* and not *P. falciparum*. The patient gradually improved and was treated with primaquine to prevent relapse.

This case shows that although unusual, severe respiratory and circulatory compromise may complicate *P. vivax* malaria. *P. vivax* should be considered if the patient's condition deteriorates despite the presence of relatively low parasite levels. As opposed to *P. falciparum*, *P. vivax* infections carry the additional risk of relapse, which warrants appropriate and adequate treatment. Finally, this case also emphasizes the importance of chemoprophylaxis and personal protective measures for anyone planning a trip to a malaria-infested region.

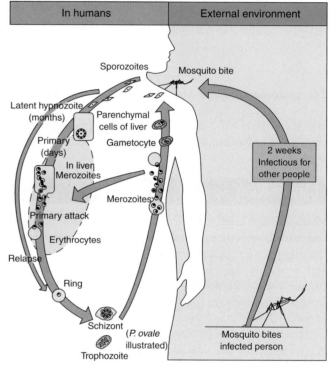

Figure 82–1. Life cycle of *Plasmodium* species.

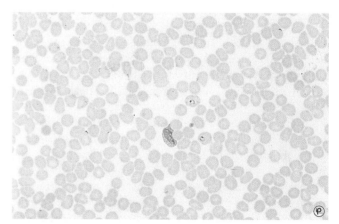

Figure 82–2. *P. vivax* ring forms and young trophozoites. Note the multiple stages of the parasite seen in the peripheral blood smear, the enlarged parasitized erythrocytes, and the presence of Schüffner dots with the trophozoite form. These are characteristic of *P. vivax* infections. (*From Marler LM, et al: Parasitology CD-ROM, Indiana Pathology Images, 2003.*)

(generally every 48 hours) as the cycle of infection, replication, and cell lysis progresses. The paroxysms may remain relatively mild or progress to severe attacks, with hours of sweating, chills, shaking, persistently high temperatures (103° F to 106° F), and exhaustion.

P. vivax causes "benign tertian malaria," which refers to the cycle of paroxysms every 48 hours (in untreated patients) and the fact that most patients tolerate the attacks and can survive for years without treatment. If left untreated, however, chronic *P. vivax* infections can lead to brain, kidney, and liver damage as a result of the malarial pigment, cellular debris, and capillary plugging of these organs by masses of adherent erythrocytes.

Laboratory Diagnosis

Microscopic examination of thick and thin films of blood is the method of choice for confirming the clinical diagnosis of malaria and identifying the specific species responsible for disease. The thick film is a concentration method and may be used to detect the presence of organisms. With training, thick films may be used to diagnose the species as well. The thin film is most useful for establishing species identification. Blood films can be taken at any time over the course of the infection, but the best time is midway between paroxysms of chills and fever, when the greatest number of intracellular organisms is present. It may be necessary to take repeated films at intervals of 4 to 6 hours.

Serologic procedures are available, but they are used primarily for epidemiologic surveys or for screening blood donors. Serologic findings usually remain positive for approximately a year, even after complete treatment of the infection.

Treatment, Prevention, and Control

The treatment of *P. vivax* infection involves a combination of supportive measures and chemotherapy. Bed rest, relief of fever and headache, regulation of fluid balance, and in some cases, blood transfusion are supportive therapies.

The chemotherapeutic regimens are as follows:

1. Suppressive—aimed at avoiding infection and clinical symptoms (i.e., a form of prophylaxis)
2. Therapeutic—aimed at eradicating the erythrocytic cycle
3. Radical cure—aimed at eradicating the exoerythrocytic cycle in the liver
4. Gametocidal—aimed at destroying erythrocytic gametocytes to prevent mosquito transmission

Chloroquine is the drug of choice for the suppression and therapeutic treatment of *P. vivax*, followed by primaquine for radical cure and elimination of gametocytes. Chloroquine-resistant forms of *P. vivax* have emerged in Indonesia, the Solomon islands, New Guinea, and Brazil. Patients infected with chloroquine-resistant *P. vivax* may be treated with other agents, including mefloquine ± artesunate, quinine, pyrimethamine-sulfadoxine

(Fansidar), and doxycycline. Primaquine is especially effective in preventing a relapse from the latent forms of *P. vivax* in the liver. Because antimalarial drugs are potentially toxic, it is imperative that physicians carefully review the recommended therapeutic regimens.

Chemoprophylaxis and prompt eradication of infections are critical in breaking the mosquito-human transmission cycle. Control of mosquito breeding and protection of individuals by screening, netting, protective clothing, and insect repellents are also essential. Immigrants from and travelers to endemic areas must be carefully screened, using blood films or serologic tests to detect possible infection. The development of vaccines to protect persons living in or traveling to endemic areas is under investigation.

Plasmodium ovale

Physiology and Structure

P. ovale is similar to *P. vivax* in many respects, including its selectivity for young, pliable erythrocytes. As a consequence, the host cell becomes enlarged and distorted, usually in an oval form. Schüffner dots appear as pale pink granules, and the cell border is frequently fimbriated or ragged. The schizont of *P. ovale*, when mature, contains about half the number of merozoites seen in *P. vivax*, and the malarial pigment is a darker brown.

Epidemiology

P. ovale is distributed primarily in tropical Africa, where it is often more prevalent than *P. vivax*. It is also found in Asia and South America.

Clinical Syndromes

The clinical picture of tertian attacks for *P. ovale* (benign tertian or ovale malaria) infection is similar to that for *P. vivax*. Untreated infections last only about a year, instead of the several years for *P. vivax*. Both relapse and recrudescence phases are similar to *P. vivax*.

Laboratory Diagnosis

As with *P. vivax*, thick and thin blood films are examined for the typical oval host cell with Schüffner dots and a ragged cell wall. Serologic tests reveal cross-reaction with *P. vivax* and other plasmodia.

Treatment, Prevention, and Control

The treatment regimen, including the use of primaquine to prevent relapse from latent liver forms, is similar to that used for *P. vivax* infections. Preventing *P. ovale* infection involves the same measures as for *P. vivax* and other plasmodia.

Plasmodium malariae

Physiology and Structure

In contrast with *P. vivax* and *P. ovale*, *P. malariae* can infect only mature erythrocytes with relatively rigid cell membranes.

Clinical Syndromes

The incubation period of *P. falciparum* is the shortest of all the plasmodia, ranging from 7 to 10 days, and does not extend for months to years. After the early influenza-like symptoms, *P. falciparum* rapidly produces daily (**quotidian**) chills and fever as well as severe nausea, vomiting, and diarrhea. The periodicity of the attacks then becomes tertian (36 to 48 hours), and fulminating disease develops. The term **malignant tertian malaria** is appropriate for this infection. Because the symptoms of this type of malaria are similar to those of intestinal infections, the nausea, vomiting, and diarrhea have led to the observation that malaria is "the malignant mimic."

Although any malaria infection may be fatal, *P. falciparum* is the most likely to result in death if left untreated. The increased numbers of erythrocytes infected and destroyed result in toxic cellular debris, adherence of red blood cells to vascular endothelium and to adjacent red blood cells, and formation of capillary plugging by masses of red blood cells, platelets, leukocytes, and malarial pigment.

Involvement of the brain (cerebral malaria) is most often seen in *P. falciparum* infection. Capillary plugging from an accumulation of malarial pigment and masses of cells can result in coma and death.

Kidney damage is also associated with *P. falciparum* malaria, resulting in an illness called **blackwater fever**. Intravascular hemolysis with rapid destruction of red blood cells produces a marked hemoglobinuria and can result in acute renal failure, tubular necrosis, nephrotic syndrome, and death. Liver involvement is characterized by abdominal pain, vomiting of bile, severe diarrhea, and rapid dehydration.

Laboratory Diagnosis

Thick and thin blood films are searched for the characteristic rings of *P. falciparum*, which frequently occur in multiples within a single cell, as well as in the accolé position (see Figure 82-3). Also diagnostic are the distinctive crescentic gametocytes (see Figure 82-4). A high-grade parasitemia (>10% of RBCs infected) consisting only of ring forms is suggestive of *P. falciparum* infection, even if no gametocytes are observed.

Laboratory personnel must perform a thorough search of the blood films, because mixed infections can occur with any combination of the four species, but most often the combination is *P. falciparum* and *P. vivax*. The detection and proper reporting of a mixed infection directly affects the treatment chosen.

Treatment, Prevention, and Control

The treatment of malaria is based on the history regarding travel to endemic areas, prompt clinical review and differential diagnosis, accurate and rapid laboratory work, and correct use of antimalarial drugs.

Because chloroquine-resistant strains of *P. falciparum* are present in all areas of endemicity (Africa, Southeast Asia, South America) with the exception of Central America and the Caribbean, physicians must review all current protocols for the proper treatment of *P. falciparum* infections, noting particularly where chloroquine resistance is known to occur. If the patient's history indicates that the origin is not from a chloroquine-resistant area, the drug of choice is either chloroquine or parenteral quinine. Patients infected with chloroquine-resistant *P. falciparum* (or *P. vivax*) may be treated with other agents, including mefloquine ± artesunate, quinine, quinidine, pyrimethamine-sulfadoxine (Fansidar), and doxycycline. Because quinine and pyrimethamine-sulfadoxine are potentially toxic, they are used more often for treatment than prophylaxis. Amodiaquine, an analogue of chloroquine, is effective against chloroquine-resistant *P. falciparum*; however, toxicity limits its use. Newer agents with excellent activity against multidrug-resistant strains of *P. falciparum* include the phenanthrene methanols, halofantrine and lumefantrine, and the artemisinins, artemether and artesunate, both sesquiterpene derivatives (see Chapter 80).

Combinations of the rapid-acting artemisinins with an existing or newly introduced antimalarial compound have been shown to be highly effective in both treatment and control of malaria due to *P. falciparum*. The rapid reduction in parasite biomass (approximately 10^8-fold within 3 days) produced by the artemisinins, leaves a relatively small number of organisms for the second agent (usually mefloquine or lumefantrine) to clear. This reduces considerably the exposure of the parasite population to mefloquine or lumefantrine, thus reducing the chance of an escape-resistant mutant arising from the infection. Combinations of artesunate and mefloquine and of artemether and lumefantrine have both been well tolerated and highly efficacious in the treatment of multidrug-resistant falciparum malaria in semi-immune and nonimmune individuals.

Although the rationale for red-cell exchange transfusion in severe malaria is compelling, there are no prospective clinical trials comparing this therapy with others. Nonetheless, red-cell exchange (or whole-blood exchange), if available, should be considered in cases of severe malaria complicated by clinical signs of cerebral malaria, acute lung injury, severe hemolysis with acidemia, shock, or a high or rising level of parasitemia despite adequate intravenous antimicrobial therapy.

When there is uncertainty whether the *P. falciparum* is chloroquine resistant, it is advisable to assume that the strain is resistant and treat the patient accordingly. If the laboratory reports a mixed infection involving *P. falciparum* and *P. vivax*, the treatment must eradicate not only *P. falciparum* from the erythrocytes but also the liver stages of *P. vivax* to avoid relapses. Failure on the part of the laboratory to detect and report such a mixed infection can result in inappropriate treatment and unnecessary delay in accomplishing a complete cure.

P. falciparum infection can be prevented and controlled exactly as for *P. vivax* and the other human malarias.

Chloroquine resistance complicates the management of these patients but can be overcome by the physician's awareness of appropriate regimens.

Babesia Species

Babesia are intracellular sporozoan parasites that morphologically resemble plasmodia. Babesiosis is a zoonosis infecting a variety of animals, such as deer, cattle, and rodents; humans are accidental hosts. Infection is transmitted by Ixodid ticks. *Babesia microti* is the usual cause of babesiosis in the United States.

Physiology and Structure

Human infection follows contact with an infected tick (Figure 82-5). The infectious pyriform bodies are introduced into the bloodstream and infect erythrocytes. The intraerythrocytic trophozoites multiply by binary fission, forming tetrads, and then lyse the erythrocyte, releasing the merozoites. These can reinfect other cells to maintain the infection. Infected cells can also be ingested by feeding ticks, in which additional replication can take place. Infection in the tick population can also be maintained by transovarian transmission. The infected cells in humans resemble the ring forms of *P. falciparum*, but malarial pigment or other stages of growth characteristically seen with plasmodial infections are not seen with careful examination of blood smears (Figure 82-6).

Figure 82–6. Ring forms of *Babesia microti*. Note the multiple ring forms *(arrows)* within the individual erythrocytes and the similarity to those of *P. falciparum* in Figure 82-3.

Epidemiology

More than 70 different species of *Babesia* are found in Africa, Asia, Europe, and North America, with *B. microti* responsible for disease along the northeastern seaboard of the United States (e.g., Nantucket Island, Martha's Vineyard, Shelter Island). *Ixodes dammini* is the tick vector responsible for transmitting babesiosis in this area, and the natural reservoir hosts are field mice, voles, and other small rodents. Serologic studies in endemic areas have demonstrated a high incidence of past exposure to *Babesia*. Presumably, most infections are asymptomatic or mild. *B. divergens*, which has been reported more frequently from Europe, causes severe, often fatal infections in people who have undergone splenectomies. Severe, persistent *B. microti* parasitemia has occurred in immunosuppressed HIV-infected patients with intact spleens. Although most infections follow tick bites, transfusion-related infections have been demonstrated.

Clinical Syndromes

After an incubation period of 1 to 4 weeks, symptomatic patients experience general malaise, fever without periodicity, headache, chills, sweating, fatigue, and weakness. As the infection progresses with increased destruction of erythrocytes, hemolytic anemia develops, and the patient may experience renal failure. Hepatomegaly and splenomegaly can develop in advanced disease. Low-grade parasitemia may persist for weeks. Splenectomy or functional asplenia, immunosuppression, HIV infection, and advanced age increase a person's susceptibility to infections, as well as to more severe disease.

Laboratory Diagnosis

Examination of blood smears is the diagnostic method of choice. Laboratory personnel must be experienced in

Figure 82–5. Life cycle of *Babesia* species.

In rodents, dogs, humans, and other vertebrates | In hard-shell ticks

Penetrates erythrocytes

Infective stage
Pyriform bodies
Salivary gland

Trophozoite
Injected by tick during bite
Transovarian transmission

Erythrocytic cycle

Reproduces in hemocytes, muscle cells

Ovary

Vermicule

Tetrad

Cell ruptures

Merozoites

Phagocytosed by intestinal epithelium, where asexual division occurs

Trophozoite
Ingested
Trophozoite
Diagnostic stage

differentiating *Babesia* and *Plasmodium* species. *Babesia* may mimic *P. falciparum*, with red blood cells multiply infected with small ring forms (see Figure 82-6). Infected patients may have negative smears because of the low-grade parasitemia. These infections can be diagnosed by inoculating samples of blood into hamsters, which are highly susceptible to infection. Serologic tests are also available for diagnostic use.

Treatment, Prevention, and Control

The drugs of choice are clindamycin combined with quinine. Other antiprotozoal regimens, including chloroquine and pentamidine, have been used with variable results. However, most patients with mild disease recover without specific therapy. Exchange blood transfusion has also been successful in patients who have had splenectomies and who have severe infections caused by *B. microti* or *B. divergens*. The use of protective clothing and insect repellents can minimize tick exposure in endemic areas, which is critical for the prevention of disease. Ticks must feed on humans for several hours before the organisms are transmitted, so prompt removal of ticks can be protective.

Toxoplasma gondii (Clinical Case 82-2)

T. gondii is a typical coccidian parasite related to *Plasmodium*, *Isospora*, and other members of the phylum Sporozoa. *T. gondii* is an intracellular parasite, and it is found in a wide variety of animals, including birds and humans. Only one species exists, and there appears to be little strain-to-strain variation. The essential reservoir host of *T. gondii* is the common house cat and other felines.

Physiology and Structure

Organisms develop in the intestinal cells of the cat, as well as during an extraintestinal cycle with passage to the tissues via the bloodstream (Figure 82-7). The organisms from the intestinal cycle are passed in cat feces and mature into infective cysts within 3 to 4 days in the external environment. These oocysts are similar to those of *Isospora belli*, the human intestinal protozoan parasite, and can be ingested by mice and other animals (including humans) and produce acute and chronic infection of various tissues, including brain. Infection in cats is established when the tissues of infected rodents are eaten.

Some infective forms (**trophozoites**) of the oocyst develop as slender, crescentic types called **tachyzoites**. These rapidly multiplying forms are responsible for the initial infection and tissue damage. Slow-growing, shorter forms called **bradyzoites** also develop and form cysts in chronic infections.

Epidemiology

Human infection with *T. gondii* is ubiquitous; however, it is increasingly apparent that certain immunocompromised

Clinical Case 82-2. Toxoplasmosis

Vincent and colleagues (Infect Med 23:390, 2006) describe a 67-year-old woman with a 3-year history of Hodgkin disease who received chemotherapy followed by autologous stem-cell transplantation. Shortly afterward, she became febrile and neutropenic, and treatment with broad-spectrum antibiotics was started. The results of blood and urine cultures were negative. Following resolution of neutropenia (1 month posttransplantation), confusion and lethargy developed. Imaging studies of the brain revealed microinfarcts in both hemispheres and the midbrain. Findings from a lumbar puncture were unrevealing. Based on the suspicion of toxoplasmosis, pyrimethamine and sulfadiazine were added to the patient's regimen. When toxic epidermal necrolysis developed, the sulfadiazine was discontinued and clindamycin was begun. Multiorgan failure ensued, and the patient died 1 week later. At autopsy, the presence of cyst forms with bradyzoites were detected in the woman's brain and heart. Histopathologic findings and immunohistochemical staining confirmed a diagnosis of disseminated toxoplasmosis.

Disseminated toxoplasmosis is rare, especially following autologous stem-cell transplantation. The likely cause of reactivation and dissemination of *Toxoplasma* in this patient was the cell-mediated immunosuppression associated with Hodgkin disease and its treatment. In addition to the brain, the heart, liver, and lungs are frequently involved in cases of disseminated toxoplasmosis.

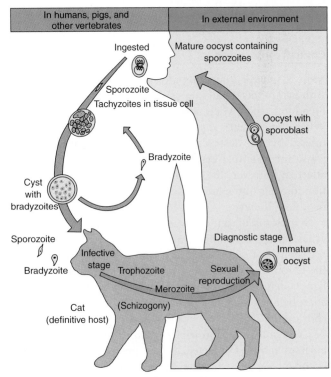

Figure 82—7. Life cycle of *Toxoplasma gondii*.

individuals (patients with acquired immunodeficiency syndrome [AIDS]) are more likely to have severe manifestations. The wide variety of animals that harbor the organism—carnivores and herbivores as well as birds—accounts for the widespread transmission.

Humans become infected from two sources: (1) ingestion of improperly cooked meat from animals that serve as intermediate hosts and (2) ingestion of infective oocysts from contaminated cat feces. Serologic studies show an increased prevalence in human populations where the consumption of uncooked meat or meat juices is popular. It is noteworthy that serologic tests of human and rodent populations are negative in the few geographical areas where cats have not existed. Outbreaks of toxoplasmosis in the United States are usually traced to poorly cooked meat (e.g., hamburger), as well as contact with cat feces.

Transplacental infection can occur in pregnancy, either from infection acquired from meat and meat juices or from contact with cat feces. Transfusion infection via contaminated blood can occur but is not common. Transplacental infection from an infected mother has a devastating effect on the fetus.

Although the rate of seroconversion is similar for individuals within a geographical location, the rate of severe infection is dramatically affected by the immune status of the individual. Patients with defects in cell-mediated immunity, especially those who are infected with the human immunodeficiency virus (HIV) or who have had an organ transplant or immunosuppressive therapy, are most likely to have disseminated or central nervous system (CNS) disease. Illness in this setting is generally believed to be caused by reactivation of previously latent infection, rather than new exposure to the organism.

Clinical Syndromes

Most *T. gondii* infections are benign and asymptomatic, with symptoms occurring as the parasite moves from the blood to tissues, where it becomes an intracellular parasite. When symptomatic disease occurs, the infection is characterized by cell destruction, reproduction of more organisms, and eventual cyst formation. Many tissues may be affected; however, the organism has a particular predilection for cells of the lung, heart, lymphoid organs, and CNS, including the eye.

Symptoms of acute disease include chills, fever, headaches, myalgia, lymphadenitis, and fatigue; the symptoms occasionally resemble those of infectious mononucleosis. In chronic disease, the signs and symptoms include lymphadenitis, occasionally a rash, evidence of hepatitis, encephalomyelitis, and myocarditis. In some of the cases, chorioretinitis appears and may lead to blindness.

Congenital infection with *T. gondii* also occurs in infants born to mothers infected during pregnancy. If infection occurs in the first trimester, the result is spontaneous abortion, stillbirth, or severe disease. Manifestations in the infant infected after the first trimester include epilepsy, encephalitis, microcephaly, intracranial calcifications, hydrocephalus, psychomotor or mental retardation, chorioretinitis, blindness, anemia, jaundice, rash, pneumonia, diarrhea, and hypothermia. Infants may be asymptomatic at birth only to develop disease months to years later. Most often these children develop chorioretinitis with or without blindness or other neurologic problems, including retardation, seizures, microcephaly, and hearing loss.

In immunocompromised older patients, a different spectrum of disease is seen. Reactivation of latent toxoplasmosis is a special problem for these people. The presenting symptoms of *Toxoplasma* infection in immunocompromised patients are usually neurologic, most frequently consistent with diffuse encephalopathy, meningoencephalitis, or cerebral mass lesions. Reactivation of cerebral toxoplasmosis has emerged as a major cause of encephalitis in patients with AIDS. The disease is usually multifocal, with more than one mass lesion appearing in the brain at the same time. Symptoms are related to the location of the lesions and may include hemiparesis, seizures, visual impairment, confusion, and lethargy. Other sites of infection that have been reported include the eye, lung, and testes. Although disease is seen predominantly in patients with AIDS, it may also occur with similar manifestations in other immunocompromised patients, in particular those undergoing solid organ transplantation.

Laboratory Diagnosis

Serologic testing is required for the diagnosis of acute active infection; the diagnosis is established by the finding of increasing antibody titers documented in serially collected blood specimens. Because contact with the organism is common, assays for different isotypes of antibodies and attention to increasing titers is essential to differentiate acute, active infection from previous asymptomatic or chronic infection. A panel of tests referred to as the *T. gondii* serologic profile (TSP) is used by specialized reference laboratories to determine whether the infection is consistent with acquisition recently or in the more distant past. The TSP consists of: (1) the Sabin-Feldman dye test to measure IgG antibodies; (2) enzyme-linked immunosorbent assays (ELISAs) to measure IgM, IgA, and IgE antibodies; (3) immunosorbent agglutination assay (ISAGA) to measure levels of IgE antibodies; and (4) differential agglutination test to measure levels of IgG antibodies.

The initial evaluation in the immunocompetent patient involves screening for IgG antibodies to *T. gondii*. Although many studies and guidelines suggest the usefulness of testing for IgM in parallel, IgM antibodies to *T. gondii* may persist for more than 12 months after an acute infection, leading to a false-positive result. If IgG titers are equivocal, serial specimens should be collected 3 weeks apart and tested in parallel. If the IgG titer is negative (less than 1:16), *Toxoplasma* infection is ruled out. A twofold rise in antibody titer indicates an acute infection, as does conversion from a negative to a positive result. A single high titer is not a sufficient basis for diagnosing toxoplasmosis, because IgG titers may remain elevated for many years after infection.

Toxoplasmosis in patients with malignancies, organ transplants, or AIDS is generally assumed to arise from reactivation of a chronic asymptomatic (latent) infection. Diagnosis can be very difficult for these patients; IgM antibody is usually undetectable, and the presence of IgG antibody only confirms past infection. In the absence of serologic evidence of acute infection, diagnosis can only be confirmed by histologic detection of the organism in tissues or detection of nucleic acids by PCR. Immunosuppressed patients who are negative for IgG antibodies are at risk for acute acquired infection, whereas seropositive patients are at risk of reactivation.

The methods used to diagnose acute toxoplasmosis in pregnant women are the same as those used for immunocompetent adults. The FDA has issued a warning to physicians against the use of *T. gondii* IgM commercial kits as the sole method of diagnosis during pregnancy due to frequent false-positive and false-negative results in these patients. Confirmatory testing at a *Toxoplasma* reference laboratory is highly recommended. If IgM and IgG antibodies are both absent, active infection can be excluded.

Prenatal diagnosis of congenital toxoplasmosis can be achieved by ultrasonography and amniocentesis. Amniotic fluid PCR analysis to detect *T. gondii* is the test of choice, offering excellent positive and negative predictive values. Since maternal IgG antibodies are present in newborns, detection of IgA and IgM antibodies is the foundation of serodiagnosis of toxoplasmosis in the newborn.

Demonstration of these organisms as trophozoites and cysts in tissue and body fluids is the definitive method of diagnosis (Figure 82-8). Biopsy specimens from lymph nodes, brain, myocardium, or other suspected tissue, as well as body fluids, including cerebrospinal fluid, amniotic fluid, or bronchoalveolar lavage fluid, can be directly examined for the organisms. Newer monoclonal antibody–based fluorescent stains may facilitate direct detection of *T. gondii* in tissue. Culture methods for *T. gondii* are largely experimental and not usually available in clinical laboratories. The two methods available are to inoculate potentially infected material into either mouse peritoneum or tissue culture. Advances in developing polymerase chain reaction–based detection methods are promising and may provide rapid and sensitive approaches for detecting the organism in blood, cerebrospinal fluid, amniotic fluid, and other clinical specimens.

Treatment, Prevention, and Control

The therapy for toxoplasmosis depends on the nature of the infectious process and the immunocompetence of the host. Most mononucleosis-like infections in normal hosts resolve spontaneously and do not require specific therapy. In contrast, disseminated or CNS infection in immunocompromised people must be treated. Before the association of *T. gondii* with HIV infection, immunocompromised patients with toxoplasmosis were treated for 4 to 6 weeks. In the setting of HIV infection, discontinuing therapy after 4 to 6 weeks is associated with a relapse rate of 25%. Such patients are currently treated with an initial high-dose regimen of pyrimethamine plus sulfadiazine and then continued on lower doses of both drugs indefinitely. Although this drug combination is the regimen of choice, toxicity (rash and bone marrow suppression) may necessitate changes to alternative agents. Clindamycin plus pyrimethamine is the best studied alternative. Atovaquone and azithromycin (each alone or with pyrimethamine) also have some activity, although their efficacy and safety compared with those of clindamycin-pyrimethamine need to be assessed. Trimethoprim-sulfamethoxazole is another alternative to pyrimethamine-sulfadiazine for treatment of disseminated or CNS toxoplasmosis. The use of corticosteroids is indicated as part of therapy of cerebral edema and ocular infections that involve or threaten the macula.

Infections in the first trimester of pregnancy are difficult to manage because of the teratogenicity of pyrimethamine in laboratory animals. Both clindamycin and spiramycin have been substituted with apparent success. Spiramycin does not appear to be effective for the treatment of toxoplasmosis in immunocompromised patients.

As more immunocompromised patients at risk for disseminated infection are identified, greater emphasis is placed on preventive measures and specific prophylaxis. Routine serologic screening of patients before organ transplantation and early in the course of HIV infection is now being performed. Individuals with positive serologic tests are at much higher risk for the development of disease and are now being considered for prophylaxis. Trimethoprim-sulfamethoxazole, which is also used as prophylaxis to prevent *Pneumocystis jirovecii* infections, also appears to be effective at preventing infections with

Figure 82–8. Cyst of *T. gondii* in tissue. Hundreds of organisms may be present in the cyst, which may become active and initiate disease with decreased host immunity (e.g., immunosuppression in transplant patients and in diseases such as AIDS).

T. gondii. Additional preventive measures for pregnant women and immunocompromised hosts should include avoiding the consumption and handling of raw or under-cooked meat and avoiding exposure to cat feces.

Sarcocystis lindemanni

S. lindemanni is a typical coccidian closely related to the intestinal forms *S. suihominis*, *S. bovihominis*, and *Isospora belli*, and the blood and tissue parasite *T. gondii*. *S. linde-manni* occurs worldwide in various animals, especially sheep, cattle, and pigs. Humans are accidentally infected only as the result of eating meat from these animals. Most infections are asymptomatic, but occasionally an infection may cause myositis, swelling of muscle, dyspnea, and eosinophilia. Infection of the myocardium has been observed but is extremely rare. There is no specific treatment for the muscle infection.

Free-Living Amoebae

Naegleria species, *Acanthamoeba* species, *Balamuthia* species, and other free-living amoebae are found in soil and in contaminated lakes, streams, and other water environments. Most human infections with these amoebae are acquired during the warm summer months by people exposed to the amoebae while swimming in contaminated water. Inhalation of cysts present in dust may account for some infections, whereas ocular infections with *Acanthamoeba* species are associated with the contamination of contact lenses with nonsterile cleaning solutions.

Clinical Syndromes (Clinical Case 82-3)

Naegleria, *Acanthamoeba*, and *Balamuthia* organisms are opportunistic pathogens. Although colonization of the nasal passages is usually asymptomatic, these amoebae can invade the nasal mucosa and extend into the brain. Acute primary **amoebic meningoencephalitis** is most commonly caused by *Naegleria fowleri*. Destruction of brain tissue is characterized by a fulminant, rapidly fatal meningoencephalitis. Symptoms include intense frontal headache, sore throat, fever, blocked nose with altered senses of taste and smell, stiff neck, and Kernig sign. The cerebrospinal fluid is purulent and may contain many erythrocytes and motile amoebae. Clinically, the course of the disease is rapid, with death usually occurring within 4 or 5 days. Postmortem findings show *Naegleria* trophozoites present in the brain but no evidence of cysts (Figure 82-9). Although all cases were fatal before 1970, survival has now been reported in a few cases in which the disease was rapidly diagnosed and treated.

In contrast to *Naegleria*, *Acanthamoeba* and *Balamuthia* organisms produce granulomatous amoebic encephalitis

Clinical Case 82-3. Amoebic Encephalitis

Rahimian and Kleinman (Infect Med 22:382-385, 2005) described a 43-year-old man, originally from the Dominican Republic, who presented after a seizure. The patient had a history of diabetes and hypertension but denied any previous history of seizures. Results of a CT scan without contrast were normal. Neurologic examination was unrevealing, and the patient was sent home. Approximately 2 weeks later, he was readmitted to the hospital because of a new, left-facial droop. A CT scan without contrast showed the new appearance of thickening and hypodensity of the right frontal gray matter. Progressive generalized weakness developed, along with paralysis of the left upper extremity. A repeat CT scan without contrast revealed an increase in the size of the right frontal hypodense area, with vasogenic edema and a new left parietal hypodense lesion. At that time, dysarthria and a bilateral occipital headache also developed. The patient was a construction worker who denied injection drug use, recent dental work, and risk factors for HIV infection. His travel history was significant only for a trip to the Dominican Republic 2 years previously. Clinical examination was remarkable for dysarthria, a left facial droop, and left upper extremity paralysis. A lumbar puncture revealed an elevated white blood count, a CSF protein level of 50 mg/dL and glucose of 145 mg/dL (serum glucose was 327 mg/dL). Gram stain of the CSF was negative. An MRI scan of the head showed two large ring-enhancing lesions with possible central necrosis. Results of an HIV test were negative. A brain biopsy showed lymphocytic infiltration, predominantly in the perivascular areas. A closer examination revealed trophozoites and amoebic cysts consistent with a diagnosis of amoebic encephalitis. Results of a PCR assay were consistent with *Balamuthia mandrillaris* infection. Therapy with pentamidine was initiated, but the patient died 3 days later.

Balamuthia encephalitis has been described in both immunosuppressed and immunocompetent individuals. Many infected patients do not have a history of swimming or exposure to contaminated water. The portal of entry is believed to be the respiratory tract or skin ulceration, with dissemination to the brain. Most cases of amoebic encephalitis have been diagnosed postmortem. Recently, a PCR assay specific for *Balamuthia* has been used for diagnosis, as was done in this case. The majority of patients have died within weeks after the onset of neurologic symptoms, despite treatment with pentamidine.

Figure 82-9. Numerous *Naegleria* trophozoites in brain tissue from a patient with amoebic meningoencephalitis. *(From Marler LM, et al: Parasitology CD-ROM, Indiana Pathology Images, 2003.)*

and single or multiple brain abscesses, primarily in immunocompromised individuals. The course of the disease is slower, with an incubation period of at least 10 days. The resulting disease is a chronic granulomatous encephalitis with edema of the brain tissue.

Eye and skin infection caused by *Acanthamoeba* organisms may also occur. Keratitis is usually associated with eye trauma that occurred before contact with contaminated soil, dust, or water. The use of improperly cleaned contact lenses is also associated with this disease. Invasion by *Acanthamoeba* species produces corneal ulceration and severe ocular pain. Cases of apparent disseminated cutaneous and subcutaneous infection with *Acanthamoeba* and *Balamuthia* organisms recently have been described in patients with acquired immunodeficiency syndrome (AIDS). These infections include multiple soft tissue nodules, which on biopsy contain amoebae. Central nervous system or deep tissue involvement may also be present with this form of infection.

Laboratory Diagnosis

For the diagnosis of *Naegleria*, *Acanthamoeba*, and *Balamuthia* infections, nasal discharge, cerebrospinal fluid, and (in the case of eye infections) corneal scrapings should be collected. The specimens should be examined using a saline wet preparation and iodine-stained smears. *Naegleria* and *Acanthamoeba* species are difficult to differentiate except by experienced microscopists. However, the observation of an amoeba in a normally sterile tissue is diagnostic (see Figure 82-9). In *Naegleria* infection, only the **amoeboid trophozoites** are found within the tissue, whereas with *Acanthamoeba* and *Balamuthia* infection, both trophozoites and cysts are found in tissues. The clinical specimens can be cultured on agar plates seeded with live gram-negative enteric bacilli. Amoebae present in the specimens use the bacteria as a nutritional source and can be detected within 1 or 2 days by the presence of the trails that form on the agar surface as the amoebae move. *Balamuthia* do not grow on agar plates used for *Naegleria* and *Acanthamoeba* but have been recovered in tissue culture using mammalian cell lines.

Treatment, Prevention, and Control

Treatment of free-living amoebic infections is largely ineffective. Amoebic meningoencephalitis due to *Naegleria*, *Acanthamoeba*, or *Balamuthia* is unresponsive to most antimicrobial agents. The treatment of choice for *Naegleria* infections is amphotericin B combined with miconazole and rifampin. *Acanthamoeba* infections may be treated with pentamidine, ketoconazole and flucytosine, whereas *Balamuthia* infections have been treated with clarithromycin, fluconazole, sulfadiazine, and flucytosine. Amoebic keratitis and cutaneous infections may respond to topical miconazole, chlorhexidine gluconate, or propamidine

isethionate. Treatment of amoebic keratitis may require repeated corneal transplantation or rarely enucleation of the eye. The wide distribution of these organisms in fresh and brackish waters makes the prevention and control of infection difficult. It has been suggested that known sources of infection be off limits to bathing, diving, and water sports, although this is generally difficult to enforce. Swimming pools with cracks in the walls, allowing soil seepage, should be repaired to avoid creation of a source of infection.

Leishmania

Leishmania are obligate intracellular parasites that are transmitted from animal to human or human to human by bites from an infected female sand fly. Depending on the geographic area, many different species can infect humans, producing a variety of diseases ranging from cutaneous, diffuse cutaneous, and mucocutaneous to visceral (Table 82-2). New species of *Leishmania* are being detected frequently. Whereas the older literature focused primarily on three species, *L. donovani* (visceral leishmaniasis), *L. tropica* (cutaneous leishmaniasis), and *L. braziliensis* (cutaneous leishmaniasis), the current taxonomy of leishmaniasis is in a state of dynamic flux. Species differentiation is currently based on molecular techniques, rather than geographic distribution and clinical presentation.

Physiology and Structure

The life cycles of all leishmanial parasites are quite similar (Figure 82-10), whereas the associated infections differ in epidemiology, tissues affected, and clinical manifestations. The **promastigote** stage (long, slender form with a free flagellum) is present in the saliva of infected sand flies. Human infection is initiated by the bite of an infected sand fly, which injects the promastigotes into the skin, where they lose their flagella, enter the **amastigote** stage, and invade reticuloendothelial cells. The change from promastigote to amastigote helps to avoid the host's immune response. Changes in the organism's surface molecules play an important role in macrophage attachment and evading the immune response, including manipulating the macrophage's signaling pathways. Reproduction occurs in the amastigote stage, and as cells rupture, destruction of specific tissues (e.g., cutaneous tissues, visceral organs such as the liver and spleen) develops. The amastigote stage (Figure 82-11) is diagnostic for leishmaniasis, as well as the infectious stage for sand flies. Ingested amastigotes transform in the sand fly into the promastigote stage, which multiplies by binary fission in the fly midgut. After development, this stage migrates to the fly proboscis, where new human infection can be introduced during feeding. The life cycles of *Leishmania* organisms are similar for cutaneous, mucocutaneous, and visceral leishmaniasis,

Table 82–2. Leishmaniasis in Humans

Parasite	Disease	Geographic Distribution
L. donovani	Visceral leishmaniasis Mucocutaneous leishmaniasis Cutaneous leishmaniasis Dermal leishmanoid	Africa, Asia
L. infantum (L. chagasi)	Visceral leishmaniasis	Africa, Europe, Mediterranean area, Southwest Asia, Central and South America
L. tropica	Cutaneous leishmaniasis Visceral leishmaniasis (rare)	Afghanistan, India, Turkey, former USSR, Middle East, Africa, India
L. major	Cutaneous leishmaniasis	Middle East, Afghanistan, Africa, former USSR
L. aethiopica	Cutaneous leishmaniasis Diffuse cutaneous leishmaniasis Mucocutaneous leishmaniasis	Ethiopia, Kenya, Yemen, former USSR
L. mexicana	Cutaneous leishmaniasis Diffuse cutaneous leishmaniasis	Texas, Belize, Guatemala, Mexico
L. braziliensis	Cutaneous leishmaniasis Mucocutaneous leishmaniasis	Central and South America
L. peruviana	Cutaneous leishmaniasis	Panama, Columbia, Costa Rica
L. garnhami	Cutaneous leishmaniasis	Venezuela
L. colombiensis	Cutaneous leishmaniasis	Colombia, Panama
L. venezuelensis	Cutaneous leishmaniasis	Venezuela
L. lainsoni, L. shawii	Cutaneous leishmaniasis	Brazil
L. amazonensis	Cutaneous leishmaniasis Diffuse cutaneous leishmaniasis	Brazil, Venezuela
L. naiffi	Cutaneous leishmaniasis	Brazil, Caribbean Islands
L. pifanoi	Cutaneous leishmaniasis Diffuse cutaneous leishmaniasis	Brazil, Venezuela

Data from Bruckner DA, Labarca JA: Leishmania and Trypanosoma. In Murray PR, et al (eds): Manual of Clinical Microbiology, 9th ed. Washington, DC, American Society for Microbiology, 2007.

except that infected reticuloendothelial cells can be found throughout the body in visceral leishmaniasis.

Epidemiology

Leishmaniasis is a zoonosis transmitted by adult female sand flies belonging to the genera *Phlebotomus* and *Lutzomyia*. The natural reservoirs include rodents, opossums, anteaters, sloths, cats, and dogs. In areas of the world where leishmaniasis is endemic, the infection may be transmitted by a human-vector-human cycle. The infection may also be transmitted by direct contact with an infected lesion or mechanically by stable flies or dog flies.

Mucocutaneous leishmaniasis most often occurs in Bolivia, Brazil, and Peru, whereas the cutaneous form is much more widespread throughout the Middle East (Afghanistan, Algeria, Iran, Iraq, Saudi Arabia, and Syria) and focal areas in South America (Brazil, Peru). Cutaneous leishmaniasis has been diagnosed among U.S. military personnel deployed in Afghanistan, Iraq, and Kuwait.

Visceral leishmaniasis (kala-azar, dumdum fever) occurs at a rate of approximately 500,000 new cases per year, 90% of which are localized to Bangladesh, Brazil, India, Nepal, and the Sudan. This infection may exist as an endemic, epidemic, or sporadic disease and is a zoonosis except for in India, where kala-azar ("black fever" in Hindi)

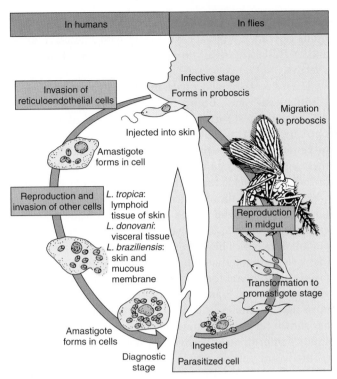

Figure 82–10. Life cycle of *Leishmania* species.

is an anthroponosis (human-vector-human). Individuals with post–kala-azar dermal leishmaniasis may be very important reservoirs for maintaining the infection in the population, owing to the high concentration of organisms in the skin. In contrast to cutaneous and mucocutaneous leishmaniasis, where a large number of leishmanial species have been implicated, only *L. donovani* and *L. infantum* (*L. chagasi*) commonly cause visceral leishmaniasis. *L. infantum* is present in countries along the Mediterranean basin (European, Near Eastern, and African) and is found in parts of China, South Africa, and the former Soviet Union,

Figure 82–11. Giemsa-stained amastigotes (Leishman-Donovan bodies) of *L. donovani* present in a touch preparation of spleen. A small, dark-staining kinetoplast can be seen next to the spherical nucleus in some parasites. *(From Connor DH, et al: Pathology of Infectious Diseases, vol 2. Stamford, Conn, Appleton & Lange, 1997.)*

whereas *L. donovani* is concentrated in Africa and Asia. Although *L. tropica* usually causes cutaneous leishmaniasis, rare viscerotropic strains have been reported in the Middle East, Africa, and India.

Clinical Syndromes

Depending on the species of *Leishmania* involved, infection can result in a cutaneous, diffuse cutaneous, mucocutaneous, or visceral disease. With the spread of the HIV pandemic, there is increasing recognition of HIV-related visceral leishmaniasis due to *L. donovani* in southern Asia and Africa and to *L. infantum* (*L. chagasi*) in South America. In these co-infected patients, leishmaniasis will manifest as an opportunistic infection, with parasites detected in atypical sites and a high associated mortality.

The first sign of **cutaneous leishmaniasis**, a red papule, appears at the site of the fly's bite between 2 weeks and 2 months after initial exposure. The lesion becomes irritated, intensely pruritic, and begins to enlarge and ulcerate. Gradually the ulcer becomes hard and crusted and exudes a thin, serous material. At this stage, secondary bacterial infection may complicate the disease. The lesion may heal without treatment in a matter of months but usually leaves a disfiguring scar. The species that is commonly associated with cutaneous leishmaniasis, *L. tropica*, also may exist in a viscerotrophic form. A disseminated nodular type of cutaneous leishmaniasis has been reported from Ethiopia, probably caused by an allergy to *L. aethiopica* antigens.

Mucocutaneous leishmaniasis is produced most often by the *L. braziliensis* complex. The incubation period and appearance of the primary cutaneous ulcers for *L. braziliensis* are similar to those found in other forms of cutaneous leishmaniasis. The essential difference in clinical disease is the involvement and destruction of mucous membranes and related tissue structures. Untreated primary lesions may develop into the mucocutaneous form in up to 80% of cases. Spread to the nasal and oral mucosa may become apparent concomitant with the primary lesion or many years after the primary lesion has healed. The mucosal lesions do not heal spontaneously, and secondary bacterial infections are common, producing severe and disfiguring facial mutilation and occasionally death.

The **visceral form of leishmaniasis** may present as fulminating, rapidly fatal disease, a more chronic debilitating process, or as an asymptomatic, self-limiting infection. The incubation period may be from several weeks to a year, with a gradual onset of fever, diarrhea, and anemia. Chills and sweating that may resemble malaria symptoms are common early in the infection. As organisms proliferate and invade the cells of the reticuloendothelial system, marked enlargement of the liver and spleen, weight loss, and emaciation occur. Kidney damage may also occur as the cells of the glomeruli are invaded. With persistence of the disease, deeply pigmented, granulomatous areas of skin, referred to as **post–kala-azar dermal leishmaniasis**, occur. In this condition, the macular or hypopigmented dermal lesions are associated with few parasites, whereas erythematous and nodular lesions are associated with abundant parasites.

Laboratory Diagnosis

Although in endemic areas, the diagnosis of visceral, mucocutaneous, or cutaneous leishmaniasis may be made on clinical grounds, definitive diagnosis depends on detecting either the amastigotes in clinical specimens or the promastigotes in culture. Demonstration of the amastigotes in properly stained smears from touch preparations or ulcer biopsy specimens and cultures of ulcer tissue determines the diagnosis of cutaneous and mucocutaneous leishmaniasis. Specimens for the diagnosis of visceral leishmaniasis include splenic puncture, lymph node aspirates, liver biopsy, sternal aspirates, iliac crest bone marrow, and buffy coat preparations of venous blood. These specimens may be examined microscopically, cultured, and subjected to molecular detection methods. Molecular techniques for the detection of leishmanial DNA or RNA have been used for diagnosis, prognosis, and species identification and are more sensitive than microscopy or culture, especially for the detection of mucocutaneous leishmaniasis. Serologic tests are available; however, they are not especially useful for the diagnosis of mucocutaneous or visceral leishmaniasis. The detection of urinary antigens has been used for the diagnosis of visceral leishmaniasis.

Treatment, Prevention, and Control

Presently, the drug of choice for all forms of leishmaniasis is the pentavalent antimonial compound sodium stibogluconate (Pentostam). In the past several years, the ubiquitous use of this agent has been threatened by the development of drug resistance. Furthermore, drug treatment can be complicated by variation in the susceptibility of *Leishmania* species to drugs, variation in pharmacokinetics, and variation in drug-host immune response interaction. The toxicity of the antimonials is also considerable, and as a result, several alternative approaches to the treatment of leishmaniasis have been developed.

Standard therapy for cutaneous leishmaniasis consists of injections of antimonial compounds directly into the lesion or parenterally. Recently both fluconazole and miltefosine have been shown to be efficacious. Other agents include amphotericin B, pentamidine, and various formulations of paromomycin. Alternatives to chemotherapy in the treatment of cutaneous leishmaniasis include cryotherapy, heat, and surgical excision.

Stibogluconate remains the drug of choice for mucocutaneous leishmaniasis, with amphotericin B as an alternative. Notably, patients clinically cured of *L. braziliensis*, which is noted for its chronicity, latency, and metastasis with mucous

membrane involvement, have been found to be PCR positive up to 11 years posttherapy. Follow-up with smears, cultures, and/or PCR is necessary to ensure that treatment has been effective.

The role of stibogluconate in the treatment of visceral leishmaniasis has been challenged in recent years. Although in most parts of the world, over 95% of previously untreated patients with visceral leishmaniasis respond to pentavalent antimonials, widespread primary failure to these agents has been reported in the North Bihar region of India. The incidence of primary response was only 54%, whereas 8% of those initially responding to treatment relapsed. Widespread misuse of the drug is blamed for this emerging resistance. Fortunately in recent years, four new potential therapies have been introduced for visceral leishmaniasis: amphotericin B liposome formulation, oral miltefosine, a parenteral formulation of paromomycin, and oral sitamaquine (an 8-aminoquinolone). In most instances, these agents remain in clinical trials; however, miltefosine has shown remarkable efficacy (>95% cure rate) and tolerability. Unfortunately, preliminary data from India suggests an increasing relapse rate in patients treated with miltefosine, indicating that drug resistance could develop and that strategies must be developed to prevent it.

Prevention of the various forms of leishmaniasis involves prompt treatment of human infections and control of reservoir hosts, along with insect vector control. Protection from sand flies by screening and insect repellents is also essential. The protection of forest and construction workers in endemic areas is most difficult, and disease in those places may be effectively controlled only by vaccination. Work to develop a vaccine is ongoing.

Trypanosomes

Trypanosoma, another hemoflagellate, causes two distinctly different forms of disease (Table 82-3). One is called **African trypanosomiasis, or sleeping sickness**, and is produced by *Trypanosoma brucei gambiense* and *T. b. rhodesiense*. It is transmitted by tsetse flies. The second infection is called **American trypanosomiasis, or Chagas' disease**, produced by *T. cruzi*. It is transmitted by true bugs (triatomids, reduviids, also called *kissing bugs*; Clinical Case 82-4).

Table 82–3. *Trypanosoma* Species Responsible for Human Diseases

Parasite	Vector	Disease
Trypanosoma brucei gambiense and *T. b. rhodesiense*	Tsetse fly	African trypanosomiasis (sleeping sickness)
Trypanosoma cruzi	Reduviids	American trypanosomiasis (Chagas' disease)

Clinical Case 82-4. Trypanosomiasis

Herwaldt and colleagues (J Infect Dis 181:395-399, 2000) describe a case in which the mother of an 18-month-old boy in Tennessee found a triatomine bug in his crib, which she saved because it resembled a bug shown on a television program about insects that prey on mammals. An entomologist identified the bug as *Triatoma sanguisuga*, a vector of Chagas' disease. The bug was found to be engorged with blood and infected with *Trypanosoma cruzi*. The child had been intermittently febrile for the preceding 2 to 3 weeks but was otherwise healthy except for pharyngeal edema and multiple insect bites of unknown type on his legs. Whole-blood specimens obtained from the child were negative by buffy-coat examination and hemoculture but positive for *T. cruzi* by PCR and DNA hybridization, suggesting that he had low-level parasitemia. Specimens obtained after treatment with benznidazole were negative. He did not develop anti-*T. cruzi* antibody; 19 relatives and neighbors were also negative. Two of three raccoons trapped in the vicinity had positive hemocultures for *T. cruzi*. The child's case of *T. cruzi* infection—the fifth reported U.S. autochthonous case—would have been missed without his mother's attentiveness and the availability of sensitive molecular techniques. Given that infected triatomine bugs and mammalian hosts exist in the southern United States, it is not surprising that humans could become infected with *T. cruzi*. Furthermore, given the nonspecific clinical manifestations of the infection, it is likely that other cases have been overlooked.

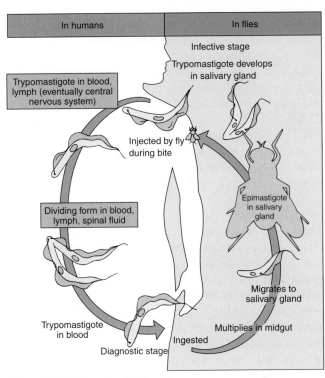

Figure 82–12. Life cycle of *T. brucei*.

Trypanosoma brucei gambiense

Physiology and Structure

The life cycle of the African forms of trypanosomiasis is illustrated in Figure 82-12. The infective stage of the organism is the **trypomastigote**, which is present in the salivary glands of transmitting tsetse flies. The organism in this stage has a **free flagellum** and an **undulating membrane** running the full length of the body (Figure 82-13). The trypomastigotes enter the wound created by the fly bite and find their way into blood and lymph, eventually invading the CNS. Reproduction of the trypomastigotes in blood, lymph, and spinal fluid is by binary or longitudinal fission. These trypomastigotes in blood are then infective for biting tsetse flies, where further reproduction occurs in the midgut. The organisms then migrate to the salivary glands, where an **epimastigote** form (with a free flagellum but only a partial undulating membrane) continues reproduction to the infective trypomastigote stage. Tsetse flies become infective 4 to 6 weeks after feeding on blood from a diseased patient.

Epidemiology

T. b. gambiense is limited to tropical West and Central Africa, correlating to the range of the tsetse fly vector. The tsetse flies transmitting *T. b. gambiense* prefer shaded stream banks for reproduction and proximity to human dwellings. Persons who work in such areas are at greatest risk of infection. An animal reservoir has not been proved,

although several species of animals have been infected experimentally.

Clinical Syndromes

The incubation period of **Gambian sleeping sickness** varies from a few days to weeks. *T. b. gambiense* produces chronic disease, often ending fatally, with CNS involvement after several years' duration. One of the earliest signs of disease is an occasional **ulcer** at the site of the fly bite. As reproduction of organisms continues, the lymph nodes are invaded, and fever, myalgia, arthralgia, and lymph node enlargement result. Swelling of the posterior

Figure 82–13. Trypomastigote stage of *T. b. gambiense* in a blood smear. *(From Marler LM, et al: Parasitology CD-ROM, Indiana Pathology Images, 2003.)*

cervical lymph nodes is characteristic of Gambian disease and is called **Winterbottom sign**. Patients in this acute phase often exhibit hyperactivity.

Chronic disease progresses to CNS involvement, with lethargy, tremors, meningoencephalitis, mental retardation, and general deterioration. In the final stages of chronic disease, convulsions, hemiplegia, and incontinence occur, and the patient becomes difficult to arouse or respond, eventually progressing to a comatose state. Death is the result of CNS damage and other infections such as malaria or pneumonia.

Laboratory Diagnosis

Organisms can be demonstrated in thick and thin blood films, in concentrated anticoagulated blood preparations, and in aspirations from lymph nodes and concentrated spinal fluid (see Figure 82-13). Methods for concentrating parasites in blood may be helpful. Approaches include centrifugation of heparinized samples and anion-exchange chromatography. Levels of parasitemia vary widely, and several attempts to visualize the organism over a number of days may be necessary. Preparations should be fixed and stained immediately to avoid disintegration of the trypomastigotes. Serologic tests are also useful diagnostic techniques. Immunofluorescence, ELISA, precipitin, and agglutination methods have been used. Most reagents are not available commercially. Referral laboratories have used PCR to detect infections and to differentiate species (*T. b. gambiense* vs. *T. b. rhodesiense*), but these methods are not routinely used in the field.

Treatment, Prevention, and Control

Suramin is the drug of choice for treating the acute blood and lymphatic stages of the disease, with pentamidine as an alternative. Suramin and pentamidine do not cross the blood-brain barrier; therefore, melarsoprol is the drug of choice when central nervous system (CNS) involvement is suspected. Difluoromethylornithine (DFMO) is a cytostatic drug with activity against the acute and late (CNS) stages of the disease. The most effective control measures include an integrated approach to reduce the human reservoir of infection and the use of fly traps and insecticide; however, economic resources are limited, and effective programs have been difficult to sustain.

Trypanosoma brucei rhodesiense

Physiology and Structure

The life cycle of *T. b. rhodesiense* is similar to that of *T. b. gambiense* (see Figure 82-12), with both trypomastigote and epimastigote stages and transmission by tsetse flies.

Epidemiology

The organism is found primarily in East Africa, especially the cattle-raising countries, where tsetse flies breed in the brush rather than along stream banks. *T. b. rhodesiense* also differs from *T. b. gambiense* in that domestic animal hosts (cattle and sheep) and wild game animals act as reservoir hosts. This transmission and vector cycle makes the organism more difficult to control than *T. b. gambiense*.

Clinical Syndromes

The incubation period for *T. b. rhodesiense* is shorter than that for *T. b. gambiense*. Acute disease (fever, rigors, and myalgia) occurs more rapidly and progresses to a fulminating, rapidly fatal illness. Infected persons are usually dead within 9 to 12 months if untreated.

This more virulent organism also develops in greater numbers in the blood. Lymphadenopathy is uncommon, and CNS invasion occurs early in the infection, with lethargy, anorexia, and mental disturbance. The chronic stages described for *T. b. gambiense* are not often seen, because in addition to rapid CNS disease, the organism produces kidney damage and myocarditis, leading to death.

Laboratory Diagnosis

Examination of blood and spinal fluid is carried out as for *T. b. gambiense*. Serologic tests are available; however, the marked variability of the surface antigens of trypanosomes limits the diagnostic usefulness of this approach.

Treatment, Prevention, and Control

The same treatment protocol applies as for *T. b. gambiense*, with early treatment for the more rapid neurologic manifestations. Similar prevention and control measures are needed: tsetse fly control and use of protective clothing, screens, netting, and insect repellent. In addition, early treatment is essential to control transmission, detect infection, and determine treatment in domestic animals. Control of infection in game animals is difficult, but infection can be reduced if measures to control the tsetse fly population, specifically eradication of brush and grassland breeding sites, are applied.

Trypanosoma cruzi

Physiology and Structure

The life cycle of *T. cruzi* (Figure 82-14) differs from *T. brucei* with the development of an additional form called an **amastigote** (Figure 82-15). The amastigote is an intracellular form with no flagellum and no undulating membrane. It is smaller than the trypomastigote, is oval, and is found in tissues. The infective trypomastigote, which is present in the feces of a **reduviid bug ("kissing bug")**, enters the wound created by the biting, feeding bug. The bugs have been called **kissing bugs** because they frequently bite people around the mouth and in other facial sites. They are notorious for biting, feeding on blood and tissue juices, and then defecating into the wound. The organisms in the feces of the bug enter the wound; penetration is usually aided when the patient rubs or scratches the irritated site.

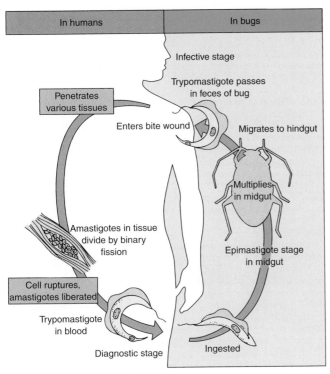

Figure 82—14. Life cycle of *T. cruzi*.

The trypomastigotes then migrate to other tissues (e.g., cardiac muscle, liver, brain), lose the flagellum and undulating membrane, and become the smaller, oval, intracellular amastigote form. These intracellular amastigotes multiply by binary fission and eventually destroy the host cells. Then they are liberated to enter new host tissue as intracellular amastigotes or to become trypomastigotes infective for feeding reduviid bugs. Ingested trypomastigotes develop into epimastigotes in the midgut of the insect and reproduce by longitudinal binary fission. The organisms migrate to the hindgut of the bug, develop

Figure 82—15. Amastigote stage of *T. cruzi* in skeletal muscle. (*From Ash LR, Orihel TC: Atlas of Human Parasitology, 2nd ed. Chicago, American Society of Clinical Pathologists, 1984.*)

into metacyclic trypomastigotes, and then leave the bug in the feces after biting, feeding, and defecating, initiating a new human infection.

Epidemiology

T. cruzi occurs widely in both reduviid bugs and a broad spectrum of reservoir animals in North, Central, and South America. Human disease is found most often among children in South and Central America, where 16 to 18 million people are infected. There is a direct correlation between infected wild-animal reservoir hosts and the presence of infected bugs whose nests are found in human homes. Cases are rare in the United States, because the bugs prefer nesting in animal burrows, and because homes are not as open to nesting as those in South and Central America.

Clinical Syndromes

Chagas' disease may be asymptomatic, acute, or chronic. One of the earliest signs is development at the site of the bug bite of an erythematous and indurated area called a **chagoma**. This is often followed by a rash and edema around the eyes and face (**Romaña's sign**). The disease is most severe in children younger than 5 years of age and frequently is seen as an acute process with CNS involvement. Acute infection is also characterized by fever, chills, malaise, myalgia, and fatigue. Parasites may be present in the blood during the acute phase; however, they are sparse in patients older than 1 year of age. Death may ensue a few weeks after an acute attack, the patient may recover, or the patient may enter the chronic phase as organisms proliferate and enter the heart, liver, spleen, brain, and lymph nodes.

Chronic Chagas' disease is characterized by hepatosplenomegaly, myocarditis, and enlargement of the esophagus and colon as a result of the destruction of nerve cells (e.g., Auerbach plexus) and other tissues that control the growth of these organs.

Megacardia and electrocardiographic changes are commonly seen in chronic disease. Involvement of the CNS may produce granulomas in the brain, with cyst formation and a meningoencephalitis. Death from chronic Chagas' disease results from tissue destruction in the many areas invaded by the organisms, and sudden death results from complete heart block and brain damage.

Laboratory Diagnosis

T. cruzi can be demonstrated in thick and thin blood films or concentrated anticoagulated blood early in the acute stage. As the infection progresses, the organisms leave the bloodstream and become difficult to find. Biopsy of lymph nodes, liver, spleen, or bone marrow may demonstrate the organisms in the amastigote stage. Culture of blood or inoculation into laboratory animals may be useful when the parasitemia is low. Serologic tests are also available. In endemic areas, xenodiagnosis is widely used. Gene amplification techniques, such as polymerase chain reaction, have been used to detect the organism in the

In humans	In bugs

Infective stage

Penetrates various tissues

Trypomastigote passes in feces of bug

Enters bite wound

Migrates to hindgut

Multiplies in midgut

Amastigotes in tissue divide by binary fission

Epimastigote stage in midgut

Cell ruptures, amastigotes liberated

Trypomastigote in blood

Diagnostic stage

Ingested

Figure 82–14. Life cycle of *T. cruzi.*

The trypomastigotes then migrate to other tissues (e.g., cardiac muscle, liver, brain), lose the flagellum and undulating membrane, and become the smaller, oval, intracellular amastigote form. These intracellular amastigotes multiply by binary fission and eventually destroy the host cells. Then they are liberated to enter new host tissue as intracellular amastigotes or to become trypomastigotes infective for feeding reduviid bugs. Ingested trypomastigotes develop into epimastigotes in the midgut of the insect and reproduce by longitudinal binary fission. The organisms migrate to the hindgut of the bug, develop

Figure 82–15. Amastigote stage of *T. cruzi* in skeletal muscle. *(From Ash LR, Orihel TC: Atlas of Human Parasitology, 2nd ed. Chicago, American Society of Clinical Pathologists, 1984.)*

into metacyclic trypomastigotes, and then leave the bug in the feces after biting, feeding, and defecating, initiating a new human infection.

Epidemiology

T. cruzi occurs widely in both reduviid bugs and a broad spectrum of reservoir animals in North, Central, and South America. Human disease is found most often among children in South and Central America, where 16 to 18 million people are infected. There is a direct correlation between infected wild-animal reservoir hosts and the presence of infected bugs whose nests are found in human homes. Cases are rare in the United States, because the bugs prefer nesting in animal burrows, and because homes are not as open to nesting as those in South and Central America.

Clinical Syndromes

Chagas' disease may be asymptomatic, acute, or chronic. One of the earliest signs is development at the site of the bug bite of an erythematous and indurated area called a **chagoma**. This is often followed by a rash and edema around the eyes and face (**Romaña's sign**). The disease is most severe in children younger than 5 years of age and frequently is seen as an acute process with CNS involvement. Acute infection is also characterized by fever, chills, malaise, myalgia, and fatigue. Parasites may be present in the blood during the acute phase; however, they are sparse in patients older than 1 year of age. Death may ensue a few weeks after an acute attack, the patient may recover, or the patient may enter the chronic phase as organisms proliferate and enter the heart, liver, spleen, brain, and lymph nodes.

Chronic Chagas' disease is characterized by hepatosplenomegaly, myocarditis, and enlargement of the esophagus and colon as a result of the destruction of nerve cells (e.g., Auerbach plexus) and other tissues that control the growth of these organs.

Megacardia and electrocardiographic changes are commonly seen in chronic disease. Involvement of the CNS may produce granulomas in the brain, with cyst formation and a meningoencephalitis. Death from chronic Chagas' disease results from tissue destruction in the many areas invaded by the organisms, and sudden death results from complete heart block and brain damage.

Laboratory Diagnosis

T. cruzi can be demonstrated in thick and thin blood films or concentrated anticoagulated blood early in the acute stage. As the infection progresses, the organisms leave the bloodstream and become difficult to find. Biopsy of lymph nodes, liver, spleen, or bone marrow may demonstrate the organisms in the amastigote stage. Culture of blood or inoculation into laboratory animals may be useful when the parasitemia is low. Serologic tests are also available. In endemic areas, xenodiagnosis is widely used. Gene amplification techniques, such as polymerase chain reaction, have been used to detect the organism in the bloodstream. These approaches are not widely available and have not been adapted for use in the field.

Treatment, Prevention, and Control

Treatment of Chagas' disease is limited by the lack of reliable agents. The drug of choice is nifurtimox. Although it has some activity against the acute phase of disease, it has little activity against tissue amastigotes and has a number of side effects. Alternative agents include allopurinol and benznidazole. Education regarding the disease, its insect transmission, and the wild-animal reservoirs is critical. Bug control, eradication of nests, and construction of homes to prevent nesting of bugs are also essential. The use of dichlorodiphenyltrichloroethane (DDT) in bug-infested homes has demonstrated a drop in the transmission of malaria and Chagas' disease. Screening of blood by serologic means or excluding blood donors from endemic areas prevents some infections that would otherwise be associated with transfusion therapy.

Development of a vaccine is possible because *T. cruzi* does not have the wide antigenic variation observed with the African trypanosomes.

Case Study and Questions

The patient, a 44-year-old heart transplant patient, complained to her primary physician about headache, nausea, and vomiting approximately 1 year after transplant. She had no skin lesions. A computed tomographic scan of the head demonstrated ring-enhancing lesions. A biopsy of the lesions was performed. All cultures (bacterial, fungal, viral) were negative. Special stains of the tissue revealed multiple cystlike structures of varying size.

1. What was the differential diagnosis of infectious agents in this patient? What was the most likely etiologic agent?

2. What other tests would have been done to confirm the diagnosis?

3. What aspects of the medical history might suggest a risk for infection with this agent?

4. What were the therapeutic options and the likelihood that therapy would be successful?

Bibliography

Baird JK: Effectiveness of antimicrobial drugs. N Engl J Med 352: 1565-1577, 2005.

Bruckner DA, Labarca JA: *Leishmania* and *Trypanosoma*. In Murray PR, et al (eds): Manual of Clinical Microbiology, 9th ed. Washington, DC, ASM Press, 2007.

Connor DH, et al: Pathology of Infectious Diseases, vol 2. Stamford, Conn, Appleton & Lange, 1997.

Conway DJ: Molecular epidemiology of malaria. Clin Microbiol Rev 20:188-204, 2007.

Croft SL, Sundar S, Fairlamb AH: Drug resistance in leishmaniasis. Clin Microbiol Rev 19:111-126, 2006.

Hotez PJ, et al: Control of neglected tropical diseases. N Engl J Med 357:1018-1027, 2007.

Jones JL, et al: *Toxoplasma gondii* infection in the United States, 1999-2004, decline from the prior decade. Am J Trop Med Hyg 77:405-410, 2007.

Karp CL, Auwaerter PG: Coinfection with HIV and tropical infectious diseases. I. Protozoal pathogens. Clin Infect Dis 45:1214-1220, 2007.

Marciano-Cabral F, Cabral G: *Acanthamoeba* spp. as agents of disease in humans. Clin Microbiol Rev 16:273-307, 2003.

Rogers WO: *Plasmodium* and *Babesia*. In Murray PR, et al (eds): Manual of Clinical Microbiology, 9th ed. Washington, DC, ASM Press, 2007.

Shiff C: Integrated approach to malaria control. Clin Microbiol Rev 15:278-293, 2002.

Talisuna AO, Bloland P, D'Alessandro U: History, dynamics, and public health importance of malaria parasite resistance. Clin Microbiol Rev 17:235-254, 2004.

Visvesvara GS: Pathogenic and opportunistic free-living amebae. In Murray PR, et al (eds): Manual of Clinical Microbiology, 9th ed. Washington, DC, ASM Press, 2007.

Zintl A, et al: *Babesia divergens*, a bovine blood parasite of veterinary and zoonotic importance. Clin Microbiol Rev 16:622-636, 2003.

Nematodes

The most common helminths recognized in the United States are primarily intestinal nematodes, although in other countries, nematode infections of blood and tissues can cause devastating disease. The nematodes are the most easily recognized form of intestinal parasite because of their large size and cylindrical, unsegmented bodies; hence the common name **roundworms**. These parasites live primarily as adult worms in the intestinal tract, and nematode infections are most commonly confirmed by detecting the characteristic eggs in feces. The identification of eggs should be approached in a systematic manner, taking into account the size and shape of the egg, the thickness of the shell, and the presence or absence of specialized structures such as polar plugs, knobs, spines, and opercula. The presence and characteristics of larvae within the eggs may also be useful. The most common nematodes of medical importance are listed in Table 83-1.

The **filariae** are long, slender roundworms that are parasites of blood, lymph, subcutaneous, and connective tissues. All of these nematodes are transmitted by mosquitoes or biting flies. Most produce larval worms called **microfilariae** that are demonstrated in blood specimens or in subcutaneous tissues and skin snips.

Enterobius vermicularis

Physiology and Structure

E. vermicularis, the **pinworm**, is a small, white worm that is familiar to parents who find them in the perianal folds or vagina of an infected child. Infection is initiated by ingestion of embryonated eggs (Figure 83-1). Larvae hatch in the small intestine and migrate to the large intestine, where they mature into adults in 2 to 6 weeks. Fertilization of the female by the male produces the characteristic asymmetrical eggs. These eggs are laid in the perianal folds by the migrating female. As many as 20,000 eggs are deposited on the perianal skin. The eggs rapidly mature and are infectious within hours.

Epidemiology

E. vermicularis occurs worldwide but is most common in the temperate regions, where person-to-person spread is greatest in crowded conditions such as in daycare centers, schools, and mental institutions. An estimated 500 million cases of pinworm infection are reported worldwide, and this is the most common helminthic infection in North America.

Infection occurs when the eggs are ingested and the larval worm is free to develop in the intestinal mucosa. These eggs may be transmitted from hand to mouth by children scratching the perianal folds in response to the irritation caused by the migrating, egg-laying female worms, or the eggs may find their way to clothing and play objects in daycare centers. They can also survive long periods in the dust that accumulates over doors, on windowsills, and under beds in the rooms of infected people. Egg-laden dust can be inhaled and swallowed to produce infestation. In addition, **autoinfection ("retrofection")** can occur, wherein eggs hatch in the perianal folds and the larval worms migrate into the rectum and large intestine. Infected individuals who handle food can also be a source of infection. No animal reservoir for *Enterobius* is known. Physicians should be aware of the related epidemiology of *Dientamoeba fragilis*; this organism correlates well with the presence of *E. vermicularis*, with *D. fragilis* transported in the pinworm eggshell.

Clinical Syndromes

Many children and adults show no symptoms and serve only as carriers. Patients who are allergic to the secretions of the migrating worms experience severe pruritus, loss of sleep, and fatigue. The pruritus may cause repeated scratching of the irritated area and lead to secondary bacterial infection. Worms that migrate into the vagina may produce genitourinary problems and granulomas.

Worms attached to the bowel wall may produce inflammation and granuloma formation around the eggs.

Table 83–1. Nematodes of Medical Importance

Parasite	Common Name	Disease
Enterobius vermicularis	Pinworm	Enterobiasis
Ascaris lumbricoides	Roundworm	Ascariasis
Toxocara canis	Dog ascaris	Visceral larva migrans
Toxocara cati	Cat ascaris	Visceral larva migrans
Baylisascaris procyonis	Raccoon ascaris	Neural larva migrans
Trichuris trichiura	Whipworm	Trichuriasis
Ancylostoma duodenale	Old World hookworm	Hookworm infection
Necator americanus	New World hookworm	Hookworm infection
Ancylostoma braziliense	Dog or cat hookworm	Cutaneous larva migrans
Strongyloides stercoralis	Threadworm	Strongyloidiasis
Trichinella spiralis		Trichinosis
Wuchereria bancrofti	Bancroft filaria	Filariasis
Brugia malayi	Malayan filaria	Filariasis
Loa loa	African eye worm	Loiasis
Mansonella species		Filariasis
Onchocerca volvulus		Onchocerciasis
Dirofilaria immitis	Dog heartworm	Dirofilariasis
Dracunculus medinensis	Guinea worm	Dracunculosis

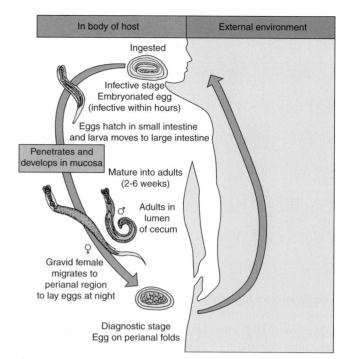

Figure 83–1. Life cycle of *E. vermicularis*.

arises and before bathing or defecation to pick up eggs laid by migrating worms during the night. Parents can collect the specimen and deliver it to the physician for immediate microscopic examination. Three swabbings, one per day for 3 consecutive days, may be required to detect the diagnostic eggs. The eggs are rarely seen in fecal specimens. Systemic signs of infection such as eosinophilia are rare.

Treatment, Prevention, and Control

The drug of choice is albendazole or mebendazole. Pyrantel pamoate and piperazine are effective, but reinfection is

Although the adult worms may occasionally invade the appendix, there remains no proven relationship between pinworm invasion and appendicitis. Penetration through the bowel wall into the peritoneal cavity, liver, and lungs has been infrequently recorded.

Laboratory Diagnosis

The diagnosis of **enterobiasis** is usually suggested by the clinical manifestations and confirmed by detection of the characteristic eggs on the anal mucosa. Occasionally, the adult worms are seen by laboratory personnel in stool specimens, but the method of choice for diagnosis involves use of an anal swab with a sticky surface that picks up the eggs (Figure 83-2) for microscopic examination. Sampling can be done with clear tape or commercially available swabs. The sample should be collected when the child

Figure 83–2. *E. vermicularis* egg. The thin-walled eggs are 50 to 60 × 20 to 30 μm, ovoid, and flattened on one side (not because children sit on them, but this is an easy way to correlate the egg morphology with the epidemiology of the disease).

common. To avoid reintroduction of the organism and reinfection in the family environment, it is customary to treat the entire family simultaneously. Although cure rates are high, reinfection is common. Repeat treatment after 2 weeks may be useful in preventing reinfection.

Personal hygiene, clipping of fingernails, thorough washing of bed clothes, and prompt treatment of infected individuals all contribute to control. When housecleaning is done in the home of an infected family, dusting under beds, on window sills, and over doors should be done with a damp mop to avoid inhalation of infectious eggs.

Ascaris lumbricoides

Physiology and Structure

A. lumbricoides are large (20 to 35 cm in length), pink worms that have a more complex life cycle than *E. vermicularis* (Figure 83-3) but are otherwise typical of an intestinal roundworm.

The ingested infective egg releases a larval worm that penetrates the duodenal wall, enters the bloodstream, is carried to the liver and heart, and then enters the pulmonary circulation. The larvae break free in the alveoli of the lungs, where they grow and molt. In about 3 weeks, the larvae pass from the respiratory system to be coughed up, swallowed, and returned to the small intestine.

As the male and female worms mature in the small intestine (primarily jejunum), fertilization of the female by the male initiates egg production, which may amount to 200,000

eggs per day for as long as a year. Female worms can also produce unfertilized eggs in the absence of males. Eggs are found in the feces 60 to 75 days after the initial infection. Fertilized eggs become infectious after approximately 2 weeks in the soil.

Epidemiology

A. lumbricoides is prevalent in areas where sanitation is poor and where human feces are used as fertilizer. Because food and water are contaminated with *Ascaris* eggs, this parasite, more than any other, affects the world's population. Although no animal reservoir is known for *A. lumbricoides*, an almost identical species from pigs, *A. suum*, can infect humans. This species is seen in swine growers and is associated with the use of pig manure for gardening. *Ascaris* eggs are quite hardy and can survive extreme temperatures and persist for several months in feces and sewage. Ascariasis is the most common helminthic infection worldwide, with an estimated 1 billion people infected.

Clinical Syndromes (Clinical Case 83-1)

Infections caused by the ingestion of only a few eggs may produce no symptoms; however, even a single adult *Ascaris* worm may be dangerous, because it can migrate into the bile duct and liver and damage tissue. Furthermore, because the worm has a tough, flexible body, it can occasionally perforate the intestine, creating peritonitis with secondary bacterial infection. The adult worms do not attach to the intestinal mucosa but depend on constant motion to maintain their position within the bowel lumen.

After infection with many larvae, migration of worms to the lungs can produce pneumonitis resembling an asthmatic attack. Pulmonary involvement is related to the degree of hypersensitivity induced by previous infections and the intensity of the current exposure and may be accompanied by eosinophilia and oxygen desaturation. Also, a tangled bolus of mature worms in the intestine can result in obstruction, perforation, and occlusion of the appendix. As mentioned previously, migration into the bile duct, gallbladder, and liver can produce severe tissue damage. This migration can occur in response to fever, drugs other than those used to treat ascariasis, and some anesthetics. Patients with many larvae may also experience abdominal tenderness, fever, distention, and vomiting.

Laboratory Diagnosis

Examination of the sediment of concentrated stool reveals the knobby-coated, bile-stained, fertilized and unfertilized eggs. Eggs are oval, 55 to 75 mm long, and 50 mm wide. The thick-walled outer shell can be partially removed (**decorticated egg**). Occasionally, adult worms pass with the

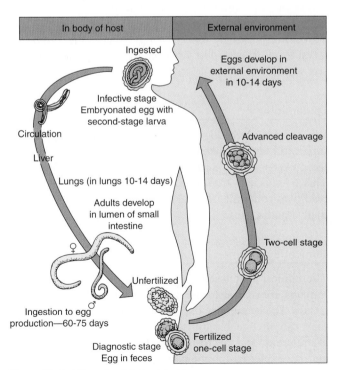

Figure 83–3. Life cycle of *A. lumbricoides.*

MEDICAL MICROBIOLOGY

Clinical Case 83-1. Hepatic Ascariasis

Hurtado and colleagues (N Engl J Med 354:1295-1303, 2006) describe a case of a 36-year-old woman who presented with recurrent right-upper-quadrant (RUQ) abdominal pain. One year earlier, she also presented with RUQ abdominal pain, abnormal liver function tests, and positive serology for hepatitis C. An abdominal ultrasonographic examination showed biliary dilatation, and endoscopic retrograde cholangiopancreatography (ERCP) showed multiple stones in the common bile duct, the left hepatic duct, and the left intrahepatic duct. The majority of the stones were removed. Examination of the bile-duct aspirate was negative for ova and parasites. One month prior to the present admission, the patient experienced recurrent RUQ pain and jaundice. Repeat ERCP again showed multiple stones in the common and left main hepatic ducts; partial removal was accomplished.

One month later, the patient was admitted with severe epigastric pain and fever. The patient was born in Vietnam and had immigrated to the United States when she was in her early 20s. She had no history of recent travel. An abdominal CT scan with contrast showed abnormal perfusion of the left hepatic lobe and dilatation of the left biliary radicles with multiple filling defects. ERCP showed partial obstruction of the left main hepatic duct, a few small stones, and purulent bile. Magnetic resonance imaging (MRI) showed diffuse enhancement of the left lobe and left portal vein suggestive of inflammation. Cultures of blood grew *Klebsiella pneumoniae*, and examination of a stool sample revealed a few *Strongyloides stercoralis* rhabditiform larvae. Biliary stents were placed, and the patient was treated with levofloxacin. Two weeks later, the patient was admitted to the hospital, where a partial hepatectomy was performed for treatment of recurrent pyogenic cholangitis. Gross examination of the left hepatic lobe showed ectatic bile ducts containing bile-stained calculi. Microscopic examination of the calculous material revealed collections of parasite eggs and a degenerated and fragmented nematode. *Klebsiella* species were identified in cultures by the microbiology laboratory. The findings were consistent with recurrent pyogenic cholangiohepatitis with infection by *Ascaris lumbricoides* and *Klebsiella* species. In addition to antibiotics for the bacterial infection, the patient was treated with ivermectin for the *Strongyloides* infection and albendazole for the *Ascaris* organisms.

The aberrant migration of *A. lumbricoides* into the pancreatobiliary tree with subsequent deposition of eggs, followed by death and degeneration of both worm and eggs, became a nidus for calculus formation and secondary bacterial infection. Although unusual in the United States, hepatic ascariasis is estimated to contribute to more than 35% of cases of biliary and pancreatic disease in the Indian subcontinent and parts of Southeast Asia.

feces, which can be quite dramatic because of their large size (20 to 35 cm long). Roentgenologists may also visualize the worms in the intestine, and cholangiograms often disclose their presence in the biliary tract of the liver. The pulmonary phase of the disease may be diagnosed by the finding of larvae and eosinophils in sputum.

Treatment, Prevention, and Control

Treatment of symptomatic infection is highly effective. The drug of choice is albendazole or mebendazole; pyrantel pamoate and piperazine are alternatives. Patients with mixed parasitic infections (*A. lumbricoides*, other helminths, *Giardia lamblia*, and *Entamoeba histolytica*) in the stool should be treated for ascariasis first to avoid provoking worm migration and possible intestinal perforation. Education, improved sanitation, and avoidance of human feces as fertilizer are critical. A program of mass treatment in highly endemic areas has been suggested, but this may not be economically feasible. Furthermore, eggs can persist in contaminated soil for 3 years or more. Certainly, improved personal hygiene among people who handle food is an important aspect of control.

Toxocara and *Baylisascaris*

Physiology and Structure

Toxocara canis, *Toxocara cati*, and *Baylisascaris procyonis* are ascarid worms that are naturally parasitic in the intestines of dogs, cats, and raccoons, respectively. These organisms may accidentally infect humans, producing disease states known as **visceral larva migrans (VLM)**, **neural larva migrans (NLM)**, and **ocular larva migrans (OLM)**. When ingested by humans, the eggs of these worms can hatch into larval forms that cannot follow the normal developmental cycle as in the natural host. They can penetrate the human gut and reach the bloodstream and then migrate as larvae to various human tissues. The *Toxocara* species are the most common causes of VLM and OLM, whereas *B. procyonis* is increasingly recognized as a cause of fatal NLM. Although the *Toxocara* species do not develop beyond the migrating larval form, *B. procyonis* larvae continue to grow to a large size within the human host.

Epidemiology

Wherever infected dogs and cats are present, the eggs are a threat to humans. Likewise, contact with raccoons or their feces presents a significant risk of infection with *B. procyonis*. This is especially true for children who are exposed more readily to contaminated soil and who tend to put objects in their mouths.

Clinical Syndromes (Clinical Case 83-2)

The clinical manifestations of VLM, NLM, and OLM in humans are related to the migration of the larvae through tissues. The larvae may invade any tissue of the body, where they can induce bleeding, the formation of eosinophilic granulomas, and necrosis. Patients may be asymptomatic and have only eosinophilia, but they can also have serious disease directly related to the number and location of the

Gavin and colleagues (Pediatr Infect Dis J 21:971-975, 2002) describe a case of a previously normal 2.5-year-old boy who was admitted to hospital with fever and recent onset of encephalopathy. Past history was significant for pica and geophagia, and he was receiving ferrous sulfate for iron-deficiency anemia. He was in good health until 8 days before admission, when a temperature of 38.5° C and mild cough developed. Three days before admission, he developed increasing lethargy and marked somnolence. He was irritable, confused, and ataxic. The family lived in suburban Chicago, and there were no sick contacts or pets at home. There was no travel history. On admission, he was febrile and lethargic but irritable and agitated when disturbed. Neck stiffness with generalized hypertonicity, hyperreflexia and bilateral extensor plantar responses were present. The white blood cell count (WBC) was elevated, and eosinophilia was present. CSF examination revealed an elevated protein and WBC with 32% eosinophils. Gram, acid-fast, and India ink stains and bacterial and cryptococcal antigen tests were all negative. Broad-spectrum antibacterial and antiviral therapy was begun empirically; however, the patient became comatose, with opisthotonus, decerebrate posturing, hypertonicity, and tremulousness. Cranial MRI demonstrated areas of increased signal involving both cerebellar hemispheres. Bacterial, fungal, mycobacterial, and viral cultures of blood and CSF were negative. Viral serologies were negative, as were tests for antibodies against *Toxocara*, cysticercosis, coccidioidomycosis, blastomycosis, and histoplasmosis. A detailed epidemiologic history revealed that 18 days before hospitalization, the family attended a picnic in a nearby suburb. Numerous raccoons were observed regularly in the vicinity, and the patient was observed playing with and eating dirt beneath the trees. CSF and serum antibodies against third-stage *Baylisascaris procyonis* were demonstrated by indirect immunofluorescent assay (IFA), with titers increasing from 1/4 to 1/1024 over a 2-week period. The patient was treated with albendazole and corticosteroids for 4 weeks but has remained severely affected with marked generalized spasticity and cortical blindness. Subsequent examination of soil and debris from the child's play site revealed thousands of infective *B. procyonis* eggs. This case underscores the devastating effects of NLM. In many regions of North America, large populations of raccoons with high rates of endemic *B. procyonis* infection (e.g., 60%-80%) live in proximity to humans, which suggests that the risk of human infection is probably substantial.

lesions caused by the migrating larvae, as well as the degree to which the host is sensitized to the larval antigens. The organs most frequently involved are the lungs, heart, kidneys, liver, skeletal muscles, eyes, and central nervous system. NLM is a common sequela of infection with *B. procyonis* and is attributed to the extensive somatic larval migration of this species. Continued growth and migration within the CNS produces extensive mechanical tissue damage. Signs and symptoms due to the migrating larvae include cough, wheezing, fever, rash, anorexia, seizures, fatigue, and abdominal discomfort. On examination, patients may have hepatosplenomegaly and nodular

pruritic skin lesions. Death may result from respiratory failure, cardiac arrhythmia, or brain damage. Ocular disease can also occur with the movement of larvae through the eye and may be mistaken for malignant retinoblastoma. Prompt diagnosis is required to avoid unnecessary enucleation.

Laboratory Diagnosis

The diagnosis of VLM, NLM, and OLM is based on clinical findings, the presence of eosinophilia, known exposure to dogs, cats, or raccoons and serologic confirmation. Enzyme-linked immunosorbent assays are available and appear to offer the best serologic marker for disease. The examination of feces from infected patients is not useful, because egg-laying adults are not present. However, examination of fecal material from infected pets often supports the diagnosis. Tissue examination for larvae may provide a definitive diagnosis but may be negative because of sampling error.

Treatment, Prevention, and Control

Treatment is primarily symptomatic, since antiparasitic agents are not of proven benefit. Anthelmintic therapy with albendazole, mebendazole, diethylcarbamazine or thiabendazole is often used. Corticosteroid therapy may be lifesaving if the patient has serious pulmonary, myocardial, or central nervous system involvement, since a major component of the infection is an inflammatory response to the organism. To date, despite anthelmintic treatment of cases of *B. procyonis* NLM, there are no neurologically intact survivors. This zoonosis can be greatly reduced if pet owners conscientiously eradicate worms from their animals and clean up pet fecal material from yards and school playgrounds. Children's play areas and sandboxes should be carefully monitored. Raccoons should not be encouraged to visit homes or yards for food, and the keeping of raccoons as pets should be strongly discouraged.

Trichuris trichiura

Physiology and Structure

Commonly called **whipworm** because it resembles the handle and lash of a whip, *T. trichiura* has a simple life cycle (Figure 83-4). Ingested eggs hatch into a larval worm in the small intestine and then migrate to the cecum, where they penetrate the mucosa and mature to adults. Some 3 months after the initial infection, the fertilized female worm starts laying eggs and may produce 3000 to 10,000 eggs per day. Female worms can live for as long as 8 years. Eggs passed into the soil mature and become infectious in 3 weeks. *T. trichiura* eggs are distinctive, with dark bile staining, a barrel shape, and the presence of polar plugs in the egg shell (Figure 83-5).

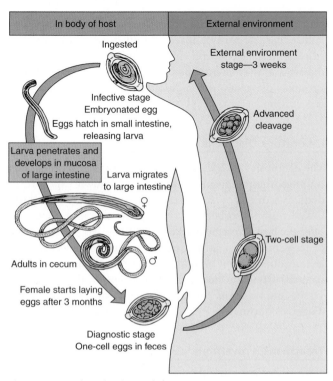

Figure 83—4. Life cycle of *T. trichiura*.

Epidemiology

Like *A. lumbricoides*, *T. trichiura* has worldwide distribution, and its prevalence is directly correlated with poor sanitation and the use of human feces as fertilizer. No animal reservoir is recognized.

Clinical Syndromes

The clinical manifestations of **trichuriasis** are generally related to the intensity of the worm burden. Most infections are with small numbers of *Trichuris* organisms and are usually asymptomatic, although secondary bacterial

Figure 83—5. *T. trichiura* egg. The eggs are barrel shaped, measuring 50 × 24 μm, with a thick wall and two prominent plugs at the ends. Internally, an unsegmented ovum is present.

infection may occur because the heads of the worms penetrate deep into the intestinal mucosa. Infections with many larvae may produce abdominal pain and distention, bloody diarrhea, weakness, and weight loss. Appendicitis may occur as worms fill the lumen, and prolapse of the rectum is seen in children because of the irritation and straining during defecation. Anemia and eosinophilia are also seen in severe infections.

Laboratory Diagnosis

Stool examination reveals the characteristic bile-stained eggs with polar plugs. Light infestations may be difficult to detect because of the paucity of eggs in the stool specimens.

Treatment, Prevention, and Control

The drug of choice is albendazole or mebendazole. As with *A. lumbricoides*, prevention of *T. trichiura* depends on education, good personal hygiene, adequate sanitation, and avoidance of the use of human feces as fertilizer.

Hookworms

Ancylostoma duodenale and *Necator americanus*

Physiology and Structure

The two human hookworms are *A. duodenale* (**Old World hookworm**) and *N. americanus* (**New World hookworm**). Differing only in geographical distribution, structure of mouthparts, and relative size, these two species are discussed together as agents of hookworm infection. The human phase of the hookworm life cycle is initiated when a filariform (infective form) larva penetrates intact skin (Figure 83-6).

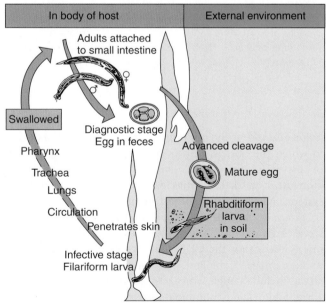

Figure 83—6. Life cycle of human hookworms.

The larva then enters the circulation; is carried to the lungs; and like *A. lumbricoides*, is coughed up, swallowed, and develops to adulthood in the small intestine. The adult *N. americanus* has a hooklike head, which accounts for the name commonly used. Adult worms lay as many as 10,000 to 20,000 eggs per day, which are released into the feces. Egg laying is initiated 4 to 8 weeks after the initial exposure and can persist for as long as 5 years. On contact with soil, the **rhabditiform** (noninfective) larvae are released from the eggs and within 2 weeks develop into **filariform** larvae. The filariform larvae can then penetrate exposed skin (e.g., bare feet) and initiate a new cycle of human infection.

Both species have mouthparts designed for sucking blood from injured intestinal tissue. *A. duodenale* has chitinous teeth, and *N. americanus* has shearing chitinous plates.

Epidemiology

Transmission of hookworm infection requires the deposition of egg-containing feces on shady, well-drained soil and is favored by warm, humid (tropical) conditions. Hookworm infections are reported worldwide in places where direct contact with contaminated soil can lead to human disease, but they occur primarily in warm subtropical and tropical regions and in southern parts of the United States. It is estimated that more than 900 million individuals worldwide are infected with hookworms, including 700,000 in the United States.

Clinical Syndromes

Skin-penetrating larvae may produce an allergic reaction and rash at sites of entry, and larvae migrating in the lungs can cause pneumonitis and eosinophilia. Adult worms produce the gastrointestinal symptoms of nausea, vomiting, and diarrhea. As blood is lost from feeding worms, a microcytic hypochromic anemia develops. Daily blood loss is estimated at 0.15 to 0.25 ml for each adult *A. duodenale* and 0.03 ml for each adult *N. americanus*. In severe, chronic infections, emaciation and mental and physical retardation may occur related to anemia from blood loss and nutritional deficiencies. Also, intestinal sites may be secondarily infected by bacteria when the worms migrate along the intestinal mucosa.

Laboratory Diagnosis

Stool examination reveals the characteristic non-bile-stained segmented eggs shown in Figure 83-7. Larvae are not found in stool specimens unless the specimen was left at ambient temperature for a day or more. The eggs of *A. duodenale* and *N. americanus* cannot be distinguished. The larvae must be examined to identify these hookworms specifically, although this is clinically unnecessary.

Treatment, Prevention, and Control

The drug of choice is albendazole or mebendazole; pyrantel pamoate is an alternative. In addition to eradication of the

Figure 83–7. Human hookworm egg. The eggs are 60 to 75 μm long and 35 to 40 μm wide, are thin shelled, and enclose a developing larva.

worms to stop blood loss, iron therapy is indicated to raise hemoglobin levels to normal. Blood transfusion may be necessary in severe cases of anemia. Education, improved sanitation, and controlled disposal of human feces are critical preventive measures. Wearing shoes in endemic areas helps reduce the prevalence of infection.

Ancylostoma braziliense

Physiology and Structure

A. braziliense, a species of hookworm, is naturally parasitic in the intestines of dogs and cats and accidentally infects humans. It produces a disease properly called **cutaneous larva migrans** but also called **ground itch** and **creeping eruption**. The filariform larvae of this hookworm penetrate intact skin but can develop no further in humans. The larvae remain trapped in the skin of the wrong host for weeks or months, wandering through subcutaneous tissue and creating serpentine tunnels.

Epidemiology

Similar to the situation with *Ascaris* worms, the threat of infection with *A. braziliense* is greatest among children coming into contact with soil or sandboxes contaminated with animal feces containing hookworm eggs. Infections are prevalent throughout the year on beaches in subtropical and tropical regions; in the summer, infection is reported as far north as the Canadian–U.S. border.

Clinical Syndromes

The migrating larvae may provoke a severe erythematous and vesicular reaction. Pruritus and scratching of the irritated skin may lead to secondary bacterial infection. About half of patients develop transient pulmonary infiltrates with peripheral eosinophilia (**Löffler's syndrome**), presumably resulting from pulmonary migration of the larvae.

Laboratory Diagnosis

Occasionally, larvae are recovered in skin biopsy or after freezing of the skin, but most diagnoses are based on the clinical appearance of the tunnels and a history of contact with dog and cat feces. The larvae are rarely found in sputum.

Treatment, Prevention, and Control

The drug of choice is albendazole; ivermectin and thiabendazole are alternatives. Antihistamines may be helpful in controlling pruritus. This zoonosis, as with animal *Ascaris* infection, can be reduced by educating pet owners to treat their animals for worm infections and to pick up pet feces from yards, beaches, and sandboxes. In endemic areas, shoes or sandals should be worn to prevent infection.

Strongyloides stercoralis

Physiology and Structure

Although the morphology of these worms and the epidemiology of their infections are similar to the hookworm, the life cycle of *S. stercoralis* (Figure 83-8) differs in three aspects: (1) Eggs hatch into larvae in the intestine and before they are passed in feces, (2) larvae can mature into filariforms in the intestine and cause autoinfection, and (3) a free-living, nonparasitic cycle can be established outside the human host.

In direct development, like the hookworm, a skin-penetrating *S. stercoralis* larva enters the circulation and follows the pulmonary course. It is coughed up and swallowed, and adults develop in the small intestine. Adult females burrow into the mucosa of the duodenum and reproduce parthenogenetically. Each female produces about a dozen eggs each day, which hatch within the mucosa and release **rhabditiform** larvae into the lumen of the bowel. The rhabditiform larvae are distinguished from the larvae of hookworms by their short buccal capsule and large genital primordium. The rhabditiform larvae are passed in the stool and may either continue the direct cycle by developing into infective **filariform** larvae

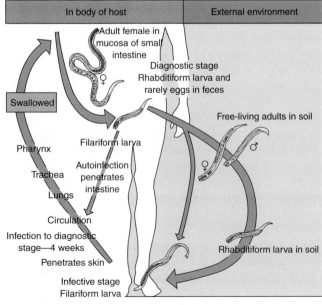

Figure 83—8. Life cycle of *S. stercoralis*.

or develop into free-living adult worms and initiate the indirect cycle.

In indirect development, the larvae in soil develop into free-living adults that produce eggs and larvae. Several generations of this nonparasitic existence may occur before new larvae become skin-penetrating parasites.

Finally, in **autoinfection**, rhabditiform larvae in the intestine do not pass with feces but become filariform larvae. These penetrate the intestinal or perianal skin and follow the course through the circulation and pulmonary structures, are coughed up, and then are swallowed; at this point, they become adults, producing more larvae in the intestine. This cycle can persist for years and can lead to **hyperinfection** and massive or disseminated, often fatal infection.

Epidemiology

Similar to hookworms in its requirements for warm temperatures and moisture, *S. stercoralis* demonstrates low prevalence but a somewhat broader geographical distribution, including parts of the northern United States and Canada. Sexual transmission also occurs. Animal reservoirs, such as domestic pets, are recognized.

Clinical Syndromes

Individuals with **strongyloidiasis** frequently are afflicted with pneumonitis from migrating larvae similar to that seen in ascariasis and hookworm infection. The intestinal infection is usually asymptomatic. However, heavy worm loads may involve the biliary and pancreatic ducts, the entire small bowel, and the colon, causing inflammation and ulceration leading to epigastric pain and tenderness, vomiting, diarrhea (occasionally bloody), and malabsorption. Symptoms mimicking peptic ulcer disease coupled with peripheral eosinophilia should strongly suggest the diagnosis of strongyloidiasis.

Autoinfection may lead to chronic strongyloidiasis that can last for years, even in nonendemic areas. Although many of these chronic infections may be asymptomatic, as many as two thirds of patients have recurring episodic symptoms referable to the involved skin, lungs, and intestinal tract. Individuals with chronic strongyloidiasis are at risk of developing severe, life-threatening hyperinfection syndrome if the host-parasite balance is disturbed by any drug or illness that compromises the host's immune status (Clinical Case 83-3). **Hyperinfection syndrome** is seen most commonly in individuals immunocompromised by malignancies (especially hematologic malignancies), corticosteroid therapy, or both. Hyperinfection syndrome has also been observed in patients who have undergone solid organ transplantation and in malnourished people. Loss of cellular immune function may be associated with the conversion of rhabditiform larvae to filariform larvae, followed by dissemination of the larvae via the circulation to

Gorman and colleagues (Infect Med 23:480, 2006) describe a case of necrotizing myositis complicated by diffuse alveolar hemorrhage and sepsis following corticosteroid therapy. The patient was a 46-year-old Cambodian man with a history of Raynaud phenomenon. He presented to the rheumatology clinic with worsening symptoms of Raynaud syndrome and diffuse muscle aches. He was employed as a truck driver and had immigrated from Cambodia 30 years earlier. Pertinent laboratory studies included markedly elevated creatine kinase and aldolase levels. Pulmonary function studies showed decreased forced vital capacity, forced expiratory volume, and carbon monoxide diffusing capacity. A high resolution CT scan of the chest showed mild ground-glass changes in both lung bases and interlobular septate thickening. Muscle biopsy showed myocyte necrosis and random atrophy but no inflammatory cells. Bronchoscopy was unremarkable, and all cultures were negative. The patient was started on prednisone for presumed necrotizing myopathy secondary to undifferentiated connective tissue disease.

He was admitted to the hospital 1 month later with profound muscle weakness and dyspnea, which improved with the administration of methylprednisolone and intravenous immunoglobulin. Three weeks later, the patient was readmitted with fever, nausea, vomiting, abdominal pain, and diffuse joint pain. A CT scan of the abdomen suggested small bowel intussusception and colitis, but his symptoms improved without treatment. Another high resolution CT scan of the chest showed early honeycombing and worsening interstitial infiltrates. The patient was scheduled for a lung biopsy; however, while awaiting the biopsy, he suffered an abrupt and fulminant deterioration, with hemoptysis and hypoxemic respiratory failure that required intubation and mechanical ventilation. Chest x-ray showed new, diffuse, bilateral infiltrates. The patient developed an acute abdomen accompanied by purpura on the lower trunk. An abdominal CT showed pancolitis. Refractory septic shock caused by *Escherichia coli* bacteremia and lactic acidosis ensued. Bronchoscopy showed diffuse alveolar hemorrhage, and numerous larvae of *Strongyloides stercoralis* were demonstrated on staining of an aspirate of endotracheal secretions. Serology was positive for anti-*Strongyloides* antibodies. Despite treatment with ivermectin, albendazole, cefepime, vancomycin, vasopressors, steroids, and dialysis, the patient died.

This case of *Strongyloides* hyperinfection syndrome emphasizes the importance of screening and treating persons at risk for latent *S. stercoralis* infection (endemic in tropical and subtropical areas) before the initiation of immunosuppressive therapy. Contact precautions should be taken in patients with hyperinfection syndrome because of the risk of infection to healthcare workers and visitors upon exposure to infectious larvae in the patient's stool and secretions.

syndrome include profound diarrhea, malabsorption, and electrolyte abnormalities. Notably, hyperinfection syndrome is associated with a mortality rate of approximately 86%. Bacterial sepsis, meningitis, peritonitis, and endocarditis secondary to larval spread from the intestine are frequent and often fatal complications of hyperinfection syndrome.

Laboratory Diagnosis

The diagnosis of strongyloidiasis may be difficult because of the intermittent passage of low numbers of first-stage larvae in stool. Examination of concentrated stool sediment reveals the larval worms (Figure 83-9), but in contrast with hookworm infections, in *S. stercoralis* infections, eggs are generally not seen. Collecting samples from three stools, one per day for 3 days (as for *G. lamblia*), is recommended because *S. stercoralis* larvae may occur in "showers," with many present one day and few or none the next. Several authors favor the **Baermann funnel gauze method** of concentrating living *S. stercoralis* larvae from fecal specimens. This method uses a funnel with a stopcock and a gauze insert. The funnel is filled with lukewarm water to a level just covering the gauze, and a specimen of stool is placed on the gauze, partially in contact with the water. The larvae in the stool migrate through the gauze into the water and then sediment into the neck of the funnel where they may be detected by low-power microscopy. When absent from stool, larvae may be detected in duodenal aspirates or in sputum in the case of massive infection. Finally, culture of the larvae from stool using charcoal cultures or an agar plate method may be used, although these are not routine in most laboratories. Demonstration of anti-*Strongyloides* antibodies in blood may be useful as a screening test or as an adjunct for diagnosis.

Figure 83–9. *S. stercoralis* larvae. The larvae are 180 to 380 µm long and 14 to 24 µm wide. They are differentiated from hookworm larvae by the length of the buccal cavity and esophagus and by the structure of the genital primordium.

virtually any organ. Most commonly, extraintestinal infection involves the lung and includes bronchospasm, diffuse infiltrates, and occasionally cavitation. Widespread dissemination that involves the abdominal lymph nodes, liver, spleen, kidneys, pancreas, thyroid, heart, brain, and meninges is common. Intestinal symptoms of hyperinfection

Treatment, Prevention, and Control

All infected patients should be treated to prevent autoinfection and potential dissemination (hyperinfection) of the parasite. The drug of choice is ivermectin, with albendazole or mebendazole as an alternative. Patients in endemic areas who are preparing to undergo immunosuppressive therapy should have at least three stool examinations to rule out *S. stercoralis* infection and thus avoid the risks of autoinfection. Strict infection-control measures should be enforced when clinicians care for patients with hyperinfection syndrome, because stool, saliva, vomitus, and body fluids may contain infectious filariform larvae. As with hookworm, control of *Strongyloides* species requires education, proper sanitation, and prompt treatment of existing infections.

Trichinella spiralis

Physiology and Structure

T. spiralis is the most important cause of human disease, but other species, such as *T. pseudospiralis* and *T. britovi* may also cause **trichinosis**. The adult form of this organism lives in the duodenal and jejunal mucosa of flesh-eating mammals worldwide. The infectious larval form is present in the striated muscles of carnivorous and omnivorous mammals. Among domestic animals, swine are most frequently involved. Figure 83-10 illustrates the simple, direct life cycle, which terminates in the musculature of humans, where the larvae eventually die and calcify.

Figure 83–10. Life cycle of *T. spiralis*.

Figure 83–11. Encysted larva of *T. spiralis* in a muscle biopsy specimen. *(From Marler LM, et al: Parasitology CD-ROM, Indiana Pathology Images, 2003.)*

The infection begins when meat that contains encysted larvae is digested. The larvae leave the meat in the small intestine and within 2 days develop into adult worms. A single fertilized female produces more than 1500 larvae in 1 to 3 months. These larvae move from the intestinal mucosa into the bloodstream and are carried in the circulation to various muscle sites throughout the body, where they coil in striated muscle fibers and become encysted (Figure 83-11). The muscles invaded most frequently include the extraocular muscles of the eye; the tongue; the deltoid, pectoral, and intercostal muscles; the diaphragm; and the gastrocnemius muscle. The encysted larvae remain viable for many years and are infectious if ingested by a new animal host. The muscle larvae of *T. pseudospiralis* do not induce the formation of a cyst and generate less inflammation than that of *T. spiralis*.

Epidemiology

Trichinosis occurs worldwide in humans, and its greatest prevalence is associated with the consumption of pork products. In addition to its transmission from pigs, many carnivorous and omnivorous animals harbor the organism and are potential sources of human infection. Notably, polar bears and walruses in the Arctic account for outbreaks in human populations, especially with a strain of *T. spiralis* (*T. natira*) that is more resistant to freezing than the *T. spiralis* strains found in the continental United States and other temperate regions. It is estimated that more than 1.5 million Americans carry live *Trichinella* cysts in their musculature and that 150,000 to 300,000 acquire new infection annually.

Clinical Syndromes

Trichinosis is one of the few tissue parasitic diseases still seen in the United States. As with other parasitic infections, most patients have minimal or no symptoms. The clinical presentation depends largely on the tissue burden of organisms and

the location of the migrating larvae. Patients in whom no more than 10 larvae are deposited per gram of tissue are usually asymptomatic; those with at least 100 generally have significant disease; and those with 1000 to 5000 have a very serious course that occasionally ends in death. In mild infections with few migrating larvae, patients may experience only an influenza-like syndrome with slight fever and mild diarrhea. With more extensive larval migration, persistent fever, gastrointestinal distress, marked eosinophilia, muscle pain, and periorbital edema occur. "Splinter" hemorrhages beneath the nails, a common finding, are probably caused by vasculitis resulting from toxic secretions of the migrating larvae. In heavy infections, severe neurologic symptoms, including psychosis, meningoencephalitis, and cerebrovascular accident, may occur.

Patients who survive the migration, muscle destruction, and encystment of larvae in moderate infections experience a decline in clinical symptoms in 5 or 6 weeks. Lethal trichinosis results when myocarditis, encephalitis, and pneumonitis combine; the patient dies 4 to 6 weeks after infection. Respiratory arrest often follows heavy invasion and muscle destruction in the diaphragm.

Laboratory Diagnosis

The diagnosis is usually established with clinical observations, especially when an outbreak can be traced to consumption of improperly cooked pork or bear meat. The laboratory may confirm the diagnosis if the encysted larvae are detected in the implicated meat or in a muscle biopsy specimen from the patient. Marked eosinophilia is characteristically present in patients with trichinosis. Serologic procedures are also available for confirmation of the diagnosis. Significant antibody titers are usually absent before the third week of illness but then may persist for years.

Treatment, Prevention, and Control

Treatment of trichinosis is primarily symptomatic, since there are no good antiparasitic agents for tissue larvae. Treatment of the adult worms in the intestine with mebendazole may halt the production of new larvae. Steroids, along with thiabendazole or mebendazole, are recommended for severe symptoms. In infections caused by *T. pseudospiralis*, albendazole may be effective. Education regarding disease transmission from pork and bear meat is essential, especially the recommendation that pork and bear meat be cooked until the interior is gray. Microwave cooking and smoking or drying meat do not kill all larvae.

Laws regulating the feeding of garbage to pigs help control transmission, as may regulations controlling the foraging of bears in garbage pits and public parks. Freezing pork, as conducted in federally inspected meat packing plants, has reduced transmission. Quick freezing of pork at −40° C effectively destroys the organisms, as does low-temperature storage at −15° C for 20 days or more.

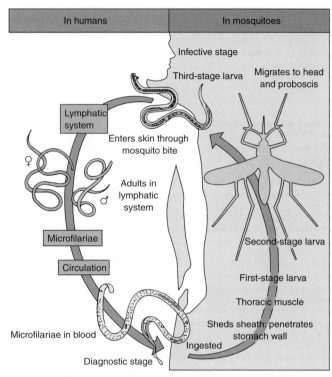

Figure 83–12. Life cycle of *W. bancrofti*.

Wuchereria bancrofti and *Brugia malayi*

Physiology and Structure

Because of their many similarities, *W. bancrofti* and *B. malayi* are discussed together. Human infection is initiated by the introduction of infective larvae, present in the saliva of a biting mosquito, into a bite wound (Figure 83-12). Various species of *Anopheles*, *Aedes*, and *Culex* mosquitoes are vectors of **Bancroft and Malayan filariasis**. The larvae migrate from the location of the bite to the lymphatic system, primarily in the arms, legs, or groin, where larval growth to adulthood occurs. From 3 to 12 months after the initial infection, the adult male worm fertilizes the female, which in turn produces the sheathed larval microfilariae that find their way into the circulation. The presence of **microfilariae** in blood is diagnostic for human disease and is infective for feeding mosquitoes. In the mosquito, the larvae move through the stomach and thoracic muscles in developmental stages and finally migrate to the proboscis. There they become infective, third-stage larvae and are transmitted by the feeding mosquito. The adult form in humans can persist for as long as 10 years.

Epidemiology

Infection with *W. bancrofti* occurs in tropical and subtropical areas and is endemic in central Africa, along the Mediterranean coast, and in many parts of Asia, including China, Korea, Japan, and the Philippines. It is also present in Haiti, Trinidad, Surinam, Panama, Costa Rica, and

Brazil. No animal reservoir has been identified. *B. malayi* is found primarily in Malaysia, India, Thailand, Vietnam, and parts of China, Korea, Japan, and many Pacific islands. Animal reservoirs such as cats and monkeys are recognized.

Clinical Syndromes

In some patients, there is no sign of disease, even though blood specimens may show the presence of many microfilariae. In other patients, early acute symptoms are fever, lymphangitis and lymphadenitis with chills, and recurrent febrile attacks. The acute presentation is thought to result from the inflammatory response to the presence of molting adolescent worms and dead or dying adults within the lymphatic vessels. As the infection progresses, the lymph nodes enlarge, possibly involving many parts of the body, including the extremities, the scrotum, and the testes, with occasional abscess formation. This results from the physical obstruction of lymph in the vessels caused by the presence of adult worms and host reactivity in the lymphatic system. This process may be complicated by recurrent bacterial infections, which contribute to the tissue damage. The thickening and hypertrophy of tissues infected with the worms may lead to the enlargement of tissues, especially the extremities, progressing to filarial **elephantiasis**. Filariasis of this type is thus a chronic, debilitating, and disfiguring disease requiring prompt diagnosis and treatment. Occasionally, ascites and pleural effusions secondary to rupture of the enlarged lymphatic vessels into the peritoneal or pleural cavity may be observed.

Laboratory Diagnosis

Eosinophilia is usually present during acute inflammatory episodes; however, demonstration of microfilariae in the blood is required for definitive diagnosis. As with malaria, microfilariae can be demonstrated in Giemsa-stained blood films in infections with *W. bancrofti* and *B. malayi* (Figures 83-13 and 83-14). Concentration of anticoagulated blood specimens and urine specimens are also valuable procedures. Buffy coat films concentrate the white blood cells and are useful for the detection of microfilariae. The presence of small numbers of microfilariae in blood can be detected by a membrane-filtration technique in which anticoagulated blood is mixed with saline and forced through a 5-μm membrane filter. After several washes with saline or distilled water, the filter is examined microscopically for living microfilariae, or it is dried, fixed, and stained as for a thin blood film.

W. bancrofti and *B. malayi* have both nocturnal and subperiodic periodicity in the production of microfilariae. Nocturnal periodicity results in greater numbers of microfilariae in blood at night, whereas with the subperiodic form, microfilariae are present at all times, with a peak in the afternoon.

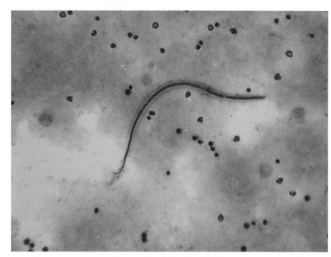

Figure 83–13. Giemsa stain of sheathed *W. bancrofti* microfilaria in blood smear; 245 to 295 μm long × 7 to 10 μm wide.

W. bancrofti, as well as *B. malayi* and *Loa loa*, demonstrate a sheath on their microfilariae. This can be the first step in identifying the specific types of filariasis. Further identification is based on study of head and tail structures (Figure 83-15). Clinically, an exact species identification is not critical, because treatment for all the filarial infections, except *Onchocerca volvulus*, is identical.

Serologic testing is also available through reference laboratories so that a diagnosis can be reached. Detection of circulating filarial antigens is promising but is not widely available as a diagnostic test.

Treatment, Prevention, and Control

Treatment is of little benefit in most cases of chronic lymphatic filariasis. The drug of choice for treatment of *W. bancrofti* and *B. malayi* infections is diethylcarbamazine (DEC). Ivermectin and albendazole may also be used, often

Figure 83–14. Giemsa stain of sheathed *B. malayi* microfilaria in blood smear; 180 to 230 μm long × 5 to 6 μm wide.

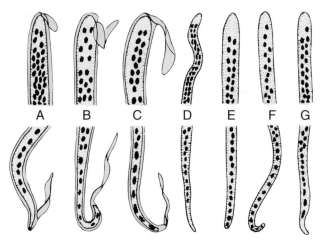

Figure 83—15. Differentiation of microfilariae. Identification of microfilariae is based on the presence of a sheath covering the larvae, as well as the distribution of nuclei in the tail region. **A,** *W. bancrofti.* **B,** *B. malayi.* **C,** *L. loa.* **D,** *O. volvulus.* **E,** *Mansonella perstans.* **F,** *Mansonella streptocerca.* **G,** *Mansonella ozzardi.*

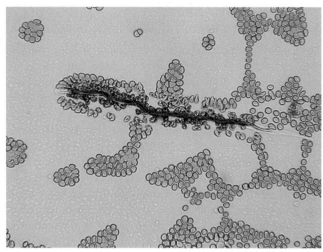

Figure 83—16. Giemsa stain of sheathed *L. loa* microfilaria in blood smear; 230 to 250 μm long × 6 to 9 μm wide.

in combination with DEC. Supportive and surgical therapy for lymphatic obstruction may be of some cosmetic help. Education regarding filarial infections, mosquito control, use of protective clothing and insect repellents, and treatment of infections to prevent further transmission is essential. Control of *B. malayi* infections is more difficult because of the presence of disease in animal reservoirs.

Loa loa

Physiology and Structure

The life cycle of *L. loa* is similar to that illustrated in Figure 83-12, except the vector is a biting fly called *Chrysops*, the mango fly. Approximately 6 months after infection, the production of microfilariae starts and can persist for 17 years or more. Adult worms can migrate through subcutaneous tissues, through muscle, and in front of the eyeball.

Epidemiology

L. loa is confined to the equatorial rain forests of Africa and is endemic in tropical West Africa, the Congo basin, and parts of Nigeria. Monkeys in these areas serve as reservoir hosts in the life cycle, with mango flies as vectors.

Clinical Syndromes

Symptoms usually do not appear until a year or so after the fly bite, because the worms are slow in reaching adulthood. One of the first signs of infection is the so-called **fugitive** or **Calabar swellings**. These swellings are transient and usually appear on the extremities, produced as the worms migrate through subcutaneous tissues, creating large, nodular areas that are painful and pruritic. Because eosinophilia

(50% to 70%) is observed, Calabar swellings are believed to result from allergic reactions to the worms or their metabolic products.

Adult *L. loa* worms can also migrate under the conjunctiva, producing irritation, painful congestion, edema of the eyelids, and impaired vision. The presence of a worm in the eye can obviously cause anxiety in the patient. The infection may be long lived and in some cases asymptomatic.

Laboratory Diagnosis

The clinical observation of Calabar swellings or migration of worms in the eye, combined with eosinophilia, should alert the physician to consider infection with *L. loa.* The microfilariae can be found in the blood (Figure 83-16). In contrast to the other filariae, *L. loa* is primarily present during the daytime. Serologic testing can also be useful for confirming the diagnosis but is not readily available.

Treatment, Prevention, and Control

Diethylcarbamazine is effective against adults and microfilariae; however, destruction of the parasites may induce severe allergic reactions that require treatment with corticosteroids. Albendazole or ivermectin (not approved by FDA) has been shown to be effective in reducing microfilarial loads. Surgical removal of worms migrating across the eye or bridge of the nose can be accomplished by immobilizing the worm with instillation of a few drops of 10% cocaine. Education regarding the infection and its vector, especially for people entering the known endemic areas, is essential. Protection from fly bites by using screening, appropriate clothing, and insect repellents, along with treatment of cases, is also critical in reducing the incidence of infection. However, the presence of disease in animal reservoirs (e.g., monkeys) limits the feasibility of controlling this disease.

Mansonella species

Filarial infections caused by *Mansonella* species are less important than those previously discussed, but physicians should be aware of the names because they may encounter patients with these infections. Infections caused by these organisms are generally asymptomatic but may cause dermatitis, lymphadenitis, hydrocele, and rarely, lymphatic obstruction resulting in elephantiasis.

All of the *Mansonella* species produce nonsheathed microfilariae in blood and subcutaneous tissues, and all are transmitted by biting midges (*Culicoides* species) or blackflies (*Simulium* species). Ivermectin is the treatment of choice for *M. ozzardi* and *M. streptocerca*, whereas DEC is used for *M. perstans*. Species identification, if desired, can be accomplished with blood smears, noting the structure of the microfilariae. Serologic tests are also available.

Prevention and control require measures involving insect repellents, screening, and other precautions as for all insect-transmitted diseases.

Mansonella perstans

M. perstans occurs primarily in parts of tropical Africa and Central and South America. It may produce allergic skin reactions, edema, and Calabar swellings like those of *L. loa* infection. Reservoir hosts are chimpanzees and gorillas.

Mansonella ozzardi

M. ozzardi is found primarily in Central and South America and the West Indies. It may produce swelling of the lymph nodes and occasional hydrocele. There are no known reservoir hosts.

Mansonella streptocerca

M. streptocerca occurs primarily in Africa, especially in the Congo basin. It may produce edema in the skin and rarely, a form of elephantiasis. Monkeys serve as reservoir hosts.

Onchocerca volvulus

Physiology and Structure

Infection occurs after the introduction of *O. volvulus* larvae through the skin during the biting and feeding of the *Simulium* or blackfly vector (Figure 83-17). The larval worms migrate from the skin to subcutaneous tissue and develop into adult male and female worms. The adults become encased in fibrous subcutaneous nodules within which they may remain viable for as long as 15 years. The female worm, after fertilization by the male, begins producing as many as 2000 nonsheathed microfilariae each day. The microfilariae exit the capsule and migrate

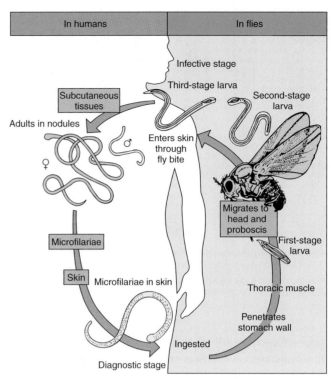

Figure 83–17. Life cycle of *O. volvulus*.

to the skin, the eyes, and other body tissues. These nonsheathed microfilariae appearing in skin tissue are infective for feeding blackflies.

Epidemiology

O. volvulus is endemic in many parts of Africa, especially in the Congo basin and the Volta River basin. In the western hemisphere, it occurs in many Central and South American countries. **Onchocerciasis** affects more than 18 million people worldwide and causes blindness in approximately 5% of infected people.

Several species of the blackfly genus *Simulium* serve as vectors but none so appropriately named as the principal vector, *Simulium damnosum* ("the damned blackfly"). These blackflies, or buffalo gnats, breed in fast-flowing streams, which makes control or eradication by insecticides almost impossible, because the chemicals are rapidly washed away from the eggs and larvae.

There is a greater prevalence of infection in men than women in endemic areas because of their work in or near the streams where the blackflies breed. Studies in endemic areas in Africa have shown that 50% of men are totally blind before they reach 50 years of age. This accounts for the common term **river blindness**, which is applied to the disease onchocerciasis. This fear of blindness has created an additional problem in many parts of Africa, because whole villages leave the area near streams and farmland that could produce food. The migrating populations then find themselves in areas where they face starvation.

Clinical Syndromes (Clinical Case 83-4)

Clinical onchocerciasis is characterized by infection involving the skin, subcutaneous tissue, lymph nodes, and eyes. The clinical manifestations of the infection are due to the acute and chronic inflammatory reaction to antigens released by the microfilariae as they migrate through the tissues. The incubation period from infectious larvae to adult worms is several months to a year. The initial signs of disease are fever, eosinophilia, and urticaria. As the worms mature, copulate, and produce microfilariae, subcutaneous nodules begin to appear on any part of the body. These nodules are most dangerous when they are present on the head and neck, because the microfilariae may migrate to the eyes and cause serious tissue damage, leading to blindness. The mechanisms for development of eye disease are thought to be a combination of both direct invasion by the microfilaria and antigen-antibody complex deposition within the ocular tissues. Patients progress from conjunctivitis with photophobia to punctate and sclerosing keratitis. Internal eye disease with anterior uveitis, chorioretinitis, and optic neuritis may also occur.

Within the skin, the inflammatory process results in loss of elasticity and areas of depigmentation, thickening, and atrophy. A number of skin conditions, including pruritus, hyperkeratosis, and myxedematous thickening, are related to the presence of this parasite. A form of elephantiasis called **hanging groin** also occurs when the nodules are located near the genitalia.

Figure 83—18. Giemsa stained unsheathed *O. volvulus* microfilaria; 300 to 315 µm long × 5 to 9 µm wide.

Laboratory Diagnosis

The diagnosis of onchocerciasis is made by the demonstration of microfilariae in skin snip preparations from the infrascapular or gluteal region. A sample is obtained by raising the skin with a needle and shaving the epidermal layer with a razor. The specimen is incubated in saline for several hours and is then inspected with a dissecting microscope for the presence of nonsheathed microfilariae (Figure 83-18). In patients with ocular disease, the organism may also be seen in the anterior chamber with the aid of a slit lamp. Serologic methods using recombinant antigens have been useful as have assays using PCR to detect onchocercal DNA in skin snip specimens.

Treatment, Prevention, and Control

Surgical removal of the encapsulated nodule is often performed to eliminate the adult worms and stop production of microfilariae (Figure 83-19). In addition, treatment with

Clinical Case 83-4. Onchocerciasis

Imtiaz and colleagues (Infect Med 22:187-189, 2005) describe the case of a 21-year-old man who immigrated from the Sudan to the United States 1 year prior to presenting with a maculopapular rash that was associated with severe pruritus. The rash and pruritus had been present for the past 3 to 4 years. In the past, the patient had undergone multiple treatments for this condition, including corticosteroids, without relief. The patient denied any systemic symptoms but did complain of blurred vision. On physical examination, his skin was somewhat thickened over different parts of the body, and he had scattered maculopapular lesions with increased pigmentation; some lesions had keloid nodules, as well as wrinkling. There was no lymphadenopathy. The remainder of his evaluation was unremarkable.

Because of the presence of intense pruritus unresponsive to treatment, blurred vision, and the prevalence of onchocerciasis in his native country, skin snips were taken from the scapular area. Microfilariae of *Onchocerca volvulus* were revealed on microscopic examination. Ivermectin was prescribed, to which the patient's condition responded. Onchocerciasis, although not common in the United States, should be considered in immigrants and expatriates with suggestive symptoms if they came from areas in which the disease is endemic.

Figure 83—19. Cross-section of an adult female *O. volvulus* in an excised nodule showing numerous microfilariae.

ivermectin is recommended. A single oral dose of ivermectin (150 mg/kg) greatly reduces the number of microfilariae in the skin and eyes, thus diminishing the likelihood of developing a disabling onchocerciasis. In endemic areas, the dose of ivermectin can be repeated every 6 to 12 months to maintain suppression of dermal and ocular microfilariae. Suppression of dermal microfilariae reduces the transmission of this vectorborne disease, and thus mass chemotherapy may prove to be a successful strategy for the prevention of onchocerciasis. At present there is no firm evidence that *O. volvulus* is becoming resistant to ivermectin; however, whenever a single agent is used for disease control with varying doses over a long period of time, it is prudent to be on guard for the possibility of resistance developing.

Education regarding the disease and its transmission is essential. Protection from blackfly bites through the use of protective clothing, screening, and insect repellents, as well as prompt diagnosis and treatment of infections to prevent further transmission, are critical.

Although control of blackfly breeding is difficult because insecticides wash away in the streams, some form of biologic control of this vector may reduce fly reproduction and disease transmission.

Dirofilaria immitis

Several mosquito-transmitted filariae infect dogs, cats, raccoons, and bobcats in nature and occasionally are found in humans. *D. immitis*, the **dog heartworm**, is notorious for forming a lethal worm bolus in the dog's heart. This nematode may also infect humans, producing a nodule called a **coin lesion** in the lung. Only very rarely have these worms been found in human hearts.

The coin lesion in the lung presents a problem for the radiologist and the surgeon because it resembles a malignancy requiring surgical removal. Unfortunately, no laboratory test can provide an accurate diagnosis of **dirofilariasis**. Peripheral eosinophilia is rare, and the radiographic features are insufficient to allow the clinician to distinguish pulmonary dirofilariasis from bronchogenic carcinoma. Serologic tests are not sufficiently sensitive or specific to preclude the surgical intervention. A definitive diagnosis is made when a thoracotomy specimen is examined microscopically, revealing the typical cross sections of the parasite.

Transmission of the filarial infections can be controlled by mosquito control and the prophylactic use of the drug ivermectin in dogs.

Dracunculus medinensis

The name *D. medinensis* means "little dragon of Medina." This is a very ancient worm infection thought by some scholars to be the "fiery serpent" noted by Moses with the Israelites at the Red Sea.

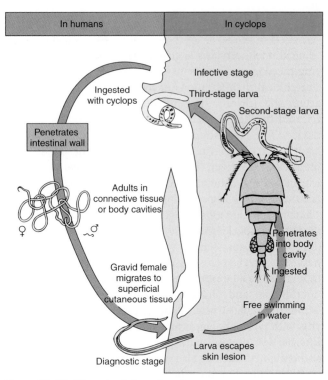

Figure 83–20. Life cycle of *D. medinensis*.

Physiology and Structure

D. medinensis is not a filarial worm but is a tissue-invading nematode of medical importance in many parts of the world. The worms have a very simple life cycle, depending on freshwater and a microcrustacean (**copepod**) of the genus *Cyclops* (Figure 83-20). When *Cyclops* species harboring larval *D. medinensis* are ingested in drinking water, the infection is initiated with liberation of the larvae in the stomach. These larvae penetrate the wall of the digestive tract and migrate to the retroperitoneal space, where they mature. These larvae are not microfilariae and do not appear in the blood or other tissues. Male and female worms mate in the retroperitoneum, and the fertilized female then migrates to the subcutaneous tissues, usually in the extremities. When the fertilized female worm becomes gravid, a vesicle is formed in the host tissue, which will ulcerate. When the ulcer is completely formed, the worm protrudes a loop of uterus through the ulcer. On contact with water, the larval worms are released. The larvae are then ingested by the *Cyclops* species in freshwater, where they are then infective for humans or animals drinking the water containing the *Cyclops* species.

Epidemiology

D. medinensis occurs in many parts of Asia and equatorial Africa, infecting an estimated 10 million people. Reservoir hosts include dogs and many fur-bearing animals that come into contact with drinking water containing infective *Cyclops* species.

Human infections usually result from ingestion of water from so-called "step wells" where people stand or bathe in

the water, at which time the gravid female worm discharges larvae from lesions on the arms, legs, feet, and ankles to infect *Cyclops* species in the water. Ponds and standing water are occasionally the source of infection when humans use them for drinking water.

Clinical Syndromes

Symptoms of infection usually do not appear until the gravid female creates the vesicle and the ulcer in the skin for the liberation of larval worms. This occurs usually 1 year after initial exposure. At the site of the ulcer, there are erythema and pain, as well as an allergic reaction to the worm. There is also the possibility of abscess formation and secondary bacterial infection, leading to further tissue destruction and inflammatory reaction with intense pain and sloughing of skin.

If the worm is broken in attempts to remove it, there may be toxic reactions, and if the worm dies and calcifies, there may be nodule formation and some allergic reaction. Once the gravid female worm has discharged all the larvae, it may retreat into deeper tissue, where it is gradually absorbed, or it may simply be expelled from the site.

Laboratory Diagnosis

Diagnosis is established by observing the typical ulcer and by flooding the ulcer with water to recover the larval worms when they are discharged. Occasionally, x-ray examination reveals worms in various parts of the body.

Treatment, Prevention, and Control

The ancient method of slowly wrapping the worm on a twig is still used in many endemic areas (Figure 83-21). Surgical removal is also a practical and reliable procedure for the patient. There is no evidence that any chemotherapeutic agent has a direct effect on *D. medinensis*, although various benzimidazoles may have an antiinflammatory effect and either eliminate the worm or make surgical removal easier. Treatment with mebendazole has been associated with aberrant migration of the worms, with the result that they were more likely to emerge at anatomic sites other than the lower limbs.

Education regarding the life cycle of the worm and avoidance of water contaminated with *Cyclops* species are critical. Protection of drinking water by prohibiting bathing and washing of clothing in wells is essential. Persons who live in or travel to endemic areas should boil water before drinking it. The treatment of water with chemicals and the use of fish that consume *Cyclops* species as food also help control transmission. Prompt diagnosis and treatment of cases also limit further transmission. These preventive measures have been incorporated into an ongoing global effort to eliminate dracunculiasis with dramatic success. The annual incidence of worldwide disease has been reduced by 98%, with complete eradication in 7 countries.

Figure 83–21. Removal of a *D. medinensis* adult from an exposed ulcer by winding the worm slowly around a stick. *(From Binford CH, Conner DH: Pathology of Tropical and Extraordinary Diseases. Washington, DC, Armed Forces Institute of Pathology, 1976.)*

Case Study and Questions

A 10-year-old boy was brought in by his father for evaluation of crampy abdominal pain, nausea, and mild diarrhea that had persisted for approximately 2 weeks. On the day before evaluation, the boy reported to his parents that he passed a large worm into the toilet during a bowel movement. He flushed the worm before the parents could see it. Physical examination was completely unremarkable. The boy had no fever, cough, or rash and did not complain of anal pruritus. His travel history was unremarkable. Examination of a stool specimen revealed the diagnosis.

1. Which intestinal parasites of humans are nematodes?
2. Which nematode was likely in this case? What organisms may be found in stool?
3. What was the most likely means of acquisition of this parasite?
4. Was this patient at risk of autoinfection?
5. Describe the life cycle of this parasite.
6. Can this parasite cause extraintestinal symptoms? What other organs may be invaded and what might stimulate extraintestinal invasion?

Bibliography

Barry M: The tail end of guinea worm - Global eradication without a drug or a vaccine. N Engl J Med 356:2561-2564, 2007.

Bruschi F, Murrell KD: New aspects of human trichinellosis: The impact of new *Trichinella* species. Postgrad Med J 78:15-22, 2002.

Cairncross S, Muller R, Zagaria N: Dracunculiasis (Guinea worm disease) and the eradication initiative. Clin Microbiol Rev 15:223-246, 2002.

Despommier D: Toxocariasis: Clinical aspects, epidemiology, medical ecology and molecular aspects. Clin Microbiol Rev 16:265-272, 2003.

Garcia LS: Diagnostic Medical Parasitology, 4th ed. Washington, DC, ASM Press, 2001.

Keiser PB, Nutman TB: *Strongyloides stercoralis* in the immunocompromised population. Clin Microbiol Rev 17:208-217, 2004.

Gavin PJ, Kazacos KR, Shulman ST: Baylisascariasis. Clin Microbiol Rev 18:703-718, 2005.

Hotez PJ, et al: Hookworm infection. N Engl J Med 351:799-807, 2004.

Hotez PJ, et al: Control of neglected tropical diseases. N Engl J Med 357:1018-1027, 2007.

McPherson T, Nutman TB: Filarial nematodes. In Murray PR, et al (eds): Manual of Clinical Microbiology, 9th ed. Washington, DC, ASM Press, 2007.

Procop GW, Neafie RC: Less common helminths. In Murray PR, et al (eds): Manual of Clinical Microbiology, 9th ed. Washington, DC, ASM Press, 2007.

Sheorey H, Biggs BA, Traynor P: Nematodes. In Murray PR, et al (eds): Manual of Clinical Microbiology, 9th ed. Washington, DC, ASM Press, 2007.

Strickland GT: Hunter's Tropical Medicine and Emerging Infectious Diseases. Philadelphia, WB Saunders, 2000.

Trematodes

The trematodes (**flukes**) are members of the Platyhelminthes and are generally flat, fleshy, leaf-shaped worms. In general, they are equipped with two muscular suckers: an oral type, which is the beginning of an incomplete digestive system, and a ventral sucker, which is simply an organ of attachment. The digestive system consists of lateral tubes that do not join to form an excretory opening. Most flukes are **hermaphroditic**, with both male and female reproductive organs in a single body. Schistosomes are the only exception; they have cylindrical bodies (like the nematodes), and separate male and female worms exist.

All flukes require intermediate hosts for the completion of their life cycles, and without exception, the first intermediate hosts are mollusks (snails and clams). In these hosts an asexual reproductive cycle is a type of germ-cell propagation. Some flukes require various second intermediate hosts before reaching the final host and developing into adult worms. This variation is discussed in the sections on the individual species.

Fluke eggs are equipped with a "lid" at the top of the shell. Called an **operculum**, the lid opens to allow the larval worm to find its appropriate snail host. The schistosomes do not have an operculum; rather, the eggshell splits to liberate the larva. The medically significant trematodes are summarized in Table 84-1.

Fasciolopsis buski

A number of intestinal flukes are recognized, including *F. buski*, *Heterophyes heterophyes*, *Metagonimus yokogawai*, *Echinostoma ilocanum*, and *Gastrodiscoides hominis*. *F. buski* is the largest, most prevalent, and most important intestinal fluke. The other flukes are similar to *F. buski* in many respects (epidemiology, clinical syndromes, treatment) and are not discussed further. It is important only that physicians recognize the relationship among these different flukes.

Physiology and Structure

This large intestinal fluke has a typical life cycle (Figure 84-1). Humans ingest the encysted larval stage (**metacercaria**) when they peel the husks from aquatic vegetation (e.g., water chestnuts) with the teeth. The metacercariae are scraped from the husk, swallowed, and develop into immature flukes in the duodenum. The fluke attaches to the mucosa of the small intestine with two muscular suckers, develops into an adult form, and undergoes self-fertilization. Egg production is initiated 3 months after the initial infection with the metacercariae. The operculated eggs pass in feces to water, where the operculum at the top of the eggshell pops open, liberating a free-swimming larval stage (**miracidium**). Glands at the pointed anterior end of the miracidium produce lytic substances that allow the penetration of the soft tissues of snails. In the snail tissue, the miracidium develops through a series of stages by asexual germ cell propagation. The final stage (**cercaria**) in the snail is a free-swimming form that, after release from the snail, encysts on the aquatic vegetation, becoming the metacercariae, or infective stage.

Epidemiology

Because it depends on the distribution of its appropriate snail host, *F. buski* is found only in China, Vietnam, Thailand, parts of Indonesia, Malaysia, and India. Pigs, dogs, and rabbits serve as reservoir hosts in these endemic areas.

Clinical Syndromes

The symptomatology of *F. buski* infection relates directly to the worm burden in the small intestine. Attachment of the flukes in the small intestine can produce inflammation, ulceration, and hemorrhage. Severe infections produce abdominal discomfort similar to that of a duodenal ulcer, as well as diarrhea. Stools may be profuse, a malabsorption syndrome similar to giardiasis is common, and intestinal obstruction can occur. Marked eosinophilia is also present. Although death can occur, it is rare.

Table 84—1. Medically Important Trematodes

Trematode	Common Name	Intermediate Host	Biologic Vector	Reservoir Host
Fasciolopsis buski	Giant intestinal fluke	Snail	Water plants (e.g., water chestnuts)	Pigs, dogs, rabbits, humans
Fasciola hepatica	Sheep liver fluke	Snail	Water plants (e.g., watercress)	Sheep, cattle, humans
Opisthorchis (Clonorchis) sinensis	Chinese liver fluke	Snail, freshwater fish	Uncooked fish	Dogs, cats, humans
Paragonimus westermani	Lung fluke	Snail, freshwater crabs, crayfish	Uncooked crabs, crayfish	Pigs, monkeys, humans
Schistosoma species	Blood fluke	Snail	None	Primates, rodents, domestic pets, livestock, humans

Laboratory Diagnosis

Stool examination reveals the large, golden, bile-stained eggs with an operculum on the top (Figure 84-2). The measurements and appearance of *F. buski* eggs are similar to that of the liver fluke *F. hepatica*, and differentiation of the eggs of these species usually is not possible. Large (approximately 1.5 to 3.0 cm) adult flukes can rarely be found in feces or specimens collected at surgery.

Treatment, Prevention, and Control

The drug of choice is praziquantel, and the alternative is niclosamide. Education regarding the safe consumption of

infective aquatic vegetation (particularly water chestnuts), proper sanitation, and control of human feces reduces the incidence of disease. In addition, the snail population may be eliminated with molluscacides. When infection occurs, treatment should be initiated promptly to minimize its spread. Control of the reservoir hosts also reduces transmission of the worm.

Fasciola hepatica

A number of liver flukes are recognized, including *F. hepatica*, *Opisthorchis sinensis*, *O. felineus*, and *Dicrocoelium dendriticum*. Only *F. hepatica* and *O. sinensis* are discussed in this chapter, although the eggs of other flukes are occasionally detected in the feces of patients in other geographical areas.

Physiology and Structure

Commonly called the **sheep liver fluke**, *F. hepatica* is a parasite of herbivores (particularly sheep and cattle) and humans. Its life cycle (Figure 84-3) is similar to that of *F. buski*, with human infection resulting from the ingestion of watercress that harbors the encysted metacercariae. The larval flukes then migrate through the duodenal wall and across the peritoneal cavity, penetrate the liver capsule, pass through the liver parenchyma, and enter the bile ducts to become adult worms. Approximately 3 to 4 months after the initial infection, the adult flukes start producing operculated eggs that are identical to those of *F. buski*, as seen in stool examination.

Epidemiology

Infections have been reported worldwide in sheep-raising areas, with the appropriate snail as an intermediate host. These areas include the former Soviet Union, Japan, Egypt, and many Latin American countries. Outbreaks are directly related to human consumption of contaminated watercress

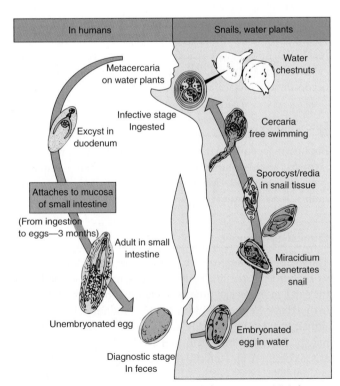

Figure 84—1. Life cycle of *Fasciolopsis buski* (giant intestinal fluke).

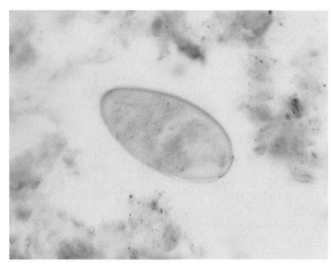

Figure 84—2. *Fasciolopsis buski* egg, 130 to 150 μm long and 65 to 90 μm wide, with a thin operculum at one end.

in areas where infected herbivores are present. Human infection is rare in the United States, but several well-documented cases have been reported in travelers from endemic areas.

Clinical Syndromes (Clinical Case 84-1)

Migration of the larval worm through the liver produces irritation of this tissue, tenderness, and hepatomegaly. Pain in the right upper quadrant, chills, fever, and marked eosinophilia are commonly observed. As the worms take up residence in the bile ducts, their mechanical irritation and

toxic secretions produce hepatitis, hyperplasia of the epithelium, and biliary obstruction. Some worms penetrate eroded areas in the ducts and invade the liver to produce necrotic foci referred to as **liver rot**. In severe infections, secondary bacterial infection can occur, and portal cirrhosis is common.

Laboratory Diagnosis

Stool examination reveals operculated eggs indistinguishable from the eggs of *F. buski*. Exact identification is a therapeutic problem because treatment is not the same for both infections. Whereas *F. buski* responds favorably to praziquantel, *F. hepatica* does not. When exact identification is desired, examination of a sample of the patient's bile differentiates the species; if the eggs are present in bile, they are *F. hepatica*, not *F. buski*, which is limited to the small intestine. Eggs may appear in stool samples from people who have eaten infected sheep or cattle liver. The spurious nature of this finding can be confirmed by having the patient refrain from eating liver and then rechecking the stool.

Treatment, Prevention, and Control

In contrast to *F. buski*, *F. hepatica* responds poorly to praziquantel. Treatment with bithionol or the benzimidazole compound triclabendazole has been effective. Preventive measures are similar to those for *F. buski* control; people who live in areas frequented by sheep and cattle should especially avoid ingestion of watercress and other uncooked aquatic vegetation.

Figure 84—3. Life cycle of *Fasciola hepatica* (sheep liver fluke).

In human, sheep, cattle | In snails, water plants

Infective stage

Ingested

Excysts in duodenum

Metacercaria on water plants

Cercaria free swimming

Penetrates intestinal wall

Migrates to bile duct

Adult in bile duct

Sporocyst/redia in snail tissue

Miracidium penetrates snail

Unembryonated egg in feces

Embryonated egg in water

Diagnostic stage

Clinical Case 84-1. Fascioliasis

Echenique-Elizondo and colleagues (JOP 6:36-39, 2005) described a case of acute pancreatitis due to the liver fluke *Fasciola hepatica*. The patient was a 31-year-old female who was admitted to the hospital because of a sudden onset of nausea and upper abdominal pain. She was otherwise healthy and gave a negative history of drug abuse, alcohol ingestion, gallstone disease, abdominal trauma or surgery. On physical exam, she was markedly tender in the epigastric region and had hypoactive bowel sounds. Serum chemistries showed elevated pancreatic enzymes (amylase, lipase, pancreatic phospholipase A2, and elastase). Her white blood count was elevated, as were tests for alkaline phosphatase and bilirubin. Serum blood urea nitrogen, creatinine, LDH and calcium were normal. Abdominal ultrasonography and CT scan showed diffuse enlargement of the pancreas, and a cholangiogram demonstrated dilatation and numerous filling defects in the common bile duct. An endoscopic sphincterotomy was performed, with extraction of numerous large flukes that were identified as *F. hepatica*. The patient was treated with a single oral dose of triclabendazole (10 mg/kg). Follow-up demonstrated normal blood chemistries and no evidence of disease 2 years postprocedure.

Opisthorchis sinensis

Physiology and Structure

O. sinensis, also referred to as *Clonorchis sinensis* in the older literature, is commonly called the **Chinese liver fluke**. (Figure 84-4) illustrates its life cycle, which involves two intermediate hosts. This trematode differs from other fluke cycles in that the eggs are eaten by the snail, and then reproduction begins in the soft tissues of the snail. *O. sinensis* also requires a second intermediate host, freshwater fish, where the cercariae encyst and develop into infective metacercariae. When uncooked freshwater fish harboring metacercariae are eaten, flukes develop first in the duodenum and then migrate to the bile ducts, where they become adults. The adult fluke undergoes self-fertilization and begins producing eggs. *O. sinensis* may survive in the biliary tract for as long as 50 years, producing approximately 2000 eggs per day. These eggs pass with feces and are once again eaten by snails, reinitiating the cycle.

Epidemiology

O. sinensis is found in China, Japan, Korea, and Vietnam, where it is estimated to infect approximately 19 million people. It is one of the most frequent infections seen among Asian refugees, and it can be traced to the consumption of raw, pickled, smoked, or dried freshwater fish that harbor the viable metacercariae. Dogs, cats, and fish-eating mammals can also serve as reservoir hosts.

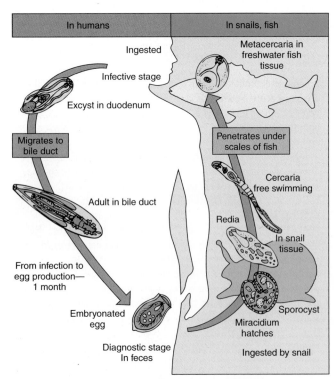

Figure 84–4. Life cycle of *Opisthorchis sinensis* (Chinese liver fluke).

Clinical Case 84-2. Cholangitis Due to *Clonorchis (Opisthorchis) sinensis*

Stunell, et al (Eur Radiol 16:2612-2614, 2006) describe a 34-year-old Asian woman who presented to a local emergency department with a 2-day history of right upper quadrant abdominal pain, fever, and rigors. She had emigrated from Asia to Ireland 18 months before and gave a history of intermittent upper abdominal pain occurring over a 3-year period. On examination, she appeared acutely ill and was clammy to the touch. She was febrile, tachycardic, and had mild scleral icterus. Her abdomen was tender, with guarding in the right upper quadrant. Routine hematologic and biochemical studies revealed a marked leukocytosis and obstructive liver function tests. Contrast-enhanced CT of the abdomen demonstrated evidence of multiple ovoid opacities within dilated intrahepatic bile ducts in the right lobe of the liver. The remainder of the liver parenchyma appeared normal. Upon stabilization of the patient, an endoscopic retrograde cholangiopancreatography (ERCP) was performed for biliary decompression. ERCP demonstrated intra- and extrahepatic bile duct dilatation, with multiple filling defects and strictures. A stool sample sent for analysis confirmed the presence of ova and adult flukes of *Clonorchis (Opisthorchis) sinensis*. The patient recovered with medical management (praziquantel) and had negative stool samples 30 days after treatment. This case, as well as Case 84-1, demonstrates the various complications of liver fluke infestation. Notably, praziquantel is the drug of choice for treating the Oriental liver fluke (*Clonorchis sinensis*), whereas triclabendazole is used to treat fascioliasis, thus emphasizing the importance of an epidemiologic history and identification of the fluke.

Clinical Syndromes (Clinical Case 84-2)

Infection in humans is usually mild and asymptomatic. Severe infections with many flukes in the bile ducts produces fever, diarrhea, epigastric pain, hepatomegaly, anorexia, and occasionally jaundice. Biliary obstruction may occur, and chronic infection can result in adenocarcinoma of the bile ducts. Invasion of the gallbladder may produce cholecystitis, cholelithiasis, and impaired liver function, as well as liver abscesses.

Laboratory Diagnosis

The diagnosis is made by recovering the distinctive eggs from stool. The eggs measure 27 to 35 μm × 12 to 19 μm and are characterized by a distinct operculum with prominent shoulders and a tiny knob at the posterior (abopercular) pole (Figure 84-5). In mild infections, repeated examinations of stool or duodenal aspirates may be necessary. In acute symptomatic infection, there are usually eosinophilia and an elevation of serum alkaline phosphatase levels. Radiographic imaging procedures may detect abnormalities of the biliary tract.

Figure 84–5. *Opisthorchis sinensis* egg. These ovoid eggs are small (27 to 35 μm long and 12 to 19 μm wide) and have a yellowish brown, thick shell with a prominent operculum at one end and a small knob at the other. *(From Marler LM, et al: Parasitology CD-ROM, Indiana Pathology Images, 2003.)*

Treatment, Prevention, and Control

The drug of choice is praziquantel. Prevention of infection is accomplished by not eating uncooked fish and by implementing proper sanitation policies, including the disposal of human, dog, and cat feces in adequately protected sites so that they cannot contaminate water supplies with the intermediate snail and fish hosts.

Paragonimus westermani

Physiology and Structure

P. westermani, commonly called the **lung fluke**, is one of several species of *Paragonimus* that infect humans and many other animals. Figure 84-6 shows a familiar fluke life cycle from egg to snail to infective metacercaria. The infective stage occurs in a second intermediate host: the muscles and gills of freshwater crabs and crayfish. In humans who ingest infected meat, the larval worm hatches in the stomach and follows an extensive migration through the intestinal wall to the abdominal cavity, then through the diaphragm, and finally to the pleural cavity. Adult worms reside in the lungs and produce eggs that are liberated from ruptured bronchioles and appear in sputum or, when swallowed, in feces.

Epidemiology

Paragonimiasis occurs in many countries in Asia, Africa, India, and Latin America. It can be seen in refugees from Southeast Asia. Its prevalence is directly related to the consumption of uncooked freshwater crabs and crayfish. It is estimated that approximately 3 million people are infected with this lung fluke. As many as 1% of all Indochinese immigrants to the United States are infected with *P. westermani*.

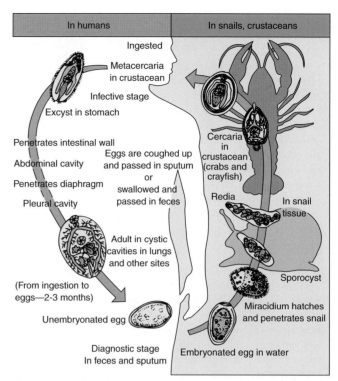

Figure 84–6. Life cycle of *Paragonimus westermani* (Oriental lung fluke).

A wide variety of shore-feeding animals (e.g., wild boars, pigs, and monkeys) serve as reservoir hosts, and some human infections result from ingestion of meat containing migrating larval worms from these reservoir hosts. Human infections endemic to the United States are usually caused by a related species, *P. kellicotti*, which is found in crabs and crayfish in eastern and midwestern waters.

Clinical Syndromes (Clinical Case 84-3)

The clinical manifestations of paragonimiasis may result from larvae migrating through tissues or from adults established in the lungs or other ectopic sites. The onset of disease coincides with larval migration and is associated with fever, chills, and high eosinophilia. The adult flukes in the lungs first produce an inflammatory reaction that results in fever, cough, and increased sputum. As the destruction of lung tissue progresses, cavitation occurs around the worms, sputum becomes blood tinged and dark with eggs (so-called *rusty sputum*), and patients experience severe chest pain. The resulting cavity may become secondarily infected with bacteria. Dyspnea, chronic bronchitis, bronchiectasis, and pleural effusion may be seen. Chronic infections lead to fibrosis in the lung tissue. The location of larvae, adults, and eggs in ectopic sites may produce severe clinical symptoms depending on the site involved. The migration of larval worms may result in invasion of the spinal cord and brain, producing severe neurologic disease (visual problems, motor weakness, and convulsive seizures) referred to as **cerebral paragonimiasis**. Migration and infection may also occur in subcutaneous sites, the abdominal cavity, and the liver.

Figure 84—5. *Opisthorchis sinensis* egg. These ovoid eggs are small (27 to 35 μm long and 12 to 19 μm wide) and have a yellowish brown, thick shell with a prominent operculum at one end and a small knob at the other. *(From Marler LM, et al: Parasitology CD-ROM, Indiana Pathology Images, 2003.)*

Treatment, Prevention, and Control

The drug of choice is praziquantel. Prevention of infection is accomplished by not eating uncooked fish and by implementing proper sanitation policies, including the disposal of human, dog, and cat feces in adequately protected sites so that they cannot contaminate water supplies with the intermediate snail and fish hosts.

Paragonimus westermani

Physiology and Structure

P. westermani, commonly called the **lung fluke**, is one of several species of *Paragonimus* that infect humans and many other animals. Figure 84-6 shows a familiar fluke life cycle from egg to snail to infective metacercaria. The infective stage occurs in a second intermediate host: the muscles and gills of freshwater crabs and crayfish. In humans who ingest infected meat, the larval worm hatches in the stomach and follows an extensive migration through the intestinal wall to the abdominal cavity, then through the diaphragm, and finally to the pleural cavity. Adult worms reside in the lungs and produce eggs that are liberated from ruptured bronchioles and appear in sputum or, when swallowed, in feces.

Epidemiology

Paragonimiasis occurs in many countries in Asia, Africa, India, and Latin America. It can be seen in refugees from Southeast Asia. Its prevalence is directly related to the consumption of uncooked freshwater crabs and crayfish. It is estimated that approximately 3 million people are infected with this lung fluke. As many as 1% of all Indochinese immigrants to the United States are infected with *P. westermani*.

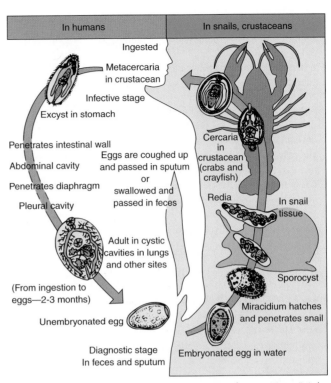

Figure 84—6. Life cycle of *Paragonimus westermani* (Oriental lung fluke).

A wide variety of shore-feeding animals (e.g., wild boars, pigs, and monkeys) serve as reservoir hosts, and some human infections result from ingestion of meat containing migrating larval worms from these reservoir hosts. Human infections endemic to the United States are usually caused by a related species, *P. kellicotti*, which is found in crabs and crayfish in eastern and midwestern waters.

Clinical Syndromes (Clinical Case 84-3)

The clinical manifestations of paragonimiasis may result from larvae migrating through tissues or from adults established in the lungs or other ectopic sites. The onset of disease coincides with larval migration and is associated with fever, chills, and high eosinophilia. The adult flukes in the lungs first produce an inflammatory reaction that results in fever, cough, and increased sputum. As the destruction of lung tissue progresses, cavitation occurs around the worms, sputum becomes blood tinged and dark with eggs (so-called *rusty sputum*), and patients experience severe chest pain. The resulting cavity may become secondarily infected with bacteria. Dyspnea, chronic bronchitis, bronchiectasis, and pleural effusion may be seen. Chronic infections lead to fibrosis in the lung tissue. The location of larvae, adults, and eggs in ectopic sites may produce severe clinical symptoms depending on the site involved. The migration of larval worms may result in invasion of the spinal cord and brain, producing severe neurologic disease (visual problems, motor weakness, and convulsive seizures) referred to as **cerebral paragonimiasis**. Migration and infection may also occur in subcutaneous sites, the abdominal cavity, and the liver.

Clinical Case 84-3. Paragonimiasis

Singh, et al (Indian J Med Microbiol 23:131-134, 2005) describe a case of pleuropulmonary paragonimiasis mimicking pulmonary tuberculosis. The patient was a 21-year-old man who was admitted to the hospital for progressive dyspnea, with a 1-month history of headache, fever, cough with scant hemoptysis, fatigue, pleuritic pain, anorexia, and weight loss. He had a history of antituberculous therapy for 6 months without improvement clinically. Two months prior to admission, after ingesting three raw crabs, he had a 3-day episode of watery diarrhea. On hospital admission, the patient was cachectic and afebrile. There was bilateral dullness to percussion and absent breath sounds in the lower two thirds of the chest. He was found to be anemic and had clubbing without lymphadenopathy, cyanosis, of jaundice. A chest radiograph showed bilateral pleural effusions that were also confirmed by CT. Ultrasound-guided thoracentesis of the right lung yielded about 200 ml of yellowish fluid. The fluid was exudative and contained 2700 WBC per ml, 91% of which were eosinophils. Gram stain of the fluid was negative, as was culture for bacteria and fungi. Sputum smears revealed operculated yellowish eggs consistent with *Paragonimus westermani* infection. The patient was treated with a 3-day course of praziquantel and responded well. Notably, the right-sided plural effusion did not recur after the thoracentesis and praziquantel treatment. This case emphasizes the importance of making an etiologic diagnosis of a pleuropulmonary process in order to differentiate paragonimiasis from tuberculosis in regions where both are endemic infectious diseases.

Laboratory Diagnosis

Examination of sputum and feces reveals golden brown, operculated eggs (Figure 84-7). Pleural effusions, when present, should be examined for eggs. Chest x-ray films often show infiltrates, nodular cysts, and pleural effusion. Marked eosinophilia is common. Serologic procedures are available through reference laboratories and can be helpful,

particularly in cases with extrapulmonary (e.g., central nervous system) involvement.

Treatment, Prevention, and Control

The drug of choice is triclabendazole; praziquantel is an alternative. Education regarding the consumption of uncooked freshwater crabs and crayfish, as well as the flesh of animals found in endemic areas, is critical. Pickling and wine soaking of crabs and crayfish do not kill the infective metacercarial stage. Proper sanitation and control of the disposal of human feces are essential.

Schistosomes

Schistosomiasis is a major parasitic infection of tropical areas, with some 200 million infections worldwide. The three schistosomes most frequently associated with human disease are *Schistosoma mansoni*, *S. japonicum*, and *S. haematobium*. They collectively produce the disease called **schistosomiasis**, also known as **bilharziasis or snail fever**. As discussed earlier, the schistosomes differ from other flukes: they are male and female rather than hermaphroditic, and their eggs do not have an operculum. They also are obligate intravascular parasites and are not found in cavities, ducts, and other tissues. The infective forms are skin-penetrating **cercariae** liberated from snails, and these differ from other flukes in that they are not eaten on vegetation, in fish, or in crustaceans.

Figure 84-8 illustrates the life cycle of the different schistosomes. Infection is initiated by ciliated, free-swimming cercaria in fresh water that penetrate intact skin, enter the circulation, and develop in the intrahepatic portal circulation (*S. mansoni* and *S. japonicum*) or in the vesical, prostatic, rectal, and uterine plexuses and veins (*S. haematobium*). The female has a long, slender, cylindrical body, whereas the shorter male, which appears cylindrical, is actually flat. The cylindrical appearance derives from folding the sides of the body to produce a groove, the gynecophoral canal, in which the female resides for fertilization. Both sexes have oral and ventral suckers and an incomplete digestive system, which is typical of a fluke.

As the worms develop in the portal circulation, they elaborate a remarkable defense against host resistance. They coat themselves with substances that the host recognizes as itself; consequently, there is little host response directed against their presence in blood vessels. This protective mechanism accounts for chronic infections that may last 20 to 30 years or longer.

After developing in the portal vein, the male and female adult worms pair up and migrate to their final locations, where fertilization and egg production begin. *S. mansoni* and *S. japonicum* are found in mesenteric veins and produce intestinal schistosomiasis; *S. haematobium* occurs in veins around the urinary bladder and causes vesicular

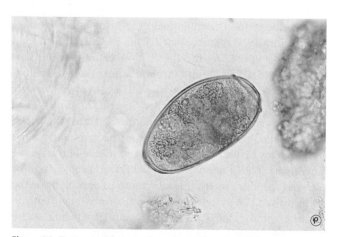

Figure 84—7. *Paragonimus westermani* egg. These large, ovoid eggs (80 to 120 μm long and 45 to 70 μm wide) have a thick, yellowish brown shell and a distinct operculum. *(From Marler LM, et al: Parasitology CD-ROM, Indiana Pathology Images, 2003.)*

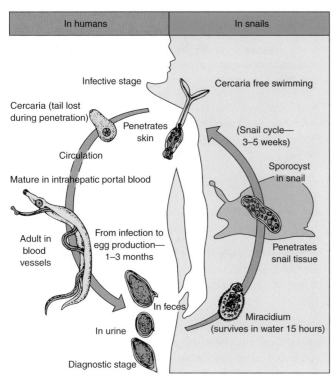

Figure 84—8. Life cycle of schistosomes.

In humans | In snails

Infective stage

Cercaria (tail lost during penetration)

Penetrates skin

Circulation

Mature in intrahepatic portal blood

Adult in blood vessels

From infection to egg production— 1–3 months

In feces

In urine

Diagnostic stage

Cercaria free swimming

(Snail cycle— 3–5 weeks)

Sporocyst in snail

Penetrates snail tissue

Miracidium (survives in water 15 hours)

schistosomiasis. On reaching the submucosal venules of their respective locations, the worms initiate oviposition, which may continue at the rate of 300 to 3000 eggs daily for 4 to 35 years. Although the host inflammatory response to the adult worms is minimal, the eggs elicit an intense inflammatory reaction, with mononuclear and polymorphonuclear cellular infiltrates and the formation of microabscesses. In addition, the larvae inside the eggs produce enzymes that aid in tissue destruction and allow the eggs to pass through the mucosa and into the lumen of the bowel and bladder, where they are passed to the external environment in the feces and urine, respectively.

The eggs hatch quickly on reaching fresh water to release motile **miracidia**. The miracidia then invade the appropriate snail host, where they develop into thousands of infectious cercariae. The free-swimming cercariae are released into the water, where they are immediately infectious for humans and other mammals.

The infection is similar in all three species of human schistosomes, in that disease results primarily from the host's immune response to the eggs. The very earliest signs and symptoms are due to the penetration of the cercariae through the skin. Immediate and delayed hypersensitivity to parasite antigens result in an intensely pruritic papular skin rash.

The onset of oviposition results in a symptom complex known as **Katayama syndrome**, which is marked by fever, chills, cough, urticaria, arthralgias, lymphadenopathy, splenomegaly, and abdominal pain. This syndrome is typically seen 1 to 2 months after primary exposure and may persist for 3 months or more. It is thought to result from the

massive release of parasite antigens, with subsequent immune complex formation. Associated laboratory abnormalities include leukocytosis, eosinophilia, and polyclonal gammopathy.

The more chronic and significant phase of schistosomiasis is due to the presence of eggs in various tissues and the resulting formation of granulomas and fibrosis. The retained eggs induce extensive inflammation and scarring, the clinical significance of which is directly related to the location and number of eggs.

Because of differences in some aspects of disease and epidemiology, these worms are discussed as separate species.

Schistosoma mansoni

Physiology and Structure

S. mansoni usually resides in the small branches of the inferior mesenteric vein near the lower colon. The species of *Schistosoma* can be differentiated by their characteristic egg morphology (Figures 84-9 to 84-11). The eggs of *S. mansoni* are oval, possess a sharp lateral spine, and measure 115 to 175 μm × 45 to 70 μm (see Figure 84-9).

Epidemiology

The geographical distribution of the various species of *Schistosoma* depends on the availability of a suitable snail host. *S. mansoni* is the most widespread of the schistosomes and is endemic in Africa, Saudi Arabia, and Madagascar. It has also become well established in the western hemisphere, particularly in Brazil, Suriname, Venezuela, parts

Figure 84—9. *Schistosoma mansoni* egg. These eggs are 115 to 175 μm long and 45 to 70 μm wide, contain a miracidium, and are enclosed in a thin shell with a prominent lateral spine.

Figure 84–10. *Schistosoma japonicum* egg. These eggs are smaller than those of *Schistosoma mansoni* (70 to 100 μm long and 55 to 65 μm wide) and have a spine that is inconspicuous. *(From Marler LM, et al: Parasitology CD-ROM, Indiana Pathology Images, 2003.)*

of the West Indies, and Puerto Rico. Cases originating in these areas may present in the United States. In all of these areas, there are also reservoir hosts, specifically primates, marsupials, and rodents. Schistosomiasis may be considered a disease of economic progress; the development of massive land irrigation projects in desert and tropical areas has resulted in the dispersion of infected humans and snails to previously uninvolved areas.

Clinical Syndromes (Clinical Case 84-4)

As noted before, cercarial penetration of intact skin may be seen as dermatitis with allergic reactions, pruritus, and

Figure 84–11. *Schistosoma haematobium* egg. These eggs are similar in size to those of *Schistosoma mansoni* but can be differentiated by the presence of a terminal, rather than lateral, spine.

Clinical Case 84-4. Schistosomiasis

Ferrari (Medicine [Baltimore] 78:176-190, 1999) described a case of neuroschistosomiasis due to *Schistosoma mansoni* in an 18-year-old Brazilian man. The patient was admitted to the hospital because of the recent onset of paraplegia. He was in good health until 33 days prior to admission, when he noted the onset of progressive low back pain with radiation to the lower limbs. During this period, he was evaluated three times in another institution, where x-ray films of the lower thoracic, lumbar, and sacral spine were normal. He received antiinflammatory agents, with only transient relief in his symptoms. Four weeks after the pain began, the disease progressed acutely with sexual impotence, fecal and urinary retention, and paraparesis progressing to paraplegia. At this time, the pain disappeared, replaced by a marked impairment of sensation in the lower limbs. On admission to the hospital, he gave a history of exposure to schistosomal infection. Neurologic examination revealed flaccid paraplegia, marked sensory loss, and absence of superficial and deep reflexes at and below the level T11. The CSF contained 84 WBC/mm^3 (98% lymphocytes, 2% eosinophils) and 1 red blood cell, 82 mg/dL total protein, and 61 mg/dL glucose. Myelography, CT-myelography, and magnetic resonance imaging (MRI) showed a slight widening of the conus. The diagnosis of neuroschistosomiasis was confirmed by the demonstration of viable and dead eggs of *S. mansoni* on rectal mucosal biopsy. The concentration of CSF IgG against soluble egg antigen of *S. mansoni* quantitated by ELISA was 1.53 μg/ml. He was treated with prednisone and praziquantel. Despite therapy, his condition remained unaltered at follow-up 7 months later. *S. mansoni* is the most frequently reported cause of schistosomal myeloradiculopathy (SMR) worldwide. SMR is among the most severe forms of schistosomiasis, and prognosis depends largely on early diagnosis and treatment.

edema. Migrating worms in the lungs may produce cough; as they reach the liver, hepatitis may appear.

Infections with *S. mansoni* may produce hepatic and intestinal abnormalities. As the flukes take up residence in the mesenteric vessels and egg laying begins, fever, malaise, abdominal pain, and tenderness of the liver may be observed. Deposition of eggs in the bowel mucosa results in inflammation and thickening of the bowel wall with associated abdominal pain, diarrhea, and blood in the stool. Eggs may be carried by the portal vein to the liver, where inflammation can lead to periportal fibrosis and eventually to portal hypertension and its associated manifestations.

Chronic infection with *S. mansoni* produces a dramatic hepatosplenomegaly with large accumulations of ascitic fluid in the peritoneal cavity. On gross examination, the liver is studded with white granulomas (pseudotubercles). Although *S. mansoni* eggs are primarily deposited in the intestine, eggs may appear in the spinal cord, lungs, and other sites. A similar fibrotic process occurs at each site. Severe neurologic problems may follow when eggs are deposited in the spinal cord and brain. In fatal schistosomiasis caused by *S. mansoni*, fibrous tissue, reacting to the eggs in the liver, surrounds the portal vein in a thick, grossly visible layer ("**clay pipestem fibrosis**").

Laboratory Diagnosis

The diagnosis of schistosomiasis is usually established by the demonstration of characteristic eggs in feces. Stool examination reveals the large golden eggs with a sharp lateral spine (see Figure 84-9). Concentration techniques may be necessary in light infections. Using rectal biopsy, the clinician can see the egg tracks laid by the worms in rectal vessels. Quantitation of egg output in stool is useful in estimating the severity of infection and in following the response to therapy. Serologic tests are also available but are largely of epidemiologic interest only. The development of newer tests using stage-specific antigens may allow the distinction of active from inactive disease and thus have greater clinical application.

Treatment, Prevention, and Control

The drug of choice is praziquantel, and the alternative is oxamniquine. Anthelmintic therapy may terminate oviposition but does not affect lesions caused by eggs already deposited in tissues. **Schistosomal dermatitis** and Katayama syndrome may be treated with the administration of antihistamines and corticosteroids. Education regarding the life cycles of these worms and molluscacide control of snails are essential. Improved sanitation and control of human fecal deposits are critical. Mass treatment may one day be practical, and the development of a vaccine may be forthcoming.

Schistosoma japonicum

Physiology and Structure

S. japonicum resides in branches of the superior mesenteric vein around the small intestine and in the inferior mesenteric vessels. S. japonicum eggs (see Figure 84-10) are smaller, are almost spherical, and possess a tiny spine. These eggs are produced in greater numbers than those of S. mansoni and S. haematobium. Because of the size, shape, and numbers of these eggs, they are carried to more sites in the body (liver, lungs, brain), and infection with a few S. japonicum adults can be more severe than infections involving similar numbers of S. mansoni or S. haematobium.

Epidemiology

This **Oriental blood fluke** is found only in China, Japan, the Philippines, and on the island of Sulawesi, Indonesia. Epidemiologic problems correlate directly with a broad range of reservoir hosts, many of which are domestic (cats, dogs, cattle, horses, and pigs).

Clinical Syndromes

The initial stages of infection with S. japonicum are similar to those of S. mansoni, with dermatitis, allergic reactions, fever, and malaise, followed by abdominal discomfort and diarrhea. Katayama syndrome associated with the onset of oviposition is observed more commonly with S. japonicum than with S. mansoni. In chronic S. japonicum infection, hepatosplenic disease, portal hypertension, bleeding esophageal varices, and accumulation of ascitic fluid are commonly seen. Granulomas that appear as pseudotubercles in and on the liver are common, along with the clay pipestem fibrosis as described for S. mansoni.

S. japonicum frequently involves cerebral structures when eggs reach the brain and granulomas develop around them. The neurologic manifestations include lethargy, speech impairment, visual defects, and seizures.

Laboratory Diagnosis

Stool examination demonstrates the small, golden eggs with tiny spines; usually, rectal biopsy is similarly revealing. Serologic tests are available.

Treatment, Prevention, and Control

The drug of choice is praziquantel. Prevention and control may be achieved by measures similar to those for S. mansoni, especially education of populations in endemic areas regarding proper water purification, sanitation, and control of human fecal deposits. Control of S. japonicum must also involve the broad range of reservoir hosts and consider the fact that people work in rice paddies and on irrigation projects where infected snails are present. Mass treatment may offer help, and a vaccine may be developed someday.

Schistosoma haematobium

Physiology and Structure

After development in the liver, these blood flukes migrate to the vesical, prostatic, and uterine plexuses of the venous circulation, occasionally the portal bloodstream, and only rarely other venules.

Large eggs with a sharp terminal spine (see Figure 84-11) are deposited in the wall of the bladder and occasionally in the uterine and prostatic tissues. Those deposited in the bladder wall can break free and are found in urine.

Epidemiology

S. haematobium occurs throughout the Nile Valley and in many other parts of Africa, including islands off the eastern coast. It also appears in Asia Minor, Cyprus, southern Portugal, and India. Reservoir hosts include monkeys, baboons, and chimpanzees.

Clinical Syndromes

Early stages of infection with *S. haematobium* are similar to those of infections involving *S. mansoni* and *S. japonicum*, with dermatitis, allergic reactions, fever, and malaise. Unlike the other two schistosomes, *S. haematobium* produces hematuria, dysuria, and urinary frequency as early symptoms. Associated with hematuria, bacteriuria is frequently a chronic condition. Egg deposition in the walls of the bladder may eventually result in scarring, with loss of bladder capacity and the development of obstructive uropathy.

Patients with *S. haematobium* infections involving many flukes frequently demonstrate squamous cell carcinoma of the bladder. It is commonly stated that the leading cause of cancer of the bladder in Egypt and other parts of Africa is *S. haematobium*. The granulomas and pseudotubercles seen in the bladder may also be present in the lungs. Fibrosis of the pulmonary bed caused by egg deposition leads to dyspnea, cough, and hemoptysis.

Laboratory Diagnosis

Examination of urine specimens reveals the large, terminally spined eggs. Occasionally, bladder biopsy is helpful in establishing the diagnosis. *S. haematobium* eggs may appear in stool if worms have migrated to mesenteric vessels. Serologic tests are also available.

Treatment, Prevention, and Control

The drug of choice is praziquantel. At present, education, possible mass treatment, and development of a vaccine are the best approaches to the control of *S. haematobium* disease. The basic problems of irrigation projects (e.g., dam building), migratory human populations, and multiple reservoir hosts make prevention and control extremely difficult.

Cercarial Dermatitis

Several nonhuman schistosomes have cercariae that penetrate human skin, producing a severe dermatitis (**"swimmer's itch"**), but these schistosomes cannot develop into adult worms. The natural hosts are birds and other shore-feeding animals from freshwater lakes throughout the world and a few marine beaches. The intense pruritus and urticaria from this skin penetration may lead to secondary bacterial infection from scratching the sites of infection.

Treatment consists of oral trimeprazine and topical applications of palliative agents. When indicated, sedatives may be given. Control is difficult because of bird migration and the transfer of live snails from lake to lake. Molluscacides such as copper sulfate have produced some reduction in the snail populations. Immediate drying of the skin when people leave such waters offers some protection.

Case Study and Questions

A 45-year-old Egyptian man was referred for evaluation of hematuria and urinary frequency of 2 months' duration. This individual had lived in the Middle East for most of his life but for the past year lived in the United States. He denied previous renal or urologic problems. His physical examination was unremarkable. A midstream urine specimen was grossly bloody.

1. What was the differential diagnosis of hematuria in this patient?
2. What was the etiologic agent of this patient's urologic process?
3. What exposures might put an individual at risk for this infection?
4. What are the major complications of this infection?
5. How is this disease treated?

Bibliography

Connor DH, et al: Pathology of Infectious Diseases, vol 2. Stamford, Conn, Appleton & Lange, 1997.

Garcia LS: Diagnostic Medical Parasitology, 4th ed, Washington, DC, ASM Press, 2001.

Jones MK, McManus DP: Trematodes. In Murray PR, et al (eds): Manual of Clinical Microbiology, 9th ed. Washington, DC, ASM Press. 2007.

Keiser J, Utzinger J: Emerging foodborne trematodiasis. Emerg Infect Dis 11:1507-1514, 2005.

Markell EK, John DT, Krotoski WA: Markell and Voges' Medical Parasitology, 8th ed. Philadelphia, WB Saunders, 1999.

Meltzer E, et al: Schistosomiasis among travelers: New aspects of an old disease. Emerg Infect Dis 12:1696-1700, 2006.

Strickland GT: Hunter's Tropical Medicine and Emerging Infectious Diseases. Philadelphia, WB Saunders, 2000.

Cestodes

The bodies of cestodes, **tapeworms**, are flat and ribbon-like, and the heads are equipped with organs of attachment. The head, or **scolex**, of the worm usually has four muscular, cup-shaped suckers and a crown of hooklets. An exception is *Diphyllobothrium latum*, the fish tapeworm, whose scolex is equipped with a pair of long, lateral, muscular grooves and lacks hooklets.

The individual segments of tapeworms are called **proglottids**, and the chain of proglottids is called a **strobila**. As new proglottids develop, existing ones mature as they become more distal. The more distal proglottids are gravid, almost completely occupied by a uterus full of eggs, which are passed with the stools of the carrier, either inside completed proglottids or free after proglottid breakage. Differentiation of the various adult cestodes may be accomplished by examination of the structure of shed proglottids (length, width, number of uterine branches) or (more rarely) of the scolex (number and placement of suckers, presence/absence of hooklets).

All tapeworms are hermaphroditic, with male and female reproductive organs present in each mature proglottid. The eggs of most tapeworms are nonoperculated and contain a six-hooked **hexacanth embryo**; the one exception, *D. latum*, has an unembryonated, operculated egg similar to fluke eggs. Tapeworms have no digestive system, and food is absorbed from the host intestine through the soft body wall of the worm. Most tapeworms found in the human intestine have complex life cycles involving intermediate hosts, and in some instances (cysticercosis, echinococcosis, sparganosis) humans serve as a form of intermediate host that harbors larval stages. The presence of extraintestinal larvae are at times more serious than that of adult worms in the intestine. The most common cestodes of medical importance are listed in Table 85-1.

Taenia solium

Physiology and Structure

The larval stage, or cysticercus ("bladder worm"), of *Taenia* species consists of a scolex, which is invaginated into a fluid-filled bladder. Larval cysts develop in the tissues of the intermediate host, are 4 to 6 mm long × 7 to 11 mm wide and have a pearl-like appearance in the tissues. After a person ingests pork muscle containing a larval worm, attachment of the scolex with its four muscular suckers and crown of hooklets initiates infection in the small intestine (Figure 85-1). The worm then produces proglottids until a strobila of proglottids is developed, which may be several meters in length. The sexually mature proglottids contain eggs, and as these proglottids leave the host in feces, they can contaminate water and vegetation ingested by swine. The gravid proglottids have a similar length and width (1 cm × 1 cm) and contain few (<12) lateral uterine branches. The eggs in swine become a six-hooked larval form called an *oncosphere* that penetrates the pig's intestinal wall, migrates in the circulation to the tissues, and becomes a cysticercus to complete the cycle.

Epidemiology

T. solium infection is directly correlated with eating insufficiently cooked pork and is prevalent in Africa, India, Southeast Asia, China, Mexico, Latin American countries, and Slavic countries. It is seen infrequently in the United States.

Clinical Syndromes

Adult *T. solium* in the intestine seldom causes appreciable symptoms. The intestine may be irritated at sites of attachment, and abdominal discomfort, chronic indigestion, and diarrhea may occur. Most patients become aware of the infection only when they see proglottids or a strobila of proglottids in their feces.

Laboratory Diagnosis

Stool examination may reveal proglottids and eggs, and treatment may produce the entire worm for identification.

Table 85–1. Medically Important Cestodes

Cestode	Common Name	Reservoir for Larvae	Reservoir for Adults
Taenia solium	Pork tapeworm Cysticercosis	Hogs Humans	Humans —
Taenia saginata	Beef tapeworm	Cattle	Humans
Diphyllobothrium latum	Fish tapeworm	Freshwater crustaceans and fish	Humans, dogs, cats, bears
Echinococcus granulosus	Unilocular hydatid cyst	Herbivores, humans	Canines
Echinococcus multilocularis	Alveolar hydatid cyst	Herbivores, humans	Foxes, wolves, dogs, cats
Hymenolepis nana	Dwarf tapeworm	Rodents, humans	Rodents, humans
Hymenolepis diminuta	Dwarf tapeworm	Insects	Rodents, humans
Dipylidium caninum	Pumpkin seed tapeworm	Fleas	Dogs, cats

The eggs are spherical, are 30 to 40 μm in diameter, and possess a thick, radially striated shell containing a six-hooked hexacanth embryo (Figure 85-2). The eggs are identical to those of *T. saginata* (**beef tapeworm**), so eggs alone are not sufficient for species identification. Critical examination of the proglottids reveals their internal structure, which is important for the differentiation of *T. solium* and *T. saginata*. Gravid proglottids of *T. solium* are smaller than those of *T. saginata* and contain only 7 to 12 lateral uterine branches, compared to 15 to 30 for the beef tapeworm.

Treatment, Prevention, and Control

The drug of choice is niclosamide. Praziquantel, paromomycin, or quinacrine are effective alternatives. Prevention of **pork tapeworm** infections requires that pork be either cooked until the interior of the meat is gray or frozen at −20° C for at least 12 hours. Sanitation is critical; every effort must be made to keep human feces containing *T. solium* eggs out of water and vegetation ingested by pigs.

Cysticercosis

Physiology and Structure

Cysticercosis involves infection of people with the larval stage of *T. solium*, the cysticercus, which normally infects pigs (Figure 85-3). Human ingestion of water or vegetation contaminated with *T. solium* eggs from human feces initiates the infection. Autoinfection may occur when eggs

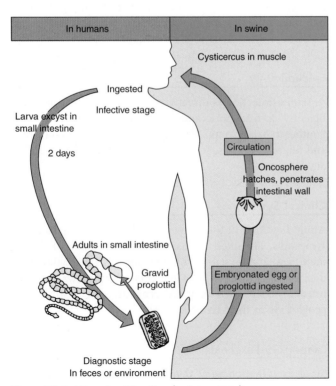

Figure 85–1. Life cycle of *T. solium* (pork tapeworm).

Figure 85–2. *Taenia* egg. The eggs are spherical, 30 to 40 μm in diameter, and contain three pairs of hooklets internally. The eggs of the different *Taenia* species cannot be differentiated.

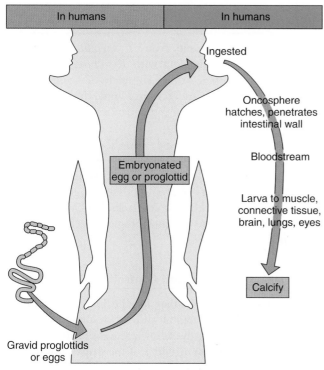

Figure 85—3. Development of human cysticercosis.

from a person infected with the adult worm are transferred from the perianal area to the mouth on contaminated fingers. Once ingested, the eggs hatch in the stomach of the intermediate host, releasing the hexacanth embryo or **oncosphere**. The oncosphere penetrates the intestinal wall and migrates in the circulation to the tissues, where it develops into a cysticercus over 3 to 4 months. The cysticerci may develop in muscle, connective tissue, brain, lungs, and eyes and remain viable for as long as 5 years.

Epidemiology

Cysticercosis is found in the areas where *T. solium* is prevalent and is directly correlated with human fecal contamination. In addition to fecal-oral transmission, autoinfection may occur when a proglottid containing eggs is regurgitated from the small intestine into the stomach, allowing the eggs to hatch and release the infectious oncosphere.

Clinical Syndromes

A few cysticerci in nonvital areas (e.g., subcutaneous tissues) may not provoke symptoms, but serious disease may follow as the cysticerci lodge in vital areas such as the brain and eyes. In the brain, they may produce hydrocephalus, meningitis, cranial nerve damage, seizures, hyperactive reflexes, and visual defects (Clinical Case 85-1). In the eye, loss of visual acuity may occur, and if the larvae lodge along the optic tract, visual field defects result. Tissue reaction to viable larvae may be only moderate, thus minimizing symptoms. However, death of the larvae results in the release of antigenic material that stimulates a marked inflammatory reaction; exacerbation of symptoms can result in fever, muscle pains, and eosinophilia.

Laboratory Diagnosis

The presence of cysticerci is usually established by the appearance of calcified cysticerci in soft-tissue roentgenograms, surgical removal of subcutaneous nodules, and visualization of cysts in the eye. Central nervous system lesions may be detected by computed tomography, radioisotope scanning, or ultrasonography. Serologic studies may be useful; false-positive results may occur in people with other helminthic infections.

Treatment, Prevention, and Control

The drug of choice for cysticercosis is either praziquantel or albendazole. Concomitant steroid administration may be necessary to minimize the inflammatory response to dying larvae. Surgical removal of cerebral and ocular cysts may be necessary. Critical to the prevention and control of human infection are the treatment of human cases harboring adult *T. solium* (to reduce egg transmission) and the controlled disposal of human feces. These measures also reduce the likelihood of infection in pigs.

Taenia saginata

Physiology and Structure

The life cycle of *T. saginata*, the beef tapeworm, is similar to that of *T. solium* (Figure 85-4), with infection resulting after cysticerci are ingested in insufficiently cooked beef. After excystment, the larvae develop into adults in the small intestine and initiate egg production in maturing proglottids. The adult worm may parasitize the jejunum and small intestine of humans for as long as 25 years, attaining a length of 10 m. In contrast with *T. solium* infections, cysticercosis produced by *T. saginata* does not occur in humans. The adult *T. saginata* worm also differs from *T. solium* in that it lacks a crown of hooklets on the scolex and has a different proglottid uterine branch structure. The gravid proglottids are longer than they are wide (18 to 20 mm × 5 to 7 mm) and contain 15 to 30 lateral uterine branches. These facts are important in differentiating between the two tapeworms but do not affect therapy.

Epidemiology

T. saginata occurs worldwide and is one of the most frequent causes of cestode infections in the United States. Humans and cattle perpetuate the life cycle: human feces contaminate water and vegetation with eggs, which are then ingested by cattle. The cysticerci in cattle produce adult tapeworms in humans when rare or insufficiently cooked beef is eaten.

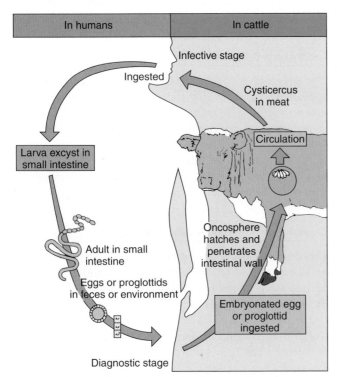

Figure 85—4. Life cycle of *T. saginata* (beef tapeworm).

Clinical Syndromes

The syndrome that results from *T. saginata* infection is similar to intestinal infection with *T. solium*. Patients are generally asymptomatic or may complain of vague abdominal pains, chronic indigestion, and hunger pains. Proglottids may pass out of the anus directly.

Laboratory Diagnosis

The diagnosis of *T. saginata* infection is similar to that of *T. solium*, with recovery of proglottids and eggs or recovery of an entire worm whose scolex lacks hooklets. Study of the uterine branches in the proglottids differentiates *T. saginata* from *T. solium*.

Treatment, Prevention, and Control

Treatment is identical to that for the intestinal phase of *T. solium*. Both praziquantel and niclosamide are highly effective in eliminating the adult worm. Education regarding cooking beef and controlling of the disposal of human feces is a critical measure.

Diphyllobothrium latum

Physiology and Structure

One of the largest tapeworms (20 to 30 feet long), *D. latum* (**fish tapeworm**) has a complex life cycle involving two intermediate hosts: freshwater crustaceans and freshwater fish (Figure 85-5). The ribbon-like larval worm in the flesh of freshwater fish is called a **sparganum**. Ingestion of this sparganum in raw or insufficiently cooked fish initiates infection. The scolex of *D. latum* is shaped like a lance and has long, lateral grooves (**bothria**), which serve as organs of attachment. The proglottids of *D. latum* are much wider than they are long (~8 by 4 mm), have a central uterine structure resembling a rosette, and produce eggs with an operculum (like fluke eggs) and a knob on the shell at the bottom of the egg. The adult worms may produce eggs for months or years. More than 1 million eggs per day are released into the fecal stream. On reaching fresh water, the unembryonated, operculate eggs require a period of 2 to 4 weeks to develop a ciliated, free-swimming larval form called a **coracidium**. The fully developed coracidium leaves the egg via the operculum and is ingested by tiny crustaceans that are called **copepods** (e.g., *Cyclops* and *Diaptomus* species); then the coracidium develops into a **procercoid** larval form. The crustacean harboring the larval stage is then eaten by a fish, and the infectious **plerocercoid**, or sparganum larvae, develop in the musculature of the fish. If the fish is in turn eaten by another fish, the sparganum simply migrates into the muscles of the second fish. Humans are infected when they eat raw or undercooked fish containing the larval forms.

Figure 85—5. Life cycle of *D. latum* (fish tapeworm).

In humans | In crustaceans, fish

Crustacean ingested by freshwater fish (development—2 weeks)

Ingested

Scolex attached to intestine

Adult in small intestine

Ingested by crustacean (development—3 weeks)

From infection to eggs—1 month

Coracidium

Undeveloped operculate egg

Diagnostic stage In feces

Mature egg (Undeveloped egg to coracidium—2-4 weeks)

Epidemiology

D. latum infection occurs worldwide, most prevalently in cool lake regions where raw or pickled fish is popular. Insufficient cooking over campfires and tasting and seasoning "gefilte fish" account for many infections. A reservoir of infected wild animals, such as bears, minks, walruses, and members of the canine and feline families that eat fish, are also sources for human infections. The practice of dumping raw sewage into freshwater lakes contributes to the propagation of this tapeworm.

Clinical Syndromes (Clinical Case 85-2)

Clinically, as is the case with most adult tapeworm infections, most *D. latum* infections are asymptomatic. Occasionally, people complain of epigastric pain, abdominal cramping, nausea, vomiting, and weight loss. As many as 40% of *D. latum* carriers may have low serum levels of vitamin B_{12}, presumably because of the competition between the host and the worm for dietary vitamin B_{12}. A small percentage (0.1% to 2%) of people infected with *D. latum* develop clinical signs of vitamin B_{12} deficiency, including megaloblastic anemia and neurologic manifestations such as numbness, paresthesia, and loss of vibration sense.

Laboratory Diagnosis

Stool examination reveals the bile-stained, operculated egg with its knob at the bottom of the shell (Figure 85-6).

Typical proglottids with the rosette uterine structure may also be found in stool specimens. Concentration techniques are usually not necessary, because the worms produce large numbers of ova.

Treatment, Prevention, and Control

The drug of choice is niclosamide; praziquantel and paromomycin are acceptable alternatives. Vitamin B_{12}

Figure 85—6. *D. latum* egg. Unlike other tapeworm eggs, *D. latum* eggs are operculated. They are 45×90 μm in size.

supplementation may be necessary in people with evidence of clinical vitamin B_{12} deficiency. The prevalence of this infection is reduced by avoiding the ingestion of insufficiently cooked fish, controlling the disposal of human feces, (especially the proper treatment of sewage before disposal in lakes), and promptly treating infections.

Sparganosis

Physiology and Structure

The larval forms of several tapeworms closely related to *D. latum* (most often *Spirometra* species) can produce human disease in subcutaneous sites and in the eye. In these cases, humans act as the end-stage host for the larval stage, or **sparganum**. Infections are acquired primarily by drinking pond or ditch water that contains crustaceans (copepods) that carry a larval tapeworm. This larval form penetrates the intestinal wall and migrates to various sites in the body, where it develops into a sparganum. Infections may also occur if tadpoles, frogs, and snakes are ingested raw or if the flesh of these animals is applied to wounds as a poultice. The larval worm leaves the relatively cold flesh of the dead animal and migrates into the warm human flesh.

Epidemiology

Cases have been reported from various parts of the world, including the United States, but the infection is most prevalent in the Orient. Regardless of location, drinking contaminated water and eating raw tadpole, frog, and snake flesh lead to infection.

Clinical Syndromes

In subcutaneous sites, **sparganosis** can produce painful inflammatory tissue reactions and nodules. In the eye, the tissue reaction is intensely painful, and periorbital edema is common. Corneal ulcers may develop with ocular involvement. Ocular disease is frequently associated with the use of frog or snake flesh as a poultice over a wound near the eye.

Laboratory Diagnosis

Sections of tissue removed surgically show characteristic tapeworm features, including highly convoluted parenchyma and dark-staining calcareous corpuscles.

Treatment, Prevention, and Control

Surgical removal is the customary approach. The drug praziquantel may be used; however, no clinical data support its efficacy. Education regarding possible contamination of drinking water with crustaceans that harbor larval

worms is essential, and contamination most likely occurs in pond and ditch water. Ingestion of raw frog and snake flesh or their use as poultices over wounds also should be avoided.

Echinococcus granulosus

Physiology and Structure

Infection with *E. granulosus* is another example of accidental human infection, with humans serving as dead-end intermediate hosts in a life cycle that occurs naturally in other animals. *E. granulosus* adult tapeworms are found in nature in the intestines of canines (dog, fox, wolf, coyote, jackal, dingo); the larval cyst stage is present in the viscera of herbivores (sheep, cattle, swine, deer, moose, elk) (Figure 85-7). The worm consists of a *Taenia*-like scolex with four sucking disks and a double row of hooklets, as well as a strobila containing three proglottids: one immature, one mature, and one gravid. Adult tapeworms in the canine intestine produce infective eggs that pass in feces. The eggs are identical in appearance to those of the *Taenia* species. When these eggs are ingested by humans, a six-hooked larval stage called an **oncosphere** hatches. The oncosphere penetrates the human intestinal wall and enters the circulation to be carried to various tissue sites, primarily the liver

Figure 85—7. Life cycle of *E. granulosus*.

and lungs but also the central nervous system and bone. This same cycle occurs in the viscera of herbivores. When the herbivore is killed by a canine predator or viscera is fed to canines, the ingestion of cysts produces adult tapeworms in the canine intestine to complete the cycle and initiate new egg production. Adult tapeworms do not develop in the intestines of herbivores or humans.

In humans, the larvae form a unilocular **hydatid cyst**, which is a slow-growing, tumor-like, and space-occupying structure enclosed by a laminated germinative membrane. This membrane produces structures on its wall called **brood capsules**, where tapeworm heads (**protoscolices**) develop. Daughter cysts may develop in the original mother cyst and also produce brood capsules and protoscolices. The cysts and daughter cysts accumulate fluid as they grow. This fluid is potentially toxic; if spilled into body cavities, anaphylactic shock and death can result. Spillage and the escape of protoscolices can lead to the development of cysts in other sites, because the protoscolices have the germinative potential to form new cysts. Eventually, the brood capsules and daughter cysts disintegrate within the mother cyst, liberating the accumulated protoscolices. These become known as **hydatid sand**. This type of echinococcus cyst is called a **unilocular cyst** to differentiate it from related cysts that grow differently. The unilocular cyst is generally about 5 cm in diameter, but some as large as 20 cm, containing almost 2 L of cyst fluid, have been reported. The cyst may die and become calcified over long periods.

Epidemiology

Human infection with *E. granulosus* unilocular cyst is directly correlated with raising sheep in many countries in Europe, South America, Africa, Asia, Australia, and New Zealand. It occurs in Canada and in the United States, with cases reported from Alaska, Utah, New Mexico, Arizona, California, and the lower Mississippi valley. Human infection follows ingestion of contaminated water or vegetation as well as hand-to-mouth transmission of canine feces carrying the infective eggs.

Clinical Syndromes (Clinical Case 85-3)

Because the unilocular cyst grows slowly, 5 to 20 years may pass before any symptoms appear. In many instances, it appears that the cyst is as old as its host. The pressure of the expanding cyst in an organ is usually the first sign of infection. In the majority of cases the cysts are located in the liver or lung. In the liver, the cyst may exert pressure on both bile ducts and blood vessels and create pain and biliary rupture. In the lungs, cysts may produce cough, dyspnea, and chest pains. Rupture of the cysts may occur in 20% of cases, producing fever, urticaria, and occasionally anaphylactic shock

---

Clinical Case 85-3. Echinococcosis

Yeh and colleagues (N Engl J Med 357:489-494, 2007) describe a 36-year-old pregnant woman at 21 weeks of gestation who presented with a 4-week history of a dry, nonproductive cough. The patient denied any constitutional symptoms, had no new pets, environmental exposures, or sick contacts. It was her first pregnancy, and there were no complications. She had no medical conditions and did not smoke or drink alcohol. She was a financial consultant and enjoyed running and hiking. She had traveled to Australia, Central Asia, and sub-Saharan Africa in the past. The patient appeared well, with appropriate weight gain for the second trimester of her pregnancy. Her physical examination, including auscultation of her lungs, was normal. Her cough did not improve with use of an inhaled bronchodilator. Imaging studies were not performed, because of her pregnancy. She had a normal, uncomplicated vaginal delivery 4 months later. She continued to have a dry cough and presented to her physician months after delivery for a reevaluation of her cough. At that time, her physical examination and laboratory studies were unremarkable. A chest radiograph revealed a soft-tissue mass, 7 cm in diameter, adjacent to the right heart border. High resolution CT scans of the chest confirmed the presence of a homogeneous and fluid-filled structure without septa, thought to be in the mediastinum. Subsequent echocardiography also confirmed a simple cystic structure with thin walls surrounding echo-free fluid that was indenting the right atrium. On the basis of the radiographic and echocardiography findings, the clinicians caring for the patient thought that the mass was most likely a benign pericardial cyst. Because she was not experiencing dyspnea, the patient declined surgical resection. However, due to worsening cough over the next few months, she consulted a thoracic surgeon for elective resection. Intraoperative findings revealed an intraparenchymal pulmonary cyst in the right lung that was not attached to the pericardium or bronchus. The cyst was removed intact without gross spillage of the contents. Staining of the cyst wall with hematoxylin and eosin after cross sectioning showed an acellular laminated layer. Microscopic examination of the cyst contents showed protoscolices with hooklets and suckers in a background of histiocytes and eosinophilic debris consistent with *Echinococcus granulosus*. CT of the abdomen after removal of the thoracic cyst revealed no hepatobiliary disease. Postoperative screening for serum antibody against *Echinococcus* was positive. Praziquantel was administered for 10 days after surgery and albendazole for 1 month after surgery, with no complications. After this course of therapy, the patient had resolution of her cough and returned to her normal level of activity. There was no evidence of recurrent disease on CT follow-up 6 months after surgery.

---

and death, which are caused by the release of antigenic cyst contents. Cyst rupture may also lead to dissemination of infection resulting from the release of thousands of protoscolices. In bone, the cyst is responsible for erosion of the marrow cavity and the bone itself. In the brain, severe damage may occur as a result of the cyst's tumor-like growth into brain tissue.

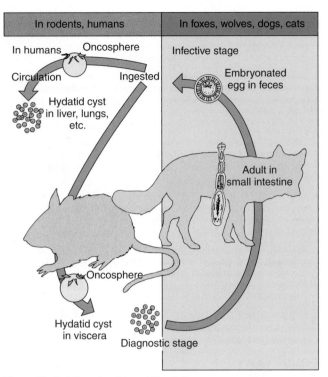

Figure 85—8. Life cycle of *E. multilocularis*.

Laboratory Diagnosis

The diagnosis of **hydatid disease** is difficult and depends primarily on clinical, radiographic, and serologic findings. Radiologic examination, scanning procedures, tomography, and ultrasound techniques are all valuable and may provide the first evidence of the cyst's presence. Aspiration of cyst contents may demonstrate the presence of the protoscolices (hydatid sand); however, it is contraindicated because of the risk of anaphylaxis and dissemination of the infection. Serologic testing may be useful, but results are negative in 10% to 40% of infections.

Treatment, Prevention, and Control

Surgical resection of the cyst is the treatment of choice. In some instances, the cyst is first aspirated to remove the fluid and hydatid sand, and then it is instilled with formalin to kill and detoxify remaining fluid; finally, it is rolled into a marsupial pouch and sewn shut. If the condition is inoperable because of the cyst's location, medical therapy with high-dose albendazole, mebendazole, or praziquantel may be considered. The most important factor in preventing and controlling **echinococcosis** is education regarding the transmission of infection and the role of canines in the life cycle. Proper personal hygiene and the washing of hands and cooking utensils in environments inhabited by dogs are critical. Dogs should not be allowed in the vicinity of animal slaughter and should never be fed the viscera of slain animals.

In some areas, the killing of stray dogs has reduced the incidence of infection.

Echinococcus multilocularis

Physiology and Structure

Like infection with *E. granulosus*, human infection with *E. multilocularis* is accidental (Figure 85-8). Adult *E. multilocularis* tapeworms are primarily found in foxes and wolves, although farm dogs and cats harbor them in some rural environments. The intermediate hosts that harbor the cyst stage are rodents (mice, voles, shrews, and lemmings). Humans become infected with the cyst stage as a result of contact with fox, dog, or cat feces contaminated with eggs. Trappers and workers who handle fur pelts may become infected by inhaling fecal dust that carries eggs.

Infective eggs hatch in and penetrate the intestinal tract to become oncospheres. These forms enter the circulation and take up residence primarily in the liver and lungs but also possibly in the brain.

The **alveolar hydatid cyst** develops as an alveolar or honeycombed structure that is not covered by a unilocular-limiting mother cyst—laminated membrane. The cyst grows via exogenous budding, eventually resembling a carcinoma.

Epidemiology

E. multilocularis is found primarily in northern areas such as Canada, the former Soviet Union, northern Japan, Central Europe, and Alaska, Montana, North and South Dakota, Minnesota, and Iowa in the United States. There is evidence that the life cycle may be extending to other Midwestern states, where foxes and mice transmit the organism to dogs and cats and eventually to humans.

Clinical Syndromes

E. multilocularis, because of its slow growth, may be present in human tissues for many years before symptoms appear. In the liver, cysts eventually mimic a carcinoma, with liver enlargement and obstruction of biliary and portal pathways. Often the growth metastasizes to the lungs and brain. Malnutrition, ascites, and portal hypertension produced by *E. multilocularis* create the appearance of hepatic cirrhosis. Among all of the worm infections of humans, *E. multilocularis* is one of the most lethal. If left untreated, the mortality rate is approximately 70% of infected people.

Laboratory Diagnosis

Unlike *E. granulosus*, the tissue form of *E. multilocularis* presents no protoscolices, and the material so resembles a neoplasm that even pathologists mistake it for carcinoma.

Radiologic procedures and scanning techniques are helpful, and serologic methods are available.

Treatment, Prevention, and Control

Surgical removal of the cyst is indicated, especially if an entire hepatic area can be resected. The same surgical approach applies to lesions in the lung wherein a lobe can be resected. Mebendazole and albendazole, as used for the treatment of *E. granulosus*, have produced clinical cures. As with *E. granulosus*, education, proper personal hygiene, and deworming of farm dogs and cats are critical. It is extremely important to treat animals that have contact with children.

Hymenolepis nana

Physiology and Structure

H. nana, the **dwarf tapeworm**, is only 2 to 4 cm in length, unlike *Taenia* organisms, which measure several meters. The life cycle is also simple and does not require an intermediate host (Figure 85-9), although mice and beetles may be infected and enter the cycle.

Infection begins when the embryonated eggs are ingested and develop in the intestinal villi into a larval cysticercoid stage. This cysticercoid larva attaches its four muscular suckers and crown of hooklets to the small intestine, and upon maturation the adult worm produces a strobila of egg-laden proglottids. Eggs passing in the feces are then immediately and directly infective, initiating another cycle. Infection may also be acquired by ingesting infected insect intermediate hosts.

H. nana also can cause autoinfection, with a subsequent increased worm burden. Eggs are able to hatch in the intestine, develop into a cysticercoid larva, and then grow into adult worms without leaving the host. This can lead to hyperinfection with very heavy worm burdens and severe clinical symptoms.

Epidemiology

H. nana occurs worldwide in humans and is also a common parasite of mice. The most common tapeworm infection in North America, it occasionally develops its cysticercoid stage in beetles; humans and mice may ingest these beetles in contaminated grain and flour. Children are especially at risk of infection, and because of the simple life cycle of the parasite, families with children in daycare centers experience problems in controlling the transmission of this organism.

Clinical Syndromes

With only a few worms in the intestine, there are no symptoms. In heavy infections, especially if autoinfection and hyperinfection occur, patients experience diarrhea, abdominal pain, headache, anorexia, and other vague complaints.

Laboratory Diagnosis

Stool examination reveals the characteristic *H. nana* egg with its six-hooked embryo and polar filaments (Figure 85-10).

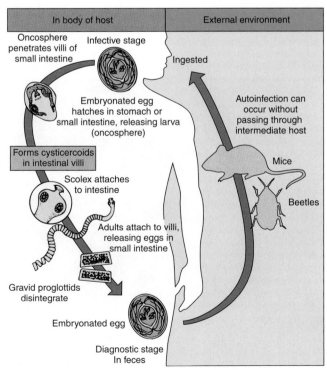

Figure 85–9. Life cycle of *H. nana* (dwarf tapeworm).

Figure 85–10. *H. nana* egg. The eggs are 30 to 45 μm in diameter and have a thin shell containing a six-hooked embryo.

Treatment, Prevention, and Control

The drug of choice is praziquantel; an alternative is niclosamide. Treatment of cases, improved sanitation, and proper personal hygiene, especially in the family and institutional environments, are essential for controlling the transmission of *H. nana*.

Hymenolepis diminuta

Physiology and Structure

H. diminuta, closely related to *H. nana*, is primarily a tapeworm of rats and mice, but it is also found in humans. It differs from *H. nana* in length, measuring 20 to 60 cm. The scolex lacks hooklets, and the egg is larger, bile-stained, and has no polar filaments (Figure 85-11). The life cycle of *H. diminuta* is more complex than that of *H. nana*, and it requires larval insects ("mealworms") to reach the infective cysticercoid stage.

Epidemiology

Infections have been found all over the world, including in the United States. Larval beetles and other larval insects become infected when they feed on rat feces that carry *H. diminuta* eggs. Humans are infected by ingesting the larval insects (mealworms) in contaminated grain products (e.g., flour, cereals).

Clinical Syndromes

Mild infections produce no symptoms, but heavier worm burdens produce nausea, abdominal discomfort, anorexia, and diarrhea.

Figure 85—11. *H. diminuta* egg. The eggs are large (70 to 85 μm × 60 to 80 μm) and have a six-hooked embryo surrounded by a membrane that is widely separated from the outer shell.

Laboratory Diagnosis

Stool examination demonstrates the characteristic bile-stained egg that lacks polar filaments.

Treatment, Prevention, and Control

The drug of choice is niclosamide, with praziquantel an alternative. Rodent control in areas where grain products are produced or stored is essential. Thorough inspection of uncooked grain products to detect mealworms is also important.

Dipylidium caninum

Physiology and Structure

D. caninum, a small tapeworm averaging about 15 cm in length, is primarily a parasite of dogs and cats, but it can infect humans, especially children whose mouths are licked by infected pets. The life cycle involves the development of larval worms in dog and cat fleas. These fleas, when crushed by the teeth of the infected pet, are carried on the tongue to the child's mouth when the child kisses the pet or the pet licks the child. Swallowing the infected flea leads to intestinal infection.

Because of the size and shape of the mature and terminal proglottids, *D. caninum* is often called the **pumpkin seed tapeworm.** The eggs are distinctive because they occur in packets covered with a tough, clear membrane. There may be as many as 25 eggs in a packet, and a single egg free of the packet is seldom seen.

Epidemiology

D. caninum occurs worldwide, especially in children. Its distribution and transmission are directly correlated with dogs and cats infected with fleas.

Figure 85—12. *D. caninum* eggs. Free eggs are rarely seen. Instead, egg packets that contain 8 to 15 six-hooked oncospheres enclosed in a thin membrane are most commonly found in fecal specimens. *(From Murray PR, et al: Manual of Clinical Microbiology, 7th ed. Washington, DC, ASM Press, 1999.)*

Clinical Syndromes

Light infections are asymptomatic; heavier worm burdens produce abdominal discomfort, anal pruritus, and diarrhea. Anal pruritus results from the active migration of the motile proglottid.

Laboratory Diagnosis

Stool examination reveals the colorless egg packets (Figure 85-12), and proglottids may be in feces brought to physicians by patients.

Treatment, Prevention, and Control

The drug of choice is niclosamide; praziquantel and paromomycin are alternatives. Dogs and cats should be dewormed and not be allowed to lick the mouths of children. Pets should be treated to eradicate the fleas.

Case Study and Questions

A 30-year-old Hispanic man entered the emergency department after a focal neurologic seizure. The patient had recently emigrated from Mexico and was in his usual state of good health before the seizure. Neurologic examination revealed no focal findings. A computed tomographic scan of the head revealed multiple small cystic lesions in both cerebral hemispheres. Punctate calcification was noted in several of the lesions.
A lumbar puncture revealed a glucose level of 65 mg/dL (normal) and a protein level of 38 mg/dL (normal) in cerebrospinal fluid. The white blood cell count was 20/mm^3 (abnormal) with a differential of 5% neutrophils, 90% lymphocytes, and 5% monocytes. A purified protein derivative skin test was negative with positive controls. Serologic test for human immunodeficiency virus was negative.

1. What was the differential diagnosis of this patient's neurologic process?

2. Which parasite or parasites may have caused this condition?

3. What diagnostic tests were available for this infection?

4. What were the therapeutic options for this patient?

5. How do people become infected with this parasite?

6. What tissue sites (besides the central nervous system) may be involved? How would these additional foci of infection be documented?

Bibliography

Budke CM, Deplazes P, Torgenson PR: Global socioeconomic impact of cystic echinococcosis. Emerg Infect Dis 12:296-303, 2006.

Cabello FC: Salmon aquaculture and transmission of the fish tapeworm. Emerg Infect Dis 13:169-171, 2007.

Eckert J, Deplazes P: Biological, epidemiological, and clinical aspects of echinococcosis, a zoonosis of increasing concern. Clin Microbiol Rev 17:107-135, 2004.

Garcia HH, Jimenez JA, Escalante H: Cestodes. In Murray PR, et al (eds): Manual of Clinical Microbiology, 9th ed. Washington, DC, ASM Press, 2007.

Garcia HH, et al: Current consensus guidelines for treatment of neurocysticercosis. Clin Microbiol Rev 15:747-756, 2002.

Garcia LS: Diagnostic Medical Parasitology, 4th ed. Washington, DC, ASM Press, 2001.

Markell EK, John DT, Krotoski, WA: Markell and Voges' Medical Parasitology, 8th ed. Philadelphia, WB Saunders, 1999.

Sorvillo FJ, DeGiorgio C, Waterman SH: Deaths from cysticercosis, United States. Emerg Infect Dis 13:230-235, 2007.

Strickland GT: Hunter's Tropical Medicine and Emerging Infectious Diseases. Philadelphia, WB Saunders, 2000.

Arthropods

The arthropods are the largest of the animal phyla, with over 1 million species. The phylum Arthropoda comprises invertebrate animals with a segmented body, several pairs of jointed appendages, bilateral symmetry, and a rigid, chitinous exoskeleton that is molted periodically as the animal grows. Characteristically, arthropods develop from egg to adult by a process known as **metamorphosis**. As they mature, the organisms pass through several distinct morphologic stages, including egg, larvae or nymph, pupa (certain insects), and adult. Five classes of arthropods are of medical importance on the basis of the number or the severity of the illnesses they cause: the Myriapoda, Pentastomida, Crustacea, Chelicerata, and Insecta (Table 86-1).

The arthropods or their larvae may affect human health in many ways. Most arthropods function indirectly in human disease; they transmit but do not produce disease. Arthropods may transmit disease mechanically, as when flies carry enteric bacterial pathogens from feces to human food. Of outstanding importance is the ability of many arthropods to act as biologic **vectors and intermediate hosts** in the transmission and developmental cycle of viruses, bacteria, protozoa, and metazoa (Table 86-2). Certain arthropods may inflict direct injury by their bites or stings. Other species, such as lice, scabies mites, and tissue-invading maggots, may act as true parasites. Still other species may function as both parasites and vectors of disease.

It is not the purpose of this chapter to consider medical entomology in detail. Rather, our purpose is to provide a brief overview of several of the more important aspects of arthropods and their relationship to human disease. More detailed information on arthropods of medical importance and the therapy and control of arthropod infestations may be found in the references listed in the Bibliography.

Myriapoda

Centipedes

Physiology and Structure

The centipedes are elongated, multisegmented (15 to more than 181 segments), many-legged, tracheate arthropods. They possess a distinct head and trunk. The body is dorsoventrally flattened, and each trunk segment bears a single pair of legs. **Maxillipeds** or poison claws are situated on the first segment and are used for capturing prey. The millipedes are sometimes classified with the centipedes; however, millipedes lack the poison claws of centipedes and have two pairs of legs per segment.

Epidemiology

Most centipedes are predaceous insectivores and are commonly found in dark, damp environments such as the areas beneath logs, among rubbish, and inside old buildings. Human bites are almost invariably the result of accidental exposure to the organism during outdoor activities.

Clinical Syndromes

Centipede bites may be extremely painful and cause swelling at the site of the bite. Reports of the effects of centipede bites on humans are conflicting. One species, *Scolopendra gigantea*, which is found in Central and South America and the Galapagos Islands, reportedly has caused several deaths. With the exception of *Scolopendra* and related tropical genera, the bite of most centipedes is harmless to humans.

Treatment, Prevention, and Control

Treatment of a centipede bite includes local measures such as the application of compresses of sodium bicarbonate or solutions of Epsom salts. Control consists of removing rubbish near dwellings.

Table 86—1. Medically Important Classes of Arthropods

Phylum	Class	Organisms
Arthropoda	Myriapoda	Centipedes
	Pentastomida	Tongue worms
	Crustacea	Copepods, decapods (crabs, crayfish)
	Chelicerata	Spiders, scorpions, mites, ticks
	Insecta	Flies, mosquitoes, lice, fleas, bugs, stinging insects

Pentastomida

Tongue Worms

The pentastomids, or **tongue worms**, are bloodsucking endoparasites of reptiles, birds, and mammals. Their taxonomic status is uncertain. Some scientists include pentastomids among the arthropods because their larvae superficially resemble those of mites. Others consider them annelids, and still others place them in an entirely separate phylum. For purposes of this discussion, they are considered with the arthropods.

Physiology and Structure

Tongue worms are degenerate, wormlike arthropods that live primarily in the nasal and respiratory passages of reptiles, birds, and mammals. Adult pentastomids are white, cylindrical or flattened parasites that possess two distinct body regions: an anterior head, or cephalothorax, and an abdomen. The adults are elongated and may attain a length of 1 to 10 cm. The head has a mouth and two pairs of hooks. Although the abdomen may appear annulated, it is not segmented (Figure 86-1). The pentastomids possess digestive and reproductive organs; however, they lack circulatory and respiratory systems.

The adult pentastomids are found in the lungs of reptiles and the nasal passages of mammals. Many vertebrates, including humans, may serve as intermediate hosts. The embryonated eggs are discharged in the feces or respiratory secretions of the infected definitive host and contaminate vegetation or water, which is in turn ingested by one of several possible intermediate hosts (fish, rodents, goats, sheep, or humans). The eggs hatch in the intestine, and the primary larvae penetrate the intestinal wall and attach to the peritoneum. The larvae mature in the peritoneum and develop into infective larvae, encyst in viscera, or die and become calcified. In tissue sections, encysted larvae can be identified by acidophilic glands, a chitinous cuticle, and prominent hooks, which are present in the anterior end of the organism. Subcuticular glands and striated muscle fibers may also be observed beneath the cuticle.

Humans may also become infected by ingesting the inadequately cooked flesh of infected reptiles or other definitive hosts or by eating the infected flesh of intermediate hosts (e.g., goats, sheep) containing infective larvae. In the latter instance, the infective larvae migrate from the stomach to the nasopharyngeal tissues, where they develop into adult pentastomids and produce the symptoms of the **halzoun syndrome** (see section on clinical syndromes). In this case, the human host is considered a temporary definitive host.

Epidemiology

Most tongue worm infections are reported in Europe, Africa, and South and Central America. The infection is common in Malaysia, where autopsy studies reveal **pentastomiasis** in up to 45% of people. As previously described, the infection is acquired by ingesting raw vegetables or water contaminated with pentastome eggs or by consuming raw or undercooked flesh of infected animals.

Clinical Syndromes

In most cases, infection is asymptomatic and is discovered accidentally during roentgenographic examination (calcified larvae), at surgery, or at autopsy. Pneumonitis, pneumothorax, peritonitis, meningitis, nephritis, and obstructive jaundice have all been ascribed to pentastomid infections; however, definitive proof of a causal relationship between disease and the presence of the parasite is frequently lacking. Localized infection of the eye has been reported, presumably secondary to direct inoculation.

Halzoun syndrome, caused by the attachment of adult pentastomes to the nasopharyngeal tissues, is characterized by pharyngeal discomfort, paroxysmal coughing, sneezing, dysphagia, and vomiting. Asphyxiation has been rarely reported.

Laboratory Diagnosis

The diagnosis is made by identifying a pentastomid in a biopsy specimen obtained at surgery or at autopsy. Occasionally, calcified larvae may be observed on x-ray films of the abdomen or chest, providing a presumptive diagnosis. There are no useful serologic tests.

Treatment, Prevention, and Control

Treatment is not usually warranted. In symptomatic patients, surgical removal of free or encysted parasites should be attempted. Preventive measures include thorough cooking of meat and vegetables and avoidance of contaminated water.

Crustacea

The crustaceans are primarily gill-breathing arthropods of fresh and salt water. Those of medical importance are found in fresh water and serve as intermediate hosts of various worms (see Table 86-2).

Table 86–2. Select Human Illnesses Transmitted by Arthropods

Primary Vector or Intermediate Host	Disease	Etiologic Agent
Chelicerata		
Mite: *Leptotrombidium* species	Scrub typhus (tsutsugamushi disease)	*Rickettsia tsutsugamushi*
Mite: *Liponyssoides sanguineus*	Rickettsial pox	*Rickettsia akari*
Tick: *Dermacentor* species	Tularemia	*Francisella tularensis*
Tick: *Dermacentor* species and other ixodid ticks	Rocky Mountain spotted fever	*Rickettsia rickettsii*
Tick: *Dermacentor, Boophilus* species	Q fever	*Coxiella burnetii*
Tick: *Dermacentor* species	Colorado tick fever	*Orbivirus*
Tick: *Ornithodoros* species	Relapsing fever	*Borrelia* species
Tick: *Ixodes* species	Babesiosis	*Babesia microti*
Tick: *Ixodes* species	Lyme disease	*Borrelia burgdorferi*
Tick: *Dermacentor variabilis, Amblyomma americanum*	Ehrlichiosis	*Ehrlichia risticii*
Crustacea		
Copepod: *Cyclops* species	Diphyllobothriasis	*Diphyllobothrium latum*
Copepod: *Cyclops* species	Dracunculiasis	*Dracunculus medinensis*
Crabs, crayfish: various freshwater species	Paragonimiasis	*Paragonimus westermani*
Insecta		
Lice: *Pediculus humanus*	Epidemic typhus	*Rickettsia prowazekii*
Lice: *Pediculus humanus*	Trench fever	*Rickettsia quintana*
Lice: *Pediculus humanus*	Louse-borne relapsing fever	*Borrelia recurrentis*
Flea: *Xenopsylla cheopis*, various other rodent fleas	Plague	*Yersinia pestis*
Flea: *Xenopsylla cheopis*	Murine typhus	*Rickettsia typhi*
Flea: various species	Dipylidiasis	*Dipylidium caninum*
Bug: *Triatoma, Panstrongylus* species	Chagas' disease	*Trypanosoma cruzi*
Beetles: flour beetle	Hymenolepiasis	*Hymenolepis nana*
Fly, gnat: *Glossina* species (tsetse flies)	African trypanosomiasis	*Trypanosoma brucei rhodesiense* and *T. b. gambiense*
Fly, gnat: *Simulium* species	Onchocerciasis	*Onchocerca volvulus*
Fly, gnat: *Chrysops* species	Tularemia	*Francisella tularensis*
Fly, gnat: *Phlebotomus* species, *Lutzomyia* species (sand fly)	Leishmaniasis	*Leishmania* species
Fly, gnat: *Phlebotomus* species	Bartonellosis	*Bartonella bacilliformis*
Mosquito: *Anopheles* species	Malaria	*Plasmodium* species
Mosquito: *Aedes aegypti*	Yellow fever	Flavivirus
Mosquito: *Aedes* species	Dengue fever	Flavivirus

Continued

Table 86—2. Select Human Illnesses Transmitted by Arthropods—cont'd

Primary Vector or Intermediate Host	Disease	Etiologic Agent
Mosquito: *Culiseta melanura, Coquillettidia perturbans, Aedes vexans*	Eastern equine encephalitis	Alphavirus
Mosquito: *Aedes triseriatus*	La Crosse encephalitis	Bunyavirus
Mosquito: *Culex* species	St. Louis encephalitis	Flavivirus
Mosquito: *Culex* species	Venezuelan equine encephalitis	Alphavirus
Mosquito: *Culex tarsalis*	Western equine encephalitis	Alphavirus
Mosquito: various species	Bancroftian filariasis	*Wuchereria bancrofti*
Mosquito: various species	Malayan filariasis	*Brugia* species
Mosquito: various species	Dirofilariasis	*Dirofilaria immitis*

The copepods, or water fleas, are represented by the genera *Cyclops* and *Diaptomus*. The larger crustaceans, called **decapods**, include crabs and crayfish. These crustaceans also serve as the second intermediate hosts of the lung fluke *Paragonimus westermani* (see Table 86-2).

Copepods

Physiology and Structure

Copepods are small, simple aquatic organisms. They lack a carapace, have one pair of maxillae, and have five pairs of biramous swimming legs. Free and parasitic forms exist. The genera *Diaptomus* and *Cyclops* are medically important.

Figure 86—1. Adult female pentastome (*Armillifer armillatus*) attached to the respiratory surface of the lung *(short arrow)* of a rock python. Note the short cephalothorax *(long arrow)* and a long, annulated abdomen. *(From Binford CH, Connor DH: Pathology of Tropical and Extraordinary Diseases, vol 2. Washington, DC, Armed Forces Institute of Pathology, 1976.)*

Copepods are an intermediate host in the life cycle of several human parasites, including *Dracunculus medinensis* (dracunculiasis), *Diphyllobothrium latum* (diphyllobothriasis), *Gnathostoma spinigerum* (gnathostomiasis), and *Spirometra* species (sparganosis). Copepods have been associated with a single case of a perirectal abscess but generally are not considered a primary cause of human infection.

Epidemiology

Copepods have a worldwide distribution and serve as intermediate hosts for helminthic diseases in the United States and Canada, as well as in Europe and the tropics. Human infection with these helminthic parasites results from ingesting water contaminated with copepods or from eating the raw or insufficiently cooked flesh of infected fish. Pseudo-outbreaks of copepods present in human stool specimens submitted for ova and parasite examination have been reported from New York. As many as 40% of concentrated stools submitted for ova and parasite examination were found to contain copepods, presumably as a result of contamination of a hospital water supply. The single reported case of apparent human infection with copepods occurred in this hospital.

Clinical Syndromes

The clinical signs and symptoms associated with helminthic infections in which copepods serve as intermediate hosts are described in Chapters 83 and 85. The single case of apparent human infection with copepods occurred in a 22-year-old man with Crohn's disease who had a perirectal abscess. Drainage of the abscess revealed purulent material that on microscopic examination contained numerous copepods surrounded by leukocytes. It was hypothesized that the copepods were introduced into preexisting perirectal lesions during sitz baths that were prepared with unfiltered tap water and may have contained copepods. Although the copepods contained within the abscess material were viable and may have been successfully feeding on body tissue, it was felt that the copepods were unlikely to have been the primary cause of the abscess.

Laboratory Diagnosis

The laboratory diagnosis of helminthic infections in which copepods serve as intermediate hosts are described in Chapters 83 and 85. In general, infection is demonstrated by detection of the infecting organism by microscopic examination of clinical material.

Treatment, Prevention, and Control

Specific treatment of copepod-associated helminthic infection is covered in Chapters 83 and 85. Prevention of these infections requires attention to standard public health measures such as the chlorination and filtration of water and thorough cooking of all fish. Infected people must not be allowed to bathe in water used for drinking, and suspected water should be avoided.

Decapods

The decapods include the prawns, shrimps, lobsters, crayfish, and crabs. The cephalothorax of these animals is always covered by a carapace. They have three anterior pairs of thoracic appendages that are modified into biramous maxillipeds and five posterior pairs that are developed into uniramous legs. Crabs and crayfish are medically important as the second intermediate hosts of the lung fluke *P. westermani*. The parasitic, epidemiologic, and clinical aspects of infection with *P. westermani* are described in Chapter 84. Thorough cooking of crabs and crayfish is the most effective means of preventing infection with *P. westermani*.

Chelicerata (Arachnida)

Spiders

Spiders have a number of characteristic features that permit easy identification. Specifically, they possess eight legs, no antennae, a body divided into two regions (cephalothorax and abdomen), and an unsegmented abdomen with spinnerets posteriorly. All true spiders produce venom and kill their prey by biting; however, few have fangs (**chelicerae**) powerful enough to pierce human skin or venom potent enough to produce more than a transitory local skin irritation. Venomous spiders may be classified as those that cause **systemic arachnidism** and those that cause **necrotic arachnidism**. This classification is based on the type of tissue damage produced.

Systemic arachnidism is primarily caused by tarantulas and black widow spiders. Tarantulas (family Theraphosidae) are large, hairy spiders of the tropics and subtropics. The tarantulas are of little importance because they are not very aggressive and avoid human habitations.

Their bite causes intense pain and a phase of agitation, followed by stupor and somnolence. The black widow spider, *Latrodectus mactans*, is widespread through the southern and western United States. Related species of *Latrodectus* are found throughout temperate and tropical regions of all continents, but none is primarily domestic; thus their contact with humans is limited.

Necrotic arachnidism is produced by spiders that belong to the genus *Loxosceles*. The bites of these spiders may produce severe tissue reaction. *Loxosceles reclusa*, the brown recluse spider, is a medically important spider of this genus.

Black Widow Spiders

PHYSIOLOGY AND STRUCTURE

The female black widow spider (*L. mactans*) is easily recognized by the presence of a globose, shiny, black abdomen bearing the characteristic orange or reddish hourglass marking on the ventral surface (Figure 86-2). Females vary from 5 to 13.5 mm in body length, but the males are much smaller.

The venom of the black widow spider is a potent peripheral neurotoxin, which is delivered by a pair of jawlike structures, or chelicerae. Only the female *Latrodectus* spider is dangerous to humans; the small, feeble male delivers an ineffective bite.

EPIDEMIOLOGY

These spiders frequent wood and brush piles, old wooden buildings, cellars, hollow logs, and privies. Given these locations, the bite is often located on the genitalia, buttocks, or extremities. Black widow spiders are common to the southern United States but are found throughout the temperate and tropical regions of both the New and Old World.

CLINICAL SYNDROMES

As is true with most cases of envenomation, the clinical picture depends on factors such as the amount of the venom injected, the location of the bite, and the age, weight, and sensitivity of the patient. Shortly after the bite, there is a sharp pain but little or no immediate

Figure 86–2. Female black widow spider (*L. mactans*). (*From Peters W: A Colour Atlas of Arthropods in Clinical Medicine. London, Wolfe, 1992.*)

swelling. This is followed by local redness, swelling, and burning. Systemic signs and symptoms generally occur within an hour of the bite and include muscular cramps, chest pains, nausea, vomiting, diaphoresis, intestinal spasms, and visual difficulties. Abdominal tetanic cramps producing a "boardlike" abdomen are highly characteristic and may mimic an acute surgical abdomen. The acute symptoms usually subside within 48 hours; however, in severe cases, paralysis and coma may precede cardiac or respiratory failure. Mortality from the bite of the black widow spider is estimated at 4% to 5%.

TREATMENT, PREVENTION, AND CONTROL

Healthy adults usually recover, but small children or weakened people suffer considerably from these bites and may die without treatment. Muscle spasms may be severe and may require the intravenous administration of calcium gluconate or other muscle relaxant agents. A specific antivenin is available and remains the treatment of choice. It is valuable if given shortly after the bite. Because it is prepared from the serum of hyperimmunized horses, patients must be tested for sensitivity to horse serum before administration. Hospitalization is advisable for the care of people with known or suspected bites.

Good housekeeping can be the simplest and most effective control for spiders in homes. This includes dusting webs and carefully removing debris from around homes and adjacent sheds. Children should be discouraged from playing on wood piles and in wood sheds.

Brown Recluse Spiders

PHYSIOLOGY AND STRUCTURE

Spiders producing necrotic arachnidism belong to the genus *Loxosceles*. These spiders are yellow to brown and are of medium size (5 to 10 mm long) with relatively long legs (Figure 86-3). They commonly display two distinguishing characteristics: a dark fiddle- or violin-shaped marking on the dorsal side of the cephalothorax, and six eyes arranged in three pairs forming a semicircle. The venom injected by the female or male spider is a necrotoxin (that may also have hemolytic properties) and causes necrotic lesions with deep tissue damage.

EPIDEMIOLOGY

Four species of the genus *Loxosceles* are found in the Americas. *L. reclusa* is found in the south and central United States, *L. arizonica* is in the western states, and *L. laeta* is in South America. *L. reclusa* is found outdoors in wood piles and debris in warmer climates and in basements or storage areas in cooler regions. *L. laeta* is found in closets and corners of rooms. Humans are bitten only when the spider is threatened or disturbed.

CLINICAL SYNDROMES

Initially, the bite of *Loxosceles* species tends to be painless; however, several hours later, itching, swelling, and soreness

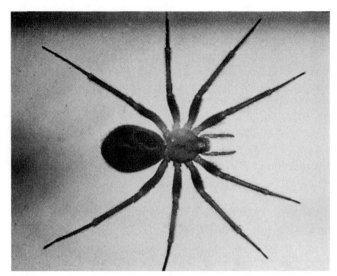

Figure 86–3. Female brown recluse spider (*L. laeta*). *(Courtesy Professor H Schenone; from Peters W: A Colour Atlas of Arthropods in Clinical Medicine. London, Wolfe, 1992.)*

may develop in the area of the bite. Frequently a vesicle or bleb may form at the site. General systemic symptoms are unusual but when present may include chills, headache, and nausea. Within 3 to 4 days, the bleb sloughs and may be followed by ulceration and radiating necrosis, which does not heal but continues to spread for weeks or months.

Intravascular coagulation and hemolysis may occur and be accompanied by hemoglobinuria and cardiac and renal failure. This hemolytic syndrome may be life threatening and occurs more commonly after the bite of *L. laeta*. In South America, this syndrome is known as **visceral loxoscelism**.

DIAGNOSIS

The discrimination of a species of spider is not possible from the appearance of the lesion alone; however, a working diagnosis is commonly based on the appearance of bleb formation around puncture marks and the nature of the developing lesion. The spider may be identified easily by the characteristic features previously described. An enzyme-linked immunosorbent assay has been developed to confirm the diagnosis of brown recluse spider bite but is not widely available.

TREATMENT, PREVENTION, AND CONTROL

The treatment of brown recluse spider bites is variable and based on the severity of the necrotic reaction. Most bites in the United States are inconsequential and require no specific therapy. Cleansing the bite wound and providing tetanus prophylaxis and antibiotics to prevent secondary infection may all be indicated. Healing is generally uncomplicated, and debridement or excision should not be performed for 3 to 6 weeks to allow natural healing to commence. Excision and skin grafting may be necessary for bites that have not healed in 6 to 8 weeks. Systemic

Figure 86—4. Scorpion (*Centruroides* species). *(Courtesy Dr JC Cokendolpher; from Peters W: A Colour Atlas of Arthropods in Clinical Medicine. London, Wolfe, 1992.)*

therapy with corticosteroids may be useful in treating the hemolytic syndrome but are of little proven value in preventing or treating cutaneous necrosis. Although not available in the United States, an antivenin is used in South America for the treatment of visceral loxoscelism.

Preventive measures are similar to those recommended for black widow spiders. *Loxosceles* (and other) spiders may be controlled in dwellings with insecticide compounds.

Scorpions

Physiology and Structure

The typical scorpion is elongated with conspicuous, pincher-like claws (or **pedipalps**) at the anterior end of the body, four pairs of walking legs, and a distinctly regimented abdomen that tapers to a curved, hollow, needle-like stinger (Figure 86-4). When the scorpion is disturbed, it uses the stinger for defense. Both male and female scorpions can sting. Venom is injected through the stinger from two venom glands in the abdomen. Most scorpions are unable to penetrate human skin or inject enough venom to cause real damage; however, a few species are capable of inflicting painful wounds that may cause death.

Epidemiology

Scorpions considered dangerous may be found in the southwestern United States, Mexico, and Venezuela. This includes several species of the genus *Centruroides*, which accounts for as many as 1000 deaths annually. Also important are several species of *Tityus*, found in Trinidad, Argentina, Brazil, Guyana, and Venezuela. Children under the age of 5 years are most likely to be fatally stung by scorpions.

Scorpions are nocturnal, and during the day they remain concealed under logs, rocks, and other dark, moist places. They invade human habitations at night, where they may hide in shoes, towels, clothing, and closets.

Clinical Syndromes

The effect of a scorpion sting in a patient is highly variable and depends on factors such as the species and age of the scorpion, the kind and amount of venom injected, and the age, size, and sensitivity of the person who was stung. Although the sting of many scorpions is relatively nontoxic and produces only local symptoms, other stings may be quite serious. Scorpions produce two types of venom: a neurotoxin and a hemorrhagic or hemolytic toxin. The hemolytic toxin is responsible for local reactions at the site of the sting, including radiating, burning pain; swelling; discoloration; and necrosis. The neurotoxin produces minimal local reaction but rather severe systemic effects, including chills, diaphoresis, excessive salivation, difficulty speaking and swallowing, muscle spasm, tachycardia, and generalized seizures. In severe cases, death may result from pulmonary edema and respiratory paralysis.

Diagnosis

Local or systemic signs and symptoms coupled with physical evidence of a single point of skin penetration are usually sufficient to establish the diagnosis. The patient may have observed the scorpion or brought it in for identification. Although scorpions are relatively easy to identify, it is important to realize that other nonpoisonous arachnids strongly resemble scorpions. An entomologist or parasitologist should be consulted if there is a taxonomic question.

Treatment, Prevention, and Control

The management of scorpion stings varies. In the absence of systemic symptoms, palliative treatment may be all that is necessary. Pain may be relieved by analgesics or local injection of Xylocaine; however, opiates appear to increase toxicity. Local cryotherapy may reduce swelling and retard the systemic absorption of the toxin. Hot packs produce vasodilatation and may accelerate toxin distribution systemically and are therefore contraindicated. Antivenin is available and is effective if administered soon after the sting. Very young children with systemic symptoms should be treated as medical emergencies. Systemic symptoms and shock should be treated supportively.

Preventive measures include the use of chemical pesticides to reduce scorpion populations. Removal of debris around dwellings can reduce hiding and breeding places.

Mites

Mites are small, eight-legged arthropods characterized by a saclike body and no antennae. A large number of mite species are free-living or are normally associated with other vertebrates (e.g., birds, rodents) and may cause dermatitis in humans on rare occasions. The number of mites that are considered true human parasites or present real medical problems is quite small and include the human itch mite (*Sarcoptes scabiei*), the human follicle mite (*Demodex folliculorum*), and the chigger mite. Mites affect humans in three ways: by causing dermatitis, by serving as vectors of infectious diseases, and by acting as a source of allergens.

Figure 86—5. Scabies mite (*Sarcoptes* species). *(From Peters W: A Colour Atlas of Arthropods in Clinical Medicine. London, Wolfe, 1992.)*

Itch Mites

PHYSIOLOGY AND STRUCTURE

The itch mite (*S. scabiei*) causes an infectious skin disease variably known as **scabies**, **mange**, or **the itch**. The adult mites average 300 to 400 μm in length with an oval, saclike body in which the first and second pairs of legs are widely separated from the third and fourth pairs (Figure 86-5). The body has dorsal transverse parallel ridges, spines, and hairs. The ova measure 100 to 150 μm.

Adult mites enter the skin, creating serpiginous burrows in the upper layers of the epidermis. The female mite lays her eggs in the skin burrows, and the larval and nymph stages that develop also burrow in the skin. The female mites live and deposit eggs and feces in epidermal burrows for up to 2 months. Characteristically, the preferred sites of infestation are the interdigital and popliteal folds, the wrist and inguinal regions, and the inframammary folds. The presence of the mites and their secretions cause intense itching of the involved areas. The mite is an obligate parasite and can perpetuate itself in a single host indefinitely.

EPIDEMIOLOGY

Scabies is cosmopolitan in distribution, with an estimated global prevalence of about 300 million cases. The mite is an obligate parasite of domestic animals and humans; however, it may survive for hours to days away from the host, thus facilitating its spread. Transmission is accomplished by direct contact or by contact with contaminated objects such as clothing. Sexual transmission has been well documented. Spread of the infection to other areas of the body is accomplished by scratching and manual transfer of the mite by the affected person. Scabies may occur in epidemic fashion among people in crowded conditions such as daycare centers, nursing homes, military camps, and prisons.

CLINICAL SYNDROMES

The outstanding clinical diagnostic symptom is intense itching, usually in the interdigital folds and sides of the fingers, buttocks, external genitalia, wrists, and elbows.

The uncomplicated lesions appear as short, slightly raised cutaneous burrows. At the end of the burrow, there is frequently a vesicle containing the female mite. The intense pruritus usually leads to excoriation of the skin secondary to scratching, which in turn produces crusts and secondary bacterial infection. Patients experience their first symptoms within weeks to months after exposure; however, the incubation period may be as little as 1 to 4 days in persons sensitized by prior exposure. Host hypersensitivity (delayed or type IV) probably plays an important role in determining the variable clinical manifestations of scabies.

Some immunodeficient people may develop a variant of scabies, so-called **Norwegian scabies**, characterized by generalized dermatitis with extensive scaling and crusting and the presence of thousands of mites in the epidermis. This disease is highly contagious and suggests that host immunity also plays a role in suppressing *S. scabiei*.

DIAGNOSIS

The clinical diagnosis of scabies is based on the characteristic lesions and their distribution. The definitive diagnosis of scabies depends on the demonstration of the mite in skin scrapings. Because the adult mite is most frequently found in the terminal portions of a fresh burrow, it is best to make scrapings in these areas. The scrapings are placed on a clean microscope slide, cleared by the addition of 1 or 2 drops of a 20% solution of potassium hydroxide, covered with a coverslip, and examined under a low-power microscope. With experience, the mite and ova may be recognized. Skin biopsy may also reveal the mites and ova in tissue sections.

TREATMENT, PREVENTION, AND CONTROL

The standard, and very effective, treatment for scabies is 1% gamma benzene hexachloride (lindane) in a lotion base. One or two applications (head to toe) at weekly intervals is effective against scabies. Lindane is absorbed through the skin, and repeated applications may be toxic. For this reason, it is not advisable to use it in treating infants, small children, or pregnant or lactating women.

Recently, a 5% permethrin cream (Elimite) has replaced lindane lotions as the treatment of choice for scabies. Clinical trials have shown permethrin to be more effective and less toxic than lindane. Other preparations used to treat scabies include crotamiton sulfur (6%) preparations, benzyl benzoate, and tetraethylthiuram monosulfide. The last two preparations are not available in the United States.

Primary prevention of scabies is best achieved with good hygiene habits, personal cleanliness, and routine washing of clothing and bed linens. Secondary prevention includes the identification and treatment of infected people and possibly their household and sexual contacts. In an epidemic situation, simultaneous treatment of all affected people and their contacts may be necessary. This is followed by thorough cleansing of the environment (e.g., boiling clothing and linens) and ongoing surveillance to prevent re-occurrence.

Human Follicle Mites

PHYSIOLOGY AND STRUCTURE

The human follicle mites include two species of the genus *Demodex*, *D. folliculorum* and *D. brevis*. These mites are minute (0.1 to 0.4 mm) organisms with a wormlike body, four pairs of stubby legs, and an annulate abdomen. *D. folliculorum* parasitizes the hair follicles of the face of most adult humans, whereas *D. brevis* is found in the sebaceous glands of the head and trunk.

EPIDEMIOLOGY

Organisms of the *Demodex* genus are obligate parasites of the human integument and are cosmopolitan in their distribution. Infestations are uncommon in young children and increase at the time of puberty. It is estimated that 50% to 100% of adults are infested with these mites.

CLINICAL SYNDROMES (Clinical Case 86-1)

The role of *Demodex* species in human disease is uncertain. They have been associated with acne, blackheads, blepharitis, abnormalities of the scalp, and truncal rashes. More recently, extensive papular folliculitis resulting from *Demodex* infestation has been described in people with acquired immunodeficiency. Factors such as poor personal hygiene, increased sebum production, mite hypersensitivity, and immunosuppression may increase host susceptibility and enhance the clinical presentation of *Demodex* infestation. Most people infested with these mites remain asymptomatic.

DIAGNOSIS

Mites may be demonstrated microscopically in material expressed from an infested follicle. They may be seen as incidental findings in histologic sections of facial skin.

Clinical Case 86-1. *Demodex* Folliculitis

Antille and colleagues (Arch Dermatol 140:457-460, 2004) reported a case of *Demodex* folliculitis in a 49-year-old man. The patient had rosacea for 12 years and presented with telangiectatic and papular rosacea on the cheeks and forehead. His condition had progressively deteriorated in spite of intermittent systemic treatments with ciprofloxacin. Six months previously, the patient had stopped all treatments except antihypertensive and antiuricemic therapies. An alternating treatment with clindamycin solution and 0.03% tacrolimus ointment once daily was initially effective and well tolerated. Three weeks later, however, he experienced an acute flare with intense erythema and extensive pustulation. A pustular smear revealed an abundance of *Demodex* mites, which were also seen in a biopsy specimen that confirmed the diagnosis of rosacea. Tacrolimus treatment was discontinued, and the flare resolved rapidly with systemic ciprofloxacin therapy. Ciprofloxacin therapy was stopped 1 month later, and there was no relapse during a 11-month follow-up. This case is an example of a situation where the immunosuppressive properties of tacrolimus facilitated the overgrowth of follicular *Demodex* mites resulting in a pustular dermatitis.

TREATMENT

Effective treatment consists of a single application of 1% gamma benzene hexachloride.

Chigger Mites

PHYSIOLOGY AND STRUCTURE

Chiggers are the larvae of mites of the family Trombiculidae. The adult trombiculid mites infest grass and bushes, and their larvae (i.e., chiggers) attack humans and other vertebrates, producing severe dermatitis. The larvae have three pairs of legs and are covered with characteristic branched, featherlike hairs.

The larvae appear as minute, barely visible, reddish dots attached to the skin, where they use their hooked mouth parts to ingest tissue fluids. Chiggers typically attach to the skin areas where clothing is tight or restricted such as the wrists, ankles, armpits, groin, and waistline. After feeding, the engorged larvae fall to the ground where they molt and undergo development into nymphs and adults.

EPIDEMIOLOGY

Chiggers that are important in North America include the larvae of *Eutrombicula alfreddugesi* and *E. splendens*. In Europe, the important species is the harvest mite, *Trombicula autumnalis*. Chiggers are a particular problem for outdoor enthusiasts such as campers and picnickers. In Europe and the Americas, they are associated with intensely pruritic lesions; however, in Asia, Australia, and the western Pacific rim, they serve as vectors of the rickettsial disease scrub typhus or tsutsugamushi fever (*Rickettsia tsutsugamushi*) (see Table 86-2).

CLINICAL SYNDROMES

Saliva injected into the skin at the time of mite attachment produces an intense pruritus and dermatitis. The skin lesions appear as small erythematous marks that progress to papules and may persist for weeks. Mite larvae may be visible in the center of the reddened, swollen area. The irritation may be so severe that it causes fever and sleep disruption. Secondary bacterial infection of the excoriated lesions may occur.

TREATMENT, PREVENTION, AND CONTROL

Treatment for dermatitis caused by chiggers is largely symptomatic and consists of antipruritics, antihistamines, and steroids. The use of insect repellents such as *N,N*-9-diethyl-m-toluamide (DEET) may be of some help in prevention for persons going into chigger-infested areas.

Ticks

Physiology and Structure

Ticks are bloodsucking ectoparasites of a number of vertebrates, including humans. Ticks are opportunistic rather than host specific and tend to suck blood from a number of large and small animals. Ticks have a four-stage life cycle

Figure 86—6. Soft tick (*Ornithodoros* species). *(From Strickland GT: Hunter's Tropical Medicine, 7th ed. Philadelphia, WB Saunders, 1991.)*

that includes the egg, larva, nymph, and adult. Although the larva, nymph, and adults are all bloodsuckers, it is the adult tick that usually bites humans.

Ticks comprise two large families, the Ixodidae, or hard ticks, and the Argasidae, or soft ticks. Soft ticks have a leathery body that lacks a hard dorsal scutum, and the mouthparts are located ventrally and are not visible from above (Figure 86-6). Hard ticks have a hard dorsal plate or scutum, and the mouthparts are clearly visible from above (Figure 86-7). Both hard and soft ticks serve as ectoparasites of humans. Soft ticks differ from hard ticks primarily in their feeding behavior. Soft ticks complete engorgement in a matter of minutes or at most a few hours; hard ticks feed slowly, taking 7 to 9 days to become engorged.

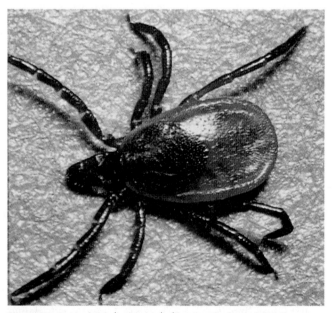

Figure 86—7. Hard tick (*I. dammini*). *(Courtesy Professor A Spielman; from Peters W: A Colour Atlas of Arthropods in Clinical Medicine. London, Wolfe, 1992.)*

Epidemiology

Ticks are found in wooded and rural areas worldwide. In North America, the important species of hard ticks include *Dermacentor variabilis* (the American dog tick), *D. andersoni* (the Rocky Mountain wood tick), *Amblyomma americanum* (the lone star tick), *Rhipicephalus sanguineus* (the brown dog tick), and *Ixodes dammini* (the deer tick). These ticks are found variably throughout the United States and are important vectors of several infectious diseases, including Rocky Mountain spotted fever (*Dermacentor* species), tularemia (*Dermacentor* species), Q fever (*Dermacentor* species), Lyme disease (*Ixodes* species), babesiosis (*Ixodes* species), and ehrlichiosis (*D. variabilis* and *A. americanum*) (see Table 86-2). Soft ticks of the genus *Ornithodoros* transmit relapsing fever spirochetes (*Borrelia* species) in limited areas in the West (see Table 86-2). In general, people at risk for tick exposure are involved in outdoor activities in wooded areas. Tick exposure may also occur during stays in rural cabins inhabited by small rodents, which commonly serve as hosts for ticks and other ectoparasites.

Clinical Syndromes (Clinical Case 86-2)

Tick bites are generally of minor consequence and are limited to small erythematous papules. More serious consequences of tick bite include the development of a type of paralysis resulting from substances released by ticks during feeding and transmission of a number of rickettsial, bacterial, viral, spirochetal, and protozoan diseases of humans and other animals.

Ticks may attach at any point on the body but typically favor the scalp, hairline, ears, axillae, and groin. The initial bite is usually painless, and the presence of the tick may not be detected for several hours after contact. After the tick has dropped off or has been removed manually, the area may become reddened, painful, and pruritic. The wound may become secondarily infected and necrotic, particularly if the mouthparts remain attached after manual removal.

Clinical Case 86-2. African Tick Bite Fever

Owen and colleagues (Arch Dermatol 142:1312-1314, 2006) describe a middle-aged woman who returned from a mission trip to Zimbabwe with an influenza-like illness and an inoculation eschar; she also had a history of travel to a game farm. Biopsy of the cutaneous lesion revealed a histopathologic pattern consistent with an infectious pathogenesis. Immunohistochemical staining confirmed the presence of rickettsial organisms. In light of the patient's history, the clinical constellation of signs and symptoms, a diagnosis of African tick bite fever was made. The patient was treated with doxycycline and had an uncomplicated course.

African tick bite fever is a rickettsial illness that has recently emerged as a significant disease among international travelers. The vector is the *Amblyomma* tick, which is endemic to sub-Saharan Africa. This is an example of just one of many rickettsial diseases transmitted by ticks.

Three species of tick, *D. andersoni*, *D. variabilis*, and *A. americanum*, have all been reported to cause **tick paralysis**. This is characterized by an ascending flaccid paralysis, fever, and general intoxication, which may lead to respiratory compromise and death. The paralysis is due to toxic substances released in the saliva of the tick and may be reversed by tick removal. Tick paralysis is observed more commonly in young children and when tick attachment is in opposition to the central nervous system (e.g., scalp, head, neck).

Ticks are also involved in the transmission of infections such as Lyme disease, Rocky Mountain spotted fever, ehrlichiosis, Colorado tick fever, relapsing fever, tularemia, Q fever, and babesiosis (see Table 86-2). The reader is referred to the appropriate sections of this book for discussion of the clinical and microbiologic aspects of these infections.

Diagnosis

The diagnosis of tick bites and tickborne diseases usually rests on the finding of a tick or a history of exposure to tick-infested areas. The identification of an organism as an adult tick is usually straightforward and based on the observations of an organism that is dorsoventrally flattened and possesses four pairs of legs and no visible segmentation (see Figures 86-6 and 86-7). An entomologist or parasitologist should be consulted if further identification is desired. The diagnosis of specific tickborne infectious diseases is covered in the respective sections of this book.

Treatment, Prevention, and Control

Early removal of attached ticks is of primary importance and may be accomplished by steady traction on the tick body, grasped with forceps as close to the skin as possible. Care should be taken to avoid twisting or crushing the tick, which may leave the mouthparts attached to the skin or inject potentially infectious material into the wound. Steady traction is superior to noxious stimuli or occlusive techniques for the removal of ticks. After removal, the wound should be cleansed and observed for secondary infection. Because ticks may harbor highly infectious agents, the clinician should use appropriate infection-control precautions (e.g., use of gloves, handwashing, proper disposal of ticks and contaminated material) during tick removal.

Preventive measures used in tick-infested areas include the wearing of protective clothing that fits snugly about the ankles, wrists, waist, and neck so that ticks cannot gain access to the skin. Insect repellents such as *N,N*-9-diethyl-m-toluamide (DEET) are generally effective. People and pets should be inspected for ticks after visits to tick-infested areas.

Insecta

The insects, or **hexapods**, constitute the largest and most important of all the classes of arthropods, accounting for approximately 70% of all known species of animals.

Insects include animals such as mosquitoes, flies, fleas, lice, roaches, bees, wasps, beetles, and moths to name just a few. The insect body is divided into three parts—head, thorax, and abdomen—and is equipped with one pair of antennae, three pairs of appendages, and one or two pairs of wings or no wings at all. The medical significance of any insect is related to its way of life, particularly its mouthparts and feeding habits. Insects may serve as vectors for a number of bacterial, viral, protozoan, and metazoan pathogens. Certain insects may serve merely as mechanical vectors for the transmission of pathogens, whereas in other insects the pathogens undergo multiplication or cyclic development within the insect host. The methods by which the insects transmit pathogens vary and are discussed here. Insects can also be pathogens themselves by causing mechanical injury through bites, chemical injury through the injection of toxins, and allergic reactions to materials transmitted by bites or stings. There are more than 30 orders of insects, but only those of major medical importance are discussed in this section.

Bloodsucking Diptera

Diptera is the large order of flying insects. All dipterans have a single pair of functional membranous wings and various modifications of the mouthparts, which have been adapted for piercing the skin and sucking blood or tissue juices. Their most important feature is their role as mechanical or biologic vectors of a number of infectious diseases, including leishmaniasis, trypanosomiasis, malaria, filariasis, onchocerciasis, tularemia, bartonellosis, and the viral encephalitides (see Table 86-2). The bloodsucking flies include mosquitoes, sand flies, and blackflies, all of which are capable of transmitting diseases to humans. Other dipterans, such as horse flies and stable flies, are capable of inflicting painful bites but are not known to transmit human pathogens. Although the common housefly does not bite, it certainly is capable of mechanical transmission of a number of viral, bacterial, and protozoan infections to human hosts. The infectious diseases transmitted by bloodsucking flies are well covered in other chapters of this book. The following section deals only with injury resulting from the bite of these insects and the effects of salivary substances introduced into the human skin and tissues.

Mosquitoes

PHYSIOLOGY AND STRUCTURE

Adult mosquitoes are small and have delicate legs, one pair of wings, long antennae, and greatly elongated mouthparts adapted for piercing and sucking. The two major families of mosquitoes (Culicidae), the Anophelinae and the Culicinae, share a number of similarities in their life cycles and development. They lay eggs on or near water, are good fliers, and feed on nectar and sugars. The females of most species also feed on blood, which they require for each clutch of 100 to 200 eggs. Females may take a blood meal every 2 to 4 days. In the act of feeding, the female mosquito injects saliva, which produces mechanical damage to the host but also may transmit disease and produce immediate and delayed immune reactions.

EPIDEMIOLOGY

Within the family Anophelinae, the genus *Anopheles* contains the species responsible for the transmission of human malaria. In the tropics, these mosquitoes breed continually in relation to rainfall. These species vary in their capacity for the transmission of malaria, and within each geographical area, the number of species that serve as malaria vectors is small. *A. gambiae* is an important vector of malaria in sub-Saharan Africa.

Mosquitoes from *Aedes*, the largest genus of the subfamily Culicinae, are found in all habitats, ranging from the tropics to the Arctic. This species may develop overwhelming populations in marsh or tundra and pasture or floodwater and have a severe impact on wildlife, livestock, and humans. *A. aegypti*, the yellow fever mosquito, usually breeds in man-made containers (flower pots, gutters, cans) and is the primary vector of yellow fever and dengue in urban environments throughout the world.

CLINICAL SYNDROMES

Mechanical damage induced by the feeding mosquito is usually minor but may be accompanied by mild pain and irritation. The bite is usually followed within a few minutes by a small, flat weal surrounded by a red flare. The delayed reaction consists of itching, swelling, and reddening of the wound region. Secondary infection may follow as a result of scratching.

TREATMENT, PREVENTION, AND CONTROL

Medical attention is usually not sought for a bite unless secondary infection occurs. Local anesthetics or antihistamines may be useful in treating reactions to mosquito bites.

Preventive measures in mosquito-infested areas include the use of window screens, netting, and protective clothing. Insect repellents such as DEET are generally effective. Mosquito-control measures that involve the use of insecticides have been effective in some areas.

Gnats and Biting Midges

PHYSIOLOGY AND STRUCTURE

Ceratopogonids represent an assortment of tiny flies with names such as **gnats, midges, and punkies**. The majority of the flies that attack humans belong to the genus *Culicoides*; they are minute (0.5 to 4 mm long) and slender enough to pass through the fine mesh of ordinary window screens. The females suck blood and typically feed at dusk, when they may attack in large numbers.

EPIDEMIOLOGY

Biting midges may be important pests in beach and resort areas near salt marshes. Those of the genus *Culicoides* are the main vectors of filariasis in Africa and the New World tropics.

CLINICAL SYNDROMES

The mouthparts of biting midges are lancet-like and produce a painful bite. Bites may produce local lesions lasting hours or days.

TREATMENT, PREVENTION, AND CONTROL

Local treatment is palliative, with lotions, anesthetics, and antiseptic measures. The treatment of breeding sites with pesticides and repellents may be useful against some of the common species of these pests.

Sand flies

PHYSIOLOGY AND STRUCTURE

Sand flies, or moth flies, belong to a single subfamily of the Psychodidae, the Phlebotominae. They are small (1 to 3 mm), delicate, hairy, weak-flying insects that suck the blood of humans, dogs, and rodents. They transmit a number of infections, including leishmaniasis (see Table 86-2). Female flies become infected when they feed on infected people.

EPIDEMIOLOGY

Phlebotomine larvae develop in nonaquatic habitats such as moist soil, stone walls, and rubbish heaps. In many areas, sand flies cause problems as pests. They also serve as vectors of infectious diseases such as leishmaniasis in the Mediterranean, the Middle East, Asia, India, and Latin America.

CLINICAL SYNDROMES

The bite may be painful and pruritic around the local lesion. Sensitized people may have allergic reactions. **Sand fly fever** is characterized by severe frontal headaches, malaise, retro-orbital pain, anorexia, and nausea.

TREATMENT, PREVENTION, AND CONTROL

Sand flies are very sensitive to insecticides, which should be applied to breeding sites and window screens. Various insect repellents may also be useful.

Blackflies

PHYSIOLOGY AND STRUCTURE

Members of the family Simuliidae are commonly called **blackflies or buffalo gnats**. They are 1 to 5 mm long, are humpbacked, and have mouthparts consisting of six "blades" that are capable of tearing skin (Figure 86-8). Blackflies are bloodsucking insects and breed in fast-flowing streams and rivers. They are of major importance as vectors of onchocerciasis (see Table 86-2).

EPIDEMIOLOGY

Blackflies are common in Africa and South America, where they serve as vectors of onchocerciasis. In North America,

Figure 86—8. Blackfly (*Simulium* species), the vector of onchocerciasis. (*Courtesy Dr S Meredith; from Peters W: A Colour Atlas of Arthropods in Clinical Medicine. London, Wolfe, 1992.*)

they are common around the lake regions of Canada and the northern United States. They are pests to hunters and fisherman in these areas. In large numbers, they may cause significant blood loss and pose a major threat to wild and domestic animals.

CLINICAL SYNDROMES

A variety of responses have been observed in humans after the bite of blackflies. The bite of the female can tear the skin surface and induce bleeding that continues for some time after the fly has departed. There is usually a distinct hemorrhagic spot at the site of the bite. Multiple bites may result in considerable blood loss. The bite is painful and accompanied by local inflammation, itching, and swelling.

The local reaction may also be accompanied by a systemic response that varies according to the number of bites and the sensitivity of the person. This syndrome is known as **blackfly fever** and is marked by headache, fever, and adenitis. It usually subsides within 48 hours and is considered a hypersensitivity reaction to the salivary secretions of the fly.

In addition to local and systemic responses to blackfly bites, a **hemorrhagic syndrome** has been described after bites of blackflies in certain areas of Brazil. This syndrome resembles thrombocytopenic purpura and is characterized by local and disseminated cutaneous hemorrhages associated with mucosal bleeding. It is thought that this hemorrhagic syndrome may be produced by a hypersensitivity phenomenon or response to a toxin caused by multiple blackfly bites.

DIAGNOSIS

The blackfly bite is marked characteristically by a point of dried blood and subcutaneous hemorrhage at the wound site. In people with the hemorrhagic syndrome, platelet counts are reduced; there is a prolonged bleeding time and poor clot retraction in about half of patients.

TREATMENT, PREVENTION, AND CONTROL

Treatment includes the usual palliative measures (e.g., anesthetics, antihistamines, lotions) to relieve local pruritus and swelling. Patients with the hemorrhagic syndrome have shown marked improvement with corticosteroid therapy.

Preventive measures include protective clothing. In general, insect repellents are ineffective against blackflies. Some control is achieved by pouring insecticides into rivers and streams.

Horse and Deer Flies

The family Tabanidae consists of species including horse flies, deer flies, gadflies, and mango flies that attack mainly animals. They are large, ranging in length from 7 to 30 mm. The males feed on plant juices, the females on blood. In the act of biting, the female fly leaves a deep wound, causing blood to flow, which the fly laps up. The fly may serve as a mechanical vector of infectious diseases when the fly's mouthparts become contaminated on one host and transfer organisms to the next. These flies are not considered important vectors of infectious disease in humans.

Muscoid Flies

Physiology and Structure

The muscoid flies include three medically important insects: the housefly, *Musca domestica*; the stable fly, *Stomoxys calcitrans*; and the **tsetse flies** of the genus *Glossina*. The stable fly, often mistaken for the housefly, is a true bloodsucker capable of serving as a short-term mechanical vector of a number of bacterial, viral, and protozoal infections. The tsetse fly (Figure 86-9) is also a biting fly and serves as the biologic vector and intermediate host for the agents of African trypanosomiasis, *Trypanosoma brucei rhodesiense* and *T. b. gambiense*. The common housefly represents a host of genera that are nonpiercing or contaminating flies. Because of their living and feeding habits, they mechanically transmit diverse agents to humans.

Epidemiology

The tsetse fly is found in the eastern and central regions of Africa, where it is of major medical and veterinary importance as the intermediate host and biologic vector of a number of trypanosomes that infect humans and animals. The housefly and stable fly are cosmopolitan in distribution and serve as indicators of poor sanitation. The housefly, *M. domestica*, lays eggs on any matter (feces, garbage, decaying plant matter) that will serve as food for developing fly larvae, or maggots. Stable flies commonly lay eggs in moist, decaying vegetable matter such as grass clippings or compost heaps found in suburban communities.

Figure 86–9. Tsetse fly, the vector of African trypanosomiasis. *(Courtesy Wellcome Foundation, Ltd, Berkhamsted; from Peters W: A Colour Atlas of Arthropods in Clinical Medicine. London, Wolfe, 1992.)*

Clinical Case 86-3. Furuncular Myiasis

Bakos and colleagues (Arch Dermatol 143:123-124, 2007) describe a 54-year-old white woman who was seen with a 2-week history of a painful inflammatory nodule on the inner aspect of her right leg. She vaguely remembered having been bitten in that area by a "bug." After 1 week of oral antibiotic treatment prescribed to relieve the surrounding inflammatory reaction, a poorly delimited nodule was observed, with a small pore on top from which a serosanguineous fluid exuded. Dermoscopy revealed a central opening surrounded by dilated blood vessels from which a yellowish structure with black barblike spines on the extremity extruded intermittently. This corresponded to the posterior extremity of *Dermatobia hominis* (human botfly) larva. The lesion was occluded with a double layer of plaster for 24 hours, and the immobile dead larva was removed with forceps and gentle squeezing. Furuncular myiasis due to *D. hominis* is a common disease in tropical American countries. The diagnosis of furuncular myiasis should always be considered in every boil-like lesion not responding to ordinary treatment, especially in travelers returning from tropical countries.

Prevention and Control

Control of tsetse fly populations has been problematic because of their widespread distribution in primarily rural and undeveloped areas. Insect repellents and insecticides may be effective against adult flies. Improved sanitation is important in controlling houseflies. Plant refuse should be protected from rain or destroyed.

Myiasis-Causing Flies (Clinical Case 86-3)

Myiasis is the term applied to the disease produced by maggots that live parasitically in human tissues. Clinically, myiasis may be classified according to the body part involved (e.g., nasal, intestinal, or urinary myiasis). The number of myiasis-producing flies and the diversity in lifestyle requirements are enormous. Only the host relations and sites of predilection of some of the more important species are covered in this section.

Specific myiasis refers to myiasis caused by flies that require a host for larval development. One important example is the human botfly, *Dermatobia hominis*, which is found in the humid regions of Mexico and Central and South America. The adult botfly attaches her eggs to the abdomen of bloodsucking flies or mosquitoes, which in turn distribute the eggs while obtaining a blood meal from an animal or human. The larvae enter the skin through the wound created by the biting insect. The larvae develop over 40 to 50 days, during which time a painful lesion known as a **warble** appears. When the larvae reach maturity, they leave the host to pupate. The resulting lesion may take weeks to months to heal and may become secondarily infected. If the larva dies before leaving the skin, an abscess forms.

Semispecific myiasis is caused by flies that normally lay their eggs on decaying animal or plant matter; it develops in a host if entry is facilitated by the presence of wounds or sores. Representatives of this group include the greenbottle fly, *Phaenicia*; bluebottle flies, *Cochliomyia*; and blackbottle flies, *Phormia*. These flies are worldwide in distribution, and their presence is encouraged by poor sanitation. They occasionally lay their eggs on the open sores or wounds of animal and humans. Another group that causes myiasis in humans is the flesh flies, or sarcophagids. These flies have a worldwide distribution and normally breed in decomposing matter. They may deposit their larvae on foods that, if ingested, may serve as a source of infection.

Flies that produce **accidental myiasis** have no requirement for development in a host. Accidental infection may occur when eggs are deposited on oral or genitourinary openings and the resulting larvae gain entry into the intestinal or genitourinary tract. Flies that may produce accidental myiasis include *M. domestica*, the common housefly.

Sucking Lice

Physiology and Structure

Although several species of lice (*Anoplura*) infest humans as blood-feeding parasites, only the body louse is important in medicine as the vector of the rickettsia of typhus and trench fevers and the vector of the spirochetes of relapsing fever (see Table 86-2). The **body louse**, *Pediculus humanus*, and the **head louse**, *P. humanus capitis*, are elongated, wingless, flattened insects with three pairs of legs and

Figure 86–10. Body louse (*P. humanus*). (*Courtesy Oxford Scientific Films, Ltd [Dr RJ Warren]; from Peters W: A Colour Atlas of Arthropods in Clinical Medicine. London, Wolfe, 1992.*)

mouthpieces adapted for piercing flesh and sucking blood (Figure 86-10). The pubic or **crab louse**, *Phthirus pubis*, has a short, crablike abdomen with clawed second and third legs (Figure 86-11).

Epidemiology

Epidemics of head lice are reported frequently in the United States, particularly among school children. The head lice

Figure 86–11. Crab louse (*P. pubis*). (*Courtesy Dr RV Southcott; from Peters W: A Colour Atlas of Arthropods in Clinical Medicine. London, Wolfe, 1992.*)

inhabit the hairs of the head and are transmitted by physical contact or sharing of hair brushes or hats. Crab lice survive on blood meals around the hairs of the pubic and perianal areas of the body. They are transmitted frequently from one person to another by sexual contact and contaminated toilet seats or clothing. Body lice are usually found on clothing. Unlike head or crab lice, they move to the body for feeding and return to the clothing after obtaining a blood meal. All of the lice inject salivary fluids into the body during the ingestion of blood, which causes varying degrees of sensitization in the human host.

Clinical Syndromes

Intense itching is the usual characteristic of infestation by lice (**pediculosis**). The patient may have pruritic, red papules around the ears, face, neck, or shoulders. Secondary infection and regional adenopathy may be present.

Diagnosis

The diagnosis is made by demonstration of the lice or eggs from a patient complaining of pruritus. Frequently the patient has noticed the insects, and the diagnosis may be made over the telephone. The eggs, or **nits**, are white, round objects that may be found attached to the hair shafts (head and crab lice) or on clothing (body lice).

Treatment, Prevention, and Control

Gamma benzene hexachloride (lindane) lotion applied to the entire body and left on for 24 hours is an effective treatment for lice. Shaving the hair of affected areas is a desirable adjunct. Adult lice in clothing must be destroyed by the application of lindane or DDT powder or by boiling. Lice may survive in the environment for up to 2 weeks; thus items such as brushes, combs, and bedding must be treated with a pediculicide or by boiling.

The best strategy for primary prevention is education and practice of good hygiene habits. Secondary prevention may be practiced by a policy of routine surveillance (e.g., scalp inspections) in schools, daycare centers, military camps, and other institutions. Repellents may be necessary for people who run a high risk of exposure in crowded conditions.

Fleas

Physiology and Structure

Fleas (*Siphonaptera*) are small, wingless insects with laterally compressed bodies and long legs adapted for jumping (Figure 86-12). Their mouthparts are adapted for sucking or "siphoning" blood from the host.

Epidemiology

Fleas are cosmopolitan in distribution. Most species are adapted to a particular host; however, they can readily feed on humans, particularly when deprived of their preferred host. Fleas are important as vectors of plague and

Figure 86–12. Flea. *(From Peters W: A Colour Atlas of Arthropods in Clinical Medicine. London, Wolfe, 1992.)*

Figure 86–13. Bedbug (*C. lectularius*). *(From Peters W: A Colour Atlas of Arthropods in Clinical Medicine. London, Wolfe, 1992.)*

murine typhus and as intermediate hosts for dog (*Dipylidium caninum*) and rodent (*Hymenolepis* species) tapeworms that occasionally infect humans.

In contrast to the majority of fleas that do not invade the human integument, the **chigoe flea**, *Tunga penetrans*, may cause considerable damage by actively invading the skin. The female chigoe flea burrows into the skin, often under the toenails or between the toes, where she sucks blood and lays her eggs. The chigoe flea is found in tropical and subtropical regions of America, as well as in Africa and the Far East. It is not known to transmit human pathogens.

Clinical Syndromes

As with the bites of other bloodsucking arthropods, flea bites result in pruritic, erythematous lesions of varying severity, which depends on the intensity of the infestation and the sensitivity of the bitten person. The irritation caused by the flea's saliva may produce physical findings that vary from small, red welts to a diffuse, red rash. Secondary infection may be a complication.

Cutaneous invasion by the chigoe flea produces an erythematous papule that is painful and pruritic. Infested tissue can become severely inflamed and ulcerated. Secondary infection is common. In severe cases, the infestation may be complicated by tetanus or by gas gangrene, resulting in amputation.

Diagnosis

The diagnosis of flea infestation is inferred in a patient with annoying bites who is also a pet (dog or cat) owner. Examination of the patient and pet usually reveals the characteristic insect. Diagnosis of tungiasis is made by detecting the dark portion of the chigoe flea's abdomen as it protrudes from the skin surface in the center of an inflamed lesion.

Treatment, Prevention, and Control

Palliative treatment with antipruritics and antihistamines is indicated for most flea bites. Surgical removal of the chigoe flea is indicated.

Commercially available insecticides may control fleas at the source. Topically applied repellents can protect people against flea bites. Flea collars or powders on pets are also effective preventive measures.

Bugs

Physiology and Structure

Bugs refer specifically to two bloodsucking insects, the **bedbug** and the **triatomid bug** (Figures 86-13 and 86-14). Both bugs are characterized by a long proboscis that is folded ventrally under the body when not in use. The bedbug (*Cimex lectularius*) is a reddish brown insect approximately 4 to 5 mm long. It has short wing pads but

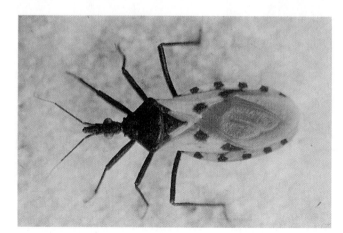

Figure 86–14. Triatomid bug. *(Courtesy Dr D Minter; from Peters W: A Colour Atlas of Arthropods in Clinical Medicine. London, Wolfe, 1992.)*

cannot fly. The triatomid, or **"kissing" bug**, has yellow or orange markings on the body and an elongated head. Triatomid bugs have wings and are aerial.

Epidemiology

Both bedbugs and triatomid bugs are nocturnal and feed indiscriminately on most mammals. Bedbugs are cosmopolitan in distribution, whereas triatomid bugs are limited to the Americas. Bedbugs hide during the day in cracks and crevices of wooden furniture, under loose wallpaper, in the tufts of mattresses, and in box springs. Triatomid bugs live in the cracks and crevices of walls and in thatched roofs. Bedbugs do not play a role in the transmission of human disease; however, triatomid bugs are important vectors of Chagas' disease (see Table 86-2 and Chapter 82).

Clinical Syndromes

The bites of bedbugs and triatomid bugs produce lesions that range from small, red marks to hemorrhagic bullae. Bedbugs tend to bite in linear fashion on the trunk and arms, whereas triatomid bugs bite with higher frequency on the face. The classic periorbital edema secondary to a triatomid bite is known as **Romaña's sign**. The intensity of reaction to a bite depends on the degree of sensitization of the patient. In addition to causing local lesions, bedbugs may be associated with nervous disorders and sleeplessness in children and adults.

Diagnosis

The pattern and location of bites suggests bedbugs or triatomid bugs. The detection of tiny spots of blood on bedding or the dead insects themselves is frequently the first sign of bedbug infestation.

Treatment, Prevention, and Control

Topical palliatives are appropriate for the relief of pruritus. Antihistamines may be indicated if dermatitis is severe. Control consists of proper hygiene and the environmental applications of insecticides.

Stinging Insects

Physiology and Structure

The order Hymenoptera comprises the bees, wasps, hornets, and ants. The modified ovipositor of the female, the apparatus for egg laying, serves as a stinging organ and is used for defense or to capture prey for food. Members of Hymenoptera are known for their complex social systems, castes, and elaborate hive or nest structures.

Epidemiology

Of the hymenopterans, the bees, or Apidae, live in complex social organizations such as hives or in less structured underground nests. Only honeybees and bumblebees are of concern to humans because of their ability to sting. The Vespidae include wasps, hornets, and yellow jackets; all are aggressive insects and a major cause of stings in humans. In the act of stinging, the aroused insect inserts the sheath to open the wound. The thrust of the stylets and injection of venom immediately follow.

One group of ants of concern in the United States is the **fire ant**, *Solenopsis invicta*. Fire ants are particularly common in the southeastern states. They are well camouflaged in large, hard-crusted mounds and attack when disturbed. They bite their victim with strong mandibles and then sting repeatedly.

Clinical Syndromes

An estimated 50 to 100 people die each year in the United States from reactions to stings of the hymenopterans. Severe toxic reactions such as fever and muscle cramps can be caused by as few as 10 stings. Allergic reactions are the most serious consequence, but others include pain, edema, pruritus, and a heat sensation at the site of the sting. Anaphylactic shock from bee stings has resulted in death in some instances.

Treatment, Prevention, and Control

No satisfactory treatment has been discovered for stings. If left in the wound, the sting apparatus should be removed immediately. The injection of epinephrine is sometimes necessary to counteract anaphylaxis. (Emergency kits are available by prescription for sensitive people.) For the relief of local discomfort, calamine lotion or a topical corticosteroid cream for more severe local lesions is helpful.

Although there are no effective repellents against these insects, their nests can be destroyed with any of several commercially available insecticidal compounds. General avoidance of areas inhabited by hymenopterans is advised for sensitive people.

Case Study and Questions

A 4-year-old child was brought in by her mother with a complaint of itchy hands. The child stayed at a daycare center during the day while her mother worked. The girl had intense itching and a rash on her hands and arms for about 2 weeks. The itching became more severe and interfered with the child's sleep. On physical examination, the child appeared well nourished and cared for. The skin on her hands, wrists, and forearms appeared red and excoriated. Raised, serpiginous "tracks" were noted on the sides of her fingers, on the ventral aspects of her wrists, and in the popliteal folds. Several of the tracks were inflamed and were beginning to form pustules. The mother stated that several other children at the daycare center were experiencing a similar problem.

1. What was the likely diagnosis?
2. How would this diagnosis have been confirmed?
3. How would this child have been treated and what advice would have been given to the mother regarding prevention?
4. Did this child require antibiotic therapy? If so, why?
5. What should have been done regarding the other children at the daycare center?

MEDICAL MICROBIOLOGY

Bibliography

Binford CH, Connor DH: Pathology of Tropical and Extraordinary Diseases, vol 3. Washington, DC, Armed Forces Institute of Pathology, 1976.

Hwang SW, et al: Bed bug infestations in an urban environment. Emerg Infect Dis 11:533-537, 2005.

Markell EK, John DT, Krotoski WA: Markell and Voges' Medical Parasitology, 8th ed. Philadelphia, WB Saunders, 1999.

Najarian HH: Textbook of Medical Parasitology. Baltimore, Williams & Wilkins, 1967.

Peters W: A Colour Atlas of Arthropods in Clinical Medicine. London, Wolfe, 1992.

Swanson DL, Vetter RS: Bites of brown recluse spiders and suspected necrotic arachnidism. N Engl J Med 352:700-707, 2005.

Telford SR III: Arthropods of medical importance. In Murray PR, et al (eds): Manual of Clinical Microbiology, 9th ed. Washington, DC, ASM Press, 2007.

Strickland GT: Hunter's Tropical Medicine and Emerging Infectious Diseases, 8th ed. Philadelphia, WB Saunders, 2000.

Van Horn KG, et al: Copepods associated with a perirectal abscess and copepod pseudo-outbreaks in stools for ova and parasite examinations. Diagn Microbiol Infect Dis 15:561-565, 1992.

Role of Parasites in Disease

A summary of the parasites (protozoan and helminths) most commonly associated with human disease is presented in this chapter. Although many parasites are associated with a single organ system (e.g., gastrointestinal tract) and therefore cause a disease process involving that system, some of the most dramatic manifestations of parasitic disease occur when the parasite leaves its "normal" location in the human body. Likewise, several different parasites may produce a similar disease syndrome. The management of a specific parasitic infection may differ tremendously depending on the etiologic agent, and many antiparasitic treatment regimens are quite toxic. So to guide both diagnostic and therapeutic efforts, it is useful to generate a differential diagnosis that includes the most likely parasites.

The development and prognosis of a parasitic infection often depend on factors aside from the innate virulence of the organism. In determining the possibility of a parasitic infection, the meaning of any microbiologic data, and the necessity to treat and with what agent, one must take into account numerous factors, such as exposure history (e.g., travel to an endemic area), the potential infectious dose and/or organism burden, the use of prophylaxis (e.g., antimalarial prophylaxis), and the immunologic status of the host. The presentation of a given parasitic infection may be quite different in a nonimmune traveler to an endemic region versus a semi-immune resident of the same region. Likewise, the treatment and prevention strategies will be different as well.

This chapter provides a very broad listing of the various parasitic agents commonly associated with infections at specific body sites and/or specific clinical manifestations (Table 87-1). This information is meant to be used in conjunction with Table 79-1 as an aid in establishing a differential diagnosis and selecting the most likely clinical specimens that will help establish a specific etiologic

Table 87–1. Summary of Parasites Associated with Human Disease

System Affected and Disease	Pathogens
Blood	
Malaria	*Plasmodium* spp.
Babesiosis	*Babesia* spp.
Filariasis	*Wuchereria bancrofti, Brugia malayi, Mansonella* spp., *Loa loa*
Bone Marrow	
Leishmaniasis	*Leishmania donovani, Leishmania tropica*
Central Nervous System	
Meningoencephalitis	*Naegleria fowleri, Trypanosoma brucei gambiense, T. b. rhodesiense, T. cruzi, Toxoplasma gondii,* Microsporidia
Granulomatous encephalitis	*Acanthamoeba* spp., *Balamuthia mandrillaris*

Continued

Table 87–1. Summary of Parasites Associated with Human Disease—cont'd

System Affected and Disease	Pathogens
Mass lesion Brain abscess	*T. gondii, Taenia solium, Schistosoma japonicum, Acanthamoeba* spp., *B. mandrillaris*
Eosinophilic meningitis Cerebral malaria	*Angiostrongylus cantonensis, Toxocara* spp. *Baylisascaris* (neural larva migrans), *Plasmodium falciparum*
Cerebral paragonimiasis	*Paragonimus westermani*
Eye	
Keratitis	*Acanthamoeba* spp., Microsporidia (*Nosema* sp., *Microsporidium* spp., *Encephalitozoon hellem*), *Onchocerca volvulus*
Chorioretinitis Conjunctivitis	*T. gondii, O. volvulus, L. loa*
Ocular cysticercosis (mass lesion)	*T. solium*
Toxocariasis	*Toxocara* spp. (ocular larva migrans; mimics retinoblastoma)
Intestinal Tract	
Anal pruritus	*Enterobius vermicularis*
Colitis	*Entamoeba histolytica, Balantidium coli*
Diarrhea/dysentery	*E. histolytica, Giardia lamblia (duodenalis),* Microsporidia, *Cryptosporidium parvum, Cyclospora cayetanensis, Isospora belli, Schistosoma mansoni, Strongyloides stercoralis, Trichuris trichiura*
Toxic megacolon	*Trypanosoma cruzi*
Obstruction Perforation	*Ascaris lumbricoides, Fasciolopsis buski*
Rectal prolapse	*Trichuris trichiura*
Liver, Spleen	
Abscess	*E. histolytica, Fasciola hepatica*
Hepatitis	Microsporidia (*Encephalitozoon cuniculi, Nosema connori*), *T. gondii*
Biliary obstruction	*A. lumbricoides, F. hepatica, Opisthorchis (Clonorchis) sinensis*
Cirrhosis/hepatosplenomegaly	*L. donovani, L. tropica, Toxocara canis* and *T. cati* (visceral larva migrans), *Schistosoma mansoni, S. japonicum*
Mass lesions	*T. solium, Echinococcus granulosus, E. multilocularis*
Genitourinary	
Vaginitis/urethritis	*Trichomonas vaginalis, E. vermicularis*
Renal failure	*Plasmodium* spp., *L. donovani*
Cystitis/hematuria	*Schistosoma haematobium, P. falciparum* (blackwater fever)
Heart	
Myocarditis	Microsporidia, *T. gondii, T. cruzi*
Megacardia/complete heart block	*T. cruzi*

Table 87–1. Summary of Parasites Associated with Human Disease—cont'd

System Affected and Disease	Pathogens
Lung	
Abscess	*E. histolytica, P. Paragonimus westermani*
Nodule/mass	*Dirofilaria immitis, E. granulosus, E. multilocularis*
Pneumonitis	*A. lumbricoides, S. stercoralis, Toxocara* spp., *P. westermani, T. gondii, Ancylostoma braziliense*
Lymphatics	
Lymphedema	*W. bancrofti, B. malayi*, other filaria
Lymphadenopathy	*T. gondii*, trypanosomes
Muscle	
Generalized myositis	*Trichinella spiralis*, Microsporidia, *Sarcocystis lindemanni, Toxocara* spp.
Myocarditis	*T. spiralis, T. cruzi*, Microsporidia, *Toxocara* spp.
Skin and Subcutaneous Tissue	
Ulcerative lesion	*Leishmania* spp., *Dracunculus medinensis*
Nodule/swellings	*O. volvulus, L. loa, T. cruzi, Acanthamoeba* spp., *Toxocara* spp.
Rash/vesicles	*T. gondii, A. braziliense*, other migrating worms, schistosomes (cercarial dermatitis)
Systemic	
General dissemination and multiple organ dysfunction	Microsporidia, *P. falciparum, T. gondii, L. donovani, T. cruzi, Toxocara* spp., *S. stercoralis, T. spiralis*
Iron deficiency, anemia	Hookworms (*Ancylostoma duodenale, Necator americanus*)
Megaloblastic anemia (Vitamin B_{12} deficiency)	*Diphyllobothrium latum*

diagnosis. Other factors that may be important in determining the relative frequency with which specific parasites cause disease (e.g., travel and exposure history, specific clinical presentations) are covered in the individual chapters in this text or in the more comprehensive infectious disease texts cited in this and other chapters.

Bibliography

Cohen J, Powderly WG: Infectious Diseases, 2nd ed. St Louis, Mosby, 2004.
Connor DH, et al: Pathology of Infectious Diseases. Stamford, Conn, Appleton & Lange, 1997.
Cook G, Zumala A: Manson's Tropical Diseases, 21st ed. London, Elsevier Science, 2003.
Garcia LS: Diagnostic Medical Parasitology, 4th ed. Washington, DC, American Society for Microbiology, 2001.

Index

Note: Page numbers followed by "f" refer to figures; those followed by "b" refer to boxes; and those followed by "t" refer to tables.

Salmonella, 307-309, 308b
  diseases caused by, 309
  drug resistance in, 315
  epidemiology of, 308-309
  pathogenic mechanisms of, 308
Salmonella Choleraesuis, 307, 308b, 309
Salmonella Paratyphi, 308-309, 308b
Salmonella Typhi, 302f, 307-309, 308b
Salmonella Typhimurium, 19f, 307, 308b
Sand flies, 904
  disease transmission by, 353, 845-847, 847f
Saprobes, 57
Saquinavir, 482, 486
Sarcocystis, 811, 844
Sarcoma, Kaposi, 538, 638
Sarcoma viruses, 641, 641t
Sarcoptes scabiei, 899-900
SARS (severe acute respiratory syndrome), 565-567
Satellite phenomenon, in *Haemophilus influenzae* culture, 348, 348f
Scabies, 900
Scalded skin syndrome, staphylococcal, 213, 215-216, 216f
Scalp, tinea infections of, 718, 719t, 720-721, 723f
Scanning electron microscopes, 157
Scarlet fever, *Streptococcus pyogenes*, 229
Scedosporium, 729, 770
Schistosoma haematobium, 876, 878f, 879-880
Schistosoma japonicum, 878f, 879
Schistosoma mansoni, 876-879, 877f
Schistosomes, 876-877, 877f. See also *Schistosoma*.
Schistosomiasis, 876-879
Schizogony
  in *Plasmodium*, 835
  in sporozoa, 828
Schleiferella, 392b
Schüffner dots
  in *Plasmodium ovale*, 837
  in *Plasmodium vivax*, 835, 836f
Scolex, of cestodes, 881. See also *specific cestodes.*
Scolopendra, 893
Scopulariopsis, 724, 770-771
Scorpions, 899, 899f
Scrapie, 661, 662t
Scrub typhus, 427, 428f, 428t, 430t, 433
Scytalidium, in onychomycosis, 724
*sec*A gene, of mycobacteria, 287-288
Secretion systems, of cell wall, 14-15, 182.
  See also Type III secretion system.
Secretory component, 103
Secretory immunoglobulin A, 103
Segmented neutrophils, 92
Selective culture media, 162t, 163
Semipermissive cells, in viral infections, 469
Semliki forest virus, 612f
Sepsis, 131, 460t
Septate hyphae, 57, 59f
Septic arthritis, staphylococcal, 219-220
Septic shock, in histoplasmosis, 745
Septicemia
  Clostridium perfringens, 381
  definition of, 189
  Erysipelothrix rhusiopathiae, 259

Septicemia *(Continued)*
  Escherichia coli, 307
  Lactobacillus, 396
  Neisseria gonorrhoeae, 295-296
  Salmonella, 309
  Vibrio vulnificus, 321
Septum formation, in cell division, 20, 20f
Serine proteases
  in cell wall synthesis, 199
  of *Pseudomonas aeruginosa*, 335
  in staphylococcal scalded skin syndrome, 213
Seroconversion
  in bacterial infections, 174
  in viral infections, 495
Serologic diagnosis, 169-175
  antibodies for, 169
  immunoassays for
    antibody and soluble antigen, 171-174, 173f, 174b, 174f
    cell-associated antigen, 170-172, 172f, 173f
  methods for, 169-170, 171f
  serology, 174-175, 174b
Serosal macrophages, 95
Serratia, 314
Sesquiterpenes, for parasitic diseases, 818
Severe acute respiratory syndrome (SARS), 565-567
Sex pili (F pili), 16, 35
Sexual spores, fungal, 58-59
Sexual transmission
  of cytomegalovirus, 536, 537
  of HIV, 636, 640
  of viral infections, 672-673, 672b
Sheep liver flukes, 872-873, 873f
Shell vial, 494
Shiga toxin
  of *Escherichia coli*, 307
  of *Shigella*, 310
Shigella, 309-311, 310b, 315
Shingles, 527, 528, 528f
Shock, in dengue fever, 616
Shunt infections, staphylococcal, 220
Shwartzman reaction, 15
Siderophores, of Enterobacteriaceae, 303
Sigma factor, in gene expression, 27
Sigmoidoscopic material, collection of, 808
Silent mutations, 32
Simian immunodeficiency virus, 635
Simian polyomavirus, 505-506
Sindbis virus, 611
Single radial immunodiffusion technique, 169-170
Sinuses
  specimen collection from, 190t, 192
  zygomycosis of, 768
Sinusitis
  Chlamydophila pneumoniae, 447
  Haemophilus influenzae, 347
  Streptococcus pneumoniae, 240
Skin
  bacterial entry through, 180-181, 181t
  barrier function of, 123, 124f
  microbial flora of, 76-77, 76b
  specimen collection from, 490t, 692t, 805t, 806t

Skin infections
  anaerobic, 402, 402f
  Ancylostoma braziliense, 859-860
  bacterial, 461t
  Bartonella, 371-373, 372b
  Blastomyces dermatitidis, 736
  Bordetella, 264
  Borrelia, 413-414, 414f
  Candida, 757, 757t, 758
  coxsackievirus, 559
  Cryptococcus neoformans, 853
  Erysipelothrix rhusiopathiae, 259
  fungal, 60, 62, 62t, 715-724, 716f, 717f, 793t
  herpes simplex virus, 520-522
  Histoplasma duboisii, 745
  human papillomavirus, 499, 501-502, 503f
  Lacazia loboi, 778, 779, 779f
  Leishmania, 846, 847
  leprosy, 282, 283f, 283t, 284f
  molluscum contagiosum, 546, 546f
  Neisseria gonorrhoeae, 295-296, 296f
  Nocardia, 270-272, 273f
  Onchocerca volvulus, 867-868
  orf, 545, 545f
  parasitic, 913t
  Prototheca, 780-781
  Pseudomonas aeruginosa, 336
  Pythium insidiosum, 781-782
  Rickettsia, 430t, 431
  scabies, 900
  schistosomal, 880
  smallpox, 544, 544f
  staphylococcal, 218-219, 218f, 219f
  Treponema, 405, 407f, 408
  varicella-zoster virus, 526-528, 527f
  zygomycosis, 768
Skin tests
  coccidioidin, 742
  tuberculin, 286-287
Slapped-cheek rash, in B19 parvovirus infections, 549, 550f
Sleeping sickness, 848-850, 849f
Slides, for parasite examination, 808
Slim disease, 638
Slime layer, 15-16, 185, 209-210, 212
Slow viruses, unconventional. See Prions.
Small intestine, microbial flora of, 75, 75b
Smallpox, 543f, 544-545, 544f
  epidemiology of, 543
  eradication of, 544-545, 544b
  history of, 541
  pathogenic mechanisms of, 543b
  vaccine for, 151-152
  variants of, 544
Snail fever (schistosomiasis), 876
Snails, as *Opisthorchis sinensis* vector, 874, 874f
Sodium stibogluconate, 798, 848
Soft-tissue infections
  anaerobic, 402, 402f
  fungal, 793t
Somatic mutation, of immunoglobulins, 103, 105
Sorbitol-containing MacConkey agar, for Enterobacteriaceae, 314
Sordarins, 709
SOS response, in DNA repair, 33